# Physiology for Nursing Practice

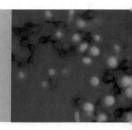

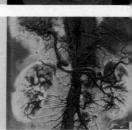

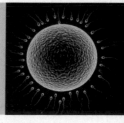

*For Elsevier*

*Commissioning Editor:* Sarena Woolfard, Ninette Premdas
*Project Development Manager:* Dinah Thom
*Project Manager:* Cheryl Brant, Naughton Project Management
*Designer:* Judith Wright

# Physiology for Nursing Practice

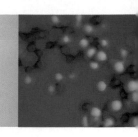

*Edited by*

## Susan E. Montague BSc(Hons) RGN HVDip RNT ILTM
Associate Head (Inter-Professional Learning), Faculty of Health and Human Sciences,
University of Hertfordshire, Hatfield, UK

## Roger Watson BSc PhD RGN CBiol FIBiol ILTM FRSA
Professor of Nursing, Faculty of Health and Social Sciences,
University of Hull, Hull, UK

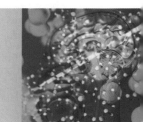

## Rosamund A. Herbert BSc(Hons) MSc RGN CertEd
Freelance Writer and Consultant in Healthcare Education,
Formerly Head of Applied Biological Sciences,
Florence Nightingale School of Nursing and Midwifery, Kings College, London, UK

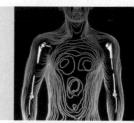

## THIRD EDITION

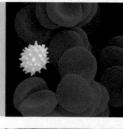

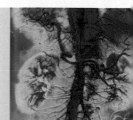

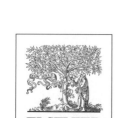

ELSEVIER

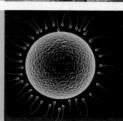

EDINBURGH  LONDON  NEW YORK  OXFORD  PHILADELPHIA  ST LOUIS  SYDNEY  TORONTO  2005

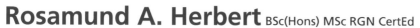

# ELSEVIER

© 1988, 1996 Baillière Tindall
© 2000 Harcourt Publishers Limited
© 2005, Elsevier Limited. All rights reserved.

First edition 1988
Second edition 1996
Third edition 2005

ISBN 0 7020 2676 X

**British Library Cataloguing in Publication Data**
A catalogue record for this book is available from the British Library

**Library of Congress Cataloguing in Publication Data**
A catalogue record for this book is available from the Library of Congress

**Note**
Knowledge and best practice in this field are constantly changing. As new research and experience broaden our knowledge, changes in practice, treatment and drug therapy may become necessary or appropriate. Readers are advised to check the most current information provided (i) on procedures featured or (ii) by the manufacturer of each product to be administered, to verify the recommended dose or formula, the method and duration of administration, and contraindications. It is the responsibility of the practitioner, relying on their own experience and knowledge of the patient, to make diagnoses, to determine dosages and the best treatment for each individual patient, and to take all appropriate safety precautions. To the fullest extent of the law, neither the publisher nor the editors assume any liability for any injury and/or damage.

*The Publisher*

Printed in Spain

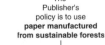

**ELSEVIER** your source for books, journals and multimedia in the health sciences

**www.elsevierhealth.com**

The Publisher's policy is to use **paper manufactured from sustainable forests**

# Contents

**Section 1** The characteristics of living matter   *1*

**Section 2** Control and coordination   *71*

**Section 3** Mobility and support  *267*

**Section 4** Internal transport  *333*

**Section 5** The acquisition of nutrients and removal of waste  *465*

**Section 6** Protection and survival  *633*

# Contributors

**Douglas Allan** BEd MN RGN RMN RNT
Senior Lecturer, School of Nursing, Midwifery and
Community health, Glasgow Caledonian University,
Glasgow, UK

**Michael G. Davis** BSc(Hons) MSc PhD
Formerly Senior Lecturer in Biochemistry, Division of
Biosciences, University of Hertfordshire, Hatfield,
Hertfordshire, UK

**Sharon L. Edwards** MSc DipN(Lon) RGN PGCEA
Senior Lecturer, School of Nursing and Midwifery,
University of Hertfordshire, Hatfield, UK

**Rosamund A. Herbert** BSc(Hons) MSc RGN CertEd
Freelance writer and consultant in Healthcare
Education; formerly Head of Biological Sciences,
Kings College, Nightingale Institute, London, UK

**Susan M. McLaren** BSc(Hons) PhD RGN
Professor of Nursing, Faculty of Health and Social
Care, London South Bank University, London, UK

**Susan E. Montague** BSc(Hons) RGN HVDip RNT ILTM
Associate Head (Inter-Professional Learning),
Faculty of Health and Human Sciences, University
of Hertfordshire, Hatfield, UK

**Carol Law** MA BSc(Hons) RNT RCNT RGN
Senior Lecturer, Department of Nursing and Midwifery,
University of Hertfordshire, Hatfield, UK

**Christine Patch** PhD BSc MA(Ed) DipEd RGN
Senior Research Fellow, Health Care Research Unit,
Southampton General Hospital, Southampton, UK

**Ann Richards** BA(Hons) MSc RGN
Senior Lecturer, School of Paramedic Science,
Physiotherapy and Radiograpy, University of
Hertfordshire, Hatfield, UK

**Mandy Sheppard**
Training and Development Consultant, Kent, UK

**Heather Skirton** MSc PhD DipPsychCounselling RN RM
Reader in Health Genetics, University of Plymouth,
Plymouth, UK

**Graeme D. Smith** BA PhD RGN
Lecturer, School of Health in Social Science,
University of Edinburgh, Edinburgh, UK

**Peter S. Vickers** BA PhD CertEd DipCD SRN RSCN
Senior Lecturer, School of Nursing and Midwifery,
University of Hertfordshire, Hatfield, UK

**Ruth Walker** BSc(Hons) RN RM ADM PGCEA
Senior Lecturer, School of Nursing and Midwifery,
University of Hertfordshire, Hatfield, UK

**William F. M. Wallace**
BSc MD FRCP FRCA FCARCSI FRCSEd
Professor Emeritus in Applied Physiology,
Queen's University, Belfast, Northern Ireland

**Roger Watson** BSc PhD RGN Cbiol FIBiol ILTM FRSA
Professor of Nursing, Faculty of Health and
Social Sciences, University of Hull, Hull, UK

**Benita Wilson** BSc MSc CertEd DNC PGCE
Lecturer, School of Nursing, Social Work
and Applied Health Studies, Hull University,
Hull, UK

# Editors' introduction

We are delighted to introduce the third edition of this successful and established textbook. The first edition of this book was published in 1988 and proved a pioneer text in supporting the development and delivery of new 'Project 2000' curricula as well as other advanced and specialist nursing and midwifery courses at diploma and degree level. The text arose directly from our experience of teaching students of nursing, midwifery and health care who were studying at diploma and degree level. We were then and remain convinced now of the need for a United Kingdom textbook which, not only presents a comprehensive review of physiology, but also indicates how physiological principles can provide a basis for understanding nursing care. The level of physiology presented in this book goes beyond that traditionally found in books written for nurses, reflecting our belief that registered practitioners require a thorough understanding of body function to practise intelligently and effectively, gain satisfaction from their work and improve standards of care.

The success of both the first and second editions, (including a second edition translation into Italian!) has confirmed this view and in this third edition of *Physiology for Nursing Practice* the underlying philosophy of the earlier editions has been retained. We do, of course, acknowledge that holistic health care does require a wider perspective of knowledge than the biosciences considered in this text. In this new edition we have not only adapted and developed the text in response to feedback from students, practitioners and lecturers, but also extended and reorganized content, both to include important new material and, to facilitate clarity and ease of use. The new content reflects current thinking in bioscience and the delivery of health care as well as the content of modern nursing and health care curricula.

We know that pre-registration nursing and other health professional students thirst for application and practice examples when learning physiology. On the other hand, registered practitioners, extending their knowledge, often have rewarding experiences in class as they suddenly understand why a patient or client has a certain problem and thus the biological rationale for his or her care. This book recognises and meets such learning needs. Like its predecessors, this third edition has been written especially for students on pre-registration diploma and degree courses in nursing and midwifery and for registered nurses and midwives following courses in specialist practice.

Although *Physiology for Nursing Practice* is written primarily for nurses, we know from experience that other health professionals also find its content useful as they learn and work within an inter-professional context. The text is most suitable for UK, European and Australasian practitioners because of its terminology and focus on care practices found in the UK, and because of its use and explanation of SI units of measurement.

In preparing the new text we had five main aims:

- to enable readers to understand the principles and mechanisms of body function, so that they can appreciate how these function in health and how they alter across the lifespan and in illness;
- to support bioscience curricula in nursing diploma and degree level courses;
- to provide readers with a rational basis for assessing a patient's health problems, and for the planning, delivery and evaluation of care;
- to convey a sense of fascination and enthusiasm, about how the body works and to motivate readers to further their studies;
- to express all of the above as clearly and as simply as possible but not at the expense of scientific accuracy.

We are aware that knowledge of any scientific discipline is continually being modified and extended through research. Every effort has been made to ensure that the physiology presented in this book reflects the consensus of opinion at the time of writing. *Physiology for Nursing Practice* is still primarily concerned with normal, healthy body function and essentially describes how the body maintains homeostasis. Throughout the text, practice applications are highlighted to demonstrate clearly how homeostasis becomes deranged by illness and how knowledge of normal function can provide a sound basis for understanding abnormality and a rationale for patient/client care.

This edition is a true evolution from the last. We have a new editor in Ros Herbert, who has been a valued author since the book was born. We also have contributions from six continuing authors, and eleven new authors. Like its predecessors, the book has six major sections which, rather than following the classical systems approach, logically illustrate the functioning of the body as a complex homeostatic system. These sections are:

1. Characteristics of Living Matter
2. Control and Co-ordination
3. Mobility and Support
4. Internal Transport
5. The Acquisition of Nutrients and Removal of Waste
6. Protection and Survival.

We have maintained the popular and useful content in Section 1 on the chemistry of life and on SI units. We know that the text of this section meets the needs of students, previously unfamiliar with the subject, equipping them with crucial foundation knowledge for their applied and integrated courses. In this edition, we have extended the content on innate and acquired defence mechanisms (Chapters 6.1 and 6.2) and added a whole new chapter on Human Genetics (Chapter 6.4), reflecting the increasing biological and clinical significance of these subjects today. All artwork in this edition is available for readers using the following url:

http://evolve.elsevier.com/Montague/Physiology

As in the previous editions, Sections 2–6 each present a major aspect of homeostasis. All chapters have been revised with requirements of modern curricula at the forefront of each contributor's attention. All our contributors – the majority of whom are nurses – were chosen because of their knowledge of biological sciences as applied to practice and for their reputation and experience in teaching and writing on their subject. The end result has been that their chapters all contain new content and focussed material which supports learning in all four branches of nursing and in midwifery.

We believe that this book will be a major new resource for those involved in learning and teaching about the nursing care of patients. We commend it to you in the hope that through its use you will experience that same sense of fascination about how the human body works that was the inspiration for its production.

Sue Montague
Ros Herbert
Roger Watson
2005

# Editors' acknowledgements

The urgently expressed learning and teaching needs of our students and professional colleagues were the inspiration for the first edition of this book. We thank them again for that and for their enthusiastic response to, and positive support for, the first two editions. This response and the excellent reviews and evaluative feedback we have received have led to the production of this further enhanced third edition.

Sincere thanks to our author colleagues and friends who were so willing to update and refocus their contributions and to produce new material. All these people have undertaken their work with characteristic professionalism and skill and with much forbearance in the face of a long and sometimes 'bumpy' production schedule!

We have also involved colleagues as critical readers for certain chapters and thank them most sincerely for undertaking this work so willingly and with such expertise, for very little reward:

**Cindy O'Malley**, PhD,
Senior Lecturer, School of Life Sciences,
University of Hertfordshire, UK

**Niall M. McMullan**, PhD,
Senior Lecturer, School of Life Sciences,
University of Hertfordshire, UK

Inevitably, with the passage of time since the second edition, some authors decided that they were unable to contribute to the third edition. Their names have been removed from the text, but we are indebted to them for their original work in the second and first editions. Notable amongst these is one of the founder editors and author of two chapters in the

first and second editions, Susan M. Hinchliff. Sue is to retire this year from her post as Head of Accreditation at the Royal College of Nursing. This book owes much to Sue's ideas, knowledge and skills and we thank her for her huge contribution and wish her well in the future. Other first and second edition authors that we also thank sincerely are:

Jennifer A. Alison
Anne V. Betts
Jennifer Boore
Margaret Clarke
Michael Hunter
Valerie Nie
Denise Knight
Janet Stocks
Jennifer Storer.

Sarena Wolfard and Dinah Thom of Elsevier Limited were instrumental in the commissioning and development of this edition and we thank them for their advice, support and patience and the publisher for their continued confidence in the text. In the latter stages of production we have been firmly 'project managed' with great tact and good spirit by Nora Naughton and her staff at Naughton Project Management.

This edition of the book is dedicated to our families: our partners, Alan Montague, Graeme Bell and Debbie Watson and our children, Sarah and James Montague, Duncan Bell and Hannah, William, Lucy, Emily, Thomas, Joseph, Charles and Rebecca Watson. They have shown huge tolerance and support.

# Publisher's acknowledgements

Figures 1.1.1 & 4.2.30. Based on *Principles of Anatomy and Physiology* 7e by Tortora, G.J. & Grabowski, S.R. Reproduced with permission from HarperCollins Publishers, Inc.

Figure 1.3.10. Reproduced with kind permission of Child Growth Foundation, London.

Figures 1.3.11 & 1.3.12. Adapted from Tanner, J.M. (1989), *Foetus into Man* 2e. Reproduced with permission from Castlemead Publications, Welwyn Garden City.

Figures 2.3.7a & b. Adapted from Davis, P. (1993) *Opening up the gate control theory*, Nursing Standard 7: 25–26, with permission from Nursing Standards Publications, London.

Figure 2.4.6. Courtesy of Clement Clarke International Ltd.

Figure 2.5.1. Adapted from Marieb, E.N. (2001) *Human Anatomy and Physiology*, 5th edn with permission from Benjamin Cummings, San Francisco.

Table 3.3.1. From *Human Anatomy and Physiology* by Carola, Harley & Noback (1992). Reproduced with permission from Peter Schwenk, Connecticut, U.S.A.

Figures 4.1.4, 4.1.8, 4.1.10. Reproduced with permission from Hoffbrand & Pettit (2002) *Color Atlas of Clinical Hematology*, 3rd edn. St Louis: Mosby.

Figures 4.1.5a & b. Adapted from Hoffbrand & Pettit, *Essential Haematology* 3/e with permission from Blackwell Scientific Publications, Oxford.

Figure 4.1.14. Reproduced with permission from Hoffbrand AV, Pettit JE & Moss PAH (2001) *Essential Haematology*, 4th edn. Blackwell Science: Oxford.

Figure 4.2.1a. Redrawn from Watson, R. (1999) *Essential Science for Nursing Students*. London: Ballière Tindall.

Figure 4.2.4. Adapted from Moore, K.L. (1993) *The Developing Human* 5/e. Reproduced with permission from WB Saunders, Philadelphia, U.S.A.

Figures 4.2.16 & 4.2.17. Courtesy Hallstrom Institute of Cardiology, Sydney, Australia.

Figure 6.1.8. Redrawn from Edwards, S.L. (2002) *Physiological insult/injury: Pathophysiology and consequences*. British Journal of Nursing, **11**(4); 263–274.

Table 6.2.1. From UK Health Department (1992) Immunization Against Infectious Diseases, HMSO, London. Crown Copyright is reproduced with the permission of the Controller of HMSO.

Figures 6.3.6a & b. Adapted from Pond C (1992). Reproductive Physiology Animal Physiology, Ou Press: Oxford.

Figure 6.4.1. Courtesy of the Paediatric Research Unit, Guy's Hospital Medical School, London.

**Section icon images**
*Section 4 icon*
Red and white blood cells, coloured SEM
Dr Yorgos Nikas/Science Photo Library
*Section 5 icon*
Coloured angiogram of kidneys
CNRI/Science Photo Library
*Section 6 icon*
Computer artwork of an egg surrounded by sperm
Alfred Pasieka/Science Photo Library

# How to use this book

The Editors' Introduction described the Sections and Chapters that make up this book. In addition, each chapter has a clear organization. This has been devised to guide you through the individual topics, to highlight key ideas and to focus on the links between physiological theory and nursing practice. All artwork is available for readers using the following url: http://evolve.elsevier.com/Montague/Physiology.

### Each chapter begins with

- A Chapter Contents List, to help you find the particular information you need.

- Learning Objectives, which identify the specific physiological principles and systems that you will learn about by studying the chapter.

- An Introduction, which provides an overview of the chapter content and discusses its significance to nursing practice.

### Within each chapter

Key concepts are highlighted not only because of their importance but also for ease of reference if you are skimming through a particular chapter.

### CLINICAL APPLICATIONS

Issues of clinical significance for nurses are highlighted throughout the chapters; these clinical applications make up a significant part of some chapters. By emphasizing the clinical implications of a disorder alongside the physiological and anatomical principles underpinning that disorder, we hope to enable readers to gain a deeper understanding of the causes, consequences and nursing requirements of different medical conditions.

We also hope that, by highlighting this material within the text, readers will be able to return to this information as and when issues arise in their practice.

### DEVELOPMENTAL ISSUES

Information on developmental issues – embryology, growth and ageing – is highlighted so that you can see how physiological processes vary across the lifespan.

### Review questions

A full list of Review Questions appears at the end of each chapter.

### At the end of each chapter

- The Clinical Review lists the main points that have been raised in the chapter in relation to clinical issues and disturbances to normal physiology.

- The annotated list of Suggestions for Further Reading will be helpful for those readers who want to pursue their studies further. This is in addition to the comprehensive list of References that appears at the end of the chapter.

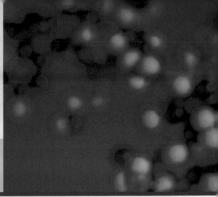

# Section 1

# The characteristics of living matter

# The human body: a framework for understanding

*Roger Watson*

## LEARNING OBJECTIVES

After studying this chapter the reader should be able to:

- Describe the basic characteristics of living matter

- Recognize the cell as the basic structural and functional unit of life

- Discuss ways in which the human body can be considered to be organized

- Demonstrate understanding of progression in levels of body organization

- Define the term 'tissue' and classify the major types of tissue that make up the human body

- Describe the two basic arrangements of tissues forming organs

- Name and state the major functions of the ten organ systems in the human body

- Define the term 'internal environment' and state its functional significance in higher animals

- State the basic requirements for and function of a homeostatic mechanism

- Discuss the concept of homeostasis and its relationship with health

- Correctly describe anatomical directional terms

- Identify the major planes of the human body

- Name and describe the major body cavities

- Demonstrate knowledge of SI units and their use in clinical practice

## INTRODUCTION

The human body is composed of billions of cells, most of which are not in contact with the outside world. Life is maintained through the coordinated activity of these cells and if that function is efficient and effective we describe the state produced as 'health'. To function effectively, each one of our cells must receive an adequate supply of oxygen and other nutrients, dispose of the waste products of its metabolism and remain within a relatively narrow range of temperature, pressure and pH. Each cell achieves this through active exchange with its immediate environment – the thin film of fluid between it and other cells. This immediate environment of our cells is called the **internal environment**. When cell function is coordinated to achieve relative stability of the internal environment, a state of **homeostasis** is achieved and this state is comparable with optimum function and health. This book describes the process through which the human being maintains homeostasis. Although it is concerned primarily with normal body function, it also contains material that demonstrates just how an understanding of structure and function underpins and provides the rationale for professional practice in nursing and health care. To this end, the book includes information that describes how health problems can arise if homeostasis breaks down, as well as explanations of the biological theory underlying important caring and therapeutic activities.

The book is divided into six sections. This section contains introductory material about the characteristics of life, the levels of organization of the human organism and units of measurement relevant to clinical practice. Chapter 1.1 also contains the important principles of homeostatic mechanisms as a foundation for the other sections, each of which presents a major aspect of homeostasis.

## The characteristics of living matter

All living matter has certain characteristics in common and these characteristics distinguish that which is living (animate) from that which is not (inanimate). The features that characterize life are:

- irritability (capable of responding to stimulation)
- respiration
- digestion and absorption
- excretion of waste
- growth and repair
- reproduction
- activity/movement.

Some of these characteristics are more evident in some organisms than others but all are vital for survival and the production of future generations.

## The organization of the human body

There are two main ways in which the body can be considered to be organized. One method of organization is grounded in **function** – or how the body works – the subject matter of **physiology**. The other has a **structural** or **anatomical** basis. These two systems of organization are not entirely distinct, in fact they are inextricably interlinked because the structure of anything determines its function.

In biology (the science of life) the basic unit of structural and functional organization is **the cell**. The structure and function of cells is described in detail in Chapter 1.3, along with a discussion of the general principles that underpin human growth, development and ageing.

Below cellular level is the chemical level of organization, and it is here that the working order of the body can really be considered to begin. It is for this reason that an understanding of the chemistry of life – the subject of the next chapter (1.2) – is so crucial as a basis for understanding human life at higher levels of organization. The increasing structural and functional complexity of chemical organization starts with simple atoms and molecules and develops through macromolecules, such as the proteins, carbohydrates, lipids and nucleic acids that are found in living matter, culminating in their organization into subcellular organelles of cells and their products.

All of the functions of life can and are carried out by single-celled (unicellular) organisms such as the amoeba. Many of the functions are present in most of the cells of higher multicellular organisms but, with increasing complexity, the organism becomes *organized* so that whole groups of cells are dedicated to specific functions, and might even lose certain functions in the process of specialization. In other words, a division of labour has evolved so that certain cells have become specialized for specific functions and, as a result, usually have a specialized structure. The cells of the human body vary considerably in both structure and function, even though they each contain an identical set of genes. The process through which cells with the same set of genetic information come to differ from each other, even when they share a similar environment, is called **differentiation**. Differentiation involves the progressive development of specialized structure and function along with the gradual loss of ability to develop in other ways.

## Tissues: societies of cells

Cells specialized for the performance of a common function are grouped together, with their associated intercellular material, to form **tissues (Fig. 1.1.1)**. For example, muscle cells have become specialized to contract and hence bring about movement. One result of cell specialization is that some cells have become so adapted to perform one particular function that they have lost the ability to perform others. A classic example of this is the mature human red blood cell, which, in becoming highly specialized for its function of oxygen transport, has lost its nucleus and many other subcellular organelles and become incapable of reproducing by cell division.

The existence of different tissues was first appreciated during anatomical dissection, but it was not until the light microscope was developed that researchers were able to recognize that these were collections of specialized cells. The study of tissues is called **histology**, and histology textbooks provide illustrated accounts of the features and functions of the various tissues. A brief classification of the major types of tissue that compose the human body is given below, and fuller descriptions of some of these tissues can be found in the relevant chapters of this book.

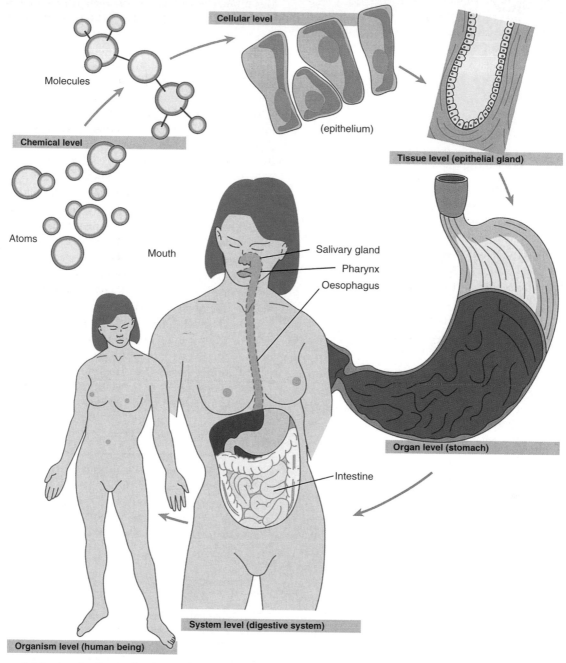

**Figure 1.1.1** Levels of organization in the human body. (After Tortora, G.J. & Grabowski, S.R. (1993) *Principles of Anatomy and Physiology*, 7th edn, with permission from HarperCollins Publishers, Inc.)

## Classification of the basic tissues

### Epithelial tissues

1. *Surface epithelia* – these cells cover or line all surfaces of the body, except the joint cavities.
2. *Glandular epithelia* – single cells, or groups of cells, specialized for secretion.
3. *Specialized epithelia* – cells specialized in sensory perception (of taste, smell, vision and hearing) and in reproduction (germinal epithelium).

### Connective tissues

1. *Connective tissues 'proper'*:
   - loose connective tissues, for example areolar connective tissue, adipose (fatty) tissue
   - dense connective tissues, for example tendons and ligaments.
2. *Blood, blood-forming tissues and lymph.*
3. *Supportive connective tissues* – cartilage and bone.

## Muscle tissue

1. *Smooth (non-striated or 'involuntary') muscle.*
2. *Skeletal (striated or 'voluntary') muscle.*
3. *Cardiac muscle.*

## Nervous tissue

1. *Neurones.*
2. *Non-neuronal cells* – for example, Schwann cells of the peripheral nervous system and glial cells of the central nervous system.

The arrangement of the specialized cells in each of the above tissues is as essential to body function as the biochemical characteristics of the molecules from which they are formed. The structure and function of the cells composing a tissue, and controlled cooperation between tissues, underlie and determine the form and function – in growth, maintenance and repair – of all parts of the body.

## Organs and organ systems

An organ is an orderly arrangement of tissues into a functional unit, for example the heart, the stomach or the kidney. Generally, organs are composed of several different types of tissue and conform to two basic arrangements:

1. tubular or hollow organs
2. compact or parenchymal organs.

### Tubular organs

An understanding of embryological development enables the body to be visualized as a large tube containing several internal tubes or tracts, such as the cardiovascular system, the respiratory system, the digestive system, the urinary system and the reproductive system. Each of these tracts, although modified for various functions – both as a whole and at different points along its length – is structurally similar to the others, in that they are all formed of layers of tissue superimposed on one another in a certain way.

Each tubular organ has three basic layers:

1. An *inner layer* composed of epithelium and its underlying connective tissue.
2. A *middle layer* composed of alternating layers of muscle and connective tissue.
3. An *external layer* composed of connective tissue and epithelium.

### Compact organs

Compact organs are characterized by their localized solid form but vary in size and shape. They may be large, such as the liver, or small, such as the ovaries.

Like tubular organs, compact organs all have a common basic pattern. They are usually enclosed by a dense, connective tissue **capsule**. If the organ is suspended in a body cavity, for example the abdominal cavity, it is covered by a serous membrane, which is a moist membrane bathed in serous fluid derived from blood plasma. On one side of the organ a thicker area of connective tissue penetrates the organ, forming the **hilus**. Compact organs have an extensive connective tissue framework, or **stroma**. Strands of connective tissue, called **trabeculae** or **septae**, extend into the organ from the capsule and hilus, sometimes dividing the organ into complete sections called **lobules**. Delicate reticular fibres interlace through the rest of the organ forming a framework for the **parenchyma**, which is the predominant functional tissue of the organ. Parenchymal cells can occur in masses, cords, strands or tubules, depending on the organ. The parenchyma can be divided into two further functionally distinct regions, a subcapsular **cortex** and a deeper **medulla**.

It might be helpful to bear in mind the general patterns of tubular and compact organs when using this book to study each body function, as knowledge of general principles such as these provides the basic plan to which the specialized structure and function of each component may be added.

## Organ systems

A 'system' is a group of organs that work together to perform a certain body function. The ten major organ systems of the human body are summarized in **Table 1.1.1**. These systems operate in a coordinated way to maintain homeostasis.

## Homeostasis

### The principle of maintaining constant cell composition

The normal function of the cells of any animal or plant depends on their ability to maintain, within relatively narrow limits, the physical and chemical properties of their constituents, such as temperature, state of hydration, concentration of nutrients, waste products, electrolytes and hydrogen ions. This is essential for normal cellular metabolism and because the cell's structural proteins and enzymes can be destroyed or inactivated by abnormal temperature and acidity.

As all cells are dynamic, open systems, continually using and producing substances as part of their metabolism, they must be able continually to exchange these substances with their immediate environment if they are to maintain constant composition.

**Table 1.1.1** Organ systems of the human body

| System | Major organs or tissues | Main functions |
|---|---|---|
| Cardiovascular | Heart, blood vessels, blood (lymphatic vessels and lymph are sometimes included in this system) | Transport of blood throughout the tissues of the body |
| Gastrointestinal | Mouth, pharynx, oesophagus, stomach, intestines, salivary glands, pancreas, liver, and gall bladder | Digestion and absorption of nutrients, minerals and water |
| Respiratory | Nose, mouth, pharynx, larynx, trachea, bronchi, lungs | Exchange of carbon dioxide and oxygen, regulation of hydrogen ion concentration |
| Renal | Kidneys, ureters, bladder, urethra | Regulation of plasma composition through controlled excretion of electrolytes, water and organic wastes |
| Musculoskeletal | Cartilage, bone, ligaments, tendons, joints, skeletal muscle | Support, protection and movement of the body. Production of blood cells |
| Integumentary | Skin | Protection against injury and desiccation. Defence against foreign invaders. Regulation of temperature |
| Immune | White blood cells, lymph vessels and nodes, spleen, thymus and other lymphoid tissues | Defence against foreign invaders, return of extracellular fluid to blood, formation of white blood cells |
| Reproductive | Male: testes, penis and associated ducts and glands. Female: ovaries, uterine tubes, uterus, vagina, mammary glands | Production of spermatozoa, transfer of spermatozoa to female. Production of ova, provision of environment for the developing embryo and fetus, nutrition of the infant |
| Endocrine | All glands secreting hormones: pancreas, testes, ovaries, hypothalamus, kidneys, pituitary, thyroid, parathyroid, adrenal, intestinal, thymus, heart and pineal | Regulation and coordination of many activities in the body |
| Nervous | Brain, spinal cord, peripheral nerves and ganglia, special sense organs | Regulation and coordination of many activities in the body, detection of changes in the internal and external environments, states of consciousness, learning and cognition |

If life is to be maintained, not only must the cell's environment be capable of supplying its requirements to maintain constant composition, but also the cell must be able to protect itself from the effects of fluctuations in aspects of its environment. The external environment of free-living, unicellular animals is usually vast in comparison with their volume. Hence, such animals have wide access to a supply of nutrients, and the dissipation of their waste products negligibly changes the composition of their environment. On the other hand, such animals are directly exposed to the effects of adverse changes in their environment and, if they are to survive these, must develop mechanisms to protect themselves.

## The consequence of increasing multicellularity

In larger, multicellular animals, certain cells are differentiated and specialized in the acquisition of nutrients and removal of waste. Such cells form the respiratory system, gastrointestinal system and renal system. To fulfil their functions, some cells in these systems communicate directly with the external environment. However, an inevitable consequence of increasing multicellularity and cell specialization is that some cells have no contact with the external environment and no contact with each other. As exchange with their immediate environment is insufficient for these cells to maintain constant composition, so there is a biological need for connecting each specialized group of cells with others and with the external environment – i.e. a need for an internal transport system. Hence, other cells became specialized to fulfil this function, forming the cardiovascular system and the fluid medium it contains, the blood. Through the function of these cells, indirect exchange between all cells and the external environment is made possible.

## Fluid compartments

In a complex, multicellular animal, then, few cells are in direct contact with the external environment. Instead, the immediate environment of the majority of cells is an 'internal' environment composed of the small amount of fluid that surrounds them – the tissue fluid or **interstitial fluid**. The watery fluid medium inside cells is, logically, called **intracellular fluid**, and that outside the cells is the **extracellular fluid**.

## Body water

Water constitutes between 50% and 70% of the total human body weight. The exact percentage depends on the amount of adipose tissue present, as this has a much lower water content relative to that of other tissues. As the amount of body fat is dependent on factors such as age, sex and dietary habits, total body water is also influenced by these variables. For example, it is lower in females and obese individuals, in whom body fat stores are greater, and is greatest in infants and children, in whom body fat stores are relatively less. After childhood, total body water gradually diminishes with age, forming, for example, about 60% of total body weight in a 70 kg adult man.

The volume of total body water is approximately 41 litres in a human adult and, together with the electrolytes and non-electrolytes that it contains in solution, this fluid is distributed between the **intracellular fluid** (25 litres) and the **extracellular fluid**

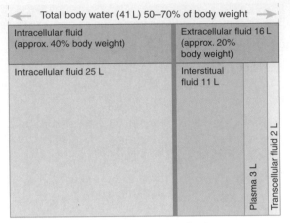

**Figure 1.1.2** Size of the major body fluid compartments in a 70 kg adult man

(16 litres) (**Fig. 1.1.2**). The human extracellular fluid compartment is therefore considerably smaller than the intracellular fluid compartment.

Blood plasma forms 3 litres of the extracellular fluid and the **interstitial fluid** forms 11 litres. Interstitial fluid directly bathes the cells and is often called **tissue fluid**. It is the medium through which exchanges between cells and the external environment occur. A further minor subdivision of the extracellular fluid compartment is provided by **transcellular fluid** (2 litres), which is separated from blood not only by the capillary endothelium but also by a layer of epithelium. It includes those fluids found in the body cavities, such as intraocular, pleural, peritoneal, synovial and cerebrospinal fluids, and the digestive secretions.

## Composition of fluid compartments

Each major fluid compartment has a unique composition but whereas plasma and interstitial fluid (both of which are extracellular) are similar, there are striking differences between these and intracellular fluid (**Fig. 1.1.3**).

In intracellular fluid the predominant positively charged ions (cations) are potassium ($K^+$) and magnesium ($Mg^{2+}$), with a very small amount of sodium ($Na^+$). The major negatively charged ions (anions) in intracellular fluid are organic phosphate (Org. $PO_4^{n-}$) and protein ($Pr^{n-}$), with very small amounts of hydrogen carbonate ($HCO_3^-$) and chloride ($Cl^-$).

In contrast, the major cation in extracellular fluid is sodium, with very small amounts of potassium, magnesium and calcium ($Ca^{2+}$). The anions chloride and hydrogen carbonate predominate in interstitial fluids, and chloride, hydrogen carbonate *and* protein predominate in plasma. Small amounts of hydrogen phosphate ($HPO_4^{2-}$), sulphate ($SO_4^{2-}$) and organic ions are also found in extracellular fluid.

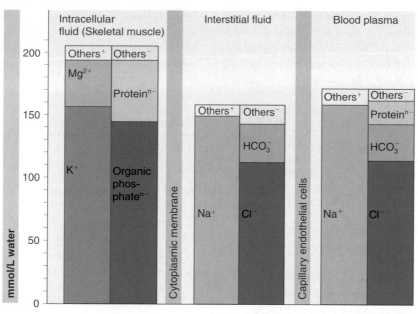

**Figure 1.1.3**   Electrolyte composition of body fluid compartments showing that total positive charges are neutralized by total negative charges within any one compartment

Thus, one of the major differences that exists between plasma and interstitial fluid is in the protein concentration, which is relatively high in plasma and low in interstitial fluid. The selective permeability of the capillary endothelium prevents large plasma protein molecules from entering interstitial fluid, although very small quantities do filter across and are returned to the vascular system via lymphatic drainage. Whereas the selective permeability of the capillary endothelium accounts for the differences in protein concentration between plasma and interstitial fluid, the differences in electrolyte concentration are explained by the fact that, because proteins are negatively charged anions (at the slightly alkaline pH of plasma 7.4), they attract diffusible cations, e.g. $Na^+$ and $K^+$, and repel diffusible anions, e.g. $Cl^-$. Because the physicochemical requirement of electroneutrality demands that in any solution the sum of the positive charges should equal the sum of the negative charges, this leads to an uneven distribution of diffusible ions across the capillary wall, with a small excess inside the capillary. This uneven distribution is referred to as the **Gibbs–Donnan membrane distribution**; the small excess of diffusible ions in plasma is known as the **Donnan excess**.

Differences in composition between intracellular and interstitial fluid are attributable to the selective permeability of the cytoplasmic membrane and the presence of an active transport, sodium–potassium ATPase pump, which continually extrudes sodium ions in exchange for potassium ions. Bearing in mind the fact that the cell contains large, non-diffusible anions such as protein and phosphate, the distribution of ions between these two compartments is also influenced by

the Gibbs–Donnan membrane equilibrium. In addition, the intracellular proteins also bind some ions, another factor that influences differences in composition between intracellular and interstitial fluid.

## The internal environment

In the middle of the nineteenth century, the French physiologist Claude Bernard realized that, in higher animals, the interstitial fluid forms the true internal environment of the cells and functions as a 'middleman' for all exchanges of matter between a cell and any other cell or with the external environment. He said that 'it is the fixity of the internal environment that is the condition of a free and independent life'. It follows that it is essential that the composition of the interstitial fluid is prevented from fluctuating widely if the cells are to be provided with the chemically stable, thermostatically controlled environment that they require. The process of preserving the constancy of the internal environment was called **homeostasis** by the American physiologist Walter Cannon (1932).

## Homeostatic mechanisms

A large number of physiological mechanisms operate to preserve the necessary conditions for life in the internal environment; such mechanisms are called homeostatic mechanisms. Homeostatic mechanisms operate via the systems that communicate with the external environment (respiratory, gastrointestinal and renal) and are controlled and coordinated by further specialized cells that comprise the nervous and endocrine systems. In addition to the body-wide homeostatic mechanisms mentioned above, locally operating mechanisms also help to maintain the stability of the internal environment; these will be considered throughout the book as each system is discussed in more detail.

A homeostatic mechanism is triggered by a change in a property of the extracellular fluid. It acts by negative feedback to restore or preserve the normal value by producing a change in the opposite direction. Some mechanisms are more complex than others. At its simplest, a homeostatic mechanism requires the following (**Fig. 1.1.4**):

1. *Detectors*. These are usually nervous receptors, which monitor the magnitude of the variables to be controlled.
2. *Effectors*. These cells, which include the muscles, glands, blood vessels, heart and kidneys, bring about the necessary compensatory changes.
3. *Coordinating mechanisms*. These can be nervous or endocrine; they couple the receptors to the effectors, ensuring that the magnitude and timing of responses are appropriate.

For example, most people drink more fluid than they require to excrete waste products in the urine (**Fig. 1.1.5**). When excess water is drunk and absorbed from the gastrointestinal tract into the circulation, the osmolality of plasma (normally about 285 mosmol/kg water) falls. This fall is detected by osmoreceptors in the hypothalamus in the brain, which transmit impulses to a controlling centre in the hypothalamus. This centre regulates the synthesis and release of antidiuretic hormone (ADH) from the posterior pituitary gland into the blood. The level of ADH in the blood determines the rate at which the kidneys excrete water. In this case, ADH secretion is reduced and so the kidneys excrete more water, restoring water

balance. This homeostatic mechanism controls the osmolality of plasma so that, in health, it fluctuates over only a narrow range. All homeostatic mechanisms can be described and explained in terms of a feedback loop similar to the one described above.

## Homeostasis and health

In health, each of the following physiological needs of a human being is kept in homeostatic balance.

1. Maintaining an adequate intake of oxygen and other nutrients.
2. Eliminating waste products and toxic substances.
3. Maintaining normal water balance, electrolyte and hydrogen ion concentration.
4. Maintaining body temperature within the normal range.
5. Maintaining intact defence mechanisms.
6. Moving and maintaining normal posture.
7. Resting and sleeping.

A supplementary physiological requirement that, although not essential for an individual's survival, is essential for the survival of the human species, is the need to reproduce.

The fulfilment of all these needs is dependent on the normal activity of the cells that perform these functions and also on the normal activity of the cells of the coordinating and integrating systems (nervous, endocrine and cardiovascular) that 'link up' homeostatic mechanisms. A malfunction in any part of these systems can have a widespread adverse effect on homeostasis and health.

The multitude of homeostatic mechanisms that maintain life and health make up a large part of the

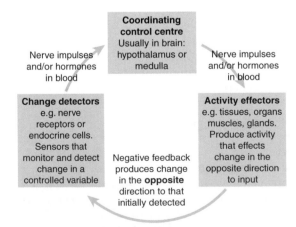

**Figure 1.1.4** A homeostatic negative feedback loop showing how negative feedback produces a change in the opposite direction to that initially detected

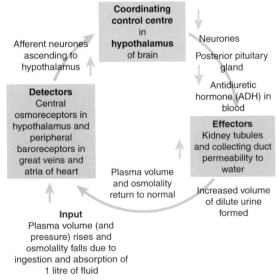

**Figure 1.1.5** Example of a homeostatic negative feedback loop: control of water balance

subject matter of physiology, and hence the content of this book. Most physical health problems can be understood as being the result of a breakdown in homeostasis. It follows that knowledge of homeostatic mechanisms, and the factors that can affect them, forms one of the major bases for the rational planning, delivery and evaluation of patient care.

## Anatomical organization

Externally, the human body has a definite and recognizable shape, and internally the organs are located in specific positions relative to one another. This constancy in the organization of the body allows its description and the location of particular parts.

The anatomical organization of the body can be considered in a number of ways, which vary in their complexity. The head, the thorax and the abdomen contain particular organs, and locations within these areas can be specified by considering the directions around these areas and the planes of the body.

Directions in the body can be considered to be anterior (towards the front), posterior (towards the rear), proximal (towards the trunk), distal (away from the trunk), medial (towards the midline of the body) and lateral (away from the midline of the body). These are shown in **Fig. 1.1.6**. The planes of the body are shown in **Fig. 1.1.7**; they are the median (midsagittal), transverse and coronal (frontal) planes.

It is sometimes necessary to be much more precise when locating areas in the body. A good example of this is the regions of the abdomen, which are shown in **Fig. 1.1.8**. These can be considered grossly, i.e. in quadrants, or much more precisely. Such precision would, for example, be required by a physician or surgeon in the diagnosis of an illness involving the abdomen or when a surgical incision has to be made.

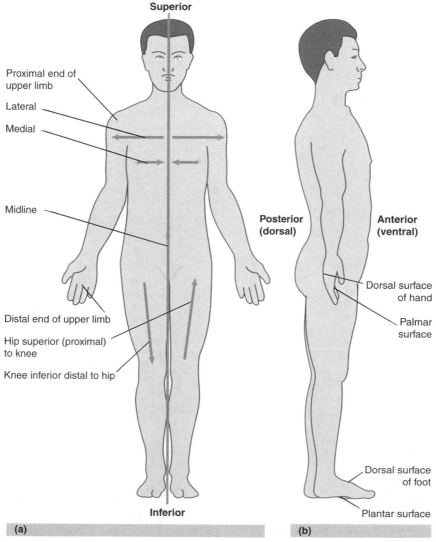

**Figure 1.1.6**   Directional terms of the body

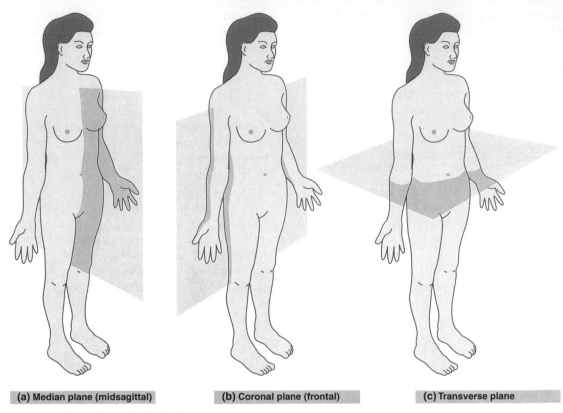

**(a) Median plane (midsagittal)**     **(b) Coronal plane (frontal)**     **(c) Transverse plane**

**Figure 1.1.7**  Planes through the body

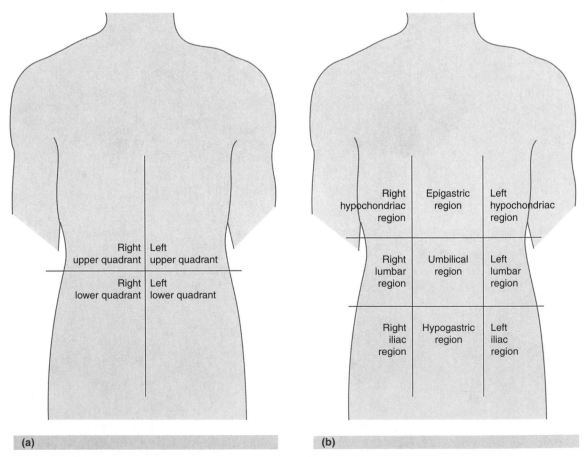

**(a)**     **(b)**

**Figure 1.1.8**  Quadrants (a) and anatomical subdivisions (b) of the abdomen

At first, anatomical terminology can seem unfamiliar and difficult to understand but once you understand the basic words, prefixes and suffixes you will discover the logical and helpful method in which structures are named. For example, once one understands that superior means 'towards the head' and anterior means 'towards the front' (see Fig. 1.1.6), and once one knows that the ilium is a bone in the pelvis (see Fig. 1.1.10), then it becomes easy to identify the 'anterior superior iliac spine of the pelvis'. Similarly, if one knows that the term 'cardium' refers to the heart and 'pulmonary' to the lungs, then the term 'cardiopulmonary function' becomes clear. Learning these terms will take time but it is well worth the effort!

## Body cavities

The cavities of the body contain the internal organs or viscera. The two main body cavities are the smaller posterior (dorsal) cavity, which contains the cranial cavity (which houses the brain), and the spinal cavity (which contains the spinal cord) (Fig. 1.1.9). The larger anterior (ventral) cavity is divided by the dome-shaped muscular diaphragm into the superior thoracic cavity and the inferior abdominopelvic cavity.

The thoracic cavity contains the pericardial membrane, which encloses the heart within the pericardial cavity, and the pleural membranes, which contain the lungs within the pleural cavities.

The abdominopelvic cavity is divided into the superior abdominal cavity and inferior pelvic cavity at the superior margin or the bony iliac crest (pelvis) (Fig. 1.1.10).

The abdominal cavity contains the stomach, small and large intestines, liver, spleen, gall bladder, pancreas and kidneys. The pelvic cavity contains the rectum,

urinary bladder and reproductive organs (Fig. 1.1.11). Both the abdominal and pelvic cavities are lined with peritoneal membrane (peritoneum), which forms the superior and inferior peritoneal cavities.

The major function of the bony adult skeleton (see Fig. 1.1.10), which consists of 206 named bones, is to support the internal organs. As well as providing this vital support, the skeleton also surrounds and protects many of these organs in bony cavities. For example, the brain is enclosed within the cranium of the skull and the lungs and heart within the thoracic rib cage. The structure and functions of bones, and their role in the lever systems that permit body movement, are described in Section 3.

## SI units in clinical practice

Système Internationale d'Unités, or the international system of units (SI for short), based on metric measurements, is now widely used in science and medicine throughout the world. In the UK the metric system replaced the Imperial system in the 1960s and 1970s; however, there was a wide variety of metric units in use at that time and so the SI system was adopted in an attempt to standardize these units. The units used in medicine are sometimes inconsistent, mainly because of tradition or the impracticality of some SI units, and also in order to avoid having to replace equipment using imperial units, e.g. sphygmomanometers for measuring blood pressure.

SI uses seven basic, so-called fundamental, units and many derived units (made from two or more of the fundamental units). Before describing the SI units and their relationship to imperial or non-SI

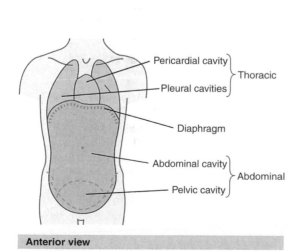

Anterior view

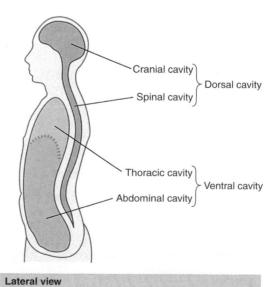

Lateral view

**Figure 1.1.9**  Anterior and lateral views of the body showing major cavities

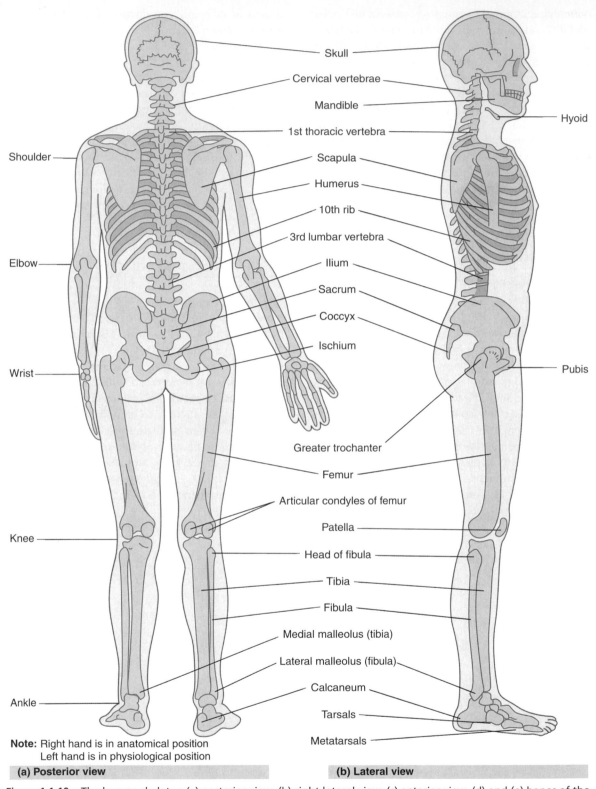

Skull
Cervical vertebrae
Mandible
Hyoid
1st thoracic vertebra
Scapula
Humerus
10th rib
3rd lumbar vertebra
Ilium
Sacrum
Coccyx
Ischium
Pubis

Shoulder
Elbow
Wrist
Knee
Ankle

Greater trochanter
Femur
Articular condyles of femur
Patella
Head of fibula
Tibia
Fibula
Medial malleolus (tibia)
Lateral malleolus (fibula)
Calcaneum
Tarsals
Metatarsals

**Note:** Right hand is in anatomical position
Left hand is in physiological position

**(a) Posterior view**

**(b) Lateral view**

**Figure 1.1.10** The human skeleton (a) posterior view, (b) right lateral view, (c) anterior view, (d) and (e) bones of the forearm

units, a brief description will be given of the accepted way of writing numbers.

Metric systems use decimal numbers, that is, numbers based on powers of 10. Very large and very small

numbers are often encountered when describing chemical and biological measurements. The scientific notation is to write such numbers in terms of a power of ten, e.g. 1000 can be written as $10^3$. This is

**Figure 1.1.10** (*contd*)

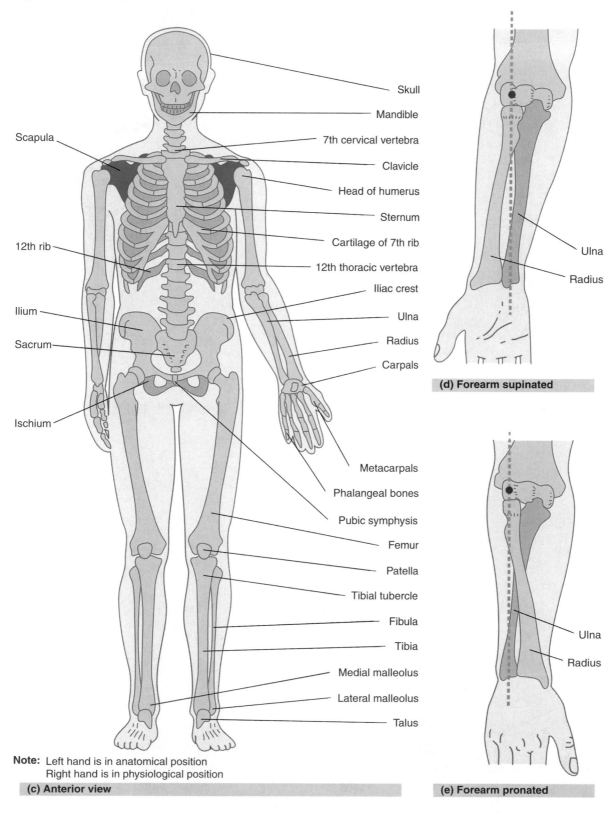

Skull

Mandible

7th cervical vertebra

Clavicle

Head of humerus

Sternum

Cartilage of 7th rib

12th thoracic vertebra

Iliac crest

Ulna

Radius

Carpals

**(d) Forearm supinated**

Scapula

12th rib

Ilium

Sacrum

Ischium

Metacarpals

Phalangeal bones

Pubic symphysis

Femur

Patella

Tibial tubercle

Fibula

Tibia

Medial malleolus

Lateral malleolus

Talus

Ulna

Radius

Ulna

Radius

**Note:** Left hand is in anatomical position
Right hand is in physiological position

**(c) Anterior view**

**(e) Forearm pronated**

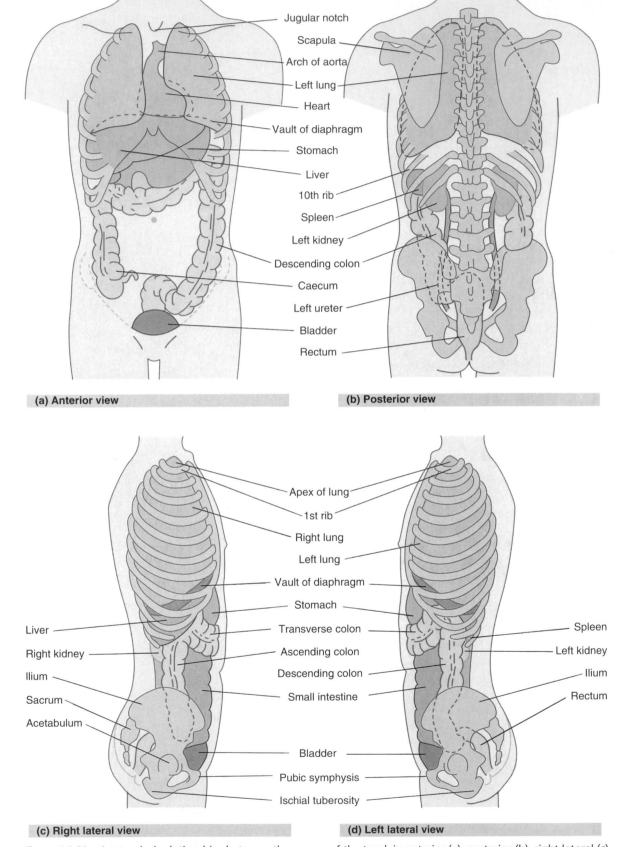

**(a) Anterior view**

**(b) Posterior view**

**(c) Right lateral view**

**(d) Left lateral view**

**Figure 1.1.11** Anatomical relationships between the organs of the trunk in anterior (a), posterior (b), right lateral (c) and left lateral (d) views

because $10 \times 10 \times 10 = 1000 = 10^3$ (i.e. ten to the power three). Similarly:

$$1000 \times 1000 = 1\,000\,000 = 10^6$$
$$10^3 \times 10^3 = 10^6$$

When a number contains other numerals, the number is written as follows:

$$5 \text{ million} = 5\,000\,000 = 5 \times 10^6$$
$$5.5 \text{ million} = 5\,500\,000 = 5.5 \times 10^6$$

The accepted form of scientific notation is to place only one numeral to the left of the decimal point.

A similar principle operates for numbers smaller than 1. For example:

$$0.001 = 1 \times 10^{-3}$$

This is equivalent to

$$0.1 \times 0.1 \times 0.1 = 1 \times 10^{-3}$$
$$\frac{1}{10} \times \frac{1}{10} \times \frac{1}{10} = \frac{1}{1000} = 1 \times 10^{-3}$$

or:

$$10^{-1} \times 10^{-1} \times 10^{-1} = 1 \times 10^{-3}$$

The negative or minus sign in front of the raised numeral indicates that the powers of 10 are being divided into the digit.

With numbers other than 1:

$$0.0004 = 4 \times 10^{-4}$$
$$0.000\,045 = 4.5 \times 10^{-5} \text{ i.e. } \frac{4.5}{100\,000}$$

Numbers with many figures are divided into groups of three digits by gaps and *not* commas as previously (e.g. earlier printing: 5,613,100; current printing: 5 613 100). The exceptions to this are 4-digit numbers, which are usually printed without a gap, e.g. 1629. Commas are no longer used because, although the decimal point is indicated by a full stop on the line in English-speaking countries (e.g. 1.96), in some other countries the decimal point is indicated by a comma (e.g. 1,96). Thus, to avoid any possible confusion, commas are no longer inserted to space large numbers (see earlier). If a number is less than 1, a zero must always be inserted before the decimal point, e.g. 0.88 and not .88.

Decimal multiples and submultiples of SI units are commonly required in everyday use of units. Powers of 1000 are preferred e.g. kilo-, milli-, micro-, but any of the prefixes in **Table 1.1.2** can be used.

| Table 1.1.2 | Prefixes indicating powers | | |
|---|---|---|---|
| **Prefic** | **Symbol** | **Value** | **Factor by which the unit is multiplied** |
| tera- | T | 1 000 000 000 000 | $10^{12}$ |
| giga- | G | 1 000 000 000 | $10^{9}$ |
| mega- | M | 1 000 000 | $10^{6}$ |
| *kilo- | k | 1000 | $10^{3}$ |
| hecto- | h | 100 | $10^{2}$ |
| deca- | da | 10 | $10^{1}$ |
| deci- | d | 0.1 | $10^{-1}$ |
| *centi- | c | 0.01 | $10^{-2}$ |
| *milli- | m | 0.001 | $10^{-3}$ |
| *micro- | μ[†] | 0.000 001 | $10^{-6}$ |
| nano- | n | 0.000 000 001 | $10^{-9}$ |
| pico- | p | 0.000 000 000 001 | $10^{-12}$ |
| femto- | f | 0.000 000 000 000 001 | $10^{-15}$ |
| atto- | a | 0.000 000 000 000 000 001 | $10^{-18}$ |

* Prefixes in common clinical use
† This symbol is the Greek letter 'mu' – however, it is read as 'micro-'

**Table 1.1.3**  Basic SI units

| Physical quantity | Name of SI base unit | Symbol of SI unit |
|---|---|---|
| Length | metre | m |
| Mass | kilogram | kg |
| Time | second* | s |
| Temperature | kelvin | K |
| Amount of substance | mole | mol |
| Electrical current | ampere | A |
| Luminous intensity | candela | cd |

\* Although the second is the basic unit for time, for general use the minute (symbol min), hour (symbol h) and day (symbol d) may be used

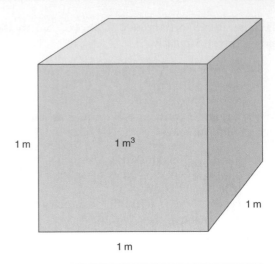

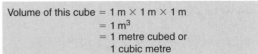
Volume of this cube = 1 m × 1 m × 1 m
= 1 m³
= 1 metre cubed or
1 cubic metre

**Figure 1.1.12**  Volume of a 1 metre cube

## Basic SI units

The seven basic units are presented in **Table 1.1.3**.

Do *not* add an 's' to the symbols to make them plural and the symbol should *not* be followed by a full stop (unless it occurs at the end of a sentence): e.g. 60 kg and *not* 60 kgs. Thus:

> Mrs Smith, who is only 1.5 m tall, weighs 80 kg and so is severely overweight.

The prefixes listed in **Table 1.1.2** are frequently combined with the basic units in **Table 1.1.3** to give workable and 'sensible sized' units. For example:

kilometre (km)     = 1000 m
centimetre (cm)    = 0.01 m
nanometre (nm)     = $10^{-9}$ m
millimole (mmol) = 0.001 mol
                         or $1 \times 10^{-3}$ mol

Where necessary, the fundamental units can be combined. For example, a fluid infusion rate of 100 millilitres per hour can be written as 100 mL/h or 100 mLh$^{-1}$. More specific combinations are possible, for example a fluid infusion rate can be described as 10 millilitres per kilogram bodyweight per hour. This can be written as 10 mL/kg/h or 10 mL kg$^{-1}$h$^{-1}$.

## Additional notes and explanations on the use of the basic units

### Length

The SI unit for length is the metre: multiples and sub-multiples of the metre replace the units of miles, yards, feet and inches (1 metre is equal to 39.37 inches).

Two metric units used in the past for very small lengths were the micron ($10^{-6}$ m) and the Ångstrom ($10^{-10}$ m). These terms are now obsolete: the micron is now referred to as the micrometre (i.e. 1 μm or $10^{-6}$ m) whereas the Ångstrom unit is equivalent to 0.1 nanometres.

### Volume

The volume of an object is found by multiplying length, breadth and depth together (**Fig. 1.1.12**). This can give a large volume and is not practical for many clinical purposes. Thus the litre (symbol 'L') is commonly used as the unit for measuring volumes of liquids and gases. The litre is not a separate fundamental unit of the SI system, but is related to both length and mass; 1 litre is equivalent to 1 cubic decimetre (1 dm³) (**Fig. 1.1.13**); 1 m³ is thus equivalent to 1000 litres.

An even smaller unit of volume is the millilitre (mL), i.e. one thousandth of a litre:

$$1 \text{ mL} = 1 \times 10^{-3} \text{ L}$$

The millilitre is familiar to most people, for instance the standard spoon for medicines is 5 mL. One millilitre is equivalent to one cubic centimetre.

The litre is also related to mass, in that one litre of water weighs approximately 1 kg.

### Mass

Although the kilogram is the basic unit for mass, the smaller unit gram (g) is used very commonly (1000 g = 1 kg). These units replace stones, pounds

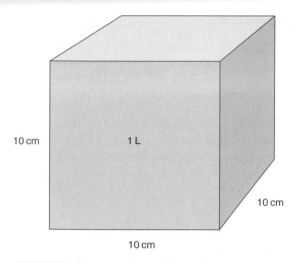

Volume of this cube = 10 cm × 10 cm × 10 cm
= 1000 cm³
= 1 dm × 1 dm × 1 dm
= 1 dm³
= 1 L

**Figure 1.1.13** Volume of a 10-centimetre cube

and ounces. The prefixes described previously are used in combination with gram, for example:

milligram (mg) = 0.001 g
*microgram (μg) = 0.001 mg or 1 × 10⁻⁶ g

(*sometimes microgram is written mcg – this is incorrect and should not be used).

Strictly speaking, the weight of an object is a measure of force, i.e. the mass multiplied by the acceleration due to gravity. However, as in most measurements, the acceleration due to gravity is constant, the weight of an object is usually expressed in kilograms, indicating its mass. This point is demonstrated by considering a person in outer space who is 'weightless' but still has a mass of, say, 75 kg.

## Temperature

The SI unit for temperature is the kelvin (symbol K) but this is not used clinically: for ordinary use the *Celsius* scale is internationally recognized. On this scale water freezes at zero degrees Celsius (0°C) and boils at one hundred degrees Celsius (100°C). These units are frequently called degrees centigrade: strictly speaking, the term 'centigrade' should not be used in SI units because in some countries it means something quite different – a measure of angle. The Celsius scale replaces the Fahrenheit scale, where water freezes at 32°F and boils at 212°F.

Absolute zero or 0 K is equal to −273°C. A change of 1 K is identical to a change of 1°C. Thus 37°C is equal to 310 K, as 37 + 273 = 310 K. Note that the symbol K is not preceded by a degree (°) symbol.

## The amount and concentration of a substance

The SI unit for the amount of a substance is the mole. For most practical purposes one mole is the molecular weight of a substance in grams. There is one mole of molecules present for every $6.023 \times 10^{23}$ molecules (an analogy to this is a ream of paper representing 480 sheets of paper).

Concentration refers to the quantity of substance present in a given volume and is usually expressed in terms of moles and litres; for example a blood glucose concentration of 4.2 mmol/L or $4.2 \, \text{mmolL}^{-1}$, or intravenous saline containing 150 mmol/L or $150 \, \text{mmolL}^{-1}$.

Proteins are of variable molecular weight and there are problems in calculating the molar concentrations, particularly when mixtures of proteins are present. Therefore it is usual to report protein concentration in grams per litre (g/L or $gL^{-1}$) rather than in moles per litre, e.g. a plasma albumin concentration of 40 g/L or $40 \, gL^{-1}$. Values for enzymes are given in international units (abbreviated as U, IU or i.u.) per litre and are a measure of enzyme activity. The values will vary from hospital to hospital if the assay procedures differ.

By convention, haemoglobin concentration is given in grams per decilitre, e.g. 14 g/dL. This is an internationally accepted inconsistency! Grams per decilitre is equivalent to grams per hundred millilitres; for example, 14 g/dL can be written as 14 g/100 mL.

Concentrations often used to be expressed in milliequivalents per litre (mEq/L) but these units have been replaced by the millimole:

$$\text{Number of equivalents (Eq)} = \frac{\text{weight in grams} \times \text{valency}}{\text{molecular weight}}$$

$$\text{Number of moles (mol)} = \frac{\text{weight in grams}}{\text{molecular weight}}$$

In the case of univalent ions (e.g. $Na^+$, $K^+$) the values will be numerically the same, i.e. a sodium concentration of 140 mEq/L becomes 140 mmol/L. For polyvalent ions (e.g. $Ca^{2+}$, $Mg^{2+}$) the old units are numerically divided by the valency, i.e. a magnesium ion concentration of 2.0 mEq/L becomes 1.0 mmol/L.

Some values were previously expressed as mg/100 mL; therefore the method of conversion to mmol/L is to divide by the molecular weight (to convert from mg to mmol) and to multiply by 10 (to convert from 100 mL to a litre).

In many clinical areas now, pH is being expressed in nanomoles of hydrogen ions per litre, i.e. pH 7.4 = 40 nmol/L.

## Derived units

The seven basic units do not cover all the parameters that need units and other units, all derived from the basic units, have been given special names and symbols of their own (**Table 1.1.4**).

## Additional explanations for derived units

### Pressure units

The SI unit for pressure is the pascal (Pa) and this replaces the Imperial unit of millimetres of mercury (mmHg). As the pascal is a very small unit of pressure, measurements are frequently given in kilopascals (kPa), i.e. 1000 Pa.

Medical science is inconsistent in its usage of pressure units. Blood gas pressure estimations are now often given in kilopascals; for example, an arterial $pO_2$ of 12.7 kPa rather than 95 mmHg. However, blood pressure recordings are still expressed in mmHg; for example, a blood pressure of 120/75 mmHg rather than 16/10 kPa.

The pressure in kilopascals = pressure in mmHg ÷ 7.5

(See **Table 4.2.3** in Chapter 4.2 to convert mmHg to kPa.)

### Energy units

The SI unit for all forms of energy is the joule (J) or, commonly, kilojoule (kJ). Thus the energy of food is usually measured in kJ and this replaces the calorie (or kilocalorie), which was a measure of units of heat.

One calorie is approximately 4.2 kJ. Thus a 2000 calorie diet is equivalent to an 8400 kJ diet.

Approximate conversion factors and formulae for conversions between SI and Imperial units are given in **Table 1.1.5**.

## Conclusion

The organization of the body can be described in both anatomical and physiological terms. The two systems of organization are closely interlinked and enable us to locate structures within the body and to understand how the cells, tissues, organs and systems of the body are organized to achieve homeostasis. The international system of units of measurement (SI) is now widely used in clinical measurement. There are seven fundamental and many more derived units, all of which might be encountered in practice.

**Table 1.1.4 SI units derived from basic units**

| Quantity/parameter | Name of derived unit | Symbol | In terms of other SI derived units |
|---|---|---|---|
| Work / Energy / Quantity of heat | Joule | J | Nm |
| Force | Newton | N | $kgms^{-2}$ ($kgm/s^2$) |
| Power | Watt | W | $Js^{-1}$ (J/s) |
| Pressure | Pascal | Pa | $Nm^{-2}$ ($N/m^2$) |
| Frequency (for periodic phenomena – replaces cycles per second) | Hertz | Hz | $s^{-1}$ (/s) |
| Electrical potential / Potential difference / Electromotive force | Volt | V | $WA^{-1}$ (W/A) |
| Absorbed dose (ionizing radiation) | Gray | Gy | $m^2s^{-2}$ ($m^2/s^2$) |
| Radionuclide activity (for measurements of numbers of nuclear transformations per second) | Becquerel | Bq | $s^{-1}$ (/s) |

**Table 1.1.5**  Approximate conversions between SI and Imperial units

| Parameter | Accepted clinical SI unit in common use | Imperial units | Approximate conversions | |
|---|---|---|---|---|
| | | | From SI units | To SI units |
| Temperature | °C | °F | (9/5)°C + 32 = °F | (5/9)°F − 32 = °C |
| Pressure | kPa | mmHg | kPa × 7.5 = mmHg | mmHg ÷ 7.5 = kPa |
| Volume | 1 (or dm³) mL | Pint Fluid ounce | l ÷ 0.57 = pint ml ÷ 28.4 = fl. oz | pint × 0.57 = L fl. oz × 28.4 = mL |
| Length | m mm | Yard Inch | m ÷ 0.91 = yard mm ÷ 25.4 = inch | yard × 0.91 = m inch × 25.4 = mm |
| Mass | kg g | Pound Pound | kg × 2.2 = lb g ÷ 454 = lb | lb ÷ 2.2 = kg lb × 454 = g |
| Concentration | mmol/L | mEq/L | see text | |
| Energy | kJ | Calorie or kilocalorie | kJ ÷ 4.2 = Cal | Cal × 4.2 = kJ |

## Clinical review

In addition to the Learning Objectives at the beginning of this chapter, the reader should be able to:

- Define the terms cell, tissue, organ, system and organism, and explain how they interrelate functionally

- Describe the structure and function of one tissue of your choice

- Describe how the various organ systems of the body function in homeostasis

- Define the term homeostasis and using examples, explain the relationship between this fundamental physiological concept and health

- Identify uses of the International System of measurement in clinical practice

## Review questions

1  How would you describe a tissue?
2  What are the main features of a hollow organ?
3  How would you describe an organ system?
4  What fluid forms the major part of the extracellular fluid?
5  Which systems control homeostasis?
6  Explain the terms anterior, posterior, medial and lateral
7  What is the position of the peritoneum?

## Suggestions for further reading

Cormack, D.H. (2001) *Essential Histology*, 2nd edn. Philadelphia: J.B. Lippincott.
*A clear introductory text that takes a fresh look at what constitutes essential subject matter.*

England, M.A. & Waddell, H. (1996) *A Colour Atlas of Life Before Birth. Normal Fetal Development*, 2nd edn. London: Mosby.
*A reduced-size, soft-cover edition of the best selling atlas, which contains a magnificent set of photographs that go a long way in aiding understanding embryology.*

Freeman, W.H. & Bracegirdle, B. (1966) *An Atlas of Histology*. London: Heinemann Educational.
*Despite its age, this book remains an excellent introductory text. It uses labelled line diagrams alongside photographs of histological specimens to aid explanation, and classifies tissue clearly.*

Fullick, A. (2000) *Heinemann Advanced Science: Biology*, 2nd edn. London: Heinemann.
*A well-presented text written to support current 'A' level syllabuses. Useful background if you have not studied biology at this level.*

Gartner, L.P. & Hiatt, J.L. (1994) *Color Atlas of Histology*, 2nd edn. Baltimore: Williams and Wilkins.
*Beautifully illustrated and organized atlas of histology.*

Kapit, W. & Elson, L.M. (2001) *The Anatomy Colouring Book*, 3rd edn. New York: Harper Collins.
*Aims to help students achieve a thorough and effective understanding of body structure and related function – and to enjoy doing so through active involvement by colouring in the parts studied!*

Larsen, W.J. (2001) *Human Embryology*, 3rd edn. Edinburgh: Churchill Livingstone.
*Excellent, concise textbook. Well organized and clearly illustrated. Written to meet the needs of first-year medical students.*

Moore, K.L. (1999) *Clinically Orientated Anatomy*, 4th edn. Baltimore: Williams and Wilkins.
*A clearly presented anatomy text, which, as its title suggests, is organized to meet the needs of clinical students, through the copious use of clinical case notes linked to the anatomy theory.*

Moore, K.L. & Persaud, T.V.N. (1998) *Before We Are Born*, 5th edn. Philadelphia: W.B. Saunders.
*Presents a clear, concise account of human embryology and birth defects. Focuses on normal development but also covers common congenital anomalies and their causes.*

Netter, F.H. (1998) *Atlas of Human Anatomy*, 2nd edn. London: Ciba-Geigy.
*Beautifully presented anatomical atlas.*

Rogers, A.W. (1983) *Cells and Tissues*. London: Academic Press.
*An unique introductory histology and cell biology text that is specifically designed to help students of health sciences understand cell structure and histological interpretation.*

Von Hagens, G., Romrell, L., Ross, M.H. & Tiedmann, K. (1991) *The Visible Human Body: An Atlas of Cross-Sectional Anatomy*. Philadelphia: Lea and Febiger.
*Another excellent anatomical atlas focusing on portraying the human body as it appears in sections through various planes.*

## Reference

Cannon, W.B. (1932) *The Wisdom of the Body*. New York: Norton.

# The chemistry of living matter

*Michael G. Davis    Roger Watson*

---

## LEARNING OBJECTIVES

After studying this chapter the reader should be able to:

- Define what an element is, know which elements are important in living matter and recognize the symbols for these elements

- Define what an atom is, know what atoms consist of, and know the difference between atomic mass (weight) and atomic number

- Define what a molecule is, know what valency means, understand how atoms join together covalently and recognize simple molecular formulae

- Define the terms 'ion', 'electrolyte' and 'salt', and understand how ionic bonds are formed

- Explain what hydrogen bonding means and understand its significance in water

- Understand the difference between the terms 'solution', 'solute' and 'solvent'

- Understand the difference between concentration and amount, and recognize the different units used to measure concentration

- Understand the difference between the terms 'hydrophilic' and 'hydrophobic'

- Explain what osmolarity means and understand the difference between hypotonic, isotonic and hypertonic solutions

- Define an acid, understand the difference between strong and weak acids and give examples of each

- Describe what a base is, understand the difference between strong and weak bases and give examples of each

- Define the term 'pH' and understand its significance for fluids of biological importance

- Explain what a buffer is and understand its function

- Define the term 'carbohydrate', recognize the structures of biologically important mono-, di- and polysaccharides, and describe their functions

- Define the terms 'hydrocarbon' and 'lipid', explain what triglycerides consist of and understand the chemical difference between saturated, monounsaturated and polyunsaturated fatty acids

- Define the term 'protein', explain what protein consists of and outline the main biological function of proteins

- Define the term 'amino acid', write the general formula for an amino acid and understand what a peptide bond is

- Understand the difference between amino acids and amines and give biologically important examples of each

- Define the terms 'nucleotide' and 'polynucleotide' and explain the chemical and biological differences between DNA and RNA

- Understand the differences between condensation and hydrolysis, hydration and dehydration, oxidation and reduction, carboxylation and decarboxylation

## INTRODUCTION

To understand how our bodies function in health and disease we need to have some understanding of the relevant medical sciences. Anatomy shows us the structure of our bodies; physiology the functions and activities of our organs and tissues; and through cell biology we discover the components of cells and their functions in living processes. However, to understand the ultimate physical basis of life we must turn to biochemistry, which has helped to explain the chemical composition of living matter and the interactions of chemicals in metabolism, energy production, biosynthesis and replication.

## The composition of living matter

Clearly there is more to life than chemistry, yet chemicals and chemical reactions make up the foundations and framework of all living processes. Therefore, some knowledge of biochemistry is essential for an understanding of human physiology. A good place to start is the chemical content and composition of the human body. **Table 1.2.1** shows that we are about two-thirds water, with roughly equal amounts of fat and protein (with considerable individual variation here!), a small residue of minerals and only tiny amounts of carbohydrate.

If a chemical analyst was to break-down these substances to their smallest components of matter or **elements**, the elemental composition of the body would be obtained, as shown in **Table 1.2.2**. An element is defined as a substance which cannot be broken down further into simpler substances, and all matter is composed of these chemical elements. Just over a hundred elements are known and each has its own **atomic symbol** for convenience (e.g. C for carbon). As **Table 1.2.2** shows, 99% of all living matter is made up from just half-a-dozen elements. Another four comprise just under 1% and a further

ten trace elements make up about 0.1% of the total body weight. So all matter (whether living or inanimate) is made from these different elements. Next we need to know what the elements themselves are made from.

## Atoms: the smallest components of elements

Elements consist of **atoms,** which can be defined as the smallest indivisible part of an element that retains the chemical and physical properties of that element. Each type of element has its own type of atom, which is distinct from all other atoms. The element carbon is made up of carbon atoms, which are quite distinct from the atoms of the elements hydrogen, oxygen and nitrogen, and so on. These atoms differ not only in their chemical and physical properties but also in size and weight. All these differences can be explained by differences in the internal composition of the atoms.

## Atomic composition and structure

Although atoms cannot be broken down chemically, atoms are in fact made up from three even smaller

| Table 1.2.1 Composition of the human body | |
|---|---|
| **Substance** | **Approximate percentage by weight** |
| Water | 65 |
| Fat | 15 |
| Protein | 15 |
| Minerals | 5 |
| Carbohydrate | <1 |

| Table 1.2.2 Elemental analysis of the human body | | |
|---|---|---|
| **Element** | **Atomic symbol** | **Approximate percentage by weight** |
| Oxygen | O | 65 ⎫ |
| Carbon | C | 18 ⎪ |
| Hydrogen | H | 10 ⎪ |
| Nitrogen | N | 3 ⎬ 99% |
| Calcium | Ca | 2 ⎪ |
| Phosphorus | P | 1 ⎭ |
| Potassium | K | 0.35 ⎫ |
| Sulphur | S | 0.25 ⎪ 0.9% |
| Sodium | Na | 0.15 ⎬ |
| Chlorine | Cl | 0.15 ⎭ |
| Magnesium | Mg | * ⎫ |
| Iron | Fe | * ⎪ |
| Zinc | Zn | * ⎪ |
| Copper | Cu | * ⎪ |
| Iodine | I | * ⎪ |
| Manganese | Mn | * ⎬ 0.1% |
| Chromium | Cr | * ⎪ |
| Molybdenum | Mo | * ⎪ |
| Cobalt | Co | * ⎪ |
| Selenium | Se | * ⎭ |
| * denotes 'trace' | | |

**subatomic particles**, named **neutrons**, **protons** and **electrons**. As shown in **Table 1.2.3**, neutrons have no charge, protons carry a positive charge and electrons have a negative charge. Protons and neutrons have the same size and weight and are present in the central **nucleus** of the atom, whereas electrons (the size and weight of which are negligible in comparison) are present in orbital layers, or shells, surrounding the nucleus (**Fig. 1.2.1**).

The electrons in these orbitals, or shells, behave rather like cloud layers of electrical charge surrounding the nucleus, and obey certain rules as to how many electrons each layer can accommodate. Electrons in outer orbitals have higher energy levels than those in the inner orbitals. Electrons are the basis of **electricity**, an electric current being caused by the movement of electrons along a conductor such as a piece of wire (and the faster they move the greater the current). Static electricity is caused by the removal of electrons from the surface of material (e.g. when brushing hair or rubbing a nylon surface). A build-up of static electrical energy can discharge in sparks or lightning.

| Table 1.2.3 Subatomic particles and their properties | | | |
|---|---|---|---|
| **Particle** | **Relative mass** | **Relative charge** | **Location** |
| Neutron | 1 | 0 | Nucleus |
| Proton | 1 | +1 | Nucleus |
| Electron | $5.4 \times 10^{-4}$ | −1 | Orbital shells |

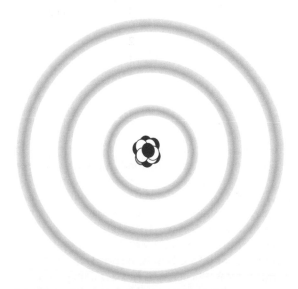

**Figure 1.2.1** Diagrammatic representation of the structure of an atom showing the nucleus surrounded by electron orbital shells

The number of negatively charged electrons in an atom equals the number of positively charged protons, so the atom as a whole is uncharged. (Later we will see what happens when atoms become charged.) This number of electrons or protons is called the **atomic number** and has a different value for each element. Neutrons contribute to the relative mass of an atom but have no effect on its charge. The sum of the number of neutrons and protons in an atom is called the **mass number**. This determines the relative **atomic mass** of an element, often referred to as its **atomic weight**. These values are shown for a number of the biologically more important elements in **Table 1.2.4**.

## Atoms with a difference: isotopes and radioactivity

Although elements always have the same atomic number (i.e. the same number of electrons and protons), the mass number can vary due to different numbers of neutrons being present in the nucleus. These different forms of the same element are called **isotopes**. **Table 1.2.4** shows that chlorine consists of two isotopes with mass numbers of 35 and 37. The resulting atomic mass of 35.5 is determined by the relative proportion of each naturally occurring isotope. In some isotopes, the presence of extra neutrons in the nucleus causes instability, resulting in atomic transformation into another, more stable, configuration, with the emission of radiation of energy and atomic particles. This phenomenon is called **radioactivity**, in which **radioactive isotopes** (also called **radioisotopes**) break down through **radioactive decay**.

Some examples of naturally occurring isotopes are shown in **Table 1.2.5**. Deuterium is a stable isotope of hydrogen with a neutron as well as a proton present in each atom. It is a component of the 'heavy water' used in the nuclear power industry, and is present as a trace in the water content of all living tissue. Carbon-14 is a radioactive isotope of carbon with two extra neutrons, and is present in all living matter in a fixed ratio to the stable and more abundant isotope, carbon-12. After death, the proportion of carbon-14 in organic material gradually decreases – at a known rate – so measuring the amount of radioactivity in a sample of wood, cloth, paper, etc. enables the age of the material to be estimated. This process, known as **radiocarbon dating**, is much used in archaeology.

Both radioactive and stable isotopes have proved valuable as tools in medical research, for example investigating the metabolism of nutrients and drugs. Radioisotopes, such as those of iodine, are used clinically in diagnostic scans, and others, such as cobalt-60, are used as sources of radiation for treating tumours during **radiotherapy**.

**Table 1.2.4** Composition of some biologically important elements

| Element | Atomic number* | Number of protons | Number of neutrons | Mass number | Atomic mass |
|---|---|---|---|---|---|
| Hydrogen | 1 | 1 | 0 | 1 | 1 |
| Carbon | 6 | 6 | 6 | 12 | 12 |
| Nitrogen | 7 | 7 | 7 | 14 | 14 |
| Oxygen | 8 | 8 | 8 | 16 | 16 |
| Sodium | 11 | 11 | 12 | 23 | 23 |
| Magnesium | 12 | 12 | 12 | 24 | 24 |
| Phosphorus | 15 | 15 | 16 | 31 | 31 |
| Sulphur | 16 | 16 | 16 | 32 | 32 |
| Chlorine | 17 | 17 | 18 or 20 | 35 or 37 | 35.5 |
| Potassium | 19 | 19 | 20 | 39 | 39 |
| Calcium | 20 | 20 | 20 | 40 | 40 |

* Also equal to the number of electrons

**Table 1.2.5** Some isotopes present in living tissue

| Element | Isotope symbol | Protons | Neutrons | Mass number |
|---|---|---|---|---|
| Hydrogen | $^1H$ | 1 | 0 | 1 |
| | $^2H$ (deuterium) | 1 | 1 | 2 |
| Carbon | $^{12}C$ | 6 | 6 | 12 |
| | $^{14}C*$ (carbon-14) | 6 | 8 | 14 |
| Chlorine | $^{35}Cl$ | 17 | 18 | 35 |
| | $^{37}Cl$ | 17 | 20 | 37 |
| Potassium | $^{39}K$ | 19 | 20 | 39 |
| | $^{40}K*$ | 19 | 21 | 40 |

* Radioactive isotopes

## How atoms join together: bonds and compounds

Although some elements, such as those in metals, exist as separate atoms, most elements in living matter are present as **compounds**, where atoms are joined together in fixed ratios through interaction between their electrons. These links between atoms are called **chemical bonds** and are formed by electrons in the outer atomic orbitals being shared, donated or received. The number of electrons available to form bonds depends on the atomic structure of the element and is called its **valency**. One bond is formed for each electron that can be shared, donated or received. Thus a valency of 1 (as in hydrogen) means that one bond is formed. A valency of 2 (as in oxygen) enables two bonds to be formed. Nitrogen has a valency of 3 and carbon has a valency of 4, so these elements form three and four bonds, respectively, as shown in **Table 1.2.6**. Phosphorus has a valency of 5 and sulphur can have valencies of 2, 4 or 6. These valency numbers are all determined by the numbers of electrons in the outer orbitals of the atoms.

**Table 1.2.6**  Atoms, valencies and molecules

| Atomic element | Valency | Examples of compounds formed | Molecular formula | Molecular structure | Bond type |
|---|---|---|---|---|---|
| H | 1 | Hydrogen | $H_2$ | H—H | Single |
| O | 2 | Oxygen | $O_2$ | O=O | Double |
| | | Ozone | $O_3$ | 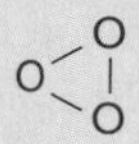 | Single |
| | | Water | $H_2O$ | 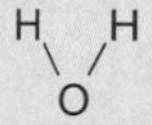 | Single |
| N | 3 | Nitrogen | $N_2$ | N≡N | Triple |
| | | Ammonia | $NH_3$ | 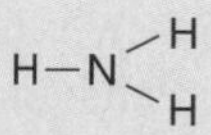 | Single |
| C | 4 | Methane | $CH_4$ | 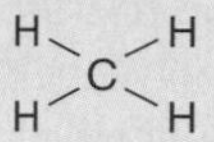 | Single |
| | | Carbon dioxide | $CO_2$ | O=C=O | Double |
| P | 5 | Phosphoric acid | $H_3PO_4$ | 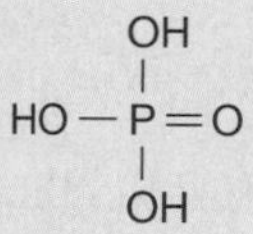 | Single and double |
| S | 2 | Hydrogen sulphide | $H_2S$ | H—S—H | Single |
| S | 4 | Sulphur dioxide | $SO_2$ | O=S=O | Double |
| S | 6 | Sulphur trioxide | $SO_3$ | 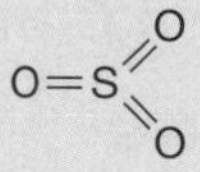 | Double |

## Covalent bonds and molecules

When two or more atoms are joined together through electrons being shared, **molecules** are formed, and the bonds between each atom in a molecule are called **covalent** bonds. For each covalent bond between two atoms, a pair of electrons are shared, one electron being provided by each atom. Examples of molecules formed by these covalent bonds are shown in **Table 1.2.6**. Hydrogen gas ($H_2$) consists of molecules of hydrogen, each molecule being built up from two atoms of hydrogen joined by a covalent bond, which consists of a pair of electrons, one from each hydrogen atom. This can be shown diagrammatically as:

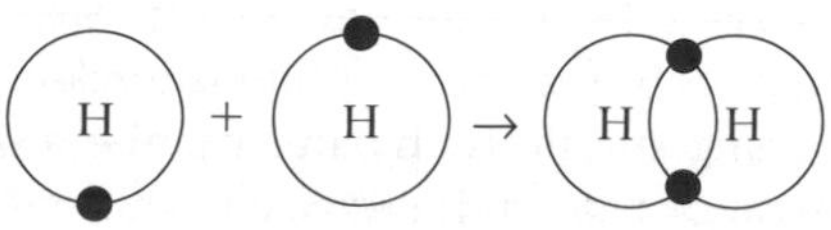

A single covalent bond (consisting of one pair of shared electrons) is normally indicated in diagrams by a short line between the atomic symbols. The oxygen atom has two electrons available for covalent bond formation, and hence a valency of 2. Atmospheric oxygen gas ($O_2$) consists of molecules of two oxygen atoms joined by a pair of covalent bonds, called a **double bond**, O=O. In the upper atmosphere, the gas ozone is formed ($O_3$), which protects the earth from damaging cosmic radiation. This consists of three atoms of oxygen per molecule but, as **Table 1.2.6** shows, the valency of 2 is still obeyed, as **single bonds** are formed between each atom. In the molecule water ($H_2O$) there is a single covalent bond between each hydrogen atom and the oxygen atom:

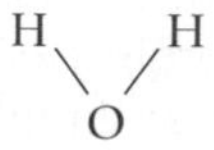

Nitrogen has a valency of 3 and can therefore form a **triple bond**, as in atmospheric nitrogen gas ($N_2$) $N \equiv N$, or three single bonds as in ammonia ($NH_3$). Carbon has four electrons available for covalent formation and hence a valency of 4. Depending on which elements it is joined to, carbon can form single, double and triple bonds, giving rise to the wide diversity of carbon-containing compounds found in living matter. Compounds containing carbon are called **organic** compounds, and some of the biologically more important of these, such as carbohydrates, hydrocarbons, proteins and nucleic acids, will be discussed later.

Molecules can be represented by a chemical shorthand known as their **molecular formulae**, for example $H_2O$ for water and $CO_2$ for carbon dioxide. The molecular formula of a molecule shows the elements present and the precise ratio in which the atoms are joined together. We saw before that each element has a relative mass number or atomic weight (e.g. H = 1, C = 12 and O = 16). We can therefore express the relative mass of a molecule in what is referred to as its **molecular weight**, more correctly known as its molecular mass. This is calculated by simply adding up the mass numbers of the component atoms. For example, the molecular mass of water is 18, derived from 16 for the single oxygen atom plus 1 for each of the hydrogen atoms. Examples of molecules and their molecular masses are shown in **Table 1.2.7**. When the molecular mass is expressed in grams this is called a **mole**, a useful unit for measuring concentrations of solutions, as will be discussed later.

### Electrovalent (ionic) bonds and ions

Not all compounds are formed through covalent bonds. Instead of electrons being shared in pairs between atoms, as in covalent bonding, electrons can be donated from one atom to another, forming an **electrovalent bond**, often called an **ionic bond**. As with covalent bonds, the number of ionic bonds that can be formed is determined by the valency. An atom (or molecular group of atoms) able to donate or receive one electron has a valency of 1, and can form one ionic bond. If the valency is 2, two electrons can be donated or received and two ionic bonds formed, and likewise for a valency of 3. When an atom (or molecular group of atoms) loses or gains an electron, it becomes an **ion** and this process is called **ionization**.

Atoms of metallic elements such as sodium, calcium and iron have the ability to lose electrons readily (which explains why they are such good conductors of electricity). One, two or three electrons can be lost according to the element's valency. Because electrons carry a negative charge, an atom gains a positive charge for each electron lost. Positively charged ions are called **cations**, because in solution they are attracted towards a negatively charged electrode, or **cathode**. The ionization of a metallic element M can be shown as follows:

$$\begin{aligned} \text{valency} = 1 \qquad & M \rightarrow e^- \; + \; M^+ \\ \text{valency} = 2 \qquad & M \rightarrow 2e^- \; + \; M^{2+} \\ \text{valency} = 3 \qquad & M \rightarrow 3e^- \; + \; M^{3+} \end{aligned}$$

$e^-$ indicates an electron and the number in front of the + sign shows the size of the positive charge. Hydrogen can behave like a monovalent metal, such as sodium, to lose an electron and form a hydrogen ion ($H^+$), which corresponds to a proton. Hydrogen ions will be discussed later when acids are considered. When dissolved in water ammonia forms positively charged ammonium ions, $NH_4^+$. These and other examples of cations are shown in **Table 1.2.8**.

Some atoms, like those of the element chlorine, are able to receive electrons and become negatively charged ions, e.g. $Cl + e^- \rightarrow Cl^-$. If two electrons are acquired, there will be a double negative charge, as in the carbonate ion $CO_3^{2-}$ and three electrons gained will give rise to a triple negative charge, as in the phosphate ion, $PO_4^{3-}$. These and other **anions** are shown in **Table 1.2.8**. Negatively charged ions are called **anions** because they are attracted to a positively charged **anode** electrode in solution.

### Salts and electrolytes

Because of their opposite charges, positively charged cations are attracted to negatively charged anions (and vice versa), giving rise to compounds called **salts**, in which cations are linked to anions by electrovalent (ionic) bonds. Unlike covalent bonds, electrons are not shared in pairs but each ionic bond is formed by an electron being effectively donated by one atom (forming the cation) and being received by the other

| Table 1.2.7 | Molecules and molecular masses | |
|---|---|---|
| **Molecular formula** | **Calculation** | **Molecular mass** |
| $H_2$ | $2 \times 1$ | 2 |
| $O_2$ | $2 \times 16$ | 32 |
| $H_2O$ | $2 + 16$ | 18 |
| $N_2$ | $2 \times 14$ | 28 |
| $NH_3$ | $14 + 3$ | 17 |
| $CO_2$ | $12 + 32$ | 44 |
| $C_2H_5OH$ (ethanol) | $24 + 6 + 16$ | 46 |
| $C_6H_{12}O_6$ (glucose) | $72 + 12 + 96$ | 180 |

### Table 1.2.8 Ions of biological importance

| Valency | Cations | Formula | Anions | Formula |
|---|---|---|---|---|
| 1 | Hydrogen | $H^+$ | Hydroxide | $OH^-$ |
| | Sodium | $Na^+$ | Chloride | $Cl^-$ |
| | Potassium | $K^+$ | Bicarbonate | $HCO_3^-$ |
| | Ammonium | $NH_4^+$ | Nitrate | $NO_3^-$ |
| 2 | Calcium | $Ca^{2+}$ | Carbonate | $CO_3^{2-}$ |
| | Magnesium | $Mg^{2+}$ | Sulphate | $SO_4^{2-}$ |
| | Ferrous | $Fe^{2+}$ | | |
| 3 | Ferric | $Fe^{3+}$ | Phosphate | $PO_4^{3-}$ |

atom (forming the anion). A simple example is the formation of common salt, sodium chloride:

$$Na \rightarrow e^- + Na^+$$
$$e^- + Cl \rightarrow Cl^-$$
$$Na^+ + Cl^- \rightarrow NaCl \text{ (salt)}$$

Salts like sodium chloride can exist as crystalline solids with the ions held together by ionic bonds in a rigid orderly lattice structure. When dissolved in water, the solid salt dissolves and **dissociates** into free ions, which are fully dispersed in solution. Some salts, such as calcium sulphate (gypsum) and calcium carbonate (chalk), have very low solubility in water and contribute to the lime scale that precipitates out from hard water. When salts are formed the cations and anions are always in a fixed ratio to one another, determined by their valencies. Salts are an important component of body fluids. Examples of these are shown in **Table 1.2.9**.

Substances that dissolve in water and dissociate into ions are called **electrolytes**. As well as salts, these include acids and bases and organic substances such as amino acids. These will all be discussed later.

### Table 1.2.9 Salts of biological importance

| Salt | Ionic composition | Formula |
|---|---|---|
| Sodium chloride | $Na^+ + Cl^-$ | NaCl |
| Potassium chloride | $K^+ + Cl^-$ | KCl |
| Sodium bicarbonate | $Na^+ + HCO_3^-$ | $NaHCO_3$ |
| Calcium chloride | $Ca^{2+} + 2Cl^-$ | $CaCl_2$ |
| Calcium carbonate | $Ca^{2+} + CO_3^{2-}$ | $CaCO_3$ |
| Calcium phosphate | $3Ca^{2+} + 2PO_4^{3-}$ | $Ca_3(PO_4)_2$ |
| Magnesium chloride | $Mg^{2+} + 2Cl^-$ | $MgCl_2$ |
| Magnesium sulphate | $Mg^{2+} + SO_4^{2-}$ | $MgSO_4$ |
| Ferrous sulphate | $Fe^{2+} + SO_4^{2-}$ | $FeSO_4$ |
| Ferric chloride | $Fe^{2+} + 3Cl^-$ | $FeCl_3$ |

## Intermolecular forces and hydrogen bonding

We have now seen how molecules are formed by atoms joining together by covalent or ionic bonds. There are also weaker bonds by which molecules are attracted to other molecules. These do not give rise to new molecules but do affect the structures and physical properties of molecules. These **intermolecular** attractions and resulting associations between molecules are caused by electronic forces arising from the outer electron shells that surround the component atoms making up the molecules. One important type of such attraction is called **hydrogen bonding**, which, as the name implies, occurs between certain molecules containing hydrogen, such as water.

As explained earlier, water is formed by covalent bonds between hydrogen and oxygen, producing the molecule $H_2O$, with each of the hydrogen atoms single electrons forming a pair with the electrons on the outer shell of the oxygen atom:

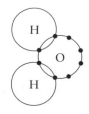

This provides oxygen with a stable octet of eight electrons but the four unpaired electrons in the outer shell carry a partial negative charge and, because the only electrons in the hydrogen atoms have been drawn towards the oxygen atom, this leaves the hydrogen atoms with partial positive charges. These partial charges are shown in diagrams as $\delta^-$ and $\delta^+$, respectively (using the lower case Greek letter delta). Hence water can be represented:

$$\begin{array}{c} \delta^+H \\ \phantom{x} \searrow \\ \phantom{xxx} O^{\delta-} \\ \phantom{x} \nearrow \\ \delta^+H \end{array}$$

Therefore although the water molecule has no net charge, the constituent atoms of the molecule carry partial charges, causing the molecule to be **polar**. This leads to interaction between neighbouring water molecules, with hydrogen atoms being attracted to adjacent oxygen atoms and vice versa.

This phenomenon of hydrogen bonding between water molecules has far-reaching effects and explains why water is a liquid at room (and body) temperature, when in theory it should be a gas, and why ice has a lower density than water (because of the crystalline lattice formed when water freezes). Insofar as all life depends on water, hydrogen bonding is clearly of major biological significance. It is also crucial for the α-helix configuration found in proteins and for the double helix of DNA.

## Solutes, solvents and solutions

We have discussed how electrolytes such as salts dissolve in water to form **solutions** of ions. Substances that dissolve are called **solutes**, and the liquid in which they dissolve is called the **solvent**. Because of hydrogen bonding, water is an excellent solvent for **polar** molecules (i.e. those carrying partial internal charges) as well as for electrolytes. Covalent molecules such as sugars dissolve in water because of hydrogen bonding between water and the hydroxyl (—OH) groups present in sugar molecules (see later for the chemical structures of carbohydrates).

Molecules that dissolve in water are said to be **hydrophilic** (from the Greek 'water-loving'). They are not usually soluble in organic solvents such as hydrocarbon oils, and are also known therefore as being **lipophobic** ('fat-hating'). By contrast, non-polar molecules, such as fats, steroids and waxes, which do not dissolve in water but do dissolve in organic solvents, are said to be **hydrophobic** and **lipophilic**. Hydrophobic interactions, rather than hydrogen bonding, enable the molecules to dissolve.

## Concentration and molarity

Most cellular processes (metabolism, respiration, etc.) take place in an aqueous environment, so solutions in water are more important physiologically than solutions in organic solvents. The amount of a solute dissolved in a solvent is measured by its concentration in units of weight (grams) per volume (in litres or millilitres) of solution. Concentration units such as grams/litre and milligrams/millilitre are frequently used in laboratories but it is often more useful to express the concentration in terms of the number of molecules dissolved. This is normally given in moles/litre, called the **molarity** of a solution. A mole is the molecular (or formula) weight in grams. Glucose has a molecular weight of 180, so a 1 molar solution of glucose will contain 180 g of glucose dissolved in 1 litre of solution. For lower concentrations of solutes, as occur in physiological solutions, millimoles/litre is often a more convenient unit to use (one millimole equals one thousandth of the gram molecular weight, that is, the gram molecular weight $\times 10^{-3}$). For even lower concentrations, micromoles can be used (one micromole equals the gram

| Table 1.2.10 | Molar concentration units | | |
|---|---|---|---|
| **Concentration** | **Units** | **Symbol** | **Example** |
| Molar | moles/litre | M | 0.05 M |
| Millimolar | moles $\times 10^{-3}$/litre (millimoles/litre) | mM | 50 mM |
| Micromolar | moles $\times 10^{-6}$/litre (micromoles/litre) | μM | $5 \times 10^4$ μM |

The correct SI unit should be the cubic decimetre ($dm^3$) but most clinical laboratories still use the term litre. Likewise, millilitre is more frequently used in the UK and USA than its SI counterpart, the cubic centimetre ($cm^3$)

molecular weight $\times 10^{-6}$ (one millionth)). It is useful to remember that micromoles per millilitre (μmol/mL) equals millimoles per litre (mmol/L) because there is a factor of 1000 between each unit. Molar concentration units are shown in **Table 1.2.10**. Molar units are now normally used to express the concentrations of glucose and electrolytes in physiological solutions such as plasma, cerebrospinal fluid and urine.

## Osmosis, osmotic pressure and osmolarity

**Osmosis** is defined as the flow of solvent (which in living things is water) across a **semipermeable membrane**, from a dilute to a more concentrated solution (or from an area of high water concentration to an area of low water concentration). This process is due to the movement of the dissolved molecules and depends on their concentration. It occurs until the concentrations on either side of the membrane are equal (**Fig. 1.2.2**).

In Fig. 1.2.2a, two solutions of equal volume but differing concentrations are separated by a semipermeable membrane. Solution I is less concentrated than solution II. Solute molecules are too large to pass through the pores in the semipermeable membrane, but solvent molecules (not illustrated) can pass through freely.

In Fig. 1.2.2b, solvent has moved across the semipermeable membrane, from solution I to solution II, until the concentration of the two solutions is equal.

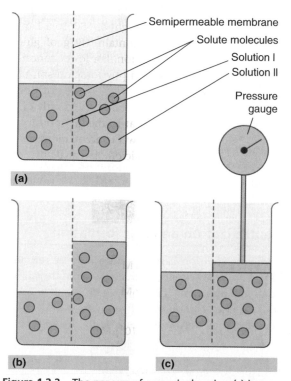

Semipermeable membrane
Solute molecules
Solution I
Solution II
Pressure gauge

(a)

(b)     (c)

**Figure 1.2.2** The process of osmosis showing (c) how the osmotic pressure can be measured. See text for further details

This movement of solvent is called osmosis. **Osmotic pressure** is the pressure required to stop the movement of solvent by osmosis (Fig. 1.2.2c). The greater the difference in concentration between the solutions on either side of the semipermeable membrane, the greater is the pressure required to halt the osmotic movement of solvent across the membrane.

A solution's ability to induce osmosis (this is the combined concentration of substances dissolved) and hence osmotic pressure is expressed by the unit the **osmole**. The number of osmoles in a solution is calculated by multiplying the molar concentration of the solution by the number of molecular components present in each molecule of solute. The unit thus reflects the number of particles present in a solution. For example, a 1 molar solution of sodium chloride contains two osmoles, as sodium chloride dissociates into one sodium and one chloride ion.

The terms **osmolality** and **osmolarity** describe the osmolar concentration of a solution. Osmolality is the number of osmoles present per kilogram of solvent; osmolarity expresses the number of osmoles per litre of solution. When, as in living systems, water is the solvent, the two values are practically identical because 1 litre of water weighs approximately 1 kilogram (1 mL water weighs 1 g). As the concentration of physiological solution is low, this is expressed in milliosmoles (mosmol).

The term **tonicity** refers to a solution's osmotic concentration compared with that of intracellular and extracellular body fluids, which are normally in osmotic equilibrium. Hence a **hypertonic** or **hyperosmotic** solution is more concentrated than body fluids, and cells placed in such a solution shrink and shrivel (crenate) because water moves out of them by osmosis, into the more concentrated hypertonic solution. Conversely, a **hypotonic (hypo-osmotic)** solution is less concentrated than body fluids and cells placed in such a solution swell, as water enters them by osmosis. They might rupture, depending on the magnitude of the osmotic gradient created.

An **isotonic (iso-osmotic)** solution is one that has the same **osmotic activity** as body fluids. Cells placed in such a solution neither gain nor lose water. A 0.9% solution of sodium chloride ('normal saline') is isotonic with blood plasma. All solutions used for intravenous infusion must be isotonic with blood plasma.

Strictly speaking, semipermeable membranes occur only in artificial membranes and in cell membranes after death. Living cell membranes such as those lining the intestinal mucosa or surrounding red blood cells are **selectively permeable** to small dissolved molecules and ions but, as they allow the movement of water, they are very sensitive to osmotic pressure. This explains why red blood cells will swell (and even burst) in hypotonic solutions (haemolysis) and shrink (due to fluid loss) in hypertonic solutions (crenation). Osmolarity also explains why nonabsorbed materials dissolved in intestinal fluid result in water being retained in the gut and hence to the diarrhoea associated with malabsorption syndromes.

## Acids, bases and buffers

## Acids

We all know that strong acids like sulphuric and nitric acids are highly corrosive and that weak acids used in the kitchen have a sour taste (e.g. acetic acid in vinegar and citric acid in lemon juice) but what are acids chemically? They are molecules that, in solution, dissociate into hydrogen ions ($H^+$), i.e. protons. If we give an acid the general formula HA, then in solution there will be dissociation (ionization) into $H^+$ and $A^-$, where $A^-$ is the anion produced, sometimes called the acid radical:

$$HA \rightleftharpoons H^+ + A^-$$

In practice, the hydrogen ion is always **hydrated** by a molecule of water due to hydrogen bonding, and the resulting ion, $H_3O^+$, is called a **hydronium** ion. The full equation for dissociation of the acid in water can therefore be written:

$$HA + H_2O \rightleftharpoons H_3O^+ + A^-$$

sometimes shown as:

$$HA_{aq} \rightleftharpoons H^+_{aq} + A^-_{aq}$$

(where aq indicates an aqueous solution). Because the proton (hydrogen ion) is *always* hydrated in solution it is normal practice to leave water out of the equation and simply write $HA \rightleftharpoons H^+ + A^-$.

The reversible arrows in the above equations indicate that the dissociation of acid is a two-way process. **The strength of an acid depends on the extent of its ability to dissociate into hydrogen ions in solution.** Strong acids are fully ionized in solution and include the inorganic (mineral) acids such as hydrochloric acid. Weak acids are only partially ionized in solution and include organic acids such as acetic acid (which chemists now call ethanoic acid). Many drugs such as aspirin (acetylsalicylic acid) are weak acids. Some well-known acids are shown in **Table 1.2.11**. Many organic acids contain the carboxyl group (—COOH), which dissociates into the carboxyl anion (—COO$^-$) and a hydrogen ion ($H^+$). These are called carboxylic acids. Acids like oxalic acid, which contain two such groups, are called dicarboxylic acids and, if three are present, as in citric acid, they are called tricarboxylic acids, as in the TCA (tricarboxylic acid) metabolic cycle (described in Chapter 2.6).

**Table 1.2.11   Some commonly occurring acids**

| Strong acids | | Weak acids | |
| --- | --- | --- | --- |
| Name | Formula | Name | Formula |
| Hydrochloric | HCl | Carbonic | $H_2CO_3$ |
| Nitric | $HNO_3$ | Acetic | $CH_3COOH$ |
| Sulphuric | $H_2SO_4$ | Oxalic | $(COOH)_2$ |
| Phosphoric | $H_3PO_4$ | Citric | $C_3H_5O(COOH)_3$ |

## Alkalis and bases

If acids can be defined as donors of hydrogen ions, then **bases** are **hydrogen ion acceptors**. When dissolved in water, bases liberate **hydroxide** ions ($OH^-$). If we give a base the symbol B, we can show its dissociation in aqueous solution as:

$$B + H_2O \rightleftharpoons BH^+ + OH^-$$

Strong bases such as sodium and potassium hydroxide are called **alkalis** (after the alkali metals from which they are derived), and dissociate completely in solution as follows:

$$NaOH \rightleftharpoons Na^+ + OH^-$$

The hydroxide ions liberated are powerful hydrogen ion acceptors,

$$H^+ + OH^- \rightleftharpoons H_2O$$

hence the strongly basic character of alkalis. They are also highly corrosive, as implied by the common name for sodium hydroxide, caustic soda.

Ammonia ($NH_3$) is an example of a weak base. Although it is a hydrogen ion acceptor, it only partially ionizes in solution to form ammonium ions and hydroxide ions:

$$NH_3 + H_2O \rightleftharpoons NH_4^+ + OH^-$$

Solutions containing hydroxide ions are commonly referred to as **alkaline**, and produce characteristic colour changes when indicators such as litmus are added.

## Neutralization and salt formation

An acidic solution can be **neutralized** by the addition of a base (or vice versa) producing the appropriate salt and water, i.e. acid + base → salt + water. For example, a solution of hydrochloric acid can be neutralized by the addition of sodium hydroxide:

$$HCl + NaOH \rightarrow NaCl + H_2O$$

If hydrochloric acid is neutralized by a weak base such as ammonia, the following reaction occurs:

$$HCl + NH_3 \rightarrow NH_4^+ + Cl^-$$

Salts such as ammonium chloride ($NH_4Cl$) derived from weak bases and strong acids produce an acidic solution. This is because the ammonium ion ($NH_4^+$) behaves as a weak acid, partially dissociating into hydrogen ions plus ammonia, i.e.

$$NH_4^+ \rightleftharpoons NH_3 + H^+$$

If sodium hydroxide is neutralized by a weak acid, such as acetic acid, the reaction is as follows:

$$NaOH + CH_3COOH \rightarrow Na^+ + CH_3COO^- + H_2O$$

The resulting salt, sodium acetate, produces an alkaline solution, due to the ability of the acetate ions to act as a weak base, accepting hydrogen ions:

$$CH_3COO^- + H_2O \rightleftharpoons CH_3COOH + OH^-$$

## Acidity, alkalinity and pH

It is clear that acidic solutions have a relatively high hydrogen ion concentration and that, the higher their concentration, the greater the acidity of the solution. By contrast, alkaline solutions have a relatively high concentration of hydroxide ions, and the higher their concentration the more alkaline the solution.

Although pure water partially dissociates into hydrogen and hydroxide ions:

$$H_2O \rightleftharpoons H^+ + OH^-$$

it is neutral, as the concentration of hydrogen ions always equals that of hydroxide ions. Solutions in which the hydrogen ion concentration is greater than the hydroxide ion concentration are always acidic, and those in which it is less are always alkaline, i.e. for acid solutions $H^+ > OH^-$ and for alkaline solutions $OH^- > H^+$. (The symbols > and < are often used to symbolize 'greater than' or 'less than', respectively.)

The acidity or alkalinity of a solution can thus be measured by the concentration of hydrogen ions. As the concentration range from a strongly acidic to a strongly alkaline solution is vast, it is convenient to use a **logarithmic** scale, in which an increase of one unit represents a tenfold increase in concentration. This logarithmic scale has been developed to denote the concentration of hydrogen ions in a solution, using water as a standard. Water can exist in two forms: either as molecules of $H_2O$ or dissociated into positive hydrogen ions ($H^+$) and negative hydroxide ions ($OH^-$)

$$H_2O \rightleftharpoons H^+ + OH^-$$

However, pure water ionizes only very slightly, in other words most of the hydrogen remains tightly bound in the water molecule. Indeed, 10 000 000 litres ($10^7$ litres) of pure water would be required to provide 1 g of hydrogen ions (or, as the molar weight of hydrogen is 1, to produce 1 mole of $H^+$). In other words, 1 litre of water contains only 0.000 000 1 mole of $H^+$. Thus the molar concentration of $H^+$ (represented as $[H^+]$) in pure water could be expressed as $10^{-7}$. In fact, $[H^+]$ is usually expressed using the pH notation, where pH is defined as the negative logarithm of the hydrogen ion concentration. As the product of two negative signs is a positive quantity, the pH of pure water is simply 7. The link between pH and hydrogen ion concentration is shown in **Table 1.2.12**.

Water is a neutral solution because, for every molecule which dissociates, 1 hydrogen ion ($H^+$) and 1 hydroxide ion ($OH^-$) are formed, each one neutralizing the other. Many other substances, such as sodium chloride, glucose and urea, do not upset the balance between $H^+$ and $OH^-$ when they are dissolved

**Table 1.2.12    The pH scale for acids and bases**

| Hydrogen ion concentration (moles/litre) | $Log_{10}$ of concentration | pH | Acidity/alkalinity |
|---|---|---|---|
| $10^{-1}$ | $-1$ | 1 | Strongly acidic |
| $10^{-3}$ | $-3$ | 3 | Acidic |
| $10^{-5}$ | $-5$ | 5 | Weakly acidic |
| $10^{-7}$ | $-7$ | 7 | Neutral |
| $10^{-9}$ | $-9$ | 9 | Weakly alkaline |
| $10^{-11}$ | $-11$ | 11 | Alkaline |
| $10^{-14}$ | $-14$ | 14 | Strongly alkaline |

in water, consequently they are said to be neutral compounds, and will not alter the pH of the solution. However, if an acid is added to water, it will increase the quantity of $H^+$ and cause a fall in pH.

The pH scale ranges from 0 to 14. A pH of below 7 is said to be acidic, whereas a pH greater than 7 (i.e. with a lower concentration of $H^+$ than in water) is called alkaline (**see Table 1.2.12**). Although all acids are alike in that they donate $H^+$, they differ in their *ability* to do so. Some acids, such as hydrochloric acid, ionize completely, donating all their $H^+$, and are said to be strong acids and have a low pH:

$$HCl \rightleftharpoons H^+ + Cl^-$$

whereas weak acids, such as carbonic acid, dissociate much less freely and therefore have a higher pH:

$$H_2CO_3 \rightleftharpoons H^+ + HCO_3^-$$

When a base (any compound that accepts $H^+$) is added to a solution, the concentration of $H^+$ falls with respect to $OH^-$, causing a rise in pH. This can be achieved either by the donation of hydroxide ions ($OH^-$), which combine with $H^+$ to form $H_2O$, or by the direct acceptance of $H^+$:

$$NaOH + H^+ \rightleftharpoons H_2O + Na^+ \quad \text{or}$$
$$NH_3 + H^+ \rightleftharpoons NH_4^+$$

## Concentration of hydrogen ions in the body

Living tissue must be maintained within a very narrow pH range because quite small fluctuations in acidity/alkalinity can inactivate the complex molecules, such as proteins and nucleic acids, which are essential to normal structure and function. The range of pH compatible with life is only 7.0–7.8.

The normal pH of blood is 7.4 and it is therefore a slightly alkaline fluid. In a healthy adult, arterial blood pH is almost always maintained between 7.35 and 7.45. The homeostatic processes that regulate and maintain the pH of the cells, body fluids and blood are mainly effected through respiratory and renal function.

Despite the advantages of the pH scale, the logarithmic instead of linear relationship between pH and the actual $[H^+]$ can cause confusion. Looking at **Fig. 1.2.3**, it can be seen that the change in $[H^+]$ per unit fall in pH is proportionately much greater than per unit rise in pH. Thus, if pH changes from 7.4 to 7.2, $[H^+]$ increases by 23 nmol/L, whereas an increase in pH from 7.4 to 7.6 represents a reduction of only 15 nmol/L of $[H^+]$. Consequently, the clinical use of the pH scale could be replaced by expressing $[H^+]$ directly in nanomoles per litre (nmol/L), where 1 nanomole $= 10^{-9}$ moles. Arterial blood normally

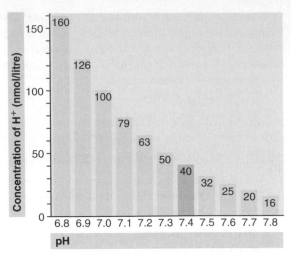

**Figure 1.2.3** The effect of changing pH on hydrogen ion concentration. The normal pH of blood (7.4) is indicated in darker blue

has a $[H^+]$ of 40 nmol/L (range 36–45 nmol/L). The range compatible with life lies between 16 and 100 nmol $H^+$/L.

Examples of pH values and their corresponding hydrogen ion concentrations are shown in **Table 1.2.12**.

## Buffers and buffering

We have seen that small changes in pH can have a marked effect on the degree of acidity of a solution and that living tissue can therefore tolerate only small variations in pH. pH therefore has to be stabilized for cellular processes to be maintained. This stabilization of pH is achieved by a process called **buffering**. Buffers are substances that, in solution, resist changes in pH when either an acid or a base is added. They consist of a mixture of a weak acid and its salt, or a weak base and its salt. Mixtures of acetic acid and sodium acetate, or of ammonia and ammonium chloride, are examples of buffers used in laboratories.

When an acid is added to such a mixture, hydrogen ions are 'mopped up' by the following reactions:

$$CH_3COO^- + H^+ \rightarrow CH_3COOH$$
$$NH_3 + H^+ \rightarrow NH_4^+$$

When a base is added, hydroxide ions are 'mopped up' as follows:

$$CH_3COOH + OH^- \rightarrow CH_3COO^- + H_2O$$
$$NH_4^+ + OH^- \rightarrow NH_3 + H_2O$$

Obviously there is a limit on the extent to which pH can be thus stabilized. This depends on the amount of buffer present, and is called the **buffer capacity** of the solution. The pH of blood plasma is stabilized through the buffering properties of amino acids and proteins present in solution. These contain a carboxyl (—COOH) and amino (—NH$_2$) group which ionize (to —COO$^-$ and —NH$_3^+$ respectively) in response to pH changes. Thus an increase in acidity causes the following changes:

$$H^+ + —COO^- \rightarrow —COOH$$
$$H^+ + —NH_2 \rightarrow —NH_3^+$$

Likewise an increase in alkalinity can be overcome by the following changes:

$$OH^- + —COOH \rightarrow —COO^- + H_2O$$
$$OH^- + —NH_3^+ \rightarrow —NH_2 + H_2O$$

The pH of urine is stabilized by the presence of ammonia and ammonium ions, which are excreted by the kidney (see Chapter 5.4).

## Chemical features of biologically important substances

The different chemical components of living tissue must run into many thousands. Fortunately, we do not need to know about all these! It is useful, though, to identify the major groups of biologically important substances present in living matter and to be aware of their chemical characteristics. This is essential for an understanding of the more biochemical aspects of physiology such as nutrition, respiration and metabolism, and also to keep up with the new and ever-increasing discoveries of the molecular basis of disease.

As a starting point we will look at the chemical structures and related properties of the three main groups of energy providing nutrients, namely **carbohydrates** (sugars and starch), **lipids** (fats and oils) and **proteins**. By investigating their structures and features we will come across the main groups of atoms (called **functional groups**) that are found within many other substances making up living tissue.

## Carbohydrates

This chemical term is used to describe the sugars and starches in our diet, as well as blood glucose and the glycogen stored in liver and muscle. Literally, the name means hydrated carbon, which is not a bad description as we can write the general formula for simple carbohydrates as $C_n(H_2O)_n$ where $n$ equals the number of carbon atoms present in each molecule. Although this general formula implies there is an equal number of water molecules, this, as we shall see, is an oversimplification. However, this formula does give us the correct ratios of carbon, hydrogen and oxygen atoms present in simple sugars called **monosaccharides**.

## Monosaccharides $C_n(H_2O)_n$

Monosaccharides include such sugars as glucose, fructose and galactose, all of which have the general formula $C_6H_{12}O_6$, and are therefore called **hexose** monosaccharides. Monosaccharides with five carbons are called **pentoses**, of which ribose is a well-known example, and these are important components of nucleic acids. Other monosaccharides with three, four and even seven carbons occur in metabolic processes but have no dietary importance. We need be concerned here only with the structures of the hexoses, and the three major ones are shown in **Fig. 1.2.4**, which also shows the structure of the pentose ribose for comparison.

It is apparent that these structures have much in common but close inspection shows that they also have certain differences. For convenience, the carbon atoms are given numbers to help us identify the different parts of each molecule. The number one carbon (C1) in ribose, glucose and galactose is shown as CHO, which is chemical shorthand for:

$$\underset{H}{\diagdown}\underset{C}{\overset{O}{\diagup\diagup}}$$

This is called an **aldehyde** group, as found also in other chemicals such as formaldehyde and acetaldehyde.

Fructose has a similar structure for its number two carbon (C2):

$$C = O$$

This is called a **ketone** group, as found in acetone and other chemically related substances. Monosaccharides containing an aldehyde group are called **aldoses** and those containing ketone groups are called **ketoses**. All sugars contain either aldehyde or ketone groups, which give them characteristic chemical properties.

The only difference between glucose and galactose is in the arrangement of the number four carbon, H—C—OH for glucose, and HO—C—H for galactose. Molecules with the same formula but different structures are called **isomers**. Glucose, galactose and fructose are all isomers, but clearly glucose and galactose are more closely related and have similar chemical properties.

Monosaccharides are hydrophilic due to the presence of **hydroxyl** (—OH) and aldehyde or ketone groups, and are therefore soluble in water. In solution, the chain structures shown in **Fig. 1.2.4** spontaneously close in on themselves to form the more stable ring structures.

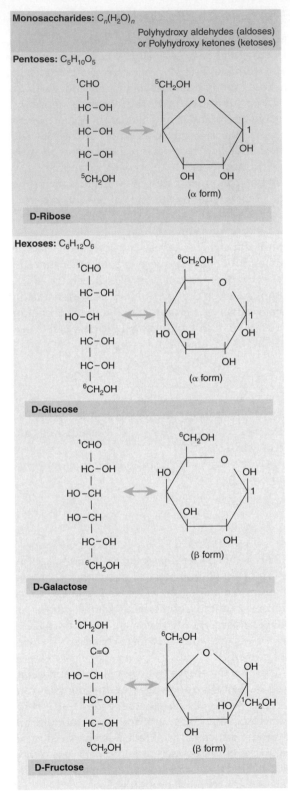

**Figure 1.2.4** Biologically important monosaccharides

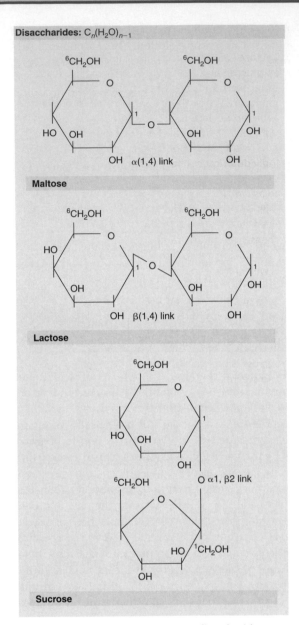

**Figure 1.2.5** Biologically important disaccharides

monosaccharides have the general formula $C_{12}(H_2O)_{11}$. A molecule of water is lost when the two monosaccharides join together, a process called **condensation**. The reverse of this process, as occurs in the digestion of disaccharides, is called **hydrolysis**, and involves the restoration of a molecule of water:

$$2\ C_6H_{12}O_6 \underset{hydrolysis}{\overset{condensation}{\rightleftharpoons}} H_2O + C_{12}H_{22}O_{11}$$

The structures of three nutritionally important disaccharides are shown in **Fig. 1.2.5**. **Maltose** is formed from two glucose molecules linked together by condensation. Maltose is produced during the breakdown of starch and is broken down to glucose by the intestinal enzyme **maltase**.

## Disaccharides $C_n(H_2O)_{n-1}$

These are formed when two monosaccharides are linked together by a covalent bond called a **glycosidic** bond. Disaccharides derived from two hexose

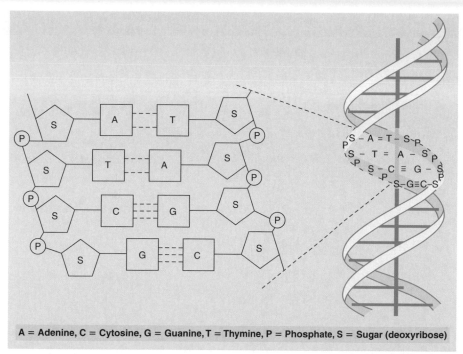

A = Adenine, C = Cytosine, G = Guanine, T = Thymine, P = Phosphate, S = Sugar (deoxyribose)

**Figure 1.2.18**    The double helical structure of DNA showing base pairing between adenine and thymine, and guanine and cytosine, respectively

**Table 1.2.15**    Functional groups found in molecules of biological importance

| Group | Structure | Class of compounds containing group | Examples of compounds containing group |
|---|---|---|---|
| Aliphatic (alkyl) | $CH_3(CH_2)_n-$ | Hydrocarbons | Fatty acids |
| Phenyl | ⬡— | Aromatic | Phenylalanine |
| Hydroxyl | $HO^-$ | Alcohols Carbohydrates | Ethanol, glycerol Glucose |
| Carbonyl | $O=C\backslash$ | Aldehydes Ketones | Acetaldehyde, glucose Acetone, fructose |
| Carboxyl | $-C{\overset{O}{\diagdown}}_{OH}$ | Carboxylic acids | Acetic acid Fatty acids |
| Amino | $H_2N^-$ | Amines Amino acids | Histamine Glycine |
| Sulphydryl | $HS^-$ | Thiols | Cysteine |

text (such as one of those suggested in Further Reading) should be consulted for further study of enzymes and metabolism. The types of reactions we are concerned with involve changes to functional groups, the removal or addition of components to a compound and the making or breaking of bonds

within the compound. Some of the types of reaction most frequently occurring in metabolism are shown in **Table 1.2.17**.

We have already encountered **condensation** and **hydrolysis** when considering the composition and digestion of nutrients such as polysaccharides,

**Table 1.2.16**  Types of bonds in compounds of biological importance

| Bond type | Structure | Examples of compounds in which found |
|---|---|---|
| Ionic (electrovalent) | $A^- B^+$ | Salts (sodium chloride, etc.) |
| Carbon–carbon single bond | $-\overset{\mid}{\underset{\mid}{C}}-\overset{\mid}{\underset{\mid}{C}}-$ | Fatty acid chains (saturated) |
| Carbon–carbon double bond | $\diagup\!\!\!\diagdown C = C \diagdown\!\!\!\diagup$ | Unsaturated fatty acid chains |
| Glycosidic (ether) | $-\overset{\mid}{\underset{\mid}{C}}-O-\overset{\mid}{\underset{\mid}{C}}-$ | Disaccharides, polysaccharides |
| Ester | $-\overset{O}{\overset{\|}{C}}-O-R$ | Triglycerides |
| Phosphate ester | $HO-\overset{O}{\overset{\|}{\underset{\underset{OH}{\mid}}{C}}}-O-R$ | Sugar phosphates, phospholipids |
| Peptide (amide) | $-\overset{O}{\overset{\|}{C}}-NH-$ | Proteins |

**Table 1.2.17**  Types of chemical reaction occurring in metabolism

| Type | Reaction | Processes in which occurring |
|---|---|---|
| Condensation | Combining molecules with elimination of water | Formation of glycosidic, ester and peptide bonds |
| Hydrolysis | Splitting a molecule through addition of water | Digestion of carbohydrates, triglycerides and proteins |
| Dehydration | Removal of water from a molecule | Carbohydrate and fatty acid metabolism |
| Hydration | Incorporation of water into a molecule | Carbohydrate and fatty acid metabolism |
| Oxidation | Removal of hydrogen (or electrons) | Conversion of alcohols into aldehydes |
| Reduction | Addition of hydrogen (or electrons) | Biosynthesis of fatty acids |
| Carboxylation | Incorporation of $CO_2$ | Carbohydrate synthesis |
| Decarboxylation | Elimination of $CO_2$ | Fermentation, amine formation |
| Amination | Incorporation of amino group ($-NH_2$) | Amino acid biosynthesis |
| Deamination | Elimination of ammonia | Amino acid degradation |
| Methylation | Incorporation of methyl ($-CH_3$) group | Synthesis of DNA and adrenaline |
| Demethylation | Removal of methyl group | Amino acid degradation |

triglycerides and proteins. These types of reaction also occur frequently in cellular processes such as glycogen synthesis and degradation. Condensation and hydrolysis should not be confused with **dehydration** and **hydration**, which are illustrated in **Fig. 1.2.19**. Although these latter reactions also involve either removal or addition of water, molecules are *not* joined together or split. These types of reaction frequently involve the saturation or desaturation of carbon–carbon bonds and are therefore important in fatty acid metabolism.

Another pair of reaction types of major biological importance are **oxidation** and **reduction**. Chemically, oxidation occurs when oxygen is added to an atom or a molecule (as when metals oxidize), when hydrogen is removed from a molecule or when electrons are removed (as when ferrous ions are oxidized to ferric ions, $Fe^{2+} \rightarrow e^- + Fe^{3+}$). Biologically, removal of hydrogen (**dehydrogenation**) is the most common form of oxidation and it is **catalysed**

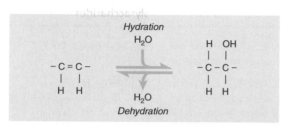

**Figure 1.2.19** Hydration and dehydration reactions

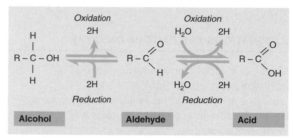

**Figure 1.2.20** Oxidation and reduction reactions between an alcohol, an aldehyde and an acid

# Review questions

1 Which chemical particles comprise the nucleus of an atom?
2 What is the atomic number of an element?
3 What is the atomic mass of an element?
4 How do isotopes differ from one another?
5 What does valency refer to?
6 What type of bond is formed between shared pairs of electrons between atoms?
7 What are organic compounds?
8 How do you calculate the molecular mass of a compound?
9 What is the basis of ionic bonding?
10 What is a salt?
11 What does the polar nature of the water molecule give rise to?
12 What is a mole?
13 How does a strong acid differ from a weak one?
14 What is formed when an acid is neutralized by a base?
15 What is the pH scale?
16 What do buffers do?
17 How do hexoses and pentoses differ?
18 Why are glucose and galactose described as isomers?
19 What is a condensation reaction?
20 How do amylose and amylopectin differ?
21 What is glycogen?
22 How do saturated and unsaturated fatty acids differ?
23 What kind of covalent bond is formed between an alcohol and an organic acid?
24 How do phospholipids differ from triglycerides?
25 Where is DNA found?
26 Which base is not found in RNA?

(facilitated) by **dehydrogenase** enzymes. These enzymes require organic **coenzymes**, called NAD or FAD, which are derived from the B-complex vitamins niacin or riboflavin, to accept the hydrogen removed. Examples of dehydrogenation occur in the oxidation of alcohols to aldehydes, and aldehydes to carboxylic acids, as shown in **Fig. 1.2.20**. The reverse of this process is called **hydrogenation**, and is the most common form of reduction to occur in biological systems. It is of major importance in the photosynthesis of carbohydrate in plants and in the biosynthesis of fatty acids.

Other types of reaction shown in **Table 1.2.17** involve the addition or removal of small molecular groups, such as carbon dioxide, amino groups or methyl ($—CH_3$) groups. These, like the other types of reaction discussed, are essential for the overall process of metabolism on which life depends.

## Suggestions for further reading

Bender, D.A. (1997) *Introduction to Nutrition & Metabolism*, 2nd edn. London: UCL Press.
*Contains a good summary of the relevant chemistry and is excellent for subsequent courses in nutrition and metabolism. Strong clinical emphasis.*

Bettelheim, F.A. & March, J. (1995) *Introduction to General, Organic and Biochemistry*, 4th edn. Philadelphia: Saunders.
*An interesting and well illustrated lead-on into biochemistry, with a bias towards health services.*

Campbell, M.K. (1995) *Biochemistry*, 2nd edn. Philadelphia: Saunders College Publishing.
*Superbly illustrated introductory text. Chemical structures are shown very clearly and biological applications well explained.*

Davis, M.G. (1993) *Structure and Catalytic Properties of Enzymes*: In *Medicinal Chemistry*, 2nd edn. Ganellin, C.R. & Roberts, S.M. (eds) London: Academic Press.
*An introduction to enzymes, with emphasis on their relevance to physiology and medicine.*

Masterton, W.L. & Hurley, C.N. (2000) Chemistry: Principles and Reactions, 3rd edn. Philadelphia: Saunders.
*For those who need to take chemistry further, this is a non-threatening and easily accessible text. Packed with colour pictures and interesting anecdotes.*

Rose, S. (1999) *The Chemistry of Life*, 4th edn. London: Penguin.
*Inexpensive best seller, used by the Open University. Provides an excellent introduction to chemistry, cell biology and biochemistry. Not a conventional textbook. A useful book to buy.*

Sackheim, G.I. & Lehman, D.D. (1997) *Chemistry for the Health Sciences*, 8th edn. New York: Macmillan.
*A comprehensive, user-friendly, well illustrated chemistry text aimed at nurses, dietitians, etc. Useful for reference.*

# Cell structure and function, growth and development

*Roger Watson*

---

## LEARNING OBJECTIVES

After studying this chapter the reader should be able to:

- Describe the components of a 'typical' cell, relating structure to function

- Describe mechanisms by which substances are transported across the cytoplasmic membrane

- Distinguish between a prokaryotic and a eukaryotic cell type

- Describe the process of mitosis and explain its functional significance

- Compare and contrast the processes of mitosis and meiosis, after also studying Chapter 6.4

- Explain how DNA functions as the genetic material in controlling cellular protein synthesis

- Describe the mechanism of protein synthesis, briefly stating how abnormalities can occur

- State the phases of the cell cycle and their characteristics

- Demonstrate understanding of the biological basis of clinical conditions, responses and therapies relating to cell structure and function

- Outline normal patterns of growth and development

- Describe factors influencing and regulating growth and development

- Discuss the biological basis of ageing

- Distinguish between an ageing change and a pathological change

- Describe physiological decline in body systems with increasing age and relate this to homeostatic capability and quality of life

---

## INTRODUCTION

The concept of the cell as the basic structural and functional unit of life was introduced and developed in Chapter 1.1. In this chapter, the structure and function of cells will be described in more detail and the fundamental concepts of growth, development and ageing will be discussed.

Each cell belonging to an organism of a particular species contains, at some stage of its development, all the genetic material required to produce that organism.

## Cell structure and function (Fig. 1.3.1)

A cell comprises its outer limiting membrane and its contents. Typically, a cell is a semifluid mass of microscopic dimensions – most mammalian cells are 7–20 μm in diameter – completely enclosed within a thin, selectively permeable cell surface or plasma membrane. The cell usually contains two distinct regions, the **nucleus** and the **cytoplasm**. The nucleus is enclosed by a nuclear membrane and contains the chromatin (genetic material) and one or more dense areas called nucleoli. Within the cytoplasm are many

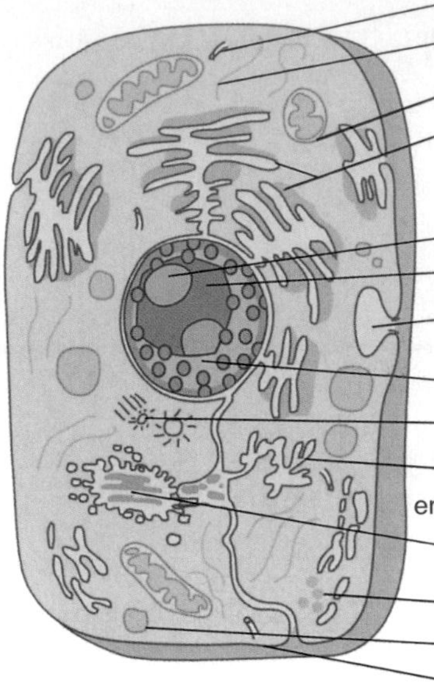
Microtubule
Microfilament
Mitochondrion
Rough surfaced endoplasmic reticulum
Nucleolus
Chromatin
Endocytotic invagination
Nuclear membrane
Centriole
Smooth surfaced endoplasmic reticulum
Golgi apparatus
Free ribosomes
Lysosome
Cell membrane

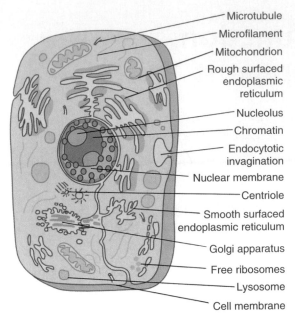

**Figure 1.3.1** Diagram of the ultrastructure of a eukaryotic cell

organelles – such as the mitochondria, the Golgi apparatus, the endoplasmic reticulum, lysosomes and centrioles – held in an aqueous fluid medium called **cytosol**.

The variety of different shapes assumed by cells is related to their particular function. Although many cells, because of surface tension forces, will assume a spherical shape if freed from restraining influences, other cells retain their shape under most conditions because of their characteristic cytoskeleton or framework of microtubules and/or microfilaments.

## DEVELOPMENTAL ISSUES

At birth the human baby has about $2 \times 10^{12}$ cells. This immense number has come from a single fertilized egg, which, by repeated cell divisions, develops into a baby usually weighing more than 2.5 kg. Cells do not divide at the same rate and some stop dividing altogether at various points in the life cycle. The growth of an organism is not merely due to an increase in the number of cells but also involves increase in cell size. Principles of human growth and development are described at the end of this chapter. A human adult has approximately $6 \times 10^{13}$ cells.

The lifespan of different human cells varies. For example, some nerve cells persist throughout life whereas a red blood cell lives for about 120 days. Extensive cell death is constantly occurring within the organism because of the wear and tear of existence and as a part of development. Some parts of the body require a constant replacement of cells: friction wears away the outer cells of the skin and the movement of food along the gastrointestinal tract removes lining cells. This loss is made up by rapid cell division. Cells also undergo a process of ageing. At some point in the life cycle of most cells there is a decrease in the chemical activity of their enzymes, a slowing down of metabolism, a breakdown of cell substance and the formation of inert material. In certain cases parts of the cell persist after its death, for example, the keratin of hair, fingernails and toenails.

The structure of cells is characterized by both membranous and non-membranous components. The limiting boundary of the cell, its outer barrier, is known as the **cell surface membrane** or **plasma membrane**. Within the limits of the cell surface membrane there are structurally and functionally distinct units. Generally, cells have certain basic features in common, but there are exceptions. For example, the cell nucleus is a characteristic structure of most cells but mature red blood cells do not contain nuclei.

To understand the general structure of the cellular subunits (organelles), it is useful to consider a brief definition of each. This is followed by a more detailed description.

The **cell surface membrane** is the outer limiting boundary of each cell, separating the intracellular area from the extracellular environment.

The **nuclear membrane** is the outer limiting boundary of the nucleus, separating the nucleoplasm from the cytoplasm.

**Cytoplasm** is the cellular fluid between the cytoplasmic membrane and the nuclear membrane.

The **nucleus**, defined by the nuclear membrane, is the cell structure that contains the genetic information.

**Nucleoplasm** is the cellular substance within the nuclear membrane.

**Chromatin** is the substance in the nucleus containing the chromosomes in an extended and diffuse state, permitting their maximum contact with the surrounding nucleoplasm.

**Chromosomes** are structures within the nucleus containing hereditary information in the form of the chemical substance deoxyribonucleic acid (DNA).

The **endoplasmic reticulum** is a network of membranous channels within the cytoplasm involved in the synthesis and transport of proteins.

**Ribosomes**, composed of ribonucleic acid (RNA) and protein, appear as free granules in the cytoplasm, giving the endoplasmic reticulum a rough appearance.

**Mitochondria** are small cytoplasmic structures with outer and inner membranes. They produce energy in the form of the chemical substance adenosine triphosphate (ATP).

The **Golgi apparatus** is a collection of smooth membranes found in the cytoplasm, near the nucleus, which stores cell secretions.

**Lysosomes** are membranous sacs of varying size and shape that contain enzymes capable of breaking down protein, carbohydrate, DNA, RNA and other large molecules.

**Microtubules** are very small tubes (20 nm in diameter) within the cytoplasm. They provide an organizational framework for coordinated cellular actions, such as cell division, and supporting structures, such as cilia (**see Fig. 5.3.4** in Chapter 5).

**Microfilaments** are very small rods (4–6 nm in diameter). They have contractile properties and facilitate cellular cohesion and events such as muscle contraction.

**Centrioles** are structures near the nucleus. They are active in cell division.

## The cell surface membrane

The cell surface membrane (plasma membrane) has a protective function and plays a vital role in the transfer of substances between the intracellular and extracellular fluids. The properties of the membrane surface also influence cell to cell recognition and immunological responses.

Biochemically, cell surface membranes are composed of protein and lipid with some carbohydrate. The fluid mosaic model of membrane structure was proposed by Singer and Nicolson in 1972 and is well supported by experimental evidence. The fluid mosaic model stresses the dynamic aspects of membrane structure and function, in that protein and lipoprotein complexes are mobile within the membrane. According to the fluid mosaic model, cell membranes consist of phospholipid molecules, which are aligned in two layers (**Fig. 1.3.2**) so that their hydrophobic (water-repellent) ends are turned inwards and their hydrophilic (water-attracting) ends face outwards. This structure is not rigid, the interior of the membrane being in an almost fluid state. Protein molecules are closely associated with the lipid bilayer. Some proteins extend right through the bilayer and others are located on only the outer or inner surface (**see Fig. 1.3.2**). Thus the membrane proteins appear to float, like icebergs, in a sea of lipid and form a mosaic pattern on the surface of the membrane.

Some glycoproteins and glycolipids associated with the outer surface of cell membranes are probably involved in the cell's recognition of, and response to, factors in its environment.

No holes or pores in the membrane have been identified but the proteins that extend all the way through the membrane provide the channels that allow ions, for example, sodium ($Na^+$), potassium

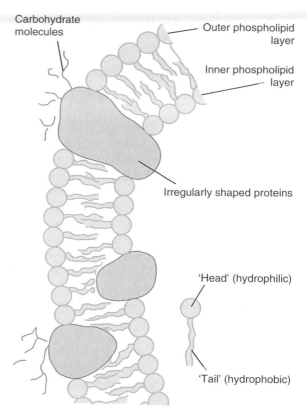

**Figure 1.3.2** Diagram of the fluid mosaic model of cell surface membrane structure

($K^+$) and chloride ($Cl^-$), and other lipid-insoluble substances, for example urea, to cross cell membranes. Lipid-soluble substances can pass through the lipid bilayer.

The outer surface of the cell membrane can be structurally modified in relation to adjoining cells. There are variable distances between adhering surfaces, a tight junction or a gap junction, which physiologically provide degrees of cellular adhesion and communication. Gap junctions can allow small molecules to pass between cells but block the passage of large molecules.

Areas of the cell surface membrane that form the surface of a tissue are specifically modified to facilitate its function. For example, the fine microvilli (brush border) of intestinal epithelium and kidney tubule cells increase their surface area, thereby accelerating the process of absorption with which these cells are involved.

**Cilia**, which are motile processes, extend from the surfaces of the cells of certain epithelial linings. They occur in the respiratory tract and the uterine tubes and, in a somewhat more elaborate form, in the spermatozoon tail. A single cilium is covered by cell surface membrane. Internally, it is composed of microtubular filaments in a constant arrangement. The cilia of surface cells, orientated in the same direction, move rapidly forward and very slowly backward, effecting movement of fluid lying adjacent to the cells.

## Mechanisms by which substances are transported across the cell surface membrane

**Diffusion** is the passive movement of a substance from an area of high concentration to an area of low concentration. It is the result of the spontaneous movement of molecules. This process can cause the movement of substances through the extracellular fluid to the cell surface membrane. Some of the substances are soluble in the lipid whereas others are soluble in the protein. By diffusion through the medium in which the substance is soluble, the required substances enter the cell. The same mechanism allows diffusion in the opposite direction when a concentration gradient is established by the accumulation of metabolic wastes. Diffusion also acts as a transport system within the cell.

**Facilitated diffusion** is transport involving carrier molecules. Although this type of diffusion is more rapid, there must be a concentration gradient similar to that required for simple diffusion. Glucose is transported into erythrocytes and liver cells in this manner. The carrier molecule is specific for the transported substance.

**Osmosis** is the flow of solvent (which in living things is water) across a selectively permeable membrane from a dilute to a more concentrated solution (or from an area of high water concentration to an area of low water concentration). This process occurs until the concentrations on either side of the membrane are equal. The cell surface membrane functions as a selectively permeable membrane, that is, *as if* it contained pores that permit only the passage of selected substances of, or below, a certain molecular weight. Recently, specific protein sites on the plasma membrane have been identified as aquaporins which allow water to pass in both directions across the plasma membrane in response to osmotic pressure (Krane and Kishore, 2003). The role of aquaporins is described in more detail in Chapter 5.4.

Energy is necessary to transport substances when there is no concentration gradient, or when transport against a concentration gradient is necessary. The movement of substances using energy is called **active transport**. Substances actively transported through cell surface membranes include the ions of sodium, potassium, calcium, iron, hydrogen, chlorine, iodine and urea, some simple sugars and amino acids. The mechanism of active transport requires energy and a carrier molecule with an affinity for the substance to be transported. In primary active transport the energy requirement is met by a chemical source such as adenosine triphosphate (ATP). This occurs in the transport of sodium. In secondary active transport the energy source is the membrane potential and/or ion gradients. For example, monosaccharides and some amino acids are transported across intestinal epithelial cell membranes, coupled with the active transport of sodium ions providing an ion gradient (see Chapter 5.1).

The process of **endocytosis**, often referred to as **bulk transport**, includes **phagocytosis**, which is the engulfing of particulate substances, and **pinocytosis**, which is the engulfing of water. Endocytosis enables larger molecules and substances to enter the cell. Phagocytosis involves the folding of the cell surface membrane around macromolecules or microorganisms and occurs in some motile cells, for example polymorphonuclear leucocytes. Particles engulfed in this manner form intracellular vesicles. Small drops of fluid containing protein can be engulfed in a similar fashion during pinocytosis. The fate of the phagocytic and pinocytic vesicles formed involves the lysosomes – enzyme-containing vesicles within the cell (see later). Each endocytotic vesicle fuses with lysosomes to form a digestive vesicle in which enzymatic breakdown of the engulfed substances occurs. The inner lining of the vesicles (which was the outer lining of the cell surface membrane) alters physiologically to provide increased permeability, which allows the products of digestion to be transferred more readily into the cytoplasm. The indigestible components of the vesicle are released into the extracellular fluid. **Exocytosis** is the bulk transport of material out of cells and is described in the section on the Golgi apparatus. Glandular cells secrete proteins (e.g. digestive enzymes) or the hormone insulin and nerve cells release their chemical messengers (neurotransmitters e.g. acetylcholine) by exocytosis.

## The nuclear membrane

The nucleus is surrounded and defined by a double membrane, each layer of which is similar in structure to the cell surface membrane. The inner and outer membranes are separated from one another by a space of 10–15 nm. The outer membrane might be continuous with the endoplasmic reticulum of the cytoplasm and have ribosomes attached on its cell surface. As a result, it can appear wrinkled or corrugated. Fusion occurs between the outer and inner membrane components around 'nuclear pores' (60–90 nm in diameter). Transport mechanisms through the nuclear membrane are not as well understood as those of the plasma membrane. There is evidence that compounds of low molecular weight diffuse through the membrane readily, and that large molecules, such as proteins and nucleic acids, pass through the nuclear pores. Binding sites for specific molecules inside the nucleus determine the concentration of certain materials within it. During the events of cell division the nuclear membrane disappears and later reforms by rearrangement of the endoplasmic reticulum.

## CLINICAL APPLICATIONS

Nuclear changes seen in cells infected with viruses or altered by carcinogens include increases in size, structural distortions of various kinds and invagination of the nuclear membrane, which can produce inclusions containing cytoplasmic organelles. Ultraviolet and ionizing radiation, viruses and a variety of other toxic substances also bring about nuclear aberrations.

## The nucleolus

The nucleolus has two major structural components. The core is a dense spherical collection of structural bars rich in DNA; the bars are called nucleonemas. The core is thought to be the structure concerned with organizing the functions of the nucleolus. In the peripheral area, filaments and granules seem to be stages in the synthesis of ribosomal RNA. There is no definite limiting membrane. The number of nucleoli per cell varies, but generally there are two per diploid cell.

During cell division the nucleoli disperse and reform in the new cells.

## The endoplasmic reticulum

A system of interconnecting membranes (5 nm in diameter) is found throughout the cytoplasm of all nucleated cells. The membranes form a loose-meshed, irregular network of branching and anastomosing tubules with saccular expansions, called cisternae, and isolated vesicles. The exact configuration and number of each element (tubules, cisternae or vesicles) vary between cell types and during cellular activity.

If the outer surface of the endoplasmic reticulum bears large numbers of ribosomes (see later), it is called **rough-surfaced** or **granular endoplasmic reticulum** because of its appearance. Glandular cells have a high proportion of rough-surfaced endoplasmic reticulum. Proteins assembled at the ribosomal sites are transported via the system of cavities within the endoplasmic reticulum to the Golgi apparatus of the cell, where they are concentrated and coated to form granules or droplets. Some carcinogenic chemicals cause prolonged detachment of ribosomes from membranes, leaving sites of unusual enzymatic activity exposed. This results in a change in the control of protein synthesis.

**Smooth-surfaced** or **agranular endoplasmic reticulum** lacks ribosomes and seldom forms cisternae. It

is often associated with the Golgi apparatus and its functions include metabolic detoxification and lipid and cholesterol metabolism in liver cells, and lipid transport in intestinal epithelium. The sarcoplasmic reticulum in skeletal and cardiac muscle cells is identical to smooth endoplasmic reticulum. The amount of smooth endoplasmic reticulum and the activity of related metabolic enzymes are increased with barbiturate administration. Some of these enzymes inactivate barbiturates, which results in barbiturate tolerance and the need for increased dosage.

## Mitochondria

Numerous small organelles, the mitochondria, show active movement within the cytoplasm. There is great variation in shape, size, mobility, orientation and number. Mitochondria have an inherent plasticity and appear as long, slender or rounded structures, with gradation of shapes between these forms. They all have the same basic structure (**Fig. 1.3.3**).

The outer boundary membrane (6–8 nm) has a smooth surface separated by a space (8 nm) from an inner membrane (6–8 nm) whose thin folds, called **cristae**, project into the cavity. Enzymes are present on the inner membrane surface. This structure provides a large area of membrane, spatially arranged to facilitate sequential chemical reactions. Mitochondria are the site of aerobic (in the presence of oxygen) cellular respiration. During cellular (or internal) respiration, energy is produced from the breakdown of nutrients and is stored in the high-energy phosphate bonds of ATP. The production of ATP takes place in mitochondria during a process called **oxidative phosphorylation.**

The number and inner complexity of the mitochondria in a cell vary directly with that cell's metabolic activity. The more metabolically active the cell,

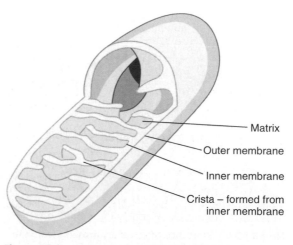

**Figure 1.3.3**  Diagram of a mitochondrion

- Matrix
- Outer membrane
- Inner membrane
- Crista – formed from inner membrane

the more mitochondria you would expect to find in its cytoplasm. Apart from their important metabolic function in cells, mitochondria contain DNA and are self-replicating (see Chapter 6.4).

## The Golgi apparatus

The Golgi apparatus of the cytoplasm is a compact network of membranes near the nucleus. It is a system of canals and has connections with the smooth endoplasmic reticulum. The components are arranged in parallel layers of flat saccules (cisternae) whose continuous ends form the boundary of a closed cavity. Small vesicles cluster around the outer convex surface and the inner cisternae might be partially distended and associated with spherical vacuoles containing secretory products. The Golgi apparatus in secretory cells is larger and has more cisternae.

Cell secretions move from the smooth endoplasmic reticulum to the Golgi apparatus prior to leaving the cell by the process of **exocytosis (Fig. 1.3.4)**. Its functions are the transport, concentration, temporary storage and channelling of these secretions. It is also involved in synthesizing glycoproteins in some mucus-secreting cells. The Golgi apparatus also has a role in the production of lysosomes at its surface.

## Lysosomes

Lysosomes are found in the cytoplasm. They are sacs formed of membrane and their role is to break down and recycle large organic molecules in the cell. They contain enzymes and appear in diverse shapes of variable internal density. The enzymes are hydrolytic, that is, they act to break down substances. It is essential that these enzymes remain separated from the cytoplasm within their membranous sacs otherwise their enzymatic action could digest the cell itself. They arise either from the Golgi apparatus or from the endoplasmic reticulum.

The lysosomes act on pinocytotic and phagocytic vesicles, as described earlier. For example, thyroglobulin (from the thyroid follicles) is taken into the thyroid cells by pinocytosis and degraded by the action of lysosomes, resulting in the release of thyroid hormones.

Phagocytic cells discharge the contents of their lysosomes to digest engulfed bacteria. Lysosomes also function to clear damaged parts of cells or entire cells (**autolysis**) if required. The lysosomes of injured or dying cells are thought to rupture spontaneously.

## Peroxisomes

Peroxisomes (microbodies) are dense structures, 0.5–1 μm in diameter, which are bounded by a single membrane. New peroxisomes are produced by the growth and subdivision of existing peroxisomes. Peroxisomes absorb and break down fatty acids and other organic compounds. As they do so, they generate hydrogen peroxide, which in turn is broken down to oxygen and water. The role of the peroxisomes is to protect the cell from the potentially damaging effects of free radicals produced during catabolism.

## Microtubules

Microtubules are fine, straight, tubular structures, 20–24 nm in diameter and of indefinite length, found in the cytoplasm. They are arranged in bundles and give structural support, maintaining cell shape. Microtubules are found in the core of the flagella of spermatozoa, within cilia and in the axoplasm of neurones, where they lie parallel to the long axis of each cell. Their hollow appearance is due to the lower density of the central protein material.

They form the spindle apparatus of the dividing cell and are found randomly dispersed in the cytoplasm of many cells and at the periphery of red blood cells and platelets. The microtubules of the spindle apparatus, which appear during cell division, are dispersed

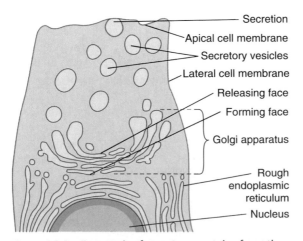

Secretion
Apical cell membrane
Secretory vesicles
Lateral cell membrane
Releasing face
Forming face
Golgi apparatus
Rough endoplasmic reticulum
Nucleus

**Figure 1.3.4** Exocytosis of secretory proteins from the Golgi apparatus

by the cytotoxic drugs vincristine and vinblastine, and hence these drugs inhibit cell division.

## Microfilaments

A network of fine filaments, 4–6 nm in diameter and of indefinite length, is found in the cytoplasm of most cells. In the periphery of the cell these filaments function to prevent the nucleus from impinging on the cell surface membrane. Microfilaments are of great significance in the physiology of striated muscle, in which they are composed of the proteins myosin and actin and called **myofibrils**.

Their function is linked with the potential contractility of the cell, the separation (cleavage) stage of cell division, cell motility and the movement of segments of cell surface membrane which occurs during endocytosis. The extrusion of the nucleus during the maturation of red blood cells is associated with the disappearance of contractile microfilaments.

Cell organelles are surrounded by intracellular fluid within the cell surface membrane. Outside the cell membrane, extracellular fluid surrounds the cell populations providing a homeostatically controlled physical and chemical environment. Living cells distinguish themselves from inanimate, non-living entities by their organized structure and the balance of physiological processes maintained in each cell and between cells.

## Eukaryotic and prokaryotic cells

The type of cell described in this chapter is known as an **eukaryotic cell**. These are neither the smallest, nor the simplest (in terms of structure) of cells. The **prokaryotic cell** type, typical of bacteria, is in many ways less complex than the eukaryotic cell that is typical of animals and plants. However, it is not correct to think of prokaryotic cells as being biochemically more simple as this is often not the case. They are not less efficient or more primitive but they are different; Table 1.3.1 indicates the major differences.

## Cell division: mitosis

### DEVELOPMENTAL ISSUES

Cells arise from the division of pre-existing cells. All the cells of the human body originate from the division of a single cell, the **zygote**, formed from the fusion of an ovum and a spermatozoon. The mechanism of cell division (mitosis) is one of the basic functions of living cells. It provides for the growth of the organism from one to many millions of cells.

There are two distinct phases of mitosis: the division of the nucleus and the division of the cytoplasm. These two phases usually occur at the same time.

The nucleus contains **chromatin**. This substance is the form that chromosomes take between cell divisions. Chromosomes carry the hereditary information in the form of DNA. During cell division the structure of each chromosome becomes well defined. At the beginning of mitosis each chromosome is a double structure because the DNA content of chromatin has replicated during the period (**interphase**) prior to cell division. Replication of DNA occurs when the double-stranded helical molecule unwinds (**Fig. 1.3.5**) and enzymes catalyse the formation of new strands precisely complementary to the old ones. Two identical double helices are therefore formed at the end of the process.

During mitosis the shape and size of the chromosomes are constant, and each chromosome has structural characteristics that enable it to be identified. For example, the shape of a double chromosome depends on the location of the **centromere** (see **Fig. 1.3.6II**).

| **Table 1.3.1** Major features of prokaryotic and eukaryotic cells | | |
|---|---|---|
| Feature | Prokaryotic cell, e.g. a bacterium | Eukaryotic cell, e.g. an animal or plant cell |
| Cell membrane | + | + |
| Cell wall | + | + |
| | Does not contain cellulose | In plants only, contains cellulose |
| Membranes in cytoplasm | − | + |
| Cytoplasmic organelles | − | + |
| Cytoskeleton | − | + |
| Membrane-bound nucleus | − | + |

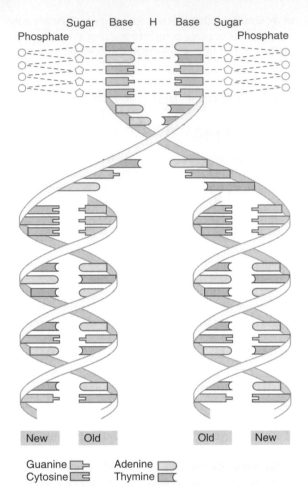

Sugar   Base   H   Base   Sugar
Phosphate                      Phosphate

New     Old        Old     New

Guanine      Adenine
Cytosine      Thymine

**Figure 1.3.5**   The replication of DNA showing the unwinding of the double helix and the formation of new strands with complementary base pairs

This is the point at which the two **chromatids**, which constitute each double chromosome, are joined. Some chromosomes have their centromeres at the midpoint, and are classified as 'metacentric'; in others the centromeres are close to one end and the chromosome has limbs of unequal length. These are called 'acrocentric'.

With the exception of the ovum and spermatozoon (the gametes), the cells of the human body each contain 46 chromosomes. The gametes each contain 23 – a half set or **haploid number**. This reduction in chromosome number is achieved during **meiosis**, a type of cell division that occurs only in the production of gametes in sexual reproduction and which is described in Chapters 6.3 and 6.4.

The 46 chromosomes of human cells can be matched into 23 pairs. The chromosomes of a cell are called its **karyotype**. The karyotype of a human male is shown in **Fig. 6.3.3 on page 729**. One chromosome of each pair has come from the person's mother and the other from his or her father. Twenty-two of the pairs are called 'autosomes' and one pair constitutes the 'sex chromosomes', which are called X and Y. The presence of the sex chromosomes determines genetic sex: a female has two identical X chromosomes and a male has one X and one – smaller – Y chromosome.

The ovum and spermatozoon each provides a haploid set of chromosomes (23) and so, with their union at fertilization, a somatic or **diploid number** (46) is established.

Mitosis ensures that each daughter cell receives an identical chromosome complement to that of the parent cell. A cell usually functions abnormally if it fails to receive a normal chromosome complement.

One of the factors that trigger cells to divide is the attainment of a critical mass and/or nuclear : cell surface ratio. However, some cells can divide without prior growth in size. It is also known that factors external to the cells, known as **growth factors**, play a crucial role and the growth factors include some hormones, erythropoietin (see Chapter 4.1), prolactin (see Chapter 2.6) and a variety of peptide (see Chapter 1.2) molecules. Cells can be prevented from dividing by administration of the drug colchicine, and exposure to radiation can cause nuclear abnormalities and prevent division. Many other factors influence the process of cell division, including nutrition and the degree of cell specialization. Generally, the more specialized the cell, the less likely it is to divide and so reproduce itself.

Whatever other factors might be operating, a cell must complete certain preparations before it can undergo mitosis. All these occur during the period between cell divisions, which is called interphase. These preparations include:

- replication of the DNA complement of the chromosomes
- replication of the centrioles
- synthesis of the proteins from which the fibres of the mitotic spindle are formed
- metabolic production of adequate energy to undergo cell division.

During interphase, a pair of highly organized structures is present in the cytoplasm, near the nuclear membrane and Golgi region; these are the centrioles. Each centriole is composed of nine groups of three protein rods, arranged in a circle, giving a cylindrical shape. The two centrioles lie with their axes at right angles to each other. Just before cell division, each centriole replicates and, at the beginning of mitosis, one of each resulting pair migrates to opposite poles of the cell (**see Fig. 1.3.6III**). Protein fibres, structures identical to microtubules, then form between the pairs of centrioles (**see Fig. 1.3.6III**). The structure formed is called the **division spindle** or **mitotic apparatus**.

Mitosis is divided, for ease of description, into four stages, although, in reality, each stage merges into the next (**see Fig. 1.3.6**).

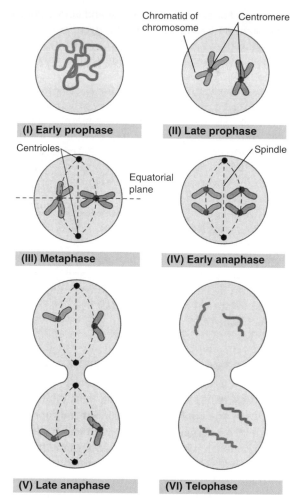

**Figure 1.3.6** The stages of mitosis. Only one chromosome pair is shown

## Prophase (Fig. 1.3.6I and 1.3.6II)

At the beginning of prophase the centrioles migrate to opposite sides of the nucleus. At the same time the spindle fibres begin to aggregate, eventually resulting in the formation of the division spindle. The nuclear membrane disappears and the nucleolus disperses. Each chromosome condenses into a visible unit and can be seen to be made up of a double filament. Each longitudinal half-chromosome (chromatid) has the identical nucleic acids of the chromosome before duplication occurred. The paired chromatids of a chromosome are joined at a single point by a centromere.

## Metaphase (Fig. 1.3.6III)

The nuclear membrane has now disappeared and the spindle fibres make connections with the centromere of each double chromosome. Each chromosome moves to a central position in the cell, and the centromeres are evenly and precisely spaced along the equatorial plane.

## Anaphase (Fig. 1.3.6IV and 1.3.6V)

Up to this time, each double chromosome has contained a single centromere holding the two chromatids together. Now the centromere splits so that two independent daughter chromosomes, each with its own centromere, are formed. The two chromatids of each double chromosome now separate. The same tension, exerted by the attached spindle fibres, that pulled the double chromosomes into the equatorial plane now pulls the daughter chromosomes (former chromatids) towards opposite poles. One set of chromosomes can be seen moving towards one pole and the other set moves to the opposite pole along the spindle fibres.

## Telophase (Fig. 1.3.6VI)

When the daughter chromosomes reach their respective poles, telophase has begun. A cleavage furrow encircles the surface of the cell, eventually constricting the cell into two daughter cells. The disappearance of the spindle fibres, gradual reappearance of the chromatin network from the distinct chromosomes, reformation of the nuclear membrane, recondensation of the nucleolus and the division of the cytoplasm all occur, in each daughter cell, during this final phase of mitosis.

The result of cell division is the formation of two daughter cells, each with an identical set of genes and each potentially the same as the initial parent cell. Cell division is essential for growth and replacement of damaged tissue, as in wound healing. It involves the assimilation of materials from the cell's environment, their transformation through breakdown and synthesis into new cellular components, and the utilization of energy.

## The cell cycle

The cell cycle is the period from the beginning of one cell division to the beginning of the next. It involves three major stages:

1. **Interphase**: a period of cell growth during which the DNA in the nucleus replicates. This stage is sometimes, incorrectly, described as a period of rest. There are actually three quite distinct phases in interphase, called $G_1$, S and $G_2$.
   - *$G_1$ phase*: this occurs immediately after a new cell has been produced. G stands for 'gap' and $G_1$ is the period between the end of cell division and DNA replication. This is a period of growth in which one centriole pair begins to replicate as do other cell surface organelles.
   - *S phase*: S stands for synthesis. It is in this phase that DNA replicates precisely,

duplicating every chromosome. During this phase the other centriole pair also replicates. The phase is induced through enzyme activity.

- $G_2$ *phase*: this is the second gap phase and growth continues. Before mitosis can begin, the parent cell must approximately double its mass and contents. The centriole pairs begin to move apart, the nuclear membrane starts to disintegrate, chromosomes begin to condense and the spindle to form as the cell moves into early prophase of mitosis.

2. **Division of the nucleus (mitosis)**: the period during which the nucleus and its constituent chromosomes divide.

3. **Cytokinesis**: the division of the cytoplasm.

## The regulation of cellular activity

The cell cycle is affected by the cell's environmental conditions, such as nutrient levels, presence or absence of growth factors and the availability of space into which to grow. If these factors are not at optimal levels, the cycle might slow or even cease. (This is one reason why tissue injury stimulates growth – because it creates a new space in which to grow. In contrast, malignant cancer cells have lost their 'space limitation' control and multiply regardless of lack of space.)

Just as environmental factors have a general influence on cellular activity, so hormones (see Chapter 2.5) and neurotransmitters (see Chapter 2.1) have specific actions in regulating cell function. These substances have several modes of action, many through the activation of second messengers, for example, calcium and cyclic adenosine monophosphate (cAMP). Some chemical regulators bind to receptors inside the cell and then enter the nucleus, where they are able directly to modify gene transcription. This action alters the balance of protein synthesis and so alters cellular function.

The lifespan of cells (the length of the cell cycle) varies considerably between cell types (tissues). At one extreme, a neurone does not reproduce in a lifetime, whereas an epithelial cell lining the gut might reproduce each day. Other cell types lie somewhere in between these two extremes. Typical cell lifespans are given in the individual chapters in which their function is described.

## Cytotoxic and radiation therapy in cancer

### CLINICAL APPLICATIONS

Cytotoxic drugs, used to treat widespread malignant disease (cancers) affect rapidly dividing cells such as those that comprise malignant tumours. For example, vincristine and vinblastine are plant-derived alkaloids that prevent mitosis by blocking the assembly of the mitotic spindle. Mustines, derived from nitrogen mustard gas, prevent DNA replication (see Chapter 1.2). Unfortunately, these drugs are non-specific in their effect and so they also destroy other rapidly dividing cells, such as those in bone marrow and the epithelial cells that form hair and those lining the mouth and gastrointestinal tract. The effects of damage to these cells produces the unpleasant side-effects associated with treatment such as hair loss, anaemia, susceptibility to infection, sore mouth and gastrointestinal disturbance.

Ionizing radiation (radiotherapy) breaks down molecules in chromatin and in the cytoplasm, so preventing cell division. Radiation can be directed specifically at the malignant tumour and great care must be taken to protect all other vulnerable tissues of the client (and therapist) from its damaging effects.

## Nucleic acids and protein synthesis

The deoxyribonucleic acid (DNA) in the nucleus of a cell is the species-specific, inherited, genetic material. To understand how DNA functions as the genetic material, it is necessary to understand how it controls the synthesis and metabolism of the cell. This is a complex problem, which scientists have not yet fully explained, but the control of cellular protein synthesis by DNA is now largely understood. Proteins can be enzymes, catalysing cellular reactions, or structural proteins. Because the metabolic activity of a cell depends on the regulated synthesis of its enzymes, by controlling protein synthesis, the nuclear genes of DNA control cellular function.

## The genetic code

The sequence of the nitrogenous bases (adenine [A], thymine [T], guanine [G] and cytosine [C]) in a DNA molecule makes up the letters of the genetic code for cellular protein construction by specifying the amino acid sequence in a protein molecule. Each nitrogenous base is a 'letter' in the code and the 'words' formed consist of groups of three bases, known as **triplets**.

As there are three bases in a 'word' and four bases in both DNA and RNA, there are $4^3 = 64$ different 'words' available to encode the 20 amino acids found in proteins. A two-letter codeword would be inadequate to specify 20 alternatives; it would give only $4^2 = 16$ different words. The triplet code, with its 64 alternatives, has more than one word specifying a given amino acid. There are also triplets of bases coding for 'initiate' and 'terminate', so defining the limits of a particular DNA message. Thus, if a protein contains 300 amino acids, the part of the DNA molecule that codes for its synthesis must have 300 codewords or base triplets – a total of 900 nitrogenous bases in linear sequence.

## Protein synthesis

Most protein synthesis takes place in the cytoplasm on the **ribosomes.** These small granules are composed of 60% RNA and 40% protein. Ribosomes are usually found attached to the endoplasmic reticulum (giving the latter a 'rough' appearance), although they can also be free in the cytoplasm.

The precise replication of DNA, prior to cell division, was described in the preceding section. As well as acting as a template to replicate itself, DNA can act as a template to synthesize an RNA molecule, because the nitrogenous bases of RNA can pair with those of DNA. That is:

| DNA base | pairs with | RNA base |
|----------|-----------|----------|
| Adenine | | Uracil |
| Thymine | | Adenine |
| Guanine | | Cytosine |
| Cytosine | | Guanine |

This enzymatically catalysed process, which is called **transcription**, occurs in the nucleus. It produces a molecule of RNA that is a precise mirror image of the DNA template. Transcription is illustrated in **Fig. 1.3.7**. The information content of the RNA so formed is identical to that of the DNA on which it was transcribed because each triplet codeword of the DNA is reproduced by a corresponding 'anti-word' or **codon** of the RNA by the base-pairing rule.

The RNA molecule so formed then leaves the nucleus and moves into the cytoplasm, where it becomes attached to the surface of ribosomes. This type of RNA is called **messenger RNA (mRNA)** because it acts as a messenger between nucleus and cytoplasm.

Just as a strand of DNA functions as a template for the synthesis of mRNA, so an mRNA molecule functions as a template for the synthesis of a particular protein. Whereas a DNA molecule can be visualized as being divided into many regions, each of which codes for the synthesis of a particular protein, the mRNA molecule encodes a single protein. As described above, the code upon which this template is based has been discovered. **Figure 1.3.8** shows the mRNA codons now known to code for specific amino acids for the initiation and termination of a polypeptide chain.

Thus the alignment of amino acids in a polypeptide chain of a protein is dictated by the base sequence in the mRNA, which is, in turn, a direct replica of the base sequence of the DNA.

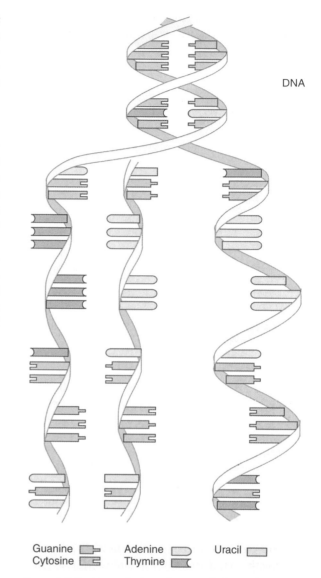

DNA

Guanine ▭ Adenine ▭ Uracil ▭
Cytosine ▭ Thymine ▭

**Figure 1.3.7** Transcription of a strand of DNA by messenger RNA. Note how uracil is substituted for thymine in the messenger RNA strand

Amino acids in the cytoplasm of the cell become bound to amino-acid-specific activating enzymes, a process that requires energy in the form of ATP. They are then attached to a small molecule of RNA called **transfer RNA (tRNA)**. There is a specific tRNA for each type of amino acid. The function of tRNA molecules is to carry their specific amino acid to the ribosomal site of protein synthesis and allow it to become aligned at the correct position on the mRNA molecule. This occurs because a region of each tRNA molecule contains a base triplet complementary to a specific mRNA codon. The tRNA triplet of bases that binds to a codon of mRNA is called an **anticodon**. The tRNA lines up on the mRNA template and so places its amino acid correctly in sequence with others also brought into position by their tRNAs. As a result, the

| First base of codon | Second base of codon: U | | C | | A | | G | | Third base of codon |
|---|---|---|---|---|---|---|---|---|---|
| U | UUU | Phenylalanine | UCU | Serine | UAU | Tyrosine | UGU | Cysteine | U |
| | UUC | | UCC | | UAC | | UGC | | C |
| | UUA | Leucine | UCA | | UAA | Terminate | UGA | Terminate | A |
| | UUG | | UCG | | UAG | | UGG | Tryptophan | G |
| C | CUU | Leucine | CCU | Proline | CAU | Histidine | CGU | Arginine | U |
| | CUC | | CCC | | CAC | | CGC | | C |
| | CUA | | CCA | | CAA | Glutamine | CGA | | A |
| | CUG | | CCG | | CAG | | CGG | | G |
| A | AUU | Isoleucine | ACU | Threonine | AAU | Asparagine | AGU | Serine | U |
| | AUC | | ACC | | AAC | | AGC | | C |
| | AUA | Methionine | ACA | | AAA | Lysine | AGA | Arginine | A |
| | AUG | + initiate | ACG | | AAG | | AGG | | G |
| G | GUU | Valine + initiate | GCU | Alanine | GAU | Aspartic acid | GGU | Glycine | U |
| | GUC | | GCC | | GAC | | GGC | | C |
| | GUA | | GCA | | GAA | Glutamic acid | GGA | | A |
| | GUG | | GCG | | GAG | | GGG | | G |

**Figure 1.3.8** Coding triplets of bases (codons) in messenger RNA showing the amino acids which are coded for incorporation into protein chains

order of amino acids in the protein is established and it only remains for enzymes to catalyse the formation of the peptide bonds to connect them together. When the polypeptide chain is complete it is released from the ribosome and becomes folded into its active configuration. The synthesis of part of the molecule of the protein hormone glucagon is illustrated in **Fig. 1.3.9**.

It is essential that the genetic code contained in DNA can transfer its 'blueprint' for protein construction into the product with both speed and accuracy. An error such as a change (mutation) in the code, altering the sequence of bases, can result in the production of a protein with one or more incorrect amino acids and resultant abnormal function. This is how genetic abnormalities are produced.

There are, then, two major steps in the synthesis of proteins. The first is the transcription of the DNA code by RNA; the second is the transformation of that information into the correct amino acid sequence of a protein.

The same diploid set of genes (DNA) is found in the nucleus of all cells except the gametes, which contain a haploid set. A single gene can be considered to be the segment of DNA that encodes a particular protein.

It is probable that, in addition to vital information, human genes also contain obsolete information that is in the process of being modified. The selection of genes to be actively expressed is crucial in determining cell function and is controlled by sophisticated mechanisms that select and activate parts of the DNA molecule, thereby limiting and determining functional gene sequences.

## CLINICAL APPLICATIONS

It is, of course, essential that a cell's DNA complement is passed on unchanged from parent to new daughter cell. A change in DNA base sequence is called a genetic **mutation**. If a mutation is not corrected it will be transmitted to all daughter cells of the parent in which the change occurred. Sometimes these mutations are repaired by enzyme action but it only takes a mutation of one base pair of DNA to produce an abnormal gene capable of producing conditions of the severity of phenylketonuria. This is a disease in which the abnormal DNA cannot synthesize the enzyme that converts the amino acid phenylalanine into tyrosine. Phenylalanine therefore accumulates in the blood and tissues. It is toxic and damages brain cells, producing mental retardation. Affected babies must have a phenylalanine-free diet to protect their brain from damage. Newborn babies are screened for the disease through the Guthrie heel-prick blood test.

Sickle-cell anaemia (see Chapter 4.1) is another life-threatening condition brought about by the mutation of just one DNA base pairing (see Chapter 6.4 for further discussion of genetic mutations).

Researchers have also found that by interfering with sections of mRNA they can interfere with, and even switch off, the production of some protein building blocks that are implicated in diseases such as cancer, Huntington's disease and Alzheimer's disease. This process is known as RNA interference (RNAi).

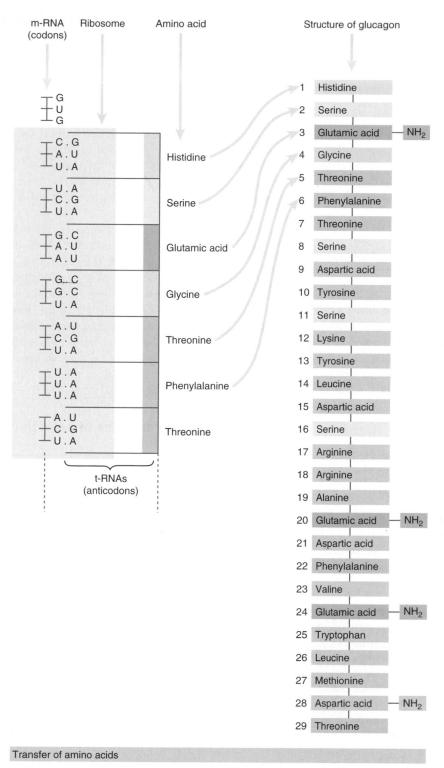

**Figure 1.3.9** The synthesis of a protein (glucagon) showing how the sequence of bases in messenger RNA is translated into a sequence of amino acids

## Cell differentiation and specialization

The process through which cells become specialized, in structure and function, is called **differentiation**. Although each nucleated cell of the body contains the same genetic material, they differ from each other because each type of cell (tissue) expresses different sections of the genetic code. The result of this is that a different array of proteins will be synthesized by different cell types and, as already explained, this has major effects on the structural appearance of the cell and on its function; consider the range of differentiation and specialization in the body. To name but a few there is the neurone, specialized for the transmission of electrical impulses (see Chapter 2.1), the muscle cell, specialized to contract and produce movement (see Chapter 3.2), the red blood cell, packed so full of the haemoglobin needed to transport oxygen that it has lost its nucleus (see Chapter 4.1) and the secretory cells of the enzyme-producing glands in the gastrointestinal tract (see Chapter 5.1). You will learn about these and other specialized cells in subsequent chapters.

## Growth, development and ageing

Growth of a human being involves an increase in size and weight of the body tissues and is thus a measurable quantitative change. By contrast, development occurs through a series of coordinated qualitative changes that affect the complexity and function of body tissues. Developmental change is most rapid when the individual is young and it results in a normally developed adult individual.

Growth and development depend on a continuous and complex interaction of inherited and environmental factors. A strong positive correlation is therefore found in the height measurements of monozygotic (identical) twins when the twins are reared together (Wilson, 1976). This correlation is more marked than in dizygotic (non-identical) twin pairs (**Table 1.3.2**). Identical twins, who develop from the same fertilized ovum, have the same genetic make-up (genotype; see

Chapter 6.4), whereas non-identical twins develop from different fertilized ova and share no more of their genes (50%) than do other siblings. If twins are reared together one would expect each individual's environment to be very similar and so any difference measured could be attributed to inherited factors – this explains the results shown in **Table 1.3.2**. Tanner (1989) describes how identical twins reared apart, with one twin raised in adverse environmental circumstances, can show marked differences in their adult height, demonstrating how environmental effects can be superimposed on genetically determined features.

Several environmental factors affect growth and development. These include diet, illness, socioeconomic factors and the emotional environment in which the child is raised. In particular, undernutrition impairs growth – the severity of the effect depends on the degree and length of the period of malnutrition. Improved nutrition has been suggested as the cause of the secular trend in growth where, for the last hundred years or so, each generation has been taller on average than the preceding one (see, for example, Chinn and Rona, 1984).

## Normal patterns of growth and development

The normal rate and pattern of growth are regulated through the endocrine system and vary at different times of life. Growth is most rapid at about four months gestation, i.e. before birth. The exact pattern of endocrine control and development in utero is not fully established. Growth and development remain rapid through the first two years of life. The average child doubles its birth length and triples its birth weight by one year of age. During childhood the rate of growth decreases substantially, with the height of the average child increasing by 5–7.5 cm/year and his or her weight by 2–2.5 kg/year. Accurate measurement and assessment of a child's height is recommended as a valuable means of monitoring the general health and progress of a child (Hall, 1989). The normality of a child's growth is checked by plotting the measurements on special graphs, or percentile charts, which include 95% confidence limits for a large number of children. **Figure 1.3.10** shows a typical growth chart for a normal baby.

Growth becomes rapid once again just before the onset of puberty, when the adolescent growth spurt occurs (**see Fig. 1.3.11**). This happens typically between the ages of 10.5 and 13 years in girls and 12.5 and 15 years in boys, although there is a large degree of individual variation in time of onset. Generally, the younger the growth spurt starts, the less the final height achieved (Tanner, 1989).

**Table 1.3.2** Mean differences between lengths (measured in cm) of monozygotic twin pairs (2140 pairs) and same sexed dizygotic twin pairs (290 pairs), reared together from birth to four years (Wilson, 1976)

|  | MZ pairs | DZ pairs |
| --- | --- | --- |
| Birth | 1.8 | 1.6 |
| 3 months | 1.4 | 1.6 |
| 6 months | 1.3 | 1.9 |
| 1 year | 1.3 | 1.8 |
| 2 years | 1.1 | 2.4 |
| 3 years | 1.1 | 2.9 |
| 4 years | 1.1 | 3.2 |

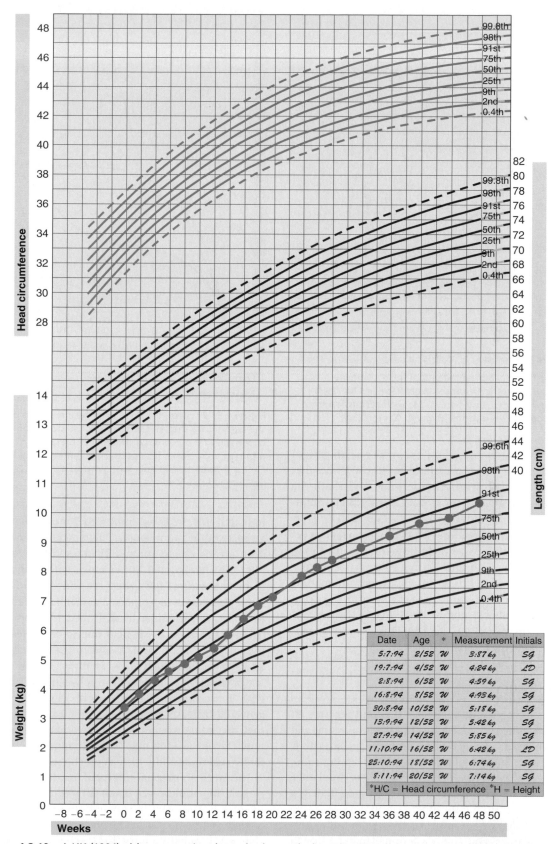

| Date | Age | * | Measurement | Initials |
|---|---|---|---|---|
| 5:7:94 | 2/52 | W | 3:87 kg | SG |
| 19:7:94 | 4/52 | W | 4:24 kg | LD |
| 2:8:94 | 6/52 | W | 4:59 kg | SG |
| 16:8:94 | 8/52 | W | 4:93 kg | SG |
| 30:8:94 | 10/52 | W | 5:18 kg | SG |
| 13:9:94 | 12/52 | W | 5:42 kg | SG |
| 27:9:94 | 14/52 | W | 5:85 kg | SG |
| 11:10:94 | 16/52 | W | 6:42 kg | LD |
| 25:10:94 | 18/52 | W | 6:74 kg | SG |
| 8:11:94 | 20/52 | W | 7:14 kg | SG |

*H/C = Head circumference  *H = Height

**Figure 1.3.10**   A UK (1994) girls cross-sectional standard growth chart showing early weight recordings for one infant of birth weight 3.43 kg. (A growth chart is also available for boys.) Length and head circumference, in relation to gestational age, may also be recorded. (© Reproduced with permission from the Child Growth Foundation, London)

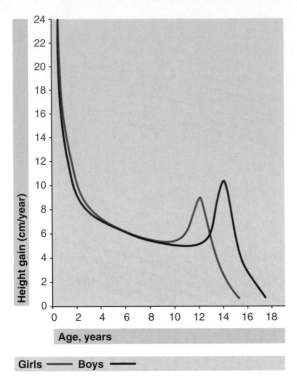

Girls ——— Boys ———

**Figure 1.3.11** Typical individual height velocity curves for boys and girls. (Adapted from Tanner, J.M. (1989) *Foetus into Man*, 2nd edn, p. 14, with permission from Castlemead Publications, Welwyn Garden City)

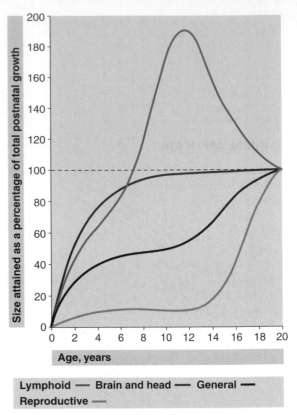

Lymphoid ——— Brain and head ——— General ———
Reproductive ———

**Figure 1.3.12** Growth curves of different tissues of the body. Note that all curves are of the size attained expressed as a percentage of the eventual size attained at 20 years. (Adapted from Tanner, J.M. (1989) *Foetus into Man*, 2nd edn, with permission from Castlemead Publications, Welwyn Garden City)

Most body tissues follow the same growth pattern as that described for overall height. Those tissues that deviate from this include the brain and skull, the lymphoid tissues of the tonsils, adenoids and intestine and the reproductive organs (**Fig. 1.3.12**). Thus the brain (including the skull, eyes and ears) achieves virtually adult size by three years of age and shows little, if any, growth spurt during adolescence. By contrast, the lymphoid tissue reaches its maximum mass before adolescence and then declines to the adult amount, probably due to the influence of sex hormones (Tanner, 1989). Reproductive tissues show little increase in size until adolescence.

## Adolescence

This is the period during which the child becomes an adult. It is accompanied by a number of physical and psychological changes that culminate in a mature, fully-grown individual who is capable of reproduction.

Growth, as we have seen, becomes very rapid once again during adolescence, leading to a gain in height of about 25 cm in girls and 28 cm in boys. It is also accompanied by a number of changes in body composition and shape. This is a period of marked growth and development of the reproductive organs. These changes are also discussed in Chapter 6.3. During the adolescent growth spurt, the limbs begin to increase

in length first, followed some 6 to 9 months later by an increase in trunk length. This unequal growth in stature can lead to some difficulties with coordination. The facial dimensions change, with an increase in prominence of the lower jaw and the forehead. These changes are more marked in males than females. In males, the shoulder breadth increases and there is overall increase in strength due to an increase in muscle mass. Limb fat decreases in the male during adolescence, although there is little gain in body fat. In females, the width of the pelvic inlet increases, with an accompanying increase in width. Body fat generally increases in females during adolescence so that the adult woman has approximately twice as much fat as the adult man. These changes give rise to the typical male and female adult shape.

The precise hormonal control of the changes occurring during adolescence is not fully understood. An increase in androgen activity in both sexes from five to eight years seems to be the precursor to adolescent changes. As puberty approaches there is an increase in circulating gonadotrophic releasing hormones, either because of an increase in secretion or a withdrawal of inhibition of endocrine activity. Growth hormone probably results in the increase in limb length and the sex hormones are responsible for the changes in trunk length and width of shoulders and hips. Testosterone secretion prevents the female pattern of fat distribution in the male.

## Adult growth

### CLINICAL APPLICATIONS

Tissues composed of relatively undifferentiated cells, for example liver and bone, are generally able to regenerate with ease. By contrast, tissues composed of cells that have become very specialized, for example nerve cells, are less able to regenerate. Some cells have become so specialized that they are not able to reproduce at all. A classic example of such a cell is the erythrocyte (red blood cell), which has lost its nucleus in the process of becoming a highly effective oxygen transporter.

Growth in the adult is normally limited to the repair and renewal processes. A change in any of the hormones controlling growth and development can lead to impaired healing. For example, high levels of circulating cortisol, such as those that occur in steroid therapy, delay the healing of wounds, as does deficiency of thyroid hormone as in myxoedema (see Chapter 2.6).

## Regulation of growth and development

Normally, growth is a well-regulated and ordered process that allows development of the human being and ensures that growth of the appropriate tissues only occurs when there is a need for repair and renewal. (These ideas have already been introduced in relation to cellular activity and cell division in growth on p. **00**). For example, liver cells grow only after partial hepatic resection, and there is growth of the contralateral (opposite) kidney following nephrectomy. There is also normally strict control over the extent to which cells proliferate in any given body tissue. Loss of this control can lead to the growth of tumours. Growth therefore depends on the integrated action of several hormones and other growth factors, which are summarized here in **Table 1.3.3** and discussed in detail in Chapter 2.6.

## Ageing

**Ageing** refers to 'the regular changes that occur in mature genetically representative organisms living under representative environmental conditions as they advance in chronological age' (Birren and Renner, 1977, p. 4). **Senescence** refers to the decline in physical abilities that frequently, but not inevitably, accompanies ageing.

**Life expectancy** figures refer to the average length of survival for members of a species, whereas **life span** denotes the maximum age achieved by these members. Life span appears to be a genetic characteristic of a species but life expectancy is largely determined by environmental factors. Thus, since the year 1900, life expectancy in human populations has increased by 20 years whereas life span has remained unchanged. This reflects the improved control of disease and improved social circumstances achieved during this period.

It is unlikely that there are genes for ageing but ageing might be genetically determined through the interaction of the genome with other factors such as nutrition and the environment (Kirkwood, 2002).

The genetic basis for ageing is also seen in studies comparing the age of death of monozygotic and dizygotic twins. Monozygotic twins show an average difference in age of death of about 37 months whilst dizygotic twins die, on average, about 78 months apart (Bank and Jarvik, 1978; Kellerman and Sander, 1979). Similarly, individuals whose parents and grandparents live to a great age, die, on average, 6 years later than those individuals whose parents and grandparents die before the age of 50 years (Murphy, 1978).

### CLINICAL APPLICATIONS

The genetic basis for ageing is also supported by the existence of certain inherited conditions that have accelerated ageing as a central feature. In the Hutchinson–Gilford progeria syndrome, for example, individuals appear normal at birth but soon show many signs associated with ageing. Weight and height decrease, hair is lost and the skin becomes inelastic. Generalized atherosclerosis and associated cerebrovascular accident and myocardial infarction rapidly become central features. Most patients die at about the age of 12 years (Schneider and Bynum, 1983).

Although it might seem desirable that life expectancy figures approach those of life span, this is only acceptable when accompanied by improved health in elderly people and when senescence is minimized. There is great individual variation in the rate and extent of senescence and changes due to ageing. It is thus difficult to predict age-related changes with certainty.

## Ageing at the cellular level

Studies of in vitro tissue cultures suggest that individual cells have a predetermined life span. Cells thus divide a certain number of times followed by a period during which no further cell division occurs. The cell then undergoes changes in its protein composition before cell death ultimately occurs. It is perhaps during this period that senescence occurs. Studies in

**Table 1.3.3** Main hormonal influences on growth

| Hormone | Effects |
| --- | --- |
| **Growth hormone** | • Stimulates growth in many tissues<br>• Stimulates protein synthesis<br>• Mainly secreted during sleep<br>• Many effects mediated through somatomedins |
| **Thyroid hormones** | • Permissive for action of growth hormone<br>• Deficiency in early childhood leads to irreversible small stature and mental retardation<br>• Essential for normal development of the central nervous system |
| **Parathyroid hormone vitamin D, and calcitonin** | • Essential for normal bone formation and growth |
| **Glucocorticoids (cortisol)** | • Regulatory effect on tissue growth<br>• In excess inhibit growth in height |
| **Insulin** | • Stimulates protein synthesis and inhibits protein breakdown<br>• Two somatomedins, the insulin-like growth factors (IGF) have similar molecular structure to proinsulin |
| **Oestrogens: oestradiol** | • Growth of female organs at puberty<br>• Stimulates female pattern of fat distribution |
| **Androgens: testosterone** | • Widespread anabolic effects on reproductive organs and somatic tissues<br>• Stimulates protein synthesis via direct influence on cellular DNA and RNA<br>• Stimulates development of typical male physique and characteristics |

which the nucleus of cells close to completing their active dividing phase are placed in young cytoplasm, and vice versa, suggest that the ageing clock is situated in the nucleus of the cells. A cell with a young nucleus and old cytoplasm will, for example, behave as a young cell, whereas young cytoplasm will not rejuvenate an old nucleus.

Several theories have been proposed to explain how cellular ageing occurs. Non-genetic theories of cell ageing suggest that age-related changes are due to the wearing-out of cell components or to the cell being deprived of essential nutrients with age. The pigment lipofuscin, which accumulates in cells as age increases, has also been implicated in the ageing process. It is, however, difficult to establish whether these changes are the cause of ageing in the cell or are caused by the ageing process.

Genetic theories of cellular ageing seem more promising, in view of the strong genetic influence on life span. There is, however, no single cellular theory of ageing that can adequately explain ageing at the present time (Kirkwood, 2002). Genetic theories suggest that repair of DNA becomes less efficient with age or that there is an increase in somatic mutations with ageing, with subsequent alteration of the genetic sequences in DNA.

It might be that, in ageing, errors occur in the way that proteins are synthesized, so that rogue amino acids occur in the protein molecules. The body might treat these different proteins as foreign and manufacture antibodies against them – an autoimmune response. The altered proteins will be unable to act as receptors for hormone molecules and this could have widespread effects throughout the body. Similarly, the altered protein molecules might change enzyme activity within the body. Changes in the physical properties of some proteins have been demonstrated in older cells. However, clear evidence of widespread errors in protein synthesis with ageing has not been demonstrated.

## Age-related changes in body function

Most studies of changes in bodily functioning with ageing tend to emphasize the negative nature of these changes (Brookbank, 1990; Sinclair, 1998). It is, however, important to remember that some of these negative changes might be due not simply to age alone but also to pathological states existing

**Table 1.3.4** Approximate percentage of functions or tissues remaining to the average 75-year-old man, taking the value found for the average 30-year-old as 100 per cent

| Function | Percentage |
| --- | --- |
| Nerve conduction velocity | 90% |
| Basal metabolic rate | 84% |
| Body water content | 82% |
| Cardiac output (at rest) | 70% |
| Number of glomeruli in kidney | 56% |
| Brain weight | 65% |
| Hand grip strength | 55% |
| Number of taste buds | 36% |
| Speed of return to equilibrium of blood acidity | 17% |

maintain homeostasis rather than to consider changes in individual systems. The person's homeostatic capabilities are perhaps more predictive of their ability to withstand illness, surgery or other invasive procedures.

## CLINICAL APPLICATIONS

Most homeostatic mechanisms are adversely affected by age and this is particularly apparent when the individual is facing physiological stressors, such as extremes of temperature, exercise or illness and associated treatments. Thus resting blood glucose levels in older people are similar to those in younger individuals. After administration of glucose, however, blood glucose levels are elevated higher and remain above resting levels for a longer period of time in elderly people.

The physiological changes that can accompany ageing can substantially affect several aspects of the individual's experience of illness. The illness itself might present in different ways, as, for example, is found in painless myocardial infarction and infections that occur without any accompanying fever.

Reduced alveolar gas exchange and decreased efficiency in the circulatory system mean that the individual is more prone to postoperative complications. Older people are more adversely affected by even short periods of immobility, with increased muscle wasting and increased likelihood of the development of pressure sores.

Drug metabolism is altered in elderly people because reduced lean body mass means that drugs can more easily become concentrated in the tissues. The increase in body fat levels means that fat-soluble drugs such as anaesthetics and benzodiazepines are metabolized more slowly leading, perhaps, to confusional states in those affected.

Several other aspects of the nurse's involvement with the older patient or client might also be altered by the changes associated with ageing. For example, hearing loss can result in impaired communication; a decrease in the number of taste buds can alter the individual's taste sensitivity and can lead to loss of appetite. Disinterest in food can be further aggravated by problems with dentition, and all these can contribute to the constipation difficulties, which might be present due to reduced peristalsis in the gastrointestinal tract.

It is extremely important that health care workers are aware that individuals vary greatly in the extent to which they experience difficulties as a result of the ageing process. It is also imperative that assessment should be based on individual needs rather than chronological age.

within the individual or to a lack of use of the particular system. Thus, impaired mobility in older people might be caused by a combination of osteoarthritis and too little exercise of the muscular system, in addition to the changes directly due to ageing.

The decline in physiological functioning of several of the body systems is summarized in **Table 1.3.4**. Herbert (1999) points out, however, that many of the physiological changes occurring with age actually cancel each other out. Thus, although the secretion of certain hormones is reduced, plasma levels of the hormones remain unchanged because there is reduced blood clearance of these substances. Similarly, although cerebral blood flow declines, cerebral ischaemia is minimized because oxygen extraction from blood is actually increased.

In this book, ageing changes in a particular physiological function are discussed and highlighted appropriately within each chapter. Generalized changes with ageing involve all organ systems within the body. There is a loss of reserve within the systems and an increasing probability of system failure and death. However, senescence proceeds at different rates within different systems and within different individuals. Many individuals are able to adapt to and overcome the functional losses found with ageing, and continue to lead productive lives. For some, however, senescence is accompanied by increasing ill health and disability.

Herbert (1999) suggests that it might be more useful to consider changes in the individual's ability to

## Clinical review

In addition to the Learning Objectives at the begining of this chapter, the reader should be able to:

- Describe the features of a cell or tissue type of your choice, relating structure to function
- After reading this chapter and Chapter 6.4, discuss the functional significance of mitotic and meiotic cell division
- Explain how proteins are synthesized
- Give an account of the normal rate and pattern of human growth
- Discuss factors that might influence growth and development
- Define the terms 'life span', 'life expectancy' and 'senescence' and briefly outline biological explanations of ageing.

## Review questions

1 What is the cell surface membrane composed of?
2 What is the function of the mitochondria?
3 How does the nucleus of prokaryotic cells differ from the nucleus of eukaryotic cells?
4 How would you describe the structure of DNA?
5 What is the product of mitotic cell division?
6 What is the cell cycle?
7 What functions does messenger RNA perform?
8 How is growth distinct from development?
9 What happens at adolescence?
10 How are homeostatic mechanisms influenced by ageing?

## Suggestions for further reading

Christiansen, J.L. & Grzybowski, J.M. (1993) *Biology of Ageing*. St Louis: Mosby.
*This has become a standard text in this area, it is short, readable and well illustrated.*

Cohen, N. (ed) (1991) *Cell Structure, Function and Metabolism*. Sevenoaks: Hodder and Stoughton; Buckingham: Open University Press.
*Focuses on how cell metabolism can be understood in terms of the structure and function of subcellular components. Designed for first- and second-year undergraduates.*

Cox, L.A. (1993) *A Guide to the Measurement and Assessment of Growth in Children*. Welwyn Garden City: Castlemead Publications.
*Concise handbook detailing current techniques of growth assessment.*

England, M.A. & Waddell, H. (1996) *A Colour Atlas of Life Before Birth. Normal Fetal Development*, 2nd edn. London: Wolfe Medical Publications.

*A reduced-size, soft-cover edition of the best-selling atlas, containing a magnificent set of photographs that go a long way in aiding understanding of embryology.*

Kirkwood, T.B.L. (2002) *The End of Age*. London: BBC Books.
*The prestigious Reith Lectures delivered by one of the foremost authorities on ageing. Very readable and informative.*

Lewis, V. (1987) *Development and Handicap*. Oxford: Blackwell Press.
*Provides a comprehensive account of the effects of different handicaps on children's development. Reprinted 1992.*

Lewontin, R.C. (1991) *The Doctrine of DNA: Biology as Ideology*. London: Penguin Science Books.
*Fascinating paperback discussing the biological implications of the DNA doctrine.*

Moore, K.L. & Persaud, T.V.N. (1998) *Before We Are Born*, 5th edn. Philadelphia: W.B. Saunders.

*Presents a clear, concise account of human embryology and growth defects. Focuses on normal development but covers common congenital anomalies and their causes.*

Redfern, S.J. & Ross, F.M. (eds) (1999) *Nursing Older People*, 3rd edn. Edinburgh: Churchill Livingstone.
*A comprehensive guide to the nurse's role with people who are elderly. Includes a sound introduction to the physiology of ageing.*

Sinclair, D. (1998) *Human Growth After Birth*, 6th edn. Oxford: Oxford University Press.

*This has become a classic text of postnatal growth and ageing.*

Tanner, J.M. (1989) *Foetus into Man*, 2nd edn. Ware: Castlemead Publications.
*Classic text detailing physical growth from conception to maturity.*

Watson, J.D. (1968) *The Double Helix*. New York: Atheneum.
*The fascinating story of the discovery of the structure of DNA, told by one of its discoverers!*

## References

Bank, L. & Jarvik, L.F. (1978) A longitudinal study of ageing twins. In: Schneider, E.L. (ed) *Genetics of Ageing*. New York: Plenum Press.

Birren, J.E. & Renner, V.J. (1977) Research on the psychology of ageing. In: Birren, J.E. & Schaie, K.W. (eds) *Handbook of the Psychology of Ageing*. New York: Van Nostrand.

Brookbank, J.W. (1990) *The Biology of Ageing*. New York: Harper and Row.

Chinn, S. & Rona, R.J. (1984) The secular trend in the height of primary school children in England and Scotland from 1912–1980. *Annals of Human Biology*, II; 1–16.

Cohen, N. (ed) (1991) *Cell Structure, Function and Metabolism*. Sevenoaks: Hodder and Stoughton; Buckingham: Open University Press.

Hall, D.M.B. (ed) (1989) *Health for All Children: A Programme for Child Health Surveillance*. Oxford: Oxford University Press.

Herbert, R. (1999) The biology of human ageing. In: Redfern, S. & Ross, F. (ed) *Nursing Older People*, 3rd edn. Edinburgh: Churchill Livingstone, pp. 55–77.

Kellerman, F.J. & Sander, G. (1979) Twin studies on senescence. In: Cunningham, W.R. & Brookbank, J.W.

(1988) *Gerontology: The Biology, Psychology and Sociology of Ageing*. New York: Harper and Row.

Kirkwood, T.B.L. (2002) Evolution of ageing. *Mechanisms of Ageing and Development*, **123**(7); 737–745.

Krane, C.M. & Kishore, B.K. (2003) Aquaporins: the membrane water channels of the biological world. *The Biologist*, **50**; 81–86.

Murphy, E.A. (1978) Genetics of longevity in man. In: Schneider, E.L. (ed) *The Genetics of Ageing*. New York: Plenum Press.

Schneider, E.L. & Bynum, G.D. (1983) Diseases that feature alterations resembling human ageing. In: Blumenthal, H.T. (ed) (1983) *Handbook of Diseases of Ageing*. New York: Van Nostrand.

Sinclair, D. (1998) *Human Growth After Birth*, 6th edn. Oxford: Oxford University Press.

Singer, S.J. & Nicolson, G.L. (1972) The fluid mosaic model of the structure of cell membranes. *Science*, **175**, (18 Feb); 720–731.

Tanner, J.M. (1989) *Foetus into Man*, 2nd edn. Ware: Castlemead Publications.

Wilson, R.S. (1976) Concordance in physical growth for growth for monozygotic and dizygotic twins. *Annals of Human Biology*, **3**; 1–10.

# Section 2

# Control and coordination

# Structure and function of nervous tissue

*Douglas Allan*

## LEARNING OBJECTIVES

After studying this chapter the reader should be able to:

- Identify the major structural features of a nerve cell

- Describe the structure of a mixed nerve

- Explain why a resting potential difference exists across a neuronal cell membrane and describe how the resting potential is maintained

- Outline the mechanism by which an action potential is generated and propagated along a nerve fibre

- Illustrate the major structural features of a chemical synapse

- Give an account of the mechanism of chemical transmission at a synapse

- Describe the electrochemical events constituting excitatory and inhibitory post-synaptic potentials

- Define the terms temporal summation and spatial summation

- Identify the principal structural components of a reflex arc

## INTRODUCTION

The maintenance of the human body in a healthy state depends on the body's ability to respond appropriately to environmental changes in a coordinated and organized fashion. A rapid means of communication is essential for this coordination.

There are two systems for communication within the body: the nervous system and the endocrine system. The nervous system is capable of transmitting electrical signals very rapidly – up to 120 m/s. The endocrine glands secrete hormones into the bloodstream which then modify the action of target organs which are often distant from the gland itself. This chapter is concerned with the structure and function of nervous tissue.

The nervous system is not only important as an internal system of communication, it also provides the individual with conscious awareness and the ability to communicate with others. Thus, the nervous system plays a vital role in establishing the relationship between nurse and patient and in directing the care that is provided.

## Organization of the nervous system

The human nervous system is divided into the **central nervous system (CNS)** and the **peripheral nervous system (PNS)**. The CNS comprises the brain, which is protected by the bones of the skull, and the spinal cord, which lies within the vertebral column or backbone. The CNS integrates and interprets signals received from all parts of the body, and controls signal output. The PNS includes all nerve tissue other than the brain and spinal cord, that is, all the nerves that run between the CNS and other organs of the body.

Some of the peripheral nerve fibres terminate at specialized structures that are capable of detecting environmental changes. These structures are called **sensory receptors**. Receptors can respond to light, heat, mechanical energy or chemical energy. They might lie near the surface of the body (i.e. close to the external environment) or be deeper within the body, where they detect internal environmental changes such as those of blood pressure. Each receptor responds preferentially to one kind of energy and converts it into tiny electrical signals that are transmitted to the CNS via the **sensory nerve fibres**. Sensory nerve fibres conveying information to the CNS are called **afferent nerve fibres**.

Other peripheral nerve fibres transmit signals in the opposite direction, that is, away from the CNS and towards distant body organs. These nerve fibres are called **efferents** or **motor nerve fibres**. Motor efferent nerve fibres terminate in structures called **effector organs**, which are capable of making a response. Most effector organs are muscles, which respond the signal brought by the efferent nerve fibres by contracting and developing force. However, some efferent nerve fibres terminate in glands, which respond by increasing their secretions.

Part of the PNS controls the activities of the viscera (heart, gut, etc.). The visceral nervous system is referred to as the **autonomic nervous system (ANS)**. The strictest definition of the ANS is that it is the motor nerve supply to visceral muscle, including cardiac muscle, and associated glands. Both visceral and cardiac muscle differ from skeletal muscle in structure and are not generally under conscious voluntary control. Motor signals are transmitted to the viscera in response to sensory signals. However, these sensory nerve fibres are included as part of the remainder of the PNS, the **somatic nervous system**. The ANS can be subdivided into two anatomically distinct parts, the **sympathetic** and the **parasympathetic nervous systems**. The parasympathetic system maintains the body in a normal resting state, while the sympathetic system prepares it to cope with (or adapt to) stress. The ANS is considered in greater detail in Chapter 2.5.

## Components of nerve tissue

The brain, spinal cord and peripheral nerves are organs that are composed principally of nervous tissue.

However, in addition, they are permeated by blood vessels and connective tissue. The blood supply provides nutrients and oxygen, and connective tissue provides mechanical strength and support.

Nervous tissue, in common with other tissues, comprises cellular elements in a small amount of fluid matrix, the extracellular fluid. Two types of cell can be identified: **neurones**, which generate and propagate the electrical signals, and **neuroglia**, or satellite cells, which provide support and protection.

## Neurones

Although the shape of the neurone adapts it to transmit electrical signals over long distances, the ultrastructure is essentially the same as that of any animal cell (see Section 1).

The integrity of the neurone is maintained by a lipoprotein semipermeable unit membrane. This separates intracellular from extracellular fluid and permits differences in the composition of each.

The neurone has a cell body (also called the soma) from which a number of fine processes arise. Cell body size is quite variable, ranging from 5 $\mu$m to 120 $\mu$m in diameter. The processes are called **dendrites** – because they resemble the branches of a tree (*dendron* is the Greek for tree) – and they increase the surface area available for connections with other neurones. Dendrites themselves bear tiny processes called dendritic spines, which are visible with high-powered electron microscopes. The soma bears one longer process, the **axon**, or nerve fibre, which might be branched. The axon conducts electrical signals from the neurone soma towards the axonal terminations.

The soma contains organelles typical of any animal cell: a nucleus, mitochondria, Golgi apparatus and lysosomes are all clearly visible. Light microscopy reveals fibres in the cytoplasm called **neurofibrillae**. Neurofibrillae and mitochondria are also found in axoplasm (the cytoplasm of the axon). **Nissl granules**, which are ribosomal in nature, are visible in the cytoplasm of the soma but are not found in axoplasm.

Neurologlial cells are associated with the axons of neurones. In the CNS these cells are called **oligodendrocytes**, whereas in the PNS they are referred to as **Schwann cells**. Oligodendrocytes and Schwann cells associate with neuronal axons in one of two ways. In the first case, the neurone is said to be **myelinated**. The Schwann cells (or oligodendrocytes) wrap their cell membranes around an axon a number of times (**Fig. 2.1.1**). The Schwann cell (or oligodendrocyte) membranes form a segmented sheath around the axon, the **myelin sheath**. Myelin is white in colour, which accounts for the appearance of white matter in the CNS. **White matter** is largely composed of myelinated nerve fibres, as opposed to the **grey**

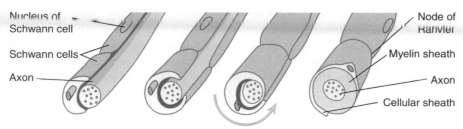

**Figure 2.1.1**  Myelination of a nerve

**matter**, which consists mainly of non-myelinated cell bodies. The gaps between segments of the myelin sheath represent junctions between adjacent neuroglial cells and are approximately 1 mm apart. The tiny gaps of naked membrane are called **nodes of Ranvier**. A myelin sheath forms a relatively good electrical insulator and in part determines the efficiency of transmission of electrical signals along a nerve fibre.

The second type of relationship between an axon and Schwann cells (or oligodendrocytes) is found in a **non-myelinated** neurone. In this case, the axon is enveloped by neuroglial cells but a myelin sheath is not formed. Each neuroglial cell can envelop a number of nerve fibres. In both myelinated and non-myelinated neurones the Schwann cell membrane surrounding the axon is termed the **neurilemma**.

Neurones can be classified on a functional or a structural basis. They can be classed as **sensory** or **motor neurones**, with interconnecting neurones in the CNS being termed **interneurones**. Or they can also be categorized according to the physical dimensions that determine their functional efficiency in conducting nerve signals. This will be referred to again later.

Neurones are easily classified according to the number of processes that arise from the soma. Three groups can be identified: **unipolar, bipolar** and **multipolar neurones**.

Unipolar neurones have only one true process arising from the cell body. Sensory neurones conveying information from the body surface (e.g. temperature, touch) are of this type. The cell bodies of these neurones are collected in groups called **ganglia**, which lie on the dorsal nerve roots of the spinal cord. The axon of a unipolar cell divides into two branches; one enters the spinal cord and transmits information to the brain and the other terminates at a sensory receptor near the body surface.

Bipolar neurones have two processes arising from the soma, a central axon and a peripheral dendrite. Bipolar neurones are found in the eye and in the ear. The peripheral dendrite transmits signals from the light receptor in the eye or sound receptor in the ear through the cell body to the central axon. The central axon terminates on another neurone, which conducts the signal to the brain.

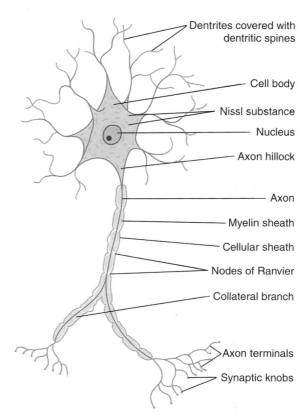

**Figure 2.1.2**  Structure of a whole nerve fibre

Multipolar neurones are found throughout the peripheral and central nervous system. A multipolar neurone has three or more processes (two or more dendrites and an axon) arising from the neuronal cell body; it can be myelinated or non-myelinated. For example, all motor neurones supplying skeletal muscles are myelinated and multipolar. They vary in shape and size, and in spread and number of dendritic processes. Axons can vary from a few micrometres up to a metre in length. **Figure 2.1.2** illustrates a multipolar neurone.

## Neuroglia

Neuroglial cells are found in large numbers in the CNS; they outnumber neurones by a ratio of 10 to 1. Estimates of the number of neurones in the human brain vary considerably, but 10 000 million is probably the minimum for a young person. The numbers of neuroglial cells are therefore enormous, but despite this their functions are still not clearly understood.

Neuroglial cells are subdivided on the basis of their size, shape and structural relationship with neurones. An **astrocyte**, as the name suggests, is a star-shaped cell with fine, long processes arising from the cell body. In preparations of brain tissue, astrocytes are commonly observed to have one or more cell processes in close proximity to neurones, and other processes closely applied to blood capillary walls. That is, astrocytes appear to 'span' gaps between neurones and capillary endothelium.

**Oligodendrocytes** in the CNS and **Schwann** cells in the PNS are somewhat smaller than astrocytes and have fewer, shorter cell processes. They are found in rows lying adjacent to neuronal axons throughout the nervous system. Their function in producing myelin has already been discussed.

**Ependyma** form a continuous layer of epithelial cells lining the ventricles of the brain and central canal of the spinal cord. They are thought to assist in the production of cerebrospinal fluid (CSF).

**Microglia** are small neuroglial cells, found throughout the CNS, which are probably tissue macrophages and uncommitted stem cells.

## Functions of neuroglia

Neuroglial cells have been implicated in a wide range of functions associated with the nervous system. Evidence indicates that neuroglial cells do not contribute to electrical signalling in the CNS. However, studies have shown that these cells might undergo electrical disturbances if surrounding neurones are active. Some of the functions are briefly considered below.

## Secretion and uptake of neurotransmitters

Neurotransmitters are chemicals that influence the passage of electrical signals across the gaps between adjacent neurones in a nerve net. One such transmitter is gamma-aminobutyric acid (GABA). GABA is an inhibitory transmitter, that is, it reduces the likelihood of a signal passing from one neurone to the next. GABA, and other neurotransmitters, can be taken up and stored in neuroglial cells. There is also some evidence to suggest that neuroglial cells secrete neurotransmitters or, at least, are necessary for the synthesis of transmitters in neurone terminations.

## Neuroglial cells in the development and maintenance of the nervous system

Differentiated neurones are not capable of cell division and cannot therefore replace damaged or ageing tissue. However, neuroglial cells can divide and increase in number to occupy atrophied areas in the brain. Indeed, brain tumours generally occur in neuroglial cells rather than in neurones; the names of such tumours are related to their glial cell of origin, e.g. oligodendrocytoma, astrocytoma.

It is thought that damaged neurones can regenerate, provided the cell bodies remain intact; however, this remains unproved. In this case, the course of axonal regeneration is directed along a pathway marked out by Schwann cells. Thus, neuroglial cells apparently aid regeneration of damaged axons as well as the establishment of precise neuronal connections during fetal development.

## Mechanical support and electrical insulation

Neuroglial cells form a packing tissue around neurones, providing support and preventing electrical interference between neurones.

## Blood–brain barrier

Blood–brain barrier, is a term used to describe a functional concept based on observations that certain chemicals transported in the blood, which gain access to soft tissues such as liver and kidney, are preferentially excluded from the brain. The normal functional importance of the blood–brain barrier seems to rest more with its role in preventing substances from getting out of the CNS rather than with its role in preventing the entry of neurotoxins. However, the latter cannot be ignored.

### DEVELOPMENTAL ISSUES

The relative immaturity of the blood–brain barrier in young children permits the accumulation of lead in the brains of exposed individuals. This can cause serious brain damage and behavioural deficits. The blood–brain barrier might also be important for the exclusion of potentially neurotoxic therapeutic agents. However, it is almost certainly of importance in rigidly maintaining the composition of the extracellular environment of neurones and in maintaining neurotransmitters within the vicinity of neuronal connections.

Astrocytes have been proposed as structural correlates of the blood–brain barrier based on histological evidence demonstrating close association between astrocyte processes, capillary endothelium and neurone membranes. Experiments have also identified the sites of the blood–brain barrier at specialized tight junctions between endothelial cells of brain capillaries. Such sites are associated with many astrocytic processes and it might be that astrocytes induce the tight endothelial junctions during early development.

## Structure of a nerve

Nerve fibres (axons) are bound together by connective tissue to form whole nerves, which vary in length and diameter. The term 'mixed nerve' is often employed. This refers to the fact that a nerve can contain both afferent and efferent nerve fibres innervating a number of different muscles or glands.

Each single nerve fibre is embedded in a delicate fibrous connective tissue, the **endoneurium**. Groups of nerve fibres are held together in bundles by a connective tissue sheath called **perineurium**. Finally, the bundles of nerve fibres are all enclosed in an outer fibrous sheath, the **epineurium (Fig. 2.1.3)**. The connective tissue framework provides mechanical support for both nerve fibres and blood capillaries within the whole nerve.

## The nerve impulse

Nerve fibres and muscle fibres are both capable of conducting electrochemical signals in the body. For this reason, both are referred to as **excitable tissues**. The ability to conduct nerve signals is dependent upon the integrity of both the intra- and extracellular environments.

The significant feature that permits electrochemical signalling to occur is the difference in ionic concentration between the outside and inside of the cell. This

difference is partly the result of an unequal distribution of potassium and sodium ions on either side of a selectively permeable membrane. In resting neurones, the intracellular potassium ion concentration is about 30 times greater than it is outside, and the sodium ion concentration is about 14 times greater in the extracellular fluid. Proteins are also found inside the cell and are large non-diffusible, negatively charged ions.

The maintenance of the difference between the intracellular and extracellular fluid of a resting neurone is principally due to the action of the sodium–potassium pump. The precise nature of this ionic pump is not known but it uses ATP as an energy source. Even when a nerve cell is not conducting an impulse, it is actively transporting ions across its membrane, via the pump. Sodium ions are actively transported out and potassium ions are actively transported in but this occurs unequally, that is, three sodium ions are exchanged for two potassium ions.

A large number of negative ions, which are mostly protein anions, are found in the inside of the cell and these diffuse very poorly or not at all across the membrane to the outside. Because sodium ions are positive and are actively transported outside by the sodium–potassium pump, the extracellular fluid is positively charged. Despite the fact that potassium ions are also positively charged and actively transported to the inside of the cell, there are insufficient potassium ions to equalize the larger number of non-diffusible negative ions trapped in the cell.

Additionally, a concentration and electrical gradient for sodium and potassium ions is created by the functioning of the sodium–potassium pump, and potassium ions tend to diffuse into the cell. This occurs through membrane proteins called potassium and sodium **channels**. As membrane permeability to potassium ions is 100 times greater than that to sodium ions, the number of potassium ions that leave the cell is 100 times greater than the number of sodium ions that enter. The sodium–potassium pump not only actively transports sodium and potassium ions but also establishes concentration gradients for the ions. This results in a difference in charge on either side of the membrane, that is, the outside is positive and the inside negative. This difference in the charge on either side of the membrane of a resting neurone is known as the **resting potential**. Such a membrane is described as being polarized.

A voltage of about 70 millivolts (mV) can be measured electrically in a polarized membrane and as this means that the inside of the membrane is 70 mV less than the outside, the membrane potential is $-70$ mV.

**Table 2.1.1** illustrates the characteristics of a resting neurone with a resting membrane potential of $-70$ mV.

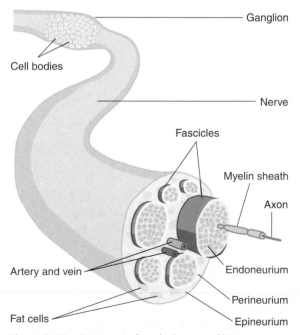

**Figure 2.1.3**   Structure of a whole nerve fibre

**Table 2.1.1** Characteristics of a resting nerve cell with a resting potential of −70 mV

| Ions | Large organic anions | Chloride (Cl⁻) | Potassium (K⁺) | Sodium (Na⁺) |
|---|---|---|---|---|
| Distribution | Intracellular | More concentrated extracellularly | More concentrated intracellularly | More concentrated extracellularly |
| Membrane permeability | Impermeable | Freely permeable | Freely permeable | Resting nerve cell membrane has a very low permeability for Na⁺ |
| Passive diffusion through membrane | Nil: ions cannot pass through membrane | Ions can pass through membrane and influx equals efflux | The resting potential is not quite large enough to prevent a small loss of K⁺ from the cell (i.e. passive efflux is slightly greater than passive influx) | Passive influx of Na⁺. Only a small amount of Na⁺ diffuses into the cell because of the low sodium membrane permeability, despite the large electrochemical gradient |
| Active transport through membrane – ionic pumping | No pump for organic anions | No pump for Cl⁻ | Actively pumps K⁺ into the cell against the concentration gradient, tending to restore the passive outward leak | Actively pumps Na⁺ out of the cell against the concentration gradient, tending to restore the passive inward leak |

## The action potential

Viable cells – nerve, muscle, blood or skin – generally exhibit resting potentials across their membranes. However, nerve and muscle fibres are able to alter the transmembrane potential difference reversibly. When this occurs, the membrane is **depolarized** and the inside of the cell transiently becomes positive with respect to the outside. This shift in the potential difference is referred to as the **action potential**. It has an amplitude of approximately 110 mV and lasts for about 1 millisecond (1 ms), after which time the resting potential is restored. The time frame of events is illustrated in **Fig. 2.1.4**.

### Generation of a nerve action potential

The initiating event in the generation of an action potential is the **stimulus**, which represents the delivery of energy to the nerve cell membrane. This energy can take the form of light, heat, mechanical force, chemical energy or electrical energy.

Essentially, the action potential reflects a change in the permeability characteristics of the nerve membrane (muscle membrane also behaves in such a way: see Chapter 3.1).

The characteristics of resting nerve membrane have already been considered. The membrane is polarized, with a potential difference across it of approximately

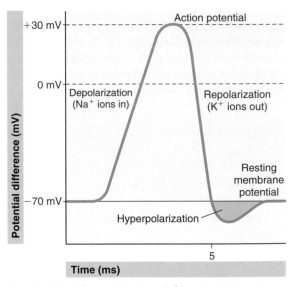

**Figure 2.1.4** The action potential in a neurone

−70 mV (inside negative). When stimulus energy is applied to nerve membrane it is depolarized, that is, the potential difference across it decreases. This depolarization appears to result in an increase in the sodium permeability of the membrane; sodium therefore enters the nerve fibre according to the electrochemical gradient. This transference of positive charge depolarizes the membrane further, which then results in a further increase in sodium permeability.

In other words, there is a positive feedback between the depolarization of the membrane and the increase in sodium permeability. There is an explosive increase in the sodium current into the cell such that sodium movement dominates other ionic movements. The potential difference across the membrane approaches the equilibrium potential for sodium.

The inside of the cell briefly becomes positive to about 40 mV. At the peak of the action potential, the membrane is in fact polarized in the opposite direction to the resting potential. That is, the depolarization is followed by a positive polarization. The changes in sodium permeability last for only a very short time, normally less than 1 ms. At the peak of the action potential the inward sodium current rapidly reduces, and the increase in sodium permeability is said to be inactivated. Meanwhile, potassium permeability increases. This rise in potassium permeability, beginning just before the peak of the action potential, and the reduced sodium permeability explain why the sodium equilibrium potential is not quite reached. As the inside of the cell is now positive with respect to the outside, and because potassium has a concentration gradient favouring an outward potassium current, potassium rapidly moves out of the cell. Movement of potassium now becomes dominant and the resting potential is rapidly restored by the transference of positive charge out of the cell. In fact, the repolarization commonly overshoots the resting potential and the equilibrium potential for potassium is approached (i.e. there is a transient overshoot hyperpolarization, see **Fig. 2.1.4**). The relationship between the action potential and sodium and potassium membrane permeability changes is demonstrated in **Fig. 2.1.5**. The rising phase of the action potential is associated with a rise in sodium permeability, whereas the falling phase of repolarization is associated with a rise in potassium permeability.

A millisecond or so after the delivery of a stimulus to nerve membrane, the resting potential is restored. However, there has been a very small change in the composition of both intra- and extracellular fluids. A small amount of sodium has been transferred into the cell and a small amount of potassium has been transferred to the extracellular field. After a single action potential, the resultant change in intra- and extracellular concentrations of these ions is negligible. Many action potentials can be transmitted before a noticeable alteration occurs in the composition of intra- and extracellular fluid. However, the sodium/potassium exchange pump normally restores the resting ionic concentrations.

Metabolic energy is not required for the generation of an action potential because the ions move through the membrane under the influence of electrochemical forces. However, metabolic energy

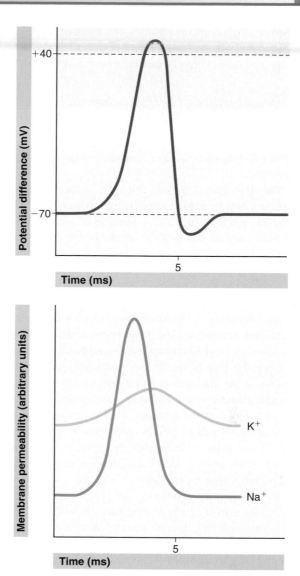

**Figure 2.1.5**  Time course of changes in membrane permeability to sodium and potassium during an action potential

is required for the exchange pump and the re-establishment of normal ionic concentrations. This is important if nerve cells are to respond continuously for long periods of time.

The reversible changes in ionic permeability associated with an action potential are peculiar to excitable tissue membrane. The membrane behaves as though it contains gated channels for sodium and potassium, such that the gates can be opened and closed in response to certain specified conditions. Thus, when the membrane is stimulated, gates across sodium channels in the membrane appear to open, permitting the entry of sodium, as directed by the electrochemical gradient. This opening of the gates is only transient. At the peak of the action potential the gates apparently close again and sodium entry is inactivated. Gates across potassium channels, which are normally closed under resting conditions, then appear to open and potassium flows out of the cell. These gates are also open for only a short period of time, and close when the resting potential is restored.

## Characteristics of action potentials

Action potentials are said to obey the **all-or-none law**. That is, they are not graded responses and are either full sized or absent, depending on stimulus strength.

The size of an action potential varies slightly between neurones but generally has an amplitude of approximately 110 mV and a duration of 1 ms or less. However, action potentials produced by any one axon are of more or less constant size provided that the neurone remains healthy.

Neither the amplitude nor the duration of an action potential varies with the strength of the stimulus. Stimulus intensity will affect the frequency of action potential generation and might also influence the number of neurones that are activated but it will not change the size of the action potentials produced. However, the stimulus must be sufficiently strong to permit a threshold level of membrane depolarization to be reached. If the stimulus is only very weak, the changes in membrane polarity and permeability might be too small to set in motion the positive feedback mechanism linking membrane depolarization with increased sodium permeability. The weak stimulus will only slightly depolarize the membrane, which will then return to the resting state without producing the explosive changes associated with an action potential. On the other hand, if the stimulus is sufficiently large to allow the threshold level of depolarization to be exceeded, then a full-sized action potential is always produced.

The **threshold** refers to a critical level of depolarization of the membrane rather than to the strength of stimulus required to reach it, although these two factors are linked.

The ease with which nerve fibre membrane reaches threshold can vary. For example, if an action potential has just been generated then a stronger than normal stimulus might be required to elicit a second one, i.e. the threshold is temporarily raised (see 'Refractory period' below).

In terms of ion movements, the threshold represents an unstable equilibrium between the sodium transfer into the cell and potassium loss from the cell. At this point, the potential difference across the membrane is of the order of 10 mV less than the resting potential. If extra sodium ions then diffuse into the cell, the positive feedback loop is set in motion such that entry of sodium depolarizes the membrane, which then increases sodium permeability, permitting still further depolarization of the membrane and producing the explosive changes of an action potential. If this occurs, threshold is exceeded and the neurone is said to fire an impulse. However, if extra potassium ions diffuse out of the cell, the potential difference across the membrane increases again towards the resting potential and resting conditions will be restored. Therefore, to fire an impulse, the stimulus must be of sufficient intensity to cause the unstable equilibrium of threshold to shift in the direction of increased influx of sodium (**Fig. 2.1.6**).

If a second stimulus is delivered to the neurone membrane while it is undergoing the events of an action potential, a second impulse will not be produced. That is, a second action potential cannot be generated during the time course of the first spike. Action potentials therefore cannot summate and become superimposed on each other. During this period of unresponsiveness the nerve membrane is said to be in a **refractory state**. While a spike is taking place, a second impulse will not be produced regardless of the intensity of the second stimulus. This time interval is referred to as the **absolute refractory period**. It generally lasts for no more than 1 ms and can be considerably shorter (e.g. 0.5 ms) in some large, myelinated mammalian nerve fibres.

Following the absolute refractory period is an interval of some 3–5 ms when it is more difficult than normal to elicit a second action potential, i.e. a stronger stimulus than that normally required to reach threshold is necessary. This time interval is referred to as the **relative refractory period**. Action potentials produced during this interval are somewhat distorted in amplitude and duration. The rate of depolarization of the membrane and the final amplitude of the action potential are both reduced below the norm. The increase in stimulus intensity that is required to fire the neurone represents a rise in the threshold level of depolarization.

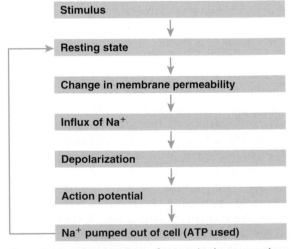

**Figure 2.1.6** The sequence of events in the generation of an action potential

It might at first sight appear as though the 'all-or-none law' is not obeyed here, because action potentials of variable amplitude can be produced during the relative refractory period. However, for any specified degree of refractoriness, the action potential amplitude and duration will be constant. Under these specified conditions the stimulus is either large enough to produce all of the response or too small to elicit a propagated impulse.

Changes occurring in the membrane permeability to sodium and potassium, associated with an action potential, can explain the phenomenon of the refractory state of nerve membrane. During the rising phase of the action potential, sodium gates are open and there is a positive feedback operating between the degree of membrane depolarization and the increase in sodium permeability. If a second stimulus is delivered during the course of these events, any effects it might have on membrane permeability will be masked, because sodium channels are already open. The second stimulus cannot open up another quite separate set of sodium gates. Thus, a stimulus occurring during the rising phase of the spike (the first stage of the absolute refractory period) can have no detectable effect on the changes in membrane polarity and permeability. During the falling phase of the action potential, sodium permeability is inactivated and potassium permeability is increased. Both of these changes tend to restore the resting potential and therefore oppose any attempt to depolarize the membrane. In fact, sodium inactivation is not simply the closure of gates in the membrane but appears to be a separate physicochemical event analogous to locking the gates. If membrane depolarization in response to a stimulus is to exceed a threshold level, then sodium current into the cell must exceed potassium current out of the cell. Sodium inactivation associated with the falling phase of the spike coupled with the corresponding increase in potassium permeability makes it impossible for such a threshold to be reached (the second stage of the absolute refractory period). During the ensuing interval of the relative refractory period, sodium inactivation wears off and potassium permeability also reduces, thereby increasing the ease with which threshold can be reached. An increased stimulus intensity during this time can overcome the opposing factors and permit sodium entry to exceed the net potassium flux. At the end of the refractory period, sodium and potassium permeabilities return to normal and a normal action potential can be generated.

## Propagation of action potentials

Nerve impulses can be generated at one end of an axon and recorded at the other end. That is, impulses can be propagated along the axon. The mechanism by which action potentials apparently move along nerve fibres will now be considered.

When a stimulus is delivered to a nerve fibre it elicits local changes in membrane permeability, which then give rise to an action potential. In other words, the stimulus opens sodium gates only at the point of stimulation and not over the whole surface area of the axon. A tiny segment of membrane is activated and this lies adjacent to the remaining resting membrane. The transmembrane potential is quite different in the active and resting segments. In the active region the inside of the axon is positive with respect to the outside by about $+40\,mV$, whereas the normal resting potential of around $-70\,mV$ exists elsewhere. Similar changes occur in the extracellular fluid. These potential differences cause currents in the form of ions to flow. Current (denoted as positive charge) flows through the cytoplasm from the active to the resting segment of the axon and in the reverse direction through the extracellular fluid. These local currents are shown in **Fig. 2.1.7a**. In fact, recorded electrical changes associated with local current flow occur much more rapidly than can be explained by the actual physical transfer of ions between active and resting segments of the axon. The local current flow really represents a 'knock-on' effect whereby the entry of a positive charge ($Na^+$) through the active segment membrane causes a realignment of ions already in the axoplasm, because unlike charges tend to attract and like charges to repel each other. Thus, the inside surface of adjacent membrane becomes more positive and the outside more negative, both of which tend to depolarize the membrane. This depolarization is normally sufficient to reach threshold and the adjacent membrane then generates an action potential. In other words, the action potential itself is not propagated but is generated anew at each point on the membrane. The active segment then repolarizes, during which time it is refractory. These changes are illustrated in **Fig. 2.1.7b**.

Local currents, as the name implies, do not travel long distances down the axon. Local current flow decreases rapidly as the distance from the point of stimulation increases. This is principally because the membrane is not a perfect electrical insulator; indeed, if it were completely impervious to current flow, action potentials would not occur at all. The membrane is said to be leaky. Current flows out of the membrane and is dissipated in the relatively large volume of extracellular fluid. However, current is only required to travel very short distances in order to stimulate adjacent resting membrane.

Action potentials are always propagated **away** from the point of stimulation. This is because each activated region subsequently becomes refractory and cannot be restimulated by local currents (**see Fig. 2.1.7c**). Within the nervous system, impulses are generally conducted in only one direction along a nerve fibre. This is not because of any inherent property of axons, indeed, in isolated tissue signals can be transmitted in either direction. However, the anatomy of the nervous system results in stimuli being delivered to one particular end of each fibre. Moreover, the junctions between neurones allow transmission in only one direction. These junctions, called synapses, are described later (see pp. 86–93).

The mechanism of action potential propagation in myelinated nerve fibres is essentially the same as in non-myelinated fibres. However, the segmented myelin sheath alters the electrical properties of the fibre. The sheath increases the electrical resistance of the membrane, which is only appreciably leaky to

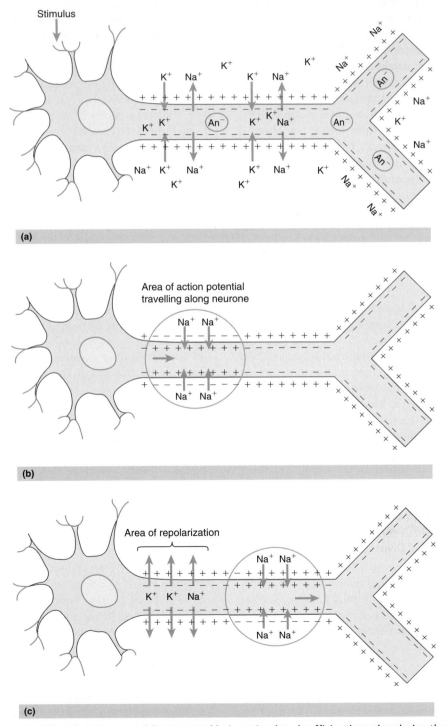

**Figure 2.1.7** Transmission along an axon (a) at rest and being stimulated sufficiently to depolarize the membrane; (b) and (c) show the conduction of the wave of depolarization along the axon. An⁻ = large anions

charge at the nodes of Ranvier. An action potential sets up a local current flow but in myelinated fibres the circuit is completed only when current leaks out through the membrane at an adjacent node of Ranvier. In other words, the impulse is transmitted by means of local current flow along the myelinated segments of the axon and action potentials are only generated at the nodes (**Fig. 2.1.8**). Action potentials therefore appear to jump from node to node and impulse conduction in myelinated nerve fibres is referred to as **saltatory conduction** (from the Latin *saltare*, meaning to leap). Saltatory conduction is considerably faster than conduction in non-myelinated neurones. In non-myelinated axons new action potentials have to be generated across each adjacent segment of membrane. That is, for a given length of axon the impulse has to be regenerated more times in the non-myelinated than in the myelinated neurone. The process of impulse generation involves the physical transfer of ions across the membrane, which is a much slower process than the charge realignment consequent on local current flow. Thus, an important consequence of myelination in the nervous system is that it speeds up nerve signalling. Rates of up to 120 m/s can be recorded in large myelinated motor neurones.

The **velocity** at which nerve impulses are conducted is variable and depends primarily on two factors, myelination and axon diameter. Myelinated nerve fibres conduct impulses faster than non-myelinated fibres of comparable diameter. In addition, impulse conduction velocity depends on the diameter of the nerve fibre. Large fibres conduct impulses more rapidly than small fibres. This is because the longitudinal resistance to current flow decreases as axonal diameter increases and so current flows more readily and more rapidly in large fibres.

## Classification of nerve fibres according to their conduction speed

### Velocities

Group A fibres are all myelinated and conduct impulses at speeds of up to 120 m/s. They are subdivided into alpha, beta, gamma and delta fibres. Group B fibres are also myelinated and are all preganglionic fibres of the autonomic nervous

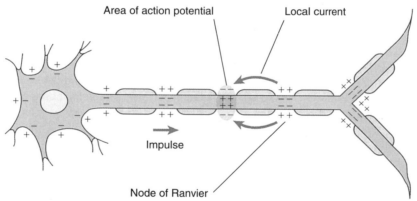

**Figure 2.1.8**  Saltatory conduction in a myelinated axon showing how the impulse leaps from one node of Ranvier to the next

| Table 2.1.2 Classification of nerve fibres according to conduction velocity | | | | |
|---|---|---|---|---|
| **Group** | **Divisions** | **Function** | **Diameter (μm)** | **Conduction velocity (m/s)** |
| **A: all myelinated** | Alpha (α) Beta (β) Gamma (γ) Delta (δ) | Motor and sensory nerve fibres. Largest fibres innervate muscle; smallest fibres convey pain and temperature | α and β 5–20  γ and δ 1–7 | α fastest and δ slowest  α and β 45–120 γ and δ 2–45 |
| **B: myelinated** | – | Preganglionic nerve fibres of ANS | Up to 3 | 3–15 |
| **C: non-myelinated** | – | Some sensory nerve fibres; postganglionic fibres of ANS | approx. 0.2–1.5 | Up to 2.5 |

system (see Chapter 2.5). Group C fibres are all non-myelinated and conduct impulses at speeds as low as 1 m/s. This classification system is summarized in Table 2.1.2.

## STRUCTURAL DISORDERS OF NERVE TISSUES

Neurones and neuroglia can become damaged from a wide range of factors, including malignancy, dietary deficiencies and exposure to heavy metal. Damage can occur in the CNS or in the PNS and can affect sensory pathways and/or motor pathways and/or higher functions such as memory and intellect.

Malignancy of the nervous system is usually due to abnormal reproduction of neuroglia; hence the term 'gliomas'. However, in an attempt to clarify the classification of primary brain tumours this term has been superseded. Table 2.1.3 summarizes the main types of tumour. Tumours can occur at any site in the brain and their effect can be widespread. The area of the brain in which the tumour is located will determine the disturbed function the

**Table 2.1.3** Signs and symptoms of brain tumours related to specific areas

| Area | Effects |
|---|---|
| Frontal lobes | Inappropriate behaviour, loss of ability to concentrate, emotional lability, loss of social control and impairment of recent memory<br>Expressive dysphasia (unable to communicate thoughts)<br>Generalized seizures<br>Frontal headaches<br>Contralateral hemiparesis or hemiplegia (weakness or paralysis in the limbs on the opposite side) |
| Parietal lobes | Impaired sensory discrimination<br>Loss of right–left discrimination, agraphia and disorientation<br>Receptive speech problems (difficulty understanding what is being said)<br>Focal seizures (motor seizure begins in one part of the body, the focus, and spreads to other muscle groups)<br>Visual deficits, e.g. homonymous hemianopia (partial or complete loss of vision in the nasal quadrant of one eye and the temporal quadrant of the opposite eye) |
| Temporal lobes | Temporal lobe epilepsy<br>Receptive aphasia (unable to put any meaning to words though other forms of communication such as miming, drawing or writing may be understood)<br>Visual deficits |
| Occipital lobes | Visual deficits<br>Generalized or focal seizures |
| Brainstem | Cerebellar dysfunction, i.e. ataxia (unsteadiness) and lack of coordination<br>Diplopia (double vision)<br>Dysphagia (difficulty in swallowing)<br>Vomiting |
| Midbrain | Hydrocephalus (excess of cerebrospinal fluid within the ventricles of the brain)<br>Ptosis (drooping of the eyelid)<br>Cerebellar dysfunction |
| Cerebellum | Cerebellar dysfunction – more marked on standing<br>Raised intracranial pressure (ICP), headache, vomiting and papilloedema (oedema of the optic disc)<br>Hydrocephalus<br>Cranial nerve deficits – 5th, 6th and 7th most common |
| Pituitary region | Headache<br>Visual disturbances<br>Hormonal disturbances |

person experiences; for example, the person might experience speech difficulties with a frontal tumour or a visual field defect with a parietal tumour. **Table 2.1.3** describes these more fully. The assessment and planning of care for these patients will be determined by the degree of disturbed function.

Investigations, including skull X-ray, computerized tomography (CT) and/or magnetic resonance imaging (MRI), will detect most tumours. Medical treatment consists of drug therapy – steroids to reduce the surrounding cerebral oedema and anticonvulsants (if indicated) to control seizures. Burr hole biopsy, where a small piece of tissue is removed for laboratory examination to determine the grade and type of tumour might be performed, followed by surgical removal of the tumour (if possible) and/or radiotherapy.

Assessment of patient needs will necessitate taking account of the information patients might have regarding diagnosis. It is important to establish the level of a patient's knowledge and to plan care accordingly. Explanations will help the patient through the investigative period.

Precautions regarding the use of drug therapy are required. The usual steroid used is dexamethasone, one of the most powerful, and its side-effects include adrenocortical insufficiency and electrolyte imbalance; fluid balance and serum electrolyte levels should be monitored. To overcome the problem of increased gastric acidity, antacids are routinely prescribed. The most frequently prescribed anticonvulsant is phenytoin sodium, which is normally well tolerated in the short term. It is imperative that patients continue to take their medication even when seizure-free.

Neurological deficits such as hemiplegia will result in balance problems affecting the patient's ability to mobilize freely. In assessing the patient's needs, consideration should be given to their safety and, when planning care, it might be necessary to ensure that a patient does not mobilize unaided.

Patients who are confused or disinhibited (as the result of a frontal tumour) can pose a danger to their own safety. They might not understand why they cannot leave the hospital and considerable diplomacy and patience is required. Relatives can help in this situation, as a familiar face and voice can sometimes exert a calming influence, although in some cases relatives become so upset by a patient's behaviour that they cannot bear to stay with the patient for more than a few minutes.

Loss of visual, hearing or tactile sensation will require compensation. If able, patients can be taught techniques to overcome these losses, e.g. demonstrating the area of remaining visual field and teaching them to make full use of it will help prevent accidents and retain a degree of independence.

Patients might experience communication difficulties such as **dysphasia**, in which they have difficulty in being understood and/or being understood by others. Care planning will necessitate the inclusion of alternative methods of communication, such as the provision of pen and paper, ensuring that patients have the means to summon help if needed or the use of sophisticated electronic communication aids. Non-verbal communication can be useful; a reassuring touch or a smile can convey a lot to a patient.

Assessment of a patient's ability to eat and drink should be considered. Neurological deficits that can interfere with this process include hemiplegia (the patient is unable to cut food with one hand), facial palsy (prevents the patient chewing food properly) and loss of the swallow reflex (the patient might choke). Care should be planned to intervene in each deficit appropriately, for example, it might be necessary to use specially adapted cutlery and non-slip mats or to modify the diet (Hickey, 2002).

Peripheral neuropathy results from degeneration of the nerves, principally in the feet. It can be a complication of diabetes mellitus, alcoholism, vitamin B deficiency and other systemic disorders. Trauma can similarly cause neuropathy, e.g. a radial nerve might be trapped following the prolonged use of crutches. These patients will be in danger as a result of the loss of protective sensory input and therefore must avoid contact with extremes of temperature, e.g. hot-water bottles. Nurses should be aware of this vulnerability when planning nursing care and should pay particular attention to the skin over the affected area.

**Multiple sclerosis (MS)**, a demyelination disorder of the nervous system, is manifested by the presence of hardened plaques in the myelin sheath. The cause is unknown but is probably multifactorial. In other words, genetic predisposition, environmental exposure (virus), an abnormal immune regulatory response and the age of the individual are all conditions more likely to result in the development of MS (Lindsay & Bone, 2004). MS is a disorder of early adulthood, often presenting between the ages of 20 and 30, and showing a slight female bias. As the plaques occur at random, their presence will affect different functions of the nervous system to varying degrees in each individual, hence the illness is characterized by a series of remissions and relapses. This diversity of presentation can make diagnosis difficult and the outcome is often impossible to predict. Some patients will quickly become wheelchair bound and fully dependent, whereas others remain in remission for a prolonged period of time. The potential nursing problems this presents are wide ranging. Psychological care is of the utmost importance; fears about the disease and for the future, based on limited knowledge, can result in patients regressing. They might refuse to communicate with other patients or staff, and adopt an attitude of complete helplessness despite the fact that they might be capable of performing many physical tasks. This can be very distressing for the family and it is essential that nurses ensure that there is always an opportunity to discuss the situation both with the relatives and with the patient, and that all their answers to questions are answered as honestly as possible within the bounds of nursing responsibility.

Physical care for patients with MS will focus on managing urinary and bowel problems and those related to skin care. Incontinence with overflow often occurs, along with the attendant problem of infection. Management will include the use of simple external urinary collection devices or bladder catheterization. Female patients are more difficult to manage, as no satisfactory external devices yet exist. Some patients respond to bladder training programmes. Constipation frequently occurs and management of this does not vary from that of any other patient. Loss of sensation in the skin expose patients to the danger of breakdown and infection. Patient education with regard to the dangers will help to obviate the situation, with the emphasis being placed on regular relief of pressure.

A patient and family teaching programme should be considered. The timing of this is crucial; some patients will want to know immediately how they can help themselves; others will not. The most usual pattern is to provide the information in small quantities at the appropriate stages in the development of the disease. Such a programme needs to include advice on care of the bladder, bowels and skin, e.g. teaching the relatives how to transfer the patient safely from chair to bed and emphasizing the need for scrupulous personal hygiene. An explanation of the drug regimen and any side-effects should be provided, together with advice about returning to work and following as normal a social life as possible. The plan should also deal with problems relating to sexuality and personal relationships, and availability of financial assistance. This advice should be available in the ward or can be obtained from a self-help group such as the Multiple Sclerosis Society, which provides support for sufferers and their families and publishes useful information leaflets.

## Synaptic transmission

For a nerve impulse to travel from one nerve cell to another, a mechanism that allows the nerve impulse to be transmitted across the small interstitial gap between the two cells is required. The specialized junctions between nerve cells or between nerve and muscle cells are called **synapses**, and the process by which a nerve impulse is transferred across a synapse is referred to as **synaptic transmission**.

## Electrical transmission

Essentially, what is required of synaptic transmission is for the action potential generated in one nerve cell to be transferred to the next excitable cell. Conceptually, the simplest scheme for such a process would be passive current flow. The process of passive current flow, which is responsible for conduction along axons, might also be capable of transferring a nerve impulse directly across a synapse. Such a mechanism would require the unit membranes of both cells to possess a very low resistance, and for the distance between the two cells – the synaptic gap or cleft – to be very narrow. The latter is necessary if the current flow is not going to be diffused away from the next cell by the extracellular fluid, which has a relatively low electrical resistance.

Electrical synaptic transmission of this kind has been described at synapses in which the outer layers of the unit membranes of the two cells are separated by as little as 2 nm. Indeed, the unit membranes might even be fused at these tight gap junctions. The process of electrical synaptic transmission assumes that the properties of axons that account for the passive transmission of signals along the nerve fibre will be sufficient to explain the transmission of signals between neurones. However, such assumptions do not seem to be acceptable for the vast majority of synapses. For example, the distance between cells at a synapse will normally be 20 nm or more, rather than the 2 nm of the tight-gap junctions. Observations such as these suggest that some other process is involved in transmission at synapses.

## Chemical transmission

The vast majority of synaptic connections seem to depend on a process involving chemical transmission of the nerve signal. The arrival of an impulse at the terminal of the presynaptic nerve fibre causes the release of a small amount of chemical agent called the **chemical transmitter**. The chemical transmitter diffuses across the synaptic cleft and, when it reaches the postsynaptic cell, it has the effect of altering the potential difference that exists across the postsynaptic cell membrane. This alteration in the transmembrane potential difference then gives rise to an action potential.

## Structure of a chemical synapse

The major features of a synapse are illustrated in **Fig. 2.1.9**. In addition to components of the synapse that have already been mentioned, such as the separation of the unit membranes of the cells by the synaptic cleft, other important features can be seen. For example, the spindly fibre of the presynaptic axon swells into a round or oval-shaped knob at its end. This is commonly referred to as the **terminal bouton** or **knob**. It is the flattened membrane of the terminal bouton that is juxtaposed to the next cell and which forms the presynaptic membrane. The area covered by the presynaptic membrane is something of the order of 1–2 μm. Other intracellular structures have been identified within the terminal bouton. In particular, mitochondria are commonly observed and their presence suggests that the cellular activities of nerve terminals require energy.

An important and distinctive cellular organelle of the terminal bouton is the **synaptic vesicle**. Synaptic vesicles are tiny sacs that occur in great profusion at the nerve ending and are formed by pinocytosis, the pinching-off of segments of the unit membrane of

the cell. They show a tendency to move towards the presynaptic membrane, where they fuse with the membrane and extrude their contents into the synaptic cleft by the process of exocytosis. Synaptic vesicles range in size from 40 nm to 200 nm.

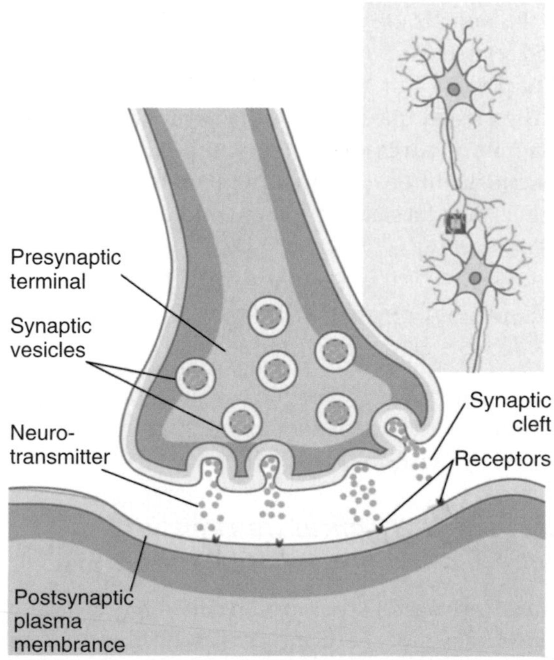

## Mechanism of chemical transmission

Electrical signals are passed from one cell to the next across a synaptic cleft by means of an intermediate stage of chemical transmission. It is possible to identify stages of the transmission and these are summarized in **Fig. 2.1.10**. A chemical is released from the

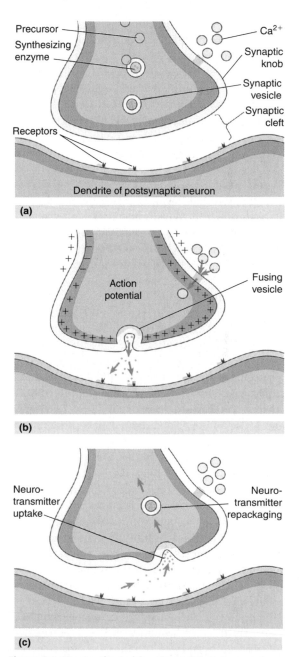

**(a)**

**(b)**

**(c)**

**Figure 2.1.10** Synthesis (a), release (b) and reuptake (c) of neurotransmitter at a synaptic knob

**Figure 2.1.9** Transmission of an impulse between two neurones or from a neurone to an effector. The electrical impulse cannot cross the synaptic cleft and transmission is achieved by release of a chemical neurotransmitter

presynaptic membrane in response to the nerve impulse; the chemical moves from the presynaptic to the postsynaptic membrane, to which it attaches and where it exerts its effects. Finally, a state of readiness to transmit another signal is re-established by reuptake and synthesis.

In discussing these stages, reference will be made to the synapse at the skeletal neuromuscular junction, because much of the detail of synaptic transmission has emerged from experiments involving the neuromuscular synapse. However, it must be noted that a nerve-to-muscle synapse differs in certain ways from the typical nerve-to-nerve synapse. For example, the morphology of the neuromuscular synapse is distinctive. The motor nerve terminals run in specialized channels that invaginate the muscle cell membrane. Such channels are not seen in the postsynaptic cell of a nerve-to-nerve synapse. Nevertheless, it can be assumed that the processes involved in neural synaptic transmission follow a similar pattern to those that have been found at the neuromuscular synapse.

## Neurotransmitters

One aspect of the synapse at the skeletal neuromuscular junction that has been clearly demonstrated is the nature of the **neurotransmitter** involved. It is known that this transmitter is **acetylcholine**. Similarly, it is known that acetylcholine and noradrenaline (norepinephrine) are both neurotransmitters in the autonomic nervous system (see Chapter 2.5).

Acetylcholine is considered to act as a central transmitter in addition to its role at the neuromuscular junction. It belongs to a group of compounds referred to as monoamines (so called because each chemical contains only a single amine group). Other monoamines that have been identified as central excitatory transmitters (i.e. chemicals promoting impulse transmission) include serotonin (5-hydroxytryptamine), dopamine and noradrenaline (norepinephrine). The last two of these belong to a subgroup of monoamines called catecholamines.

Certain amino acids have also been identified as central neurotransmitters. Gamma-aminobutyric acid (GABA), an amino acid that is not incorporated into proteins, appears to be a common inhibitory transmitter (i.e. a chemical inhibiting impulse transmission) in the brain. Glycine has been shown to act as an inhibitory transmitter in the spinal cord. Other amino acids considered to act as neurotransmitters include glutamic acid and aspartic acid.

In addition to the above, an increasing number of **neuropeptides** have been identified and are regarded, with varying degrees of certainty, as central neurotransmitters. These substances, which consist of short chains of amino acids, have been located at neural synapses, although some are found in other body areas as well as within the nervous system. This group of substances includes adrenocorticotrophic hormone (ACTH), leucine enkephalin, methionine enkephalin, endorphin, angiotensin II, luteinizing hormone releasing hormone, somatostatin and substance P. More recently, neuropeptides with longer chains have been discovered; these include beta-endorphin, vasoactive intestinal peptide and neurotensin. Reference will be made to some of these in later chapters.

## Stage 1 of chemical transmission: transmitter synthesis, storage and release

Biosynthesis of the transmitter substance within the terminal bouton has been described for several neurotransmitters, e.g. acetylcholine and the catecholamines.

Release of the chemical transmitter from the presynaptic membrane is achieved by the alteration of membrane permeability caused by the arrival of an action potential at the terminal bouton. The arrival of a nerve impulse at the terminal bouton is followed by an influx of calcium ions from the interstitial fluid. The sharp but brief rise in free calcium levels within the terminal bouton leads to the fusion of synaptic vesicles with the presynaptic membrane. The fusion of the synaptic vesicles with the presynaptic membrane and the extrusion of their contents into the synaptic cleft are seen as the way in which the presynaptic cell releases its transmitter substance.

The vesicles are responsible for transmitter storage and release. Transmitters are secreted in multimolecular packets – or **quanta** – rather than in a continuously graded quantity. In other words, the smallest amount of a transmitter that can be released would be one quantum, perhaps 10 000 molecules of transmitter, the next smallest amount would be two quanta, and so on.

## Stage 2 of chemical transmission: diffusion of transmitter

The second stage of synaptic transmission is the passage of the transmitter across the synaptic cleft; this occurs by means of passive diffusion.

## Stage 3 of chemical transmission: action at the postsynaptic cell

The third stage of synaptic transmission is the action of the transmitter at the postsynaptic cell membrane. On arrival at the postsynaptic cell, the chemical transmitter initiates a change in the potential difference across the membrane. This change can either depolarize the cell, that is, reduce the potential difference and increase the likelihood of action potential generation, or it can hyperpolarize the membrane so that the resting potential is increased and the chance of an action potential occurring is reduced.

It seems that there are at least two processes whereby a chemical transmitter can cause an alteration to the postsynaptic membrane potential. First, and most importantly, the transmitter substance can act at specific **receptor sites** on the postsynaptic membrane, directly opening ionic gates. The alteration in the membrane potential is thus attributed to the passive diffusion of ions through these opened gates. For example, the excitatory effects of acetylcholine at the neuromuscular junction are attributed to simultaneous increases in permeability of the postsynaptic membrane to potassium and sodium. As sodium ions are far from equilibrium at rest, sodium movement will dominate, despite the increase in potassium permeability, and depolarization occurs. Again, the hyperpolarizing effects of the inhibitory transmitter GABA are attributed to the opening of chloride gates. A rise in chloride permeability will maintain the resting potential and resist any tendency towards depolarization, although an actual increase in the transmembrane potential difference might not be seen.

The second mode of action of the transmitter substance is less direct and is still not fully understood.

Receptors are those molecules on the postsynaptic membrane that are responsible for recognizing the chemical involved in synaptic transmission. Recognition of the transmitter will be the first event occurring at the postsynaptic cell, regardless of whether that cell is another nerve cell or a muscle cell. A receptor needs to be specific in its recognition of a particular chemical compound, yet any one cell can respond to a number of different kinds of receptor distributed throughout its membranes. Any one neurotransmitter can act on more than one type of receptor. For example, acetylcholine has been found to act on muscarinic and nicotinic receptors. **Muscarinic receptors** are so called because at these sites muscarine has actions similar to those of acetylcholine. These sites occur in smooth muscle, cardiac muscle and exocrine glands. The receptors can be competitively blocked by atropine. On the other hand, **nicotinic receptors**, which occur in the autonomic ganglia and in skeletal muscle, are insensitive to muscarine but respond to nicotine as well as to acetylcholine. A further complication arises because the nicotinic receptors in the autonomic ganglia and in skeletal muscle are not identical. The effects of acetylcholine in the autonomic ganglia are blocked by hexamethonium, whereas the receptors at the skeletal neuromuscular junction are blocked by *d*-tubocurarine. *d*-Tubocurarine is used clinically as a muscle relaxant during surgery, or when a patient requires assisted ventilation.

The binding of neurotransmitter with receptors on the postsynaptic membrane leads to a change in the potential difference across that membrane. These effects can be recorded in the postsynaptic cell and are called **postsynaptic potentials**. Postsynaptic potentials can be excitatory or inhibitory, and are consequently referred to as **excitatory postsynaptic potentials (epsps)** or **inhibitory postsynaptic potentials (ipsps)**. The excitatory postsynaptic potentials recorded at the neuromuscular junction are known as **endplate potentials (epps)**. Certain features of a postsynaptic potential should be noted. First, it shows a continuously graded response up to a maximum; second, it spreads for only short distances, perhaps 1 mm or less, before becoming severely attenuated; and third, it has a relatively long duration, lasting 10–15 ms.

Excitatory postsynaptic potentials and endplate potentials represent a simultaneous increase in sodium and potassium permeability of the postsynaptic membrane, caused by the binding of transmitter molecules with receptors. The fact that membrane permeability to both sodium and potassium occurs simultaneously distinguishes this process from the time-locked changes in membrane permeability to sodium and potassium that lead to action potential generation. It might be thought that the simultaneous opening of sodium and potassium gates would lead to no change in transmembrane potential, because both ions would flow down their concentration gradients and consequently cations would flow into and also out of the cell. However, under resting conditions potassium is much nearer its equilibrium than sodium and, as a consequence, there will be a tendency for sodium entry to dominate. This will lead to a net gain of positive charge by the cell and a corresponding tendency to depolarize the postsynaptic membrane. By contrast, an inhibitory postsynaptic potential results from changes in membrane permeability to potassium and chloride. These changes will stabilize the transmembrane potential difference at its resting level and might even hyperpolarize the postsynaptic cell.

The continuous gradation of synaptic potential amplitude implies that the size of the change in potential difference across the postsynaptic membrane is a function of the number of receptors affected by the transmitter and hence the amount of transmitter release. In other words, the greater the number of postsynaptic membrane receptors that are affected, the greater the potential change.

At the neuromuscular junction, one impulse travelling along the motor neurone will be sufficient to depolarize the muscle fibre. This will not be the case at a neural synapse, where the situation is more complicated. Any one nerve cell can have many hundreds or even thousands of other nerve cells making contact with it. Moreover, some contacts will be inhibitory and some excitatory, and they will not all be active at the same time. The activity of the cell will therefore depend on the aggregate effects of all the excitatory and inhibitory influences operating on it at any one time. For example, if it is assumed that the cell is dominated by excitatory influences, then the spread of depolarization from the excitatory synapses will tend to be along the dendrites towards the axon hillock (axonal bulge adjacent to neuronal soma). The cell membrane of the axon hillock has a much lower threshold than the rest of the cell membrane. Consequently, action potentials are produced more readily and more rapidly here. The axon hillock is therefore the site of generation of action potentials in the postsynaptic cell. However, if inhibitory influences dominate then any depolarization will be countered and will not be sufficient to reach threshold level.

Because the axon hillock is remote from the synaptic connections on the dendrites it permits all epsps and ipsps occurring at any one time to be algebraically added together. At the dendrites, the transmembrane potential changes reflect the activity of local synapses rather than all of the synapses acting on the cell. The much lower threshold of the axon hillock membrane ensures that action potentials are generated at the axon hillock, where all synaptic activity can be taken into account.

## Stage 4 of chemical transmission: recovery

The final stage of chemical neurotransmission is that of recovery. Recovery is the process involved in preparing for another impulse to arrive at the synapse. In order that each impulse remains a discrete signal, the transmitter substance released as a result of each impulse must be inactivated or removed by the time the next one arrives at the synapse. The major components of the process of re-establishing a state of readiness are biochemical deactivation of transmitter and reuptake of transmitter by the presynaptic neurone.

Deactivation of the transmitter substance by enzymatic action has been described for several neurotransmitters. For example, **acetylcholinesterase**, which is localized in postsynaptic neuronal membranes, hydrolyses and hence deactivates acetylcholine. This process transforms acetylcholine into choline plus acetate. The choline is then available for reabsorption by the presynaptic neurone, where it will be used once more for the synthesis of acetylcholine.

It has been suggested that an active reuptake mechanism, an amine pump, in the presynaptic neurone can account for the removal of most of the noradrenaline released at adrenergic synapses. The portion of noradrenaline that is not accounted for in this way will be deaminated by monoamine oxidase.

## Synaptic integration

The nervous system is responsible for selecting and integrating information, enabling the individual to make sense of the world and to respond appropriately. This process necessitates the careful channelling and filtering of information, as can be seen in many aspects of everyday behaviour. For example, people living in houses beside a busy road tend to be less aware of the traffic noise than their visitors. The noise is a constant background and is presumably filtered out of their conscious awareness. Again, when someone accidentally touches a hot saucepan the immediate response is a reflex withdrawal of the hand. In addition to this, several other responses occur: the individual orientates his or her gaze towards the saucepan, alters posture to compensate for the sharp withdrawal of the hand and might utter a scream or an appropriate verbalization. These separate components of the behavioural response are controlled by different parts of the nervous system and, for them to be integrated into a complete piece of behaviour, the relevant information must be channelled appropriately.

The process of integrating information depends on the synapse, because the synapse represents the basic switching mechanism of the nervous system. This mechanism yields great flexibility. For example, the human brain consists of something of the order of $10^{11}$ nerve cells, and any one of these cells can have many hundreds of synaptic contacts impinging on it. This demonstrates the immense capacity that the nervous system possesses for integrating information. The following discussion considers how this integration takes place.

## Temporal and spatial summation

A single epsp at a single synapse will almost never cause an action potential in the postsynaptic cell. However, one epsp might not be completed before another action potential arrives at the synapse. Consequently, the change in the transmembrane potential caused by the second epsp will be added to what is left of the change caused by the first. The effects of the two epsps will summate over time, a process known as **temporal summation**. Although a single epsp at any single synapse might not be sufficient to generate an action potential in the postsynaptic cell, a train of several epsps coming quickly one after the other might be able to do so. Therefore temporal summation depends on the frequency of firing of the presynaptic cell.

In addition to temporal summation, **spatial summation** can also occur. A single nerve cell might have many hundreds of synaptic contacts impinging on it and hence it is likely that many excitatory synapses will be operating at the same time. Although a single epsp alters the postsynaptic cell's transmembrane potential by only a small amount in a localized manner, the effects of many epsps occurring at different synapses at the same time might summate to reach the threshold level.

It seems, then, that at any particular time a nerve cell membrane is being shifted either towards or away from its threshold potential by the effects of all its excitatory and inhibitory influences, and that these are combining by the processes of temporal and spatial summation. The generation of an action potential at the axon hillock will depend on these summated inhibitory and excitatory potentials.

## Sensitization

When a neuronal pathway is consistently and regularly stimulated, the synapses along the circuit appear to transmit the nerve impulses with increasing ease. In other words, the repetition of firing of a pattern of neuronal connections leads to the synapses becoming sensitized to impulses travelling along that pathway. As a neurone becomes sensitized to a particular pattern of impulses, the influx of calcium ions into the presynaptic membrane apparently increases. This in turn leads to an increase in the release of the transmitter, which improves the chances of firing the postsynaptic cell. It is likely that sensitization of neuronal circuits takes place during learning.

## Reflexes

Some of the basic mechanisms whereby neurones influence the behaviour of other neurones and muscles have now been considered. In general, the nervous control of behaviour involves the transmission of nerve signals through complex networks of fibres. However, some aspects of behaviour can be broken down into components that can be investigated to illustrate the relationship between anatomical connections and function. A reflex is such an example of behaviour that can be examined to see how the events occurring at synapses are integrated to produce a response.

A reflex can be defined as an innate involuntary response to peripheral stimulation requiring the presence of part of the CNS. This definition immediately presents some difficulties in deciding whether a particular response is reflex or not. So-called conditioned reflexes would be excluded because the relationship between the stimulus and the response develops after a period of training or conditioning. That is, it develops after birth. Pavlov's famous experiments with dogs illustrate the difference. Dogs salivate when food is placed in the mouth, a reflex response that is innate. Dogs can be conditioned to salivate in response to a ringing bell if, during training, the bell rings at the time that food is presented. Salivation to the bell is a **conditioned reflex response** and the training process is known as **classical conditioning**. The response of salivation is the same in both cases but the stimuli eliciting the responses differ. Distinguishing between the two can be useful when examining patterns of behaviour but is less useful when considering the underlying physiology of the response.

The involuntary nature of a reflex response is also not always clear cut. The withdrawal reflex that occurs in response to pain stimulation is involuntary but it can be modified, depending on the individual's perception of the circumstances in which stimulation occurs. If a hot object is accidentally picked up, the withdrawal reflex generally results in the object being dropped. However, if the object happens to be an expensive piece of pottery, the reflex might be overridden and conscious voluntary control exerted to replace the object without damaging it. Eye blinking will occur reflexly and involuntarily in response to a threatening gesture. However, the same response can occur entirely voluntarily or involuntarily without an obvious stimulus eliciting it.

The stimulus that elicits the reflex response might occur at the body surface or in an internal organ. Strong stimuli that give rise to the sensation of pain can elicit withdrawal reflex responses when applied to the skin. Light directed through the pupil of the eye will cause a reflex constriction of the pupil, and visual stimuli that are subconsciously interpreted as a threatening gesture can cause reflex blinking. There are many examples of reflexes arising from internal stimulation. These include the reflex maintenance of muscular tone (which will be considered in more detail below), cardiovascular reflexes involved in the maintenance of arterial blood pressure, coughing, swallowing, vomiting and salivary secretion. Some of these responses are quite complex and involve the coordination of a number of muscles. In some cases the response is an increase in a glandular secretion rather than a change in the degree of muscle contraction.

Reflex pathways operate via the CNS. In some cases, the CNS component is the brain. For example, coughing, swallowing, vomiting and blinking all involve the medulla, which is the part of the brain adjacent to the spinal cord. However, a number of reflexes operate via the spinal cord and do not involve the brain at all. The withdrawal reflex, which is of importance in protecting the body from harm, involves a pathway through the spinal cord. The maintenance of muscle tone (i.e. normal stage of contraction of muscle) is another spinal reflex that is of considerable importance in posture control.

When considering reflexes, it is important to bear in mind that they rarely operate as isolated systems. Nerve axons characteristically branch and the sensory signal that initiates the reflex response might also be conveyed to other parts of the nervous system. Thus, the activation of a reflex pathway can lead to the activation of other reflexes and also to the activation of the cerebral cortex, the part of the brain that provides for conscious awareness. For example, when a withdrawal reflex operates via the spine to cause the removal of the foot from a sharp object, nerve impulses are also directed along other pathways to initiate maintenance of posture and to elicit conscious awareness of pain. Other actions might follow. The individual might vocalize, grimace, rub the affected area and so on. These other actions, and the conscious perception of pain, are not part of the reflex as such but they do form part of the total behaviour of the individual and represent a complex level of integration by the nervous system.

## Component structures in a reflex pathway

The term **reflex arc** is often employed to describe the pathway from the sensory receptor that detects the stimulus to the CNS and, via synapses, to the effector organ that produces the response. Indeed, the term 'reflex' indicates that the sensory signal is **reflected** to the muscles.

The component structures in a reflex pathway obviously vary depending on the particular reflex concerned, but some general features can be identified:

- **Sensory receptor.** Because a reflex is a response to peripheral stimulation, it is clear that receptors must be present, as these are the only structures that can transduce stimulus energy into nerve signals.
- **Sensory afferent nerve fibre.** Nerve impulses, once generated at receptors, must be conveyed to the CNS by sensory afferent fibres.

- **Synapse in the CNS.** Sensory nerve fibres cannot directly synapse on to muscle, therefore nerve impulses generated in receptors must be passed through at least one synapse in the brain or spinal cord before reaching the motor neurones. In general, reflex pathways involve more than one synapse and interneurones form part of the pathway through the CNS.
- **Motor efferent fibre (motor neurone).** Nerve signals pass out of the CNS via the motor neurones to the effector organs that will make the reflex response.
- **Effector organs.** The reflex response itself is a change in either muscular contraction or glandular secretion. Muscles or glands form the final structures in the reflex pathway.

The anatomical relationship between these structures is illustrated in **Fig. 2.1.11**. It is worth noting that a reflex response normally involves many receptors, sensory afferents and motor efferents. Summation therefore occurs at the CNS synapses. The diagrammatic representation of a reflex pathway in **Fig. 2.1.11** is therefore an oversimplification.

## Characteristics of reflex activity

The majority of reflexes are excitatory and result in increased muscle contraction or glandular secretion. However, some reflexes are inhibitory and, when stimulated, cause a discharge of nerve impulses that pass from the sensory afferents to interneurones, which then inhibit motor neurones innervating the effector organs. Reflex inhibition of antagonist muscles generally accompanies reflex excitation of protagonist muscles. For example, when flexor muscles attached to a limb contract reflexly, the corresponding extensor muscles relax, thereby facilitating movement of the limb. This pairing of excitation and inhibition illustrates the principle of **reciprocal inhibition**.

## Withdrawal (flexion) reflex

Noxious stimuli applied to receptors in the skin can give rise to the sensation of pain. Pain can be regarded as protective because it directs attention to a potentially harmful situation that the affected individual might then be able to control. The perception of pain and the interpretation of the circumstances giving rise to it require the activation of a number of different systems in the brain. This activation must take place before the individual can consciously respond to the stimulus. A more immediate response is the subconscious reflex withdrawal of the part of the body affected. This is a very important protective reflex because it permits a more rapid removal from the

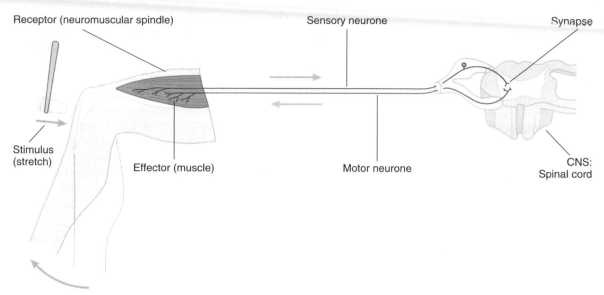

Figure 2.1.11    A monosynaptic reflex (the patellar reflex) illustrating the component structures of a reflex arc involving only two neurones and one synapse. A sensory neurone transmits the message to the spinal cord and a motor neurone transmits the message back to the muscle

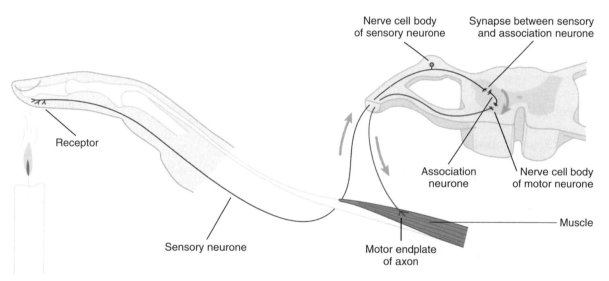

Figure 2.1.12    A polysynaptic reflex involving a chain of neurones and two synapses. A sensory neurone transmits the message to the central nervous system where it synapses with an associated neurone. This synapses with a motor neurone, which transmits the message to the muscle which withdraws the hand from the flame

source of harm than could occur via conscious control of the body.

The withdrawal reflex operates via a pathway through the spinal cord and it exhibits many of the general properties of reflex action that have already been described. The nature of the response depends in part on the site of stimulation but generally involves a flexion movement, hence the name flexion reflex. It involves more than one synapse in the spinal cord and is termed a **polysynaptic reflex arc**. Temporal and spatial summation occur at these synapses. The number of muscles involved in the response and the tension developed by each muscle therefore depend on the area, intensity and duration of the stimulus.

The flexion reflex pathway is illustrated diagrammatically in **Fig. 2.1.12**. When the pain receptor is stimulated, nerve impulses are generated. These pass through interneurones in the spinal cord and then excite motor neurones supplying the flexor muscle. The muscle contracts, thereby removing the body from the source of stimulation.

A simple flexion reflex results in contraction and flexion together with reciprocal inhibition and relaxation of antagonist muscles. If the intensity of the stimulus is increased, other muscle groups might also contract reflexly. For example, if a person stands on a drawing pin, flexion can occur at the ankle, knee and hips. Even the trunk of the body might flex under these conditions. Moreover, extensor muscles might contract reflexly, resulting in extension of other parts of the body. In the example of standing on a drawing pin, it is of course important that posture is maintained at the same time as the foot is withdrawn, otherwise the person might fall back onto the drawing pin. The opposite leg therefore extends, with contraction of the extensor muscles. This associated response is termed the **crossed-extensor reflex**. The withdrawal reflex therefore has the dual function of withdrawal from the noxious stimulus and maintenance of posture.

## Crossed-extensor reflex

Nerve signals from the sensory afferents are transmitted, via interneurones, across the spinal cord to the other side of the body. These interneurones synapse with motor neurones supplying extensor muscles, which then contract. At the same time, the associated flexor muscles are reciprocally inhibited.

The crossed-extensor reflex is most easily elicited if noxious stimuli are delivered to the foot. Contraction of extensor muscles in the opposite limb to that stimulated is very important for maintenance of posture, and indeed the whole weight of the body might be acting on the extended leg. The crossed-extensor muscles and the motor neurones innervating them are therefore recruited into the withdrawal response.

## Plantar reflex and Babinski response

If the sole of the foot is stroked firmly, the toes reflexly curl downwards. This is a healthy plantar response and is said to be flexor despite the fact that the toes apparently show an extension movement downwards. It is more useful to consider this response as flexion because it is part of the normal reflex withdrawal response to noxious stimulation of the foot.

The plantar response is of considerable importance in neurological examinations. Disease of the motor pathways from the brain (the corticospinal tracts) can result in an extensor plantar response. Here, the big toe turns upwards and the other toes spread out when the sole of the foot is stroked firmly. This extensor plantar response was first described by Babinski in 1896 and is often referred to as a positive Babinski response.

### DEVELOPMENTAL ISSUES

The plantar response is also of interest in child development. Infants normally exhibit extensor plantar responses before they are able to stand and walk. The flexor response develops when myelination of the corticospinal tracts occurs, and this corresponds with the infant's ability to stand.

## The stretch reflex

The stretch reflex is a spinal reflex in which the stretching of a muscle causes contraction of the same muscle. Sensory afferent fibres from stretch receptors synapse directly onto motor neurones in the spinal cord. Interneurones are not involved and the reflex is said to be **monosynaptic**. The functional integrity of stretch reflex pathways is essential for normal maintenance of muscle tone.

The stretch receptors are spindle-shaped structures that lie embedded in skeletal muscle, parallel to the muscle fibres. The ends of these **muscle spindles** are attached to the connective tissue framework of the muscle. Thus, a change in the length of the muscle causes a corresponding change in the length of the spindles contained within it. Activation of muscle spindles causes nerve signals to be transmitted to lower centres of the brain, which might then modify stretch reflex activity. This will not give rise to a conscious sensation.

The structure of a muscle spindle is illustrated in **Fig. 2.1.13**. It contains six to ten small specialized muscle fibres, called intrafusal muscle fibres to distinguish them from the normal extrafusal fibres of the main body of the muscle. The polar ends of the intrafusal fibres are striated and contractile and in essence function like small-scale extrafusal fibres. The middle portions of the intrafusal fibres contain the nuclei and are non-contractile. Thus the centre portion of the whole spindle is also non-contractile. A large afferent nerve fibre is wrapped spiral fashion around the middle portion of the spindle. This is the primary annulospiral nerve ending. This afferent fibre belongs to the nerve fibre group A$\alpha$ (sometimes called IA). It can approach 20 $\mu$m in diameter, with a conduction velocity of over 100 m/s. Two secondary sensory nerve endings are also wrapped around the spindle, one on each side of the primary afferent. These are the secondary flower-spray endings. These secondary afferents are smaller, less than 10 $\mu$m in diameter and they conduct impulses at much slower velocities. These belong to the A$\gamma$ group (sometimes called group II). The contractile poles of the spindle have their own motor efferent supply, the gamma ($\gamma$) motor neurones, belonging to the A$\gamma$ group of fibres.

The stretch reflex pathway is illustrated in **Fig. 2.1.14**. When stretch is rapidly applied to the muscle, the spindles are stretched and this causes discharges of nerve impulses in the spindle afferents.

The spindle afferents convey nerve signals to the spinal cord, entering via the dorsal roots. The afferents synapse directly onto the alpha-motor neurones, which supply the extrafusal muscle fibres (alpha-motor neurones belong to group A$\alpha$). The alpha-motor neurones conduct the signals via the ventral roots of the

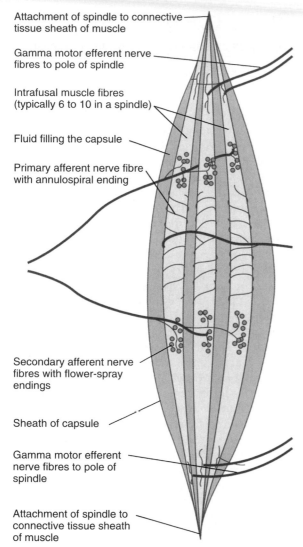

Attachment of spindle to connective tissue sheath of muscle

Gamma motor efferent nerve fibres to pole of spindle

Intrafusal muscle fibres (typically 6 to 10 in a spindle)

Fluid filling the capsule

Primary afferent nerve fibre with annulospiral ending

Secondary afferent nerve fibres with flower-spray endings

Sheath of capsule

Gamma motor efferent nerve fibres to pole of spindle

Attachment of spindle to connective tissue sheath of muscle

**Figure 2.1.13**   A muscle spindle

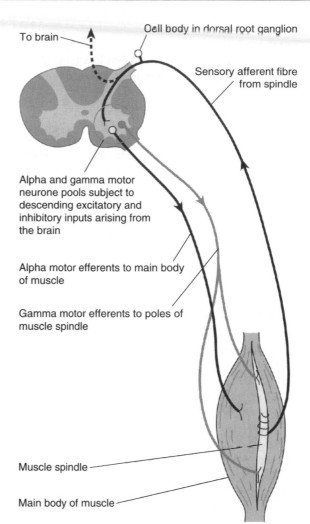

Cell body in dorsal root ganglion

To brain

Sensory afferent fibre from spindle

Alpha and gamma motor neurone pools subject to descending excitatory and inhibitory inputs arising from the brain

Alpha motor efferents to main body of muscle

Gamma motor efferents to poles of muscle spindle

Muscle spindle

Main body of muscle

**Figure 2.1.14**   The stretch reflex pathway. When the muscle spindle is stretched the sensory afferent nerve terminal is stimulated. This reflexly stimulates the alpha-motor neurone and the muscle contracts

spinal cord to the muscle, which then contracts and shortens, thereby removing the stretch. As the muscle shortens, the spindles within it shorten and the stimulation of the afferents is reduced. Some afferents terminate on interneurones, which simultaneously inhibit antagonist muscles.

This pattern of events occurs in tendon-jerk reflexes, which utilize the stretch reflex pathways. In the knee-jerk reflex, the patellar tendon is sharply tapped and this stretches the quadriceps muscle in the thigh. Muscle spindle afferents in the quadriceps are activated and impulses are conveyed to the alpha-motor neurone pool in the spinal cord. These alpha-motor neurones conduct impulses to the muscle, causing it to contract and the leg kicks forwards and upwards as the quadriceps muscle shortens. An ankle jerk can be elicited in the same way, by sharply tapping the Achilles tendon. In tendon-jerk reflexes, the rate of change of stretch is very important. Pressure slowly applied to the tendon does not cause a jerk response.

Tendon-jerk reflex responses are important in the neurological assessment of patients because they can provide information about the integrity of the stretch reflex pathways. However, the stretch reflex is not only elicited when a tendon is sharply tapped. Stretch can also be applied to muscle spindles by gravitational pull or by internal stimulation arising from the brain. It is by these means that the reflex operates in the control of muscle tone.

When an individual is standing, gravity causes some stretching of postural muscles. This activates the stretch reflex pathway and causes contraction of the muscles. The stretch reflex therefore plays a part in the maintenance of posture.

## Golgi tendon organ reflex

The muscle spindles essentially monitor the length of the muscle but normally, when a muscle contracts, it develops tension in addition to shortening. Embedded in the tendinous parts of the muscle are specialized receptors that detect tension development. These receptors are called **Golgi tendon organs**. They consist of bundles of collagen fibres around which are wrapped afferent nerve terminals. When activated, these receptors generate nerve impulses that stimulate inhibitory interneurones in the spinal cord. These interneurones synapse onto the motor neurones and decrease their activity. Golgi tendon organ activity therefore inhibits muscle contraction.

Golgi tendon organs and the tendon organ reflex pathways undoubtedly play a part in the control of muscle contraction, although their precise role is not clearly understood. Signals will also be transmitted from the Golgi tendon organs to motor control centres in the brain, and these centres might then modify the output to the motor neurones. In addition, the Golgi tendon organ reflex appears to have a protective role. If the tension in a muscle increases to an extent that could be damaging and could cause muscle tearing, then tendon organ reflex inhibition will cause a reduction in muscle contraction and a lengthening reaction. This can be demonstrated if tension is applied passively to a spastic limb in an attempt to bend it. At first the limb resists the movement and tension builds up. The limb then suddenly gives way and bends, the 'clasp-knife' response. This is caused by reflex tendon organ inhibition of the motor neurones.

## Reflexes in the control of posture

The maintenance of posture and balance is accomplished by a number of complex reflexes. The sensory afferent components include vision receptors in the eye, balance receptors in the ear, touch receptors in the skin, stretch and tension receptors in muscle, and various position sense receptors in joints. The CNS components might be in lower centres of the brain or in the spinal cord, whereas the final motor efferent component is the same in all cases, namely the motor neurones in the spinal cord.

In sighted persons, vision appears to be a dominant sensory input for balance control. A person standing on one leg will sway considerably more if the eyes are closed. However, blind persons adapt to the lack of visual input and maintain balance very well, with only a slight loss of precision. In general, it is the combination of all afferent inputs that reflexly determines muscle contraction in maintenance of posture.

### CLINICAL APPLICATIONS

#### REFLEXES IN NEUROLOGICAL ASSESSMENT

Tendon-jerk reflex testing forms part of routine neurological assessment. A tendon-jerk response will be diminished or even abolished if any part of the pathway from receptor to muscle is damaged. If a patient suffers from muscle disease, for example muscular dystrophy, then reflex responses involving affected muscles will be diminished. Similarly, if either sensory afferent nerve fibres or motor efferent nerve fibres are damaged, the reflex response will be reduced. For example, dorsal spinal nerve root damage, which can occur in association with syphilis (tabes dorsalis), causes primary afferent nerve damage with a resultant diminution of affected reflexes. Motor neurone disorders, such as poliomyelitis, damage the efferent pathway and also result in diminution or abolition of affected reflexes. Certain disorders of the brain, resulting in coma or raised intracranial pressure, can also cause a reduction in reflex responses, presumably because of a decrease in the central control of spinal motor neurone activity. A knowledge of the parts of the body affected and the extent to which reflex responses are diminished contributes to diagnosis of the disorder.

Some individuals quite normally have brisker and more readily elicited tendon-jerk reflex responses than others. However, tendon reflexes can become exaggerated under certain conditions, especially in anxiety states associated with increased muscle tension. Clinically exaggerated tendon-jerk reflexes can indicate damage to the motor pathways from the brain to the spinal motor neurone pool. In this case, the damage has caused an imbalance between excitatory and inhibitory inputs, resulting in excessive stretch reflex activity. In spasticity the stretch reflex is so powerful that the muscles are in a permanent state of extreme tension.

If the spinal cord has been transected, as can occur in road traffic accidents, reflex responses are initially abolished below the level of transection and a state of 'spinal shock' exists. It is believed that the sudden cessation of nerve signals travelling to and from the brain causes disorder of function of even spinal reflexes. However, after a period of time, spinal reflex responses not only return but are considerably exaggerated.

## Conclusion

This chapter has been concerned with the basic histology of the nervous system. We have seen how the coordinated conduction of nerve impulses is essential for homeostasis. This is achieved with a unique combination of electrical and chemical inputs resulting in smooth coordinated action via a complex system of reflexes. Structural disorders of the nervous system have also been reviewed. Review of the minute, complex chemical and electrical changes at cellular level and of the functioning of reflexes enhances understanding of how the rest of the CNS functions along with its complex interactions with other body systems. It also serves to highlight how much more of the structure and function of the nervous system has yet to be discovered.

## Clinical review

In addition to the Learning Objectives at the beginning of this chapter, the reader should be able to:

- Outline the putative function of neuroglial cells
- Identify the major features of peripheral neuropathy
- Outline the characteristic properties of reflex responses
- Describe the structural elements and the functions of the flexion reflex, the crossed-extension reflex and the stretch reflex
- Describe common disorders which affect nervous tissues and identify appropriate nursing interventions for them
- Explain the importance of the assessment of reflexes in nursing

## Review questions

1. What are the two major divisions of the nervous system?
2. What is the difference between afferent and efferent nerve fibres?
3. What are the two parts of the autonomic nervous system?
4. Of which two cell types is nervous tissue composed?
5. What are the major features of a neurone?
6. Describe the two types of 'matter' in the central nervous system
7. How are neurones classified?
8. What are ganglia?
9. Why can nerve cells not repair damaged areas of the brain?
10. Describe the system of sheaths that holds nerves together
11. What happens, in ionic terms, when a nerve cell is depolarized?
12. What part does energy (in the form of ATP) play in the depolarization of a nerve?
13. What part does stimulus intensity play in the generation of an action potential?
14. What is the difference between the absolute and relative refractory period?
15. Are nerve fibres good at transmitting electrical current?
16. What factors determine the rate of conduction of impulses in nerve fibres?
17. Describe the mechanism of chemical transmission at a synapse.
18. What is the consequence of the binding of a neurotransmitter to a postsynaptic membrane?
19. By what physiological processes can neurotransmitter action at synapses be stopped?
20. Contrast temporal and spatial summation at synapses
21. What is a reflex?
22. What are the essential components of a reflex arc?

## Useful addresses

Epilepsy Action
New Anstey House, Gate Way, Yeadon, Leeds, LS19 7XY
www.epilepsy.org.uk

Stroke Association
Stroke House, 240 City Road, London, EC1V 2PR
www.stroke.org.uk

Multiple Sclerosis Society
372 Edgeware Road, London, NW2 6ND
www.mssociety.org.uk

Parkinson's Disease Society
215 Vauxhall Bridge Road, London, SW1V 1ES
www.parkinsons.org.uk

The Meningitis Trust
Fern House, Bath Road, Stroud, GL5 3TJ
www.meningitis-trust.org.uk

Royal National Institute of the Blind
224 Great Portland Street, London, W1N 6AA
www.rnib.org.uk

Royal National Institute for the Deaf
19–23 Featherstone Street, London, EC1Y 8SL

## Suggestions for further reading

Fox, S. & Lantz, C. (1998) The brain tumour experience and quality of life: A qualitative study. *Journal of Neuroscience Nursing*, **30**(4); 245–252.
*An investigation into the quality of life of patients with brain tumours. Provides information that healthcare professionals caring for brain tumour patients can use to give care and anticipatory guidance.*

Guerrero, D. (1998) *Neuro-oncology for Nurses.* London: Whurr Publishers.
*An excellent text providing comprehensive coverage of all aspects of neuro-oncology.*

Guerrero, D. (1999) Systems and disease: brain tumours. *Nursing Times*, **95**(4); 48–51.
*Basic overview of brain tumours.*

Lepola, I., Toljamo, M., Aho, R. & Louet, T. (2001) Being a brain tumour patient: A descriptive study of patient's experiences. *Journal of Neuroscience Nursing*, **33**(3); 143–147.

*An interesting investigation on the experience of being a patient with a brain tumour. Draws important conclusions that have implications for nursing care.*

Lisak, D. (2001) Overview of symptomatic management of multiple sclerosis. *Journal of Neuroscience Nursing*, **33**(5); 224–230.
*Provides a comprehensive overview of multiple sclerosis, highlighting the crucial role of the nurse in the effort to moderate and modulate the symptomatic problems associated with multiple sclerosis.*

Madonna, M.G. & Keating, M.M. (1999) Multiple sclerosis pathways: An innovative role in disease management. *Journal of Neuroscience Nursing*, **31**(6); 332–335.
*Examines an approach to caring for multiple sclerosis patients that encompasses holistic care.*

## References

Hickey, J.V. (2002) *The Clinical Practice of Neurological and Neurosurgical Nursing*, 5th edn. Philadelphia: Lippincott, Williams and Wilkins.

Lindsay, K. & Bone, I. (2004) *Neurology and Neurosurgery Illustrated*, 4th edn. Edinburgh: Churchill Livingstone.

# The central nervous system

*Douglas Allan*

## LEARNING OBJECTIVES

After studying this chapter the reader should be able to:

- Identify the main features of the embryological development of the central nervous system (CNS)

- Locate and describe the appearance of the four ventricles and the aqueduct in the human brain

- Identify the separate layers of the meninges

- Describe the site of production, path of flow and site of reabsorption of cerebrospinal fluid (CSF)

- Describe the function and composition of CSF and demonstrate the importance of CSF analysis to the identification of disease

- Identify the major blood vessels supplying the brain

- Describe the relationship between the spinal cord, spinal nerves and the vertebral column

- Describe the structural features of grey and white matter in the spinal cord

- Name the 12 pairs of cranial nerves and describe their separate functions

- Identify the major structural features of the brain and outline their functions

- Describe the neurophysiology of sleep and how an understanding of the subject can assist the nurse in patient care

- Explain the importance of accurate assessment of conscious level

- Describe how and why the Glasgow Coma Scale is applied

- Describe and explain the significance of the brainstem death criteria

- Explain how a knowledge of the origins and effects of epilepsy can be used effectively in patient assessment and the planning and delivery of care

## INTRODUCTION

The central nervous system (CNS) is made up of the brain and spinal cord, which control and coordinate the activities of the nervous system. This chapter will examine the embryological development of the nervous system, the structure and function of the brain and spinal cord, the so-called protective functions of the meninges and ventricular system, and the cranial nerves. The latter part of the chapter will consider

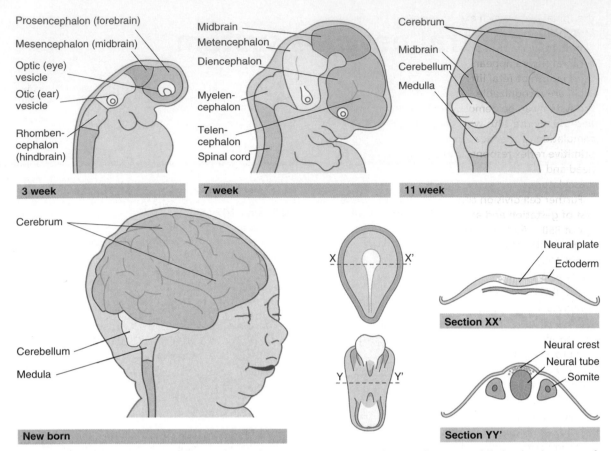

**Figure 2.2.1** Embryological development of the human nervous system showing (bottom right) the development of the neural tube

how these component parts and functions integrate to perform 'higher' functions such as motivation. Finally, states of consciousness will be outlined, as these are important in terms of brain function.

## Embryological development of the central nervous system

### DEVELOPMENTAL ISSUES

The central nervous system (CNS) comprises the brain and spinal cord. In the human embryo the CNS develops from a plate of ectodermal cells along the midline of the back of the embryo. This neural plate is at first exposed to the amniotic fluid but, as it elongates, the lateral edges of the plate rise and grow medially until they meet and unite to form a neural tube (**Fig. 2.2.1**).

An arrest in the process, leading to incomplete closure of the neural tube (and an associated malformation of the vertebral column), results in the condition of **spina bifida**. This condition varies in severity depending on the site and extent of the abnormality; it occurs in approximately 1 in every 200 pregnancies.

### DEVELOPMENTAL ISSUES

The neural tube is normally formed by about the 20th day of gestation, after which it becomes detached from the ectoderm and sinks beneath the surface layers of the developing embryo. As the neural tube elongates it also changes shape. The tube bulges at the head end to form three enlarged areas, which represent the developing brain. From the furthest forward to the one that is contiguous with the rest of the neural tube, these three enlargements are called the prosencephalon (or forebrain), the mesencephalon (or midbrain) and the rhombencephalon (or hindbrain). Early in the second month of gestation these three enlargements increase in number to five: the prosencephalon subdivides into the telencephalon (endbrain) and the diencephalon (between-brain) and the rhombencephalon subdivides into the metencephalon (after-brain) and the myelencephalon (spinal brain).

Further alterations to the structure of the brain are made by the twists, or 'flexures', of the neural tube and by the differential enlargements of parts of the developing brain. Nevertheless, the tube arrangement is retained throughout, with the cavity of the tube becoming the central canal of the spinal cord, which expands at the head end into the ventricular system of the brain.

In the third month of gestation the lateral cerebral fissure appears and by the end of the third month of fetal life the main outlines of the brain are recognizable. Indeed, the integrity of the system can be demonstrated at this stage because, by the 14th week of gestation, tactile stimulation of the face of the fetus will evoke primitive reflex responses, such as rotation of the head and pelvis, and contraction of the trunk musculature.

Further cell division continues throughout the rest of gestation and at birth the brain weighs about 350 g. By the end of the first year of postnatal life, the brain weight has increased to about 1000 g but this is not caused by any large increase in the number of nerve cells. It appears that cell division of neurones is more or less complete at birth. However, nerve tissue that is already present at birth continues to grow postnatally, especially in the first 3 years of life. The process of myelination of nerve fibres continues during infancy and adolescence; it is more or less completed by about the age of 15 years. By puberty, the brain has almost reached its full development and weighs about 1300 g. An average adult human brain weighs about 1400 g.

Definite morphological changes associated with ageing have been identified within the central nervous system. These changes include loss of cerebral volume at the rate of 2–3% per decade from the age of 20 years. This can result in a weight difference of 100 g between the brains of a young and old person. The most important change is degeneration and loss of neurones within the cortex, cerebellum and spinal cord (MacFarlane, Reid & Callander, 1999). The general changes that can occur include loss of memory, increased difficulty in learning new tasks and a decrease in the speed of processing by the brain. More specific changes include slight imbalance when walking, slower reflexes, slower pupillary responses, increased blood pressure, postural hypotension and decreased muscle strength. All of these changes need to be taken into account when assessing the neurological status of an older patient.

## The ventricular system of the brain

As mentioned above, a cavity within the neural tube is retained throughout embryological development, so that in a mature brain a central canal exists within the spinal cord. This expands into larger cavities, or 'ventricles', in the brain.

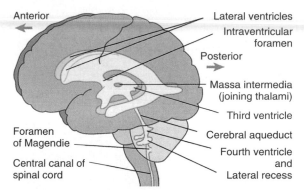

**Figure 2.2.2** The ventricular system of the brain (lateral view)

There are four **ventricles** within the brain. The most posterior, lying in the midline of the hindbrain, is called the **fourth ventricle**. This is joined by the **cerebral aqueduct**, the midbrain equivalent of the neural tube, to the **third ventricle**, which also lies in the midline. A pair of openings called the **intraventricular foramina** then joins the third ventricle with the two **lateral ventricles**, which extend in a horseshoe shape either side of the midline within each cerebral hemisphere. The third ventricle and the two lateral ventricles are the cavities of the forebrain (**Fig. 2.2.2**).

Each ventricle contains a spongy network of capillary blood vessels called a **choroid plexus**. The choroid plexuses are responsible for producing **cerebrospinal fluid** (CSF), which circulates around the brain and within the ventricular system (**Fig. 2.2.3**).

### CLINICAL APPLICATIONS

The ventricular system can be viewed using computerized axial tomography (CAT scan), a radiographic technique whereby serial sections through the brain can be viewed as X-ray plates with the aid of computer integration (**Fig. 2.2.4**). When this is done, any distortions of shape and size of the ventricles (which may be of clinical importance) can be seen. For example, hydrocephalus, which results from an abnormal build-up of the pressure of cerebrospinal fluid, can lead to enlarged and distorted ventricles. Also, a space-occupying lesion in the brain might push the ventricles away from their normal position with respect to the midline.

## The meninges of the brain and the cerebrospinal fluid

The brain and spinal cord are surrounded by three layers of connective tissue, which are collectively referred to as the brain **meninges**. The first of these

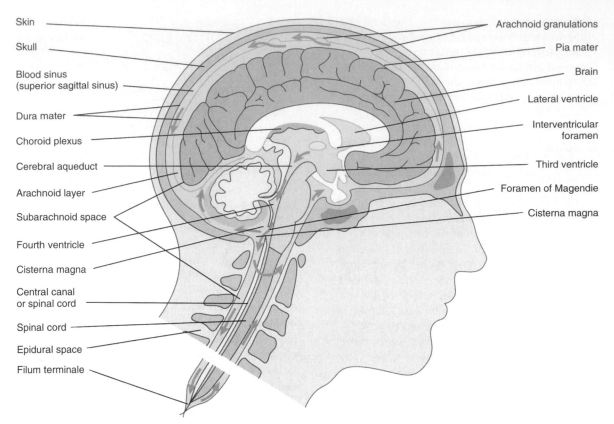

Skin
Skull
Blood sinus (superior sagittal sinus)
Dura mater
Choroid plexus
Cerebral aqueduct
Arachnoid layer
Subarachnoid space
Fourth ventricle
Cisterna magna
Central canal or spinal cord
Spinal cord
Epidural space
Filum terminale

Arachnoid granulations
Pia mater
Brain
Lateral ventricle
Interventricular foramen
Third ventricle
Foramen of Magendie
Cisterna magna

**Figure 2.2.3** Path of flow of cerebrospinal fluid

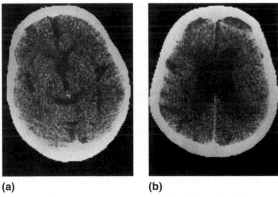

(a)                    (b)

**Figure 2.2.4** A CT (computerized tomography) scan showing (a) a normal adult brain and (b) an adult brain with enlarged ventricles

is a thin, filmy layer of connective tissue called the **pia mater**, which adheres closely to the surface of the brain and spinal cord and follows every indentation and fissure. Between the pia mater and the next layer of tissue is a space that contains circulating cerebrospinal fluid. This space is referred to as the subarachnoid space; the next meninge is called the **arachnoid layer**. The arachnoid layer surrounds the brain and spinal cord and follows the contours of the bony casing of the skull and backbone rather than the neural surface itself. The outermost meninge is a thick membrane principally composed of tough

fibrous tissue; it is called the **dura mater**. The dura lies in close association with the arachnoid layer and follows the contours of the inside of the cranium and spinal column. It also extends as a double layer into the midsagittal fissure between the cerebral hemispheres as the **falx cerebri**, and into the area between the occipital lobe and cerebellum as the **tentorium**. The dura encloses the major sinuses of the venous drainage system, such as the superior sagittal sinus, which runs in the midline above the midsagittal fissure.

**Cerebrospinal fluid** is a clear, colourless liquid that is similar in composition to blood plasma, from which it is derived. It contains small amounts of protein, glucose, sodium, potassium, calcium, chloride, bicarbonate and urea. Isolated lymphocytes are usually present but no red blood cells. The specific gravity is 1005 and the pH is 7.3.

An adult brain can have about 130–150 mL of circulating cerebrospinal fluid at any one time, of which 80–100 mL will be in the brain ventricles and the remainder in the subarachnoid space. Production of cerebrospinal fluid has been estimated to be about 500 mL per day. It is produced by the **choroid plexuses** of the brain ventricles. These plexuses are complex capillary networks covered by a specialized epithelium, the cells of which contain mitochondria and other organelles essential for active transport. Formation of cerebrospinal fluid is a selective secretory process with active transport of certain constituents, and this accounts for the differences in composition between cerebrospinal fluid and plasma.

The pressure of cerebrospinal fluid varies but is of the order of 100–150 mmH$_2$O when the subject is supine. The specific gravity of cerebrospinal fluid is approximately the same as that of brain tissue, so brain and spinal cord float in a bath of cerebrospinal fluid. The support provided by the cerebrospinal fluid and meninges protects the brain from damage caused by movements of the head. In this way the cerebrospinal fluid acts as a shock absorber between the rigid bones of the cranium and the soft malleable tissue of the brain. The cerebrospinal fluid probably fulfils other functions as well, some of which are probably related to metabolic activity and others to additional protective processes such as the blood–brain barrier. However, these latter imputed functions are not clearly understood at present.

Once secreted, the cerebrospinal fluid flows from the lateral ventricles into the third and fourth ventricles and then through three small apertures in the roof of the hindbrain into the subarachnoid space. The apertures are the two lateral **foramina of Luschka** and the medial **foramen of Magendie**. They open into an enlargement of the subarachnoid space known as the **cisterna magna (see Fig. 2.2.3)**. The cerebrospinal fluid then circulates within the subarachnoid space before diffusing into the venous blood supply. This diffusion largely occurs through **arachnoid granulations**, which are projections of the arachnoid layer into the major venous sinuses of the brain.

Towards the tail-end of the spinal column, at the level of the second lumbar vertebra, the spinal cord terminates and the associated pia mater forms the fine, hairlike **filum terminale,** which anchors the cord to the base of the vertebral column. The space between the spinal cord and the arachnoid layer forms the lumbar cisterna, which contains the roots of the lower spinal nerves (called the **cauda equina**) and cerebrospinal fluid.

## CLINICAL APPLICATIONS

The space of the lumbar cisterna is sufficient to allow the drawing-off of samples of cerebrospinal fluid without any serious threat to the neural tissue. This might be done for several reasons, for example to extract samples of cerebrospinal fluid for diagnostic analysis; for the estimation of cerebrospinal fluid pressure; and for the introduction of drugs. The procedure is referred to as **lumbar puncture** and it involves puncturing the dura with a hollow needle between lumbar vertebrae L3 and L4 or between L4 and L5. One direct result of drawing off any large sample of

cerebrospinal fluid will be the lowering of cerebrospinal fluid pressure. This procedure is contraindicated in a patient with undiagnosed raised intracranial pressure. The release of pressure at the lumbar region encourages herniation of the brainstem with subsequent loss of consciousness. If the pressure falls much below normal, the effectiveness of cerebrospinal fluid as a shock absorber between brain and skull will be lessened and, as a consequence, any head movement by the patient could result in headache. It should be noted, however, that this pain is not being mediated by the brain itself, as the brain has no sensory receptors. Rather, it is the meninges and blood vessels that will mediate the pain because they are extensively innervated by pain afferents.

Standard patient care following lumbar puncture includes a minimum of 6 hours bedrest with one pillow and administration of extra oral fluids to enhance the replacement of cerebrospinal fluid. The puncture site is checked frequently for leakage and routine neurological observations should be performed.

The circulation of cerebrospinal fluid, its hydrostatic pressure and its composition can be altered in certain pathological states of the central nervous system. For example, intracranial pressure might be raised when a cerebral tumour develops. The raised pressure might distort and partially block the apertures in the roof of the fourth ventricle and, in addition, might squash the cerebellum (part of the hindbrain) into the foramen magnum – the opening at the base of the skull through which the spinal cord passes. The resulting compression of the hindbrain and spinal cord might occlude the spinal canal, from which about a fifth of total cerebrospinal fluid is normally absorbed. As a consequence of compression, cerebrospinal fluid reabsorption will be greatly impaired.

## CLINICAL APPLICATIONS

**Hydrocephaly** is a condition in which there is a discrepancy between cerebrospinal fluid production and reabsorption, resulting in an excess of fluid. This excess causes an increase in intracranial pressure and can lead to enlargement and distortion of the brain ventricles. The condition is particularly apparent in affected infants because the suture lines of their skull bones can become widely separated, so that the whole head becomes abnormally enlarged. There are many causes of hydrocephaly, including cerebral tumour, infection and congenital and developmental abnormalities. The cerebral aqueduct is particularly vulnerable to blockage owing to its narrowness. Certain congenital disorders and infections can cause obstruction in the flow of cerebrospinal fluid through the aqueduct. A disorder such as this, which causes a blockage of the cerebrospinal fluid circulation through the brain ventricles, is referred to as 'non-communicating hydrocephalus'. Hydrocephalus caused by abnormal reabsorption of cerebrospinal fluid by the arachnoid granulations is called **communicating hydrocephalus**.

Treatment of hydrocephalus essentially involves removing or bypassing the block in the system. Congenital hydrocephalus and some forms of communicating hydrocephalus can be treated by shunting the excess cerebrospinal fluid through a valve into the peritoneum or right atrium of the heart.

The composition and appearance of cerebrospinal fluid can also become abnormal in certain diseases of the CNS. The cerebrospinal fluid is normally clear and colourless but turbidity develops when there is an excess of leucocytes, which is typically associated with meningeal irritation. The excess of cells in cerebrospinal fluid can result from a raised polymorphonuclear cell count, which is usually associated with acute infections, or a raised mononuclear cell count, which is usually associated with chronic infections. However, acute viral infections predominantly raise the mononuclear cell count, in addition to the lymphocyte count, and this typically occurs in viral meningitis.

**Meningitis** can be caused by a range of microorganisms, including bacteria, spirochaetes, fungi and viruses, but in all cases inflammation of the meninges, particularly of the pia mater and arachnoid, is the major feature. Blood is not normally present in cerebrospinal fluid unless there is a pre-existing subarachnoid haemorrhage.

A **subarachnoid haemorrhage** can result from rupture of an intracranial aneurysm, from a cerebral haemorrhage breaking into the ventricular system or, rarely, from severe head injury.

The protein content of cerebrospinal fluid is normally 0.2–0.4 g/L, with albumin and globulin being present in a ratio of about 8 : 1. Inflammatory diseases such as meningitis, encephalitis, poliomyelitis, multiple sclerosis and syphilis can all result in a moderate rise in the protein content. A large rise in protein content to 5 g/L or greater is usually indicative of either obstruction of the spinal subarachnoid space or acute infective polyneuritis.

Glucose levels in cerebrospinal fluid might also show abnormalities and, typically, the glucose content of cerebrospinal fluid is reduced in bacterial or fungal meningitis.

## Cerebral circulation

Blood flow through the adult brain is 750 mL per minute, which represents about 15% of total cardiac output at rest. The supply of blood to the brain is closely associated with metabolic activity of brain tissue, so that factors affecting metabolic activity quickly affect blood flow. For example, within limits, an increase in carbon dioxide concentration, an increase in hydrogen ion concentration or a decrease in oxygen concentration will lead to a rapid increase in cerebral blood flow. The arterial blood supply to the brain passes through two pairs of major arteries, the **vertebral arteries** and the **internal carotid arteries**. The vertebral arteries enter the base of the cranial cavity and then unite to form the **basilar artery**. The basilar artery then runs up on the underside of the structures of the brainstem until it reaches the level of the midbrain, where it again bifurcates into the two posterior cerebral arteries. The vertebral arteries supply the brainstem, the cerebellum and posterior portions of the forebrain. The internal carotid arteries enter the cranial cavity and take up a position on either side of the pituitary gland. The internal carotid arteries divide into several branches including the anterior and middle cerebral arteries. The blood flowing through these arteries supplies the remainder of the forebrain (**Fig. 2.2.5**).

Venous drainage from the brain passes through superficial venous plexuses and dural sinuses into the internal jugular veins of the neck. The dural sinuses are valveless channels formed by the dura mater. One such sinus is the midsagittal sinus, which lies in the dura above the midline fissure of the cerebrum. It drains blood from the upper lateral and medial aspects of the cerebral hemispheres.

The brain requires a constant supply of blood to maintain metabolic activity. Indeed, consciousness is lost if the blood supply is cut-off for only a few seconds. Nevertheless, neuronal activity will not be constant over all the brain at any particular time. In other words, particular areas of the brain will be relatively more or less active depending on the behaviour of the individual at the time. One consequence of this will be that cerebral blood flow will be directed more intensively towards those areas of brain that are relatively more active; the metabolic demands of the neurones in these areas will be greater. Following this line of argument, a measure of localized cerebral blood flow would indicate whether an area of brain is relatively more or less active at any one time. Radiographic techniques have been developed to record local cerebral blood flow in conscious human subjects. These techniques have enhanced our knowledge of head injury and its effects.

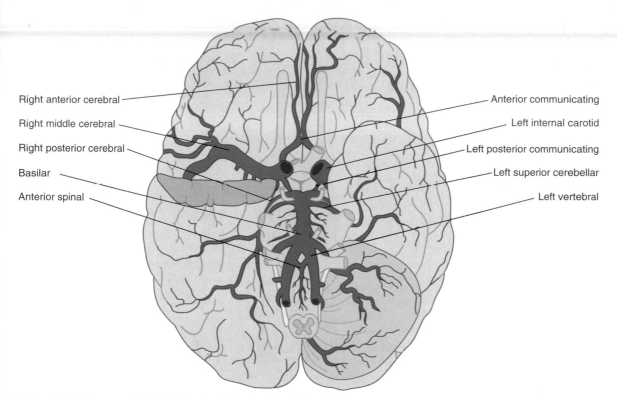

Right anterior cerebral

Right middle cerebral

Right posterior cerebral

Basilar

Anterior spinal

Anterior communicating

Left internal carotid

Left posterior communicating

Left superior cerebellar

Left vertebral

**Figure 2.2.5**   The arterial circulation in the brain. The circle of Willis – an alternative circulatory pathway – is made up of arterial anastomoses by virtue of the communicating arteries

## The spinal cord

The spinal cord lies in the flexible bony column of the vertebrae and stretches from the base of the brainstem to the level of the second lumbar vertebra. In cross-section, the spinal cord comprises a central canal surrounded by a butterfly-shaped area of grey matter, which is in turn surrounded by white matter.

Thirty-one pairs of **spinal nerves** leave the spinal cord and pass through successive intervertebral foramina. These pairs of nerves are identified according to the segment of the spinal column from which they emerge:

- 8 cervical pairs
- 12 thoracic pairs
- 5 lumbar pairs
- 5 sacral pairs
- 1 coccygeal pair.

The pairs of nerves correspond to the number of vertebrae in each region of the spine, except in the case of the cervical nerves, where there are only seven vertebrae, and the coccygeal nerve, where four coccygeal vertebrae are fused to form the coccyx. The relationship between the spinal nerves, segments of the spinal column and the vertebral column is illustrated in **Fig. 2.2.6**.

Each spinal nerve, which is surrounded by a meningeal sleeve of dura, has a dorsal root and a ventral root. The **dorsal root** consists of sensory afferent fibres, which have their cell bodies gathered together in the dorsal root ganglion that is located within the intervertebral foramen. The **ventral root** consists of motor efferents, which have their cell bodies lying within the grey matter of the ventral horn of the spinal cord. The roots of the spinal nerves below the level of the second lumbar vertebra, that is, below the caudal end of the spinal cord, gather together as the **cauda equina** (mare's tail) before they exit through lower lumbar and sacral intervertebral foramina.

Each spinal nerve is distributed to a particular part of the body. Consequently, the dorsal root of each spinal nerve conducts sensory information from a particular body area. These body areas – **dermatomes** (**Fig. 2.2.7**) – show a considerable degree of overlap. Hence, damage to a single spinal nerve need not necessarily result in any great loss of sensation. The ventral root similarly projects to localized muscle groups.

### CLINICAL APPLICATIONS

Peripheral nerves can become damaged and might degenerate, resulting in **neuropathy**. Compression, such as that resulting from a prolapsed intervertebral disc, is a common physical cause of neuropathy but some viral infections, such as herpes zoster (shingles), can

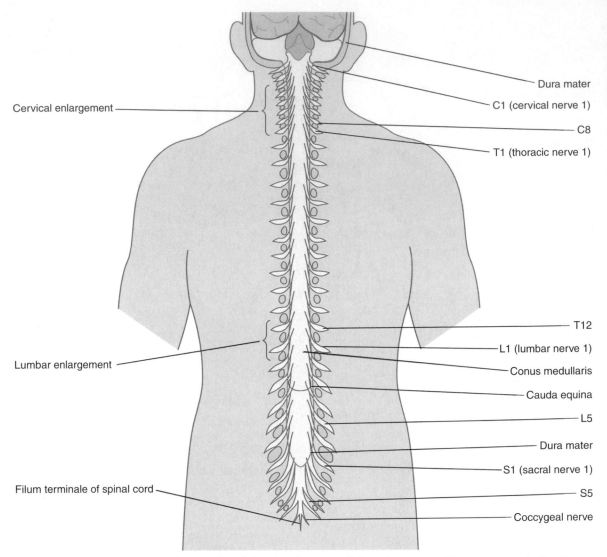

Cervical enlargement

Lumbar enlargement

Filum terminale of spinal cord

Dura mater
C1 (cervical nerve 1)
C8
T1 (thoracic nerve 1)

T12
L1 (lumbar nerve 1)
Conus medullaris
Cauda equina
L5
Dura mater
S1 (sacral nerve 1)
S5
Coccygeal nerve

**Figure 2.2.6** Posterior view of the spinal cord showing the roots of the spinal nerves. These are named after the general region of the spinal cord from which they originate

also cause neuropathy as a result of acute inflammation of a peripheral nerve. The term **'polyneuropathy'** refers to a condition in which many peripheral nerves are simultaneously impaired. This usually results in flaccid muscular weakness and sensory disturbances, which present a number of problems for the patient, who needs to be aware of the dangers of contact with extremes of temperature, e.g. sitting too close to a fire. Loss of sensory information can result in damage without the patient's knowledge. Regular skin inspection is necessary as these patients will be more prone to skin breakdown.

The use of aids may be indicated to support weakened muscles, e.g. lightweight splints might be applied to the affected arm or leg, and cutlery with padded handles might be useful for the patient with a sensory disturbance affecting the hands.

The grey matter of the spinal cord is organized into left and right dorsal (sensory) horns, intermediate zones, and left and right ventral (motor) horns. Further subdivisions can be made. The dorsal horn can be divided into three main groups of cells, which receive the major somatic sensory input. The intermediate zone includes columns of cells associated with sympathetic (thoracolumbar region, lateral horns) and parasympathetic (sacral region) autonomic control, in addition to groups of cells involved in somatic sensory and motor functions. The ventral horn can be subdivided according to the groups of muscles innervated; these will vary at different levels of the spinal cord.

The white matter of the spinal cord can also be differentiated because it is made up of bundles (or tracts) of nerve fibres travelling along the longitudinal axis of the cord. Some of these tracts are illustrated in **Fig. 2.2.8**.

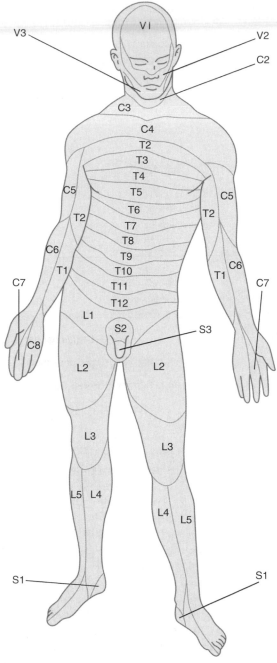

**Figure 2.2.7** Distribution of spinal nerves and branches of the trigeminal nerve to segments of the body surface. Each segment is named for the principal nerve that serves it. C = cervical segments; L = lumbar segments; S = sacral segments; T = thoracic segments; V = trigeminal segments. *Note*: anatomists do not agree entirely on the designation of specific segments, party because of the extensive overlap of the neurones that supply them

The shape of the spinal cord varies at different levels. In particular, two enlargements of the grey matter at cervical and lumbar levels reflect the greater number of cells required for innervation of the arms, legs and extremities. At higher levels, more white matter is present because ascending sensory fibres are added by progressively more rostral dermatomes and, at the same time, descending motor fibres are still coursing caudally to their target muscles and glands.

## Cranial nerves

The particular significance of the cranial nerves is that they conduct sensory information from the important special sense organs, such as the eye and the ear; they also control the voluntary muscles involved in facial expression and speech. In addition, they are involved in sensory and motor functions of visceral organs. The sensory branches of the cranial nerves are arranged in a similar manner to the dorsal roots of the spinal cord, with the cell bodies of the afferent fibres grouped in ganglia that lie outside the CNS. Thus, the cell bodies of the optic nerve are the ganglion cells of the retina and the spiral ganglion of the cochlea contains the cell bodies of the auditory nerve.

The cranial nerves can be identified with little difficulty when the brain is viewed from the inferior (ventral) aspect. **Figure 2.2.9** illustrates the points of entry of the cranial nerves and **Table 2.2.1** summarizes their individual functions.

## The brain

Before a brief outline of the various part of the brain can be considered, a number of issues regarding nomenclature need to be addressed.

The term '**cortex**' is used in association with several brain structures, as in 'cerebral cortex' and 'cerebellar cortex'. The term refers to the mantle of cell bodies (grey matter) that surrounds the agglomerated nerve axons (white matter). This arrangement of grey matter outside and white matter inside is the reverse of that found in the spinal cord, where the nerve fibres course up and down the cord in bundles, which surround the central area of grey matter. This reversal of the relative positions of grey and white matter allows ascending fibres in the spinal cord to fan out in the brain to reach the cells of higher brain structures and descending fibres from the brain to gather together as they descend to the cord.

The term '**nucleus**' is also used in a specific way when referring to parts of the nervous system. A nucleus refers to a mass of cell bodies that are grouped together because of their proximity and their structural and functional relatedness. Nuclei appear as discrete masses of grey matter embedded in the core of the brain. This use of the term 'nucleus' must be distinguished from the conventional use of the word to indicate the nucleus of an individual cell.

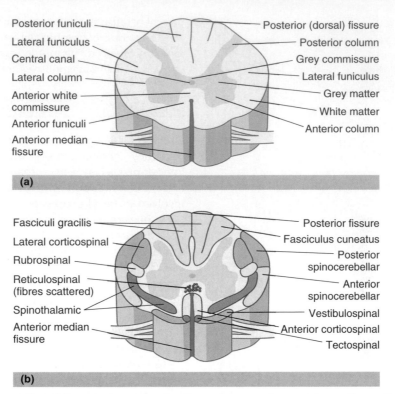

Posterior funiculi — Posterior (dorsal) fissure
Lateral funiculus — Posterior column
Central canal — Grey commissure
Lateral column — Lateral funiculus
Anterior white commissure — Grey matter
Anterior funiculi — White matter
Anterior median fissure — Anterior column

(a)

Fasciculi gracilis — Posterior fissure
Lateral corticospinal — Fasciculus cuneatus
Rubrospinal — Posterior spinocerebellar
Reticulospinal (fibres scattered) — Anterior spinocerebellar
Spinothalamic — Vestibulospinal
Anterior median fissure — Anterior corticospinal
Tectospinal

(b)

**Figure 2.2.8**  A cross-section of the spinal cord showing the major ascending and descending pathways

## The cerebrum

Looked at from the side, the human brain is dominated by the cerebrum and is shaped rather like an oversized boxing glove, with the lateral sulcus representing the separation between the thumb and the fist of the glove (**Fig. 2.2.10**). The brain shows many convolutions. The raised ridges of these convolutions are called **gyri** (singular: gyrus) and the slit-like indentations are called **sulci** (singular: sulcus). The outer surface of the cerebrum consists entirely of cortex, which follows the contours of the gyri and sulci. The corrugations of the cerebral cortex enable approximately $0.2\,m^2$ of cortex to fit inside the cranium.

If the brain is viewed from above, it can be seen that the cerebrum is composed of two halves, or **hemispheres**, with a clear line of separation running along the midline. This deep midline sulcus is called the **midsagittal sulcus**, or midsagittal fissure. In each hemisphere of the brain, another sulcus is clearly seen running at right angles to the midsagittal fissure down the convexity of the lateral surface of the brain, roughly in the midcoronal plane. This is called the **central sulcus** (see **Fig. 2.2.10**).

Each cerebral hemisphere can be subdivided into six lobes. The large area anterior to the central sulcus and superior to the lateral sulcus is referred to as the **frontal lobe**. The area inferior to the lateral sulcus (which comprises the thumb of the boxing glove) is

called the **temporal lobe**. The area posterior or to the central sulcus is called the **parietal lobe** and the area at the very back of the brain, which is posterior to a line taken roughly vertically from the preoccipital notch (**see Fig. 2.2.10**), is called the **occipital lobe**. The major portion of the occipital lobe lies within the midsagittal fissure and can be seen only when the two halves of the brain are separated. The **insula**, or central lobe of cerebral cortex, is revealed when the frontal and temporal lobes are eased apart along the line of the lateral sulcus, thus separating the thumb and the fist of the boxing glove. The insula cortex lies in the depths of the lateral sulcus. Finally, the **limbic lobe** is a ring of cortex on the medial surface of the brain; it can be seen if the brain is divided along the line of the midsagittal fissure (**see Fig. 2.2.21**).

Another gross subdivision of the cerebral cortex is the distinction made between **primary projection areas** and **association areas**. The projection areas comprise the primary sensory and primary motor areas of cerebral cortex. The primary sensory areas of the cerebral cortex receive sensory afferent inputs arising from the periphery. The strip of cortex of the postcentral gyrus, which follows the line of the central sulcus and lies posterior to it, is the projection area for somatosensation (principally touch and position sense). The area at the posterior extremity of the occipital lobe is the primary projection area for the

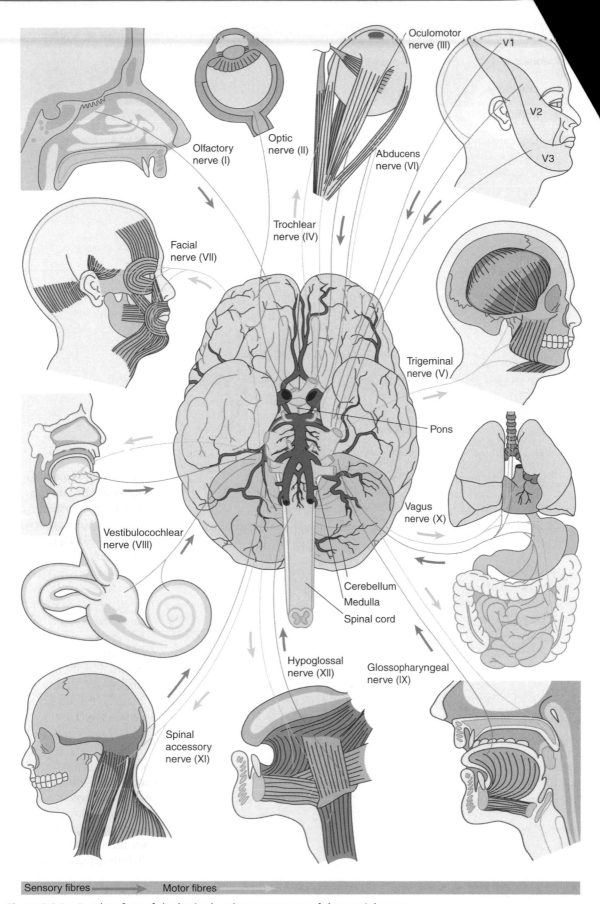

Olfactory nerve (I)

Optic nerve (II)

Oculomotor nerve (III)

Abducens nerve (VI)

V1

V2

V3

Trochlear nerve (IV)

Facial nerve (VII)

Trigeminal nerve (V)

Pons

Vagus nerve (X)

Vestibulocochlear nerve (VIII)

Cerebellum
Medulla
Spinal cord

Hypoglossal nerve (XII)

Glossopharyngeal nerve (IX)

Spinal accessory nerve (XI)

Sensory fibres ⟶   Motor fibres ⟶

**Figure 2.2.9**   Basal surface of the brain showing emergence of the cranial nerves

## ...f the cranial nerves

| | | ...unction |
|---|---|---|
| | | Afferent – smell |
| | | Afferent – vision |
| ...III | ...motor | Efferent – eye movements (to inferior and superior rectus, internal rectus and inferior oblique muscles, also to iris and ciliary muscles) |
| IV | Trochlear | Efferent – eye movements (to superior oblique muscles) |
| V | Trigeminal | Afferent – somatic sense (from anterior half of head, including face, nose, mouth and teeth)<br>Efferent – to muscles of mastication |
| VI | Abducens | Efferent – eye movements (to external rectus muscle) |
| VII | Facial | Afferent – taste and somatic sense (from tongue and soft palate)<br>Efferent – to muscles of face (controlling facial expression), plus parasympathetic outflow to salivary glands (submaxilliary and sublingual glands) |
| VIII | Vestibulocochlear | Afferent – hearing and balance |
| IX | Glossopharyngeal | Afferent – taste and somatic sense from posterior third of tongue and from pharynx<br>Efferent – to pharyngeal muscles (controlling swallowing), plus parasympathetic outflow to salivary glands (parotid gland) |
| X | Vagus | Efferent – taste (from epiglottis) and sensory nerves from heart, lungs, bronchi, trachea, pharynx, digestive tract and external ear<br>Efferent – parasympathetic outflow to heart, lungs, bronchi and digestive tract |
| XI | Accessory | Efferent – to larynx and pharynx, plus to muscles of neck and shoulder (controlling head and shoulder movement) |
| XII | Hypoglossal | Efferent – to muscles of tongue and neck |

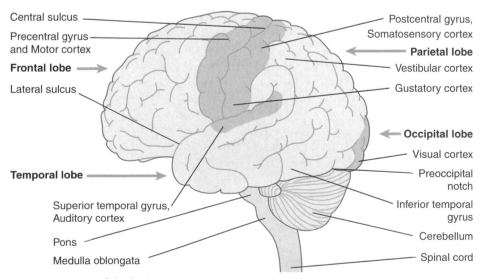

**Figure 2.2.10** Lateral aspect of the brain

sense of vision. The primary projection area for the sense of hearing lies in the depths of the lateral sulcus. Primary projection areas for taste and smell can also be identified; that for taste is illustrated in **Fig. 2.4.21**. The primary motor area of cortex is that part of the cerebral cortex that projects descending efferent nerve fibres to the motor neurones of the spinal cord. The primary motor cortex lies in the precentral gyrus – the strip of cortex which follows the line of the central sulcus and is just anterior to it.

Six horizontal cell layers can be distinguished over most of the cerebral cortex but there are only two major subtypes of nerve cells within the cortex. The two subtypes are **pyramidal cells**, which vary in size and tend to have long axons, and **stellate** (or granule) **cells**, which tend to have much shorter axons and make fewer synaptic contacts.

## Midline structures

If the brain is bisected along the line of the midsagittal fissure, a view of midline structures is revealed. This is represented in **Fig. 2.2.11**.

### Forebrain structures

It can be seen from **Fig. 2.2.11** that the cerebral cortex descends into the midsagittal fissure. In particular,

the cingulate gyrus forms part of the ring of bic lobe of the cerebral cortex. The **corpus call** is a thick band of nerve fibres that connects the cerebral hemispheres and is hence seen in cro section. The corpus callosum maintains a constant flo of information between the two halves of the cerebral cortex.

The **thalamus** is a major centre of neural integration. It can be thought of as a relay-station interpolated between the cerebral cortex and lower brain structures. The two thalami (one thalamus in each half brain) are located on either side of the third ventricle.

The **hypothalamus** is situated inferior to the thalamus and is functionally related to the autonomic nervous system (see Chapter 2.5). Cells of the hypothalamus are involved in the control of food and water intake, in body temperature regulation and in emotional expression. The hypothalamus is also directly involved in the control of the activity of the **pituitary gland**. The pituitary gland – the 'master gland' – in turn controls and integrates the activity of other endocrine glands (see Chapter 2.6).

The **pineal body** is attached to the roof of the third ventricle and lies directly in the midline. It is a secretory organ associated with the endocrine system and contains melatonin, serotonin and other biologically active amines. As yet, its functions remain unclear,

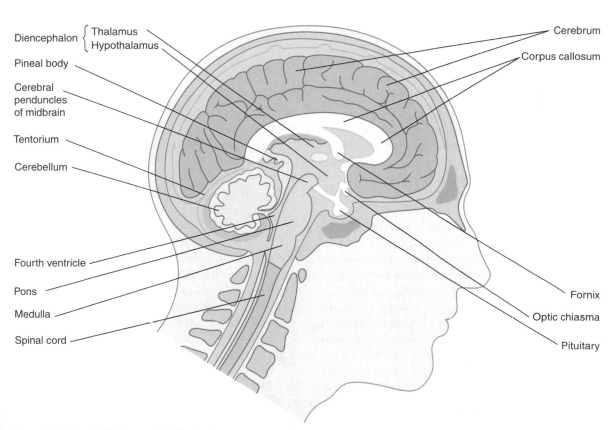

**Figure 2.2.11**    Medial aspect of the brain

SYSTEM

...exual development at

...the **inferior colliculi**
...of the midbrain. The superior
...ed with visual functions and the
...with hearing.

...to the cerebral aqueduct, the major visible
...rain structures are the **cerebral peduncles**. These
are large trunks of ascending and descending nerve
fibres lying either side of the midline.

## Hindbrain structures

The major hindbrain structures include the pons, the
medulla oblongata and the cerebellum. The **pons**
and the **medulla oblongata** lie ventral to the fourth
ventricle and are the level at which most cranial
nerves enter the brain. The pons has many clearly
defined transverse fibres crossing the midline, and
both pons and medulla contain ascending and
descending nerve fibres.

The reticular formation is a loose framework of
diffuse neurones, located in the pons, medulla and
midbrain, with connections to the cerebral cortex.
It is sometimes referred to as the reticular activating
system (RAS). Its functions include providing continuous impulses to the muscles to support the body
against gravity, as well as control of the sleep–
wakefulness cycle and the level of consciousness.

The mesencephalic portion of the reticular activating system comprises of grey matter located in
the pons and medulla. If this area is stimulated,
impulses pass to the thalamus and large areas of
the cerebral cortex, resulting in an increase in
cortical activity. The second portion of the reticular activating system is the thalamic part, which
comprises the grey matter in the thalamus. Similar
to what has already been described, stimulation of
the thalamic portion results in increased cortical
activity. The mesencephalic portion is responsible
for consciousness and the thalamic portion is concerned with awakening from deep sleep (arousal).

Arousal occurs when the reticular activating system is stimulated by a sensory signal, e.g. bright
light, which in turn raises the activity of the cortex
and the individual is roused from sleep. This state
of alertness is maintained via a feedback system in
which the reticular activating system, the cerebral
cortex and the skeletal muscles stimulate one
another continuously. The result is a state of wakefulness termed **consciousness**. The level of consciousness depends on the number of feedback
circuits operating at a given time. Sleep is the natural state that occurs when the feedback systems

are inhibited. Consciousness can be affected by a
number of other factors, such as medication and
damage to the nervous system. This is elaborated
later on in this chapter.

The pons and medulla also contain nuclei responsible for the reflex control of essential functions such
as respiration, heart rate and vasomotor activity. These
functions are termed **brainstem reflexes**.

The **cerebellum** is a large outgrowth forming the
roof of the fourth ventricle. It consists of an outer
mantle of cortex, which is highly convoluted, together
with underlying associated white matter and deeper-
lying nuclei. The cerebellum is essential for normal
motor coordination.

## Structures lateral to the midline

### Forebrain structures

The **basal ganglia** are made up of three large nuclei
that lie lateral to the thalamus (**Fig. 2.2.12**). The three
structures are the **globus pallidus**, the **putamen** and
the **caudate nucleus**. The putamen and the globus
pallidus together form the **lentiform nucleus**. The
caudate nucleus and putamen are together referred
to as the **corpus striatum**. The basal ganglia exercise
important influences on motor activity.

The caudate nucleus has a head and a long tail that
sweeps around underneath the lateral ventricle (**see
Fig. 2.2.12**). The tail of the caudate merges into the
amygdaloid nucleus (or **amygdala**). The **amygdaloid
nucleus**, deep within the temporal lobe, is associated
with the olfactory system and with emotional
behaviour.

The **hippocampus** lies on the medial wall of the
temporal lobe. It follows a path similar to that of the
tail of the caudate nucleus, curving around beneath
the lateral ventricle. The hippocampus represents that
portion of the limbic lobe that is composed of evolu-
tionarily older cortex. The hippocampus has been
associated with several different behavioural functions
such as memory, spatial orientation and emotional
responses.

The **internal capsule** is the large bundle of fibres
passing to and from the cerebral cortex and linking
the cerebrum with lower brain structures. The fibres
of the internal capsule pass to and from the cerebral
peduncles, between the thalamus and the lentiform
nucleus. They then fan out to the cortex.

### Midbrain structures

The **subthalamus** (subthalamic nucleus), the **red
nucleus** and the **substantia nigra** are all midbrain
nuclei lying lateral to the midline (**see Fig. 2.3.8**).
They are all concerned with the control of movement

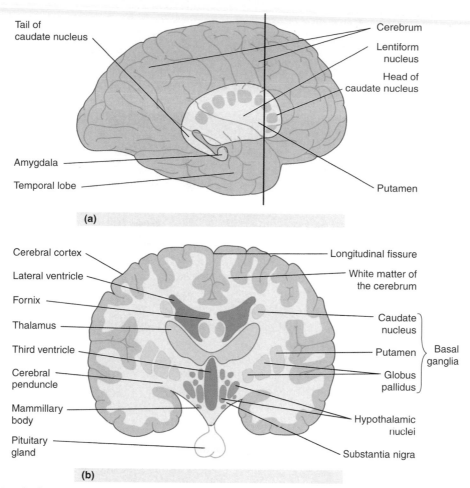

**Figure 2.2.12** The location of the principal basal ganglia (a) in lateral view and (b) in a frontal section through the cerebrum and part of the hypothalamus

and they have extensive connections with the basal ganglia.

## Somatosensation

### Cortical representation

Nerve fibres from thalamic nuclei, in particular the ventroposterolateral nucleus, project to the primary and secondary sensory areas of the cerebral cortex.

Projections to the primary sensory area maintain a strict somatotopic organization such that the representation of body parts in the postcentral gyrus forms a **sensory homunculus** of the opposite half of the body (**Fig. 2.2.13**). The size of the area of cortex receiving sensory input from any particular part of the body is a function of the degree of innervation rather than of the physical size of that body part. Consequently, the sensory homunculus appears distorted because of the greater innervation of the lips, tongue and thumb compared with that of the trunk and legs.

### CLINICAL APPLICATIONS

Extensive parietal lobe lesions are associated with sensory inattention and disturbances of the body schema. That is, patients show a disordered appreciation of their own body image. For example, they might ignore parts of their own body, feeling that the arm or leg contralateral to the lesion is not theirs. This can even extend to a patient washing and shaving only half the face and combing hair on only one side of the head. Other extensive parietal lobe lesions, especially those involving the lower portions of the parietal lobe, can lead to fairly generalized disturbances of spatial relationships. These can be demonstrated by the inability of patients to learn finger mazes, to comprehend maps and follow directions, or to assemble and compare objects and patterns in two or three dimensions.

The sensory projection areas of the cerebral cortex receive information via the pathways of the somatosensory system; this is more explained fully in Chapter 2.3.

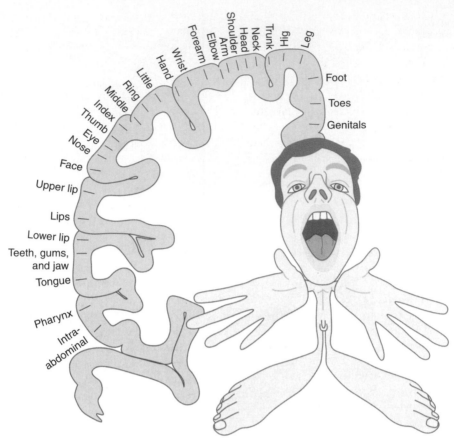

**Figure 2.2.13** The sensory homunculus showing the amount of the cerebral cortex devoted to sensory input from each part of the body

## The central nervous system and motor control

Motor activity ultimately involves the effects of peripheral motor neurones upon muscle cells. For example, the activity involved in a skilled act, such as catching a cricket ball, eventually rests upon the integration of motor units so that tension and force in various muscles are altered appropriately. The complexity of this integration can be seen when the muscle coordination necessary for a fielder to catch a cricket ball is considered in detail. The muscles directly involved in the catch, that is those of the fingers, thumb and hand, contract in a coordinated fashion at precisely the right moment. Other muscle groups that are not directly involved in the catch act synergistically. For example, the muscles of the shoulder and arm act to position the hand correctly in space. Postural muscles of the trunk and legs position the body to receive the ball and adapt to the rapid deceleration of the ball when it reaches the hand. The flight of the approaching ball is followed by smooth pursuit movements of the eyes. Moreover, if the ball is temporarily obscured from view, the fielder is able to predict its likely position when it

comes back into view, and can adjust position in relation to this predicted flightpath. In summary, the execution of this type of skilled act involves the coordination of many muscle groups in a precisely controlled manner and in such a way as to allow for the alteration and adjustment of activity in response to moment-to-moment feedback from sensory receptors.

Many aspects of the central nervous control of motor activity have been elucidated and will be discussed in this section. Many brain structures are implicated in the control of motor activity. Traditionally, motor control has been subdivided into three neural systems. First, the **pyramidal system**, which consists of a fast and direct descending pathway from the motor cortex; second, the **extrapyramidal system**, which consists of a multisynaptic pathway involving many brain structures, of which the most important are the basal ganglia; and third, the **cerebellum**, which interacts with both the pyramidal and extrapyramidal motor pathways. In addition to this division of the motor system, the traditional conception of motor control has implied a hierarchical arrangement of these various subunits. Thus, the pyramidal system has been regarded as the most important subunit because its influences on the musculature are fast, direct and concentrated particularly upon distal muscles, such as those of the fingers and hand, which perform skilled acts. The extrapyramidal system has been seen as performing a supporting role because it consists of more diffuse and slower pathways and its influences are generally more strongly concentrated upon the proximal muscle groups of the arms, legs and trunk. However, it has been argued more recently that this traditional view of central motor control underrepresents the role of the extrapyramidal system.

## CLINICAL APPLICATIONS

The problem of ascribing a subservient role to the extrapyramidal system is clear when the effects of lesions to the pyramidal system are considered. For example, damage to the hand and arm areas of the motor cortex leads to severe motor impairment of the contralateral forelimb musculature. However, this impairment is, for the most part, only temporary. After a period of time, motor control is usually regained over all but the most distal muscle groups. An inability to clasp the fingers in a grip is the only permanent disability found in experimental primates. It is assumed that the extrapyramidal motor pathways are responsible for re-establishing this high degree of motor control.

The traditional view of central motor control has stressed the overriding importance of the pyramidal tract and the motor cortex. It has even been suggested that the conscious intent, or 'will', to move develops in the motor cortex. However, clinical investigations involving the electrical stimulation of the motor cortex in conscious patients have disproved this hypothesis. Patients stimulated in this way develop twitches and movements in peripheral muscle groups but they report no feeling of any intention to make these movements. Indeed, they report that the movements seem to be outside their control. In addition, more recent evidence from experimental studies in animals has shown that a great deal of neural activity in many different areas of the brain precedes an intentional motor act. It seems reasonable to assume that this widespread preparatory neural activity is responsible for converting a conscious intention into a planned and precisely controlled coordination of muscular activity. Thus, the motor cortex rather than being the location of the intention to act, in fact appears to be involved only towards the end of the process of neural integration.

## Motor cortex

The motor cortex occupies the precentral gyrus of the cerebral cortex, extending medially into the midsagittal fissure. It is topographically organized so that the muscle groups to which its cells project can be represented as a homunculus. This homunculus (**Fig. 2.2.14**) extends from the toes and feet, represented in the depths of the midsagittal fissure, through the areas projecting to the trunk, arm and hand, and finally to the cells projecting to the face, lips and tongue, which lie at the lateral end of the precentral gyrus. The various body parts of the homunculus appear distorted in size and shape according to the relative extent of the innervation of the musculature.

The motor cortex receives inputs from the supplementary motor cortex, from somatosensory cortex, from the contralateral motor cortex of the opposite cerebral hemisphere, and from the thalamus. The thalamic nuclei concerned are those of the ventroposterolateral nucleus, the ventrolateral nucleus and the ventral anterior nucleus. The ventrolateral nucleus is of particular importance as it relays signals from the cerebellum and from the basal ganglia and thus allows for the interplay of neural signals between the various subunits of the motor system.

The efferent fibres of the motor cortex project in a topographically organized manner to the basal ganglia, the thalamus, the red nucleus, the lateral reticular formation and the spinal cord.

## Pyramidal tract neurones

Because the motor cortex contributes to extrapyramidal pathways as well as to the corticospinal tracts, it is not possible to identify the motor cortex as being exclusively part of the pyramidal system. Nevertheless, the medullary pyramids consist almost entirely of corticospinal axons and, therefore, it is possible to manipulate pyramidal tract fibres exclusively at this level.

## CLINICAL APPLICATIONS

### PYRAMIDAL DISORDERS

Damage to the corticospinal tract at the medullary pyramids reveals an uncontaminated picture of the results of pyramidal tract injury. The major difference between a section of the medullary pyramid and removal of the motor cortex is that the spasticity and exaggerated reflexes seen following damage to the motor cortex are not present with a pure section of the corticospinal tract. Instead, a decrease in muscle tone in the limbs is observed, together with a loss of reflexes. From this it can be assumed that the spasticity seen after damage to the motor cortex is the result of damage to extrapyramidal pathways. One response that is of particular clinical importance as being diagnostic of pyramidal tract damage is the Babinski response (see p. 94).

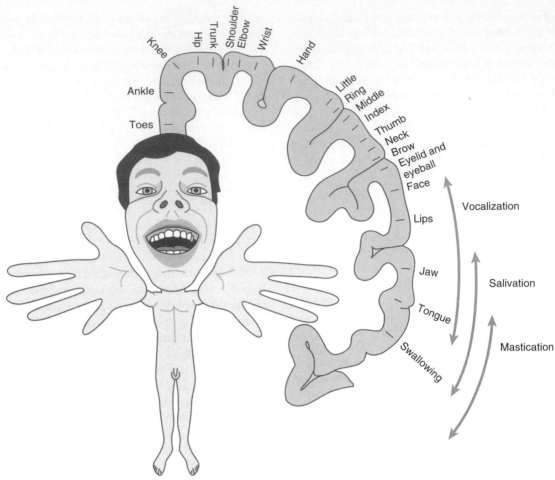

**Figure 2.2.14** The motor homunculus showing the amount of the cerebral cortex devoted to control of each part of the body.

**Cerebrovascular accident (stroke)** is the third most common cause of death in the Western world and occurs most frequently in the older population. It is characterized by a variable degree of neurological deficit produced either as a consequence of cerebral ischaemia caused by thrombus, embolism and/or atherosclerosis, or as a result of cerebral haemorrhage. It frequently occurs in the region of the internal capsule (**see Fig. 2.3.8**), causing disruption of major inhibitory and facilitatory descending motor influences. Depending on the severity of the disturbance, a weakness or paralysis of one-half of the body musculature (hemiparesis/hemiplegia) occurs contralateral to the site of the damage. If the stroke occurs in the left hemisphere, speech might also be lost because of damage to the speech motor pathways.

Initially, the paralysis is flaccid, presumably a shock response to a massive loss of descending influences, but hypertonus (spastic paralysis) of the affected muscles usually follows. Considerable recovery of motor activity can occur following a stroke, particularly in the lower limbs.

The motor deficit associated with stroke might be accompanied by sensory loss, depending on the extent to which ascending sensory pathways in the internal capsule are also damaged.

A characteristic feature of the disruption of descending motor pathways that can be caused by stroke is the persistence, and even exaggeration, of emotional facial expression, despite the loss of voluntary control of facial muscles. This occurs because the pathways controlling emotional facial expression arise from parts of the limbic lobe of the brain rather than from the motor cortex.

The physical problems that present in a patient who has suffered a major stroke, then, will include some or all of the following: alteration in conscious level, hemiparesis/hemiplegia, speech problems and visual field defects. Some stroke victims are managed at home, with support from their general practitioner and community nursing services, whereas others merit admission to hospital due to the seriousness of their condition or because of their home background.

A small number of patients are treated by surgical means: carotid endarterectomy involves the removal of atheroma from the internal carotid artery, thereby re-establishing circulation to the brain. A second procedure involves anastomosing the superior temporal artery to the middle cerebral artery, creating a bypass collateral to the brain. However, for the vast majority of patients, treatment is conservative and is aimed towards rehabilitating the individual to his or her fullest potential. Nursing management is individually tailored according to the main presenting problems.

**Alteration in conscious level**. The care appropriate for the unconscious patient is given. Emphasis must be placed on the maintenance of adequate pulmonary function, necessitating a patent airway and efficient gaseous exchange; this is a priority.

**Hemiparesis/hemiplegia** is a weakness or paralysis down one side of the body. Proper positioning and support of the affected limbs in good alignment will assist in better mobility. Frequent alteration of body position is also necessary, to avoid the development of skin breakdown.

**Speech problems** commonly involve dysphasia, which can be expressive (an inability to express oneself) or receptive (an inability to comprehend the spoken word). Specialist advice and help are obtained from the speech and language therapist, who will assess the patient's deficit and create a treatment programme. It is beneficial for the nurse to be involved in all aspects of the patient's therapy so that it can continue in the therapist's absence.

**Visual problems** can include field defects, diplopia (double vision) or blurring of vision. Diplopia can be abolished with the use of an eye patch, and the nurse should be aware of the decreased visual acuity and its attendant problems for the patient with blurred vision. Identification of the visual defect and compensating for this by approaching patients from their unaffected sides are appropriate management (this is elaborated on in Chapter 2.4). Many other problems can arise, involving intellectual and emotional deficits, e.g. lability or confusion, and other physical aspects, e.g. swallowing difficulties.

**Rehabilitation**: The active promotion and restoration of independence is the goal for all patients following stroke. Carr & Shepherd (2002) provide excellent guidance on rehabilitation following stroke. The role of the nurse with a hemiplegic patient should include consideration of the problems encountered by this patient in relation to loss of balance on the affected side, sensory disturbance that inhibits movement, spasticity and loss of free selection of precision movements.

The main nursing interventions identified during the acute period will often be continued during the rehabilitative phase, with the emphasis altering according to the patient's needs. Involving the patient's family in the recovery phase is crucial as their cooperation can result in the increased likelihood of success. The use of self-help leaflets and pamphlets from the Stroke Association should be considered along with help and support from appropriate community groups.

## Extrapyramidal motor control

### The basal ganglia

Strictly speaking, extrapyramidal motor control refers to all neural integration of motor activity occurring outside the influence of the corticospinal tracts. Nevertheless, the cerebellum is a clearly distinguishable brain structure and hence its function tends to be assessed separately. Again, the red nucleus forms a major extrapyramidal motor pathway but it is perhaps better considered alongside the pyramidal system because of the close parallels between the fuctions of the pyramidal tract and the rubrospinal tract. Consequently, the term 'extrapyramidal motor control' has come to refer to the influences upon motor activity of a group of brain structures, the most important of which are the basal ganglia.

The basal ganglia comprise the **caudate nucleus, putamen** and the **globus pallidus (see Figs 2.2.12 and 2.3.8)**. The caudate nucleus and putamen are together referred to as the **corpus striatum**, and make up by far the largest subcortical cell mass in the human brain. Caudate and putamen both consist of numerous small neurones interspersed with a scattering of a few large cells. The globus pallidus, on the other hand, contains large, widely spaced neurones and is divisible into a medial and a lateral part. The putamen lies immediately lateral to the globus pallidus and, together, these two nuclei are referred to collectively as the **lentiform** (or **lenticular**) **nucleus**.

### Extrapyramidal pathways

In each hemisphere, all areas of neocortex send fibres to both the caudate nucleus and the putamen of the same side. From the corpus striatum (caudate plus putamen), nerve axons pass through the globus pallidus and descend to the **substantia nigra**, a nucleus located in the brainstem. Axon collaterals of this pathway synapse with cells of the globus pallidus. Axons from the medial part of the globus pallidus project to the thalamus, in particular to the ventral anterior and ventrolateral nuclei. The ventrolateral nucleus of the thalamus in turn projects axons to the cortex. Together, all these synaptic connections make

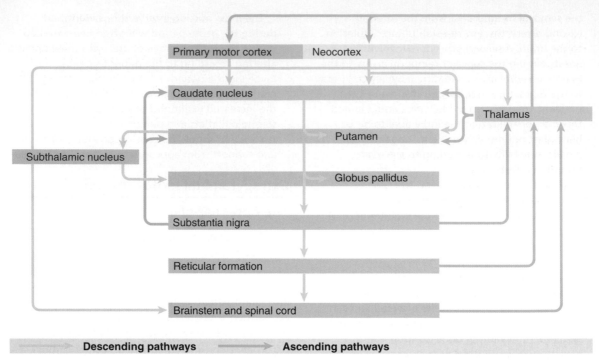

**Descending pathways** ——▶ **Ascending pathways**

**Figure 2.2.15** Schematic representation of the neural interconnections of the extrapyramidal motor system (adapted from DeLong, 1974)

up a feedback loop from cortex to striatum to globus pallidus to thalamus and back to the cortex (**Fig. 2.2.15**). The implication of this is that information from the entire neocortex can be processed and fed back to the motor cortex via the basal ganglia and thalamus in preparation for motor activity.

In addition to their contribution to the corticocortical feedback loop, the basal ganglia also make other important neural connections. For example, they receive input from the intralaminar nuclei of the thalamus, to which they also project. This connects the basal ganglia with the activity of the reticular formation, because the reticular formation provides a major source of input to the intralaminar nuclei of the thalamus. The cerebellum also has indirect access to the extrapyramidal circuits of the basal ganglia as cerebellar fibres terminate in areas of the thalamus (the ventral anterior and ventrolateral nuclei), which overlap with the areas of termination of fibres from the globus pallidus. The basal ganglia also have reciprocal connections with the **subthalamic nucleus** and the substantia nigra (**see Figs 2.2.15 and 2.3.8**). Indirect pathways via the substantia nigra also project to the superior colliculus and the reticular formation.

## Extrapyramidal function

The complexities of the extrapyramidal neural connections suggest that the basal ganglia have diffuse and widespread influences on motor control.

Unfortunately, the detailed functions of these neural connections remain largely unknown. In terms of their physiological characteristics, it is known that the caudate nucleus and putamen are generally excitatory, whereas the outflow from the globus pallidus tends to be inhibitory. It has also been found that neurones of the basal ganglia tend to fire before those of the motor cortex and cerebellum. Thus, the latencies between extrapyramidal activity and an associated muscle contraction tend to be longer than those seen in the motor cortex or cerebellum.

### CLINICAL APPLICATIONS

### EXTRAPYRAMIDAL DISORDERS

The neural connections between the striatum and the substantia nigra have been implicated in the neurological condition known as **Parkinson's disease** or Parkinsonism.

Parkinson's disease (paralysis agitans) is characterized by three features. First, patients display a rhythmical tremor at a frequency of approximately six times a second, which is usually seen most clearly in the head and hands. The tremor disappears during sleep and when an intentional act, such as reaching and grasping, is carried out. For this reason it is referred to as a **non-intention tremor**. A second feature is a unique muscular rigidity, which is clearly seen in the facial muscles and gives the patient an expressionless 'mask-like' appearance. The third feature of Parkinson's disease is a slowness in the initiation and execution of movements (bradykinesia). Parkinson's disease is progressive and is generally associated with older people.

The tremor and ridigity of Parkinson's disease are principally attributable to the loss of the inhibitory influences of the basal ganglia, leading to an exaggeration of excitatory descending cortical output. The mechanism involved in this disinhibition appears to begin with the degeneration of cells in the substantia nigra. The basal ganglia and substantia nigra have a reciprocal neural connection (**see Fig. 2.2.15**). The neurotransmitter used in the striatonigral circuit appears to be **gamma-aminobutyric acid** (GABA). The reciprocal nigrostriatal pathway uses **dopamine** as the neurotransmitter. In Parkinsonism, the cells of the substantia nigra, which synthesize dopamine, degenerate. The degeneration of these cells closely parallels a reduction in dopamine levels in the corpus striatum. Pharmacological methods of treatment for Parkinsonism can raise dopamine levels in the striatum and can significantly ameliorate patients' symptoms. Administration of the dopamine precursor, L-dopa, especially in association with the administration of carbidopa, which blocks the decarboxylation and transamination of L-dopa, has been found to result in a marked remission of the symptoms of Parkinsonism.

Despite this clinical success, it should be noted that L-dopa therapy provides only short-term relief from Parkinson's disease. Unfortunately, this therapy does not halt the degeneration of cells of the substantia nigra, and the cause and mechanism of this degeneration remain unknown. Some success has been achieved with the transplantation of fetal cells, although this treatment remains controversial.

The tremor, rigidity and bradykinesia experienced by these patients pose the main nursing problems. These can be overcome in the following ways:

- The provision of a low bed with a firm mattress, located near to toilet facilities. This will ease the problems associated with getting out of bed and poor bladder control.
- Adapted clothing, e.g. replacing buttons and zips with Velcro.
- Rising from a high-backed chair rather than a low one is easier for the patient; such a chair should be provided.
- Initiating walking can pose a problem. To overcome this, the attendant should gently rock the patient back and forward.
- Occasionally a patient will freeze up and be unable to move. This is remedied by suggesting that the patient imagines a step to get over; this can achieve recommencement of movement.

The term '**chorea**' refers to involuntary, rapid, jumpy movements of the limbs and facial muscles. These abnormal movements are associated with a number of clinical conditions, including the severe and fatal **Huntington's disease**. Huntington's disease is an hereditary condition that usually shows itself in the fourth or fifth decade of life. It is a progressive disorder involving chorea (irregular, spasmodic movements beyond the patients' control), dementia and eventual death.

Huntington's disease has been demonstrated to be associated with the degeneration of cells of the striatum. In particular, small cholinergic intrastriatal neurones are destroyed, along with others that project to the substantia nigra in the GABA-ergic striatonigral pathway. It has been suggested that the destruction of these cells disinhibits the substantia nigra. The substantia nigra, by way of its reciprocal pathway, then exerts excessive inhibitory influences upon the outflow from the basal ganglia to the thalamus. In this way the motor outflow to the cortex is affected and the abnormal movements result. At present, however, these suggestions for the mechanism of the disorder remain speculative.

Other signs of extrapyramidal disorder include athetosis and ballisms. **Athetosis** refers to slow writhing movements of the fingers, hands and arms. It has been associated with damage to the putamen and globus pallidus. **Ballisms** are violent and unexpected flailing movements, often involving the proximal muscles of one side of the body. These abnormal movements have been associated with damage to the subthalamic nucleus. **Tardive dyskinesia** is an abnormality of movement caused by exposure to antipsychotic drugs, such as chlorpromazine (Largactil). Antipsychotic drugs have an effect upon dopaminergic pathways in the brain and, consequently, these drugs can affect normal extrapyramidal activity. Tardive dyskinesia is therefore a side-effect of antipsychotic drug therapy.

## The cerebellum

### Anatomy

The cerebellum is a very large brain structure lying underneath the occipital lobes and is separated from them by a fold in the dura mater called the **tentorium** (**see Fig. 2.2.11**). The surface of the cerebellum appears as a highly convoluted mantle of cells, the **cerebellar cortex**. Beneath the cerebellar cortex lies white matter and in the depths of the white matter

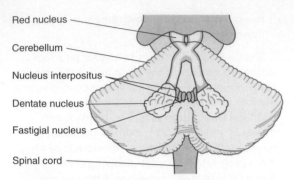

Red nucleus

Cerebellum

Nucleus interpositus

Dentate nucleus

Fastigial nucleus

Spinal cord

**Figure 2.2.16**   The cerebellum and cerebellar nuclei

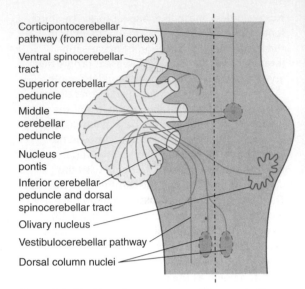

Corticopontocerebellar pathway (from cerebral cortex)

Ventral spinocerebellar tract

Superior cerebellar peduncle

Middle cerebellar peduncle

Nucleus pontis

Inferior cerebellar peduncle and dorsal spinocerebellar tract

Olivary nucleus

Vestibulocerebellar pathway

Dorsal column nuclei

**Figure 2.2.17**   Neural connections of the cerebellum showing inputs to the cerebellum

are three pairs of deep-lying cerebellar nuclei – the **fastigial**, **interpositus** and **dentate nuclei** (**Fig. 2.2.16**). These nuclei provide nearly all the efferent outflow of the cerebellum.

The cerebellum appears as a bilaterally symmetrical structure with a central portion, the **vermis**, separating the two halves. Unlike the neocortex, the cerebellum does not possess any interhemispheric nerve fibres and so does not transfer information from one side of the brain to the other.

The structure and organization of the cerebellar cortex are uniform and relatively simple. The cortical mantle contains three layers of cells. The outer layer, the molecular layer, contains small interneurones, basket cells and stellate cells. The middle layer consists of large Purkinje cells. Dendrites from the cells of the Purkinje layer extend into the molecular layer; the axons of the Purkinje cells provide the only efferent path from the cerebellar cortex. The inner layer of cortex, the granular layer, is composed of a huge number of densely packed granule (small stellate) cells.

## Cerebellar function

The cerebellum is involved in motor coordination. Essentially, it monitors both signal output from the motor cortex to muscles and the execution of a motor act via sensory inputs arising from proprioceptive and touch receptors in the periphery. It is thought that the cerebellum 'assesses' the force and rate of contraction, and the distance moved, and then feeds-back signals to the motor cortex, resulting in adjustments to the motor signal output so that the movement is executed in a smooth and coordinated fashion. For example, consider the execution of a relatively simple motor act such as drinking a cup of tea. The cerebellum monitors the muscle contraction and provides continuous feedback to the motor cortex so that, at a subconscious level, the cortex receives signals that might be expressed as 'commands', such as 'move to the right', 'move to the left', 'move up', 'move down', 'move more quickly', 'move more slowly'. These commands occur rapidly on a

moment-to-moment basis and the cup is brought to the mouth directly and smoothly, even without the aid of visual cues. It should be noted that visual and auditory inputs to the cerebellum occur via the superior and inferior colliculi.

In addition to its role in motor coordination, the cerebellum is essential for normal balance and posture control and is connected to the vestibular nuclei of the brainstem.

The **afferent inputs** to the cerebellum arise from the whole of the body as well as from higher brain centres, most importantly from the cerebral cortex (**Fig. 2.2.17**). The input from peripheral receptors carries proprioceptive and tactile information and reaches the cerebellum either directly, via the spinocerebellar pathways, or indirectly via brainstem nuclei, particularly the inferior olives. The spinocerebellar pathways arise from proprioceptive and skin afferents and project to the ipsilateral hemisphere of the cerebellum. The input from the inferior olives is contralateral and again arises from widespread sources – the olivary nuclei receive input from all quadrants of the spinal cord as well as receiving collateral branches of descending motor axons. The input from the cerebral cortex to the cerebellum arrives via the corticopontocerebellar pathway. Collaterals from descending pyramidal tract neurones, particularly those arising in the motor cortex, synapse in nuclei of the pons. From here, cells project to the contralateral hemisphere of the cerebellum.

All the **efferent fibres** of the cerebellum arise from the Purkinje cells (**Fig. 2.2.18**). Almost all these axons synapse in the deep-lying nuclei of the cerebellum. The only exception to this is the axons of those cells of the flocculonodular lobe, which pass directly and

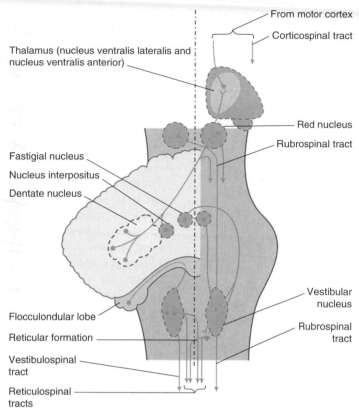

From motor cortex

Corticospinal tract

Thalamus (nucleus ventralis lateralis and nucleus ventralis anterior)

Red nucleus

Rubrospinal tract

Fastigial nucleus

Nucleus interpositus

Dentate nucleus

Vestibular nucleus

Flocculondular lobe

Reticular formation

Rubrospinal tract

Vestibulospinal tract

Reticulospinal tracts

**Figure 2.2.18**   Neural connections of the cerebellum showing outputs from the cerebellum

ipsilaterally to the vestibular nuclei of the brainstem. The cells of the fastigial nuclei project bilaterally to the vestibular nuclei, thereby complementing the cells of the flocculonodular lobe in exerting their influence upon vestibular control. Each interpositus nucleus projects mainly to the contralateral red nucleus but also sends axons to the ventrolateral nucleus of the contralateral thalamus. Cells from this thalamic nucleus project to the motor cortex. The dentate nucleus projects mainly to the ventrolateral and ventral anterior nuclei of the contralateral thalamus, and from here cells project to the motor cortex. It should be noted that although the interpositus and dentate nuclei project contralaterally, because the descending axons of the red nucleus and motor cortex also decussate in the brainstem, the influences of the interpositus and dentate nuclei are exerted over the ipsilateral musculature. This effectively constitutes a crossing and then a recrossing of nerve fibres across the midline, such that damage to one side of the cerebellum will result in dysfunction of the musculature on the same side of the body.

The cerebellar output is entirely inhibitory, with the Purkinje cells using the inhibitory transmitter gamma-aminobutyric acid (GABA). The effects of this inhibitory influence are clearly seen in the activity of vestibular nuclei after damage to the cerebellum. Such damage removes the inhibitory

influence of the cerebellum over the vestibular nuclei and, as a consequence, the increase in vestibular excitation of motor neurones leads to an exaggeration of muscle tone.

## CLINICAL APPLICATIONS

### EFFECTS OF DAMAGE

Damage to the cerebellum results in a number of disturbances of posture and movement that reflect the various neural connections of the cerebellum. Injury to the cerebellum can disturb the maintenance of balance, such that standing and walking are performed unsteadily. Patients will walk with a wide and unsteady gait, tending to deviate towards the side of the injury. Disturbance of eye movement control, such as nystagmus, might also be present, as might abnormalities of reflex movements. Disturbances of voluntary movement include an **intention tremor**. Here, a tremor develops when patients perform an intentional act. Voluntary movements are also performed in a jerky and uncoordinated fashion and misreaching can be demonstrated by asking patients to try to touch their nose. All these disturbances of fine coordination of movement can be interpreted as illustrating the cerebellum's activity as an adjuster of ongoing motor actions. For example, the neural connections between the cerebral cortex and the cerebellum relay information concerning an intended action. The information from peripheral proprioceptors to the cerebellum will in turn relay information relating the status of that action in terms of position of a limb, speed of movement and intensity of muscular contraction. The cerebellum is then able to effect the execution of the act, both via the feedback loop to the motor cortex and also by means of its outputs to rubrospinal and vestibulospinal motor neurones. It has been suggested that this intervention acts as a damping mechanism to achieve a smooth, coordinated action. Damage to the cerebellum eliminates this damping action so that an intentional movement becomes jerky. The initiation of an intentional act causes a muscle contraction and, if this is not damped by the cerebellum, it tends to overshoot. As a consequence, the cerebral cortex compensates by initiating opposing muscular contractions. However, these again overshoot and the resultant effect is that of the tremor associated with intentional acts.

## States of consciousness

A state of conscious awareness implies that the nervous system is operating at a level of functioning that allows deliberate volitional interactions with the environment. Such a broad definition covers a very wide range of states that occur in normal everyday experience – from euphoric excitement, through placid relaxation, to deep depression. All these different states will be reflected in variations in nervous activity. Beyond these, other states exist outside what is normally accepted as conscious awareness. For example, sleep, coma and hypnotic trance all reflect different levels of consciousness. Not a great deal is known at present about the neural processes that underlie states of consciousness and the concept of consciousness itself remains a baffling biological question. For example, we spend almost a third of our lives asleep and yet a comprehensive biological reason for sleep has still to be established. At present it is generally accepted that sleep serves restorative functions, although why these need to be accompanied by the dramatic changes in behaviour that are seen in sleep is not clear.

## The sleep–wakefulness cycle

### DEVELOPMENTAL ISSUES

During the first weeks of life, newborn babies demonstrate a polyphasic sleep–waking cycle (i.e. many alternating periods of sleep and waking throughout the day). This changes within weeks to a pattern of long periods of sleep at night and shorter periods of sleep during the day. By the second or third year of life the infant has adopted the typical circadian biorhythm of sleeping at night and waking during the day: the child has adapted to the rhythm of the light–dark cycle.

That the light–dark cycle plays a role in controlling the sleep–wakefulness cycle can be seen when subjects are allowed to 'free-run'. In this type of study, the subjects are kept in conditions of continuous light or continuous darkness with no knowledge of the time of day. In such circumstances, subjects tend to adopt a pattern of activity and rest that either extends beyond 24 hours or is less than 24 hours. In other words, left to themselves, subjects behave as if the 'day' is either longer or shorter than 24 hours. Much the most common finding is for subjects to behave as if the day is slightly longer than 24 hours, perhaps 25 or 26 hours. However, subjects have been reported to adopt cycles of as long as 48 hours and as short as 16 hours. From this evidence it seems that the normal cycle of activity and rest is at least partly controlled by the light–dark cycle. However, even in 'free-running' conditions all subjects maintain a typical biphasic pattern of sleep and activity. In other words, sleep is followed by activity and then sleep again and so on, in a regular diurnal pattern.

## Neurophysiology of sleep and waking

Sleep is a complex phenomenon resulting from numerous physiological processes. The pattern of sleep has been studied using electroencephalography in which the electrical activity of the brain is measured by attaching electrodes to the sleeping subject's head.

Normal sleep consists of two types: non-rapid eye movement sleep (NREM) and rapid eye movement sleep (REM). NREM sleep can be further divided into four stages:

1. A *transitional stage*, which lasts 1–7 minutes. The person is relaxed with eyes closed.
2. *Light sleep*. Dreaming commences and the subject is more difficult to rouse.
3. *Moderately deep sleep*. Occurs about 20 minutes after falling asleep. The subject is now very relaxed with blood pressure and body temperature decreasing.
4. *Deep sleep*. The subject will not respond immediately if wakened.

There are significant physiological differences between NREM sleep and REM sleep. During REM sleep muscle tone is depressed except for rapid movements of the eyes, and the subject's respirations and pulse increase in rate and become irregular. Most dreaming occurs during REM sleep.

During an 8-hour sleep, a person passes from stage 1 to stage 4 of NREM sleep, repeats stages 3 and 2 and then moves to REM sleep. This occurs within 50–90 minutes of falling asleep. REM and NREM sleep then alternate throughout the sleep period at approximately 90-minute intervals, thus the cycle repeats itself 3–5 times. The REM period initially lasts 5–10 minutes but gradually lengthens throughout the sleep period until the final REM period lasts 50 minutes. The sleep pattern of infants comprises 50% REM sleep, compared with 20% in the adult.

## CLINICAL APPLICATIONS

### NURSING IMPLICATIONS

Few patients in hospital achieve a satisfactory sleep pattern and many experience the ill-effects of this. It has been suggested, although it remains unproven, that wound healing is delayed as the result of disturbed sleep. Psychological effects include loss of the ability to concentrate, irritability, irrational thinking and distortion of sensory perception.

In assessing the needs of hospitalized patients, attention should be paid to the need for sleep. Care planning should take account of the normal pattern of sleep and external factors that might disrupt this, including:

- *Noise*: many strange and unusual noises are heard in hospital at night. These include ringing telephones, trolleys, metal bins being emptied, doors banging and people coughing.
- *Pain*: pain and discomfort, particularly in the postoperative period, will disturb sleep.
- *Hospital beds*: the design of beds and the types of mattresses and their covers are all known to interrupt sleep.
- *Temperature control*: feeling too hot or cold will prevent sleep.
- *Assessment of sleep*: assessment by nursing staff of a patient's sleep pattern is notoriously difficult.

Appropriate interventions to overcome these will include reducing the amount of noise at night over which the nurse has control; ensuring that the patient is kept pain-free and comfortable; suggesting to relatives that they can bring items such as a pillow from home for the patient to use; the use of appropriate warming and cooling measures, e.g. the use of additional bedclothes or cool fanning; and the use of a comprehensive sleep assessment tool.

## Other states of consciousness

Temporary loss of consciousness can occur because of **fainting** (syncope). This is most often caused by a reduction in cerebral blood flow and can be quickly rectified by ensuring the head is at, or below, the level of the heart. Heat syncope is caused by peripheral pooling of blood as the body tries to lose heat in a hot environment. If the patient is removed to a cooler environment, consciousness can be quickly restored. On the other hand, coma implies a relatively permanent state of unresponsiveness that can end in death.

**Coma** can be the result of large lesions of the midbrain and forebrain areas (usually distinguished as supratentorial, i.e. above the level of the tentorial membrane of dura mater), lesions of the upper brainstem (designated subtentorial lesions) or metabolic disorders. Supratentorial lesions cause coma because of the compression that they exert on brainstem areas. For example, a large space-occupying lesion, such as a tumour in the cerebrum, can cause distortion of the temporal lobe over the medial edge of the tentorial membrane and this will cause compression of upper brainstem structures. As the pressure is exerted more caudally, a progression of dysfunction occurs. Initially, the patient might be roused by verbal command or shaking; as unconsciousness deepens, the patient can be roused only by painful stimuli but the pupils of the eyes are reactive and Cheyne–Stokes respiration is present (see Chapter 5.3). As the midbrain is affected, signs of decerebrate rigidity, together with disconjugate eye movements and fixed pupils, become apparent and the patient becomes unresponsive. As the brainstem is affected, respiration becomes grossly irregular, the pupils dilate and no eye movements can be elicited. The patient is totally unresponsive and, as the respiratory centres of the medulla are affected, terminal gasping eventually ceases and death ensues.

Coma caused by subtentorial lesions is principally associated with damage to the upper brainstem and the associated reticular formation. The role of lower brainstem areas in causing coma is less clear because damage to these areas will affect the respiratory and cardiovascular centres and any such damage is likely to prove rapidly fatal.

Metabolic coma can be a symptom of many conditions, for example, brain anoxia, hypoglycaemia, uraemia, liver failure and meningitis, as well as a consequence of the ingestion of drugs such as opiates and barbiturates. In most, but not all, cases of metabolic coma the pupillary light reflex is retained and eye movements are not affected.

The ability to assess coma quickly and accurately is important. This information will help to determine deterioration or improvement in a patient's condition. The assessment of coma is most frequently performed by nurses and this can apply in any department within a hospital. No patient is immune from falling out of bed and sustaining a head injury!

The **Glasgow Coma Scale** (GCS) is a measurement tool used to assess the level of consciousness. It was devised in Glasgow in the early 1970s and is one of the most frequently used standardized assessment tools in acute neurological environments. It came about for three important reasons:

1. **The importance of conscious level**. It is well established that the most consistent clinical characteristic of the brain damage that results from acceleration/deceleration head trauma is an immediate alteration of consciousness. The depth and duration of unconsciousness are useful guides to the severity of a head injury and changes in consciousness overshadow all other clinical features in importance. It is therefore vital to be able to assess and to record changing states of altered consciousness reliably (Teasdale & Jennett, 1974).

2. **The need for a clinical scale**. Loss of consciousness can also be due to other causes, including drug or metabolic imbalances, or to the combination of remote and local effects produced by brain damage that was initially focal. Furthermore, coma of mixed origin is not uncommon, as when head injury is suspected of being associated with ingestion of drugs or alcohol, or with a vascular accident. These are good reasons for devising a generally applicable scheme of assessment (Teasdale & Jennett, 1974).

3. **The inadequacy of existing systems**. At the time of the introduction of the GCS there was an abundance of alternative terms by which levels of coma were described and recorded. The reality at the time was one of unstructured observation resulting in ambiguous descriptions and many misunderstandings when information about a patient was exchanged. There was no general agreement about what terms to use, nor were those in common use interpreted in a consistent way by different observers. The various classification systems in use at the time used terms that defied clear definition. None of the systems allowed for repeated bedside assessment of the level of consciousness (Teasdale & Jennett, 1974).

To assess conscious level, three aspects of behaviour are independently measured – motor responsiveness, verbal performance and eye opening. These responses are arranged in a scale of increasing dysfunction and are graphically displayed to illustrate the patient's progress (Woodward, 1997) (**see Fig. 2.2.19**).

To elicit a response, an appropriate stimulus of varying intensity is applied. The stimulus is verbal or, if this fails to produce a response, a painful stimulus is used. In most situations there is only one recommended method for this, fingernail bed pressure. This is achieved by applying a pen or pencil to the proximal side of one of the patient's fingernail beds. It is seldom of any value to apply varying degrees of painful stimuli.

On first approaching the patient the nurse should note whether the patients eyes are open or closed; if open, the patient is described as **eye opening spontaneously**. If closed, a stimulus needs to be applied to elicit a response and, in the first instance, the patient is roused verbally to ascertain if he or she is **eye opening to speech**.

| Name | | | | | | | | | | | | | | | | | | | | | | | | | | | | | | Date | |
| Record No. | | | | | | | | | | | | | | | | | | | | | | | | | | | | | | Time | |
| **Coma scale** | Eyes open | Spontaneously | | | | | | | | | | | | | | | | | | | | | | | | | | | | | Eyes closed by swelling = C | |
| | | To speech | | | | | | | | | | | | | | | | | | | | | | | | | | | | | | |
| | | To pain | | | | | | | | | | | | | | | | | | | | | | | | | | | | | | |
| | | None | | | | | | | | | | | | | | | | | | | | | | | | | | | | | | |
| | Best verbal response | Orientated | | | | | | | | | | | | | | | | | | | | | | | | | | | | | Endotracheal tube or tracheostomy = T | |
| | | Confused | | | | | | | | | | | | | | | | | | | | | | | | | | | | | | |
| | | Inappropriate words | | | | | | | | | | | | | | | | | | | | | | | | | | | | | | |
| | | Incomprehensible sounds | | | | | | | | | | | | | | | | | | | | | | | | | | | | | | |
| | | None | | | | | | | | | | | | | | | | | | | | | | | | | | | | | | |
| | Best motor response | Obeys commands | | | | | | | | | | | | | | | | | | | | | | | | | | | | | Usually record the best arm response | |
| | | Localizes pain | | | | | | | | | | | | | | | | | | | | | | | | | | | | | | |
| | | Flexion to pain | | | | | | | | | | | | | | | | | | | | | | | | | | | | | | |
| | | Extension to pain | | | | | | | | | | | | | | | | | | | | | | | | | | | | | | |
| | | None | | | | | | | | | | | | | | | | | | | | | | | | | | | | | | |

**Figure 2.2.19**  A coma scale observation chart

Failure to respond to a verbal stimulus means that a painful stimulus needs to be applied, as already described, and the patient's response is noted. If the patients eyes open in response to this, it is termed **eye opening to pain**. Failure to eye open despite the application of these stimuli is charted as **none**.

To ascertain the best motor response, the patient is asked to perform a simple command such as lifting an arm or sticking out the tongue. If patients comply as requested they are described as **obeying commands**. If patients fail to obey commands, they are deemed to be **localizing to pain**, i.e. they locate the source of the painful stimulus. For this to be conclusive, the stimulus is applied by pinching the opposite shoulder (trapezius pinch). Failing this, fingernail bed pressure is applied to determine the appropriate response. Bending of the arm at the elbow indicates flexion, and extension exists when the elbow straightens; this might also be accompanied by inward rotation at the shoulder and in the forearm with the wrist being flexed and the fingers straightened. **No response** is self explanatory.

To determine the best verbal response, patients are asked some simple questions to assess their degree of orientation, for example, what day is it or which year. Supplying the correct answers would indicate that a patient was **orientated**. Lack of a response to repeated questioning requires the observer to apply a painful stimulus (fingernail bed pressure) to elicit a response. The patient might respond to a physical stimulus by speaking only a word or two (often swearing) and this is defined as **inappropriate words**.

Alternatively, the observer might hear only incomprehensible sounds or no verbal response whatsoever, and this would be charted as such.

Once all these behaviours have been tested and recorded we have a clear indication of the patient's conscious level. Thus a patient's conscious level is described using Glasgow Coma Scale terminology, e.g. a patient might have eye opening to pain, be offering a confused verbal response and be flexing to a painful stimulus. Note the absence of any potentially misleading terminology such as 'stuporous' or 'slightly drowsy'.

The evaluation of each of the behaviours depends on the absence of factors that could deter assessment. Some patients might be unable to open their eyes due to localized swelling and this should be noted (**C = closed**) rather than be recorded as no eye opening. Conversely, some patients in coma with flaccid eye muscles might have their eyes open almost constantly, but clearly this is not spontaneous eye opening and merits a **no response** recording. A patient with a language disorder or deafness, or who is unable to understand the native language, will not produce an accurate verbal response. The patient with an endotracheal tube or tracheostomy will be unable to phonate. The cause of the factor that precludes these observations should be noted on the chart (**D = dysphasia, T = tracheostomy**). For the motor response, it is the best arm response that is recorded, even though there might be differences between the two sides. Leg responses are unreliable and might be due to spinal reflex action. A useful study by Edwards (2001) analysed the limitations of the Glasgow Coma Scale and provides a full perspective on its use in practice.

The assessment system described so far applies only to adults. Particular difficulties are encountered in the assessment of children under 5 years of age. The accurate assessment of conscious level in the child under 5 years of age demands the use of a scale devised specifically for such a purpose) (**see Fig. 2.2.20**).

| Name | Paediatric Neurological observation chart (0–5 years) | | | | | | | | | | | | | | | | | | | | | | | | |
|---|---|---|---|---|---|---|---|---|---|---|---|---|---|---|---|---|---|---|---|---|---|---|---|---|---|
| **Record No.** | | | | | | | | | | | | | | | | | | | | | | | | **Date** | |
| Age | Coma scale | | | | | | | | | | | | | | | | | | | | | | | **Time** | |
| **Eyes open** | | Spontaneously | | | | | | | | | | | | | | | | | | | | | | Eyes closed by swelling = C | |
| | | To speech | | | | | | | | | | | | | | | | | | | | | | | |
| | | To pain | | | | | | | | | | | | | | | | | | | | | | | |
| | | None | | | | | | | | | | | | | | | | | | | | | | | |
| **Best verbal response** | 5 years | Orientated to place | | | | | | | | | | | | | | | | | | | | | | Endotracheal tube or tracheostomy = T | |
| | 12 months | Words | | | | | | | | | | | | | | | | | | | | | | | |
| | | Vocal sounds | | | | | | | | | | | | | | | | | | | | | | | |
| | 6 months | Cries | | | | | | | | | | | | | | | | | | | | | | | |
| | | None | | | | | | | | | | | | | | | | | | | | | | | |
| **Best motor response** | | Obeys command | | | | | | | | | | | | | | | | | | | | | | Usually record the best arm response | |
| | 6 months–2 years | Localizes pain | | | | | | | | | | | | | | | | | | | | | | | |
| | 6 months | Flexion pain | | | | | | | | | | | | | | | | | | | | | | | |
| | | Extension pain | | | | | | | | | | | | | | | | | | | | | | | |
| | | None | | | | | | | | | | | | | | | | | | | | | | | |

**Figure 2.2.20**   A coma scale observation chart adapted for children

A number of modified scales exist and one is described by Westbrook (1997). One such adaptation has been researched and benchmarked, as reported by Warren (2000).

Some patients in coma never recover. Those in apnoeic coma with no prospect of recovery can be assessed for brainstem function to determine if they are brain dead. This procedure has two parts. First, the doctor, who must have been registered for at least 5 years, has to be satisfied that the patient fulfils certain preconditions prior to testing. These include confirmation of the irremediable brain damage leading to apnoeic coma. The damage might be the result of cardiac arrest, cerebral haemorrhage or head injury, which is the most common diagnosis. Testing would not normally take place less than 6 hours after the onset of coma and 12–24 hours is more usual. The examiner needs to be satisfied that temporary depression of brainstem reflexes has occurred neither as the result of ingestion of a large quantity of depressant drugs, as in attempted overdosage, nor because of the use of neuromuscular relaxant drugs to facilitate the commencement of artificial ventilation. The patient must not be hypothermic and the presence of severe metabolic or endocrinological disturbances, such as uncontrolled diabetes, must be ruled out.

Only when the patient fulfils these preconditions can the examiner proceed to testing for the presence of brainstem reflexes. These are tested as in **Table 2.2.2**.

The brain-dead patient will display a negative response to all of the tests in **Table 2.2.2**.

To eliminate observer error the entire procedure is repeated a second time by another medical examiner. Once the patient has been diagnosed as brain dead by the second examiner, the date and time is noted and, for medico-legal purposes, this is considered to be when the patient 'dies'. At this stage artificial ventilation and other interventional therapy is withdrawn. In this situation thought needs to be given to the relatives and Coyle (2000) provides some thoughtful insights into the care required.

## Epilepsy

Seizures are classified according to whether their onset is focal (partial) or generalized. Partial seizures are further subdivided according to whether consciousness is retained throughout the seizure (simple partial seizure) or impaired at some point (complex partial seizure). A partial seizure can progress to a generalized one.

| Table 2.2.2 Testing of brainstem reflexes | | |
| --- | --- | --- |
| **Reflex** | **Method of testing** | **Normal response** |
| Pupillary reaction | Shine bright light in patient's eye | Pupil constricts in response to light stimulus |
| Corneal reflex | Draw wisp of cotton wool across exposed cornea | Patient's eye blinks |
| Oculovestibular reflex | Inject 20 mL of ice cold water into each ear in turn, having previously visualized the tympanic membrane | Deviation of the eyes to the affected side (nystagmus) |
| Cranial nerve motor response | Application of painful stimulus to more than one site, e.g. fingernail bed pressure. Include stimulation to face lest the patient has a high spinal cord injury | Facial grimace or movement of arm to painful stimulus |
| Gag reflex | Move endotracheal tube back and forth or apply suction | Patient will cough or gag |
| Breathing | Disconnect patient from ventilator but administer oxygen to maintain tissue perfusion and avoid hypoxia: observe chest wall closely for any respiratory effort | Spontaneous respirations |

## Partial seizures

### Simple partial seizures

A focus within a particular part of the brain. Usually, the motor strip is irritated resulting in a disturbance in function of the affected area. Typically, a focal seizure comprises of a twitching of the thumb or side of the face. The patient does not lose consciousness. If the twitching spreads to affect other parts of the body it is referred to as a Jacksonian seizure, e.g. the twitching might start in the thumb and then spread (or march) to affect the hand and arm, and possibly include the affected side of the body.

### Complex partial seizures

These seizures, which normally originate in the temporal lobe, are usually proceded by an aura or warning. This is followed by an episode of altered behaviour in which patients perform a series of repeated movements. Automatism, in which patients continually rub their hands or pluck at their clothes, might be demonstrated. Some patients might also describe a sensory experience, e.g. a particular smell, and some describe experiencing familiarity with an unfamiliar situation, i.e. deja vu.

## Generalized seizures

### Absence seizures

As the name implies there is a brief alteration in consciousness, which onlookers often do not notice. It typically occurs in childhood and is often noticed only as the child falls further behind with school work. In complex absences, automatism as previously described, accompanies the brief alteration in consciousness.

### Myoclonic seizures

Sudden, repeated, jerking movements of one or more of the limbs during which there is a momentary loss of consciousness. Can occur repeatedly over a number of hours and is most frequently seen within 1 hour of waking from sleep. If standing, the person would fall to the ground.

### Tonic seizures

Starts with a sudden loss of body posture, characteristically the arms flex and the legs extend. Loss of consciousness usually occurs and respiration might cease for a time. Can be seen as part of a tonic clonic seizure.

### Tonic atonic seizures

The patient experiences a tonic phase, as outlined above, but then experiences atony, i.e. loss of tone. Can be repeated several times during which there is loss of consciousness.

### Tonic clonic seizures

These comprise several distinct stages. First, the patient might experience an aura. This often takes the form of a strange taste in the mouth or feeling (this does not occur in everyone with this type of seizure). The aura can act as an early warning that, once recognized, can prompt the patient to move to a safe place. This is followed by a loss of consciousness that heralds the start of the seizure proper. A patient who is standing will fall to the ground. The tonic phase is signalled by stiffening of the body. The jaw closes tight shut and the patient might utter a cry as the thoracic muscles contract and air is forcefully ejected via the vocal chords. As apnoea intervenes the patient becomes cyanosed and is often incontinent of urine/faeces.

After a period of time the patient will start to breath stertorously accompanied by rhythmic jerking of the limbs. Frothing of the mouth occurs as a result of excessive production of saliva. The patient is usually tachycardic and sweating. Once the jerking movements begin to subside coma supervenes. Most patients will fall into a deep sleep for a number of hours and are usually amnesic once they waken and display episodes of drowsiness and confusion.

### Status epilepticus

This occurs when one seizure, usually of the tonic clonic variety, is rapidly followed by another. This can continue for a prolonged period. It can be life threatening and therefore requires urgent medical intervention.

## Treatment

Treatment is aimed at achieving a seizure-free lifestyle for the sufferer. This is usually brought about with careful prescription of anticonvulsant medication such as carbamazepine, ethoxosuximide, phenytoin and sodium valporate, gabapentin, lamotrigine and vigabatrin. Success depends on the patient's understanding of the need to continue taking the medication even when seizure free. Non-compliance with medication is the most common reason for an increased number of seizures. If a primary focus can be attributed as the cause of the seizures then surgical resection of that area might be feasible, e.g. temporal lobectomy. However, only a small number of patients will be suitable for this. Epilepsy is perhaps the most misunderstood disorder of the nervous system, which serves to make resocialization of the person with epilepsy more difficult. Social rehabilitation is vital.

The nurse should assess the patient's educational, emotional and psychosocial needs together with those of family and friends. Discussion with the sufferer should cover specific themes:

- coping with epilepsy in family, social and occupational life
- knowledge about seizures
- medications
- occupational problems that sufferers associate with epilepsy
- topics on which patients feel they need to have more information.

The following points should be covered in patient/family education sessions:

1. What epilepsy is and how the diagnosis is arrived at. Dispel myths about possible brain damage, insanity or criminal tendencies!
2. The chances of passing the disorder on to children.
3. Precautions that can be taken to lessen the chance of seizures occurring. These include sleeping with a safety pillow, taking showers rather than a bath or, if using a bath is the only option, then keeping the water shallow. Knowledge of trigger factors such as stress, hunger, hyperventilation, overtiredness, premenstrual state, fever and alcohol can help to avoid attacks.
4. Sports should be encouraged, with the activity dependent on the sufferer's seizure pattern.
5. Alcohol ingestion interferes with the action of some anticonvulsants and should be avoided.
6. Driving a vehicle is illegal unless the patient has been seizure free for at least 2 years or the seizures are nocturnal.
7. The importance of maintaining drug regimes even when seizure free.

8. Educating work colleagues about the seizures and what to do in the event of one.
9. Insurance might need to be sought from specialist companies or through Epilepsy Action.
10. The condition needs to be discussed fully with the sufferer's future spouse or partner.
11. An epilepsy sufferer considering becoming pregnant should discuss this with her doctor prior to conception so that medication regimes can be monitored more closely and other complications can be fully explained. Epilepsy is not a contraindication to pregnancy.
12. Making contact with appropriate self-help group such as Epilepsy Action.

## Motivation and emotion

### Motivation

The **hypothalamus** has been identified as a brain structure of major importance in the control of motivation. It lies beneath the thalamus and forms the floor and part of the walls of the third ventricle. Several nuclei can be distinguished within the hypothalamus, although large areas consist of a diffuse neural matrix.

The hypothalamus occupies the nodal position in a series of complex, interconnecting ascending and descending pathways (**Fig. 2.2.21**). It is connected to forebrain structures such as the preoptic area, septum, thalamus, limbic lobe cortex and frontal lobe cortex, as well as to midbrain and hindbrain centres such as the reticular formation, the visceral and somatic motor centres of the brainstem, and the spinal cord. The major nerve fibre pathway passing through the hypothalamus and involved in these ascending and descending connections is the **medial forebrain bundle**.

In addition to these neural connections, the hypothalamus has a controlling influence over the activity

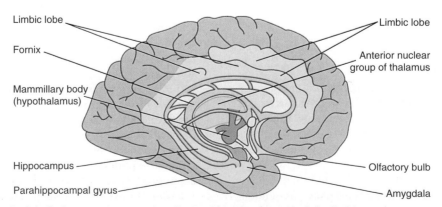

Limbic lobe
Fornix
Mammillary body (hypothalamus)
Hippocampus
Parahippocampal gyrus
Limbic lobe
Anterior nuclear group of thalamus
Olfactory bulb
Amygdala

**Figure 2.2.21** The labelled structures are generally considered to be part of the limbic system

of the pituitary gland, the major endocrine gland. The pituitary gland lies directly beneath the hypothalamus, separated from it by the infundibular stalk (see Chapter 2.6). The posterior pituitary comprises the axon terminals of two distinct hypothalamic nuclei, the paraventricular nucleus and the supraoptic nucleus. These two nuclei synthesize the hormones oxytocin and antidiuretic hormone (vasopressin), respectively. The cells of these nuclei transport the hormones along their axons, down the infundibular stalk and into the posterior pituitary for release directly into the circulatory system. Smaller cells from a much wider area of the hypothalamus indirectly control the activity of the anterior pituitary by extruding releasing hormones (or releasing factors) and inhibiting hormones. These releasing and inhibiting hormones pass from axon terminals at a position midway down the infundibular stalk (i.e. at the median eminence) into the pituitary portal blood vessels. This specialized portal system conducts the hormones to the anterior pituitary, where they effect the release of anterior pituitary hormones.

An example of the role of the hypothalamus in the control of homeostatic mechanisms can be seen in its influence over body temperature control. Stimulation of anterior regions of the hypothalamus in unanaesthetized animals results in vasodilation and a drop in body temperature. Damage to this area causes hyperthermia. By contrast, stimulation of posterior regions of the hypothalamus causes shivering and vasoconstriction consistent with conservation of body heat. Damage to the posterior regions results in chronic hypothermia. Central receptors for both sets of responses appear to lie in the anterior or hypothalamus and to be sensitive to local temperature changes, presumably caused by locally circulating blood (see Chapter 6.1). In addition, signals from peripheral temperature receptors in the skin are involved in this control.

The hypothalamus is also implicated in the control of eating and drinking. Destruction of the ventromedial nuclei of the hypothalamus in experimental animals leads to hyperphagia (overeating) and severe obesity, whereas electrical stimulation of this area suppresses feeding. Contrastingly, destruction of the lateral nuclei causes aphagia (not eating) and adipsia (not drinking) and the animals die unless they are force fed and hydrated. Again, electrical stimulation of this area has the opposite effect, causing feeding to occur. Unfortunately, recent experimental evidence has suggested that this apparently straightforward formulation of a lateral hypothalamic 'feeding centre' and a ventromedial hypothalamic 'satiety centre' is incomplete. It has been suggested that damage to some of the nerve fibres passing through the hypothalamus might contribute to the effects of these lesions. For example, lateral hypothalamic lesions could damage the trigeminal nerve pathways and the resultant sensory and motor loss might contribute to the reluctance to eat. Lesions of the hypothalamus can also affect the release of hormones and this might indirectly affect feeding behaviour. For example, damage to the medial hypothalamus can cause an increase in insulin release, which, in turn, might be partially responsible for the hyperphagia and weight gain seen in ventromedial hypothalamic lesions. It appears that the role of the hypothalamus in eating and drinking is far from clear. Nevertheless, this can hardly be regarded as surprising in view of the complex interaction of visceral cues, environmental stimuli and learned behaviour patterns that contribute to eating and drinking.

In addition to motivation related to specific behaviour patterns, the hypothalamus also appears to be involved with general mechanisms of reward and punishment. These more general mechanisms of motivation have become known as **pleasure centres** and **pain centres**. In laboratory animals, experiments using electrical stimulation as a reward have mapped pleasure centres in a large number of brain structures, from the reticular formation to the hippocampus and limbic cortex. However, the areas of brain in which stimulation is most likely to elicit these responses are the septum, the hypothalamus and their associated nerve fibre pathway, the medial forebrain bundle.

Pain centres are more accurately described as **aversion centres**, as it is not known whether stimulation actually causes pain. Aversion centres tend to be fewer in number than pleasure centres and are associated with more medial and midline areas of the brain. In these areas, stimulation leads to an immediate reduction and cessation of responding.

Stimulation of pleasure and aversion centres in humans has occurred as a consequence of some clinical procedures. Patients report that stimulation is either generally pleasurable or somewhat unpleasant, depending on whether a pleasure or an aversion centre is stimulated. However, the human experience would appear to be much less extreme and, consequently, much less highly motivating than that implied by the behaviour of laboratory rats.

## Emotion

In addition to its role in motivated behaviour, the hypothalamus, along with other brain structures, also seems to be involved in emotional responses, although its precise role is not completely understood.

The importance of the hypothalamus in emotional behaviour would appear to lie in its position at the nodal point of a complex of ascending and descending nerve pathways. The descending pathways influence both the voluntary and involuntary motor responses.

For example, the voluntary motor responses to a threatening situation will involve fight or flight. The involuntary responses will involve the associated sympathetic activity of the autonomic nervous system (see Chapter 2.5). The complexities of the ascending nerve pathways are much less clearly understood, but are often said to involve the limbic system.

The **limbic system** is not really an identifiable system at all. It comprises a large number of forebrain structures, including the limbic lobe of the cortex, which are interconnected in a very complex manner. The functional significance of most of these connections is not understood at present. It will suffice here to say that the limbic system involves links between the hypothalamus, the septal area, the thalamus, the hippocampus, the amygdala, the limbic lobe of the cortex, and inferior (orbital) areas of the frontal cortex. All these structures, which have been implicated in emotional responses, presumably operate through a complex pattern of nerve connections and feedback loops, although suggestions of how these mechanisms work are only speculative at the moment.

## Higher mental functions

Higher mental functions, such as learning, memory, language and thought, have been studied extensively by psychologists. Although insights have been gained into the nature of these important human abilities, it is impossible at the present time to relate these functions closely to physiological mechanisms. It is reasonable to assume that the nervous system subserves all these forms of mental functioning, but the mechanisms involved are not understood.

## Learning and memory

Learning implies a modification of an organism's behaviour with experience. If any such modification takes on a degree of relative permanence then we can impute the existence of a memory system. At present, little is known of the changes in nervous activity that underlie learning.

Attempts to understand where memories lie within the nervous system have so far achieved no more success than those investigations concerned with the question of how learning and memory occur. Investigations of patients with neurological problems have suggested that the hippocampus might play a role in the establishment or recall of short-term memories. However, the evidence has been obtained from patients with large bilateral temporal lobe lesions and the precise role of the hippocampus in short-term memory has yet to be elucidated.

## The cerebral cortex

The cerebral cortex constitutes a much larger proportion of the brain in humans and other primates than in lower animals. It is therefore assumed that the cerebral cortex is responsible for our highest mental activities – activities such as thinking, communicating with others, problem solving and so on. Indeed, studies of patients with neurological problems have shown that damage to the cerebral cortex can result in serious disruption of higher mental functions.

### CLINICAL APPLICATIONS

#### DISORDERS

Certain clinical conditions lead to severe disruption of higher mental functioning. For example, disturbances occurring in psychosis and dementia involve disordered thought processes, perceptions and memories. **Schizophrenia** is typically associated with thought disorder, hallucinations (particularly auditory hallucinations of voices) and disturbed emotional status, whereas the development of **dementia** can extend from minor lapses of memory to a state of utter confusion and debility in which the whole personality of the individual changes. At present, knowledge of the causes of these psychopathological states is limited. Nevertheless, some insights into physiological mechanisms have emerged recently. For example, in the case of schizophrenia it has been discovered that certain drugs, which can alleviate the symptoms of psychosis, affect dopaminergic pathways in the brain. These drugs, such as chlorpromazine, block dopamine receptors and consequently lower the activity of central dopaminergic nerves. The effectiveness of antipsychotic drugs has led to their wide use. Even so, it must be remembered that they are not effective in all cases and that they are not equally effective in the patients that are helped by them. Moreover, it has not been possible, so far, to extrapolate from treatment with antipsychotic drugs to any full understanding of the causes of the behavioural and intellectual impairments seen in schizophrenic patients.

## Conclusion

This chapter has considered the brain, spinal cord and associated structures that comprise the central nervous system. We have seen how they work together to provide smooth integrated function; this is explored further in Chapter 2.3.

## Clinical review

In addition to the Learning Objectives at the beginning of this chapter, the reader should be able to:

- Identify the major pathways for somatosensory input to the brain
- Explain the role of the cerebellum in motor coordination and control of balance
- Explain the role of the brainstem in the control of states of consciousness
- Describe the behavioural characteristics of the major types of epilepsy
- Relate the structure to function in the CNS in the control of motivation and emotion

## Review questions

1  What is the function of the choroid plexus?
2  Describe the organization of the meninges
3  What is the function of the CSF?
4  What are the two main pairs of arteries supplying the brain?
5  How do the nerves in the dorsal and ventral roots of the spinal cord differ in function?
6  Which cranial nerve is the vagus?
7  What are the gyri and sulci of the cerebral cortex?
8  Which lobes of the cerebral hemispheres are divided by the central sulcus?
9  What function is served by the corpus callosum?
10  Why does the sensory homunculus appear to have large hands and small feet?
11  Which three neural systems control motor activity?
12  What is the source of afferent input to the cerebellum?
13  How does the hypothalamus exert control over the endocrine system?

## Suggestions for further reading

Adelbratt, S. & Strang, P. (2000) Death anxiety in brain tumour patients and their spouses. *Palliative Medicine,* **14**(6); 499–507.
*Describes research carried out in this field and identified the main categories common to patients and their next of kin.*

Fairley, D. & Cosgrove, J. (1999) Glasgow Coma Scale: Improving nursing practice through clinical effectiveness. *Nursing in Critical Care,* **4**(6); 276–279.

*Demonstrates the use of audit and development of clinical guidelines in relation to the use of the Glasgow Coma Scale.*

Hickey, J.V. (2002) *The Clinical Practice of Neurological and Neurosurgical Nursing,* 5th edn. Philadelphia: Lippincott, Williams and Wilkins.
*Excellent textbook on neurological and neurosurgical nursing providing comprehensive coverage of the subject.*

## References

Carr, J.H. & Shepherd, R. A. (2002) *Stroke Rehabilitation.* Edinburgh: Churchill Livingstone.
Coyle, M.A. (2000) Meeting the needs of the family: The role of the specialist nurse in the management

of brain death. *Intensive and Critical Care Nursing,* **16**(1); 45–50.
Delong, M.R. (1974) *Motor functions of the basal ganglia: Single unit activity during movement in*

*The Neurosciences Third Study Programme* (eds Schmitt, F.O. & Worden, F.G.). Cambridge, MA: MTP Press.

Edwards, S. (2001) Using the Glasgow Coma Scale: Analysis and limitations. *British Journal of Nursing*, 10(2); 92–101.

MacFarlane, P.S., Reid, R. & Callander, R. (1999) *Pathology Illustrated*, 5th edn. Edinburgh: Churchill Livingstone.

Teasdale, G. & Jennett, B. (1974) Assessment of coma and consciousness: A practical scale. *Lancet*, ii; 81–84.

Warren, A. (2000) Paediatric coma scoring researched and benchmarked. *Paediatric Nursing*, 12(3); 14–18.

Westbrook, A. (1997) The use of a paediatric coma scale for monitoring infants and young children with head injuries. *Nursing in Critical Care*, 2(2); 72–75.

Woodward, S. (1997) Neurological observations, part 1: Glasgow Coma Scale. *Nursing Times*, 93(45); 1–2.

# Sensory receptors and sense organs

*Douglas Allan*

## LEARNING OBJECTIVES

After studying this chapter the reader should be able to:

- Describe the varieties of form of sensory receptors

- Describe the characteristics of a generator potential

- Explain how the intensity and locality of a stimulus are coded in nerve signals from sensory units

- Define the term 'lateral inhibition' and explain its importance to perception of a stimulus

- Describe in outline the structural and functional differences between tactile receptors, proprioceptors, thermal receptors and pain receptors

- Describe the cortical representation of somatosensation

- Describe the underlying physiology of pain perception

- Describe the major features of the pyramidal and extrapyramidal pathways for motor control

## INTRODUCTION

Changes in the external and internal environment of the body are detected and coded into nervous impulses by sensory receptors. The central nervous system is continuously being made aware of conditions within and outside the body; it integrates the many sensory inputs, 'compares' them with previous experience, and makes appropriate responses. Sensory signals can be integrated in parts of the brain or spinal cord that do not give rise to conscious awareness, for example in spinal and brainstem reflexes.

Sensory receptors are either adapted nerve fibre terminals or specialized cells associated with nerve terminals. They are diverse in structure and convey the many qualities of sensation that can be experienced. These include touch, pressure, pain, temperature,

light, sound, taste and smell. Sensory receptors also convey information that assists in the maintenance of balance and motor control, in regulating the chemical composition and hydrostatic pressure of arterial blood, and in regulating gut motility.

Sensory afferents arising from the body are grouped together as the **somatosensory system**. Somatosensation includes sensory information arising from the skin, the muscles and joints, and the viscera. The **special senses** are associated with specialized sense organs in the head and include vision, hearing, balance, taste and smell. These are described in Chapter 2.4.

An explanation of the classification of receptors provides a basis for the understanding of the somatosensory system. This chapter describes the structure and function of the motor system and demonstrates how these two separate systems are integrated. It also considers the physiological basis of pain, along with several associated areas of importance.

## Classification of receptors

Sensory receptors can be classified on a structural or functional basis. Anatomical studies of receptors have revealed a bewildering variety of structural types. Certain common anatomical features permit a simplified structural classification consisting of only three groups: (i) unspecialized free nerve endings; (ii) specialized or encapsulated nerve endings; and (iii) specialized non-neuronal receptor cells.

**Unspecialized free nerve endings** are found in considerable numbers in both the epidermis and the dermis of the skin; they are also found in muscles and the viscera. Free nerve endings are certainly involved in detecting painful stimuli. However, in parts of the body that contain only this type of receptor (e.g. the cornea, which covers the exposed surface of the eye) free nerve endings can also detect touch, pressure and temperature. It is unclear to what extent free nerve endings elsewhere in the body convey these other sensations. Those in the epidermis are probably associated with touch and/or temperature because the superficial epidermis apparently does not contain pain receptors and it can be peeled off without eliciting pain.

**Specialized nerve endings** are found in muscle spindles, in Golgi tendon organs and in olfactory epithelium in the nose. They are also found in abundance in the skin. Some are found in the deeper growing layer of the epidermis, notably the tactile (Merkel's) discs, which are believed to detect light touch. Various encapsulated nerve endings exist in the dermis. Meissner's corpuscles and basket nerve endings wrapped around hair bases are both thought to respond to touch, whereas the deeper-lying Pacinian corpuscles are believed to respond to deeper pressure. Krause's end-bulbs and Ruffini's endings have been associated with cold and warmth detection, respectively, but many studies have shown that free nerve endings can be temperature detectors and Krause's end-bulbs and Ruffini's endings are also candidates for pressure receptors.

**Specialized non-neuronal receptor cells** are found in the ear, the eye and in the taste buds of the mouth. In response to appropriate stimuli these cells produce electrical potential changes that influence the generation of action potentials in associated afferent nerve fibres.

Sensory receptors can be functionally classified according to the nature of the stimulus energy to which they respond. There are mechanoreceptors, chemoreceptors, thermoreceptors, electromagnetic receptors and pain receptors.

**Mechanoreceptors** are sensitive to mechanical energy and exist in many forms. Touch and pressure cause mechanical deformation and hence stimulation of mechanoreceptors found in the skin. Stretch receptors in muscle spindles, in the gut, in lung tissue and in blood vessels (baroreceptors) similarly respond to mechanical energy. Sound receptors and balance receptors in the ear respond to mechanical pressure waves in air and in gravity and head movements, respectively. Golgi tendon organs respond to muscle tension; joint receptors respond to changes of angle and position of joints.

**Chemoreceptors** are sensitive to chemical changes in the vicinity of the receptors. They include gustatory (taste) receptors; olfactory (smell) receptors; chemoreceptors that detect oxygen, carbon dioxide and acidity levels in arterial blood; and osmoreceptors detecting changes in salt concentration and hence the osmotic pressure of arterial blood.

**Thermoreceptors** respond to thermal energy. Cold and warmth receptors have been identified in the skin.

**Electromagnetic receptors** respond to light and are found in the visual receptor layer (the retina) of the eye.

**Pain receptors** might respond to more than one kind of stimulus energy, but characteristically pain is elicited only by intense and potentially damaging stimuli. Pain can be experienced after tissue damage has occurred when the tissue is inflamed and oedematous, thereby causing mechanical deformation of receptors contained within it. Inflamed tissue releases local chemicals such as histamine, bradykinin and prostaglandins. The stimulus for pain is therefore presumably either mechanical or chemical, although the tissue damage might have been caused by some other type of energy, for example ultraviolet irradiation.

Somatosensory receptors can also be classified according to their general location. Thus, there are cutaneous receptors in the skin, receptors in the viscera and receptors in muscles and joints. These latter contribute information about body position and body movement and are collectively called **proprioceptors**.

## Properties of receptors

### Specificity

In general terms, each receptor elicits only one kind of sensory experience. The various types of sensation are termed **modalities of sensation**, for example touch, pain and temperature. Hence, receptors are referred to as being modality specific. The term '**adequate stimulus**' describes the nature of the stimulus to which a receptor is normally sensitive.

Regardless of the type of energy that stimulates a receptor, it will always elicit the same modality of sensation. Modality of sensation reflects the nature of the stimulated receptor together with its terminations in the brain.

Specific pain receptors are sensitive to several kinds of stimulus energy and it is therefore difficult to define the adequate stimulus. Adequate stimuli for pain receptors can include high-intensity mechanical, electromagnetic, chemical and thermal energies. However, specific pain receptors and pathways can be identified. Free nerve endings can subserve touch, pressure and temperature in addition to pain, and there is probably some overlap of function between the many specialized nerve ending receptors. However, any single receptor, for example one free nerve ending, will transmit only one modality of sensation.

## Thresholds

Sensory receptors transduce stimulus energy into nervous impulses, which are conducted to the CNS via the sensory afferent neurones. Because a threshold level of stimulation must be reached to generate action potentials in a nerve fibre, it is clear that sensory receptors must also reach a threshold intensity of stimulation to excite nerve impulses in sensory afferents. Perception, however, depends on the transmission pathway and on brain organization, as well as on the electrophysiological properties of the receptors.

### Adaptation

All sensory receptors adapt to stimulation after a short period of time. That is, the frequency at which impulses are generated reduces or even falls to zero if the stimulus input to the receptor is maintained at a constant level. Adaptation allows receptors to signal changes in environmental conditions.

### Electrophysiological properties

When a receptor is appropriately stimulated, the transmembrane potential shifts and depolarizes. This potential change is a graded phenomenon and the amplitude of the depolarization depends on stimulus intensity, duration of stimulation and receptor adaptation. This graded potential change is called a **generator potential** if it occurs in a neuronal receptor and a **receptor potential** if it occurs in a non-neuronal receptor cell. If the generator (or receptor) potential is large enough, action potentials are generated in the associated sensory afferent nerve fibres. In general

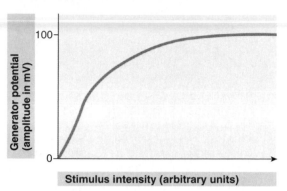

**Figure 2.3.1** The relationship between the generator potential and stimulus intensity in a sensory receptor

terms, the larger the generator potential amplitude, the greater the frequency of impulse generation.

Generator (or receptor) potentials can be compared with the postsynaptic potentials described in Chapter 2.1. Like postsynaptic potentials, they are not all-or-none events, and generator potentials can summate if stimulation is maintained or reapplied before the resting potential is re-established. The duration of the generator potential is variable, for a single stimulus application it typically lasts for 5–10 ms.

As the stimulus intensity (or rate of change of stimulus intensity) increases, so the generator potential increases to its maximum level. Increases in intensity beyond this point cannot be detected by the receptor. The relationship between stimulus intensity and generator potential amplitude is illustrated in **Fig. 2.3.1**.

Generator (or receptor) potentials have an ionic basis. The application of an adequate stimulus causes a generalized increase in membrane permeability to small ions. Because, at rest, $Na^+$ are far removed from equilibrium, a net inward flow of these positive ions occurs on stimulation, resulting in membrane depolarization.

The adequate stimulus for a skin Pacinian corpuscle (**Fig. 2.3.2**) is pressure resulting in mechanical deformation. When pressure is applied to one side of the capsule, the deformation results in a shifting of the connective tissue and enclosed fluid layers relative to one another, and this apparently results in membrane permeability changes in the unmyelinated nerve terminal, which in turn gives rise to the generator potential. The generator potential spreads passively from the site of stimulation and, if it is of sufficiently large amplitude, excites the production of action potentials at the first node of Ranvier, which has a lower threshold for action potentials than the unmyelinated portion of the nerve terminal. Generation of the action potential continues as long as the generator potential is maintained. Characteristically, a burst of impulses occurs when a Pacinian corpuscle is stimulated.

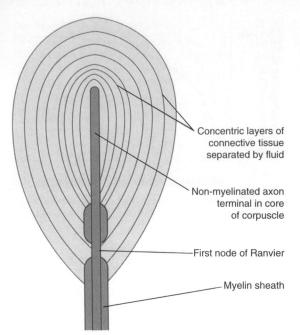

**Figure 2.3.2** Section through a Pacinian corpuscle

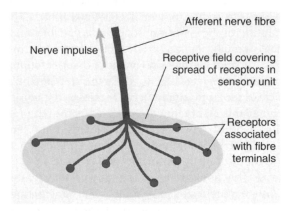

**Figure 2.3.3** The receptive field of a sensory unit

## Sensory units

A single afferent nerve fibre branches to produce a number of peripheral terminals, each of which is associated with a receptor. The area innervated by these terminals is called the **receptive field** of the neurone. The afferent neurone, together with its associated receptive field, is known as a **sensory unit** (**Fig. 2.3.3**).

## Information content of sensory signals

All sensory receptors transduce stimuli into action potentials yet each burst of impulses provides unique information regarding intensity, modality and locality of the stimulus. The transmitted elements are simple, i.e. action potentials along sensory afferents. It is

the *pattern* of transmitted elements, together with the transmission pathway, that is essential for the transfer of information in the signal.

## Intensity code

The brain can determine stimulus intensity despite the fact that the action potential is of fixed amplitude. Information about intensity is provided in three ways.

1. **Frequency of impulse generation at the receptor.** Up to a maximum, the greater the stimulus intensity, the greater the generator potential and the higher the frequency of action potential generation at each receptor.
2. **Recruitment of other receptors in the sensory unit.** As stimulus intensity increases, higher-threshold receptors in the sensory unit will be activated. These will also produce bursts of impulses, which will be conducted to the final common path of the receptive field – the sensory afferent fibre. Provided the membrane is not refractory, the recruited receptors will increase the frequency of impulses in the sensory afferent fibre.
3. **Recruitment of other sensory units.** High-intensity stimuli usually stimulate larger areas of tissue than low-intensity stimuli. Thus, higher-intensity stimuli can stimulate more than one sensory unit; recruitment of sensory units can be indicative of an increase in intensity of stimulation.

## Modality code

The modality code of the sensory input is a function of the receptor type together with its particular pathway to, and termination point in, the brain.

## Location code

The transmission pathway from receptor to brain is also important for localizing a stimulus. In general terms, the greater the degree of overlap of receptive fields and the smaller the individual fields, the more precise the location of the stimulus. Thus, touch can be precisely located when applied to the skin of the fingers, where receptive fields are small and overlap considerably, but precision is lost if the skin of the back is so stimulated because receptive fields here are larger and overlap less. This is illustrated in **Fig. 2.3.4**.

In **Fig. 2.3.4**, stimulation occurs at the centre of field Y and on the periphery of fields X and Z. As low-threshold receptors generally occur at the centres of receptive fields and high-threshold receptors occur at the edges, it follows that action potentials will be elicited more readily in sensory afferent Y than in X

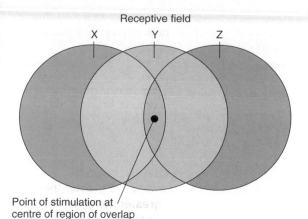

Receptive field

Point of stimulation at centre of region of overlap

**Figure 2.3.4** Overlapping receptive fields enable localization of the stimulus (see text)

and Z. The pattern of discharge in the three sensory units therefore permits a fairly precise location of the stimulus, and the higher rate of discharge in Y compared with the other two fields indicates that the stimulus is nearer the centre of field Y and towards the periphery of fields X and Z.

## Coding of boundaries

Weaker signals tend to be filtered out and inhibited and stronger signals boosted, thereby providing sharp boundaries of stimulation. The term '**lateral inhibition**' describes the process of inhibition of weak signals arising from peripheral areas of stimulation. This can be readily demonstrated by pressing a pointed object firmly into the skin of a fingertip. The point is clearly felt and localized, despite the fact that surrounding tissue is also deformed and indented. Pressure receptors are stimulated in all deformed areas but the weaker signals from the tissues surrounding the point are inhibited at synapses in the transmission pathway to the brain. The same phenomenon is also demonstrated in the visual system, where edges to shapes and patterns are clearly seen. Again, signals from visual receptors that are only weakly stimulated and which surround strongly stimulated areas are laterally inhibited.

## Somatosensation

Somatosensory signals arise from the skin, muscles, joints and viscera. Somatosensory receptors can be classed as tactile, proprioceptive, thermal and pain receptors. In addition, there are stretch receptors in the viscera. Stretch receptors in the gut are chiefly concerned with the initiation of *local* reflex contractions of the gut muscle, whereas stretch receptors in the arterial tree detect changes in blood pressure and send signals

to the lower centres of the brain only. The major somatosensory input terminates in higher centres of the brain. Afferent fibres conveying somatosensory input from the trunk and limbs arise from unipolar cell bodies, which are aggregated together in ganglia on the dorsal roots of the spinal cord. These unipolar neurones give rise to central afferents that convey the sensory signals to the higher centres of the brain.

## Tactile receptors

Tactile receptors respond to touch, pressure or vibration. In each case the stimulus energy is mechanical. Pressure simply implies a greater intensity of stimulation than touch. Vibration is rapid, repetitive mechanical deformation.

Tactile receptors vary in structure. **Meissner's corpuscles** consist of spiral nerve endings embedded in corpuscles of epithelial tissue. They are found just beneath the epidermis of the skin, especially in hairless areas such as the fingertips. They respond to light touch and adapt readily to zero if stimulation is maintained. They therefore respond best to light movements across the skin. By contrast, **Merkel's discs**, which are also found in abundance in hairless areas of skin, adapt more slowly and respond to continuous touch stimuli. **Basket nerve endings** around hair bases are found in all other areas of the skin. They are sensitive to touch and respond when the hair is bent. Like Meissner's corpuscles, they adapt readily to stimulation.

Pressure receptors generally lie deeper within the tissues. For example, **Pacinian corpuscles** are found deep within the dermis, in joints and also in parts of the viscera. They adapt very rapidly to pressure stimuli and can therefore signal vibration. **Ruffini's endings**, which are also found in deeper tissues, adapt more slowly and can signal continuous deformation.

Most of the tactile receptors send signals along larger diameter sensory fibres belonging to group Aβ. However, free nerve endings and most tactile nerve endings associated with hair bases transmit signals in Aδ and C fibres. These slower-conducting pathways transmit rather poorly localized stimuli when compared with the Aβ fibre group.

## Proprioceptors

Proprioceptors transmit signals that provide information about body position and movement. Muscle spindles and Golgi tendon organs signal muscle length and muscle tension, respectively.

Receptors in joints also signal important information about movement. Ruffini's endings are abundant in joints. They maintain a steady discharge in response to continuous stimulation, although the initial firing rate at the onset of stimulation is much greater. As the angle of a joint is changed, so particular Ruffini's endings are switched on or off. Each receptor responds maximally to a particular angle or position of joint. *Rate of change* of angle at the joint is probably detected, at least in part, by the initial strong rate of firing before the Ruffini's receptors adapt to the lower steady rate of activity. The *initial* receptor response to stimulation is certainly proportional to the rate of movement. In addition, rapidly adapting Pacinian corpuscles in the joints probably aid in the detection of rate of movement. Proprioceptor signals are transmitted in the larger-diameter $A\alpha$ and $A\beta$ fibres.

## Thermal receptors

The many gradations of temperature that an individual can detect seem to depend on the relative activities of two populations of receptors, namely cold and warmth receptors. In addition, pain receptors can be stimulated in extremes of cold or heat. Cold and warmth receptors are probably free nerve endings, although specialized Krause's end-bulbs and Ruffini's endings have been associated with cold and warmth, respectively. In any case, there are more cold receptors than warmth receptors.

The stimulus for temperature receptors is apparently thermal energy. However, it is probable that a change in temperature that causes a change in the metabolic rate of a receptor is acting indirectly only as a stimulus, and the receptor is in fact activated directly by chemical stimulation resulting from the changed metabolic rate.

Thermal signals are transmitted to the brain largely in $A\delta$ fibres but also in small C fibres.

## Pain receptors

Pain receptors are all free nerve endings. They are located in the skin, muscles, joints, arterial walls, membranes surrounding the brain, and also in the hollow organs of the gut. Pain is variously described as pricking, cutting, burning, aching, stabbing or crushing. The quality of the pain experienced seems to depend on the part of the body affected and on the nature and extent of the injury that causes it. The perception of pain depends partly on the physiological response of the receptors and partly on a psychological reaction to the pain itself. This section is restricted to a consideration of the physiology of pain receptors. Other aspects of the topic are dealt with later in the chapter.

The stimulus for pain can be physical or chemical. Physical stimuli can be thermal, mechanical or electrical energy of high intensity. For example, excessive mechanical stretching can elicit pain and this might contribute to the pain of inflammation. Excessive dilation of intracranial arteries can cause headache.

It is possible that physical stimuli actually act through chemical mediators. Certainly, it is known that a number of chemicals can elicit pain when applied to tissues. Severe physical blows or burns produce immediate pain but pain might well continue after cessation of physical stimulation and it is thought likely that chemical factors are responsible for this. Prostaglandins, histamine, bradykinin and 5-hydroxytryptamine (serotonin) are all chemicals produced by the body when tissue damage occurs and will all elicit pain if experimentally applied to a blister on the skin.

Pain receptors do not appear to adapt and, while stimulation is maintained, pain continues to be transmitted to the CNS. Pain is transmitted in unmyelinated C fibres or in slightly larger myelinated $A\delta$ fibres. The $A\delta$ fibres conduct signals more rapidly than the C fibres, and painful stimulation of skin elicits a double pain, a fast pricking sensation transmitted by $A\delta$ fibres and a slower burning sensation transmitted by C fibres.

## The somatosensory system

The pathways of the somatosensory system within the CNS connect the primary afferents from receptors to the sensory projection areas of the cerebral cortex. The pathways involve synapses at several levels including the spinal cord, the nuclei of the lower brainstem and the sensory relay nuclei of the thalamus. Axons from the thalamic nuclei then project to the primary sensory cortex, which lies along the postcentral gyrus, and to secondary sensory cortex. There are also descending pathways from the cerebral cortex, which terminate in the main relay nuclei of the sensory projection pathways.

The ascending sensory pathways can be divided into the **dorsal column medial lemniscal pathway** and the **spinothalamic tract**. This division has functional relevance because the two pathways transmit information that has qualitative differences. The spinothalamic tract transmits important information concerning pain and temperature but provides rather poor localization and poor discrimination of the stimulus. Sensory information of this somewhat diffuse, all-or-none kind is referred to as **protopathic**. The dorsal columns mediate tactile and **kinaesthetic** information, which is highly discriminatory and can be precisely localized. This more discriminative type of information is referred to as **epicritic**.

### The dorsal column–medial lemniscal pathway (Fig. 2.3.5)

The dorsal columns are large bundles of nerve fibres lying in the dorsal (posterior) quadrant of the spinal cord. The columns consist of ascending branches of dorsal root fibres. As the dorsal root fibres enter the

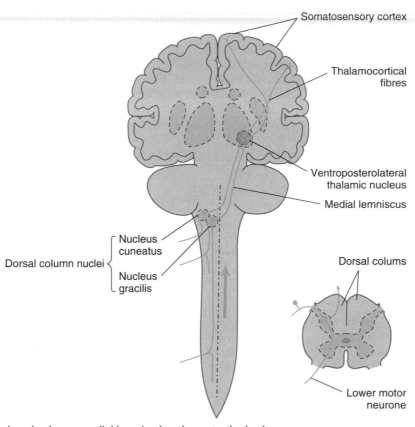

**Figure 2.3.5** The dorsal column: medial lemniscal pathway to the brain

dorsal horn, they immediately enter the dorsal columns without synapsing, although collateral branches synapse with cells of the dorsal horn. The dorsal root fibres of the dorsal columns tend to be large-diameter myelinated A fibres, which can transmit impulses at relatively high velocities (around 70 m/s). The nerve fibres are arranged somatotopically, such that nerve fibres from sacral and lumbar roots take up a medial position and those from higher levels of the spinal cord assume a more lateral position. As the cord is ascended, the nerve fibres from higher levels are added to the lateral aspect of the dorsal columns so that the higher the level of origin, the more lateral will be their position within the dorsal columns.

The first synapse of the dorsal column nerve fibres is at the level of the lower medulla. Here, the axons terminate on cells of the two dorsal column nuclei, called the **nucleus gracilis** and the **nucleus cuneatus**. The cells of these brainstem sensory nuclei then project **second-order nerve fibres** to the thalamus.

The second-order fibres cross the midline and join a large fibre bundle called the **medial lemniscus**. Crossing the midline results in the projections from one half of the body travelling to the contralateral half of the brain. Consequently, at the level of the cerebral cortex, the left side of the body is represented in the right sensory projection area of the cortex and the right side of the body is represented in the left

sensory cortex. The second-order nerve fibres ascend in the medial lemniscus to terminate in the **sensory relay nucleus** of the thalamus – the ventroposterolateral nucleus (VPL). Cells of this nucleus then project to the sensory projection areas of cerebral cortex, principally to the primary sensory area.

## The spinothalamic tract (Fig. 2.3.6)

The dorsal root fibres of the protopathic pathway tend to be of the smaller-diameter myelinated Aδ or unmyelinated C fibre type. The conduction velocities of these nerve fibres are consequently slower than those typical of the dorsal column fibres.

The dorsal root fibres enter the spinal cord and can either ascend or descend for a few segments (usually from one to six segments) before terminating on cells of the dorsal horn. In the dorsal horn, the cells of the intermediate grey matter, the cells of the **substantia gelatinosa** (which caps the dorsal horn) and the marginal cells lying outside the substantia gelatinosa all receive input from dorsal root fibres either directly or via interneurones lying within the dorsal horn itself. Dorsal horn cells then project fibres that usually ascend for a few segments before crossing the midline in the ventral (anterior) commissure of the spinal cord. These fibres then ascend the spinal cord as the spinothalamic tract. The nerve fibres of the spinothalamic tract travel in the ventrolateral (antero-lateral) quadrant of the cord, maintaining a roughly somatotopic organization.

Most of the fibres terminate on cells of the ventro-posterolateral nucleus of the thalamus, although some synapse with cells of the posterior group of thalamic nuclei. Cells of the thalamic relay nuclei then project fibres to both the primary and second-ary sensory projection areas of the cerebral cortex, but mainly to the primary sensory area.

It is worth noting here that another pathway ori-ginates from groups of cells in the dorsal horn similar to those giving rise to the spinothalamic tract. This pathway arises mainly from cells of the intermediate grey matter and also ascends the spinal cord in the ventrolateral quadrant. This is the **spinoreticular tract**, which projects fibres to the reticular formation of the brainstem. The ascending influences of the retic-ular formation have widespread effects on the arousal level of the brain and upon conscious awareness. The closeness of the association between the spinothala-mic tract and the spinoreticular tract presumably rests on the necessity for a protopathic input, such as a noxious stimulus, to be responded to immediately. Control and direction of such a rapid response might require a generalized increase in arousal level, proba-bly associated with a shift in the direction of attention.

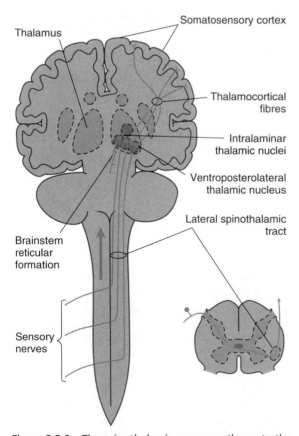

Thalamus

Somatosensory cortex

Thalamocortical fibres

Intralaminar thalamic nuclei

Ventroposterolateral thalamic nucleus

Lateral spinothalamic tract

Brainstem reticular formation

Sensory nerves

**Figure 2.3.6**   The spinothalamic sensory pathway to the brain

## The trigeminal nerve

The somatosensory fibres of the trigeminal nerve, the fifth cranial nerve, transmit sensory information from the face. The peripheral fibres synapse with cells of two brainstem nuclei. Second-order fibres then join the spinothalamic tract and the medial lemniscus. The fibres joining the spinothalamic tract mostly cross to the opposite side of the brain but a portion of the fibres joining the medial lemniscus remain uncrossed.

## CLINICAL APPLICATIONS

### SPINAL CORD LESIONS

Lesions of the spinal cord can be caused by physical insult or disease. Motor car, industrial and other accidents account for the majority of cases of spinal cord lesion but clinical conditions such as tumours, cervical spondylosis (associated with degeneration of intervertebral discs), syringomyelia (which involves the development of elongated cavities close to the central canal of the cord) and myelitis (inflammation of the cord) can all cause compression or lesions of the spinal cord.

### PAIN

#### The function of pain

The sensation of pain provides an important defence mechanism against tissue damage and is therefore essential for survival, even though the experience of pain is distressing. In the very rare cases of congenital analgesia or the more common cases of analgesia caused by lesions of nervous pathways, patients can sustain extensive tissue damage without being aware of any noxious stimulus. Such patients constantly have to be wary of potential harm and nursing such patients requires special procedures. For example, it is necessary regularly to move and alter the position of paraplegic patients to avoid constant pressure on parts of the body, such as the back and the sacrum, which could result in pressure ulcers.

Pain as a protective mechanism has some shortcomings. Irradiation of the body with either ionizing or non-ionizing radiation frequently does not elicit pain at the time of stimulation, although extensive tissue damage can occur. Many people will have experienced painful sunburn following an apparently pleasant and comfortable spell of sunbathing; pain in this instance does not serve any warning function. Similarly, pain is not generally associated with many cancers until a tumour is quite extensive. Indeed, the tumour might have metastasized and produced 'secondaries' elsewhere before pain is appreciated. Chronic pain associated with degenerative disorders, such as arthritis, can also hardly be regarded as protective.

## Perception of pain

The perception of pain depends on both physiological and psychological factors. The location and intensity of the stimulus will affect the quality and severity of the perceived pain. Cutaneous pain can be described as pricking or burning pain and can readily be distinguished from pain arising from joints or muscles and from that arising from the gut. In general, the greater the intensity of the stimulus, the more severe the perceived pain. Pain perception is also determined by the non-physiological functions described in McCaffery & Beebe (1989) and Sofaer (1992).

Culture also appears to play a part in the tolerance of pain. This aspect of the psychological reaction might be so powerful as to cause pain where there is no obvious physiological stimulation. In certain cultures, childbirth is associated with apparent 'labour pains' in the father while the mother – quietly and seemingly without undue discomfort – produces the infant.

## Transmission of pain signals

Pain signals appear to be transmitted in both myelinated A$\delta$ and unmyelinated C fibres. It has been suggested that the division of painful stimuli into those causing sharper, pricking sensations and those causing the duller, burning or aching sensations is associated with these two nerve fibre types. Sharp, pricking sensations are thought to be transmitted by the faster-conducting A$\delta$ fibres, whereas aching sensations are conducted by the slower C fibres. Certainly, experiments in which nerve fibres are subjected to ischaemia induce a block of fast, pricking pain first. Ischaemia blocks larger myelinated fibres before unmyelinated ones. On the other hand, experiments utilizing local anaesthetics, such as procaine, block the burning or aching pain preferentially, and local anaesthetics are known to have a predilection for small, unmyelinated C fibres. Nevertheless, it is still not clear whether different receptors as well as different types of nerve axon are responsible for the differentation of pain into these two qualitatively separable experiences.

## The gate control theory

The **gate control theory** of pain proposed by Melzack and Wall in 1965 (see Melzack & Wall, 1988) suggests that there is a relationship between the inputs from touch receptors and pain receptors at the level of the spinal cord. In particular, it suggests that interneurones in the substantia gelatinosa of the dorsal horn can regulate the conduction of ascending afferent input. The theory proposes that large-diameter fibres from touch receptors normally presynaptically inhibit small-diameter fibres from pain receptors. This constitutes a 'gate', which inhibits the transmission of input from pain receptors unless a great deal of small-diameter fibre activity forces open the gate to allow transmission along pain pathways in the spinothalamic and spinoreticular tracts. Melzack and Wall also propose that descending fibres from the brain synapse in the same area of the dorsal horn of the spinal cord and can modify the transmission of pain signals (**Fig. 2.3.7**).

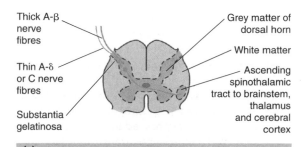

**(a)**

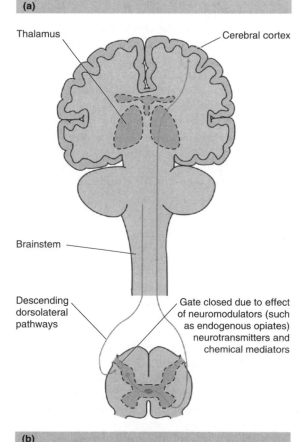

**(b)**

**Figure 2.3.7**   The gate control theory showing (a) a diagrammatic cross-section of the spinal cord and (b) internal influences on the gate mechanism (adapted from Davis (1993) with permission of Nursing Standard Publications, London)

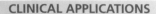

## CLINICAL APPLICATIONS

The gate control theory helps to explain a number of observable pain phenomena. For example, the destruction of large-diameter afferents following amputation of a limb and the consequent release of inhibitory influences over small-diameter nerve fibres might account for the experience of **phantom limb pain**. Similarly, the destruction of, or damage to, touch fibres in inflamed tissue could in part account for the phenomenon of hyperalgesia, whereby inflamed tissue is more sensitive to pain. The presence of descending influences from the brain also helps to explain the relationship between psychological factors and pain perception.

Since their original paper, research relating to Melzack and Wall's gate control theory has indeed established the existence of inhibitory interactions between large- and small-diameter afferent nerve fibres in the dorsal horn, although these interactions now appear to be rather more complicated than was at first suggested. Despite this, there is no doubt that the theory has led to many important developments. For example, **transcutaneous electrical stimulation (TENS)** as a means of relieving pain is now a well established and widely used technique. This development owes much to Melzack and Wall's ideas, even though the effectiveness of the treatment might not lie entirely in the action of stimulated large-diameter afferents inhibiting the activity of small-diameter pain fibres. In addition to the interactions of dorsal horn cells, the presence of a powerful descending inhibitory pathway from nuclei in the brainstem is now firmly established, and stimulation of these nuclei causes marked analgesia.

### Representation of pain in the brain

Many parts of the brain contribute to the pain experience. The thalamic nuclei seem to influence the conscious appreciation of pain, and damage to the thalamus can cause severe and intractable pain. This pain is experienced as arising from those parts of the body that normally transmit afferent input of the damaged areas of the thalamus. Extensive damage to the somatosensory cortex on the postcentral gyrus does not abolish pain and it appears that the adjacent area of cortex is more important for the integration and interpretation of pain signals.

### Referred pain

The phenomenon of 'referred pain' has attracted considerable attention in pain research. The term describes the way in which pain arising from damage in one part of the body is actually experienced as though it were arising in a different part of the body. It is thought to result from the fact that the pain fibres from the damaged visceral organs enter the spinal cord at the same level as afferents from the referred area of the body.

### Pain transmitters

A major recent development in the study of pain has been the discovery of various peptides that have been implicated in pain transmission and pain relief.

**Substance P** is a neurotransmitter, or neuromodulator, which has been identified in various parts of the nervous system, including the substantia gelatinosa of the dorsal horn. Noxious stimulation causes the release of substance P from dorsal root afferents and consequently it has been suggested that substance P acts, at least partly, as a transmitter for pain.

Whereas substance P is implicated in the transmission of pain, other peptides seem to possess analgesic properties. The discovery of these peptides, the **enkephalins and endorphins**, stemmed from research into the powerful analgesic action of opiate derivative drugs such as morphine (Hughes et al., 1975). In performing its analgesic action, morphine binds to receptors on the nerve cell membrane. These receptors are, at least partly, located presynaptically. The existence of receptors to which morphine can attach implied the existence of some endogenous substance, similar to morphine, to which receptors would bind under normal conditions (i.e. without the presence of morphine). The search for this endogenous opiate-like substance led to the discovery of the enkephalins. Hughes and colleagues were the first to isolate and identify these endogenous opiates in 1975. They identified two peptide chains, comprising just five amino acids each, which they called methionine and leucine enkephalin. These peptides are very unstable and have a half-life of 1 minute or less in brain tissue, but they are fragments of a much longer peptide chain, beta-endorphin. Beta-endorphin comprises 30 amino acids and is a much more stable molecule, and it too binds with opiate receptors. In turn, beta-endorphin is a fragment of the pituitary hormone beta-lipotrophin, which is itself derived from the same precursor as adrenocorticotrophic hormone (ACTH).

The endogenous opiates have been shown to inhibit prostaglandin formation and **prostaglandins** are putative chemical stimuli for pain. In addition, endogenous opiates have been shown experimentally to inhibit the actions of a number of transmitters, including substance P, the suggested transmitter for pain.

The enkephalins and endorphins have an analgesic action similar to that of morphine, and it is thought that the analgesia of acupuncture might be attributable to enkephalin activity. Despite the many questions that still remain about the precise mode of action and range of influence of enkephalins and endorphins in the central and peripheral nervous systems, their existence does go some way to explain phenomena such as the **placebo response**, where an individual perceives pain relief even though no analgesic agent is administered. It is possible that in such cases the mere expectation of pain relief is sufficient to release, psychogenically, the endogenous opiates, which would then cause genuine analgesia even without the administration of an analgesic drug.

## Management of pain

The approach to the management of pain will vary considerably depending upon a number of factors, including:

- **Identification of the cause.** For example, is the pain due to an underlying disease requiring treatment, the direct result of a known painful clinical procedure in hospital (e.g. surgery) or trauma (e.g. a fracture)?
- **Whether the pain is acute or chronic.** Acute pain is defined as pain that has an identifiable cause and is of short duration (e.g. as a result of injury or surgery). Chronic pain does not necessarily have an obvious cause and is unremitting, affecting the patient's lifestyle. Treatment for each of these will vary enormously.
- **Curative versus palliative.** If pain is caused by an underlying disorder, is this curable with treatment or will the condition become terminal?
- **The patient's perception.** What do patients understand of the pain that they are experiencing? Do they know the reasons for it? What are their expectations as to the duration, implications and significance of the pain?
- **The nurse's biases.** Can the nurse accept the patient's reactions to the painful experience in a non-judgmental way? It is now widely accepted that pain is what the patient says it is and that it exists when a patient says it does.

The patient should be assessed prior to implementing interventions to relieve pain. The subjective nature of an individual's experience of pain makes it difficult to assess but clearly, if

therapies are to be evaluated and the patient kept comfortable and pain free, then assessment is crucial.

In some situations it will be immediately obvious that the patient is profoundly distressed and requires urgent intervention, e.g. the person suddenly admitted to hospital with a perforated ulcer. Intervention in these circumstances should be immediate and only a brief assessment of the situation is required. In other circumstances a more detailed assessment is both possible and desirable and the initial approach to this is to obtain a pain history during the interview immediately following admission (if appropriate). The following questions should be addressed:

- Can you describe your pain?
- When did you last experience it?
- How long does it last?
- What do you do to relieve it? Does it work?
- Does anything make the pain worse?
- Are you on medication for the relief of your pain?
- Are you in pain at the moment?
- Is there a pattern to your pain, e.g. does it come at a particular time of day?
- Do you feel it is getting worse?
- Does the pain interfere with your day-to-day life?

Assessment of the patient's needs is a continuing process and this equally applies to the assessment of pain. A patient admitted for minor surgery may be pain free on admission and not experience any pain until the postoperative period. Equally, a patient may be admitted for management of a painful condition, such as trigeminal neuralgia, in which case ongoing assessment is crucial to measure the efficacy of therapy. One way to achieve this is to use an appropriate pain assessment tool (McCaffery, 2002).

Examples of pain assessment tools include the simple linear scale on which the patient places a cross on a line indicating the severity of the pain. The scale can be numerical, with 0 indicating no pain and 10 severe pain, or descriptive, with 'no pain' at one end of the line and 'severe pain' at the other.

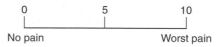

Interventions intended to achieve pain relief are varied and should be selected according to the assessment of the patient's needs and the situation. Appraisal of the selected intervention(s)

is essential to gauge effectiveness and, if necessary, to alter the approach. Measures to relieve pain include the use of drugs, and in particular analgesics, and the use of therapies such as cutaneous stimulation (e.g. massage), which adopt a drug-free approach. Alternative methods, such as therapeutic touch, might also be considered. For some patients the only solution to their pain is to undergo surgical procedures to achieve relief. An example is cordotomy, in which sensory fibres of the spinothalamic tract are divided.

A number of interventions can be implemented by the nurse to enhance the effectiveness of the strategies outlined here. These include:

- **Comfort measures.** Repositioning the patient, maintaining proper body alignment, ensuring adequate rest, immobilizing a painful part and elevating an affected extremity.
- **Environmental considerations.** Eliminating noxious stimuli and providing quiet surroundings.
- **Patient teaching.** Providing information to reduce the patient's anxiety and fear and inform of the options available for pain relief.
- **Emotional support.** Spending time with the patient, displaying an accepting and open approach to his or her feelings and explaining to family and friends how best they can help.

### Analgesic drugs

These are drugs specifically intended to abolish pain. A wide range is now available. They can be delivered by a variety of routes, including orally, intramuscularly, subcutaneously, intravenously, rectally, epidurally, by inhalation and by topical application.

Patient-controlled analgesia (PCA) is now commonplace and permits patients to take responsibility for their pain management if they so wish and are able (Jackson, 1999). One group of oral drugs commonly used in the treatment of mild to moderate pain is the non-steroidal anti-inflammatory drugs (NSAIDS). These include aspirin, ibuprofen and mefenamic acid. Along with their analgesic properties, these drugs are also antipyretic and anti-inflammatory, which enhances relief of pain. Severe pain is effectively treated with narcotics, which act by binding to opiate receptors in the CNS and altering both pain perception and the emotional response to pain. The best-known of these is morphine, which can be delivered by a variety

of routes; others include codeine and pentazocine.

The use of adjuvant (a substance that aids another) drugs is an important aspect in the use of analgesics. Examples include sedatives, tranquillizers, muscle relaxants and steroids, all of which enhance the action of the analgesia. The careful use of adjuvant therapy can even result in the need for a smaller dose of analgesia.

One final aspect in relation to the use of drugs is that of the placebo. This is an inert preparation or form of treatment that nevertheless produces a response in the patient. About one-third of patients who are given a placebo and who are told beforehand that this is an effective method of abolishing pain will experience relief. It does not, however, mean that the patient did not experience pain in the first place and it is therefore not advocated as a means of detecting whether pain actually exists.

'Non-drug' approaches to relieve pain can incorporate the use of cutaneous stimulation. The application of a sensory stimulus to the skin can result in inhibition of the painful impulses. Parents who rub the hurt away from their child's arm to achieve relief are using this strategy. Methods that can be used include:

- topical applications (which usually contain a local anaesthetic)
- massage
- application of heat and/or cold
- acupuncture.

### Other strategies

Transcutaneous electrical nerve stimulation (TENS) works by applying or implanting small electrodes that can be activated to supply a low electrical current. This results in stimulation of nerve fibres and reduction of pain impulses. This technique can be controlled by the patient.

Cognitive strategies encompass the harnessing of mental powers to block pain at the cortical level. These include distraction, in which patients learn to focus attention on something other than their pain (e.g. reading a book or listening to music). Another technique is relaxation, in which the patient learns progressive muscle relaxation such as that used in yoga. Finally, using the patient's imagination to evoke an image in his mind of, for example, a favourite place, can be effective. The patient is instructed to imagine every detail of the place – the sights, sounds, smells, etc. This is known as guided imagery. Hypnosis is effective for some people but requires the patient's active cooperation.

Some patients need to resort to surgical interventions to obtain relief. Techniques available to them include:

- **Nerve block.** Peripheral nerves are temporarily interrupted by injection of a local anaesthetic or destroyed by a neurolytic agent such as phenol. Traumatic brachial plexus pain can respond to this technique.
- **Rhizotomy.** Division of sensory nerve roots at the level of the pain and at neighbouring segments. Motor function is preserved but other sensations are lost. This can be combined with injection of alcohol to prevent regeneration of the axons. Rhizotomy is useful for intractable pain caused by degenerative conditions.
- **Cordotomy.** Division of sensory fibres in the lateral spinothalamic tract. The most common levels at which this is performed are the thoracic and cervical levels. Again, it is useful for intractable pain caused by degenerative conditions.
- **Thalamotomy.** Stereotactic (a technique for locating structures in the brain) destruction of pain fibres in the thalamus can be performed as a last resort in patients with intractable pain due to malignancy of the face or head.
- **Sympathectomy.** Resection of part of the sympathetic trunk. Carried out in patients with causalgia (an intense burning sensation).

## The motor system

### Upper and lower motor neurones

The section on the CNS and motor control in Chapter 2.2 (pp. 114–122) should be read in conjunction with this section.

At the level of the spinal cord, motor nerve cells are divided, by convention, into 'upper' and 'lower' motor neurones. Strictly speaking, the term 'upper motor neurone' is a misnomer because only nerve fibres innervating muscle cells can truly be described as motor neurones. Nevertheless, the division of the nerve pathways into upper and lower motor neurones is valuable clinically and hence the terms continue to be used.

The term '**lower motor neurone**' is applied to cells of the ventral horn of the spinal cord and their associated nerve fibres that innervate muscle fibres. The axon of a single lower motor neurone branches at its distal end so that it innervates a number of muscle fibres – anything from a few to a few hundred.

The muscle fibres innervated by a single motor neurone are referred to collectively as a **motor unit**.

### CLINICAL APPLICATIONS

Damage to the lower motor neurone effectively disconnects the muscle from its nerve supply. This results in a **flaccid paralysis**, in which muscle tone is lowered (hypotonia). A marked reduction in resistance to passive movement occurs, and a loss of spinal reflexes ensues. In addition, denervation of the muscle can result in twitches, called fasciculations, and the muscle might also show signs of atrophy.

The term '**upper motor neurone**' is applied to the nerve fibres of the spinal cord that descend to synapse on lower motor neurones or upon spinal cord interneurones. Upper motor neurone fibres make up the long descending spinal tracts of the central motor system. Damage to upper motor neurones tends to cause dysfunction in muscle groups rather than in individual muscle units and, consequently, the motor deficit tends to involve disruption of whole movements. This contrasts with lower motor neurone damage, which affects single muscles. In addition, upper motor neurone damage does not cause the disconnection of the muscle from its nerve supply because upper motor neurone damage is not necessarily accompanied by lower motor neurone damage. Consequently, upper motor neurone damage is not associated with the muscle atrophy seen in lower motor neurone injury, although prolonged lack of use of affected muscles will cause wastage in the longer term.

### CLINICAL APPLICATIONS

Upper motor neurone damage is also normally associated with **spastic paralysis**. Spastic paralysis involves an increase in muscle tone (hypertonus), which is assumed to be caused by a reduction or removal of descending inhibitory influences following an upper motor neurone lesion. This same removal of descending inhibitory influences would also account for the exaggeration of spinal reflexes that occurs below the level of the lesion following upper motor neurone injury. An increased resistance to passive movement also occurs after upper motor neurone injury, resulting in the **claspknife response**. The **Babinski response** is also associated with upper motor neurone lesions in adults (see p. 94).

The cell bodies of lower motor neurones lie within the ventral horn of the spinal cord. It can be seen at

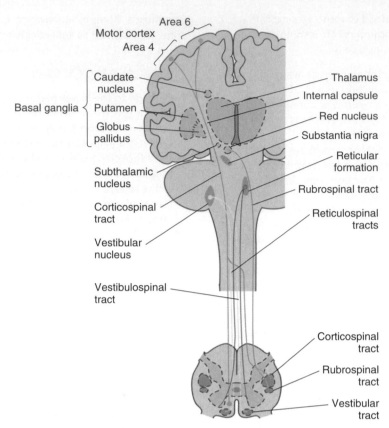

**Figure 2.3.8**  Descending motor pathways from the brain

the segmental level that the motor neurones are arranged within the ventral horn in an organized manner such that those cells projecting to proximal muscles are located medially and those projecting to more distal muscles are located progressively more laterally.

Upper motor neurones can synapse directly on α and γ lower motor neurones, or they might terminate on spinal interneurones. Direct termination on lower motor neurones will allow for immediate changes in muscle tension following alterations in the descending upper motor neurone discharge. On the other hand, spinal interneurones can act as gating mechanisms, so that peripheral sensory input via spinal reflexes such as the stretch reflex can be switched on or off, thereby enhancing or inhibiting the reflex activity. In fact, the major proportion of descending influences are integrated with ongoing sensory events via spinal interneurones. These spinal interneurones are referred to as propriospinal neurones.

## Descending pathways (Fig. 2.3.8)

The corticospinal, rubrospinal, vestibulospinal and reticulospinal tracts constitute the major descending nerve pathways of the spinal cord.

The **corticospinal tracts**, which are also referred to as the cerebrospinal or pyramidal tracts, originate from widespread areas of the cerebral cortex. The

nerve fibres descend in the internal capsule to the brainstem, where they form easily identifiable lumps (or pyramids) on the ventral surface of the medulla. The term 'pyramidal tract' derives from this anatomical feature. Approximately 90% of the nerve fibres cross the midline (i.e. decussate) and descend further as the lateral corticospinal tract of the spinal cord. This tract extends throughout the length of the spinal cord. The other 10% of nerve fibres descend ipsilaterally as the ventral (anterior) corticospinal tract. Although the nerve fibres of the ventral corticospinal tract descend ipsilaterally, most of them cross the midline before synapsing in the spinal grey matter.

The **rubrospinal tract** originates from cells of the red nucleus of the midbrain. This nucleus forms one of the final integrating centres in the extrapyramidal motor pathway. It is topographically organized and receives major inputs from the cortex, via collaterals of pyramidal tract axons, and also from the cerebellum. Additional inputs come from the reticular formation and from the spinal cord. The red nucleus projects descending nerve fibres, which comprise the rubrospinal tract. Rubrospinal fibres decussate and then descend the spinal cord alongside lateral corticospinal fibres to terminate in the grey matter of the cord. Functionally, the rubrospinal pathway closely mirrors the pyramidal tract system. For example, research in primates has shown that removal of the red nucleus and the closely surrounding reticular formation results in motor dysfunction that is similar to that seen following pyramidotomy. The only major difference seems to be in the control of the most distal musculature, in particular the ability to grip with the fingers.

The **vestibulospinal tracts** originate from cells of the vestibular nuclei of the brainstem. The lateral vestibulospinal tract projects from the lateral vestibular nucleus and descends, uncrossed, throughout the length of the spinal cord. The medial vestibular tract originates from the medial vestibular nucleus and comprises both crossed and uncrossed nerve fibres, which terminate at cervical levels of the spinal cord. Stimulation of vestibulospinal fibres has a facilitatory effect and enhances muscle tone.

The **reticulospinal tracts** comprise the descending projections of cells of the brainstem reticular formation. The medial reticulospinal tract projects from cells of the pons and descends, as an uncrossed tract, the length of the spinal cord. The lateral reticulospinal tract projects from cells of the medulla and descends, both as a crossed and uncrossed pathway, the entire length of the cord. These two tracts appear to function in a reciprocal manner through their indirect influences on α and γ motor neurones. The medial reticulospinal tract facilitates extensor and inhibits flexor muscle reflexes, whereas the lateral reticulospinal tract inhibits extensor and facilitates flexor reflexes. However, the precise nature of reticular control over motor activity might be more complex than this description implies, because the reticular formation receives descending input from many brain structures, including the cerebral cortex (particularly the premotor area) and limbic forebrain structures as well as from extrapyramidal motor fibres. It also receives ascending sensory input.

## CLINICAL APPLICATIONS

Complete or partial spinal transection has marked effects on motor activity. A complete section through the spinal cord results in **spinal shock**, in which there is no activity below the level of transection. Subsequently, spinal reflex activity recovers. Loss of voluntary control of muscle activity persists, owing to the sectioning of all upper motor neurones.

Paraplegia describes a paralysis of the lower half of the body, whereas quadriplegia is a paralysis from the neck downwards. The degree of motor deficit following partial spinal transection depends on the location and extent of the lesion. For example, a hemisection results in paralysis of the muscles on the side of the lesion and below the level of the lesion. A patient suffering from paraplegia or quadriplegia relies, in the acute phase, on skilled nursing care to

exploit residual ability to the full. Meticulous care must be taken when positioning the patient in bed, to ensure that paralysed limbs are maintained in good alignment and properly supported. The patient's position also needs to be changed frequently to prevent ischaemic damage to the tissues from unrelieved pressure.

Bladder and bowel dysfunction can also be common features. A high-fibre diet and the use of stool softeners usually suffice to produce a formed bowel movement every other day. Urinary catheterization is often used in the early stages but the aim is to remove the catheter as soon as possible and retrain the patient's bladder to empty reflexly. This requires perseverance on the patient's part and encouragement from the nurse. However, the achievement of continence is a major morale booster. Every opportunity should be taken to educate the patient, who will need to accept responsibility for a lot of his or her future care.

## The pyramidal system

### Pyramidal tract

The terms 'pyramidal tract' and 'corticospinal tract' are used interchangeably. The term 'pyramidal' in this context refers to the appearance of the descending tracts at the level of the medulla, rather than to the pyramid-shaped neurones, the axons of which make up the tracts.

Primary motor cortex lies along the precentral gyrus and contains very large pyramid-shaped cells, called **Betz cells**, which are exclusive to this area of cortex and which give rise to a small proportion of the nerve fibres of the pyramidal tracts. However, by far the greatest proportion (approximately 50%) of nerve fibres in the corticospinal tracts project from smaller, pyramid-shaped cells in the larger anterior portion of the motor cortex.

The pyramidal tract is commonly represented as consisting of nerve fibres that project directly from motor cortex to motor neurones or spinal cord interneurones. In fact, most axons leaving the motor cortex do not reach the spinal cord. Moreover, those fibres that do enter the pyramidal tracts project axon collaterals to many other brain structures. For example, axon collaterals of pyramidal fibres project to the red nucleus, the basal ganglia the thalamus and the brainstem reticular formation.

## Conclusion

This chapter has outlined the importance of an integrated sensory/motor system and discussed its application in relation to the phenomenon of pain.

## Clinical review

In addition to the Learning Objectives at the beginning of this chapter, the reader should be able to:

- Explain how spinal cord lesions can arise

- Outline the gate control theory of pain transmission

- Explain how the gate control theory is useful in explaining some phenomena associated with pain e.g. 'phantom limb'

- Describe the difference between upper and lower motor neurone damage

## Review questions

1  How can sensory receptors be classified on the basis of function?
2  Are generator potentials at neuronal receptors linearly related to stimulus intensity?
3  From which areas of the body do somatosensory signals arise?
4  What kind of information do proprioceptors provide?
5  Why might pain from a mechanical stimulus persist after the stimulus has been removed?
6  Explain the somatotopic arrangement of fibres in the dorsal column.
7  Which structure forms a 'cap' on the dorsal horn?
8  What is referred pain?
9  Distinguish between flaccid and spastic paralysis

## Further reading

McCaffery, M. & Pasero, C. (1999) *Pain: Clinical Manual,* 2nd edn. St Louis: Mosby.
*Definitive text on all aspects of pain management.*

Melzack, R. & Wall, P. (1988) *The Challenge of Pain,* 2nd edn. London: Penguin.
*Classic text that explores several aspects of pain from two of the foremost experts on the subject.*

## References

Davis, P. (1993) Opening up the gate control theory. *Nursing Standard,* **7**; 25–26.
Jackson, C. (1999) Postoperative care and patient controlled analgesia. *Assignment,* **5**(4); 3–10.

McCaffery, M. (2002) Controlling pain. Teaching your patient to use a pain rating scale. *Nursing,* **32**(8); 17.
Melzack, R. & Wall, P. (1988) *The Challenge of Pain,* 2nd edn. London: Penguin.

# The special senses

*Douglas Allan*

## LEARNING OBJECTIVES

After studying this chapter the reader should be able to:

- Describe the mechanism of the production and drainage of tear fluid in the eye

- Draw a labelled diagram of a cross-section through a human eyeball and describe the functions of the labelled parts

- Account for the direction and extent of refraction of light as it passes through the eye to the retina

- Define the term 'power of accommodation' and explain its role in normal vision

- Distinguish the difference in the optics of normal vision, myopia, hypermetropia and astigmatism

- Describe the structure of the retina

- Described in outline the photochemical reaction between light and rhodopsin

- Define the term 'visual acuity' and describe a method of its measurement

- Describe how changes in electrical potential of photoreceptors are transmitted and processed by cells of the intermediate layer of the retina

- Identify the visual pathway from the retinae to the brain and explain how the visual input is processed by the cerebral cortex

- Describe the pathways involved in visual reflexes and eye movements

- Identify and describe the functions of the major components of the auditory apparatus of the ear

- Describe the structure of a taste-bud and illustrate the distribution of taste-buds in the mouth

## INTRODUCTION

In Chapter 2.3 we learned of the importance of the sensory system and general sensation; this chapter will examine the more specialized senses of smell, taste, sight, hearing and equilibrium. These are described as the special senses because the structures involved are more complex than those for general sensation.

## The eye and vision

### Anatomy of the eye

Each eyeball is 1.5–2 cm in diameter and is located in a conical bony orbit of the skull. The exposed surface of the eye and the inner surfaces of the eyelids are covered with a delicate membrane, the conjunctiva, which helps to prevent drying-out of the tissues.

The eye is also protected by reflex blinking, by the eyelashes and eyebrows, and by the production of tear fluid, which bathes the surface of the eye.

The more or less regular blinking that occurs every few seconds throughout life aids in washing tear fluid across the surface of the eye. If this process is impaired, for example as sometimes occurs with the wearing of contact lenses, then the transparent exposed suface of the eye, the **cornea**, can become inflamed and even ulcerated. An inability to blink effectively can also occur in patients who have had a stroke or in unconscious patients who receive inadequate eye care. If the problem is severe, the patient's eyelids can be sewn together, a procedure referred to as tarsorrhaphy. Blinking is normally initiated by stimulation of the conjunctiva, the cornea or of the eyelid itself. Blinking can also operate as a protective reflex response to a threatening gesture or in response to bright light.

The production of **tear fluid** is of considerable importance to the maintenance of a healthy cornea. Tear fluid contains salts and protein but very little glucose. It also contains oil secreted by sebaceous glands, which affects its physical properties and helps to prevent overflow of tears at the lid margins. Tears also contain an enzyme, lysozyme, which is responsible for the mild bacteriocidal action of tear fluid. Tears are produced by the **lacrimal apparatus**, which is located in the upper outer corner of each bony orbit, partly by the lacrimal gland itself and partly by microscopic accessory glands. The production of tears by the lacrimal gland is normally a reflex response to irritation or drying of the cornea and/or conjunctiva. It is controlled by the parasympathetic nervous system. However, there is also a sympathetic nervous system input to the lacrimal gland that is involved in emotional weeping. Tear fluid is produced continuously by the accessory glands and the eyes will not normally suffer dryness even if the lacrimal gland itself is removed.

Adequate drainage of tear fluid is also important. Tears normally drain into small channels, **canaliculi**, which open at a number of small holes, the **puncta**, at the inner ends of the lid margins. The canaliculi drain tears into the **lacrimal sac**, which is located on the medial surface of the orbit. The lacrimal sac is continuous with the **lacrimal duct**, which finally drains the tears into the nasal cavity.

### CLINICAL APPLICATIONS

The tear drainage system can become blocked, causing a watery eye condition called **epiphora**. Apart from the nuisance aspect of epiphora, dermatitis and secondary infections can ensue if it is untreated. Blockage of tear ducts can occur in newborn babies, where it can be caused by maldevelopment or by blockage with mucus. Massage can clear a plug of mucus but surgery might be necessary to clear the duct adequately.

Dacryocystitis is an inflammation of the lacrimal sac that can also result in obstruction of the tear drainage system. This condition is more common in older women and might require surgery to open-up a bypass passage into the nose.

Many older people also suffer from watery eyes. This commonly occurs because the lids are malaligned and turn outwards or inwards such that the puncta cannot adequately collect the tear fluid. Surgical repair of the lids is necessary in severely affected individuals.

The eyeball is attached to the skull bones by three pairs of extraocular muscles, which permit rotational, horizontal and vertical movements of the eye. The lateral and medial rectus muscles move the eye from side to side. They are controlled by the VIth and IIIrd cranial nerves, respectively. Normal positioning of the eye in the horizontal plane depends on the relative activities of these muscles. For example, weakness or paralysis of the lateral rectus leads to excessive medial (nasal) movement of the eye and a squint develops. The superior and inferior rectus muscles cause upward and downward movement of the forward-facing eye and are controlled by the IIIrd cranial nerve. The superior and inferior oblique muscles cause rotational movements of the forward-facing eye and are controlled by the IVth and IIIrd cranial nerves, respectively.

The structure of the eye is illustrated in **Fig. 2.4.1**. The outer layer of the wall of the eyeball is composed of mechanically strong fibrous tissue. It is white in colour over most of the eyeball and forms the **sclera**, the visible part of which forms the 'white of the eye'. The most anterior part of the wall of the eye is transparent and forms the **cornea**. The cornea is a protective window through which light can pass into the globe of the eyeball. Because its surface is curved it acts as a 'fixed lens', and considerable bending (refraction) of light rays occur at the cornea.

The sclera is lined by a very vascular layer of tissue called the **choroid**, which contains the pigment melanin and absorbs scattered light. Over the posterior two-thirds of the wall of the eye is an inner, photosensitive layer of tissue called the **retina**. Lying immediately adjacent to the choroid is the retinal pigmented epithelium. This is heavily pigmented with melanin and absorbs light that has passed through the photoreceptors of the retina. The receptor layer, which is attached to the pigmented epithelium, is stimulated by light energy. The receptors transmit visual signals through other cells in the retina.

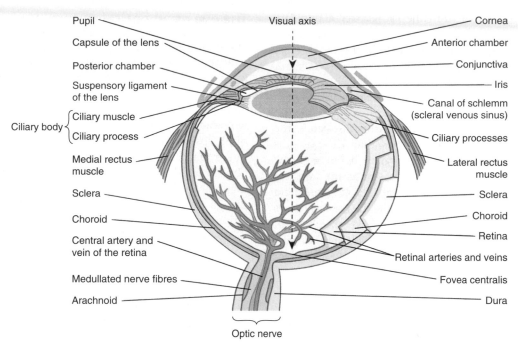

**Figure 2.4.1** Structure of the eye (transverse section)

The surface of the retina is covered with a 'mat' of nerve fibres, which arise from retinal cells and are collected together to form the **optic nerve**. The optic nerve leaves the bony orbit of the skull from a position that is slightly medial to the optical axis of the eye. The point where the optic nerve leaves the eyeball is called the **optic disc** or **blind spot**. The blind spot does not contain any receptors and is therefore insensitive to light.

### CLINICAL APPLICATIONS

If the intracranial pressure is raised, for example as a result of a brain tumour, the optic disc bulges and appears oedematous when observed with an ophthalmoscope. This condition is known as **papilloedema**. Optic neuritis, an inflammation of the optic nerve, can also cause papilloedema but if the inflammation occurs central (brain side) to the optic disc, papilloedema is not seen and the condition is known as retrobulbar neuritis. Unlike the papilloedema associated with raised intracranial pressure, papilloedema resulting from optic neuritis is associated with immediate rapid deterioration in vision.

The blind spot is not apparent in normal vision. This is largely because the image falling on the blind spot of each eye is not exactly the same. Thus, the left eye can provide the visual information that is missing from the right eye and vice versa. The brain also assists in 'filling in' missing detail.

There is a small depression in the retina lying lateral (temporal) to the blind spot. This depression is about 0.4 mm in diameter and is called the **fovea centralis**. In this part of the retina the receptor layer is exposed directly to the light, whereas elsewhere in the retina light is filtered through several layers of retinal cells. The fovea is important for detailed discrimination of visual images.

Anteriorly, the choroid layer bulges to form a ring of smooth muscle called **ciliary muscle**, to which the lens is attached. Anterior to this the choroid projects into the eye as the **iris**. The iris is the coloured part of the eye; its colour is determined genetically. The iris forms a variable aperture, the **pupil**, through which light is directed into the eye. It contains circularly arranged smooth muscle fibres, which are innervated by the parasympathetic nervous system. Contraction of these muscle fibres makes the iris aperture smaller and the pupil constricts.

### CLINICAL APPLICATIONS

Parasympathetic stimulation can be blocked if eye-drops containing homatropine, an atropine derivative, are administered. This drug blocks the action of acetylcholine, the parasympathetic transmitter, and the pupils then dilate, facilitating clinical examination of the eye.

The iris also contains radially arranged smooth muscle fibres, which are innervated by the sympathetic nervous system. Activation of these muscle fibres causes pupillary dilation. Emotional arousal is associated with activation of the sympathetic nervous system and it results in dilated pupils.

**151**

Shining a light into the eye evokes a pupillary reflex response in which the pupil constricts. It is a bilateral response, that is, if light is directed through only one eye, the pupils of both eyes constrict.

The **lens** of the eye is attached to the ciliary muscle by means of radially orientated suspensory ligaments. The lens has convex surfaces and causes refraction and convergence of light rays passing through it. The anterior surface is more curved than the posterior surface and therefore causes more bending of the light. The lens is composed of concentric layers of epithelial cells in an elastic capsule. It is not rigid and, when it is detached from the ligaments, it takes up a more or less spherical shape. The central core of the lens has a higher refractive index than other parts of the lens and therefore has the greatest potential for bending light passing through it.

### DEVELOPMENTAL ISSUES

The lens is normally transparent but old age or exposure to infrared radiation can cause coagulation of lens protein resulting in cloudiness. This condition is known as **cataract**. It can also present as a congenital disorder or as a complication of diabetes mellitus.

The narrow space between the iris and the lens forms the **posterior chamber** and the space between the iris and the cornea forms the **anterior chamber**. Both chambers are filled with a fluid derived from plasma called **aqueous humour**. Aqueous humour supplies oxygen and nutrients to the lens, which does not have an independent blood supply. Aqueous humour is secreted in the posterior chamber by blood vessels in ciliary processes at the base of the ciliary muscle. It is formed at the rate of 2 or 3 mm$^3$ per min and it then passes through the pupil into the anterior chamber. It is reabsorbed into ocular veins at the **angle of Schlemm**, which is the angle formed between the iris and the cornea. The rate of secretion and reabsorption of aqueous humour determines the intraocular pressure.

### CLINICAL APPLICATIONS

In glaucoma, the reabsorption of aqueous humour is impaired and intraocular pressure increases. If untreated, the raised pressure is transmitted to the retinal artery and blindness can ensue because of impaired oxygen and nutrient supply to the retina.

The space between the lens and the retina does not communicate directly with the posterior or anterior chambers of the eye. It is filled with a gelatinous mass called **vitreous humour**.

## The eye as an optical system

The primary function of the eye is to convert light energy into nervous impulses that can be 'interpreted' by the brain as visual images. To do this, the eye behaves like a camera so that light radiating from an object is brought into sharp focus on the photoreceptor layer of the retina. The retina is the equivalent of photosensitive film in the back of a camera. The image that is being viewed is reproduced, without blurring, on the retina and the pattern of stimulation of photoreceptors therefore accurately reflects the pattern of light radiating from the object. Thus, clear vision depends not only on the neurophysiological properties of the eye but also on its optical properties.

### Light

The behaviour of light can be described in terms of straight lines or rays of energy, which enter the eye through the pupil. Light rays from distant points appear to be parallel, whereas those from near points appear to diverge.

Regardless of whether light arrives at the surface of the eye as divergent, parallel or convergent rays, it passes through the cornea, the aqueous humour, the lens, the vitreous humour and the surface layers of the retinal cells before impinging on the photoreceptors. As light passes through these layers it will be **refracted** to varying degrees, ultimately to be focused on the receptors.

Biconvex lenses cause refraction and convergence of light rays passing through them, and parallel rays of light are brought together to a point at a finite distance behind the lens. This is known as the **focal length** (**Fig. 2.4.2a**). Concave lenses cause refraction and divergence of light rays passing through them, such that parallel rays of light passing through a biconcave lens appear to originate from a point, a fixed distance in front of the lens (**Fig. 2.4.2b**).

Refraction of light occurs at several points in the transmission pathway through the eye. When the eye is focused on a near object, the curvature of the lens increases to cause greater refraction of the diverging rays of light so that they will be brought to a focus on the retina. The refractive power of the lens increases, thus reducing the focal length of the lens so that when it is focused on near objects, parallel rays of light from distant points are focused in front of the retina and images of distant objects are then blurred (**Fig. 2.4.3**).

Convex lenses cause an inversion of the image of the object in both vertical and horizontal planes (**Fig. 2.4.3**). The visual world is therefore upside down and laterally reversed on the retina. This is of no importance to visual perception because the brain

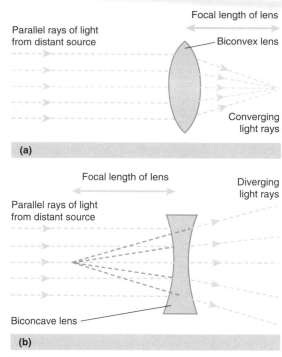

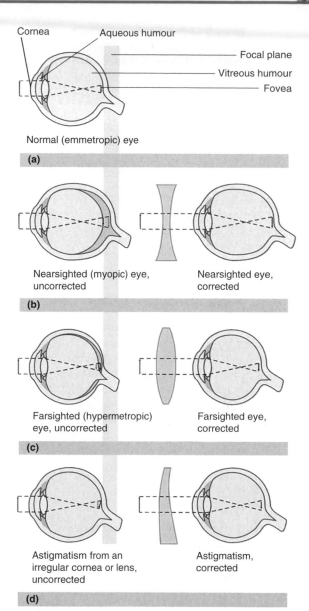

Figure 2.4.2  Refraction of light through a lens:
(a) refraction through a biconvex lens and (b) refraction
through a biconcave lens

Figure 2.4.3  (a) A clear image is focused on the fovea
centralis in the normal (emmotropic) eye. (b) In myopia
the image is focused in front of the retina. A concave
lens corrects this condition. (c) In hyperopia the image is
focused behind the retina. A concave lens is corrective.
(d) Astigmatism from irregular cornea or lens

effectively 'learns' to organize the visual signals from
the inverted retinal image into a view of the world
that is the right way up.

## Accommodation

The ability of the lens to change shape is termed the
**power of accommodation**. When distant objects are
viewed, the lens is flattened and the ciliary muscle
to which it is attached is relaxed. When the eye
focuses on a near object, the ring of ciliary muscle
reflexly contracts in response to parasympathetic
stimulation. The ciliary muscle is largely composed
of circularly arranged fibres, so that when they contract
the ring of muscle constricts and less tension is applied
to the attached suspensory ligaments. The slackening
of the ligaments slackens the pull on the lens. Because
the lens is flexible and relatively elastic, it takes up a
more curved shape in response to ciliary muscle contraction and it therefore increases its refractive power.
The refractive power increases so as to focus divergent
light rays from near objects onto the retina.

In addition to the circular muscle fibres, some ciliary muscle fibres have radial attachments to the cor-
neoscleral junction. Contraction of these fibres tends
to pull forwards on the ring of muscle, which facilitates
increased curvature of the anterior surface of the lens.

When near objects are viewed, accommodation
is accompanied by reflex pupillary constriction.
Parasympathetic stimulation of circular muscle fibres
in the iris accompanies contraction of ciliary muscle.

The resultant pupillary constriction serves to shut
down the periphery of the lens so that light rays
entering the eye are directed through the most curved
central part of the lens. The combination of contraction of ciliary muscle and pupillary constriction
forms the **accommodation reflex**.

## Near-point and presbyopia

The nearest source of light that can be brought into
focus on the retina is determined by the maximum
increase in refractive power of the lens achievable by
accommodation.

**Table 2.4.1** Changes in the near-point with age

| Near-point (cm from eye) | Age (years) |
|---|---|
| 9 | 10 |
| 10 | 20 |
| 12.5 | 30 |
| 18 | 40 |
| 50 | 50 |
| 100 | 70 |

### DEVELOPMENTAL ISSUES

The power of accommodation reduces with increasing age, slowly at first and then rapidly from age 40 to 50 years onwards. This condition is called presbyopia. Thus, with increasing age, the nearest point that can clearly be focused on the retina recedes. Normally, most older people require correcting spectacles with biconvex lenses for close work such as reading or sewing. Some examples of typical near-points at various ages are given in **Table 2.4.1**.

## Optical defects of the eye

The most common are short-sightedness, long-sightedness and astigmatism.

Short sight (**myopia**) describes the condition in which only near objects can be focused on the retina. It usually occurs because the eyeball is 'too long' for the refracting power of the lens (see **Fig. 2.4.3**). Myopia can be corrected with an appropriate biconcave lens, which will cause divergence of distant rays of light, enabling them to be focused on the retina instead of in front of it (see **Fig. 2.4.3b**).

In contrast to short sight, long sight (**hypermetropia**) normally occurs when the eyeball is 'too short' for the refractive power of the lens and divergent light rays from near objects are then focused behind the retina. A person with hypermetropia might even require some accommodation of the lens to focus on distant objects, and hence hypertrophy (enlargement) of ciliary muscle might be evident. Even with a maximally accommodated lens, the hypermetropic person cannot focus on near objects and requires correction with a biconvex lens to cause some convergence of light rays before they enter the eye (see **Fig. 2.4.3a and b**).

**Astigmatism** is a defect of the eye in which the curvature of the cornea in the horizontal plane is not the same as that in the vertical plane. Less commonly, the astigmatism can affect the lens rather than the cornea. An astigmatism results in blurring of parts of a visual image.

## Physiology of the retina

### Structure

The retina is a complex layer of tissue lining the eye. It is responsible for the conversion of light into visual nervous signals. The structure of the retina is schematically illustrated in **Fig. 2.4.4**.

Light passes through the mat of optic nerve fibres and two major layers of retinal cells before impinging on the photoreceptors. This might appear to be a rather 'back to front' arrangement. However, the photoreceptors lie adjacent to the pigment epithelium, which is intimately associated with the photochemistry of the receptors, and this probably accounts for the positioning of the photoreceptor layer. Clearly, the retinal cell layers and the mat of optic nerves do not prevent the transmission of light.

### CLINICAL APPLICATIONS

The photoreceptor layer can separate from the pigmented epithelium, leading to the condition of **retinal detachment**. The retina, especially the photoreceptor layer, depends on the choroid and pigmented epithelium for much of its nutrient and oxygen supply. Consequently, retinal detachment, if prolonged, can lead to inadequate nutrition and to deterioration of the retina. However, in the short term the retina might remain viable because nutrients can diffuse across from the choroid.

The photoreceptor layer of the retina contains two types of receptors called **rods** and **cones**. Their structures are illustrated in **Fig. 2.4.5**. Each receptor has an outer segment containing stacked piles of membranous discs on which are located the photosensitive chemical pigments. The outer segment of each receptor lies directly adjacent to the pigmented epithelium. Note that the outer segment of a cone is, as its name suggests, cone shaped, whereas that of a rod is rod shaped. The photochemical itself is manufactured in the inner segment before transfer to the outer segment, and hence the inner segment is characterized by the presence of mitochondria.

Rods and cones differ with respect to the organization of the outer segment. In rods, the membranous discs are produced continuously at the base of the outer segment and removed at the apex, where they are absorbed into the pigmented epithelium. In cones, the membranous discs are not replaced

Choroid layer & sclera

Retina

Vitreous body

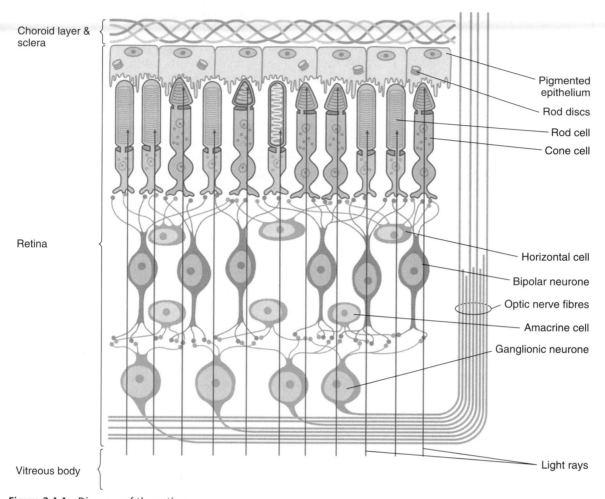

Pigmented epithelium
Rod discs
Rod cell
Cone cell
Horizontal cell
Bipolar neurone
Optic nerve fibres
Amacrine cell
Ganglionic neurone
Light rays

**Figure 2.4.4**   Diagram of the retina

continuously and the same complement of discs remains throughout life.

The nature of the photosensitive chemical is also different in the two types of receptors. Rods all contain the same photopigment, **rhodopsin**, which is purple in colour and is often referred to as 'visual purple'. Because they all contain the same photosensitive chemical, the rods can respond in only one way to light, that is, they can either be stimulated or not. Different rods cannot respond differentially to light of various wavelengths and hence cannot respond differentially to colour. Cones, on the other hand, do not all contain the same pigment. One group contains a pigment called **erythrolabe**, which is most reactive to light at the red end of the spectrum. A second group contains **chlorolabe**, which responds best to green light, and a third group contains **cyanolabe** and responds preferentially to blue light. Cones are essential for colour vision.

Adjacent to the inner segment of each receptor is the cell nucleus, which is attached to a synaptic ending. Rods and cones are not true neurones but they do make synaptic contacts with other retinal cells

and the synapses are characterized by the presence of vesicles. The synaptic ending of a cone is broad and flattened and is called a **pedicle**, whereas the synapse of a rod forms a smaller, bulbous contact called a **spherule**.

Rods and cones are not distributed randomly across the retina. The fovea centralis contains only cones, whereas there are no cones at all in the most peripheral parts of the retina. Foveal cones are structurally distinct and appear to be longer and thinner than cones elsewhere. Altogether there are approximately 6 or 7 million cones in each human retina. Rods are found in greatest numbers in the periphery of the retina. There are many more rods than cones, with estimates varying over a range of 120–125 million rods per retina.

The intermediate layer of retinal cells consists of bipolar cells, horizontal cells and amacrine cells. Bipolar cells principally transmit signals from rods and cones to the third retinal layer of cells, which consists of ganglion cells. The ganglion cells give rise to optic nerve fibres, and all signals from other retinal cells are finally transmitted to the ganglion cell layer.

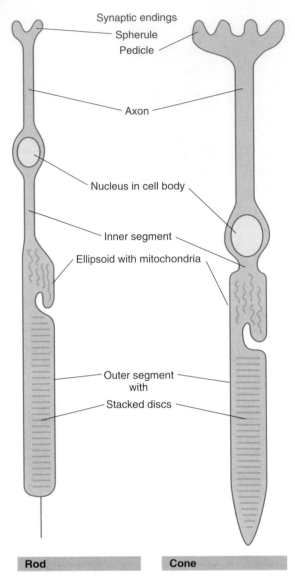

Rod | Cone

**Figure 2.4.5** Structure of the photoreceptor cells

## Receptor photochemistry

The photosensitive chemicals in both rods and cones are stored on the membranous discs of the outer segments of the receptors. The stacked disc arrangement maximizes the exposure of the contained photopigments to incident light. This process involves a chemical change in the photopigment that is brought about by light energy, the chemical change then induces a receptor potential in the rod or cone.

Rods contain the photopigment rhodopsin, which consists of vitamin A aldehyde, called **retinene**, combined with a protein referred to as **opsin**. When light is directed onto rhodopsin, the retinene portion of the molecule *isomerizes*, that is, it undergoes a change in shape from a curly to a straight form, without a change in chemical composition. The curly form of retinene, termed the all-*cis* form, fits snugly onto its attachment site on the protein opsin. However,

the straight form, the all-*trans* form of retinene, is the wrong shape for the attachment and so the isomerization induced by light makes the photopigment unstable until finally the opsin splits completely from the retinene. The final products of the conversion are lighter in colour when compared to the purple of rhodopsin, and light is therefore said to bleach the photopigment. Bleaching actually takes several seconds, whereas receptor potentials are produced within a fraction of a second of light exposure. Clearly, the chemical change inducing the receptor potential must occur during the decay process and before complete bleaching of the pigment occurs.

For rods to continue to function, rhodopsin must be reformed so that it can once again 'capture' light and induce a receptor potential. The first stage in its reformation involves the reconversion of all-*trans* (straight) retinene into all-*cis* (curly) retinene. This reaction requires an isomerase enzyme and energy. Once the all-*cis* retinene is formed, it readily recombines with opsin and the reconstituted rhodopsin is then stable until light energy is again absorbed.

Retinene is formed from vitamin A by a dehydrogenation reaction. Normally both *cis* and *trans* forms of vitamin A are present, as well as *cis* and *trans* forms of retinene. Large stores of vitamin A are located in the pigment epithelium. In conditions of darkness, virtually all the retinene is converted into rhodopsin and much of the stored vitamin A is then converted first into retinene and then into rhodopsin.

Cone photopigments are similar to rhodopsin. They all contain retinene but it is bound to different opsins. Thus, erythrolabe, chlorolabe and cyanolabe represent three different opsins bound to retinene. Essentially the same process of decomposition of the pigment is thought to occur, and vitamin A is essential for cone as well as rod function.

## Functional differences between rods and cones

Rods and cones are functionally as well as structurally distinct. Their relative contributions to colour vision have already been referred to, and colour vision depends on the integrity of cones rather than of rods. Rods and cones also differ in their relative sensitivities to light. Rods have low thresholds to light and are easily stimulated, even by quite low light intensities. However, in bright light rods appear to adapt to stimulation and they no longer respond. On the other hand, cones have higher thresholds to light. They require a greater intensity of light to be stimulated and they therefore operate under conditions of bright light when rod function is reduced.

Because rods function best under conditions of relatively low light intensity when cones are not stimulated, and as rods do not contribute to colour vision, it is to be expected that vision in semidarkness will depend on rods and will provide information on relative brightness but not colour of the objects viewed. In moonlight, everything appears in shades of silvery grey, with those objects that appear lighter in shade reflecting more light than apparently dark grey or black objects.

Rods and cones also respond differentially to different wavelengths and hence colours of light. This was first described by Purkinje, following observations that the relative brightness of colours changes as daylight fades to dusk. Reds look less bright whereas blue–greens increase in brightness in dusk conditions. This shift in spectral sensitivity is now known as the Purkinje shift, and it reflects a change from predominantly cone vision in daylight to predominantly rod vision at dusk. In daylight, all wavelengths of light are absorbed by cone pigments but peak absorption and peak sensitivity occur with yellow–green light. Cone vision in daylight is termed **photopic vision**. As dusk falls, rods take over from cones. Rhodopsin maximally absorbs blue–green light and therefore rod sensitivity is maximal for light of this wavelength. Thus, blue–green objects appear brighter with rod vision than with cone vision. Rod vision at dusk is termed **scotopic vision**.

Night blindness is a condition associated with a severe deficiency of vitamin A. Vitamin A is essential for the formation of photopigments and a severe deficiency might therefore be expected to impair both rod and cone function. However, the 'blindness' is most apparent in conditions of low light intensity when vision is dependent on rod function. If vitamin A deficiency is very prolonged and severe, cone function also deteriorates and blindness progresses. It is thought that cones are less susceptible than rods because they operate under daylight conditions of relatively high light intensity, when sufficient light is available to elicit a response despite the reduction in available photopigment.

## Visual acuity

The ability to discriminate visually between two separate points of light is called **visual acuity**. Visual acuity permits detail to be appreciated.

An emmetropic eye (one with normal accommodation and refraction) can generally distinguish between two separate light sources provided that the angle that they subtend at the eye, the visual angle, is at least 1 minute of arc (1′). However, some individuals have much better visual acuity than this. Visual acuity is most acute when the visual image falls on the fovea. It has been suggested that visual acuity is at its limit when two stimulated foveal cones are separated by one unstimulated cone.

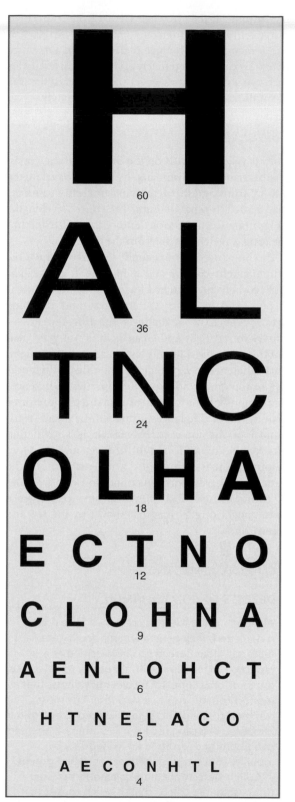

**Figure 2.4.6** An example of Snellen's type (Courtesy of Clement Clarke International Ltd)

Visual acuity is measured using **Snellen's type**, an example of which is shown in **Fig. 2.4.6**. Snellen's type usually consists of rows of letters with each row being of a different size. The letters subtend an angle of 1 minute at the eye when viewed from a specified distance. Typically, there are 60, 36, 24, 18, 12, 9, 6 and 5 metre lines. The type is viewed from a distance of 6 m by each eye separately and the visual acuity for each eye is expressed as 6 over the number of the line of smallest letters that is recognized accurately.

## Colour vision

Colour vision depends on the integrity of the cones. The human eye is stimulated by light of wavelengths 400–750 nm and this represents an ability to recognize 150–200 separate hues. The short wavelengths of light are from the violet end of the spectrum and the long wavelengths are from the red end.

The human eye is not equally sensitive to the three primary light colours and if blue light, green light and red light are matched for intensity, the red light is perceived as being the brightest and the blue light appears to be the dimmest. The difference in sensitivity to red light and green light is not very great but the eye is considerably less sensitive to blue light. This difference in sensitivity might reflect differences in photopigment absorption properties, differences in amounts of photopigment contained in the three cone types, or differences in the numbers and distribution of the three cone types. It is known that blue cones are not found in the fovea and therefore colour vision is dichromatic here. Furthermore, the pattern of distribution and connection of blue cones is more diffuse and shows greater convergence onto ganglion cells than that shown by the red and green cones.

### CLINICAL APPLICATIONS

#### DEFECTS OF COLOUR VISION

Although colour defects can occur if the retina is damaged, they generally result from genetic factors. Colour defects can be classified as a reduction of, or absence of, the ability to detect red, green or blue light. Total **colour blindness**, that is, monochromatic vision, is very rare. The most common colour defect is so-called red–green colour blindness. This can arise from a number of inherited conditions and results in an inadequacy or inability to distinguish between reds and greens.

Colour defects are most commonly assessed using Ishihara's colour charts, which consist of arrays of coloured dots with a figure or pattern picked out in different colours from the background. For example, a number might be picked out in red dots on a green dot background. The number can be recognized by a person with normal colour vision but not by someone with red–green colour blindness.

## Adaptation

All sensory receptors adapt to stimulation to some extent and cones and rods adapt to light energy. The phenomenon of dark adaptation is readily appreciated when one enters a dark room, such as a cinema auditorium, from a well-lit area. Initially, considerable difficulty is experienced in seeing anything but, as the eyes adapt to the darkness, vision improves. Complete dark adaptation can take over half an hour, by which time the sensitivity of the eye to light can be increased by up to a million times.

# Electrophysiology of retinal cells

Light falling on retinal receptors induces an electrical change that is transmitted by cells in the intermediate layer of the retina. The signal might undergo modification here before transmission to a ganglion cell and its associated optic nerve fibre, which finally transmits the signal to the brain.

## Electrical changes in receptors

Neither rods nor cones can generate action potentials and the predominant electrical response to light stimulation in a visual receptor is a slow, graded membrane **hyperpolarization**. Retinal receptors in the dark are partially depolarized to around $-30$ mV because there is a steady leak of sodium ions into the cells. When a receptor is stimulated by light, the sodium permeability is reduced and fewer sodium ions leak into the cell. The membrane potential then increases to a more negative value and is hyperpolarized. Thus, retinal receptors are partially excited in the dark and are inhibited by light. However, in the dark the receptors spontaneously release transmitters that can inhibit intermediate retinal cells. Thus, in the dark, partial excitation of receptors can result in inhibition of bipolar cells. Stimulation by light then reduces this inhibition because the receptor hyperpolarization reduces the release of inhibitory transmitter. The disinhibition so caused then results in increased activity of the bipolar cells.

## Processing of visual signals in the intermediate layer

In common with visual receptors, the cells of the intermediate layer of the retina do not appear to transmit action potentials. Instead, they produce slow, graded membrane potential changes, some of which are depolarizing and some of which are hyperpolarizing.

## Electrical changes in ganglion cells

Ganglion cells constitute the final stage in retinal processing of visual signals. Ganglion cell axons carry the signals in the optic nerves to further processing centres in the brain.

## The visual pathways

The ganglion cells of the retina project their axons towards the posterior pole of the eye when they converge and pass out of the eye as the **optic nerve**. Upon leaving the eye, the cells of the optic nerve acquire a myelin sheath.

The optic nerves pass to the **optic chiasma**, which is situated at the base of the brain, anterior to the pituitary stalk. At the optic chiasma, a proportion of the nerve fibres cross the midline in a partial decussation. The fibres from the nasal halves of the retinae cross to the opposite side of the brain, whereas fibres from the temporal halves of the retinae maintain their ipsilateral (same-sided) projection (**Fig. 2.4.7**). Consequently, fibres from the temporal half of one retina are joined by fibres from the nasal half of the other and, in this way, fibres leaving the right side of each eye project to the right half of the brain and fibres from the left side of each eye project to the left side of the brain. As a result, the right visual hemifield is projected to the left cerebral hemisphere and the left visual hemifield is projected to the right cerebral hemisphere.

After the partial decussation of the optic chiasma, the axons of the retinal ganglion cells continue as two diverging optic tracts before terminating on cells of the **lateral geniculate nuclei** (LGN). These thalamic relay nuclei contain six layers of cells receiving ipsilateral and contralateral input from the eyes.

The nerve fibres from the lateral geniculate nuclei constitute the optic radiations, which arc around the lateral ventricles and terminate on cells of the striate cortex of the occipital lobe, the primary visual cortex. The strict organization of the projection from the retina is maintained at the level of the primary visual cortex, with the lower halves of the retinae (representing the upper halves of the visual field) projecting to the visual cortex below the calcarine sulcus and the upper halves of the retinae projecting to the visual cortex above the calcarine sulcus. Retinal projections from the fovea, which represent vision in the centre of the visual field, project to the posterior part of the primary visual cortex.

## Visual processing

The way in which the nervous system interprets the visual world is still far from being clearly understood. Nevertheless, the use of single-cell electrophysiological recording techniques has led to considerable advances since its introduction in the 1960s, revealing details of the function of nerve cells at different levels of the visual system.

### CLINICAL APPLICATIONS

In humans, the inability to recognize objects visually in the absence of any obvious peripheral sensory loss is called **visual agnosia**. This dysfunction is associated with lesions in posterior parts of the brain. Patients are unable to recognize and name an object when it is presented in the visual modality, even though they might be able to recognize the same object if they are allowed to touch it or experience it in some other non-visual way. Visual agnosia can vary greatly in severity but one particularly severe, although rare, form is **prosopagnosia**. In this condition, patients are unable to recognize faces and, consequently, are disturbingly unable to recognize family or friends by sight.

## Visual perception

It is necessary to relate the way in which the visual system processes visual signals to the way in which the visual world is perceived.

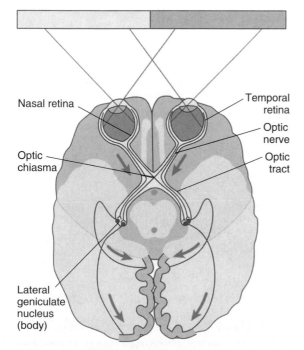

Nasal retina
Temporal retina
Optic nerve
Optic chiasma
Optic tract
Lateral geniculate nucleus (body)

**Figure 2.4.7**   Visual pathways to the brain

## Pattern recognition

The basis of pattern recognition is laid down in the sensitivity of the cells of the visual cortex. These cells can detect the barriers to areas of light and dark that lie in particular orientations and in particular parts of the visual field. Separating the visual world into blocks of light and shade provides a first step to identifying objects. The visual system also seems to enhance the distinction between areas of light and dark at the boundaries. For example, if you observe a large sheet of white paper against a blackboard, the paper appears to be whiter at the edges than it does in the centre. In other words, the visual system responds vigorously to contrast.

## Movement

At the level of the retina, the perception of movement in the visual scene is probably linked with the activity of the γ-type ganglion cells. These cells produce fast, transient responses and the axons project both to the LGN and also to the superior colliculus, where they presumably have some effect on the control of eye movements.

## Stereoscopy and depth perception

Several factors contribute to the perception of depth. The relative sizes of objects can provide one clue. For example, a person standing 50 m distant will provide an optical image that is much smaller than that of a person standing only 5 m away. However, we do not interpret such a visual image as meaning that one person is only a fraction of the size of the other, because memory suggests very strongly that objects show a constancy of size. Consequently, we assume that the two people are of roughly the same height but are at different distances from us.

Shadows can also play a part in depth perception. The casting of a shadow of one object onto another provides information about the relative positions of the objects in space.

Movement might also play a role in depth perception. As we travel in a car or train, stationary objects outside, such as trees or fences, which are close to the vehicle, pass across the visual field very quickly, whereas distant objects pass across the visual field much more slowly. This is referred to as **motion parallax**.

Another very important factor in depth perception is that we observe the visual world binocularly and are thus able to decipher information about the relative positions of objects from the disparity of the images presented to the two eyes. It has been reported in some animal experiments that some binocular cortical cells do respond preferentially to the disparity between the images of an object presented to the two eyes.

## Colour

A variety of colour-sensitive cells has been described at various levels of the visual system. The opponent colour coding found in the retina is also present at the LGN. The colour-sensitive cells are concentrated in the area of cortex receiving information from the fovea (see Chapter 2.2).

## Visual reflexes and eye movements

The **pupillary light reflex** refers to the constriction of the pupil in response to the illumination of the eye. The reflex pathway is multisynaptic and bilateral (**Fig. 2.4.8**). The reflex arc begins with retinal ganglion cells, which project via the optic nerve to the pretectal area of the midbrain. Axons of pretectal neurones project bilaterally to the accessory oculomotor nuclei

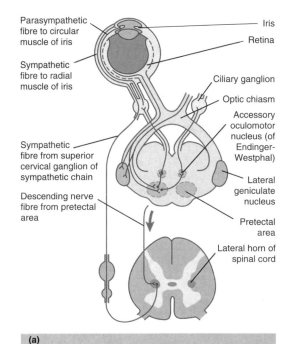

(a)

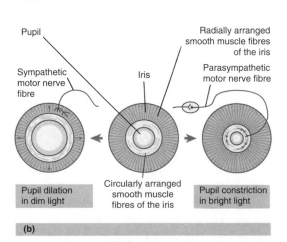

(b)

**Figure 2.4.8** (a) Nerve pathway of the pupillary reflex and (b) autonomic stimulation affecting the pupil

and, in turn, axons from these nuclei join the oculo-motor nerve (IIIrd cranial nerve) to the ciliary ganglia lying just behind the eyes. Here, they make contact with postganglionic parasympathetic neurones, which innervate the circular muscle fibres of the iris of the eye and cause the pupillary constriction.

Dilation of the pupil acts through descending sympathetic pathways, which stimulate the preganglionic sympathetic neurones of the lateral horns of the upper thoracic spinal cord. These preganglionic fibres then ascend in the sympathetic chain and synapse in the superior cervical ganglion. From here, postganglionic fibres project anteriorly along the branches of the internal carotid artery before terminating on the radial muscle fibres (dilator muscle) of the iris.

The **accommodation reflex** alters the curvature of the lens of the eye to focus the eye on objects at different distances. Movements of the eyes within the orbits are effected by the six extraocular muscles and these are innervated by the IIIrd, IVth and VIth cranial nerves. The frontal eye fields and the occipital eye fields of the cerebral cortex influence the cranial nerve nuclei via the superior colliculus and the pretectal area. The frontal eye fields are concerned with voluntary scanning of the visual scene and the larger occipital eye fields are associated with pursuit movements, which occur in the voluntary pursuit of a moving visual target.

## CLINICAL APPLICATIONS

### TESTING

#### Ophthalmoscopy

**Papilloedema** (swelling of the optic disc) occurs in many medical conditions and, consequently, examination of the fundus of the eye with an ophthalmoscope is of great importance. Papilloedema can be caused by the raised intracranial pressure associated with brain abscesses, intracranial tumours or meningitis. It also occurs in optic neuritis (inflammation of the optic nerve), which might be associated with demyelinating diseases such as multiple sclerosis.

#### Visual field defects

Reduction of the normal size of the visual fields or the development of areas of blindness (scotomas) within the visual field can be assessed by **perimetry**. The patient is asked to fixate each eye successively on a central target and then to indicate when a stimulus enters the peripheral

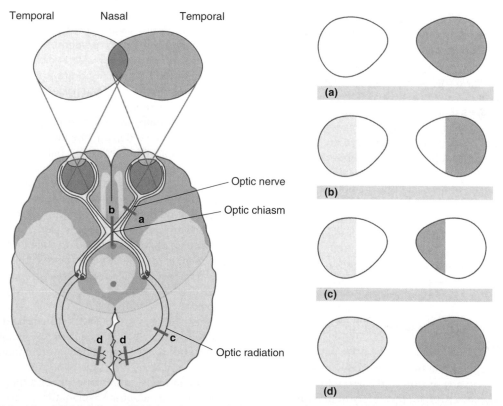

**Figure 2.4.9** Visual field defects related to damage of the visual pathways. (a) The right optic nerve is cut resulting in blindness in the right eye. (b) The optic chiasma is cut causing blindness in the temporal half of the visual fields of each eye. (c) The right optic radiations are cut causing blindness in the left half of the visual field of each eye. (d) The visual input to the cortex is cut bilaterally leading to complete blindness

vision. The stimulus, usually a small white or coloured disc, is then moved inwards from various points around the periphery of the visual field. Damage to the visual pathway at various stages will result in the visual field defects illustrated in **Fig. 2.4.9**.

Lesions of the optic chiasma resulting in a bitemporal hemianopia (half visual field loss) can occur in association with a pituitary tumour. Damage to one optic tract posterior to the chiasma causes a crossed homonymous hemianopia. That is, damage to the left optic tract will cause a loss of vision in the right half of the visual field, and damage to the right optic tract will cause a visual defect in the left half of the visual field.

### Eye movement defects

Defects in the control of eye movements can result from damage to the nerve pathways involved in controlling the ocular muscles or from damage to the muscles themselves. For example, paralysis of the ocular muscles, **ophthalmoplegia,** can be caused by subcortical damage, by brainstem lesions associated with the IIIrd, IVth and VIth cranial nerves, or by muscular disorders such as myasthenia gravis. However, cases of ophthalmoplegia caused by muscle disorders are rare.

Disorders of eye movement control can result in conjugate ophthalmoplegia, strabismus or diplopia. **Conjugate ophthalmoplegia** refers to an impairment of conjugate eye movements. In other words, the patient loses the ability to move both eyes harmoniously together. **Strabismus**, or **squint**, refers to a condition in which one eye moves normally but, owing to some weakness in the ocular muscles, the other eye does not. **Diplopia**, or double vision, occurs when a dysfunction of ocular muscle control results in the image of a visual object falling on non-corresponding parts of the retinae of the two eyes. For example, a target in the centre of the visual field will fall on the fovea in the normal eye but might be displaced to the side in the weaker eye. Consequently, a double image is perceived. Diplopia might be a presenting feature in the early stages of multiple sclerosis.

### VISUAL DEFECTS: IMPLICATIONS FOR NURSING

'Hemianopia' is the term used to describe a visual loss in any section of the visual field, and 'homonymous hemianopia' refers to a complete or partial loss of the nasal half of vision in one eye and of the temporal half in the other. This type of defect can arise in several disorders affecting the nervous system, including stroke and intracranial tumour. In the latter, encroachment on the visual pathways by the tumour will produce a defect, the extent of which will depend on the location and size of the offending tumour. The stroke victim's visual field defect is a consequence of the deprivation of the blood supply to the affected area of the brain.

To assist patients with a defect such as hemianopia, the nurse should always approach from the unaffected side and remind patients to turn their head to compensate for visual defects. Impairment of vision can pose a safety threat and nurses need to be aware of dangers within the ward and home environments. Establishing and maintaining communication is essential and, to this end, the position of the patient's bed is important. Visually impaired patients should be allocated a bed that permits maximum use of the unaffected field of vision; to do otherwise would essentially render them 'blind' and reduce contact with other patients and members of staff to a minimum.

Double vision can often be abolished with the use of an eye patch and blurring of vision, which will result in decreased visual acuity, is dealt with as it arises.

Complete blindness, when it occurs, rarely happens in both eyes at the same time but it is common for blindness in one eye to be followed by that in the other. Humans depend on visual images for sensory input and stimulation and a loss of these will pose considerable problems for the affected person. Blind inpatients require to be orientated to new surroundings; this could be by verbal description or, if the patient's condition permits, providing a conducted tour. Once the patient is familiar with the new layout, alterations should not be made, e.g. moving furniture to a new location. When escorting blind people, allow them to take your arm; they can follow your body movements more easily if you gently squeeze your arm against your body. The nurse should enquire how patients normally cope with the activities of living at home, and attempt as far as possible to accommodate their normal prehospital routine. It might be that this is not always possible and, when a new arrangement is proposed, adequate explanation must be provided beforehand.

The blind person should be addressed on approach and nurses should identify themselves and state what they are doing, even though this might not directly affect the blind person. When performing nursing care directly concerned with the blind patient, adequate explanation is absolutely crucial. A recently blinded person will require a lot of support, reassurance and explanation. A return to independence is encouraged as soon as possible, with guidance being provided on all aspects of the activities of daily living.

The Royal National Institute of the Blind provides a comprehensive welfare service, supplying information and facilities to the blind person. Being registered as blind or partially sighted will allow the person to become eligible for local and national services and for additional tax relief and supplementary benefit.

## The ear and audition

### Structure of the auditory apparatus

The human ear is sensitive to an enormous range of sounds. The auditory apparatus of the ear is able to code the various characteristics of sound into patterns of nervous signals, which the brain can interpret.

The ear is subdivided into three main compartments, the outer ear, the middle ear and the inner ear (**Fig. 2.4.10**). The outer ear funnels the sound energy into the middle ear, which serves to transmit the sound to the auditory apparatus of the inner ear, which transduces the mechanical energy of sound vibration into electrical energy. An electrical potential change is produced in the inner ear and this gives rise to patterns of action potentials in the auditory branch of the VIIIth cranial nerve. The auditory nerve transmits the signals to the brain.

### The outer ear

The two ears are cartilaginous outgrowths covered by skin. They are called the **pinnae** or **auricles**. In humans, the pinna plays a minor role in protection by surrounding the opening to the **external auditory meatus** (the auditory canal, which transmits sounds to the middle ear), and so helping to prevent hair and skin debris from entering the ear.

The external auditory meatus is 'S' shaped and about 25 mm in length. It terminates in the **tympanic membrane** (the eardrum). The shape of the canal does not impair the transmission of sound; indeed, it aids sound amplification. It probably also plays a defensive role. The 'S' shape will help to prevent the ingress of particulate matter and also to reduce the effects of air currents, which could otherwise damage the eardrum. The external auditory meatus is lined by skin, which contains the **ceruminous glands**. These glands secrete a waxy substance that prevents drying-out of the tissue. Ear wax is sticky; sloughed-off skin cells and dust stick to it and are removed from the ear. However, excess production of ear wax can impair sound transmission through the outer ear, especially if a plug of wax attaches to the eardrum.

The tympanic membrane is composed of connective tissue and stretches across the aperture of the inner end of the auditory canal, separating the outer ear from the middle ear. It is covered by skin on the outer ear side and by mucous membrane on the middle ear side and is slightly conical in shape, with the apex of the cone pointing into the middle ear. The shape aids funnelling of sound. The tympanic membrane vibrates and moves in and out in response to sound. It can easily be observed with an otoscope.

### Middle ear

The middle ear is an air-filled cavity containing three tiny bones – the **ossicles** – which are, individually, the **malleus**, the **incus** and the **stapes**. The ossicles transmit sound energy from the tympanic membrane to a much smaller membrane, the **oval window**, which separates the middle ear from the inner ear.

The malleus is hammer shaped and the handle of the hammer is attached by ligaments to the tympanic membrane. The head of the hammer is firmly attached to the incus (the anvil), which articulates with the stapes (the stirrup). The face-plate of the stapes is attached by an annular ligament to the oval window (**Fig. 2.4.11**). The ligaments between the malleus and the incus effectively prevent relative movement

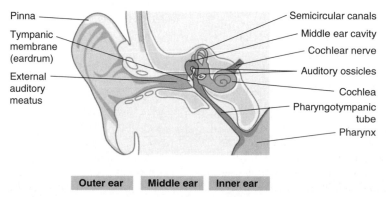

| Pinna | Semicircular canals |
| Tympanic membrane (eardrum) | Middle ear cavity |
| | Cochlear nerve |
| External auditory meatus | Auditory ossicles |
| | Cochlea |
| | Pharyngotympanic tube |
| | Pharynx |

**Outer ear**  **Middle ear**  **Inner ear**

**Figure 2.4.10**  Structure of the ear

between the two bones and they act as a single unit. When the tympanic membrane vibrates, the malleus and incus are displaced. The displacement is such that the hammer head acts as a pivot and the long process of the incus alternately pushes and pulls against the stapes, which in turn acts as a plunger on the oval window. The oval window, like the tympanic membrane, is flexible. It vibrates in phase with the plunging action of the stapes and transmits the sound vibration to the contents of the inner ear. The plunging action of the ossicles can be damped by two small muscles: the **tensor tympani** muscle pulls on the tympanic membrane and the **stapedius** muscle pulls on the neck of the stapes (**see Fig. 2.4.11**). Both muscles reflexly contract in response to loud sound, although the tensor tympani is now also thought to be important in controlling the relative positions of the ossicles in relation to head and body movement. The stapedius reflex, that is, the reflex contraction of the stapedius muscles, occurs with a latency of about 30 ms in response to high-intensity sound. It stiffens the ossicles and damps-down transmission of sound vibration to the inner ear. It therefore has a protective function in attenuating high-intensity sound vibration, which is potentially damaging. High-intensity sound can cause destruction of auditory receptors in the inner ear, resulting in a hearing loss. However, the latency of the reflex is such that it does not afford any protection against loud impulsive sound, such as that produced by hammering.

It has already been noted that the middle ear is air filled. For the tympanic membrane to 'follow' the vibrations of sound, the air pressures on the two sides of the membrane need to be equalized. The air on the outer ear side is continuously open to the atmosphere. However, the middle ear chamber is open to the atmosphere only periodically. A narrow tube, the **pharyngotympanic tube** (formerly called the Eustachian tube), passes between the middle ear cavity and the pharynx but the pharyngeal opening is normally sealed (**see Fig. 2.4.10**). It opens during yawning and swallowing and at these times the air in the middle ear achieves equilibrium with the atmosphere. This explains why yawning or swallowing relieves the feelings of pressure in the ear that occur during rapid changes in altitude. The change in atmospheric pressure that occurs with a change in altitude causes an air pressure difference across the tympanic membrane and deliberate swallowing or yawning then allows the pressure in the middle ear to equilibrate with the atmosphere. Catarrh can block the pharyngotympanic tube and 'popping' of the ears will not then be possible. Furthermore, the air in the middle ear might be absorbed and the tympanic membrane will then bulge inwards, causing pain and loss of hearing.

### Inner ear

The inner ear is composed of several fluid-filled chambers encased in a bony labyrinth in the temporal bone. The semicircular canals are important for balance. The inner ear auditory apparatus is the **cochlea**, which is a closed-ended tube, coiled like a snail's shell. There are about two and a half turns in the spiral of the cochlea, with the basal turn connecting to the middle ear chamber. The cochlea is coiled around a central bony core, the **modiolus**.

For simplicity, the cochlea can be 'unwound' and illustrated as an uncoiled straight tube (**Fig. 2.4.12**). It is divided into two main chambers along most of its length by a structure called the **basilar membrane**. The upper chamber is the **scala vestibuli**, which is sealed at its basal end by the oval window. The lower

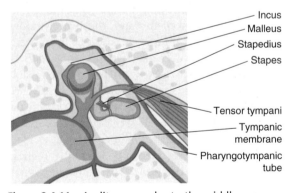

**Figure 2.4.11** Auditory muscles to the middle ear (medial view)

*Labels:* Incus, Malleus, Stapedius, Stapes, Tensor tympani, Tympanic membrane, Pharyngotympanic tube

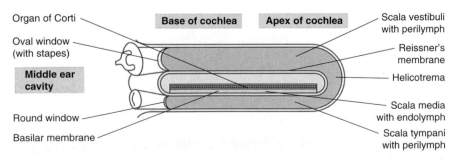

*Labels:* Organ of Corti, Oval window (with stapes), Middle ear cavity, Round window, Basilar membrane, Base of cochlea, Apex of cochlea, Scala vestibuli with perilymph, Reissner's membrane, Helicotrema, Scala media with endolymph, Scala tympani with perilymph

**Figure 2.4.12** Schematic diagram of the cochlea

chamber is the **scala tympani**, which is sealed at its basal end by another flexible membrane, the **round window**. Like the oval window, the round window separates the inner ear from the middle ear. The scala vestibuli and scala tympani are continuous with each other at the **helicotrema**, which is at the apex of the cochlea. Both chambers therefore contain fluid of the same composition. They are both filled with **perilymph**, which is similar in ionic composition to other extracellular fluids. Perilymph is secreted by arterioles in the periosteum and it drains into the subarachnoid space via the perilymphatic duct.

The scala vestibuli is actually separated from the basilar membrane by another very thin membrane, **Reissner's membrane**. Reissner's membrane and the basilar membrane enclose a third chamber, the **scala media** or **cochlear duct**. The scala media is roughly triangular in cross-section, the sides of the triangle being formed by Reissner's membrane, the basilar membrane and the **stria vascularis**. The latter is vascular tissue located in the outer wall of the cochlear spiral (**Fig. 2.4.13**). The scala media is quite separate from the scala vestibuli and scala tympani and contains a fluid called **endolymph**, which is very different in composition from perilymph, being much more like intracellular fluid; endolymph is believed to be formed by the stria vascularis. It also fills the vestibular apparatus (described later) and drains into the venous sinuses of the brain via the endolymphatic duct.

The scala media contains the receptor mechanism for audition. Auditory receptor cells are situated on the basilar membrane in a structure called the **organ of Corti**, which extends the length of the cochlea as far as the helicotrema. The organ of Corti is innervated by terminals of bipolar cells, the cell bodies of which are located in the **spiral ganglion**, which extends through the bony core of the modiolus. The central axons of the bipolar cells give rise to the auditory branch of the VIIIth cranial nerve, which transmits to the brainstem. The organ of Corti also has an *efferent* nerve supply and these descending nerve fibres arise from structures in the brainstem called the **olives**. These olivocochlear fibres modify the afferent output from the organ of Corti.

When the oval window vibrates with the plunging action of the stapes, the column of perilymph in the scala vestibuli is displaced. As the oval window moves inwards, so the fluid in the scala vestibuli is displaced towards the apex of the cochlea. If movements of the oval window are slow, fluid is pushed through the helicotrema into the scala tympani and the result of fluid displacement here is that the round window bulges towards the middle ear cavity. However, sound vibrations generally occur too quickly to allow fluid to be pushed all the way round from base to apex and back to the base again. Thus, as the oval window vibrates, the vibration is transmitted to the basilar membrane, which is flexible and moves up and down in phase with the displacement of perilymph in the scala vestibuli. Reissner's membrane is so thin that it does not impede transmission of vibration. As the basilar membrane vibrates, it stimulates auditory receptors, which signal sound to the brain. Movement of the basilar membrane causes displacement of fluid in the scala tympani and consequent movement of the round window. Thus, under normal conditions, the sound vibration effectively takes a 'short-cut' from the scala vestibuli through the basilar membrane to the scala tympani and little flow of perilymph occurs through the helicotrema.

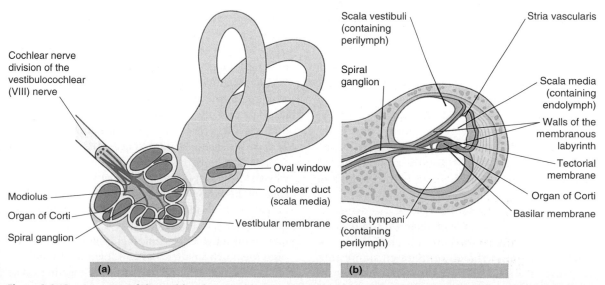

**Figure 2.4.13**　Anatomy of the cochlea showing (a) cross-section of the cochlea and (b) an enlargement of the chambers

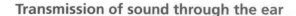

## Transmission of sound through the ear

The primary function of the outer and middle ear chambers is the transmission of sound to the auditory receptors of the inner ear.

### Characteristics of sound and sound perception

Sound is produced by mechanical vibration and the audibility of a sound is determined by how strongly and how rapidly the vibration occurs. The sound is transmitted away from the source because of a 'knock-on' effect whereby the disturbed molecules of air adjacent to the sound source in turn cause displacement of air molecules next to them.

The rate at which a sound source vibrates determines the spacing of bands of compression (and rarefraction). The distance between two adjacent compressions is a measure of the wavelength of the sound and it is directly related to the frequency of vibration. Conventionally, sound waves are described in terms of frequency of vibration rather than wavelength. The unit of frequency is the hertz, where 1 hertz (Hz) equals one complete cycle of vibration that occurs between two compression (or rarefraction) bands.

Speech is a complex sound composed of many frequencies, particularly those in the 400–500 Hz range. Noise is a mixture of a wide range of frequencies and the term 'white noise' is employed to describe the sound produced by a mixture of all frequencies detectable by the human ear.

The term '**pitch**' describes the perception of the frequency of a sound. High-frequency vibration produces a high pitch, and low-frequency vibration a low pitch. The human ear is able to hear sounds covering an enormous frequency range, approximately 20 Hz to 20 000 Hz. The audible range shows individual variability and is particularly affected by age. In old age there is a loss of sensitivity to high frequencies, a phenomenon referred to as **presbyacusis**. In older people, the audible range might be foreshortened at the high-frequency end to 5000 Hz, depending on the intensity of the sound.

Although the range of audible frequencies is large, the human ear is not equally sensitive across the whole range. The greatest sensitivity occurs for frequencies in the range 1000–4000 Hz and the audibility threshold intensity of sound is lowest for this frequency band.

The intensity of a sound reflects the degree to which the molecules of the medium are compressed. When sound is transmitted through air, the compression bands represent bands of increased air pressure, the change in air pressure being related to the intensity (strength) of vibration of the sound source. A large difference in pressure, which is associated with a high-intensity sound, causes more displacement of the eardrum than a small difference in pressure. The intensity of a sound can therefore be described in terms of pressure. The intensity of a sound is actually a measure of the magnitude of the energy flow from a sound source to the surrounding medium.

Changes in intensity of sound are perceived as changes in loudness. As intensity increases, so the difference threshold for a detectable change in loudness increases. Thus, a change in apparent loudness appears to depend on a relative change in intensity, and a logarithmic scale of relative intensity better reflects perception of loudness.

### Resonance in the ear

When a solid object or column of air or liquid is struck it vibrates with its own natural frequency. In other words, the material can become a sound source emitting a sound of a characteristic frequency. This phenomenon of 'natural vibration' causes structures to amplify or resonate sound waves of the same frequency. The air-filled chambers of the ear have their own characteristic resonance frequencies. The shape and size of the chambers are such that specific frequencies are amplified. Resonance in the outer and middle ears probably plays a large part in determining the frequency characteristics of the ear, the sensitivity of which is greatest for sounds of 1000–4000 Hz.

### Impedance matching in the middle ear

The middle ear serves to conduct sound travelling in air from the outer ear to the fluid-filled cochlea of the inner ear. The fluid in the cochlea has much greater inertia than the air in the outer and middle ear chambers. Owing to its greater mass, more force is required to displace the fluid. Consequently, a mechanism is needed to overcome the inertia of cochlear fluid to effect a displacement of the oval window equivalent to that of the tympanic membrane.

The middle ear ossicles are vital for the transmission of sound to the auditory receptor mechanism of the inner ear. First, the lever system operating round a pivot on the malleus head has some mechanical advantage because the stapes is attached nearer to the pivot than is the vibrating tympanic membrane. Consequently, when a force is applied to the tympanic membrane, the effect of the ossicle lever system is to amplify the vibration at the oval window. The second important advantage of the ossicle system is that it permits all of the force applied to the tympanic membrane to be directed onto the much smaller oval window membrane.

The advantages of the lever system together cause an approximate twentyfold increase in pressure on the oval window and this is sufficient for virtually perfect impendance matching. Sound vibration is transmitted to the basilar membrane of the cochlea with little loss.

## Frequency selectivity in the middle ear

The presence of one sound reduces the ability of the ear to respond to other less intense sounds; this phenomenon is referred to as **masking**. The extent to which a sound is masked depends not only on its intensity but also on its frequency, and particularly on the degree to which its frequency differs from the masking sound.

## Bone conduction of sound

Because the cochlea is situated in a bony labyrinth, vibration of the temporal bone can induce cochlear fluid displacement and stimulation of auditory receptors. Thus, sound vibration can be transmitted through bone. Indeed, bone conduction is used diagnostically to assess whether a hearing impairment is the result of primary damage to the auditory receptor mechanism of the inner ear or is secondary to impaired transmission of sound through the outer and middle ears. Under normal circumstances, bone conduction plays only a very small part in the transmission of sound because sound waves in air will only cause slight vibration of the skull bones.

## Neurophysiology of audition

### The organ of Corti

The organ of Corti is situated in the scala media of the cochlea. Its structure is illustrated in **Fig. 2.4.14**.

The 'floor' of the organ of Corti is formed by the basilar membrane, which is composed of laterally orientated fibres that run between the bony modiolus and the spiral ligament of the cochlea. The basilar membrane is narrow and stiff at the basal turn of the cochlea but progressively widens and becomes more elastic towards the apex. This is despite the fact that the chambers of the cochlea actually get smaller towards the apex.

The auditory receptors are called **hair cells**. They are arranged in orderly rows and are attached to the basilar membrane by supporting **Deiter's cells**. There is a single row of inner hair cells, which lies nearest to the central core of the cochlear spiral, and three to five rows of outer hair cells. The inner and outer hair cells are separated by a triangular-shaped tunnel, the tunnel of Corti, which is bounded by the rods of Corti. The tunnel of Corti contains perilymph, whereas the main chamber of the scala media contains endolymph.

The hair cells are so called because prominent hairs, or cilia, project from their upper surfaces. The hairs project through the dense granular layer of the **reticular lamina** and into the **tectorial membrane**. The tectorial membrane is gelatinous in texture and is composed of glycoprotein. On the inner side of the cochlear spiral the tectorial membrane is attached to the modiolus and on the outer side to the upper surfaces of supporting cells situated on the basilar membrane (**see Fig. 2.4.14**). Thus the tectorial membrane effectively forms the 'roof' of the organ of Corti.

The projecting hairs of the hair cells are quite stiff and bristle like. Mechanical bending of the hairs occurs when the basilar membrane vibrates in response to sound. This movement is the mechanical event that induces receptor potentials in the hair cells and hence action potentials in the cochlear nerve fibres.

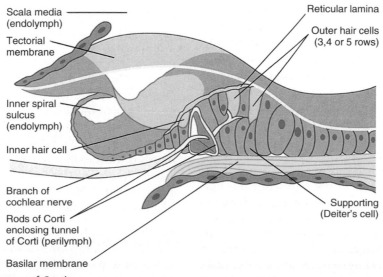

Scala media (endolymph)
Tectorial membrane
Inner spiral sulcus (endolymph)
Inner hair cell
Branch of cochlear nerve
Rods of Corti enclosing tunnel of Corti (perilymph)
Basilar membrane
Reticular lamina
Outer hair cells (3,4 or 5 rows)
Supporting (Deiter's cell)

**Figure 2.4.14** The organ of Corti

The afferent nerve supply to the organ of Corti is the cochlear nerve branch of the VIIIth cranial nerve. Intimately associated with the base of each hair cell is one or more afferent nerve terminals derived from the dendrites of bipolar cells. The bipolar cell bodies are located in the spiral ganglion. The central axons of these cells form the cochlear nerve, which ascends to the brainstem and then to the auditory cortex. The afferent 'wiring' of the hair cells differs for inner and outer hair cells. There are over 3000 inner hair cells, each of which is innervated by approximately 10 afferent nerve fibres, which do not overlap or converge up to the level of the brainstem. Inner hair cells receive fibres from approximately 90% of the total afferent supply to the cochlea. By contrast, the outer hair cells converge on to the bipolar cells. Typically, 10 outer hair cells receive terminals from one single afferent nerve fibre and there is considerable overlap of innervation. The outer hair cells receive only about 10% of the total afferent supply to the cochlea, despite the fact that they outnumber inner hair cells by a ratio approaching 4 : 1.

The efferent nerve supply to the cochlea, provided by the olivocochlear fibres, also shows a differential pattern of input to inner and outer hair cells. Most efferent fibres appear to terminate on the outer hair cells, although some efferent fibres make close contacts with the afferent dendritic supply of the inner hair cells. The precise role of the efferent nerve supply is not understood at present. However, increased activity in efferent fibres appears to result in an inhibition of afferent activity in the cochlear nerve. The efferents therefore apparently influence the sensitivity of auditory detection of sound.

## The endolymphatic potential

The scala media contains endolymph, which contains sodium and potassium ions in concentrations similar to those found in intracellular fluid. In contrast, the scalae vestibuli and tympani contain perilymph, which has a higher sodium ion and lower potassium ion concentration than endolymph. The composition of perilymph is similar to that of extracellular fluid.

The difference in composition between perilymph and endolymph is maintained because Reissner's membrane and the reticular lamina are impermeable to sodium and potassium ions. These ions can readily penetrate the basilar membrane and so it is assumed that endolymph surrounds the organ of Corti but only penetrates it between the tectorial membrane and the reticular lamina. This means that the nerve terminals associated with the hair cell bases are surrounded by perilymph.

When no sound is impinging on the ear, a steady potential difference exists between endolymph and perilymph. This potential difference is referred to as the endolymphatic potential. It is normally of 50–80 mV amplitude, with endolymph being positive with respect to perilymph. The sign of the endolymphatic potential is somewhat surprising: typically, intracellular fluid is negative with respect to extracellular fluid and, hence, the endolymphatic potential cannot result from the differences in distribution of sodium and potassium ions between endolymph and perilymph. The endolymphatic potential is maintained metabolically by the stria vascularis.

## Transduction of the mechanical vibration of sound into electrical signals

When sound waves impinge on the ear, the energy is transmitted to the cochlea and the basilar membrane vibrates. As the basilar membrane moves up and down, so the hairs of the cells bend. In effect, the basilar membrane, which is attached on both sides, alternately bows upwards and dips downwards, and the change in the curvature of its surface causes changes in the orientation of the hairs on the hair cells. Because the tips of the hair cells are embedded in the relatively firm, gelatinous mass of the tectorial membrane, the vibration of the hair cell bases results in a shearing or bending of the projecting hairs. This shearing movement then results in the generation of receptor potentials.

## Frequency coding in the ear

The human ear can discriminate small changes in the frequency of sound, an ability that appears to depend primarily on the nature of the mechanical displacement of the basilar membrane.

The most widely accepted theory to explain frequency coding of a sound is the place theory, first proposed by Helmholtz in 1863 and later refined by Georg von Békésy in the 1920s. In essence, the place theory states that different parts of the basilar membrane resonate at different frequencies. The basal end of the basilar membrane is narrow, stiff and composed of short lateral fibres. This favours fast-frequency vibration. In contrast, the apical end of the basilar membrane is wider and more elastic and it vibrates maximally in response to low-frequency sounds.

The place theory proposes that the hair cells in the region of the basilar membrane that is maximally displaced will produce the greatest response in the afferent fibres associated with them. The pattern of afferent input to the brain is then interpreted as a sound of a specific frequency.

## Intensity coding in the ear

The intensity of a sound is primarily coded by the frequency of impulse discharge in stimulated afferents.

High-intensity (loud) sounds produce a higher frequency of discharge than low-intensity sounds. In addition, high-intensity sounds produce a greater displacement over a wider area of the basilar membrane, although the region of maximal displacement remains a function of the frequency of the sound source.

## Localization of a sound source

The majority of people can locate the source of a sound reasonably accurately. This ability depends on two factors. First, the timing of the arrival of a sound wave at the two eardrums will differ, depending on the position of the sound source. This will in turn influence the timing of the impulse discharge in the afferents from the two ears and this discrepancy can be interpreted by the brain to enable localization of the sound. Second, the head casts an 'acoustic shadow' such that sounds originating from the left side produce marginally higher intensity vibrations in the left ear when compared with the right ear. Again, the discrepancy in intensity will result in a small difference in the frequency of impulse discharge arising from the two ears.

### CLINICAL APPLICATIONS

#### HEARING LOSS

Impaired hearing can result from impaired conduction of sound through the outer and middle ear, from damage to the cochlea or from damage to the auditory pathway beyond the ear. It is important to distinguish between deafness that is conductive (the most common) and sensorineural, which could indicate important neurological disease.

Complete deafness is uncommon; the adult labelled 'deaf' is much more likely to have a markedly reduced sense of hearing. This often develops gradually and can be well advanced before the person realizes. Some children are born deaf, the most common cause being contraction of rubella by the mother during the first trimester of pregnancy.

Intact hearing is essential for proper communication and maintaining a safe environment. When communicating with a deaf patient, nurses should not speak until they have the person's attention. Having achieved this, the nurse should speak slowly and clearly, ensuring that the deaf person can see the lips moving. Exaggerated lip movements are not necessary. If the patient has a 'good' ear, this should be identified and utilized. If the patient has difficulty understanding, it is better to rephrase your statement rather than to

repeat the same misunderstood phrase. As a general rule, vowels are more readily heard than consonants.

It is imperative to take your time and display patience and tolerance while the deaf person communicates with you. Any outward displays of irritability or impatience on the part of the nurse will serve only to discourage contact with the deaf person.

Some patients will be trained to lip read and others will benefit from the use of an appropriate and properly fitted hearing aid. People with impaired hearing benefit from receiving advice and guidance from the Royal National Institute for the Deaf, an organization that specializes in the welfare of the deaf person.

## Auditory pathways (Fig. 2.4.15)

Axons from cells of the spiral ganglion of the cochlea leave the inner ear as the VIIIth (auditory) cranial nerve and terminate on cells of the cochlear nucleus in the medulla. Afferent fibres from the base of the cochlea, signalling high frequencies, penetrate deep into the nucleus before dividing. Afferent fibres from the apex of the cochlea, signalling low frequencies, divide at more superficial levels. In this way the strict organization of the frequencies of sound that exists in the cochlea is maintained at the level of the cochlear nucleus.

The cells of the cochlear nucleus give rise to axons that cross the midline in either the acoustic stria or the trapezoid body. The nerve fibres of the acoustic stria arise from the dorsal part of the cochlear nucleus, cross the midline and ascend in the lateral lemniscus to terminate on cells of the inferior colliculus. The fibres of the trapezoid body arise from the cells of the ventral part of the cochlear nucleus, cross the midline and synapse in the superior olive. This nucleus in turn projects axons that join the lateral lemniscus and terminate in the inferior colliculus (Fig. 2.4.15).

Although the majority of nerve fibres cross the midline, a sizeable minority synapse in the ipsilateral superior olive. Some cells of the superior olive receive input from ipsilateral and contralateral axons and these 'binaural' cells are sensitive to the differences in the time of arrival of auditory signals from the two ears. Such time differences, although very small, are an important cue for the localizing of a sound source in the environment.

The inferior colliculus retains the tonotopic organization of the sensory input. The probable function of the inferior colliculus is the orienting response when a sound is being attended to. The connections between the inferior colliculus and the superior colliculus are presumably important in performing this role. The cells of the inferior colliculus project axons

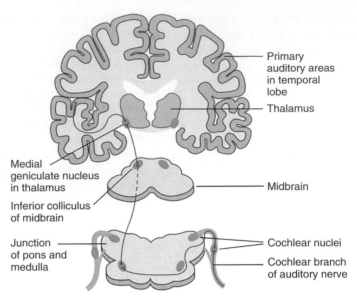

**Figure 2.4.15**   Auditory pathways

to the thalamic sensory relay nucleus of the auditory pathway, the medial geniculate nucleus (MGN).

The cells of the MGN project to the primary auditory cortex in the superior temporal gyrus, also known as the transverse gyri of Heschl. Here, too, an ordered tonotopic map of the sensory input is retained.

There is asymmetry in function between the two cerebral hemispheres. The left hemisphere contains an area referred to as **Wernicke's area**, which is concerned with the analysis of speech. Damage to this area causes a sensory (or receptive) aphasia such that the patient is able to hear sounds but cannot interpret speech. Speech sounds seem to become as unintelligible as listening to the gabble of an unfamiliar foreign language. Damage to the corresponding area in the right hemisphere will leave the perception of language intact but will cause dysfunction in the recall, recognition and discrimination of non-verbal sounds. Such dysfunctions, called **amusias**, lead to the inability to discriminate between melodies.

### CLINICAL APPLICATIONS

Speech problems will lead to impairment of the patient's ability to communicate. The speech therapist should be involved at an early stage so that the best possible recovery is achieved. A skilled assessment is performed to establish the extent of the disorder and an individualized therapy programme is then devised. This could range from the use of exercises and massage to the use of sophisticated microcomputer systems. It is imperative that the nurse attempts to communicate with the dysphasic patient on a day-to-day basis to restore the patient's self-esteem and avoid any feelings of isolation.

## The ear and balance

The inner ear contains the **vestibular apparatus** in addition to the cochlea. The vestibular apparatus signals rotational movements of the head and changes in its position relative to the pull of gravity. These sensory signals are involved in the reflex control of posture and in the control of eye movements.

## Anatomy of the vestibular apparatus

The vestibular apparatus consists of a **membranous labyrinth** contained within the **bony labyrinth** of the temporal bone. The major features of the vestibular apparatus are illustrated in **Fig. 2.4.16**.

There are three **semicircular canals** oriented at right-angles to each other. The membranous labyrinth of the canals is filled with endolymph and is surrounded by perilymph contained within a bony cavity in the temporal bone. At the base of each canal is a swelling, the **ampulla**, which contains a ridge called the **crista**. Hair cells are situated on the crista and the hairs project into a gelatinous mass, the **cupola**, which divides the semicircular canal into two parts (**Fig. 2.4.17**). The bases of the hair cells are innervated by afferent nerve terminals of bipolar vestibular nerve cells. The cell bodies of these afferents are located in the vestibular ganliona. The central axons of the fibres project to the brainstem as part of the VIIIth cranial nerve.

The semicircular canals communicate with the **utricle**, which in turn communicates with the **saccule**. The utricle and saccule are filled with endolymph and are connected directly to the scala media of the cochlea by the ductus reuniens. The utricle and saccule

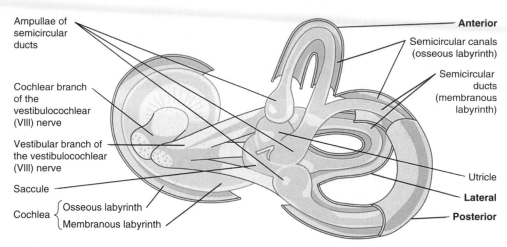

Ampullae of semicircular ducts

Cochlear branch of the vestibulocochlear (VIII) nerve

Vestibular branch of the vestibulocochlear (VIII) nerve

Saccule

Cochlea { Osseous labyrinth
Membranous labyrinth

**Anterior**

Semicircular canals (osseous labyrinth)

Semicircular ducts (membranous labyrinth)

Utricle

**Lateral**

**Posterior**

**Figure 2.4.16**   Posterior view of the labyrinths of the inner ear. The outer purple colour shows the bony labyrinth and the inner yellow colour shows the membranous labyrinth

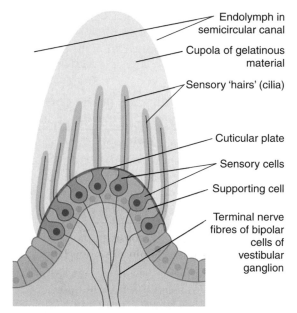

Endolymph in semicircular canal

Cupola of gelatinous material

Sensory 'hairs' (cilia)

Cuticular plate

Sensory cells

Supporting cell

Terminal nerve fibres of bipolar cells of vestibular ganglion

**Figure 2.4.17**   Structure of the ampulla of a semicircular canal

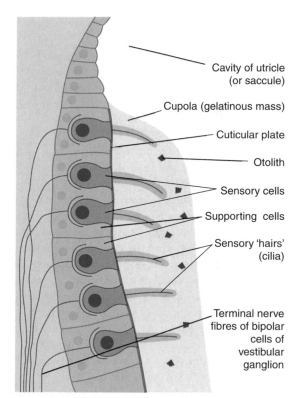

Cavity of utricle (or saccule)

Cupola (gelatinous mass)

Cuticular plate

Otolith

Sensory cells

Supporting  cells

Sensory 'hairs' (cilia)

Terminal nerve fibres of bipolar cells of vestibular ganglion

**Figure 2.4.18**   Structure of the macula of an otolith organ

each contain a ridge, the **macula**, from which hair cells project into a gelatinous cupola in much the same way as in the ampullae of the semicircular canals. However, the cupolae in the utricle and saccule contain calcium carbonate particles called **otoliths** (**Fig. 2.4.18**). When posture is erect the macula of the utricle projects horizontally, whereas in the saccule the macula projects vertically. As in the semicircular canals, the hair cells of the utricle and saccule are associated with afferent terminals of the vestibular nerve.

The hair cells of the vestibular apparatus are the receptors that detect head movement. Bending of the projecting hairs initiates an impulse discharge in the vestibular nerve. The mechanism is assumed to be similar to the receptor mechanism in the cochlea.

## The semicircular canals

Receptors in the three **semicircular canals** in each ear are stimulated by rotational movements of the head. Because the canals are oriented at right angles to each other, they can respond to rotation in any plane. Thus, the receptors in the horizontal canal are primarily stimulated when the head is rotated from side to side, as when gesturing 'no'; those in the superior canal are stimulated when the head is rotated up and down, as when gesturing 'yes'; and those in the posterior canal are stimulated when the head is

**171**

rotated in a transverse plane, tilting the head towards one shoulder.

When the head is rotated laterally, the hair cells of the two horizontal canals are stimulated. As the head moves, the semicircular canals move with it. However, the endolymph contained within each canal is unattached and, because of its own inertia, its movement lags behind movement of the head. Thus, the relatively stationary columns of endolymph displace the cupolae in the two ampullae and this in turn causes bending of the projecting hairs. In each cupola, bending of the hairs in one direction causes an increase in the impulse discharge in the associated afferent nerve terminal, whereas bending in the opposite direction reduces the discharge. As the head is rotated to the left, the impulse discharge in the vestibular nerve from the left ear decreases but that from the right ear increases, and vice versa. This imbalance in input to the brain is presumed to form the basis for interpretation of direction of movement.

The bending of the hairs occurs only when the rotational movement accelerates or decelerates. During acceleration the endolymph rapidly overcomes its inertia and it then moves in unison with the semicircular canals. The cupolae then resume their normal orientations and the bending force on the hair cells is removed. The impulse discharge then returns to its resting level. During deceleration, the events occur in reverse. The endolymph continues to move under its own momentum after cessation of movement of the head. Thus, the hair cells are again bent until the endolymph also becomes stationary. The nervous discharge to the CNS from the two ears also reverses because deceleration is equivalent to movement in the opposite direction. Thus, as a rotational movement to the left decelerates, the left ear impulse discharge increases and the right ear discharge decreases.

As the semicircular canals are only stimulated during acceleration or deceleration, they can perform a predictive function. The impulse discharge from the semicircular canals signals a rate of change of position of the head, and the brain can therefore predict the position of the head in advance of the movement. This is thought to be an important afferent input enabling the brain to modify the output to postural muscles to effect coordinated movement without loss of balance.

The events described can occur in the three pairs of semicircular canals, depending on the plane of rotation of the head.

### The utricle and saccule

The utricle and saccule are stimulated by changes in position of the head relative to the pull of gravity. They are collectively referred to as the **otolith organ**.

When the head is tilted away from its normal upright position, the otoliths in the cupolae tend to move under the influence of the gravitational pull and this causes bending of the projecting hairs of the hair cells. The projecting hairs differ in their orientations and therefore movement of the otoliths causes maximal stimulation of only some of the hair cells, depending on the direction of tilt of the head. Stimulation of hair cells gives rise to an impulse discharge in the associated afferent terminals. Bending of the hairs in one direction causes an increased impulse discharge, whereas bending in the opposite direction results in a decrease in impulse discharge. The pattern of impulse discharge arising from the otolith organ codes the direction of movement of the head. The frequency of the impulse discharge is primarily dependent on the distance moved by the head.

The nervous discharge shows little adaptation, in contrast to the rapidly adapting signal transmitted from the semicircular canals. The otolith organ therefore continually appraises the CNS of the position of the head in space.

## The vestibular apparatus in the control of posture and eye movements

The vestibular apparatus signals changes in position of the head in space and, together with the visual input and proprioceptor input, contributes to the reflex maintenance of posture and balance during movement.

The otolith organ continuously signals the position of the head even when the body is not moving; this signal is involved in the reflex control of postural muscles. When linear acceleration occurs, the otolith organ is again stimulated. The otoliths in the utricles and/or saccules experience a thrust in the opposite direction to that of the movement, and this can also initiate stimulation of hair cells. The utricle and saccule provide important afferent inputs for posture control during the linear acceleration that occurs when an individual starts to walk forwards.

The otolith organ also contributes to the control of eye movements that occur when the head position is changed. Eye movements occur to enable visual fixation of an image despite head movement. Thus, as the head is tilted upwards, the eyes are lowered, and vice versa. (Visual input from the eyes also contributes to the reflex control of the extrinsic eye muscles.)

During rapid rotational movements, reflex compensatory eye movements also occur in an attempt to maintain a fixed visual reference point. The eyes move back and forth, a **rotational nystagmus**. The nystagmus results from the input to the brain from stimulated semicircular canals. When rotation occurs to the left, the slow component of the nystagmus is towards the right in an attempt to keep a fixed visual reference point. The fast component occurs towards the left, the direction of rotation, to pick up a new visual reference point. When rotation ceases, the semicircular canals will at first be stimulated as though rotation were occurring in the opposite direction, and a postrotational nystagmus occurs.

In addition to the reflex control of eye movements, the semicircular canals also provide an input for posture and balance control. Thus, when rotating to the left, extensor muscles in the left limbs contract to maintain balance. When the rotation stops, the initial effect on the semicircular canals is as though the body is rotating to the right, and the right limb extensors therefore reflexly contract. However, because the body has in fact stopped rotating, extension of the right limbs causes the body to fall towards the left and there is a temporary loss of balance. Dancers can overcome the effects of postrotational nystagmus and loss of balance by making short sharp movements of the head in the opposite direction to that of rotation, thereby preventing movement of endolymph in the semicircular canals.

## CLINICAL APPLICATIONS

### DISTURBANCES OF THE VESTIBULAR APPARATUS

Ear infections can cause abnormalities of vestibular function, resulting in disturbances of balance and dizziness. **Ménière's disease** is a condition in which there is excessive production of endolymph. This can cause auditory disturbances but it also commonly causes dizziness and nausea as a result of impaired function of the vestibular apparatus. Patients with these distressing symptoms are advised to rest in bed in a quiet, darkened room. This is a frightening time for the sufferer and the nurse will need to stay with the patient, to provide reassurance during the worst stages of the attack.

A relatively common disturbance associated with vestibular function is that of **motion sickness**. This appears to result when movement is erratic and there is poor correlation between movement detected by the vestibular apparatus and movement detected by the eyes. People vary in their susceptibility to motion sickness.

## Pathways of the vestibular system

The central representation of the vestibular system begins with the bipolar cells of the vestibular ganglion. These cells are peripherally connected with the hair cells of the vestibular apparatus of the inner ear and project centrally along the VIIIth cranial nerve to the four vestibular nuclei of the medulla (**Fig. 2.4.19**). However, some fibres ascend directly to terminate in the cerebellum. The four brainstem nuclei – the superior, inferior, lateral and medial vestibular nuclei – comprise the vestibular nuclear complex.

The lateral vestibular nucleus receives relatively few primary vestibular fibres but has input from the cerebellum and also from the spinal cord. The cells of this nucleus then project axons that descend as the vestibulospinal tract in the ventral columns of the spinal cord and terminate in the ipsilateral ventral horn of the cord at all levels from cervical to lumbar regions. This pathway has a facilitatory influence on muscle tone and spinal reflex activity.

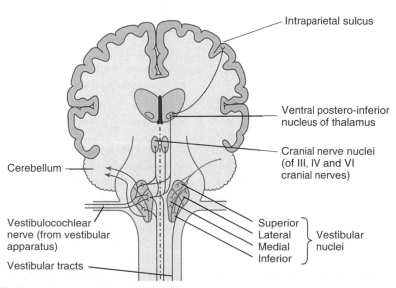

Intraparietal sulcus

Ventral postero-inferior nucleus of thalamus

Cranial nerve nuclei (of III, IV and VI cranial nerves)

Cerebellum

Vestibulocochlear nerve (from vestibular apparatus)

Vestibular tracts

Superior
Lateral
Medial
Inferior

Vestibular nuclei

**Figure 2.4.19** Vestibular pathways: note that for clarity some inputs are indicated on the left and some on the right side of the brain only

The medial and superior vestibular nuclei send axons that ascend to terminate bilaterally on the nuclei controlling the extraocular muscles, that is, the nuclei of the IIIrd, IVth and VIth cranial nerves. The connections between the vestibular fibres and the oculomotor centres are concerned with the reflex pathway, which produces eye movements compensating for head movements.

The medial and inferior vestibular nuclei project descending fibres to the cervical segments of the spinal cord. These axons are concerned with the control of head and neck muscles. In addition, these nuclei project ascending axons to the cerebellum.

As yet, there is no clear understanding of how vestibular sensation reaches conscious experience. A small thalamic nucleus, which projects to the parietal lobe, might be involved in this but there is little clear evidence at present.

## CLINICAL APPLICATIONS

Disturbances of the central vestibular system can cause dysfunctions in the control of eye movements and the control of balance. For example, a disturbance of ocular muscle control leading to nystagmus can be caused by peripheral or central damage to the vestibular system. **Vertigo**, which implies a disorientation of the body in space and which might be accompanied by nausea, sweating, pallor and changes in heart rate, might also be a sign of vestibular damage.

## The chemical senses of gustation and olfaction

Taste (gustation) and smell (olfaction) are both chemical senses that depend on the detection of a local change in the chemical environment of appropriate receptors.

## Gustation

Taste results from stimulation of chemical receptors, which are located primarily on the tongue (**Fig. 2.4.20**). Four primary tastes appear to be detected by these receptors: sour, sweet, salt and bitter. All the flavours that a human being can experience depend on the relative activation of these four primary taste receptor types and on associated olfactory sensations. The involvement of olfaction in taste is demonstrated by the reduction in ability to taste food when a heavy cold interferes with smell. Olfaction is an important component for the identification of particular tastes. It is also possible that texture and chewiness contribute to the recognition of foods.

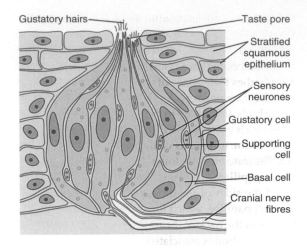

**(a)**

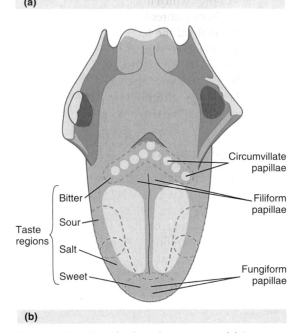

**(b)**

**Figure 2.4.20** Taste buds and taste zones. (a) Structure of a taste bud and (b) location of taste zones on the tongue

Taste identification might therefore involve several sensory areas in the brain.

### Taste receptors

Taste receptors are grouped together in oval-shaped structures called **taste buds**, which are located primarily on the tongue; a few are found on the soft palate and at the back of the throat. There are up to 10 000 taste buds in the mouth. The structure of a taste bud is illustrated in **Fig. 2.4.20a**. Each bud is about 70 $\mu$m long and up to 40 $\mu$m wide and contains up to 20 functioning taste receptor cells. The taste receptor cells are derived from epithelial cells. At the exposed tip of the bud, microscopic taste hairs, which arise from the taste cells, project through a pore. The hairs (or microvilli) bear receptor sites for the attachment of chemicals that stimulate the cells. The taste pore is the route of access for the receptors. All substances that are tasted are dissolved in saliva, which bathes the surface of the taste buds and penetrates the taste pores.

Taste buds are located in the sides of small connective tissue elevations called **papillae**, which give the surface of the tongue its characteristic rough appearance. The taste buds are found in the fungiform knob-shaped papillae, which are located primarily at the tip and the sides of the tongue, and in circumvallate (circular) papillae, which form a prominent inverted 'V' shape at the back of the tongue (**see Fig. 2.4.20b**).

Each taste bud is associated with two or three large afferent nerve fibres, which branch to form a network of fine unmyelinated fibres innervating the receptor cells. The terminals of the fibres lie in folds in the taste receptor cell membranes so there is intimate contact between the receptors and the sensory afferent fibres. There is some overlap of innervation of taste buds; one large afferent fibre might have branches supplying more than one taste bud.

## The mechanism of taste

Electrophysiological studies of taste afferents have shown that any single taste bud can respond to several, even up to four, of the primary tastes of sourness, saltiness, sweetness and bitterness. However, each taste bud shows differential sensitivity to the four tastes such that a maximum sensitivity is shown to only one taste type. In addition, single taste receptor cells within a bud might respond to more than one taste. Each cell might therefore bear receptor sites on microvilli for more than one of the primary tastes.

## Distribution of sensitivity to the primary tastes

There is a distinct pattern in the distribution of taste buds in terms of the predominant taste to which they are sensitive. Thus, taste buds that are maximally sensitive to sour chemicals are located on the sides of the tongue, those that respond primarily to sweetness are found at the tip, and those for bitterness at the back of the tongue (**see Fig. 2.4.20**). Buds that respond predominantly to saltiness are found in all of these areas, but particularly at the tip of the tongue.

## Threshold and sensitivity to taste

The threshold concentration required to elicit a taste sensation is an individual characteristic of a chemical. However, there do appear to be general differences in threshold between the four primary tastes.

Very much weaker concentrations of bitter substances are required to elicit a bitter sensation than threshold concentrations for sweet or salt chemicals; receptor cells for sourness tend to have intermediate thresholds.

Sensitivity to the four primary tastes is influenced by a number of factors, chiefly individual variability, age and temperature. Individual variability among people is clearly to be expected, but one particular aspect is of interest genetically determined variability. About 3% or 4% of the Caucasian population has a very high threshold for the taste of a bitter chemical, called phenylthiourea. Their measured thresholds are of the order of 400 times that expected for the rest of the population. The ability to taste phenylthiourea is determined by a single dominant gene. This is of particular interest because it is so specific to one chemical and there is no apparent shift in threshold to other bitter substances, nor to the other primary tastes.

### DEVELOPMENTAL ISSUES

Age has an effect on sensitivity to taste. Newborn infants are apparently relatively insensitive to taste, whereas young children are often very sensitive to, and indeed intolerant of, bitter or salty substances. Adult sensitivity is less than that found in children and it decreases further in old age. These changes in sensitivity could contribute to the differences in food preferences that are often exhibited by children and adults.

Temperature also appears to alter sensitivity to tastes but the effect is quite complex. Salt and bitter tastes are generally stronger at lower temperatures, and an adequately salted hot casserole might seem oversalted as it cools a little. By contrast, sweetness sensitivity appears to increase to a maximum at a temperature of about 40°C. Sensitivity to sourness is relatively unaffected by temperature changes.

## Adaptation

Adaptation to sapid (taste-producing) substances occurs rapidly, although the reduction in sensation is minimized if the food is moved continuously around the mouth. The adaptation appears partly to reflect receptor adaptation to stimulation but also to depend on central brain mechanisms.

### CLINICAL APPLICATIONS

#### TASTE AND HEALTH

Taste is probably of greatest clinical significance in terms of changes that occur secondarily to other

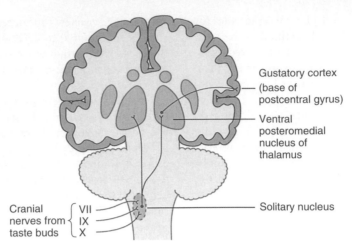

**Figure 2.4.21**  Gustatory pathways of the brain

disorders or conditions. Poor oral hygiene can be a direct cause of an impaired taste sensation and loss of appetite. This serves to emphasize the importance of assessment of the patient's mouth during illness. Those most at risk of developing a dry mouth are patients receiving oxygen therapy or those constantly breathing through their mouths. Patients with a swallowing difficulty, who might be leaving food debris in the mouth, and infected or dehydrated patients are all at risk. Effective oral hygiene should be performed as each individual patient's needs demand. Patients with an impaired sense of taste will need to be tempted to eat, and this can be enhanced by proper presentation and service of meals.

### Gustatory pathways

The peripheral afferent nerve fibres from the taste buds travel from the tongue via the VIIth (facial), IXth (glossopharyngeal) and Xth (vagus) cranial nerves to the solitary nucleus of the medulla. From here, cells project axons, which ascend to the ventral posteromedial nucleus of the thalamus, and cells from this nucleus in turn project to the gustatory area of cortex at the bottom of the postcentral gyrus (**Fig. 2.4.21**). Little is known about the central integration of gustatory information and the status of taste, as a relatively minor sensory experience, has meant that little experimental work has been undertaken in this area. However, dysfunctions of the gustatory system do occur. For example, some epileptic patients report an aura of a distinctive taste in the mouth preceding an epileptic seizure. The aura might be caused by abnormal firing of cells in the area of the gustatory cortex or the closely neighbouring temporal cortex. In particular, these hallucinations of taste are associated with irritative lesions of part of the limbic lobe of the cortex.

## Olfaction

The sense of smell is even less well understood than taste. So far, primary odour types have not been identified. Smell might play a role in survival as many, although by no means all, noxious volatile materials have characteristic odours.

Smell might also be involved in sexual attraction. Certainly, humans, insects and animals secrete attracting chemicals as a forerunner to mating. There is currently debate as to whether humans are subconsciously attracted by body odours (see Chapter 6.3) but sexual secretions do have characteristic odours.

### Olfactory receptors

The olfactory receptors are found in olfactory epithelial tissue, which is located in the roof of the nasal cavity. It extends down to cover the superior turbinate bone in each nostril and also the upper part of the walls of the dividing nasal septum.

The olfactory receptors are derived from dendritic terminals of bipolar cells, the central axons of which unite to form the olfactory nerves. The olfactory nerves transmit to the two olfactory bulbs, which lie under the frontal poles of the brain. The dendrites of the olfactory bipolar cells extend as olfactory rods that bear microscopic hairs, or cilia. The olfactory hairs bear receptor sites for chemical attachment and they are embedded in the mucous lining of the nasal cavity (**Fig. 2.4.22**).

### Mechanism of olfaction

The olfactory cilia bear receptor sites for the attachment of odoriferous chemicals, which are brought into contact with the olfactory epithelium by the passage of air through the nose. Because the epithelium is situated in the roof of the nasal cavity, sniffing

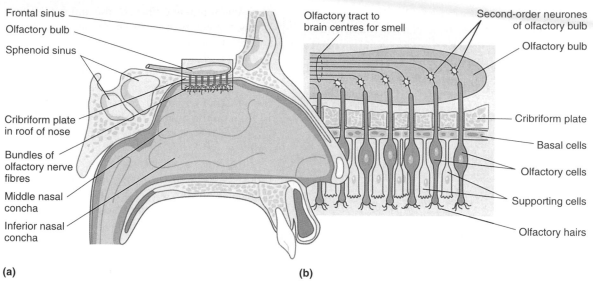

**Figure 2.4.22** Olfactory receptors. (a) Location of olfactory receptors in the nasal cavity and (b) magnification of the olfactory receptors

helps to draw air up across the surface of the sensory cells. Any odoriferous chemical must clearly be sufficiently volatile to produce a vapour that can be carried in the airstream through the nasal cavity. To gain access to receptor sites on the olfactory cilia, a chemical must be able, at least partially, to dissolve in the aqueous mucous lining of the nasal cavity. Lipid solubility is probably also important because the olfactory cilia membranes largely consist of lipoprotein.

The olfactory epithelium appears to show regional variations in terms of the type of odoriferous chemicals to which the receptors respond (cf. the distribution of the primary tastes on the tongue). However, as no primary odour types can be identified, the pattern of distribution of receptors in relation to odour is not precise.

## Olfactory pathways

Central representation of olfaction occurs in the olfactory bulb and in several areas of the limbic lobe. The pathway begins with the olfactory bipolar cells, the peripheral terminations of which serve as olfactory sense receptors. Centrally, the thin unmyelinated axons of the bipolar cells pass through the cribriform plate into the skull cavity and synapse in the olfactory bulb (see Fig. 2.4.22).

The **olfactory bulb** is the primary integrating centre for olfactory impulses. It is a small, oval-shaped structure containing a multiplicity of cells and synaptic contacts grouped together in bundles called **olfactory glomeruli**. The olfactory glomeruli contain the terminations of descending efferent nerve fibres as well as the terminations of the bipolar cells. There are numerous interneurones within the glomeruli, including large cells called mitral cells, which form

the main outflow from the olfactory bulb. The axons of the mitral cells pass posteriorly along the olfactory tract, which lies underneath the frontal lobe of the brain and attaches to the base of the brain at its posterior end. Some axons synapse in the anterior olfactory nucleus. This nucleus is in fact made up of small groups of neurones strung out along the olfactory tract. Other olfactory afferents terminate in the olfactory tubercle, which lies at the posterior end of the tract. However, the main branch of the olfactory tract passes posteriorly and laterally as the lateral olfactory stria, to terminate in the amygdala and in the olfactory cortex of the limbic lobe, which lies adjacent to the anterior hippocampus.

The olfactory system is unique as a sensory system in that it does not have a specific relay nucleus within the thalamus. However, both the olfactory cortex of the limbic lobe and the olfactory tubercle send large numbers of fibres to the medial nucleus of the thalamus. In turn, this projects to a wide area of the frontal lobes.

### Threshold and sensitivity to smell

Different chemicals will require different concentrations in air to achieve the threshold level for odour detection. Moreover, the pattern of breathing will influence the quantity of chemical that is brought into contact with the olfactory epithelium.

As with taste, odour sensitivity is not a constant and individuals vary widely in their sensitivities to different odoriferous chemicals.

### Adaptation

Adaptation to odour occurs very rapidly and an odour might not be detectable seconds or minutes after the beginning of exposure, the time to extinction depending on the particular chemical. Most people have experienced how even a very unpleasant smell rapidly fades and apparently disappears. As with taste adaptation, olfactory adaptation apparently partly depends on central brain mechanisms.

## Olfaction and health

As with taste, changes in olfactory sensitivity are chiefly of clinical importance as secondary signs of disorder. The main problem encountered is decreased stimulation of appetite, as taste is enhanced by the sense of smell. The person who lives alone, and whose sense of smell is not acute, runs the risk of being exposed to noxious gases and needs to be warned of this potential danger.

### DEVELOPMENTAL ISSUES

The ageing process invokes a number of changes in the special senses. Hearing becomes gradually impaired and there is a particular decline in sensitivity for higher frequencies, which results in greater difficulty in understanding speech. A number of changes have been noted in the ear that contribute to this, including rigidity of the tympanic membrane and the bones of the middle ear along with some loss of muscle fibres, changes to the Reissner's and basilar membranes, loss of hair cells in the organ of Corti and a gradual loss of ganglion cells and fibres of the auditory nerve. Finally, the ability to locate sound becomes slower and less accurate with age.

Vision is affected in many ways, resulting in the loss of ability to accommodate for near vision (presbyopia). This is due to the loss of flexibility of the lens altering how and where the image is focused on the retina. The size of the visual field is reduced due to loss of receptors from the retina.

The number of taste buds on the tongue is reduced and those remaining undergo degeneration with age. This results in impaired taste, which might be exacerbated by a reduced flow of saliva. The sense of smell will undergo similar changes.

Maintenance of balance relies on the integration of appropriate responses. This will include those from the visual system, the vestibular system and from proprioceptors in the muscles and joints. Older people require greater angular movements for this to be achieved. This explains the exaggerated sway seen in an older person when asked to stand and close their eyes.

## Conclusion

Each of the senses has been described, along with its functions. We have seen that some are more sensitive than others and that the special senses allow us to detect changes in our external environment.

## Clinical review

In addition to the Learning Objectives at the beginning of this chapter, the reader should be able to:

- Describe the structure and innervation of the organ of Corti

- Define the term 'endolymphatic potential'

- Explain how perceived pitch and loudness relate to the frequency and intensity of sound vibration impinging on the ear

- Describe the structure of the vestibular apparatus of the ear

- Explain the mechanism by which the vestibular apparatus responds to rotational movements of the head and changes in position of the head relative to gravitational pull

- Outline the contribution of the vestibular apparatus to the control of posture and eye movement

- Describe the structure of olfactory epithelium

- Describe and outline the mechanisms of taste and smell

## Review questions

1. Which enzyme is contained in tears?
2. Why is it sometimes possible to taste chemicals that are applied topically to the eye?
3. What is the blind spot in the eye?
4. What kind of muscle is the ciliary muscle?
5. Which structures does light pass through in the eye before reaching the photoreceptors?
6. How do the functions of rods and cones differ?
7. How are rods and cones able to respond to light?
8. What electrical events in rods and cones are stimulated by light?
9. What happens at the optic chiasma?
10. Outline the functions of the outer, middle and inner ears
11. What are the muscles of the inner ear and what do they do?
12. Where are the endolymph and the perilymph respectively found in the cochlea?
13. How are intensity of sound and air pressure related?
14. What does the lever system of the inner ear achieve?
15. How is the effect of sound waves in the middle ear converted into action potentials in the cochlear nerve fibres?
16. What is made possible by the arrangement of the semicircular canals?
17. How does the function of the utricle and sacule differ from the semicircular canals?
18. What is rotational nystagmus?
19. What are the primary tastes?
20. Are the taste buds sensitive to the primary tastes evenly distributed over the surface of the tongue?
21. What is the key difference between the way in which chemicals are presented to the sensory systems of taste and smell?

## Suggestions for further reading

Todd, F. (2001) Keep in touch: How would you cope if your patient was deaf and blind? *Nursing Standard,* **16**(11); 21.
*Helpful article that provides practical guidelines.*

Walsh, M. (2002) *Watson's Clinical Nursing and Related Sciences,* 6th edn. London: Baillière Tindall.
*Helpful chapter on caring for the patient with a disorder of the senses.*

# The autonomic nervous system

*Ann Richards*

## LEARNING OBJECTIVES

After studying this chapter the reader should be able to:

- Recognize the importance of the autonomic nervous system to the maintenance of homeostasis

- Classify the autonomic nervous system into its divisions

- Relate the autonomic nervous system to the central nervous system and the peripheral nervous system

- Enumerate the anatomical differences between the two divisions of the autonomic nervous system

- Name the neurotransmitters involved in the autonomic nervous system and the way in which they are inactivated

- Explain the function of the sympathetic nervous system

- Explain the functions of the parasympathetic nervous system

- Describe the structural reasons for the diffuse nature of sympathetic activity

- Discuss the complexity of interactions between the two divisions of the autonomic nervous system

- Describe the mechanism of action of some drugs acting on the autonomic nervous system

## INTRODUCTION

The primary role of the autonomic nervous system (ANS) is to maintain optimal homeostasis through the monitoring and regulation of the internal environment. This involves the contribution of all body systems, with the ANS playing the most crucial role of all.

The anatomical circuitry of the ANS is broadly dispersed, creating a general response, quite unlike the highly specific pathways and responses of the central nervous system (CNS). This enables the ANS to mediate overall changes in state.

The ANS regulates the contraction of smooth muscle and cardiac muscle, as well as controlling glandular secretion and thus, in health, it is able to maintain key physiological variables (e.g. blood pressure, body temperature) within safe limits, often by negative feedback mechanisms.

The main processes regulated by the ANS are:

- contraction and relaxation of smooth muscle
- all exocrine and certain endocrine secretions
- the heartbeat
- certain steps in intermediary metabolism.

A degree of autonomic control influences many other processes, including the function of the immune system and the somatosensory system, although the physiological importance of autonomic control in such systems is not yet clear (Rang et al., 1999).

The ANS is an extensive network of cells and fibres, which are widely distributed inside the body. It was defined by Langley in 1898 as the visceral efferent nervous system and thus, by definition, the ANS includes no sensory components. Its activities, however, are modified by sensory inputs and nowadays the term 'ANS' can be used more widely to include functionally related visceral afferents.

Unlike the somatic motor system, which has the single job of innervating and commanding skeletal muscle fibres, the ANS has the complex task of commanding every other tissue and organ in the body that is innervated. The somatic motor system can excite only its peripheral targets, whereas the ANS is capable of balancing synaptic excitation and inhibition to achieve widely coordinated and graded control (Bear et al., 1996). Some differences between

the autonomic and somatic motor systems are shown in **Table 2.5.1**.

'Autonomic' is from the Greek, *automania*, meaning 'independence' or 'self-government'. The term is apt, because the ANS usually operates without conscious awareness and has no cognitive component (Longstaff, 2000). Control of visceral organs by the ANS is usually regarded to be automatic and involuntary, but this might be misleading as it is possible for some individuals to use biofeedback techniques to exert some control of variables regulated by the ANS, e.g. blood pressure. By contrast, control of skeletal muscle by the somatic nervous system is regarded as voluntary and willed. However, the respective control exerted by the autonomic and somatic nervous systems over visceral and skeletal muscular functioning is not totally independent. For example, the activity of skeletal muscle does require the autonomic nervous system to divert blood from the gastrointestinal tract to skeletal muscle. These two systems are coordinated

| Table 2.5.1 A comparison of the somatic and autonomic motor systems | |
|---|---|
| **Somatic nervous system** | **Autonomic nervous system** |
| Innervates and commands skeletal muscle | Commands every other tissue in the body that is innervated |
| Upper motor neurone in brain | Upper motor neurone in brain |
| Cell bodies of all LMNs lie within CNS | Cell bodies of LMNs lie outside the CNS in clusters called ganglia |
| Monosynaptic pathway – single neurone with single axon extends from CNS to effector | Disynaptic pathway – preganglionic neurone and postganglionic neurone |
| Neurones are heavily myelinated | Preganglionic neurones are lightly myelinated Postganglionic neurones are unmyelinated |
| Conduction is faster than ANS | Conduction slower than somatic nervous system |
| Pinpoint accuracy | Actions often multiple and widespread |
| Neurotransmitter is acetylcholine | Main neurotransmitters are acetylcholine and noradrenaline (norepinephrine) |
| Control is willed and voluntary | Control is automatic and mostly involuntary |
| Only able to excite peripheral targets | Balances synaptic excitation and inhibition to achieve widely coordinated and graded control |
| CNS, central nervous systems; LMN, lower motor neurone. | |

at the higher level of central control, and these higher centres can be influenced by both the external environment and emotion. The results of autonomic nervous activity frequently impinge in a very real way on our conscious awareness. Many of these effects accompany strong emotions, for example, we become aware of the increased force and rate of the heartbeat during strong emotions such as fear. There is a very complex relationship between the action of the ANS, emotion and our experience of physiological actions within our own bodies.

The ANS is organized on the basis of a reflex arc. Subconscious sensory signals from visceral organs enter the CNS and autonomic nerves make adjustments as necessary to ensure optimal support for body activities. In response to changing conditions, the ANS is able to alter the flow of blood to an organ, increase the heart rate, adjust blood pressure and body temperature and increase or decrease gastrointestinal secretions. Most of this 'fine-tuning' occurs without our being aware of it (Marieb, 2004). Many adjustments do involve negative feedback but some might change physiological variables in response to altered demand rather than defending a set point. The functions of the ANS underlie physiological aspects of coping during stress and form one of the links between the nervous and endocrine control of behaviour. In response to a wide variety of stressors, the sympathetic nervous system is activated and organs such as the heart, liver, airways and blood vessels respond, allowing increased cardiac output, increased airflow through the respiratory passages, raised blood glucose levels and regional alterations in blood flow to enable us to combat stress. Occasionally, the ANS works by positive feedback, which carries the system away from its normal stable state – an example is sexual arousal.

## Divisions of the ANS

There are two subdivisions of the ANS, the sympathetic and the parasympathetic, with both structural and functional differences between them. Although they operate in parallel, they use structurally distinct pathways and transmitter systems. In very general terms, the two branches are antagonistic. The sympathetic nervous system (SNS) is associated with the 'flight or fight' response of emergencies, stress and the expenditure of energy, whereas the parasympathetic is associated with 'resting and digesting' and the production and conservation of energy. They are typically described as having opposite effects on target organs and what one subdivision stimulates, the other is likely to inhibit. An example here is the effect of the ANS on the heart rate. Stimulation of the SNS speeds up the

cardiac rate whereas stimulation of the parasympathetic division slows down the cardiac rate. This is an oversimplification of the situation and it is more realistic to think of the two divisions as cooperating together constantly to control the internal balance of the body.

One of the most striking features of the ANS is the rapidity and intensity with which it can change visceral functions. The SNS is activated by many stimuli including feelings, noise, light, drugs and chemicals. In response to the stimulus an immediate anticipatory state is generated. Within 3–5 seconds it can increase the heart rate to twice normal and within 10–15 seconds the arterial blood pressure can be doubled. At the other extreme, arterial pressure can be decreased low enough within 4–5 seconds to cause fainting (Guyton & Hall, 2000). Sweating can begin within seconds and the urinary bladder can empty involuntarily, also within seconds. It is these extremely rapid alterations that are measured by the lie detector polygraph, and they reflect the inner feelings and emotions a person might be experiencing. Unlike the somatic motor system, the neurones of which can rapidly excite skeletal muscle with pinpoint accuracy, the actions of the ANS are always multiple and widespread.

## Structure of the ANS

In common with the rest of the nervous system, the ANS is composed of neurones, neuroglia and other connective tissue. Structurally, however, it displays many distinctive features. For descriptive purposes, it can conveniently be dealt with in the traditional two divisions, the **sympathetic division** and the **parasympathetic division**. This anatomical classification coincides with a functional differentiation between the two divisions (Table 2.5.2).

The ANS originates with cell bodies in the brainstem and spinal cord. These give rise to preganglionic myelinated axons, which secrete **acetylcholine**. The preganglionic neurones synapse with unmyelinated postganglionic fibres in autonomic ganglia, as shown in **Fig. 2.5.1**. The sympathetic division arises from the thoracic spinal cord and the first two lumbar spinal segments and has its ganglia close to the cord in the paravertebral chains. Its long postganglionic fibres secrete **noradrenaline** (norepinephrine). The parasympathetic division originates from the brainstem and the sacral spinal cord and its autonomic ganglia are located on, or close to the innervated organ. The short postganglionic fibres secrete acetylcholine. Based on their origins in the brainstem and spinal cord, the sympathetic division is sometimes called the **thoracicolumbar division** and the

**Table 2.5.2** Anatomical and physiological comparison of the sympathetic and parasympathetic nervous systems

| Parasympathetic nervous system | Sympathetic nervous system |
| --- | --- |
| Emerges from the brainstem and sacral spinal cord | Emerges from thoracolumbar section of spinal cord |
| Long preganglionic fibres | Short preganglionic fibres |
| Short postganglionic fibres | Long postganglionic fibres |
| Ganglia located in or close to the visceral effector organ | Ganglia located close to the spinal cord |
| Minimal branching of preganglionic fibres | Extensive branching of preganglionic fibres |
| Function involves production, conservation and storage of energy – maintenance role – 'resting and digesting' | Function involves energy expenditure and intense muscular effort – emergency response role – 'flight or fight' |
| **Neurotransmitters** Preganglionic fibres release acetylcholine | **Neurotransmitters** Preganglionic fibres release acetylcholine |
| Postganglionic fibres release acetylcholine | Postganglionic fibres to the sweat glands and some blood vessels release acetylcholine |
| | Most postganglionic fibres release noradrenaline (norepinephrine) |
| | Neurotransmitter activity augmented by release of adrenal medullary hormones |

parasympathetic division is occasionally known as the **craniosacral division**.

## Sympathetic division (Fig. 2.5.2)

The sympathetic division innervates more organs than the parasympathetic – some glands and smooth muscle structures (e.g. sweat glands and arrector pili muscles, which cause the hair to stand on end) are served only by sympathetic fibres. All arteries and veins have smooth muscle in their walls that is innervated only by sympathetic fibres. This partly explains why the sympathetic division of the ANS is more complex than the parasympathetic.

The system is formed from the unit structure of two neurones in series, the **presynaptic neurone** and the **postsynaptic neurone**. The cell bodies of the presynaptic neurones lie in the intermediolateral horn of grey matter of their respective spinal segments T1 to L2 (**Table 2.5.3**). These preganglionic sympathetic neurones in the grey matter of the spinal cord produce the lateral horns – the visceral motor zones (**see Fig. 2.5.2**) – which are absent in the sacral region of the spinal cord because there are fewer parasympathetic preganglionic neurones. The nerve fibres pass first into the **sympathetic chain of ganglia** and then to the

tissues or organs that are stimulated by the sympathetic nerves. A more detailed description now follows and is shown in **Fig. 2.5.2**.

The sympathetic fibres leave the spinal cord through the ventral (anterior) roots into the corresponding spinal nerve. Immediately after the spinal nerve leaves the spinal canal, the preganglionic sympathetic fibres leave the nerve and terminate in the paired **paravertebral ganglia**, which run either side of the spinal column, or the unpaired **prevertebral (collateral) ganglia** (e.g. the coeliac plexus). The presynaptic nerve fibre is myelinated and the short branches of the spinal nerve running to the sympathetic chain are called the **white rami communicans**, reflecting the appearance of the myelination. The paravertebral ganglia are joined together by nerve strands to form a chain on both sides of the vertebral column, extending from the base of the brain to the sacrum, and look rather like a string of beads. Within the sympathetic chain of ganglia, most of the presynaptic fibres synapse, although some pass upward or downward in the chain and synapse with other ganglia and a few run through the chain intact, to synapse within the prevertebral (collateral) ganglia lying nearer to the visceral organs, which the postsynaptic fibre will ultimately supply.

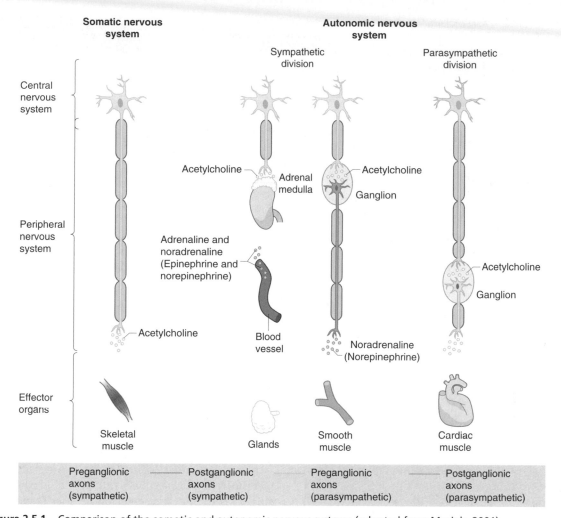

**Figure 2.5.1** Comparison of the somatic and autonomic nervous systems (adapted from Marieb, 2001)

## Sympathetic nerve fibres in skeletal nerves

Postsynaptic fibres are mainly unmyelinated and, on leaving the paravertebral sympathetic chain, many enter the ventral (dorsal) ramus of adjoining spinal nerves by way of communicating branches called the **grey rami communicantes**. Parasympathetic fibres never run in spinal nerves and so rami communicantes are associated only with the sympathetic division. Grey rami issue from every chain ganglion from the cervical to the sacral region, allowing sympathetic output to reach all parts of the body. These postsynaptic fibres are distributed to effector tissues (blood vessels, sweat glands and piloerector muscles), with the appropriate spinal and peripheral nerves to each dermatome. About 8% of the fibres in each skeletal nerve are sympathetic fibres, demonstrating their importance (Guyton & Hall, 2000). Each preganglionic fibre synapses on average with eight or nine postganglionic neurones, each of which supplies numerous effector cells. This arrangement means that **sympathetic activity tends to be diffuse** and there is much

divergence of stimuli, unlike the parasympathetic system, which acts in localized and discrete regions.

## Segmental distribution of sympathetic nerves (summarized in Table 2.5.3)

The **paravertebral chain of ganglia** extends superiorly to the level of the cervical vertebrae **(Fig. 2.5.3)**. Some of the postganglionic fibres that arise from this cervical extension are distributed to the head. Within this cervical extension there are three ganglia: the **superior, middle and inferior cervical ganglia.** Postganglionic fibres arising from the superior cervical ganglion are distributed to the blood vessels and skin of the head, the pupil of the eye and the salivary glands. Postganglionic fibres arising from all three cervical ganglia are distributed to the lungs and heart.

## Sympathetic nerve endings in the adrenal medulla

As a general rule, the characteristic anatomy of the sympathetic division is the relative shortness of the

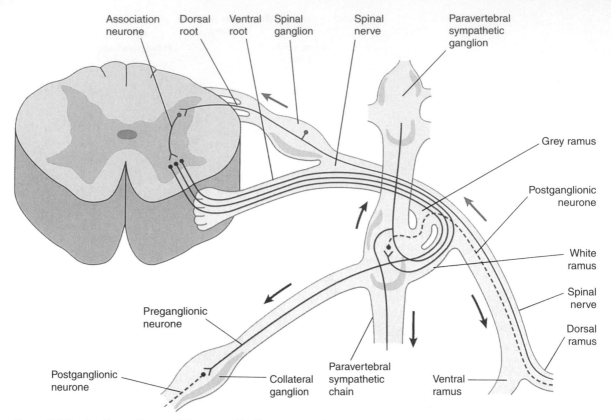

**Figure 2.5.2** A reflex pathway of the sympathetic nervous system

| Table 2.5.3 Segmental distribution of the sympathetic nerves | |
| --- | --- |
| **Spinal cord segment** | **Organs served** |
| T1–T5 | Head and neck, heart |
| T2–T4 | Bronchi and lungs |
| T2–T5 | Upper limb |
| T5–T6 | Oesophagus |
| T6–T10 | Stomach, spleen and pancreas |
| T7–T9 | Liver |
| T9–T10 | Small intestine |
| T10–L1 | Kidney, reproductive organs |
| T10–L2 | Lower limb |
| T11–L2 | Large intestine, ureters, urinary bladder |

preganglionic fibres and the relative length of the postganglionic fibres. There are exceptions to this characteristic pattern, the most important and striking being the case of the adrenal medulla. Here, an exceptionally long preganglionic set of fibres runs to the organ itself. Fibres travel in the thoracic splanchnic nerve and pass through the coeliac ganglion without synapsing. The **adrenal medulla** is considered to be a sympathetic ganglion in which the postganglionic cells have lost their axons and become highly specialized,

secreting adrenaline (epinephrine) and noradrenaline (norepinephrine) directly into the bloodstream. This leads to widespread excitatory effects, such as a raised heart rate, that most people will recognize as being due to 'a rush of adrenaline'. The stimulus for this secretion is the acetylcholine released by the preganglionic fibres arriving at the adrenal medulla.

## Collateral (prevertebral) ganglia

The preganglionic fibres from T5 down enter and leave the sympathetic chains without synapsing. They form several nerves, called the splanchnic nerves, that contribute to a number of nerve plexuses, known collectively as the **abdominal aortic plexus.** The **collateral sympathetic ganglia** within serve the entire abdominopelvic viscera and include the coeliac, superior mesenteric, inferior mesenteric and hypogastric ganglia, which are named after the arteries they associate with. The postsynaptic sympathetic fibres normally travel alongside the arteries and are distributed diffusely to the thoracic and abdominal visceral organs.

As well as a cervical extension, there is also an inferior extension of the sympathetic ganglionic chain. Preganglionic fibres originating from T10 to L2 innervate the pelvis. They descend in the sympathetic trunk to lumbar and sacral chain ganglia and most leave the cord via lumbar and sacral splanchnic nerves,

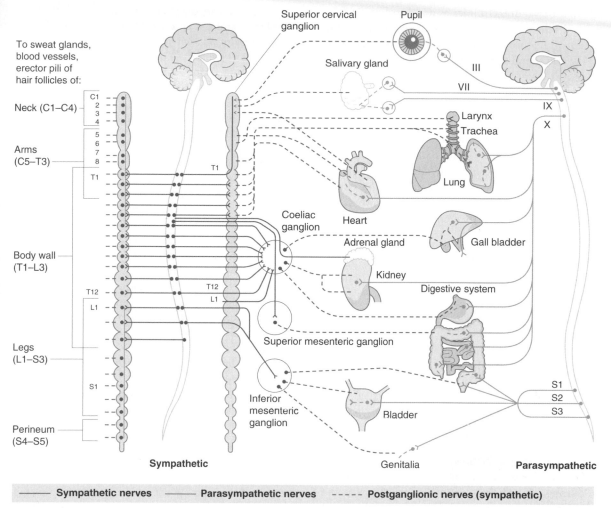

To sweat glands,
blood vessels,
erector pili of
hair follicles of:

Neck (C1–C4)

Arms
(C5–T3)

Body wall
(T1–L3)

Legs
(L1–S3)

Perineum
(S4–S5)

**Sympathetic**

Superior cervical
ganglion

Pupil

Salivary gland

III

VII

IX

X

Larynx

Trachea

Lung

Coeliac
ganglion

Heart

Adrenal gland

Gall bladder

Kidney

Digestive system

Superior mesenteric ganglion

Inferior
mesenteric
ganglion

Bladder

S1
S2
S3

Genitalia

**Parasympathetic**

——— **Sympathetic nerves** ——— **Parasympathetic nerves** ----- **Postganglionic nerves (sympathetic)**

**Figure 2.5.3** Sympathetic and parasympathetic nervous systems. For clarity, peripheral and visceral nerves of the sympathetic system are shown on separate sides of the spinal cord

which send their fibres to the inferior mesenteric and hypogastric ganglia. From there, the postganglionic fibres are distributed to the anal and bladder sphincters, and to the sexual organs.

The sympathetic division is by no means simple in its structure. This complexity is inevitable when one realizes that effector organs are found in the most peripheral areas of skin as well as core visceral organs, and that the originating preganglionic cells occur within the limits of the thoracic spinal cord segments and two lumbar spinal cord segments. The effectors supplied by the SNS are smooth muscles of all organs, the heart and the salivary, sweat and digestive glands as well as adipose cells, liver cells and the renal tubules.

### CLINICAL APPLICATIONS

The anatomical distinctiveness of the sympathetic chain of ganglia lying on either side of the vertebral column has led to the possibility of the operation **sympathectomy** being performed. This

is very occasionally carried out for the congenital idiopathic condition of hyperhidrosis (excessive sweating), as the sympathetic nerves innervate the sweat glands. It is now possible to use endoscopic surgery to perform the procedure with only very small incisions but there are complications and there might be compensatory increased sweating in other areas of the body.

### The parasympathetic division

The basic unit of the structure of the parasympathetic division (see Fig. 2.5.3) is also that of two neurones in series. As described above, the preganglionic nerve cells are situated at opposite ends of CNS, either in the brainstem (as one component of some cranial nerve nuclei) or in the medial lateral grey matter of sacral segments.

Preganglionic fibres of the parasympathetic division are long: ganglia lie close to, or within, the effector organ; postganglionic fibres are very short.

Again, the system is complex as it is distributed to the eye and salivary glands in the head region and to the viscera of the thoracic, abdominal and pelvic cavities. Unlike the sympathetic division, it is not distributed to blood vessels, sweat glands and piloerector muscles of the skin.

From this we can see that most of the organs of the thoracic, abdominal and pelvic cavities have both a sympathetic and a parasympathetic nerve supply and that they act as effector organs to *both* divisions.

The length of the preganglionic fibres of the parasympathetic division means that the parasympathetic component of peripheral nerves tends to be preganglionic for the most part.

## Parasympathetic division and cranial nerves

Parasympathetic fibres are found as a component of the **IIIrd cranial nerve (oculomotor)**. They run to the ciliary ganglia in the orbit of the eye, where they synapse. The postganglionic fibres innervate the ciliary muscle of the pupil, causing pupillary constriction (miosis).

The **facial (VIIth cranial) nerve** also contains parasympathetic fibres. Some innervate the lacrimal glands and others supply the submaxillary and sublingual salivary glands. The parotid salivary gland, however, derives its parasympathetic innervation from a branch of the **glossopharyngeal (IXth cranial) nerve**.

Although these three cranial nerves supply the parasympathetic innervation of the head, the distal ends of their preganglionic fibres join branches of the **trigeminal nerve (V)** to synapse. This means that the postganglionic fibres can travel with the trigeminal nerve, which has the widest distribution of all the cranial nerves to the facial area.

The most complex and important parasympathetic outflow is that contained in the **vagus (Xth cranial) nerve**; 75% of all parasympathetic fibres run in the vagus nerve and these form a substantial proportion of its substance.

Ganglionic synapses include the cardiac plexus, from whence postganglionic fibres proceed to the heart. From the pulmonary plexus, postganglionic fibres run to the bronchi. Other branches of the vagus nerve carry preganglionic fibres to intramural plexuses within the oesophagus, stomach and intestines. Short postganglionic fibres innervate these organs.

### CLINICAL APPLICATIONS

A **lower motor neurone lesion** of the facial nerve can cause loss of lachrymation (tear formation) on the affected side, although salivation still occurs

because salivary glands have two sources of innervation. A lesion affecting the IIIrd (oculomotor) cranial nerve, as in early tentorial herniation, causes the dilatory action of the sympathetic supply to act unopposed, giving a dilated pupil on the affected side. Tentorial herniation is a potential outcome when there is dangerously increased intracranial pressure, as can occur, for example, in extradural haematoma complicating a head injury. The dilating pupil (together with an increasingly sluggish response to light) should be reported immediately it is observed so that emergency action may be taken.

The operation of **vagotomy** does not, as its name implies, involve the whole of the vagus nerve but refers instead to a division of the branch that supplies the pyloric muscle of the stomach and the secretory glands of the stomach (thus the term **selective vagotomy** is sometimes used). This prevents the vagus nerve from stimulating the secretion of digestive juice; consequently, acidity is reduced. The operation also allows more rapid emptying of the contents of the stomach into the duodenum. This operation might be carried out to treat peptic ulceration in the few cases that do not respond to drug therapy with ulcer-healing drugs.

## Parasympathetic sacral outflow

The preganglionic fibres arising from spinal cord segments S2–S4 branch off to run with the pelvic splanchnic nerve and then to the vesicular plexus, from which they continue to synapse in ganglia within those organs that are innervated from the sacral part of the parasympathetic division, namely, the distal part of the large intestine including the rectum and anus, the ureters, the urinary bladder and its sphincter, and the reproductive organs. It is particularly important to note that these organs also have a sympathetic nerve supply and, in addition the sphincter muscles, have a voluntary nerve supply as well. Normal function of the emptying of the bladder and bowel relies not only on an intact nervous supply but also on coordinated control of the input to the organs from the various types of nervous supply. This is also true of sexual activity, as both parasympathetic and sympathetic activities are involved in erection and ejaculation.

## Visceral reflexes and the enteric nervous system

The presence of sensory fibres, mostly visceral pain afferents, in autonomic nerves is often not described because anatomists consider the ANS to be only a visceral motor system.

## CLINICAL APPLICATIONS

The visceral pain afferents travel along the same pathways as somatic pain fibres and this partly explains how referred pain occurs. This is when pain originating in the viscera is felt as being somatic in origin, e.g. gall bladder pain is referred to the area between the shoulder blades.

The visceral sensory neurones send information regarding stretch, irritation and chemical changes, and form the first link in autonomic reflexes. Complete three-neuronal reflex arcs with sensory, motor and intrinsic neurones exist entirely within the walls of the gastrointestinal tract in the enteric nervous system.

At the beginning of the twentieth century, Langley recognized the **enteric nervous system** as the third division of the ANS, distinct from the sympathetic and parasympathetic divisions. It consists of neurones whose cell bodies lie in the intramural plexuses within the walls of the alimentary canal and is sometimes called a collection of 'little brains'. It is estimated that there are more cells in this unique system than in the spinal cord, and it is pharmacologically more complex than either the sympathetic or parasympathetic branches of the ANS, involving many neurotransmitters.

The enteric nervous system is embedded in the lining of the alimentary canal and consists of two complicated networks each with sensory nerves, interneurones, and autonomic neurones. They make up the intrinsic nerve plexuses of the gastrointestinal tract:

- **myenteric plexus** – responsible for coordinating gut motility
- **submucosal plexus** – responsible for controlling secretion and absorption.

Enteric sensory neurones monitor tension and stretch of gastrointestinal walls, the chemical status of the stomach and intestinal contents, and the hormone levels in the blood. The information is used by the enteric interneuronal circuits to control the activity levels of enteric output motor neurones, which govern smooth muscle motility, production of mucous and digestive secretions, and the diameter of the local blood vessels (Bear, 1996).

## CLINICAL APPLICATIONS

Consider a partially digested meal moving through the small intestine. The enteric plexus will ensure that there is sufficient mucus to lubricate the partially digested food and that there are digestive enzymes available to finish digestion. It will also control the rhythmic muscular action that works to mix food and enzymes and will ensure a good flow of blood through the intestine to allow adequate absorption of the digested nutrients.

The enteric nervous system has sufficient integrative capacity to allow it to function independently, whereas the sympathetic and parasympathetic divisions are essentially agents of the CNS and cannot function without it. However, the enteric nervous system is not entirely independent and does receive some input from the sympathetic and parasympathetic divisions of the ANS.

## DEVELOPMENTAL ISSUES

In the fifth week of fetal development, cells originating from the neural crest of the thoracic region migrate to form a bilateral chain of sympathetic ganglia interconnected by longitudinal nerve fibres. These are the sympathetic chains, located either side of the spinal cord. Some of the sympathetic neuroblasts migrate in front of the aorta to form the coeliac and mesenteric ganglia; others migrate to the heart, lungs and gastrointestinal tract. Once these sympathetic chains have been established, nerve fibres penetrate the ganglia of the chain and form synapses around the developing neuroblasts. These are the preganglionic fibres and pass from the spinal nerves to the sympathetic ganglia, forming the white communicating rami.

Neural crest cells also invade the medial aspect of the adrenal glands to give rise to the medulla of the gland that will secrete adrenaline (epinephrine) and noradrenaline (norepinephrine).

The origin of the parasympathetic ganglia is still controversial and some believe the cells migrate out of the central nervous system along the preganglionic fibres of the oculomotor, facial, glossopharyngeal and vagus nerves, whereas others believe they arise from neuroblasts within the sensory ganglia of the V, VII and IX nerves (Sadler, 2003). Failure of neural crest cells to migrate into the wall of the colon results in a lack of formation of parasympathetic ganglia in this area. This is Hirschsprung's disease or congenital megacolon, where the baby has decreased peristalsis, usually in the sigmoid colon and rectum, resulting in abdominal distension and severe constipation. This condition usually presents in the first month of life and can cause delayed passage of meconium (the first sticky stools of a newborn baby). Older children present with chronic constipation that has been present since very early childhood. A variety of surgical procedures are possible for the treatment of Hirschsprung's disease and the aim is to bring the ganglionic bowel down to the anus.

## Neurotransmitters and receptors

All nervous system communication to connecting nerves or other tissues is achieved via the release of chemical transmitter across a synapse and not by direct contact. The chemical transmitters are synthesized and stored in nerve endings, released on stimulation and interact with highly specific **surface receptors** on the receiving nerve or tissue. Activation of these receptors can cause changes in membrane permeability or induce the enzyme-mediated formation of a second messenger in effector cells.

The receptor is on the outside of the cell membrane, bound as a prosthetic group to a protein molecule that penetrates the cell membrane. Binding of the chemical transmitter to the receptor causes a conformational change in the structure of the protein molecule. The altered protein molecule now **excites** or **inhibits** the cell, usually causing a change in the permeability of the cell membrane to one or more ions or affecting an enzyme attached to the other end of the receptor protein where it protrudes into the cell interior. Activation of the receptor thus brings about the observed effect caused by stimulation of that nerve (e.g. glandular secretion, muscle contraction).

Historically, the ANS has probably taught us more than any other part of the body about how neurotransmitters work. The anatomical distinctiveness of the ANS in having synapses within ganglia outside the CNS has allowed its neurotransmitters to be studied with more ease than those within the CNS, and the accessibility of the ANS has led to the development of drugs that can mimic transmitters (agonists) or block their effects (antagonists).

The ANS comprises two sets of neurones in series with one another and it follows that there are two sets of neurotransmitters involved at its synapses: one set at the presynaptic nerve ending, affecting the postsynaptic neurone and situated within the ganglia, and the other set released from the postganglionic nerve ending at the effector organ **(see Fig. 2.5.3)**.

## Cholinergic receptors

The neurotransmitter released from the preganglionic nerve ending in *both* divisions of the autonomic nervous system is **acetylcholine** (which can be abbreviated to **ACh**), and the receptors it binds to are **cholinergic receptors.** The transmission at these ganglionic synapses is characterized as **nicotinic** because the cholinergic receptor on the postganglionic membrane responds to nicotine in a way that is similar to its response to acetylcholine. When the acetylcholine binds to the nicotinic cholinergic receptor

it immediately evokes a fast excitatory postsynaptic potential (EPSP), which usually triggers an action potential in the postganglionic cell. This can be likened to the action of acetylcholine at the skeletal neuromuscular junction and drugs such as curaré, which paralyses skeletal muscle by blocking the nicotinic acetylcholine receptors, also block autonomic output.

It is at the postganglionic nerve ending that the two divisions differ from one another. Within the effector organs, the neurotransmitter at the postganglionic nerve ending of the parasympathetic division is again acetylcholine; however, there is a difference between the action of acetylcholine at this site and its action at the preganglionic site and it has been found that it is muscarine, the active component of the poisonous mushroom *Amanita muscaria*, which mimics the action of acetylcholine release at the effector organs. This is because of the presence of a different type of cholinergic receptor, the muscarinic cholinergic receptor, which responds to muscarine and not nicotine. The effects of stimulation of the muscarinic receptor can be blocked by the administration of small doses of atropine, a drug that is used in anaesthesia to dry secretions and in bradycardia to speed up the heart rate. **Atropine** blocks the muscarinic effects of acetylcholine without affecting the nicotinic effects. It is a **muscarinic antagonist**, blocking the parasympathetic stimulation of the effector organs without affecting the sympathetic effects of the nicotinic action of acetylcholine at the preganglionic nerve ending.

## Adrenergic receptors

In the sympathetic division of the ANS, the neurotransmitter released onto tissue receptors at the effector organ in the majority of postganglionic nerve endings is **noradrenaline (norepinephrine)**. Here, at least two different classes of membrane receptor have been identified, and these respond differently to drugs. These have been called **alpha($\alpha$)- and beta ($\beta$)-adrenergic receptors**. Organs that respond to noradrenaline (norepinephrine) have one or both types of receptor; $\alpha$-adrenergic receptors are stimulated by noradrenaline (norepinephrine) to a greater extent than adrenaline (epinephrine), whereas $\beta$-adrenergic receptors are stimulated by adrenaline (epinephrine) to a greater extent than by noradrenaline (norepinephrine). Noradrenaline (norepinephrine) excites mainly the $\alpha$-receptor but does also excite the $\beta$-receptor to a lesser extent, whereas adrenaline (epinephrine) excites both types of receptor approximately equally.

Preganglionic sympathetic nerve endings act directly upon cells within the adrenal medulla. These nerve endings release acetylcholine, which stimulates the release of the hormones adrenaline (epinephrine) and noradrenaline (norepinephrine) directly into the blood flowing through the gland. Both catecholamines can thus reach the peripheral receptor sites of the sympathetic nervous system from the bloodstream, reinforcing its widespread and diffuse action. On average, about 80% of the secretion of the chromaffin cells of the adrenal medulla is adrenaline (epinephrine) and the other 20% is noradrenaline (norepinephrine).

A small number of sympathetic nerve endings are not adrenergic but **cholinergic**. These nerve endings act on the sweat glands of the skin (the sweat glands in the palm of the hand are an exception to this, because the sympathetic nerve endings here are adrenergic) and some peripheral blood vessels associated with the skin of the face and neck where stimulation brings about vasodilation, resulting in blushing or flushing. These sympathetic cholinergic nerve endings are muscarinic in type.

## Receptor subtypes

The effects of acetylcholine and noradrenaline (norepinephrine) are not consistently either excitation or inhibition, and the response of the visceral effectors to these neurotransmitters depends not only on the transmitter released but also on the receptors they attach to. The existence of different types of receptor for both acetylcholine and noradrenaline (norepinephrine) mean that they can exert different effects of excitation or inhibition at different targets within the body. The effects of acetylcholine binding to nicotinic receptors is always stimulatory and results in the excitation of the neurone or effector cell. The effects of acetylcholine at the muscarinic receptor can be either stimulatory or inhibitory, and three important types of muscarinic receptor make this possible: the $M_1$-, $M_2$- and $M_3$-receptors. $M_1$- and $M_3$-receptors produce mainly **excitatory effects**, e.g. increased acid production in the stomach ($M_1$) and stimulation of glandular secretions ($M_3$), whereas $M_2$-receptors are found in the heart and exert **inhibitory effects** – they are responsible for vagal inhibition of the heart, slowing the heart rate.

The effect of noradrenaline (norepinephrine) at the **α-receptor** is usually **stimulatory** and its effect at the **β-receptor** is usually **inhibitory** but there are exceptions to this, which are made possible by the existence of two main α-receptor subtypes ($\alpha_1$ and $\alpha_2$) and three β-receptor subtypes ($\beta_1$, $\beta_2$ and $\beta_3$). The different physiological effects of the catecholamines at various tissues depend on the presence of these different adrenoreceptor subtypes. The distinction between $\beta_1$- and $\beta_2$-receptors is an important one: $\beta_1$-receptors are found mostly in the heart, where they are excitatory and are responsible for the positive chronotropic (increased rate) and positive inotropic (increased force) effects of catecholamines; $\beta_2$-receptors are responsible for smooth muscle relaxation in many organs (e.g. the respiratory tract) – an effect that is utilized by drugs, such as salbutamol, that are agonists at the $\beta_2$-receptors and are used as bronchodilators.

## Agonists and antagonists

An **agonist** is an agent that binds to a receptor and mimics the action of the natural neurotransmitter. An **antagonist** binds to a receptor but does not produce the necessary conformational change within the receptor for the usual response to stimulation to occur. The antagonist can be thought of as a receptor 'blocker', for example drugs called 'β-blockers' block the β-adrenergic receptor and so compete with noradrenaline (norepinephrine) at the receptor, reducing its usual effects. These drugs therefore slow the heart rate in exercise or emotion when the sympathetic nervous system is usually active.

## Non-adrenergic, non-cholinergic transmission in the ANS

Acetylcholine and noradrenaline (norepinephrine) are not the only autonomic transmitters, a fact that was first discovered when it was realized that drugs that abolish these transmitters could not completely block autonomic transmission. Compounds believed to function as non-adrenergic, non-cholinergic (NANC) transmitters include nitric oxide, adenosine triphosphate (ATP), vasoactive intestinal peptide (VIP) and neuropeptide Y (NPY) at postganglionic nerve terminals. Other substances, such as dopamine, γ-aminobutyric acid (GABA), substance P and 5-hydroxytryptamine (5-HT, also known as serotonin) play a role in ganglionic transmission. Cholinergic and adrenergic drugs do not work well at these receptor sites.

## Termination of transmitter action

Acetylcholine is **rapidly inactivated** in the synaptic cleft by the enzyme **acetylcholinesterase**. The inhibition of this enzyme by drugs such as neostigmine allows the accumulation of acetylcholine at the mucosal endplate and can be used to treat **myasthenia gravis**, a condition in which there is a reduction in acetylcholine receptors on the skeletal muscle cells at the neuromuscular junction.

The action of noradrenaline (norepinephrine), which is released at postganglionic sympathetic nerve endings, is terminated in a very different manner. There is no synaptic enzyme to inactivate noradrenaline (norepinephrine) and reuptake by the noradrenergic nerve terminals and other cells is the chief method of disposal. Circulating adrenaline (epinephrine) and noradrenaline (norepinephrine) are **degraded by enzymes** that include monoamine oxidase (MAO), which is bound to the surface membrane of mitochondria in the postganglionic cells. Some drugs prescribed as antidepressants work by blocking this enzyme.

## Functions of the ANS (Table 2.5.4)

The importance of the ANS in the maintenance of homeostasis has already been mentioned. It provides the automatic neural control within vital organs, which is the background to the voluntary and purposeful activity of daily life. For example, unless the ANS aided the maintenance of a blood supply to the brain on standing and increased blood supply to the skeletal muscles in exercise, voluntary actions would be impossible even with an intact somatic nervous system.

## Interactions of the sympathetic and parasympathetic divisions in the control of homeostasis

Implicit in the description of the anatomy of the ANS is one of its unique features, that of the **dual innervation** (involving both sympathetic and parasympathetic fibres) to many of the effector organs. It follows from this that the interaction of the two divisions is extremely complex. The standard physiological model of the ANS is of reciprocal tension, with the two parts keeping each other in check – when sympathetic activity goes up, parasympathetic activity goes down.

**Table 2.5.4**  The effects of the autonomic nervous system

| Effector organs | Noradrenergic impulses | Cholinergic impulses |
|---|---|---|
| **Eyes** | | |
| Pupil | $\alpha_1$ Dilates (mydriasis) | Constricts (miosis) |
| Ciliary muscle | $\beta_2$ Slight relaxation for far vision | Contraction for near vision |
| **Blood vessels** | | |
| Vascular smooth muscle | $\alpha_1$ Constriction | Most often little or no effect |
| | $\beta_2$ Dilation | |
| Coronary arterioles | $\alpha_1$ Contraction – vasoconstriction | Contraction – vasoconstriction |
| | $\beta_2$ Relaxation – vasodilation | |
| Viscera, skin, brain arterioles | $\alpha_1$ Constriction | No known effect |
| Skeletal muscle arterioles | $\beta_2$ Dilation | No known effect |
| | $\alpha_1$ Constriction | |
| Kidney arterioles | $\alpha_1$ Constriction and decrease in urine volume | No known effect |
| Erectile tissue | $\alpha_1$ Constriction | Dilatation |
| Systemic veins | $\alpha_1$ Constriction | No known effect |
| | $\beta_2$ Dilation | |
| **Heart** | | |
| Sinoatrial node | $\beta_1$ Increase in heart rate | Decrease in heart rate |
| Atrial muscle | $\beta_1$ Increased force of contraction | Decrease in contractility |
| Atrioventricular node | $\beta_1$ Increased automaticity | Decreased conduction velocity Atrioventricular block |
| Ventricular muscle | $\beta_1$ Increased automaticity Increased force of contraction | No effect |
| Coronary vessels | $\beta_2$ Dilation | Dilation |
| | $\alpha_1$ Constriction | |
| **Glands** | | |
| Nasal, lacrimal, salivary, gastric, pancreatic | $\alpha_1$ Vasoconstriction and slight secretion | Stimulation of copious secretion containing many enzymes if produced |
| Endocrine pancreas | $\alpha_2$ Inhibits insulin secretion | Secretion of insulin |
| | $\beta_2$ Promotes glucagon secretion | |

*(Contd)*

**Table 2.5.4** *(Contd)*

| Effector organs | Noradrenergic impulses | Cholinergic impulses |
|---|---|---|
| Posterior pituitary | $\beta_1$ Secretion of antidiuretic hormone | No known effect |
| Sweat glands | Copious sweating (cholinergic) | |
| | $\alpha_1$ Sweating on palms of hands and feet | No effect |
| **Lungs** | | |
| Bronchial smooth muscle | $\beta_2$ Relaxation – airway dilation | Contraction – airway constriction |
| Blood vessels | Mildly constricted | Dilated |
| **Gastrointestinal tract** | | |
| Lumen | Decreased peristalsis and tone | Increased peristalsis and tone |
| Sphincter | $\alpha_1$ Increased tone (most times) | Relaxed (most times) |
| Liver | Glucose release | Glycogen synthesis |
| Gall bladder | $\beta_2$ Relaxation | Contraction |
| Kidney | $\beta_1$ Renin secretion | No known effect |
| **Bladder** | | |
| Detrusor | $\beta_2$ Relaxation (slightly) | Contraction |
| Sphincter | $\alpha_1$ Contraction | Relaxation |
| Sex organs | $\alpha_1$ Ejaculation of semen in males | Vasodilation; erection of clitoris (females) and penis (males) |
| **Uterus** | | |
| Non-pregnant | $\beta_2$ Relaxation | Minimal effect |
| Pregnant | $\alpha_1$ Contraction | Minimal effect |
| Coagulation | Increased | None |
| Blood glucose | Increased | None |
| Blood lipids | Increased | None |
| Basal metabolism | Increased up to 100% | None |
| Adrenal medullary secretion | Increased | None |
| Mental activity | Increased | None |
| Arrector pili muscles | $\alpha_1$ Contraction (goose bumps) | None |
| Hair follicles | Erection of hairs | |
| Skeletal muscle | Increased glycogenolysis | None |
| | Increased strength | |
| Adipose tissue | $\beta_1$ Lipolysis | None |
| | $\beta_3$ Release of fatty acids into bloodstream | |

Normally, both are continually active and the basal rates of activity are known as sympathetic and parasympathetic tone. **Neurogenic tone** allows a single nervous system to increase and decrease the activity of a stimulated organ. The best example to illustrate this is the **sympathetic tone** that keeps systemic arterioles constricted to about half their maximum diameter. They can be constricted even more by increasing sympathetic stimulation and can be dilated by decreasing stimulation. Without background tone the vessels could only be constricted, and not dilated because they would have no opposing parasympathetic innervation. If ganglionic transmission to sympathetic efferent fibres innervating this vascular smooth muscle is blocked throughout the body by the ganglion-blocking agent hexamethonium, there is a profound fall in peripheral resistance and a catastrophic reduction in arterial blood pressure.

The chief role of the ANS is maintaining homeostasis and although the sympathetic nervous system has a role in 'fight or flight' responses, most of the time there is no emergency but the needs of the body still have to be met, for example in response to postural change or exercise rather than in response to extreme fear. Neurogenic tone is a maintained low frequency of nerve impulses under resting conditions that aids the maintenance of homeostasis within the body. An example of parasympathetic tone is the impulse activity in the vagal nerves that normally produce a tonic slowing of the heart rate to about 65–75 beats per minute. If this vagal tone is blocked by the administration of the drug atropine, the heart rate rises to about 120 beats per minute.

In organs such as the heart and the gut, where there is dual innervation, the sympathetic and parasympathetic systems do usually **produce opposite effects**. This is done by **reflex activity** to maintain homeostasis. An example is sympathetic activity speeding-up heart rate and constricting vascular beds, thus leading to an increase in blood pressure. This increase is detected by vagus (Xth cranial) nerve baroreceptors in the aortic arch and other sites. The visceral afferents in the vagus can now reflexively stimulate vagal parasympathetic efferents that slow heart rate. When a more sustained rise in blood pressure is needed (as in the flight or fight response) sympathetic activation is not nullified by parasympathetic response to dampen the needed activation (Zigmond et al., 1999). We thus should not think of the sympathetic and parasympathetic branches of the ANS as always being opponents but as having their own physiological functions and changing their activity in a particular organ according to the need at the time. It is the balance between the two divisions that achieves the desired outcome. **Coordinated autonomic control** is exemplified by the dual innervation of the urinary bladder, where tonic sympathetic activity allows the bladder to fill and urination is achieved by a spinal reflex when the stretch receptors in the bladder wall activate parasympathetic relaxation of the internal sphincter of the bladder. In adults this reflex is normally under conscious control via neurones in the pons. If the spinal cord is severed, urination is entirely reflexive.

In given circumstances, it is usually one division or the other that exerts the predominant effects and in a few circumstances the divisions cooperate with each other. Most organs are **dominantly controlled** by one or other of the two systems and there are other areas where only one division of the autonomic nervous system operates. The sweat glands, the arrector pili muscles of the skin, the kidneys and the adrenal glands have **only sympathetic innervation**. Most blood vessels have only sympathetic innervation and resistance arteries have only sympathetic vasoconstrictor innervation. They have no parasympathetic innervation but the constrictor tone is opposed instead by the release of nitric oxide from the endothelial cells. Bronchial smooth muscle has only a parasympathetic innervation but its tone is extremely sensitive to circulating adrenaline (epinephrine), which relaxes the smooth muscle.

## The sympathetic division (see Table 2.5.2)

As an oversimplification, the sympathetic division can be characterized as underlying many of the physiological coping mechanisms during threat – those of the **fight and flight response** (described by Cannon, 1932), which is a response of the sympathetic nervous system and the endocrine system. The parasympathetic division can be characterized as underlying relaxed, restful, sleepy circumstances. It is also involved in the digestion of food and anabolic metabolism – **resting and digesting** – a system of maintenance and energy conservation.

The **sympathetic nervous system** is stimulated by physical exertion and by many emotions, such as fear, pain, anger, embarrassment, anxiety and fear. Sympathetic activity favours body functions that can support **intense physical activity** and the rapid production of ATP. In a stressful situation, whether of physical or mental origin, the body's response is dominated by the sympathetic nervous system:

- The body is prepared for an emergency and sympathetic nerves to the cardiovascular system, enhanced by the secretion of adrenaline (epinephrine) and noradrenaline (norepinephrine) from the adrenal glands, ensure increased heart rate, increased conduction velocity of the specialized conducting tissue of the heart, and increased contractility of cardiac muscle – all of which contribute to increased cardiac output.
- Coronary blood vessels and the blood vessels within skeletal muscle are dilated. However, blood vessels supplying the gastrointestinal organs are constricted – the body is not concerned with digestion in an emergency.
- Motility and tone of the muscles of the oesophagus, stomach and intestine are reduced and secretion of digestive juice is inhibited. The anal sphincter is (usually) contracted.
- Skin arterioles are in a state of constriction, which can be seen as pallor.
- The spleen contracts, ejecting blood into the system. This is of little significance in man but in some animals, such as dogs, it does play an important role in combating hypovolaemia.
- Renin secretion from the juxtaglomerular apparatus in the kidney is enhanced, leading to the activation of angiotensinogen and the production of angiotensin II, a powerful vasoconstrictor that increases the production of aldosterone. The latter aids the direct conservation of sodium chloride and the indirect conservation of water. Together, the net effect of these adjustments increases the blood pressure.
- In general, respirations will be quiet because bronchial muscles are relaxed. An increase in the rate and depth of respirations is less a direct effect of sympathetic stimulation than an indirect effect

of the other changes, in particular the cardiovascular changes.

- The detrusor muscle of the bladder will be in a state of relaxation and the bladder sphincter will (usually) be contracted.
- Stimulation of the adrenal gland enhances all the effects of the sympathetic system. Adrenaline (epinephrine) and noradrenaline (norepinephrine) increase the arousal effect of the ascending reticular system.
- Insulin secretion is depressed and blood glucose levels are increased through glycogenolysis.
- Lipolysis increases the free fatty acid levels in the blood.
- The tendency of blood to clot is enhanced, aided by the constriction of peripheral blood vessels mentioned above.
- Other effects of sympathetic arousal include contraction of the piloerector muscles. This might be insignificant in humans but in furry animals it leads to an apparent increase in size.
- There is a slight localized secretion of the sweat glands in the palm of the hand (adrenergic sweating). In addition, the normal insensible fluid loss through the skin can stand out as 'sweat' in the absence of heat from the blood to evaporate this fluid during the 'shut down' of skin blood vessels.

These physiological adjustments have **great survival value** when an individual is **under physical threat**. However, many or all of them can occur in humans when there is psychological, but no physical, threat. Far from having survival value, such 'useless' action of the sympathetic division, if it occurs frequently or is prolonged, can be detrimental. This will be further considered in Chapter 2.7.

## The adrenal medulla

The presence in the bloodstream of adrenaline (epinephrine) and noradrenaline (norepinephrine) released by the adrenal gland ensures that stimulation by the sympathetic nervous system is widely diffused, because these hormones attach to the adrenergic receptors. The circulating adrenaline (epinephrine) and noradrenaline (norepinephrine) have almost the same effects on organs as those caused by direct stimulation of the SNS, except the **effect lasts about five to ten times as long** because of the slow removal of these hormones from the bloodstream. They are potently active for approximately 10–30 seconds, with this effect decreasing over a period of 1–3 minutes. Adrenaline (epinephrine) has a greater stimulatory effect on the $\beta_2$-receptor and a greater metabolic effect than noradrenaline (norepinephrine). It can increase the metabolic rate of the body by up to 100%

above normal when secreted by the adrenal gland. This increases the overall activity and excitability of the body, as well as increasing glucose release into the bloodstream. Noradrenaline (norepinephrine) and adrenaline (epinephrine) from the adrenal medulla can stimulate structures that are not directly innervated by the sympathetic fibres. There is a basal secretion of adrenaline (epinephrine) and noradrenaline (norepinephrine) from the adrenal gland too – about $0.2\,\mu g/kg/min$. This is sufficient to maintain blood pressure almost up to normal even if all direct sympathetic pathways to the cardiovascular system were removed and much of the overall sympathetic tone is due to this secretion by the adrenal gland.

## The parasympathetic division
### (see Table 2.5.2)

Unlike the sympathetic division, during activity of the parasympathetic division, the postsynaptic neurotransmitter (acetylcholine) is not found in the bloodstream and **no widespread autonomic stimulation occurs**. Therefore, in general, the effects of the parasympathetic division of the ANS are discrete and of **short duration**. This is not only due to the more discrete release of acetylcholine but also to the highly effective action of cholinesterase in splitting acetylcholine and deactivating it. This can be contrasted with the case of the sympathetic system, in which the destruction of catecholamines is less prominent than their reuptake by postsynaptic nerve endings. This mechanism of reuptake not only prolongs the effect of sympathetic activity but contributes to a significant extent to the level of noradrenaline (norepinephrine) in the circulation. It is not surprising, then, to note the more diffuse effect of sympathetic activity.

As parasympathetic activity is discrete, it is less accurate to portray a global abstracted picture of an individual during parasympathetic activity, and instead more helpful to consider its effects on the different effector tissues:

- Parasympathetic stimulation of the gastrointestinal tract aids the digestion and absorption of food by increasing the motility of the muscle, increasing the amount of digestive secretions and relaxing the pyloric sphincter. The gall bladder contracts, releasing bile, and insulin secretion from the pancreas is favoured. The salivary glands are stimulated to produce profuse watery secretions and the blood vessels supplying them are dilated.
- The vagus (Xth cranial) nerve has an important role in carrying parasympathetic fibres and distributing them widely to the thoracic and abdominal organs; its role in the functions related to digestion and

absorption has already been dealt with. In relation to the respiratory system, parasympathetic stimulation increases the secretion from nasopharyngeal and bronchial glands and favours the contraction of bronchial muscle.

- Parasympathetic stimulation via the vagus nerve decreases the heart rate and also decreases the contractility of muscle and the conduction velocity through the specialized conducting tissue of the cardiac muscle. Under resting conditions, vagal inhibitory effects predominate, slowing the heart rate.
- In the eye, parasympathetic stimulation acts on the sphincter muscle of the iris to constrict the pupil. It also contracts the ciliary muscle, allowing the lens to become more convex and thus aiding near vision. It is activity of the parasympathetic division which leads to weeping, through stimulation of the lacrimal glands.
- Turning to the function of those parasympathetic fibres with their origin in the sacral segments of the spinal cord, those supplying the bladder stimulate contraction of the detrusor muscle and relaxation of the sphincter, bringing about micturition, although after infancy voluntary control also plays a very important part in this act. Similarly, relaxation of the anal sphincter at an involuntary level is a function of the parasympathetic supply to the muscle.
- Parasympathetic stimulation causes vasodilatation of the blood vessels in the external genitalia and is responsible for erection in the male penis and the female clitoris. Ejaculation of semen and reflex contraction of the vagina are a response to sympathetic stimulation. Anxiety, by stimulating the sympathetic division of the nervous system, can thus affect sexual performance.

Overall, it can be seen that, on the one hand, the sympathetic division activates the body for a short-term emergency, but that this is at the expense of certain processes that keep us healthy over the long term. The parasympathetic division, on the other hand, works calmly for the long-term good. Both cannot be stimulated strongly at the same time because their general goals are incompatible (Bear et al., 1996). In practice, it can sometimes be difficult to distinguish the role of stimulatory effects of the parasympathetic division from the absence of stimulation by the sympathetic division.

## Integration and control of autonomic functions

We are usually unaware of the autonomic reflexes that regulate the many controlled conditions in the body, such as blood pressure, breathing, digestion and core temperature. The activity of these reflexes is controlled at several hierarchical levels of the CNS, including the spinal cord, the brainstem, the hypothalamus and even the cerebral cortex (usually at a subconscious level). The main integration centre for the ANS is the hypothalamus and from here commands flow to lower CNS centres.

Simple reflexes controlling the contraction of a full bladder and defaecation are integrated at the level of the spinal cord but are subject to conscious inhibition in adulthood. More complex reflexes controlling heart rate and respiration are integrated in the brainstem, which exerts a direct influence over heart rate (cardiac centre), blood vessel diameter (vasomotor centre) and respiration (respiratory centres in the medulla and the pons). The sensory inputs involved in these reflex actions often travel to the brainstem via the vagus nerve. Centres within the hypothalamus coordinate body temperature, water balance and endocrine activity, and these are discussed in the relevant sections of this text.

The final control of all voluntary behaviour is exerted by the cerebral cortex; recently, meditation and biofeedback techniques have shown that a certain degree of voluntary control of visceral activities, such as heart rate and blood pressure, is possible.

## Ageing and the ANS

Ageing is associated with the inefficient maintenance of body homeostasis, especially under stress, and it is probable that many aspects of normal ageing are mediated via the ANS. The demonstration of specific lesions to explain changes is difficult but tonic parasympathetic outflow declines and although overall sympathetic neural activity might increase, there is a reduced response to β-adrenergic stimulation. This means that, although the resting heart rate might not change much, the maximal attainable heart rate and cardiac output are reduced. Common reported problems in older people are constipation, which can be due to reduced motility of the gastrointestinal tract, and dry eyes due to lack of tear production, which can result in eye infections. Older people are also less able to cope with perioperative stress.

### CLINICAL APPLICATIONS

#### AGEING AND THE ANS

Most disorders of the ANS in young people are due to injury. However, the function of the ANS declines with age and the most common presentation of this is postural (orthostatic) hypotension, which can cause fainting episodes.

## Postural hypotension

This is an abnormal fall in systolic blood pressure (of more than 20 mmHg) on moving from a supine to an upright position. Blood pressure is not immediately corrected by autonomic reflex action via the baroreceptors, which would usually rapidly produce vasoconstriction. The fall is the result of loss of sympathetic reflexes and occurs typically on getting out of bed in the morning or jumping up suddenly. Symptoms due to decreased cerebral perfusion can follow, with dizziness, light-headedness and even loss of consciousness. Postural hypotension occurs in approximately one in five older people and repeated falls can lead to loss of confidence as well as possible trauma. Other factors are often present, including immobility, dehydration and arrhythmias. Drugs such as antihypertensives, anti-Parkinson agents and some antidepressants are frequently implicated. Postural hypotension is not usually life-threatening and the person should not rise to the standing position rapidly. Management includes the removal of any precipitating factors, especially drugs, and advice to patients to modify their lifestyle so that postural changes are always slow.

## Accidental hypothermia

The ability to regulate body temperature decreases in older people. This is due to changes in the ANS that impair heat conservation by the skin and a failure to increase heat production by metabolic processes. There are other contributing factors such as immobility, poor nutrition and drugs such as hypnotics (sleeping tablets) and antidepressants. Maintenance of a core temperature of 37°C is vital for metabolic processes and, if the core temperature drops below 35°C, hypothermia is present. Prevention is better than cure and those at risk should be kept in a warm environment and encouraged to mobilize when this is possible.

## ABNORMALITIES OF AUTONOMIC FUNCTIONING

Autonomic dysfunction of one kind or another is present in very many diseases, including such common disorders as hypertension and heart failure. This will become more visible later, when drugs that act on the ANS are discussed.

As many organs have a dual autonomic innervation, it is possible that an interruption of the nerve supply from one ANS division leaves the supply from the other division acting unopposed. An example of this in relation to the pupil of the eye has already been mentioned. When the IIIrd cranial nerve nucleus is subjected to pressure during very early tentorial herniation, it leaves the sympathetic innervation to the pupil acting unopposed (producing dilation).

## Horner's syndrome

Unopposed action of the parasympathetic supply to the pupil can occur in **Horner's syndrome**, which arises when there is a lesion of the cervical sympathetic ganglion supplying the eye, head and neck. The features of Horner's syndrome are: constriction of the pupil (miosis); drooping of the eyelid (ptosis); slight retraction of the globe of the eye within the orbit (enophthalmos); and loss of sweating on the affected side of the head and neck (anhidrosis). An aneurysm or thrombosis of the internal carotid artery affecting the sympathetic nerve can occasionally cause all these signs, with the exception of anhidrosis, because the nerve fibres affecting sweating are carried with the external carotid artery.

## Lesions of the cauda equina and spinal cord

A severe lesion of the cauda equina affects bladder and bowel function as a result of damage to the sacral parasympathetic outflow. The detrusor muscle of the bladder is affected and reflex contraction no longer occurs in response to distension. The bladder wall has a certain amount of elasticity and, as pressure mounts, the elasticity forces some urine into the urethra. However, the unopposed sympathetic supply to the sphincter muscle keeps it contracted and closed, and dribbling incontinence occurs. A similar situation arises with regard to the bowel and anal sphincter.

A lesion of the spinal cord itself, in which voluntary control of the bowel and bladder is affected but in which the parasympathetic outflow is not affected, leads to an automatic bladder (once spinal shock has worn off). Such lesions can affect the sympathetic innervation to the skin. Initially, during spinal shock, the skin below the level of the lesion is dry, pale and cool, but at a later stage, profuse sweating in the affected area is common and can be provoked by many cutaneous or other stimuli.

## Autonomic dysreflexia

This syndrome is caused by uncontrolled sympathetic discharge in those with a spinal cord injury usually above the level of T6. The condition is seen after recovery from spinal shock and is usually triggered by noxious stimulants to areas below the level of spinal injury. The most common example is stretching of the full bladder wall – the sensory impulse cannot ascend the spinal cord and mass stimulation of the sympathetic nerves below the injury occurs. The condition is potentially life-threatening and results in severe vasoconstriction and hypertension. It is characterized by a pounding headache and a flushed warm skin with profuse sweating above the injury but a pale, cold, dry skin below. There is increased parasympathetic output via the vagus nerve and bradycardia results.

### Raynaud's disease

This produces intermittent attacks of exaggerated vasoconstriction of the arteries supplying the fingers and toes. It is usually bilateral and fingers are affected more commonly than toes. Pallor occurs due to vasoconstriction and then cyanosis due to sluggish blood flow. Redness follows due to hyperaemia. The duration of the attacks varies but some can last for hours. Pain can be severe and in some cases gangrene occurs. Sympathectomy can be used to eliminate vasoconstriction in severe cases.

### Hirschprung's disease

This is a congenital abnormality whereby the parasympathetic nerve supply to the distal part of the colon fails to develop adequately. It was described earlier in this chapter (see p. 189).

### The ANS in diabetes mellitus

Peripheral nerve damage and autonomic defects are very common in patients with long-standing diabetes but not all have actual symptoms. The dysfunction is attributed to metabolic consequence of a chronically raised blood glucose level (hyperglycaemia) and patients with both types of diabetes (type 1 and type 2) can be affected. The incidence of neuropathy increases with the duration of the disease, especially in those where there has been poor control of blood glucose levels. Symptoms include postural hypotension, cardiovascular reflex abnormalities, impotence and a reduced awareness of hypoglycaemia (low blood glucose). Damage to sympathetic nerves also causes changes in blood flow, which are related to some of the foot problems that can occur in diabetes. Vasomotor denervation causes a large rise in peripheral blood flow and the foot is warm and often oedematous. This should not be confused with ischaemia (a lack of blood supply), which can also occur in diabetes when there is a reduction of blood flow to the foot secondary to narrowing of the arteries caused by the deposition of fatty deposits (atherosclerosis).

### SYMPATHECTOMY

This operation was referred to earlier in relation to the anatomy of the sympathetic division of the ANS, because the paravertebral chain of ganglia are rendered relatively accessible for surgical intervention. There are several reasons for considering such an operation, in addition to the condition of hyperhidrosis already referred to:

- Vascular:
  - to improve the blood flow to peripheral areas whose physiological integrity is threatened by vasospasm
  - to reduce blood pressure more generally in hypertension.
- In chronic pain:
  - for causalgia (burning pain in the cutaneous distribution of an injured peripheral nerve)
  - for phantom limb pain.

It is important to note, however, that with the increased knowledge available today, this operation is carried out only as a last resort because less drastic and non-invasive methods of opposing the action of the sympathetic nervous system are available.

Vascular effects of sympathetic stimulation can be opposed with drugs having very specific effects upon the blood vessels (see below).

In the case of chronic pain, behavioural methods have been developed to help patients (McCaffery, 1989).

Before sympathectomy is carried out, the effect of an injection of local anaesthetic into the paravertebral sympathetic ganglionic chain at the required level is checked to ensure that the operation is likely to be successful.

Sympathectomy can alter vasomotor tone because the smooth muscle in blood vessel walls is entirely innervated by sympathetic fibres, which control the extent of contraction of muscle and hence the calibre of blood vessels. Removal of the impulses stimulating constriction leads to vasodilation. Postoperatively, hypotension is a potential problem.

The rationale for sympathectomy in the treatment of causalgia and phantom limb pain is much more complex and not entirely understood. However, the afferent peripheral pathway for visceral sensation runs with the efferent autonomic nerves, the sympathetic ones in particular. Visceral sensory fibres, having entered the posterior nerve roots, then travel centrally within the spinal cord with somatic afferents. It is believed that the phenomenon of referred pain is related to this close anatomical relationship between sensory nerve fibres in the spinal cord. An example with which many nurses will be familiar is the referral of cardiac pain (visceral) to the somatic areas of the left arm and substernal region.

It is believed that afferent visceral fibres provide an alternative path for pain from areas deprived of somatic sensory nerves. Certainly, pain can be carried by afferents accompanying the autonomic supply to blood vessels. This occurs in migraine, for example.

Following an incomplete lesion of a peripheral nerve, a syndrome of causalgia can arise in which there is excessive sweating, excessive sensitivity to touch and pain in the area normally supplied by the nerve. Afferent stimuli responsible for this are carried with the autonomic nerve and removal of the sympathetic supply to the area relieves the pain.

Phantom limb pain appears to be a special example of causalgia and can be relieved by sympathectomy in the same way. Prior to operation the stump might be cold, cyanotic and covered with perspiration, and exposure to cold and excessive emotional stress increase the pain. Postsympathectomy, the stump becomes warm, dry and non-tender.

## DRUGS AND THE ANS

The importance of the ANS in the control of such a wide range of the body's vital functions, plus the ease of accessibility of its effector organs, have resulted in the development of many pharmacological agents, both naturally occurring and synthetic, that modulate its action. Receptor subtypes within the ANS produce specific effects and this has allowed the development of agonists to stimulate, and antagonists to block, these effects. Drug action in the ANS can involve:

- agonists or antagonists at adrenergic or cholinergic receptors
- release, storage or synthesis of neurotransmitters
- enzymes inactivating neurotransmitters.

### Drugs affecting the sympathetic division

#### Sympathomimetic agents

These drugs stimulate the sympathetic nervous system. They might act **directly**, e.g. adrenoreceptor agonists such as adrenaline (epinephrine), noradrenaline (norepinephrine), isoprenaline and dopamine, or **indirectly** by causing a release of noradrenaline (norepinephrine) from stores at nerve endings, e.g. amphetamines. Sympathomimetic agents are classified according to the receptor sites on which they have their major effect. This might be the $\alpha$- or $\beta$-receptor site. $\beta$-receptor sites in turn can be further subdivided into $\beta_1$ and $\beta_2$, the former being present in the heart.

Two **naturally occurring** and powerful sympathomimetic agents are adrenaline (epinephrine) and noradrenaline (norepinephrine). Adrenaline (epinephrine), with comparatively more $\beta$-receptor activity, is used as **a cardiac stimulant** in cardiac arrest and can be of value in the relief of bronchospasm, as in acute asthma. It is also used in acute anaphylaxis (see Chapter 6.2), for its mix of actions – it causes relief of bronchospasm, increased cardiac contractility and stabilizes the mast cells, thus preventing further release of histamine. Adrenaline (epinephrine) can be life-saving in this situation. It is occasionally used for its vasoconstrictor effects as an additive to some local anaesthetics, thus prolonging their effectiveness because the anaesthetic is removed from the area, by the blood, more slowly.

$\alpha_1$-**receptors** are located on blood vessels and influence both blood pressure and tissue perfusion. Stimulation of the $\alpha$-receptors produces vasoconstriction. **Noradrenaline** (norepinephrine), with its comparatively greater $\alpha$-receptor effects, is a very **powerful vasoconstrictor**. The vasoconstriction produced by an intravenous infusion of noradrenaline (norepinephrine) increases the peripheral resistance of the circulation and so raises blood pressure. If it comes into contact with tissue other than the endothelial lining of blood vessels, it causes tissue necrosis. It is occasionally used in critical care to treat acute hypotension when other measures have failed and is given as a dilute solution by intravenous infusion via a central venous catheter.

**Dopamine** is the naturally occurring precursor to noradrenaline (norepinephrine) and is used in critical care to **increase renal output**. It stimulates dopamine receptors in the kidney at low doses and increases renal blood flow. It is also a **selective $\beta_1$-receptor agonist** and, at larger doses, is a potent agent in increasing the force of cardiac contraction, thereby improving cardiac output. At higher doses this selectivity is lost and the $\beta_2$-receptors are also stimulated; at still greater doses it will also stimulate the $\alpha$-receptors.

### Selective agonists at adrenergic receptors

Other drugs have been developed for their more selective effects upon the different adrenergic receptors:

- $\beta_1$-**receptors**: a synthetic $\beta_1$-receptor agonist, dobutamine, is more commonly used to stimulate the $\beta_1$-receptor in cardiogenic shock than the naturally occurring dopamine, which has little effect on cardiac rate or blood pressure. Dobutamine has to be given by intravenous infusion because it is destroyed very rapidly and removed from the circulation.
- $\beta_2$-**receptors**: these receptors are distributed on the smooth muscle of the bronchioles, skeletal

muscle, blood vessels supplying the heart, lungs, kidneys and skeletal muscle and on the uterus:

- Stimulation of the $\beta_2$-receptor relieves bronchospasm in asthma and chronic bronchitis. **Salbutamol** is a synthetic agonist drug that is relatively selective for $\beta_2$-receptors. It has been developed for its bronchodilatory effect and can be given by inhalation for a more direct effect on the respiratory tract.
- Stimulation of the $\beta_2$-receptor will also result in increased skeletal muscle excitability, resulting in a fine muscle tremor. This is seen as a side-effect of drugs such as salbutamol, especially if large doses are prescribed or if the patient overuses their salbutamol inhaler or nebulizer.
- Stimulation of the $\beta_2$-receptor can also lead to hypokalaemia carrying with it an arrhythmogenic potential.

### Selectivity for adrenoreceptors

Selectivity for receptors is always relative and not absolute. Some agents are more selective for specific receptors than others but in high doses this selectivity often disappears. This also applies to drugs that block certain receptors (antagonists; discussed later). A cardioselective $\beta_1$-adrenergic antagonist will not be totally cardiospecific and its blocking effects are likely to affect the $\beta_2$-receptors, but to a much lesser degree than the $\beta_1$-receptors.

### Adrenoreceptor antagonist drugs

The action of adrenaline (epinephrine) and noradrenaline (norepinephrine) can be blocked by drugs that prevent their access to receptor sites. Again, the effect can be selective for particular types and subtypes of receptor:

- **α-adrenoreceptor antagonists:**
  - Drugs that block the α-receptor effects of sympathetic stimulation have a vasodilator action and thus decrease blood pressure. They might be non-selective or selective $\alpha_1$-antagonists. **Phenoxybenzamine** is an example of a powerful non-selective α-blocker with many side-effects that is occasionally used to reduce blood pressure in phaeochromocytoma (a rare benign tumour of the adrenal medulla) and can produce marked compensatory tachycardia.
  - α-antagonists can cause quite severe **postural hypotension** (the blood pressure falls on standing). There are drugs now developed that are selective $\alpha_1$-antagonists and do not have these side-effects to any degree. Prazosin, doxazosin and indoramin are

examples, and are used in the treatment of hypertension.
  - **Labetalol** blocks both α- and β-receptors. It is a particularly effective hypotensive agent because the peripheral vascular dilation is not counteracted by increased cardiac output. It is used occasionally to reduce blood pressure in pregnancy.
- **β-adrenoreceptor antagonists**: these drugs were first discovered in 1958 and have since been developed so that they are now one of the most frequently prescribed classes of drug in cardiovascular disease. They can be effective against both types of β-receptor, or might be selective. The effects produced depend on the degree of sympathetic activity, and are less in subjects at rest:
  - The most important actions of these drugs are on the cardiovascular system, where they decrease heart rate, myocardial contractility, cardiac output and conduction velocity within the heart (Johnston, 1999).
  - When administered over a period of time, β-adrenoceptor antagonists also result in a reduction in blood pressure by complex actions not totally understood but including a reduction in the release of renin from the kidney and alterations in baroreceptor activity.
  - Due to the wide distribution of the β-receptor these drugs have many uses, including cardiac disease, hypertension, migraine prophylaxis, anxiety and hyperthyroidism.
  - They should not be given to patients with asthma, as they will be antagonistic at both the $\beta_1$- and the $\beta_2$-receptor and can provoke severe bronchoconstriction.
  - Other side-effects include bradycardia, fatigue, cold extremities (due to loss of $\beta_2$-receptor-mediated vasodilation in cutaneous vessels) and nightmares in some patients.
  - **Propranolol** is a non-selective agent and so is effective against both $\beta_1$ and $\beta_2$ activity. Some drugs, such as **atenolol**, are $\beta_1$-selective (cardioselective) and so have fewer side-effects. They are also less likely to provoke an asthma attack. They are used for their action on the cardiovascular system both in angina and hypertension.
  - The use of β-adrenergic antagonists is increasing as research now shows them to be of value both following a myocardial infarction and in stable heart failure. Stimulation of the cardiovascular system by the sympathetic nervous system, and thus the renin–angiotensin–aldosterone system, can be damaging in these instances and a β-adrenergic antagonist can improve the outlook for many patients.

## Drugs that affect noradrenaline (norepinephrine) synthesis

The drug methyldopa exerts its hypotensive effects by interfering with the metabolic pathway through which noradrenaline (norepinephrine) is produced. It used to be used in hypertension but is little used now as there are other drugs available with fewer side-effects. It is, however, still used in hypertension in late pregnancy because it is known to be safe.

## Indirectly acting sympathomimetic drugs

**Amphetamine** displaces noradrenaline (norepinephrine) from its vesicles, allowing it to escape. It also prevents the neuronal reuptake of several monoamines, which produces stimulation of the central nervous system. It is a drug that increases mental activity and can cause hallucinations and seizures. There are many derivatives of amphetamine and these drugs have been used as aids to weight loss, for attention deficit syndrome and also socially as drugs of abuse because of their stimulant action on the central nervous system.

## Inhibitors of noradrenaline (norepinephrine) uptake

These drugs interfere with the termination of action of noradrenaline (norepinephrine). They include the tricyclic antidepressants, such as amitriptyline, that have their major effects on the central nervous system but can also cause tachycardia and cardiac arrhythmias, especially if an overdose of drug is taken. **Cocaine**, known mainly as a drug of abuse and as a local anaesthetic, enhances transmission in the sympathetic nervous system by this method. It produces central effects of euphoria and excitement and causes drug dependency. Withdrawal leads to depression, anxiety and craving.

## Inhibitors of the enzymic destruction of noradrenaline (norepinephrine)

These drugs are monoamine oxidase inhibitors (MAOIs). Dopa, dopamine and serotonin are central neurotransmitters and are all dependent on monoamine oxidase for their degradation. The MAOIs (for example, phenelzine) are psychoactive drugs and have the effect of lifting depression. Patients who take them should avoid food and drink containing large amounts of the amine tyramine, such as cheese and yeast products, as these cannot be properly metabolized. Unpleasant and potentially dangerous symptoms and effects such as headaches, cardiac dysrhythmias and severe hypertension through excess stimulation of adrenergic receptors can result.

## Drugs affecting the parasympathetic division

Drugs can influence cholinergic transmission either by acting on the cholinergic receptors or by affecting the release or destruction of endogenous acetylcholine.

### Drugs acting on the acetylcholine receptor – cholinergic agonists

The naturally occurring parasympathetic postsynaptic neurotransmitter acetylcholine is broken down so rapidly by the action of the enzyme cholinesterase that it is of no therapeutic value itself, and so similar substances, which are less easily degraded, are used instead:

- Carbachol is a drug that has most of the properties of acetylcholine at its receptor but is stable and effective orally. It has the effect of causing contraction of both bladder and intestinal muscle and was used to treat retention of urine but is potentially dangerous as a ruptured bladder could result. It has been superseded by catheterization as the treatment for retention of urine.
- Pilocarpine is a cholinergic agonist used, for its production of pupillary constriction, as eye drops for glaucoma. In acute glaucoma the intraocular pressure increases and a dilated pupil impedes the drainage of aqueous humour into the canal of Schlemm, which runs around the eye close to the outer margin of the iris (see Chapter 2.4). Abnormally raised intraocular pressure damages the eye and is one of the most common causes of blindness. Activation of the *constrictor pupillae* muscle by muscarinic agonists lowers the intraocular pressure in these cases. Alternatively, an adrenergic antagonist could be used, and timolol is a β-receptor antagonist commonly used as eye drops for glaucoma.

### Cholinergic antagonists

These include agents that are antagonists at the nicotinic receptor and those that are antagonists at the muscarinic receptor. Nicotinic antagonists block neuromuscular transmission and are used as muscle relaxants in anaesthesia. Examples include pancuronium and vecuronium. They are of relevance in the somatic, not the autonomic, nervous system.

### Muscarinic antagonists

Atropine and hyoscine are two naturally occurring agents that block the muscarinic acetylcholine receptor. They block the access of acetylcholine to its postsynaptic receptors and so decrease the effects of parasympathetic activity. The effects of muscarinic antagonists include:

- Reduction of smooth muscle tone and gastrointestinal activity in general. By virtue of this activity, muscarinic antagonists are particularly useful in the relief of renal, biliary and intestinal colic. Hyoscine is often given as injection or tablets of Buscopan.
- Relaxation of bronchial smooth muscle and inhibition of salivary, lacrimal and bronchial secretions. Used in anaesthesia, atropine prevents reflex bronchoconstriction (relaxation of smooth muscle) and also decreases bronchial and salivary secretions. Ipratropium (Atrovent) is a muscarinic antagonist given as an inhaler or nebulizer in obstructive airway disease; it bronchodilates and reduces secretions.
- Increased heart rate due to block of cardiac muscarinic receptors. Atropine causes a modest tachycardia (rapid heart rate) of 80–90 beats per minute. It does not have an effect on the sympathetic nervous system but inhibits the parasympathetic tone mentioned earlier. It is used as a treatment for bradycardia (slow heart rate).
- Dilation of the pupil: atropine eye drops are used in ophthalmology to dilate the pupil, but cause impairment of near vision due to relaxation of the ciliary muscle. They can also produce a rise in intraocular pressure that is dangerous in glaucoma.
- Atropine has an excitatory effect upon the CNS: this can be observed in atropine poisoning, seen usually in children who have eaten deadly nightshade (*Atropa belladonna*) berries. There is hyperactivity and a rise in body temperature, which can be treated by anticholinesterase drugs such as physostigmine.
- Hyoscine is similar in its effects on secretions and smooth muscles but has a depressant effect upon the CNS. For this reason it is sometimes preferred over atropine if used as a premedication prior to surgery. Hyoscine also has an antiemetic effect (stops vomiting) and is used to treat motion sickness.

### Drugs affecting the destruction of acetylcholine

Natural cholinergic activity can be enhanced by the use of drugs (**anticholinesterases**) that interfere with the activity of cholinesterases. Neostigmine is an example of such a drug, and is used chiefly for its stimulating effect upon the voluntary motor endplate, another site where acetylcholine is active. It is used in **myasthenia gravis**, a condition leading to weakness of certain muscles due to autoimmune destruction of the nicotinic receptors for acetylcholine. Physostigmine

is another example and has already been mentioned as an antidote in atropine poisoning.

**Alzheimer's disease** is the most common cause of dementia, affecting 2–3% of people over the age of 65 years. The onset of symptoms is gradual, with progressive deterioration. There is marked loss of cholinergic neurones in the cerebral cortex and, although the muscarinic receptor density appears normal, the nicotinic receptor density is reduced. The drugs now being used to treat this condition act by increasing cholinergic transmission in the brain by inhibiting cholinesterases. They produce modest improvement in cognitive function and memory in up to 40% of sufferers (Waller et al., 2001). Examples of these drugs are donepezil, galanthamine and rivastigmine.

### Irreversible anticholinesterases

Most of these are organophosphate compounds and are very poisonous. They are used as insecticides and in chemical warfare. They totally block the enzyme acetylcholinesterase, sometimes for weeks, and so affect the autonomic cholinergic synapses, the neuromuscular junction and the central nervous system. In anticholinesterase poisoning severe bradycardia results, hypotension and difficulty in breathing. There is twitching of muscle followed by paralysis. Excitement of the central nervous system is followed by depression and convulsions occur, followed by unconsciousness and respiratory failure. Soldiers in danger of chemical attack carry injections of atropine as an antidote to the muscarinic effects of these gases.

## The ANS and stress

The occurrence of and effects of stress are described in some detail in Chapter 2.7, but it is important to note here that activity of the ANS is a major component of the physiological stress response. In particular, sympathetic nervous activity (the fight and flight response) produces the rapid response to acute stress and forms an important part of the *alarm reaction* which is the initial stage of the *triphasic stress response* first described by Selye in 1976 (see Chapter 2.7).

## Shock

### DEVELOPMENTAL ISSUES

The adaptive (coping) nature of the sympathetic nervous response and the accompanying secretion of adrenaline (epinephrine) and noradrenaline (norepinephrine) from the adrenal medulla can be seen in the signs and symptoms of *shock* following accidental or surgical trauma involving blood or fluid loss. Together, the responses to sympathetic nervous activity function to maintain the blood pressure and hence blood flow to the vital organs – the brain and heart. This response is crucial to survival and occurs largely through an increase in heart rate and contractility and because vasoconstriction occurs in non-vital areas such as the skin (causing pallor) and gut, diverting blood to the vital organs. It is only if homeostasis is not restored and intense vasoconstriction continues that the response becomes non-adaptive and irreversible shock ensues.

Shock can be defined as a dynamic syndrome in which there is inadequate tissue and organ perfusion. This inadequate perfusion seriously reduces the delivery of oxygen and other essential substances to a level below that required for normal cellular function. Shock is associated with very severe stress. The stressor is usually predominantly physiological in nature, e.g. trauma.

The signs of shock include the signs of sympathetic nervous system arousal. Such arousal is part of the physiological response to a stressor, which will restore homeostasis if the response is successful. If the physiological response is unsuccessful the condition becomes progressive. In the absence of effective treatment for progressive shock, irreversible shock occurs. This is fatal.

Signs of shock are not identical with those of sympathetic nervous arousal but are more complex because they include signs associated with the impact of the stressor upon the body. Therefore the signs of shock are a result of:

- sympathetic nervous arousal
- the effects of the stressor upon the body (e.g. burns, haemorrhage, dehydration)
- hormonal changes, which are part of the body's stress response.

It is important to recognize the early signs of shock because there are occasions when shock occurs in individuals not apparently at risk (e.g. after a minor operation) and it is essential for the condition to be recognized so that appropriate action can be taken.

In compensated shock the vital signs (temperature, pulse, respiration and blood pressure) might not reveal any deviation from normal and in such cases the clinical signs assume greater importance. Increased vulnerability to shock can occur because of pre-existing states such as chronic stress and anxiety, infection and dehydration, for example. The very young and very old are also likely to be particularly vulnerable to shock. It is important to treat early shock to prevent the condition from becoming progressive.

The clinical signs of early shock are as follows: the individual appears to be very ashen and pale and the skin will feel cold to the touch. It is also likely to be moist and clammy because there is no heat at the skin surface to evaporate insensible perspiration. The pulse rate will be increased and the pulse will feel rather weak and thready. The rapid pulse rate is of course a reflection of an increase in heart rate. The individual's blood pressure may be normal or slightly lower than normal. The respiratory rate is likely to be increased in both rate and depth. The core body temperature may be either reduced or increased depending upon the cause of the shock. If the shock is caused by an infection then it is likely that the temperature will be higher that the normal. Urinary output will be reduced and bowel sounds will be reduced. The individual may be confused as to time and place. Subjectively the patient will feel restless, apprehensive and anxious and may complain of thirst and is likely to have a dry mouth. In addition the pupils will be dilated.

## HYPOGLYCAEMIA

This is a low level of glucose in the blood usually giving symptoms when the glucose level is less than 3 mmol/L. Some of the early symptoms are due to increased activity of the sympathetic nervous system. Hypoglycaemia is a very common condition in patients with type 1 diabetes who are receiving insulin, but can also occur in those with type 2 diabetes if they are taking sulphonulurea drugs (e.g. glibenclamide, gliclazide) as hypoglycaemic agents. It does not occur if the patient is diet controlled or taking only metformin tablets. It is a major hazard of insulin treatment and can cause rapid loss of consciousness.

The effects of sympathetic nervous activity usually precede signs of CNS involvement with tremulousness and sweating often being the first signs. Other effects are pallor, piloerection, tachycardia and palpitations. These usually occur when the blood glucose falls to about 2 mmol/L. Severe mental confusion occurs when the blood glucose falls to 1 mmol/L or less and is due to deprivation of glucose to the brain. The patient might be uncharacteristically aggressive because of this and if untreated fits can follow with loss of consciousness.

The condition is easily treatable by the administration of sugary food or a glucose drink if the patient is fully awake or by the injection of glucagon or intravenous dextrose if unconscious. This should always be followed by a longer-lasting carbohydrate snack to prevent recurrence of the hypoglycaemia.

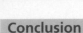

## Conclusion

The autonomic nervous system controls the internal environment and the viscera, keeping physiological variables at the level necessary to support the body's varying activities in a given environment. It is divided into three divisions: sympathetic, parasympathetic and enteric. In some situations the sympathetic and parasympathetic divisions have opposing actions (e.g. control of heart rate, control of gastrointestinal activity) but not in other situations (e.g. salivary glands). Parasympathetic activity is dominant when the body is relaxed following eating, whereas the sympathetic activity increases in 'fight and flight' situations as a response to stress. When the body is not at either of these extremes, both systems are exerting continuous control of the internal organs, ensuring the maintenance of homeostasis.

---

### Clinical review

In addition to the Learning Objectives at the beginning of this chapter, the reader should be able to:

- Explain the signs of shock in terms of autonomic activity
- Discuss the relationship of autonomic activity with the overall experience of stress
- State how drugs acting on the ANS exert their effect
- Identify risk factors for the development of shock

---

### Review questions

1. Briefly describe the role of the autonomic nervous system in the maintenance of homeostasis.
2. Draw a diagram to illustrate the relationship of the autonomic nervous system to the central nervous system, showing the divisions of each.
3. Give one example of the sympathetic and parasympathetic divisions of the autonomic nervous system apparently working in opposition to one another.
4. Describe the anatomical differences between the two divisions of the ANS.
5. Where and what is the enteric nervous system?
6. Name the main neurotransmitters released at the effector organs of the sympathetic and parasympathetic branches of the ANS.
7. How can the adrenergic receptor be subdivided?
8. Give one example of a sympathomimetic drug and list its possible uses.
9. Describe how noradrenaline (norepinephrine) and acetylcholine are inactivated in the body.
10. What is an antagonist? Describe the action of one drug that acts as an antagonist within the autonomic nervous system.

---

### Suggestions for further reading

Canon, W.B. (1932) *The Wisdom of the Body.* New York: Appleton.

Galbraith, A., Bullock, S., Manias, E., Richards, A. & Hunt, B. (1999) *Fundamentals of Pharmacology.* Harlow: Addison Wesley Longman.

Guyton, A.C. & Hall, J.E. (2000) *Medical Physiology,* 10th edn. London: W.B. Saunders.

Johnston, G.D. (1999) *Fundamentals of Cardiovascular Pharmacology.* Chichester: Wiley.

Longstaff, A. (2000) *Neuroscience – Instant Notes*. Oxford: BIOS Scientific Publishers.

McCaffery, M. (1989) *Pain: Clinical Manual for Nursing Practice*. St Louis: Mosby.

Rang, H.P., Dale, M.M. & Ritter, J.M. (1999) *Pharmacology*, 4th edn. Edinburgh: Churchill Livingstone.

Sadler, T. (2003) *Langman's Medical Embryology*, 9th edn. Philadelphia: Lippincott, Williams and Wilkins.

Selye, H. (1976) *The Stress of Life*. New York: McGraw-Hill.

Waller, D.G., Renwick, A.G. & Hillier, K. (2001) *Medical Pharmacology and Therapeutics*. Edinburgh: Saunders.

Zigmond, M.J., Bloom, F.E., Landis, S.C., Roberts, J.L. & Squire, L.R. (eds) (1999) *Fundamental Neuroscience*. London: Academic Press.

## References

Bear, M., Connors, B. & Paradiso, M.A. (1996) *Neuroscience – Exploring the Brain*. Baltimore: Williams and Wilkins.

Marieb, E.N. (2004) *Human Anatomy and Physiology*, 5th edn. San Francisco: Benjamin Cummings.

# Endocrine function

*William F. M. Wallace*

## LEARNING OBJECTIVES

After studying this chapter the reader should be able to:

- Describe the general organization of the endocrine system and the relationship between the nervous and endocrine systems

- Describe the two main groups of hormones, steroids and peptides, and discuss the methods of action of hormones on target cells

- Discuss the secretion, transport, metabolism and excretion of hormones and indicate how these factors affect the timescale of the activity of different hormones

- Discuss the role of the thyroid hormones in the control of metabolic rate and contrast the effects of secretion of inadequate and excessive amounts of these hormones

- Describe the metabolic changes that take place to maintain the blood glucose level within normal limits, and the role of hormones in controlling these changes

- Describe the endocrine regulation of fluid and electrolyte balance

- Indicate the roles played by calcium and phosphate in the body and discuss how the blood calcium level is controlled

- Discuss the involvement of the endocrine system in coordinated growth and development

- Discuss the role of the endocrine system in responding to life-threatening challenges such as a car crash or severe infection

## INTRODUCTION

The nervous and endocrine systems are the major controllers and organizers of the body. They both coordinate activities in widely scattered parts of the body and they both act by releasing chemicals. The nervous system acts with speed and specificity – a signal can be sent along nerves from the brain to a small group of distant muscles in well under a tenth of a second. By contrast, endocrine signals travel in the bloodstream and produce responses that take minutes to build up and can last for hours. Because the signals travel in the blood, all cells of a particular type receive it, no matter where they are located.

The term **endocrine** (from the Latin *endo*, meaning within) arose when it was found that some glands secrete chemicals within the body; these chemicals are then carried in the bloodstream. This activity contrasts with **exocrine** glands (*exo*, to the outside), which secrete to the outside of the body. Exocrine secretions include sweat secreted on to the surface of the skin and digestive secretions secreted into the gut cavity, as, strictly speaking, this is outside the body proper.

The endocrine system plays a major part in **homeostasis**. It does this in several ways. First, it controls the rate at which cells are provided with energy for all their functions, including generating heat to maintain body core temperature. This energy is used in the body's chemical reactions (**metabolism**) and the rate of use of energy is the **metabolic rate**. Second, the endocrine system regulates the supply of raw materials (**substrates**), mainly glucose and fatty acids, for this metabolism. Third, it controls the volume and electrolyte composition of the **extracellular fluid** that bathes our cells. Fourth, it regulates the **calcium and phosphate** that not only comprise much of our bones but that also, in ionic form, control the **excitability of nerves and muscles**. If excitability is too low, we are weak and lethargic, if too high, we suffer from spasms.

This chapter deals with the above topics in the order given. It also looks at growth and development and with how the body responds to life-threatening challenges, such as a severe car crash and subsequent admittance to intensive care. Such incidents could be regarded as dramatic examples of homeostasis but they are included because first, in conjunction with the reproductive system (considered elsewhere), growth and development contribute to the maintenance of the human race by replacing one generation of individuals by the next, and second, an adequate response to life-threatening challenge ensures survival of function on a shorter timescale.

A list of major endocrine glands is given in **Table 2.6.1**. At the head of the list is the hypothalamus, a region of the brain. This is where the nervous and endocrine systems interact. The hypothalamus is part of the brain and is open to all the influences of brain activity. Its neurones secrete hormones into the bloodstream and these travel to the nearby pituitary gland, which in turn regulates major body organs either directly or via endocrine glands such as the thyroid, ovary and testis. At the bottom of the list are organs like the kidneys, better known for nonendocrine functions, but which also secrete hormones. In fact, the first hormone isolated came from the gut, the hormone secretin, which stimulates exocrine secretion by the pancreas. The skin is

| Table 2.6.1 | Major endocrine glands of the body and positions |
|---|---|
| Hypothalamus | Base of brain |
| Pituitary gland (hypophysis) | |
| Posterior pituitary gland (neurohypophysis) | Pituitary fossa of cranium |
| Anterior pituitary gland (adenohypophysis) | |
| Thyroid gland | Neck, below larynx |
| Parathyroid glands (4) | Posterior surface of thyroid gland |
| Adrenal glands (2) | Superior pole of kidneys |
| Adrenal cortex | Outer layers of adrenal gland |
| Adrenal medulla | Inner core of adrenal gland |
| Islets of Langerhans | Embedded in pancreas |
| Ovaries (2) (female) | Pelvic cavity |
| Testes (2) (male) | Scrotum |
| Trophoblast (followed by placenta) | Pregnant uterus |
| Pineal gland | Cranial cavity, behind midbrain |
| Thymus | Mediastinum |
| Kidneys | Retroperitoneal position |
| Gastric and intestinal mucosa | Gut wall |
| Skin | Areas exposed to sunlight |

| Table 2.6.2 | Endocrine glands involved in aspects of body function |
|---|---|
| **Gland** | **Function** |
| Thyroid gland, adrenal medulla | Control of metabolic rate |
| Pancreas, adrenal cortex, anterior pituitary, adrenal medulla | Control of glucose metabolism |
| Anterior pituitary, thyroid, gonads, adrenal cortex, pancreas, skin, kidneys | Growth and development |
| Posterior pituitary, adrenal cortex, kidneys | Fluid and electrolyte balance |
| Parathyroid glands, thyroid, skin, kidneys | Calcium and phosphate balance |
| Adrenal cortex, adrenal medulla, thymus | Responses to life-threatening challenge |
| Anterior pituitary, ovaries, testes, placenta, ?pineal gland | Reproduction and nurturing (see Chapter 6.3) |

included in the list because it can synthesize vitamin D, which is then modified in liver and kidneys to form a hormone that regulates absorption of calcium in the upper intestine.

Table 2.6.2 summarizes the functions of the main endocrine glands. These are listed in the order used in this chapter, with the addition of reproductive glands, which are considered in Chapter 6.3.

Other related secretions that can be mentioned briefly at this stage include chemical messengers, which travel from one cell to other nearby cells. This is described as **paracrine** control (*para*, beside) as opposed to endocrine control. The chemical might even stimulate another part of the secreting cell (**autocrine** control; *auto*, self).

We now consider some details of the endocrine system as a whole, before passing to specific glands.

## Organization of the endocrine system

At this stage we look first at the key roles of the hypothalamus and pituitary as organizers of many, but not all, of the other endocrine glands. We then consider some general principles of hormone structure and action, including factors determining hormone level in the circulation.

## The hypothalamus

The hypothalamus plays a major role in the maintenance of the internal environment in two main ways – by nervous system reflexes and through the endocrine system. The reflexes include vital behavioural effects. Core temperature regulation includes behaviour aimed at avoiding uncomfortably cold or hot environments, and one of the fundamental nursing functions has always been to assist patients in this way. Hunger, satiety and thirst are also generated in the hypothalamus to ensure an appropriate intake of food and fluids, again a fundamental nursing function. Having ensured an intake of food and fluids, the hypothalamus then acts through the pituitary to control endocrine responses that ensure homeostasis. This is done by controlling the metabolism of food products and by renal retention of appropriate amounts of fluid and electrolyte and excretion of unwanted items. Hypothalamic control of the endocrine system is shown in **Fig. 2.6.1**.

Notice that in **Fig. 2.6.1** there are three initial arrows leading from the hypothalamus. These summarize nicely the interactions between nervous and hormonal control. The arrow on the left represents sympathetic nerves passing from the hypothalamus to the adrenal medulla, an endocrine gland involved in emergency situations requiring rapid strenuous

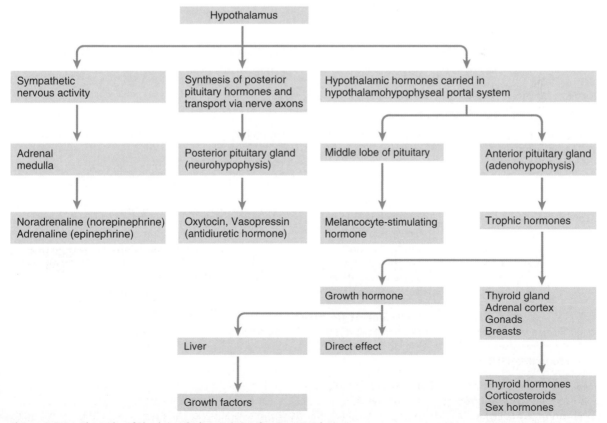

**Figure 2.6.1** The role of the hypothalamus in endocrine regulation

activity ('fight or flight'). This endocrine gland secretes the catecholamines adrenaline (epinephrine) and noradrenaline (norepinephrine), which act on the same receptors as the noradrenaline released by other sympathetic nerves in a direct path from the hypothalamus to vital organs such as the heart. In this way, the nervous system initiates the emergency response and the endocrine system augments and maintains it.

The middle arrow from the hypothalamus indicates that the hypothalamus contains cells that send axons down the pituitary stalk to the posterior pituitary gland, where they release chemicals – not beside the target cells but into the circulation, where they are classed as hormones. These hormones then travel to target cells in the uterus (oxytocin) and in the kidney (vasopressin, otherwise known as antidiuretic hormone, ADH).

The third arrow, on the right, indicates control of several major endocrine effects, including some described later in this chapter. These effects are mediated almost entirely through the anterior pituitary (adenohypophysis). Effects mediated through the middle lobe of the pituitary are not normally of much significance, because the melanin in our skin is determined mainly genetically and by exposure to sunlight. **Table 2.6.3** lists the hypothalamic hormones that influence pituitary secretion of further hormones.

## The pituitary gland

The development of this gland in the embryo is shown in **Fig. 2.6.2** and helps us to understand its role as the link between the hypothalamus and the major endocrine glands (see **Fig. 2.6.1**). Note that another term for the pituitary is the hypophysis: something that grows (*physis*) below (*hypo*) the brain. The anterior part originates from an upgrowth of the primitive mouth and is known as the **adenohypophysis**, because of its glandular nature (*adeno-*, gland). The posterior pituitary is

**Table 2.6.3** Hypothalamic hormones influencing pituitary secretion, and organs affected

| Hypothalamus | Anterior pituitary | Tissues affected | Action |
|---|---|---|---|
| Corticotrophin-releasing hormone or factor (CRH or CRF) | Adrenocorticotrophic hormone (ACTH) ↑ | Adrenal cortex | Glucocorticoid secretion ↑ Aldosterone secretion ↑ temporarily |
| Thyrotrophin-releasing hormone (TRH) | Thyroid stimulating hormone (TSH) ↑ | Thyroid gland | Thyroid hormones secretion ↑ |
| Growth hormone releasing hormone (GRH) | Growth hormone (GH) ↑ | Most body tissues, particularly liver | Growth factors secretion ↑ Growth increased |
| Growth hormone release-inhibiting hormone (GI) | Growth hormone ↓ | | |
| Prolactin releasing hormone (PRH) | Prolactin (luteotrophic hormone, LH) ↑ | Breasts | Development of breasts |
| Prolactin release-inhibiting hormone (PIH) | Prolactin ↓ | | Secretion of milk |
| Gonadotrophin releasing hormone (GnRH) | Luteinizing hormone (LH)/interstitial cell stimulating hormone (ICSH) ↑ Follicle stimulating hormone (FSH) ↑ | Ovaries or testes Ovaries or testes | Ovulation, development of corpus luteum (females) Testosterone secretion (males) ↑ Ovarian follicle growth Spermatogenesis ↑ |
| Melanocyte stimulating hormone releasing hormone (MSHRH) | *Middle lobe of pituitary* Melanocyte stimulating hormone (MSH) ↑ | Skin | Deposition of melanin by melanocytes |
| Melanocyte stimulating hormone release inhibiting hormone (MSHRIH) | Melanocyte stimulating hormone (MSH) ↓ | | |

derived from the base of the brain and is known as the **neurohypophysis** because it consists of nervous tissue – the axons of hypothalamic neurones, down which antidiuretic hormone and oxytocin pass after they are synthesized in the hypothalamus.

The anterior pituitary has no direct (nervous) link with the hypothalamus, instead, the link is provided by capillaries in the hypothalamus, from which blood passes into small veins in the pituitary stalk. These veins break-up into a second set of capillaries in the anterior pituitary. Hypothalamic hormones are secreted into the first set of capillaries and are taken up by the second set to control the pituitary glandular cells. A system that unites two sets of capillaries in series like this is known as a **portal** circulation, and this one has the grandiose title of the hypothalamohypophyseal portal system.

## CLINICAL APPLICATIONS

Disorders of the pituitary gland can have extremely varied and dramatic results. Destruction of the anterior pituitary gland will result in hypopituitarism, with loss of function in the glands to the right in **Fig. 2.6.1**. Such patients lose thyroid and reproductive function and fail to secrete cortisol in emergencies. They might need very careful nursing and medical care. Tumours of the pituitary gland, however, can sometimes cause increased secretion of a hormone. A dramatic, but fortunately very rare, example of this is excessive secretion of growth hormone in a child, causing the child to grow into a giant.

## Homeostatic regulation of the pituitary gland

As well as control by the hypothalamus above, the pituitary is also influenced by the circulating level of hormones from the endocrine glands it controls. In true homeostatic fashion this is by negative feedback (**Fig. 2.6.3**). Most of this negative feedback is via the anterior pituitary and it serves to keep

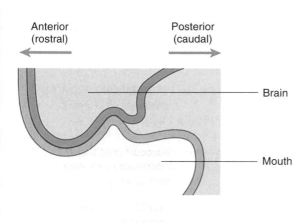

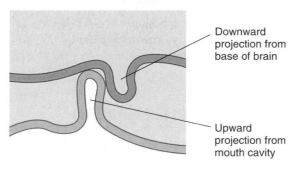

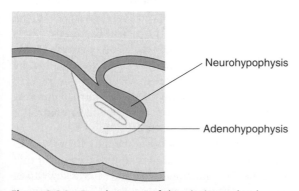

**Figure 2.6.2**  Development of the pituitary gland (adapted from Passmore & Robson, 1976)

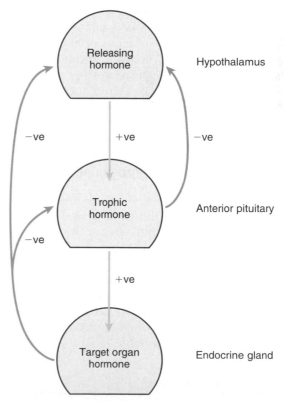

**Figure 2.6.3**  Negative feedback control of endocrine systems involving the hypothalamus, anterior pituitary and target endocrine organs

**Table 2.6.4**   Endocrine function directly controlled by the condition of the internal environment (i.e. the extracellular fluid)

| Endocrine organ | Hormone secreted | Regulation of release | Activity |
|---|---|---|---|
| Pancreas β-cells<br>α-cells | Insulin<br>Glucagon | ↑ in blood glucose<br>Inhibited by ↑ in blood<br>glucose | Regulation of blood<br>glucose level |
| Parathyroid glands (4)<br>Kidneys<br>Thyroid parafollicular<br>cells | Parathormone<br>1,25-dihydroxycholecalciferol<br>Calcitonin | ↑ when blood calcium low<br><br>↑ by parathormone<br>↑ when blood calcium high | Regulation of plasma<br>concentration of<br>calcium ions ($Ca^{2+}$) |
| Adrenal cortex | Aldosterone | ↑ when low serum sodium<br>↑ when high serum<br>potassium<br>↑ by action of renin from<br>kidney | Regulation of sodium<br>and potassium<br>concentration in<br>plasma |
| Kidney | Erythropoietin | ↑ by hypoxia | Production and<br>release of erythrocytes |

hormonal levels constant. The role of the hypothalamus is to override this constancy when a change is needed. There are two interesting examples of this for the hormone cortisol, one of the hormones produced by the adrenal cortex. Cortisol shows a marked daily (circadian) rhythm, being lowest during night-time sleep and several times higher during daytime activities. This rhythm results from a similar rhythm in the production by the hypothalamus of one of its releasing hormones. The hypothalamus can do this because it has an 'internal clock', which is synchronized with our daily rhythm of daylight and darkness, activity and sleep. A second example is when cortisol is released in large amounts during life-threatening stress, after the hypothalamus has been 'made aware' of injury by inputs through nerves from damaged areas.

## Hormones outside hypothalamic–pituitary control

Some endocrine glands are not influenced directly by the hypothalamus and pituitary but by a combination of factors, particularly by the condition of the internal environment, the interstitial component of the extracellular fluid. This is generally reflected in the blood, as small particles such as, glucose and sodium ions, exchange readily between blood and interstitial fluid through capillary walls. This type of control is summarized in **Table 2.6.4**.

### Hormone structure

Hormones fall into two main groups: one group comprises the steroid hormones, which are formed from cholesterol and the second group comprises peptides (chains of amino acids) of greatly varying length and complexity. **Figure 2.6.4** shows the structure of cholesterol and some of the steroid hormones secreted by the body. As can be seen, they are very similar in structure, with only small chemical differences leading to the varied actions of the different hormones. The similarities in structure of these hormones explain the overlap in activity that occurs between the different steroid hormones. This group includes all the hormones of the adrenal cortex, the glucocorticoids, mineralocorticoids and sex hormones, and the sex hormones secreted by the ovaries and testes.

## Methods of action of hormones

Hormones vary in the way they act on their target organs, with some having a very rapid action and others taking a considerable time to have any noticeable effect. A number of methods have been identified whereby hormones cause an alteration in the activity of specific cells. The metabolism of the cell is modified largely through regulation of enzyme activity, which can occur in two main ways: either by increasing the amount of enzyme present or by regulating the level of activity of already formed enzyme. In addition, cell activity can be altered by control of entry of substances into the cell.

The point at which a hormone initially influences cellular function is referred to as the receptor for that hormone. The hormone acts rather like a key, fitting into or reacting with the receptor to start a chain of effects that constitutes the target cell's response. The

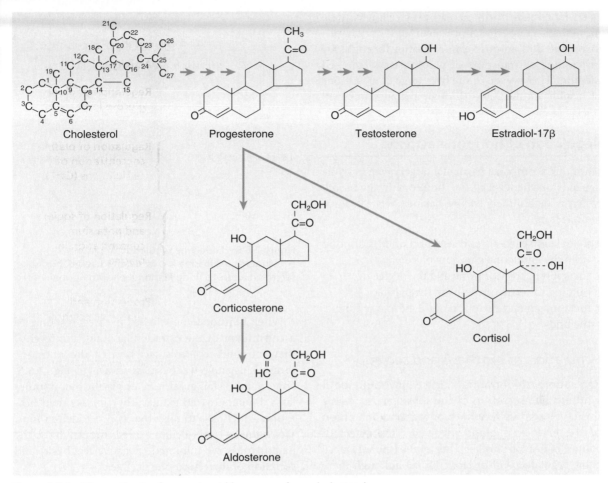

**Figure 2.6.4** The synthesis of some steroid hormones from cholesterol

two main types of hormone, steroid and peptide, tend to act via receptors at different sites in the cell.

**Steroid hormones** are fat soluble, so penetrate the cell wall readily and act on internal receptors. **Thyroid hormones**, the smallest of the peptide group, also act internally. Most other hormones do not enter the cell readily so have to act on receptors in the cell membrane. The steroids and thyroid hormones, having entered the cell, act by increasing the synthesis in the nucleus of messenger ribonucleic acid (mRNA), which then passes into the cytoplasm of the cell and acts as a template for the formation of a specific enzyme. The synthesis of that enzyme is thus increased. A considerable period of time (hours or even days) of exposure to the hormone might be needed before any effect can be detected. Another way of increasing enzyme synthesis is by stimulation at the ribosome in the cell cytoplasm, where the enzyme is synthesized against the already formed mRNA template.

Most **peptide hormones**, and some smaller hormones that are not fat soluble, act by binding to specific receptors in the cell membrane. Examples are insulin and the catecholamines (adrenaline (epinephrine) and noradrenaline (norepinephrine)), which alter the transport of molecules and ions across the cell membrane into the cell by direct binding to membrane receptors. Finally, also through membrane receptor binding, hormones can act by regulating the level of intracellular messengers that start a cascade of chemical reactions leading to the definitive effect. In such cases the hormone is regarded as the 'first messenger' and the chemical whose intracellular concentration it alters is called the 'second messenger'. An example of such a second messenger is cyclic adenosine monophosphate (cAMP). Cyclic AMP is a fairly small molecule, synthesized from adenosine triphosphate, which activates a large variety of enzymes that regulate a number of metabolic pathways. The level of cAMP can be increased or decreased by the action of hormones, depending on the tissue involved.

Another second messenger is the calcium ion. Many hormones and neuronal transmitters act by opening calcium channels in the cell membrane (or in intracellular membrane-bound stores that concentrate the ion). As intracellular calcium is normally much lower than extracellular calcium, calcium ions pour through the channels and a rise in the level of intracellular calcium ions triggers the cell's response.

213

An individual hormone can alter cell activity by more than one of the above methods. For example, in muscle and adipose tissue, insulin functions by increasing the transport of glucose across the cell membrane. However, in the liver some of the actions of insulin are mediated through a change in cAMP levels.

## Regulation of hormone activity

Hormone action on a particular target organ or tissue depends on the level of free hormone in the blood, which is determined by the balance between three main factors:

- the rate of synthesis and secretion of the hormone from the endocrine gland involved
- transport of the hormone and the degree of binding to carrier proteins in the plasma
- metabolism and excretion of the hormone from the body.

### Regulation of synthesis and secretion

Regulation of hormone release, involving both synthesis and secretion of the substance, is mainly through **negative feedback** or **feedback inhibition** of the endocrine gland involved. This system of control endeavours to keep the level of the substance being regulated within close limits, although there will be some vacillation within those limits. However, as mentioned earlier, through the action of the hypothalamus and its links with other parts of the nervous system, the endocrine system can also respond to environmental and emotional change.

Those hormones released through the action of the hypothalamus and anterior pituitary gland on a target organ act in negative feedback fashion on one or both of these organs to reduce the secretion of the appropriate hypothalamic and pituitary hormones (see **Fig. 2.6.3**).

When a disorder of an endocrine gland prevents secretion of a hormone, the levels of the trophic hormone involved in its release are not inhibited and might become very high. An example is Addison's disease. In this condition there is atrophy of the adrenal cortex, so corticosteroids are not secreted and cannot, therefore, inhibit the secretion of adrenocorticotrophic hormone (ACTH). The level of ACTH greatly increases. Such rises in the trophic (controlling) hormone help in the diagnosis of target organ failure: they are the body's own diagnosis of target organ failure. A curious additional effect is that excessive ACTH is also associated with stimulation of the pituitary cells that form melanocyte-stimulating hormone (see **Fig. 2.6.1**). Progressive pigmentation of the skin develops due to the action of melanocyte-stimulating hormone.

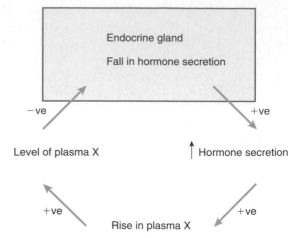

**Figure 2.6.5** Endocrine regulation of plasma constituents. As Plasma X is raised or lowered, hormone secretion alters to bring Plasma X back to normal level

When hormones are released in direct response to a constituent of the extracellular fluid, the level of that substance controls secretion of the hormone through negative feedback, as shown in **Fig. 2.6.5**. For example, a fall in calcium ions in the blood stimulates the parathyroid glands. They release their hormone, which acts to raise the level of calcium ions. When the level of calcium exceeds the 'set' level, the parathyroids are inhibited (negative feedback) and secretion of their hormone declines.

### Transport and protein binding

Hormones are secreted into the capillaries passing through an endocrine gland and transported through the circulation. The circulation time taken for a bitter substance injected into an arm vein to reach the tongue, where it is tasted, is about 15 seconds, which gives an indication of the speed with which hormones can reach the various organs of the body. The free hormone in the blood is available to act on the target organ but is also exposed to metabolizing enzymes, which degrade it into an inactive form.

The **half-life** of a hormone is the time taken for half of it to be removed from the plasma. To put it another way, it is the time taken for the plasma concentration to fall by half. For many common hormones the half-life is around 10 minutes. This allows them to disappear quickly so that their effects do not persist for long after secretion stops. As the concentration falls by half each 10 minutes, the levels will be:

| Time 0 | 100% |
|---|---|
| 10 minutes | 50% |
| 20 minutes | 25% |
| 30 minutes | 12.5% |
| 40 minutes | 6.25% |

Thus, by 20–30 minutes the effect will be down to a very low level, and by 30–40 minutes it will be negligible. This is important for many actions that must terminate promptly. For example, if the insulin level remained high for several hours after a meal it would lead to a profound fall in blood glucose, leading to coma.

Hormones such as the catecholamines, anti-diuretic hormone and insulin have short half-lives (as in the above example), and tend to be transported through in the bloodstream in the free state. However, some hormones, e.g. thyroxine and the corticosteroids, are transported in the plasma bound to specific proteins, and these hormones have a longer half-life. The bound hormone is in a state of equilibrium with the free hormone:

$$\text{free hormone} + \text{protein} \rightleftharpoons \text{hormone–protein}$$

As the free hormone is used up, more is released from the protein-bound state.

## Metabolism and excretion

The major organs involved in metabolism and excretion of hormones are the liver and kidneys. Some hormones are inactivated by the tissues on which they act but the liver plays the major role in hormone degradation. Protein-bound hormones are protected from destruction.

Enzymes in the endoplasmic reticulum of the liver cells catalyse a number of chemical reactions that reduce the endocrine activity of the hormones and, by making them water soluble, enable them to be more readily excreted from the body. Some hormones are conjugated (combined) with other chemicals (mainly glucuronate or sulphate) before excretion and this also increases the water solubility of the hormone molecules. Excretion takes place in the bile from the liver and in the urine through the kidneys. Patients with liver disease might be unable to metabolize hormones normally and will show signs of high levels of particular hormones. For example, a male patient with cirrhosis of the liver might develop enlargement of the breasts (gynaecomastia) due to high levels of oestrogens (female sex hormones) in his blood.

Other enzymes, found widely in the body, tend to inactivate circulating compounds by altering their composition by oxidation, breaking down peptide links, etc. These scavenging enzymes ensure that no active compound – hormone or drug – can linger long in the blood. Overall, this tendency to remove active compounds is very important in homeostasis because it 'switches off' effects, allowing the body to 'switch on' again as and when required.

## Disturbances in endocrine function

Many of the functions of the endocrine system have been established by studying patients who have disturbances of hormone secretion. There might be overactivity of the hormone (e.g. hyperthyroidism, too high a level of thyroid hormones) or underactivity (hypothyroidism, too low a level of thyroid hormones). Understanding such conditions will help the nurse not only to deal appropriately with the patients concerned but also to understand what the hormone in question contributes to the everyday life of healthy people.

Many endocrine disorders are due to hypo- or hypersecretion by a gland; these can be primary or secondary in nature. Primary alteration relates to an altered ability of the endocrine gland itself whereas secondary dysfunction is the result of an alteration in the control of the secretion of the gland. This is normally due to a disturbance of the pituitary gland or the hypothalamus.

Some endocrine disturbances are caused by substances that antagonize or inactivate the hormone, others are the result of target cell resistance. The end result is the same as inadequate hormone production – inadequate hormone activity.

### DEVELOPMENTAL ISSUES

Changes in endocrine function occur in old age and play a part in loss of homeostasis in old age – deviations from the normal are less promptly and completely corrected. These changes are not simply due to a decrease in endocrine function and, indeed, with some hormones there is no alteration of levels in the blood. There is some evidence that decreased sensitivity of the nerve cells in the hypothalamus, which regulate the secretion of the pituitary gland, account for some of the changes seen. However, changes in the responsiveness of the target organs to the hormones would also account for some of the variation seen.

### Control of metabolic rate

**Metabolism** consists of all the chemical reactions taking place in the body cells. It includes catabolism and anabolism. In **catabolic reactions**, carbohydrates, amino acids and fatty acids are broken down through oxidation into smaller molecules, mainly water and carbon dioxide, and energy is produced. The energy is released in small amounts, which is stored within the body in high-energy phosphate compounds, the major one of which is adenosine triphosphate (ATP). Some of the energy at this stage, however, is liberated in the form of heat. In **anabolic reactions**, energy is required for the formation of more complex molecules.

During catabolism the total energy ultimately liberated (when the ATP releases its energy, largely for muscle contraction and ionic pumps) appear as heat. This heat energy is the same as the amount of heat energy that would be liberated if the original food were burnt outside the body. We get an idea of the heat produced by metabolism when we exercise vigorously, particularly in a fairly warm room. The amount of energy released and used by the body in a given time is called the **metabolic rate**. It equals the heat energy produced by the body in a given time and can be calculated from the rate of oxygen consumption (or carbon dioxide production) in a given time.

The SI units of energy are the joule (J), the kilojoule (kJ = 1000 J, or $10^3$ J), or the megajoule (MJ = 1 000 000 J, or $10^6$ J). The alternative unit, often used outside Europe and still sometimes used clinically, and almost invariably by the general public, is the calorie (the heat required to raise 1 g of water through 1°C), or the kilocalorie (kcal), usually known in nutrition as the Calorie, with a capital C (1 Cal = 1000 calories). One Calorie equals 4.2 kJ.

Energy is released during the breakdown of nutrients, and oxygen is required for these reactions to occur with maximum efficiency. The energy released from the different types of nutrients varies somewhat, but the amount of energy released per litre of oxygen utilized is approximately 20 kJ. Therefore, by measuring the quantity of oxygen used in a given time it is possible to calculate, with an acceptable degree of accuracy, the amount of energy released, i.e. the **metabolic rate**. The **basal metabolic rate** is the rate at which energy is used in the body while the person is awake but is: (i) at complete rest; (ii) emotionally tranquil; (iii) in a comfortable temperature; and (iv) not digesting and assimilating a meal. The four parallel conditions that raise the metabolic rate are: (i) physical exercise; (ii) excitement; (iii) responding to an uncomfortable cold or hot environment; and (iv) carrying out the chemical reactions and ionic pumping involved in processing a meal. In disease conditions when the metabolic rate is altered, such as in thyrotoxicosis or myxoedema, it is expressed as plus or minus a percentage from normal for an individual of that age, sex and size.

## Factors influencing metabolic rate

A number of factors that influence the metabolic rate are shown in **Table 2.6.5**. Of these, gender, age and size (indicated by height, weight and surface area) determine the basic metabolic rate. In most cases, the others raise the metabolic rate above the basal level. In practice, people normally produce most increases in metabolic rate by exercise. Moderate walking can treble the basal rate, brisk walking can raise it about half as much again. When exercising maximally, the average young adult can increase metabolism (and heat production) tenfold; athletes can raise it to as much as 15 or 20 times the basal rate.

### CLINICAL APPLICATIONS

Patients in hospital taking little exercise will often have a low daily metabolic rate and feel the cold. Anaesthetized patients in theatre have even lower metabolic rates and their core temperatures tend to fall even in the heat of the theatre. Steps are taken to avoid this as far as possible, as even a modest fall in temperature impairs body functions, including the clotting mechanism and maintenance of arterial blood pressure. By contrast, patients with fever and some patients in intensive care who are responding to severe injury have an increased metabolic rate and hence nutritional requirements.

**Table 2.6.5** Factors influencing metabolic rate

| Factor | Effect |
|---|---|
| Gender | Females lower than males |
| Age | Declines with increasing age |
| Emotional state | Anxiety → ↑ adrenaline (epinephrine) secretion → ↑ metabolic rate |
| | Depression → ↓ metabolic rate |
| Pregnancy or menstruation | ↑ metabolic rate |
| Muscular exertion | ↑ metabolic rate |
| Ingestion of food | Specific dynamic action of food → ↑ metabolic rate (protein greater effect than carbohydrates and fat) |
| | Starvation → ↓ metabolic rate |
| Environmental temperature | Cold → ↑ metabolic rate |
| | Heat → ↑ metabolic rate |
| Fever | Rise of 1°C → ↑ metabolic rate of 14% |
| Height, weight, surface area | Allowed for in calculation of metabolic rate |

Thyroid hormones markedly affect the basal, or resting, metabolic rate of the body, as well as being essential for normal growth and development. The metabolic rate might be as low as $-40\%$ to $-50\%$ when there is a complete lack of thyroid secretion, or as high as $+60\%$ or $+100\%$ when excessive thyroid hormones are secreted. In healthy people, metabolic activity of the tissues of the body is maintained at the optimal level by regulated secretion of the thyroid hormones.

## Role and disorders of thyroid hormones

As with some other hormones, the thyroid hormones exist in more than one form. The main forms are thyroxine and tri-iodothyronine. These are sometimes referred to as $T_4$ and $T_3$, respectively, because thyroxine has four iodine atoms and tri-iodothyronine has three. Further details of their formation and actions are given later. Together, they play a major role in the regulation of the metabolic rate of most body tissues. They increase the resting metabolic rate and thus increase oxygen consumption and heat production. They also play a vital role in normal development during childhood, and this will also be discussed later.

The thyroid hormones readily cross the cell membrane to act within the cell by binding to receptors within the nucleus. This is followed by increased synthesis of mRNA, leading to increased production of respiratory enzymes within the mitochondria of the cell. This mode of action explains the considerable lag period before any observable effect when administering thyroid hormones to hypothyroid patients. Some effects will probably be seen within a week but the full benefit of treatment might take several months to develop.

The effect of increased stimulation by thyroid hormones is that mitochondria speed up the oxidation of substrate and generation of adenosine triphosphate (ATP), the high-energy compound that circulates in the cell to provide energy. The increased cell activity also leads to increased heat release from mitochondrial metabolism. The overall effects are that more substrate is consumed, more oxygen is consumed, more energy is available to and used by the cell, and more heat is produced.

### CLINICAL APPLICATIONS

To understand the effects of thyroid hormones in normal people it is particularly helpful to consider the effects of deficiency (hypothyroidism, myxoedema) and compare them with the effects of excess (hyperthyroidism, thyrotoxicosis, Graves' disease). These conditions (more common in women than men) are of considerable importance

in nursing practice because they are the second most common group of endocrine disorders in patients (diabetes mellitus being the most common endocrine disorder).

## HYPERTHYROIDISM

### Metabolic changes

Due to the increased mitochondrial activity, more energy is available in the cells and heat production is increased. The sufferer therefore feels warm, even in cold conditions, and the body temperature may be raised. This '**heat intolerance**' is a major feature. Typically, the hyperthyroid patient will want to have windows opened and will tolerate only light clothing or bedclothes. This resembles the situation in pregnant women, who also have increased heat production, in this case due to the developing baby. Increased metabolism causes increased utilization of oxygen and an increase in the amount of carbon dioxide formed. The rise in carbon dioxide produced stimulates an increase in the rate and depth of respiration. This might be interpreted by the patient as **shortness of breath**. There is also an increased demand for nutrients, with an **increased appetite** and rate of absorption of these nutrients, but the patient still tends to report **loss of weight**.

### Patient care

The nurse should encourage the patient to eat a high-protein, high-carbohydrate diet, and should remember that an increase in the motility and secretion of the gastrointestestinal tract leads to **increased frequency and bulk of stools**, which the patient might report as diarrhoea. Excessive protein breakdown causes muscle weakness and fatigue, and **muscle tremor** is commonly seen in the outstretched arms. With increased available energy the hyperthyroid patient might at first seem to be in an enviable position. However, the energy is above that required for normal activity, it is not efficiently used and the overall effect is of fatigue, nervousness and generally feeling hot and bothered and sweaty.

### Cardiovascular disturbances

The changes described result in an increased demand on the cardiovascular system to supply the nutrients and oxygen required and to remove the increased waste products of metabolism. In addition, the increased heat production demands increased heat elimination by increased blood flow to the skin. The resulting rise in pulse and blood pressure indicates the resultant increase in cardiac output. The circulation is described as hyperdynamic and is associated with an increased gap between systolic and diastolic pressures. Tachycardia persisting during sleep is one of the earliest signs of thyrotoxicosis but it might be difficult to measure a sleeping pulse as these patients wake from sleep very easily.

Cardiac arrhythmias can develop, particularly atrial fibrillation in older people. The nurse should plan care to encourage rest and reduce the demand on the cardiovascular system, but as these patients have considerable difficulty in resting, nursing measures alone might be insufficient to ensure relaxation and so sedative drugs may be necessary.

### Nervous and reproductive disturbances

The effect of excessive thyroid secretion on the nervous system is particularly marked. Patients often demonstrate increased rapidity of thought; tend to be irritable, nervous and agitated and might show exaggerated and purposeless movements (hyperkinesis). They might also show symptoms of an anxiety state and suffer from insomnia. Menstrual irregularities (a tendency for scanty periods) sometimes occur and the patient might become infertile.

### Graves' disease (Fig. 2.6.6)

Graves' disease is a form of hyperthyroidism. It is an autoimmune disease in which the patient forms antibodies against the thyroid-stimulating hormone (TSH) receptors in the thyroid cells. These antibodies also stimulate activity of the thyroid cells and are known as **thyroid-stimulating immunoglobulins**. In this condition, **exophthalmos** (protrusion of the eyeballs, as in **Fig. 2.6.6**) also develops; this gives a typical staring appearance. The cause of the eyeball protrusion is uncertain. It does not seem to be due to an excess of thyroid hormones because it does not occur in all cases where the level is raised.

Compare **Figs 2.6.6** and **2.6.7**. Notice the hyperalert expression, reduced subcutaneous fat and smooth skin in **Fig. 2.6.6**, in contrast to the dull expression and coarser skin in **Fig. 2.6.7**. Picture in your mind the normal healthy appearance in between these two extremes.

### Treatment

Treatment of hyperthyroidism can be by antithyroid drugs, by surgery or by the use of radioactive iodine. As the thyroid has a great capacity to take up iodine (which it uses to synthesize its hormones) the dose of radioactive iodine is almost all taken into the gland and the

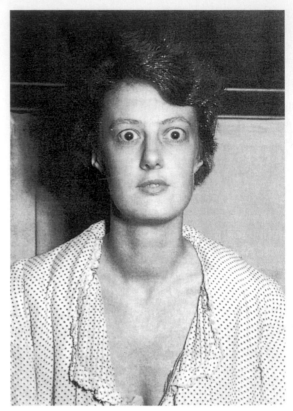

**Figure 2.6.6**　A person with Graves' disease

radioactivity then selectively attacks and reduces the amount of active thyroid tissue.

In carrying out the assessment and implementing the care planned it is extremely important that the nurse remains calm and interacts in a way that soothes the hyperthyroid patient. A quiet, cool environment is necessary to make the patient as comfortable and relaxed as possible in the face of an increased metabolism.

### HYPOTHYROIDISM (MYXOEDEMA)

Patients with reduced thyroid activity demonstrate opposite signs and symptoms from hyperthyroid patients. The term 'myxoedema' refers primarily to the tissue swelling that contributes to the coarsening of the features (**Fig. 2.6.7**). However, it is often used to describe the general condition of hypothyroidism. The individual suffers from '**cold intolerance**' and might even develop hypothermia as the body metabolism produces less heat than normal. A warm environment is therefore required for comfort. The patient's mental processes become slowed and most other body functions become sluggish. This is seen in slow, lethargic movements and rather slow

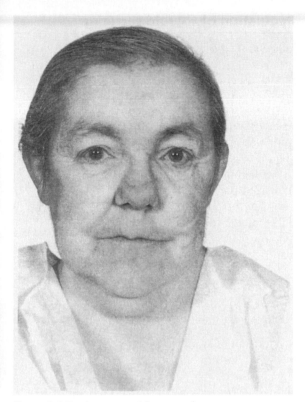

**Figure 2.6.7** A person with myxoedema

speech, slow pulse and respiratory rates, and a tendency to become constipated (a diet high in fibre should be encouraged). The skin becomes thickened and coarse, hair becomes thin and the patient puts on weight. In the adult, changes due to lack of thyroid hormones are readily reversed with the administration of exogenous hormones provided the condition is diagnosed at an early stage. The diagnosis can be made on biochemical grounds when the patient complains of typical but mild features of the disease long before developing the marked effects seen in **Fig. 2.6.7**. Treatment is more difficult when the tissues, including the heart, have been damaged by long-established hypothyroidism.

## DEVELOPMENTAL ISSUES

### THYROID DISORDERS IN INFANTS AND CHILDREN

These are relatively uncommon but it is particularly important to recognize them so that they can be treated at an early stage to avoid permanent damage. **Hypothyroidism** in the infant born with an absent or much impaired thyroid can be catastrophic if not diagnosed and remedied at

an early stage. This is because adequate thyroid hormones are essential for normal development of the brain and normal growth of the body. Certain anatomical, physiological and mental problems occur in addition to those described for adults. Without thyroid hormone replacement the child will be mentally retarded and dwarfed (**cretinism**), retaining the proportions of an infant, with a large head and short arms and legs. The eyes tend to be far apart, the tongue protrudes, the bridge of the nose is depressed and an umbilical hernia is common. Bone development is delayed and the posterior fontanelle is large. The child is sluggish, sleeps more than a normal baby and has poor muscle power. Replacement hormone at an early stage ensures normal development.

**Hyperthyroidism** is uncommon in children. Its presentation is similar to that in adults with the addition that behaviour problems might occur and active, restless movements might cause difficulties in achieving a diagnosis. Radioactive iodine is not used in treatment at this early age because of the increased risk of cancer developing later in life due to the late effects of the radioactivity. The alternative options are antithyroid drugs or surgical removal of part of the overactive gland.

## Formation and release of thyroid hormones

The thyroid gland is in the form of two lobes lying either side of the trachea just below the larynx; the lobes are connected by a bridge, called the **isthmus**, passing in front of the trachea. It originates in fetal life from a pouching in of the epithelium forming the pharynx and moves down from the base of the tongue to its normal position in the neck. Occasionally, this migration is interrupted and parts of the thyroid tissue are left along the track of the descent. The gland is composed of many follicles lined with epithelial cells and filled with colloid, a substance secreted by the lining epithelial cells. The amount of colloid present varies with the degree of activity of the gland, being reduced when large amounts of thyroid hormones are released.

The epithelial cells of the thyroid secrete a complex protein molecule, **thyroglobulin**, into the colloid within the follicles of the gland. The amino acid tyrosine is one of the component parts of this molecule and it is this amino acid that is the basis for the formation of **thyroxine** ($T_4$) and **tri-iodothyronine** ($T_3$), the thyroid hormones. Each molecule of hormone is formed from two molecules of tyrosine, with added iodine. Thyroxine contains four atoms of iodine, whereas tri-iodothyronine only contains three atoms of iodine per molecule of hormone. It is now suggested that thyroxine is a form of prohormone because much of it is converted into tri-iodothyronine in the tissues, and it is this that is available to the tissues and is active at the cellular level.

The thyroid hormones are stored in the follicles of the gland before release into the bloodstream. The secretion of the thyroid hormones begins at about the twelfth week of gestation and increases steadily until the end of the pregnancy.

The iodine required for the formation of the thyroid hormones is obtained in the diet, approximately 1.2 mmol being required daily, and is carried in the bloodstream. The cells of the thyroid gland have a particular affinity for iodine and are able to transfer iodine from the blood into the cells, by means of the iodide pump, and concentrate it in the follicles of the gland in combination with thyroglobulin. As well as the treatment of hyperthyroidism mentioned above, this ability to concentrate iodine is used in treatment of carcinoma of the thyroid gland with radioactive iodine, which is similarly concentrated in the thyroid gland and thus the effect is localized.

Transport mechanisms within the thyroid cells engulf thyroglobulin from the colloid. Enzymes split the thyroid hormones off the large protein molecule and they are released into the blood capillaries for transport around the body.

## Transport and breakdown of thyroid hormones

On entering the blood, both hormones combine with plasma proteins, particularly thyroxine-binding globulin, and can be measured as protein-bound iodine. Thyroxine has a greater affinity for plasma proteins than has tri-iodothyronine. Only about 0.05% of thyroxine and 0.3% of tri-iodothyronine are in the free form in the plasma. However, the amount of $T_4$ secreted daily is greater than that of $T_3$, and the concentrations free in the plasma are 75–150 mmol/L of $T_4$ and 1.1–2.2 mmol/L of $T_3$. $T_3$ has a half-life of 24 hours and $T_4$ a half-life of 6 days. It is only the free hormone that is available for its action on the tissues, and for metabolism and excretion.

The thyroid hormones are broken down in many tissues and the iodine returned to the bloodstream. Some of this is taken up again by the thyroid gland and reused; the rest is excreted in the urine. Thyroid hormones are conjugated in the liver and excreted in the bile, although some might be reabsorbed from the gut and then excreted by the kidneys.

## Regulation of thyroid secretion

This follows the general pattern of **Fig. 2.6.3**, and the details for regulating the secretion of thyroid hormones are shown in **Fig. 2.6.8**. To maintain the metabolic rate within normal limits, it is essential that the level of thyroid hormones available to the tissues is precisely controlled, and this is achieved mainly through negative feedback from $T_3$, mainly to the anterior pituitary, thus regulating the amount of **thyroid-stimulating hormone** (TSH, thyrotrophin or thyrotropin). As with other anterior pituitary functions, **thyrotrophin-releasing hormone** (TRH; produced by the hypothalamus) can also influence the amount of TSH secreted from the anterior pituitary gland. The TSH stimulates the secretion of thyroid hormones by increasing the production of cAMP in the thyroid cells, thus influencing the activities of the thyroid gland. High levels of TSH secretion lead to the following changes in thyroid function:

- extraction of iodine from the blood is increased
- thyroid hormone release from thyroglobulin is increased
- thyroid cells increase in size and secrete more hormone.

When the thyroid gland is unable to produce enough thyroid hormones for some reason, e.g. inadequate supply of iodine, lack of feedback inhibition results in a continued high level of TSH. This leads to an enlarged thyroid gland, or simple **goitre**.

## Control of glucose metabolism

Glucose is a special source of energy for body function. Many cells, including exercising muscle, use fatty acids or ketones for energy. However, they can only do so efficiently when blending them with glucose as a mitochondrial energy source. About half the energy must be derived from glucose for efficient cell function. Otherwise, unused fatty products tend to accumulate, producing a degree of ketoacidosis. This leads to mild poisoning so that the patient feels lethargic, as during a period of fasting when glucose stores have been used up.

The brain and a few other tissues, however, rely solely on glucose for energy. Furthermore, the brain, unlike skeletal and cardiac muscle, has no glycogen stores so relies entirely on the circulating blood glucose. When the blood glucose falls (**hypoglycaemia**) to about half, brain function is impaired and the patient becomes confused and drowsy. A more severe fall can cause coma and death. It is, therefore, essential that a continuous supply of glucose is available. Prolonged hypoglycaemia can result in permanent

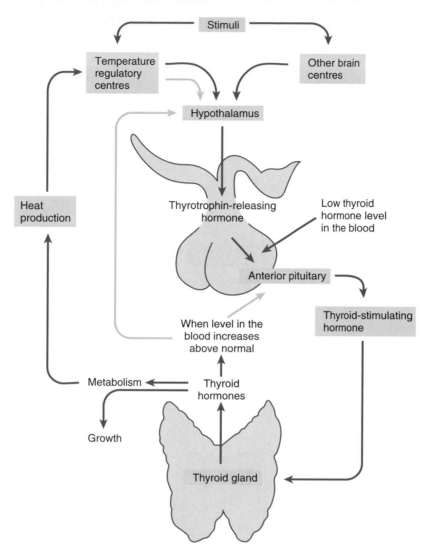

**Figure 2.6.8** Regulation of thyroid hormone secretion; yellow arrows indicate inhibition

brain damage. Only in exceptional circumstances, such as lack of sufficient food for some weeks, when the body is living largely on its fat stores, can brain cells begin to form the enzymes to utilize ketones as an energy source. The normal fasting blood glucose level is around 4 to 6 mmol/L, rising to around 7–9 mmol/L after a meal and then falling to the fasting level again over a period of about 2 hours. **Figure 2.6.9** summarizes the events involved in the maintenance of the blood glucose concentration within normal limits (**blood glucose homeostasis**). The processes involved are mainly regulated by hormonal activity.

## Glucose metabolism

### After a meal

Glucose is obtained from the digestion of carbohydrates in the diet. The simple sugars (monosaccharides) released are absorbed through the intestinal wall and transported in the hepatic portal system to the liver. Here, fructose and galactose are converted into glucose, although some fructose can be metabolized directly. After a meal, the blood glucose level rises and then begins to fall as it is stored as glycogen in the muscles for use during exercise and in the liver for release into the circulation when the blood glucose tends to fall. A major function of the hormone **insulin** is to stimulate storage of glucose as glycogen, but it also stimulates cellular uptake of other products of digestion, especially fatty acids in fat stores, and amino acids and potassium into cells generally. Depending on activity, the glycogen stores will last for several hours to about a day. Thus the pattern of eating several times a day means that we maintain adequate glucose reserves most of the time.

### Use of glucose for energy

Glucose taken up by the cells goes through a series of chemical reactions, mainly in the mitochondria to

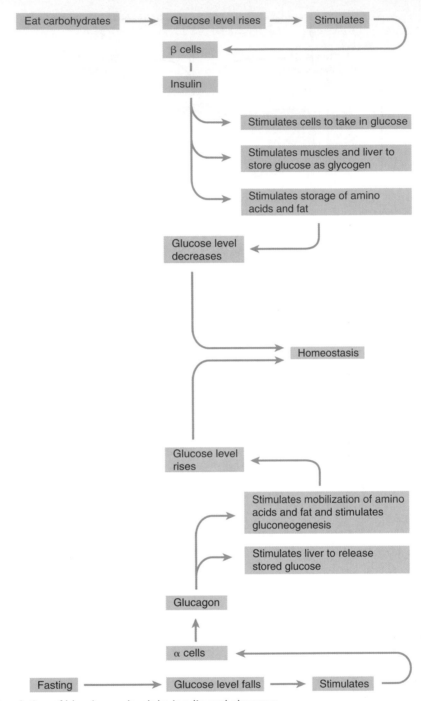

**Figure 2.6.9** Regulation of blood sugar levels by insulin and glucagon

extract the energy within its molecular structure. The energy made available is stored in the high-energy molecule **adenosine triphosphate (ATP)**, and is then available for use throughout the cell. The first stage in the catabolism of glucose is the **glycolysis pathway (Fig. 2.6.10)**, which takes place in the **cytoplasm** of the cell. During the series of reactions making up this pathway, the 6-carbon molecule (glucose) is split into two 3-carbon molecules of glyceraldehyde and then converted into pyruvate. Under anaerobic conditions, when adequate oxygen is not

available, pyruvate is converted into lactate and a net total of only two molecules of ATP are formed from the one molecule of glucose.

Under aerobic conditions, however, the pyruvate is transported into the **mitochondria** of the cell where very much more energy can be extracted. Here it is converted into acetate (a 2-carbon molecule) and, in combination with coenzyme-A, to acetyl-CoA. The mitochondria have been described as the 'powerhouses' of the cell and metabolic pathways concerned mainly with the extraction of energy from

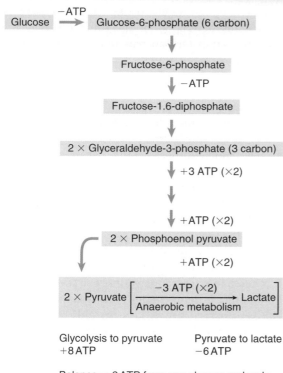

**Figure 2.6.10** A summary of glycolysis under anaerobic conditions. ATP, adenosine triphosphate

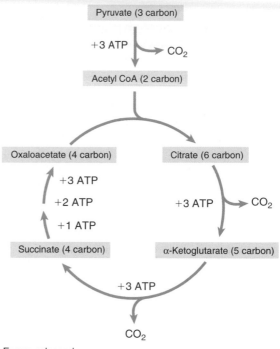

**Figure 2.6.11** A summary of the Krebs' cycle. ATP, adenosine triphosphate

substances and the storage of that energy in the form of ATP are located here. Acetyl-CoA is at the junction of these major metabolic pathways. Particularly important amongst these is the **Krebs' cycle** (or **citric acid** or **tricarboxylic acid** (TCA) cycle), which is the major route for the formation of ATP. A brief outline of the Krebs' cycle is shown in **Fig. 2.6.11**. Ultimately, the breakdown of one glucose molecule, with adequate oxygen available, produces 38 molecules of ATP. The difference between this and the two molecules formed under anaerobic conditions helps to explain the lethargy and rapid tiring of patients with tissue hypoxia, whether due to respiratory, cardiac or blood disease. It also emphasizes the crucial importance of appropriate and careful administration of oxygen to critically ill patients.

Another situation when lactate is formed is during severe exercise. When someone pushes strenuous exercise to the limit, maximal uptake of oxygen will be reached and further energy is derived, relatively briefly, from anaerobic glycolysis involving lactate production. It is striking that two contrasting groups of people can develop high levels of lactate – athletes performing at an exceptionally high level and severely ill patients in intensive care, where even the resting oxygen requirements of the tissues cannot be met, despite optimal supportive treatment.

## Fasting

During fasting there are two main considerations in metabolism. First, it is essential to maintain the blood glucose level for brain function to continue. Second, it is necessary to supply an adequate energy source for all tissues of the body.

The blood glucose level is maintained in two ways. First, liver glycogen is broken down to glucose (by a process known as **glycogenolysis**); the glucose is released into the bloodstream. However, the hepatic glycogen store is relatively small – about 0.15 kg of glycogen, representing about 600 kcal (2.5 MJ). This will be supplemented by fat for energy source, but even so will become depleted rapidly, possibly even overnight and certainly within 24–36 hours. At this stage hunger becomes marked.

However, people can survive in famine conditions for long periods with an energy deficit – using more energy than is available in their food. Healthy people can survive complete deprivation of food (but not fluid) for around 2–3 months. They make use of the second source of blood glucose, through **gluconeogenesis** (the formation of new glucose) from glycerol (released from triglycerides) and amino acids (from protein breakdown). This maintains a reduced daily supply of glucose that is adequate to maintain life.

However, most of the body's energy is now derived directly from the fat stores (mainly subcutaneous).

A non-obese 70-kg man has fat stores equivalent to about 15% of his body weight. This works out at 10.5 kg of fat, which liberate around 100 000 kcal (about 420 MJ). During prolonged starvation people are not usually capable of doing much physical work, so the energy from the fat can be spread over 2–3 months. Obese people can probably survive a little longer. However, as well as the ketosis of starvation, prolonged starvation is also associated with depletion of vitamins not stored in the body (e.g. vitamin C). So the person gradually becomes weaker and is afflicted by the effects of severe vitamin deficiency.

One of the body's methods of surviving prolonged starvation or undernutrition is to adapt to relatively large-scale use of ketones, including in the brain. Pathways for maintaining glucose supplies are shown in **Fig. 2.6.12** – on the left when glucose from the diet is adequate, and on the right when it is not.

## Endocrine regulation of blood glucose level

Two hormones play a major role in blood glucose homeostasis: **insulin**, produced by the β cells of the islets of Langerhans in the pancreas, and **glucagon**,

produced by the α cells of the islets. The islets of Langerhans develop from the same tissue as the exocrine part of the pancreas and, as islets of tissue with a good blood supply, become separated from the lumen of the smaller pancreatic ducts. The two hormones released by the islets function in opposite directions; insulin acts to lower the blood glucose level, mainly during absorption of a meal, and glucagon to cause an increase, mainly after absorption is complete. Before birth, when nutrition is obtained steadily from the placenta and the gut is inactive, the secretion of glucagon prevents hypoglycaemia in the fetus. The normal regulatory pattern involving the two hormones begins with oral feeding after birth.

Although the blood glucose level is maintained steady for much of the time there are situations when it is raised, e.g. in dealing with severe stress. A number of other hormones contribute to a rise in blood glucose, particularly glucocorticoids, adrenaline (epinephrine), thyroxine and growth hormone.

### Insulin

The effects of insulin are anabolic in nature and it has been described as 'the hormone of nutrient storage'. Insulin is secreted in large amounts during

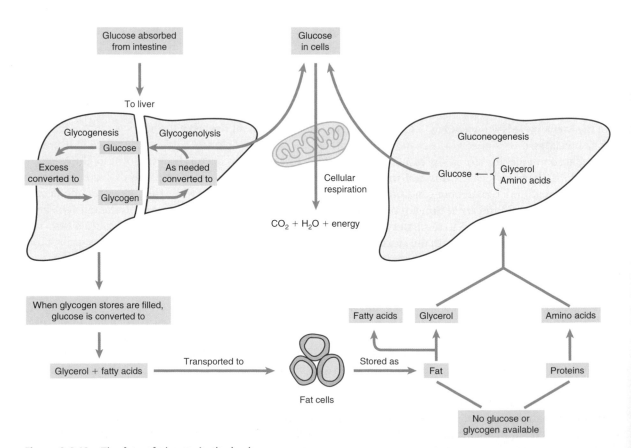

**Figure 2.6.12** The fate of glucose in the body

a meal and is essential for adequate uptake into cells of glucose, amino acids and potassium. After absorption and storage of the products of digestion, much less insulin is secreted until the next meal. The major metabolic effects of insulin are in skeletal muscle, adipose tissue and the liver.

Insulin binds firmly to a receptor site on the cell membrane and it appears that it carries out most of its functions without entering the cell. The effects of insulin on muscle and adipose tissue are not the same as its effect on the liver. One of the main results of the action of insulin on muscle and adipose tissue is the stimulation of the transport of glucose and a number of other substances, including amino acids and potassium, across the cell membrane into the cell. The increased glucose entry into the cell leads to an increase in all glucose metabolism within the cell, so that glycogen is laid down in muscle cells and the catabolism of glucose to acetyl-CoA is increased. Insulin also stimulates the synthesis and deposition of triglycerides in adipose tissue and inhibits the release of fatty acids. It also appears to stimulate protein formation from the amino acids entering the cell and has been shown to reduce protein breakdown. Insulin is not needed for the uptake of fats into cells as the largely lipid membrane is freely permeable to other lipids.

In the liver, the cell membrane is not a barrier to the passage of glucose but insulin increases the synthesis and hence storage of glycogen in the liver. It also favours hepatic synthesis of protein and lipid and decreases gluconeogenesis from protein breakdown.

## Biosynthesis and metabolism of insulin

Insulin is made up of two chains of 21 and 30 amino acids. These chains lie alongside each other and are linked by chemical bonds. Insulin can thus be regarded as a fairly large peptide or a fairly small protein. Insulin synthesis starts in the endoplasmic reticulum of the β cells of the pancreas, which produce proinsulin, which has no, or very little, endocrine activity. Proinsulin is then converted into insulin in the Golgi body of the β cell, and is stored in secretory granules until released.

The pancreas stores about five times the amount of insulin that is secreted daily; daily secretion being about 40 international units (iu). When the pancreas is stimulated, secretory granules containing the insulin move to the cell membrane, fuse with it, and liberate the free hormone into the extracellular fluid, from which it moves into the capillaries to be transported round the body to its sites of action. During prolonged secretion of insulin after a meal, much of the released insulin has been newly synthesized.

Insulin shares the short half-life (about 5 minutes) of many hormones, which favours prompt withdrawal of its action when nutrient absorption ceases. It is broken down by a protease found mainly in the liver and kidneys.

## Regulation of insulin secretion during assimilation of food

It is important that secretion of insulin is related closely to the flood of nutrients entering the circulation with absorption of a meal. Three main controlling mechanisms help to fit insulin secretion to insulin requirements.

First, when we begin a meal there is nervous release by the vagus (X) nerve (parasympathetic), which mobilizes insulin to deal with the absorption that begins soon after food enters the stomach. Second, the gut is galvanized into action by digestive hormones such as gastrin and secretin, and these same hormones also stimulate release of insulin from the pancreas. Third, as the major nutrients, such as glucose and amino acids, build up in the circulation, they further stimulate the release of insulin. Thus, although glucose is the dominant stimulator of insulin release, it has been found that oral glucose leads to more release of insulin than intravenous injection of the same amount of glucose. In the fasting state (when no more nutrients are being absorbed) secretion of insulin is closely related to the blood glucose level, in true homeostatic fashion.

It has been found that a high-fibre diet reduces the amount of insulin required for diabetic control. This may be related to a slowing in the rate of absorption of nutrients, thus requiring lower levels of insulin.

## Glucagon

Glucagon in many ways has opposite effects to insulin. Whereas insulin favours blood glucose homeostasis by lowering it when it rises, glucagon favours homeostasis by raising it when it falls. Glucagon, a smaller peptide than insulin, is a single chain of 29 amino acids. It is released from the α cells of the pancreas, particularly in response to a low blood glucose level (hypoglycaemia) and causes a rapid increase in the blood glucose level. It acts mainly on the liver and causes a rapid rise in cAMP within the cells. This leads to an increase in glycogenolysis and inhibition of glycogenesis. Thus, there is a rise in the amount of glucose released from the breakdown of glycogen. Gluconeogenesis and the formation of ketones are also enhanced. Within adipose tissue, glucagon stimulates fat breakdown and the liberation of fatty acids.

Glucagon has a half-life of 5 to 10 minutes and is broken down largely in the liver.

## Coordinated regulation of glucose metabolism

A number of hormones are involved in regulating or modifying glucose metabolism. Insulin alone acts to reduce the blood glucose concentration, whereas glucagon, catecholamines, glucocorticoids, growth hormone and thyroxine all contribute to a rise in blood glucose level. These apparently contradictory effects become clearer when we realize that insulin has the main positive effect of storing or assimilating nutrients after absorption. It thus avoids severe hyperglycaemia (raised blood glucose) after a meal, with the consequent spilling-over of nutrients into the urine where they would be lost to the body. The hormones that raise the blood glucose tend to be involved in situations where body metabolism must increase, notably during strenuous exercise and response to severe injury. Overall, this is a typical example of homeostasis, where body properties such as the blood glucose level are kept within tight limits most of the time but where they can move outside the normal level when unusual circumstances require it.

Regulation of glucose metabolism becomes less effective with increasing age. Decreased sensitivity to insulin develops, possibly due to a reduction in the number of insulin receptors on the body cells. Some individuals will maintain blood glucose within normal limits by increasing their secretion of insulin. Others will be unable to achieve this and will show impaired glucose homeostasis. It seems that demands on the pancreatic cells for insulin are increased when people eat more than they need and become obese. Virtually all countries of the world are experiencing an epidemic of decreased activity (hence decreased nutritional requirements), excessive eating (as food becomes more available in most countries) and increasing obesity at all ages. In this situation, the form of diabetes mellitus associated with overweight is rapidly becoming more common.

### CLINICAL APPLICATIONS

#### DIABETES MELLITUS

This – by far the most common of the endocrine disorders – is a condition in which there is an absolute or relative lack of insulin for the requirements of the tissues. If untreated, severe forms can cause extreme body wasting and eventual coma and death, and before insulin became available for treatment about eighty years ago the disease was often fatal.

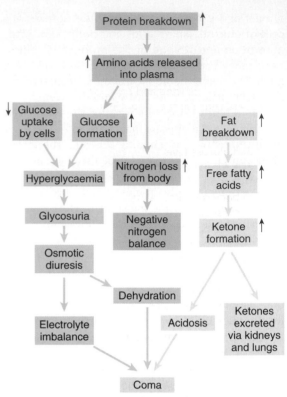

**Figure 2.6.13** The physiological effects of diabetes mellitus

Abnormalities affect metabolism of carbohydrates, proteins and fats as shown in **Fig. 2.6.13**. There are many potential long-term complications.

For centuries, long before the advent of biochemical tests for glucose, diabetes mellitus was recognized by the passing of copious sweet urine. The word 'diabetes' refers to copious urine and 'mellitus' means sweet – taste being the only way the presence of glucose in the urine could then be detected. Diabetes mellitus (there is also a rare disease called diabetes insipidus, in which the copious urine is not sweet, or 'insipid') is still often diagnosed by finding glucose in the urine, although more precise diagnosis requires measuring the blood glucose level.

Although there are various ways of classifying diabetes mellitus, probably the most useful practical way is to divide it into insulin-dependent diabetes mellitus (IDDM) and non-insulin-dependent diabetes mellitus (NIDDM).

**Insulin-dependent diabetes** is also called type I or juvenile-onset, because it often starts in the first two or three decades of life, quite commonly in young children. It is the type in which life-threatening coma (ketoacidosis) can rapidly develop and it requires regular injections of insulin for its control. The pancreatic β cells are severely damaged.

**Non-insulin-dependent diabetes** (type II) is also called maturity-onset because it most often starts in late middle age or old age. There is a *relative* lack of insulin due to the development of insulin resistance, most commonly due to obesity. When the diet is restricted and body weight returns towards normal the condition is usually improved or cured. Although insulin is not required, oral drugs might be needed to maintain a normal blood glucose level.

The fundamental problem in all forms of diabetes mellitus is that assimilation of nutrients into body cells after a meal is impaired. This has two consequences – cellular metabolism is abnormal and nutrients accumulate in the circulation, giving high levels of glucose in particular. When people without diabetes have a meal their blood glucose level rises from about 5 to about 7–8 mmol/L glucose. In diabetics, the level rises above 10 and may reach 30–40 mmol/L. A high blood glucose is termed **hyperglycaemia**. A blood level of 10 mmol/L is crucial because above this level the kidneys can no longer reabsorb the filtered glucose and it spills over into the urine to be lost. The level of 10 mmol/L is called the **renal threshold** for glucose, and glucose in the urine is termed **glycosuria**. Other nutrients, including amino acids, are similarly lost. Thus much of the ingested nutrition does not benefit the body and there is a state of partial **tissue starvation**.

At the same time, the particles of glucose and other nutrients in the urine retain water osmotically, so that the diabetic has an increased urinary volume (**osmotic diuresis**). This depletes the body fluids (**dehydration**), causing excessive thirst and, in severe cases, collapse of the circulation (**shock**). The passage of glucose-laden urine can lead to pruritus; it is important, therefore, that patients who have glycosuria are encouraged to be scrupulous in their personal hygiene.

Some of the most severe effects of uncontrolled diabetes mellitus are due to the abnormal cellular metabolism. The fundamental cause is lack of insulin but the effects are complex and include unbalanced actions of the hormones that mobilize glucose and particularly the production of large amounts of toxic products of fat metabolism. These include **ketones**, which spill over into the urine (where they can be detected biochemically), and **excess hydrogen ions** – hence the term 'ketoacidosis'. Arterial blood pH falls rapidly to low levels. These biochemical changes cause progressive confusion and drowsiness in the patient and eventually life-threatening **coma**.

However, it is important to realize that most older people developing diabetes do not have dramatic symptoms and that their hyperglycaemia is often diagnosed at routine testing, when they present with problems that arise as general complications of diabetes. These complications can affect most body systems. Many arise from damage to blood vessels so that the organ involved has an inadequate blood supply. These common complications will be considered shortly.

## COMA IN DIABETICS

Patients with diabetes are prone to two contrasting causes of coma, one (described above) due to too little insulin and the other due to too much insulin. The nurse should be able to differentiate between these two. In general, patients with too little insulin have **ketoacidotic coma**, with a combination of hyperglycaemia, ketoacidosis and dehydration in various proportions. Patients with severe acidosis tend to have deep, rapid breathing in an attempt to reduce the acidosis by excreting carbon dioxide. This type of coma usually takes several days to reach a severe level.

Diabetics can also go into coma much more rapidly because an excess insulin, in relation to diet, causes an abnormal fall in blood glucose – **hypoglycaemic coma**. In this situation the patient is not dehydrated or acidotic and breathes normally. The condition occurs almost entirely in diabetics treated with insulin. The problem is that the insulin level is temporarily much higher than needed. The blood glucose level plummets and, when it has fallen to about half the normal level, the brain is deprived of its energy source and can no longer function normally. An early warning sign is mildly abnormal behaviour by the patient, who might appear confused, drowsy or perhaps aggressive. Physiological functions try to restore the blood glucose level. A fall in blood glucose stimulates the patient's sympathetic system. As well as mobilizing glucose from glycogen stores, this produces other typical signs that help confirm the diagnosis of hypoglycaemia – sweating, tremor and a rapid bounding pulse. Treatment to raise the blood glucose level must be given urgently to prevent deterioration and brain damage. Giving the patient something sweet by mouth can terminate the attack but if the patient is unconscious then intravenous glucose will be necessary. It is essential that patients and their relatives are taught to identify the onset of hypoglycaemia and to take immediate action. In some cases, relatives and friends are particularly important when impaired brain function due to hypoglycaemia prevents the patient from recognizing the problem.

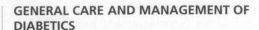
## GENERAL CARE AND MANAGEMENT OF DIABETICS

A major nursing role in the care of the diabetic patient is to educate him or her: (i) to adapt to and cope with the problems that the disease can present; and (ii) to be aware of and, where possible, prevent potential complications.

Long-term complications can be minimized by optimizing control of the condition. The patient needs to be able to balance three components – dietary intake of energy, the amount of insulin injected and the amount of exercise taken. Strenuous exercise is possible and generally desirable, but it is important to realize that it can greatly increase nutritional energy requirements and greatly decrease insulin requirements. Less insulin is needed because exercise facilitates the uptake and use of glucose. To be able to adjust these three factors safely to maintain the blood glucose level in balance, the patient must be able to monitor blood glucose regularly. Multiple daily injections of insulin are also needed to cover meals and to avoid hypoglycaemia when exercising or fasting, particularly overnight. This can be very demanding for patients and families.

A number of complications can develop as a result of long-standing diabetes, particularly if poorly controlled. Blood vessels, including small vessels, are liable to fatty deposits in their walls (**atherosclerosis**). This can arise in many sites, increasing the risk of blocked arteries in the heart or brain. Disease of small blood vessels can be the cause of damage to nerves (**neuropathies**). A disabling complication is **ulceration of the feet**, which can be very slow to heal. This might be related to a combination of poor circulation (**ischaemia**) and damage due to ill-fitting shoes, undetected because neuropathy has impaired perception of pain locally. Meticulous foot care is therefore essential and regular care by a podiatrist desirable. Cutting the toe nails needs particular care.

Diabetics tend to be vulnerable to infection of the urinary tract and skin, probably due to the higher-than-normal glucose levels in both blood and urine. The nurse should assist the patient to recognize signs of impending infections and to take appropriate action. Both nurse and patient should feel confident in recognizing the clinical features of hypoglycaemic and hyperglycaemic comas. Education towards self-care must be a priority in the nursing care of all patients with this chronic condition.

**Insulin for injection** can come from various sources. For many years insulin was obtained as a byproduct of the meat industry from cows (bovine) or pigs (porcine). Some patients still receive these forms, which differ from human insulin in having several different amino acids, although the effects are virtually identical to human insulin. Developments in biotechnology have now made it possible to obtain insulin identical in structure to human insulin by inserting the genes for insulin synthesis into bacteria.

Insulin is prepared in short-, medium- and long-acting forms and several subcutaneous injections of different types of insulin can be given throughout the day. It is also possible to administer insulin continuously through an infusion pump with additional amounts administered at meal times. A possible disadvantage of these methods is that the insulin enters the general bloodstream. By contrast, insulin released normally from the pancreas passes directly to the liver in the hepatic portal circulation, to act there and be partially broken down. Efforts are being made to find an effective means of transplanting islet cells into patients to avoid some of these complications.

Patients started on regular treatment with insulin need to be taught how to monitor their blood glucose levels. A drop of blood is obtained and the glucose level measured in a glucometer. When the patient is a child, working with all members of the family, particularly the parents, becomes extremely important.

## Fluid and electrolyte balance

The function of the kidneys in fluid and electrolyte balance is considered in Chapter 5.4. Here, the role of the endocrine system in controlling renal function is discussed. Two major hormones are involved and will be considered in detail. Although a number of other hormones have a role in regulating fluid and electrolytes (see the regulation of calcium ions, discussed in the next section of this chapter, p. 234), two major hormones dominate the picture. These are **antidiuretic hormone** (ADH), also known as vasopressin, and **aldosterone**. They control, respectively, total body water and extracellular fluid volume, the regulation of which is crucial to homeostasis.

### Total body water

The cells of the human body are highly complex, with many delicate structures (receptors, ion channels) in the membrane and highly organized intracellular organelles, such as the mitochondria and the Golgi system for packaging secretions. These all function in a fluid medium, which in total constitutes the intracellular fluid – between a third and a half of the body mass. If body water is depleted, the cells shrink, like withered flowers, and function gradually grinds to a halt. If there is too much water in the cells, they swell up and the delicate cellular structures become distorted and again cease to function. To avoid these twin disasters we have a major detector system and two major effector systems for maintaining water homeostasis. The effector systems are well known – if we are short of water we develop **thirst** and are compelled to drink; if we have too much water we produce a greatly increased urinary volume, a **diuresis**.

The major detector system consists of cells in the hypothalamus known as **osmoreceptors**. These cells, like other body cells, shrink when we are short of water and swell when we have too much. When they **shrink** they send messages to higher parts of the brain to make us **thirsty**. They also secrete **antidiuretic hormone** from their nerve terminals in the posterior pituitary, so that we do not have a diuresis but retain most of our body water.

When the osmoreceptor cells **swell**, they send signals to make us want to **stop drinking** and they stop secreting antidiuretic hormone. The hormone (half-life about 5 minutes) falls rapidly in concentration so that in half an hour or less we start to produce large volumes of urine (a **diuresis**).

The detector cells are called osmoreceptors because they are responding to changes in the dilution of the body fluids. This can be measured in a sample of the plasma and is described as **osmolality**. It is a measure of the number of dissolved particles. When the number of particles is high, the osmolality is high. The osmolality is the same inside and outside the body cells because water moves freely so that if there is even a slight gradient in osmolality, the water moves towards the more concentrated area to dilute it. Body osmolality, measured in plasma, is normally around 290 milliosmoles per kg of water. It is the sum of all dissolved particles, mainly sodium, chloride, bicarbonate and potassium ions, but also glucose and urea molecules. Because, as an approximation, millimoles and milliosmoles are similar for many dissolved particles, plasma solutes can be combined to estimate osmolality as follows:

| | |
|---|---|
| sodium | 140 mmol/L |
| chloride | 100 mmol/L |
| bicarbonate | 25 mmol/L |
| potassium | 5 mmol/L |
| glucose | 5 mmol/L |
| urea | 5 mmol/L |
| others | 10 mmol/L |
| **Total** | 290 mmol/L, equivalent to approximately 290 mosmol/L. |

Thus a major rise in glucose can increase osmolality, disturbing cellular function as discussed earlier.

## Extracellular volume

The extracellular fluid volume is about half that of total cell volume. It is the bathing fluid that surrounds the body cells (**interstitial fluid**) plus the **plasma** in the blood. If the extracellular volume falls, the tissues begin to look shrunken (and babies have sunken fontanelles) and the blood volume falls. In severe cases, the lowered blood volume has the same effect as after serious haemorrhage and patients suffer circulatory failure (**shock**) with low blood pressure, weakness and inability to stand up without fainting. A relatively complicated system (considered shortly) recognizes this disturbance of the circulation and leads to increased secretion of **aldosterone**. Aldosterone acts on the kidneys to retain more than usual of the filtered salt (sodium chloride). Retention of this salt is accompanied by an equivalent amount of water to maintain normal osmolality, so the end effect is to restore the body's extracellular volume.

The signs and symptoms of disturbances of fluid and electrolyte balance in patients are rather non-specific, particularly in the early stages, and diagnosis depends partly on suspicion. A clear understanding by the nurse of the normal physiology and the possible disturbances that can occur, and a knowledge of the circumstances when they are most likely to develop is essential.

It is important to realize that no amount of hormonal activity can restore body fluids if there is a deficit and the patient cannot take fluids – hence the need for intravenous infusion in serious disturbances. In these cases, accurate monitoring of fluid intake and output is essential. The nurse is responsible for recording **fluid output** in the form of urine, vomiting, faeces (particularly when fluid content is increased in diarrhoea) and losses from surgical drains and other sites. In working out fluid requirements, allowance also needs to be made for fluid lost by evaporation from the respiratory tract and skin (even in the absence of sweating) – this is called **insensible water loss** and amounts to about a litre a day. Precise management of serious disturbances of body fluids is a major roll of high-dependency and intensive care units.

The major hormones that regulate the body fluids – antidiuretic hormone and aldosterone will now be considered.

## Antidiuretic hormone (ADH, vasopressin)

As mentioned above, antidiuretic hormone is one of the hormones synthesized in the hypothalamus and released from the posterior pituitary gland. As its name suggests, it prevents diuresis by increasing the reabsorption of water from the renal tubules back into the body. Water is retained within the body and the plasma osmolality is maintained at about 290 milliosmol/kg of water (normal range 285–295 mosmol/kg). Antidiuretic hormone also has a direct constrictor effect on the smooth muscle of blood vessels, leading to a rise in blood pressure, but only at levels above those required for fluid balance regulation. Thus the name vasopressin is less appropriate than antidiuretic hormone, although it is commonly used.

Antidiuretic hormone regulates the amount of water retained in the body by increasing the permeability to water of the distal region of each renal nephron. It does this by opening water channels and the water in the nephron is drawn into the interstitial fluid of the kidney by powerful osmotic forces. These exist for two reasons (see Chapter 5.4). First, the fluid entering the distal nephron (collecting duct) is very dilute, with an osmolality well below the normal body value. Second, cells more proximal in the nephron (loop of Henle) create a highly concentrated interstitial fluid in the renal medulla and particularly in the inner medulla near where urine leaves the kidney. The gradient is normally at least tenfold, with the collecting duct osmolality 100 mosmol/kg or below and the interstitial fluid osmolality 1000 mosmol/kg or more.

In the **absence of antidiuretic hormone** the collecting ducts are impermeable to water and **large volumes of dilute urine** are lost. The urine in these circumstances is almost colourless, because the urochrome that gives urine its colour is so highly dilute. When there is a **high level of antidiuretic hormone** the water channels are open and nearly all the fluid in the collecting ducts is absorbed into the body, leading to a **small volume of highly concentrated urine**. This urine is dark yellow. The ability to vary the urine between these two extremes – from about 20–30 mL/hour to several hundred mL/hour in an adult – is a sign of healthy kidneys.

## CLINICAL APPLICATIONS

**Diabetes insipidus** (large volumes of tasteless urine) is a rare condition in which antidiuretic hormone is not secreted (or the kidney cannot respond to it). Patients produce 5–10 or more litres of very dilute urine in a 24-hour period (the normal volume with an average fluid intake in temperate climates is 1–2 L per day). This results in a raging thirst and patients have to drink huge amounts of fluid for replacement. If for any reason this fluid is not available, the body water will be rapidly depleted and a patient could die, rather like someone lost in a burning desert. With age, the range of urinary concentration contracts, due to gradual decline in renal function. Older patients are less able to withstand fluid loss for any reason, including poor intake because of intestinal disturbances including obstruction and food poisoning. When dehydrated, patients may require 2-hourly pressure area care to prevent damage to their skin, and frequent mouth care to refresh their dry mouths.

Diabetes insipidus can be treated effectively by administration of the antidiuretic hormone by nasal spray (the small peptide of nine amino acids, hence 'nonapeptide', is easily absorbed here).

## Secretion and metabolism of antidiuretic hormone

Antidiuretic hormone has a very similar structure to oxytocin, the other nonapeptide hormone secreted from the posterior pituitary gland; they differ by only two amino acids. Both are synthesized in nerve cell bodies in the hypothalamus and pass down the axons of the nerves to the posterior pituitary gland, where they are stored in neurosecretory granules in combination with a protein, neurophysin. The release of either hormone from the axon of the specific neurosecretory cell is triggered by nerve impulses passing down the axon.

Antidiuretic hormone has a short half-life of about 10 minutes. It is not bound to plasma proteins and hence is rapidly inactivated in the liver and kidneys.

## Regulation of secretion (**Fig. 2.6.14**)

As already mentioned, **osmoreceptors** in the anterior hypothalamus shrink when the body is short of water and there is a rise in osmotic pressure. As we know, taking a large amount of salt produces thirst, and this operates by a similar mechanism. The salt is retained mainly in the extracellular fluid, drawing water out of cells osmotically, again stimulating the activity of the nerve cells containing the hormone. If the osmotic pressure falls, secretion of the neurosecretory cells is inhibited. So in general, the higher the osmolality, the more ADH is secreted, the hormone being 'switched off' as the osmolality falls below normal. The urgency with which the body treats a serious drop in osmolality is seen when more fluid than is needed is drunk. A diuresis results in about half an hour and continues until the excess fluid has been eliminated. If for any reason a patient cannot respond in this way, or perhaps has a tumour secreting inappropriate antidiuretic hormone, the body, especially the brain, becomes waterlogged and confusion and coma can result – 'water intoxication'.

So far, body osmolality has been described as the controlling factor in the secretion of antidiuretic hormone, and this is the case in normal life. However, there are a number of situations (**Fig. 2.6.14**) in which antidiuretic hormone is released in much higher amounts and then helps to maintain blood pressure, the name vasopressin becoming appropriate. One such situation is a blood loss sufficient to cause a fall in blood pressure. Arterial baroreceptors detect a fall in pressure, the signal is passed neuronally to the hypothalamus and secretion of antidiuretic hormone rises markedly.

## CLINICAL APPLICATIONS

The pain and stress caused by injury and a surgical operation also increase secretion of antidiuretic hormone, as do exercise and certain drugs, including nicotine and morphine. This is of particular relevance when nursing surgical patients who might be producing large amounts of antidiuretic hormone after operation and will, therefore, form small amounts of urine. This needs to be borne in mind in patients receiving an intravenous infusion, to avoid excess volumes and possible water intoxication. Electrolyte monitoring might indicate this by the presence of a low serum sodium level (hyponatraemia).

## Aldosterone

Aldosterone is the major **mineralocorticoid hormone** secreted from the adrenal cortex. Its name does not help in remembering its function but refers to its chemical structure – an aldehyde steroid. Its function is to raise the body's salt content and hence control extracellular volume. It does this mainly by stimulating the active pumping of sodium ions from the nephron lumen back into the body in the distal convoluted tubule where the final amount of sodium excretion is determined. Associated effects are somewhat complex but the following are the main events:

1. To maintain electrical neutrality, the sodium ions are accompanied by large numbers of chloride ions.
2. To maintain normal osmolality, the sodium and chloride ions are accompanied by appropriate volumes of water. Thus the main function of regulating extracellular volume (largely isotonic saline) is accomplished.
3. The action of aldosterone overlaps with regulation of other ions and it also increases the absorption of sodium in exchange for the excretion of potassium and/or hydrogen ions.

Overall then, aldosterone increases extracellular volume but also tends to increase excretion of potassium and hydrogen ions in the urine. These latter

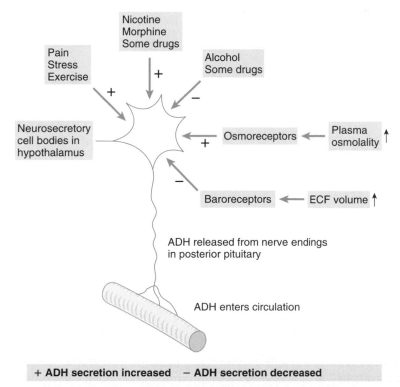

**+ ADH secretion increased    – ADH secretion decreased**

**Figure 2.6.14**  The regulation of antidiuretic hormone (ADH) secretion

231

effects explain some features of excessive aldosterone secretion:

### CLINICAL APPLICATIONS

The effect of **excessive aldosterone secretion** is seen in Conn's syndrome – **primary hyperaldosteronism** (Conn, 1977), in which the adrenal cortex secretes inappropriately large amounts of the hormone. The excessive aldosterone stimulates excessive reabsorption of sodium in the renal tubules. Thus, as explained above, the extracellular fluid volume becomes abnormally large. This increases the blood volume and favours hypertension. The condition can be treated by removal of the affected adrenal gland.

More common than primary hyperaldosteronism is **secondary hyperaldosteronism.** The condition can be secondary to either cardiac or liver failure. In cardiac failure, the weakness of the heart's pumping leads to a poor circulation and a drop in blood pressure, which acts through the normal control of aldosterone secretion (see below) to increase secretion of aldosterone. This can be regarded as a normal body response but, instead of favouring homeostasis, it further disturbs it by

increasing the extracellular fluid volume and making oedema worse. It also adds to the load on the failing heart and impairs its output further – a kind of vicious circle. In liver failure there is impaired breakdown of aldosterone so that oedema (and also fluid accumulation in the peritoneal cavity – ascites) gets worse. In both cases, diuretic therapy improves symptoms by breaking the vicious cycle of increasing extracellular fluid.

Aldosterone is one of the many vital hormones formed from cholesterol (**see Fig. 2.6.4**). The CH=O group at the top left of the molecule is the aldehyde group, which gives the hormone its name. It is metabolized in the liver and kidneys and mainly excreted in the urine. Other corticosteroids, including cortisol, share some of the salt-retaining effect of aldosterone.

## Regulation of secretion

Although adrenocorticotrophic hormone plays a permissive role in the secretion of aldosterone, it is relatively unimportant at physiological levels in controlling the amount of aldosterone secreted. A fall in

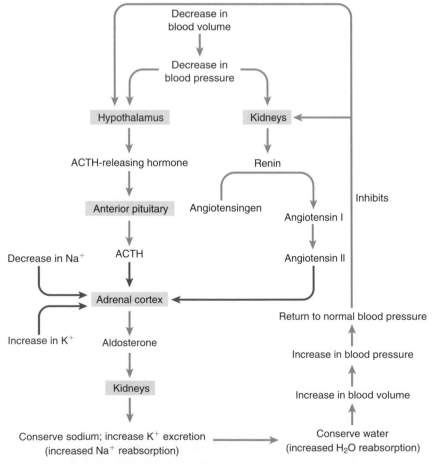

**Figure 2.6.15** Regulation of aldosterone secretion. ACTH, adrenocorticotrophic hormone

serum sodium or a rise in potassium increases the release of aldosterone from the adrenal cortex. In addition, a fall in the extracellular fluid volume increases the secretion of aldosterone through its effect on the kidney and the **renin–angiotensin–aldosterone system**. **Figure 2.6.15** outlines the complex negative feedback systems that contribute to homeostasis of blood volume via extracellular fluid volume.

The renin–angiotensin–aldosterone system is the term used for the major regulation of aldosterone. This system can be modified, with excellent effect, in a number of conditions, including hypertension and heart failure, two conditions in which it is particularly helpful to reduce extracellular fluid volume. The system is controlled mainly by a baroreceptor system within the afferent arteriole of the renal glomerulus. This arteriole is particularly subject to changes in pressure as blood volume fluctuates. It is linked in the **juxtaglomerular apparatus** with cells that release **renin** (nothing to do with digestive rennin, which coagulates milk) when there is a fall in the arteriolar pressure. Causes of a fall in pressure include haemorrhage and cardiac failure.

**Renin**, a proteolytic enzyme, acts on **angiotensinogen** (a plasma protein formed in the liver) to form angiotensin I. Angiotensin I is inactive but is converted into the active angiotensin II (an octapeptide) by a converting enzyme found in endothelial cells widely distributed through the body, particularly in the lungs. The enzyme is generally referred to as ACE – angiotensin converting enzyme.

Angiotensin II has two actions that help to restore arterial blood pressure. It stimulates the secretion of aldosterone from the adrenal cortex and is also a potent vasoconstrictor. Some of the most effective drugs used to treat hypertension and heart failure are angiotensin-converting-enzyme inhibitors.

## Coordinated regulation of water and electrolyte balance

The two hormones, antidiuretic hormone and aldosterone, interact to maintain the balance of water and sodium in the body, as shown in **Fig. 2.6.16**. For example, a fall in extracellular fluid (ECF) volume (**Fig. 2.6.16a**) due to loss of body fluids causes an increase in renin secretion, which leads to a rise in aldosterone release. This increases the reabsorption of salt in renal tubules, thus raising the osmolality of the blood plasma. This stimulates secretion of antidiuretic hormone (also stimulated directly by the fall in extracellular fluid volume) which causes reabsorption of water. Thus the extracellular fluid volume and osmolality are both restored to normal.

**Figure 2.6.16b** illustrates responses when the primary disturbance is a change in osmolality. For example, a fall in osmolality accompanied by a rise in extracellular fluid volume due to drinking a large volume of water is rapidly corrected by a fall in antidiuretic hormone secretion. However, a rise in extracellular fluid volume without an alteration in osmolality, as

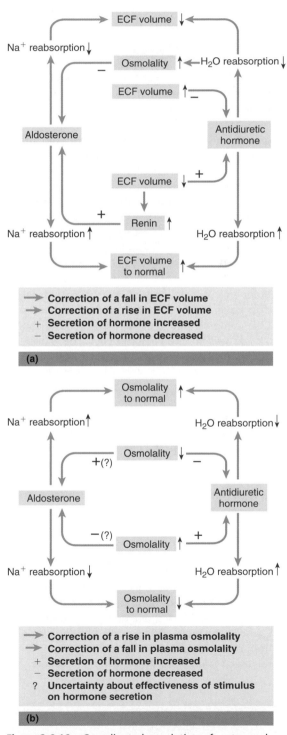

**Figure 2.6.16**   Coordinated regulation of water and electrolyte secretion showing (a) correction of changes in extracellular fluid volume and (b) correction of changes in osmolality. ECF, extracellular fluid

can occur in a patient receiving excessive intravenous 0.9% sodium chloride solution (which is isotonic with plasma), is corrected more slowly. The change in osmolality is a more potent regulator of anti-diuretic hormone secretion than is a change in extracellular fluid volume. A rise in osmolality is rapidly corrected both by release of antidiuretic hormone, increasing water reabsorption, and by thirst, increasing water consumption.

## CLINICAL APPLICATIONS

Changes in fluid balance can be assessed by accurate measurement of the patient's weight and this method is used when the fluid balance is a crucial factor in adjustment of treatment, as in a patient undergoing dialysis. The usual fluid intake and output charts only take account of the liquid taken in and the urine eliminated. Even if accurately completed, they do not take account of either insensible losses, or the water content of food and water formed through metabolism.

During treatment of severe oedema with potent diuretics, the patient might lose five or more litres from the excessive interstitial fluid (oedema is excessive interstitial fluid). As the density of body fluids is close to 1, a litre of interstitial fluid weighs close to one kilogram. Thus a patient who loses 5 L of oedema fluid (a good response) loses about 5 kg of weight, often in a few days. This is well within the range that can be detected by daily weighing of patients. Nutritional causes of change in weight, act over a much longer period. Another hormone that plays a part in controlling body salt in some situations is **atrial natriuretic hormone**. Its name implies its action – it increases urinary loss of sodium (*natrium*, Na) just as a diuresis consists of increased water loss. It is released into the circulation from the atria when they are stretched (and so is sometimes called atrial natriuretic peptide). Stretching is increased when the blood volume increases and so the hormone action plays a part in homeostasis of blood volume. It can be useful in assessing the severity of cardiac failure – the worse the failure, generally the more the atria are stretched and the higher the level of the natriuretic hormone. Confusingly, this hormone exists in several forms, one of which was first found in the brain and so is called brain natriuretic hormone, or peptide (BNP) even though it is released mainly from the atria in heart failure.

## Control of calcium and phosphate metabolism

Calcium is the most common mineral in the body (about 1 kg in an adult), with at least 90% of the total in the bones and teeth. However, the relatively small amount in the extracellular and intracellular fluids and cells plays a vital role in most body functions, ranging from muscular contraction to nerve impulses and coagulation of blood. Phosphate is also crucial in body function. Again, most of it is found in the skeleton but it is also a major constituent of intracellular fluid and an important buffer, including in urine.

In the skeleton, most of the calcium and phosphorus is present as crystals of hydroxyapatite, $Ca_{10}(PO_4)_6(OH)_2$, forming the matrix of the bone. This matrix imparts hardness to the structure, and collagen fibres act like the steel reinforcing in concrete. Importantly, the deposition of the hydroxyapatite crystals, and their orientation, are influenced by the mechanical stresses on the bone, which allows adaptation to varied forces. Thus, in people who have little force acting on their bones for a period of time, for example astronauts in space and patients on bedrest, a reduction in the mineral content of the skeleton occurs, leading to a fall in bone density and reduced strength. This is a condition known as **osteoporosis** (see p. 238).

The skeletal minerals are in a continual state of flux as the bone is being remodelled all the time. The minerals in bone are derived from and return to the calcium and phosphorus in the extracellular fluid. Normally, there is an equilibrium between calcium and phosphate released from bone by **osteoclast** activity and calcium and phosphate deposited following **osteoblast** activity.

The normal plasma concentration of calcium is around 2.5 mmol/L, and that of phosphate is about 1.25 mmol/L. The total calcium represents about equal amounts of free ion and of calcium bound to plasma proteins. The free calcium and phosphate are in equilibrium between plasma (where they are measured) and interstitial fluid (where calcium level plays a vital role in excitation of nerves and muscles). The concentration in extracellular fluid of both these minerals is determined by the balance between the amounts: (i) absorbed from the gut; (ii) excreted by the kidneys; and (iii) deposited in and released from the bone (**Fig. 2.6.17**). By contrast, although cells have membrane-bound stores of calcium, the calcium ion level in intracellular fluid is hugely less than in extracellular fluid, and increases in intracellular fluid often act as second messengers to switch on cellular function.

## Calcium

Calcium is present in the plasma about equally bound to protein (albumin and globulin) and in ionized form, with a small amount combined with

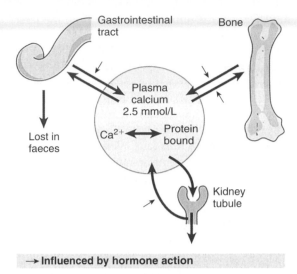

**Figure 2.6.17** Calcium metabolism

other substances such as citrate. In terms of physiological activity, it is the ionized calcium ($Ca^{2+}$) that is important. A fall in the plasma (and hence interstitial) concentration of calcium leads to increased activity of motor units (motor nerves and the associated muscle fibres), resulting in **tetany** when the skeletal muscles go into spasm.

## Phosphate

Phosphates – phosphate ($PO_4^{3-}$), hydrogen phosphate ($HPO_4^{2-}$), dihydrogen phosphate ($H_2PO_4^-$) – play a vital role in intracellular fluid, contributing a large proportion of the anions that balance intracellular potassium cations. Phosphates are components of nucleic acids, ATP (adenosine triphosphate), cAMP (cyclic adenosine monophosphate), other nucleotides, phospholipids and some proteins. Extracellular phosphate levels are regulated less precisely than extracellular calcium levels.

Three different hormones are involved in the control of calcium and phosphorus homeostasis – parathyroid hormone, vitamin D and calcitonin. Parathyroid hormone is vital in maintaining the level of calcium ions in the extracellular fluid within normal limits. Its actions raise the calcium level to correct for a fall. Vitamin D controls absorption of calcium from the gut (mainly upper small intestine), thus regulating the total body calcium, mostly found in hard tissues such as bone. Calcitonin seems to have a much less important role in decreasing high calcium levels.

## Parathyroid hormone (parathormone)

Parathyroid hormone (also called parathormone) is secreted from the four parathyroid glands, which lie embedded within the thyroid gland. The main effects of parathyroid secretion are to elevate the concentration of $Ca^{2+}$ in the extracellular fluid and to depress the plasma phosphate concentration.

Parathyroid hormone secretion is regulated directly by the concentration of calcium ions in the extracellular fluid. As the level of calcium ions falls, more parathyroid hormone is secreted and acts to restore the calcium level to normal. At the same time, it favours phosphate excretion in the kidneys.

Parathyroid hormone achieves these effects mainly by acting on the bones and kidneys. In bone it increases bone reabsorption by osteoclasts, thus causing a rapid release of calcium and phosphate ions into the interstitial fluid. The extra calcium ions restore the level to normal, correcting the risk of serious hypocalcaemia. However, the phosphate ions inevitably released from bone at the same time as the calcium ions, present a problem. According to the Law of Mass action, the product of calcium and phosphate ions determines the likelihood of deposition of the salt. So the extra phosphate ions could lead to deposition of harmful calcium phosphate crystals in the tissues.

This is counteracted by a second action of parathyroid hormone – this time in the kidney. Here, it depresses the reabsorption of filtered phosphate, so the excretion of phosphate is greater and the phosphate level in the interstitial fluid and plasma falls.

A third action of parathyroid hormone compensates for the steady loss of calcium salts from the bones and from the body that would result from the above activities. The hormone increases the activation of vitamin D in the kidneys to form the hormone-activated (hydroxylated) vitamin D that increases absorption of calcium from the gut.

Parathyroid hormone is a large polypeptide of 84 amino acids. It is synthesized in the chief cells of the parathyroid gland. Only small amounts of the hormone are stored in the cell, thus it is continually being synthesized and secreted. It has a half-life of 15–20 minutes and is degraded in the liver.

Overactivity of the parathyroid gland (**primary hyperparathyroidism**) produces an exaggeration of the above effects, raising the ionized calcium above normal. Whereas a low calcium level causes hyperexcitability of nerves and muscles, including muscle spasms, a high level calcium causes weakness. Excessive removal of bone salts causes weak bones and a tendency to painful cracks in the bones. Finally, excessive phosphate in the urine is accompanied by excessive calcium, because so much is being filtered. The product of the two ions often rises to the level where the salt is deposited in the urinary tract as renal stones (calculi). Renal calculi can cause impairment of renal function and nurses should encourage such patients to increase their fluid intake to 2–2.5 L per day.

The level of plasma calcium in chronic renal failure is chronically low because vitamin D is not activated by the diseased kidney. This stimulates the parathyroid glands and leads to hypertrophy and **secondary hyperparathyroidism**. Although this helps to maintain the vital calcium level, it does so at the expense of the bones, which become weakened.

## Hypoparathyroidism and tetany

In contrast to the above, **hypoparathyroidism** causes a fall in plasma $Ca^{2+}$ and a rise in phosphate levels, which results in **tetany** – overexcitability in the neuromuscular system. This involves increased excitability in three situations. Overexcitable sensory nerves can cause tingling (paraesthesia); overexcitable cerebral neurones can cause epileptic fits; but most often, overexcitable motor nerves cause skeletal muscle spasm. **Carpopedal spasm** (spasm of the hands and feet) is the most common finding in adults, with laryngeal spasm occurring in children. The development of tetany is a possible complication of thyroidectomy as the parathyroid glands or their blood supply might be inadvertently damaged. Another cause of tetany is alkalosis. A rise in plasma pH, from whatever cause, leads to an increase in the amount of calcium bound to protein, and again there is a fall in the concentration of the ionized form of calcium in plasma. In an emergency, tetany is treated with intravenous calcium gluconate.

It is worth noting that a level of extracellular calcium ions low enough to cause tetany is still adequate for the requirements of blood clotting. Also, intracellular calcium levels are not depressed, so muscle activity is unimpaired, apart from the interfering spasms of tetany.

## Vitamin D

The term 'vitamin D' refers to a group of closely related steroid substances (cholecalciferol), the active form of which (**1,25-dihydroxycholecalciferol**) is the second hormone involved in the regulation of calcium and phosphate metabolism. This active form of vitamin D is produced in the kidney and transported as a hormone in the circulation to its target cells, mainly in the upper small intestine. Here, as another steroid hormone, it enters cells and stimulates calcium absorption from the gut.

There are two sources of vitamin D – ingestion in the diet and the action of sunlight, which forms cholecalciferol in the skin (**Fig. 2.6.18**). Whichever the source, the vitamin is protein bound and transported to the liver, where it is converted into **25-hydroxycholecalciferol**. This has no physiological action and is the main storage form of vitamin D (dietary fish and mammal liver is a rich source of the vitamin). This substance is further hydroxylated in the kidney into **1,25-dihydroxycholecalciferol**, the active hormone, or 24,25-dihydroxycholecalciferol, which is less active.

The formation of the active hormone is regulated indirectly by the plasma calcium level and directly by parathyroid hormone. Hypocalcaemia increases the secretion of parathyroid hormone and this increases the renal production of 1,25-dihydroxycholecalciferol. The hormone increases the plasma concentration of calcium, and – by negative feedback – the secretion of parathyroid hormone and activation of vitamin D then fall.

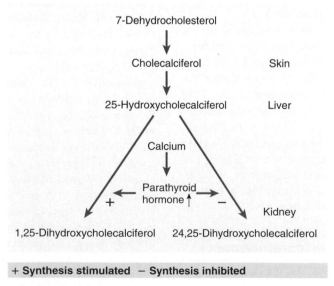

**+ Synthesis stimulated — Synthesis inhibited**

**Figure 2.6.18**  Formation and activation of vitamin D

## CLINICAL APPLICATIONS

**Rickets** is a serious disease of the bones that occurs particularly in children. It is due to deficiency of active vitamin D, caused by a combination of an inadequate amount of vitamin D in the diet and insufficient formation of cholecalciferol in the skin. As darkly pigmented skin shields the skin from sunlight, this factor increases the risk of rickets, as does lack of exposure to sunlight. Deficiency of active vitamin D means that inadequate calcium is absorbed from the gut so the bones are poorly calcified and soft, and become deformed. These deformities become marked when the child begins to sit, crawl and walk, so knock knees or bow legs and deformities of the spine develop. Distortion of the pelvis can occur and this results in serious difficulties during childbirth in women who had rickets as children. The equivalent condition in adults is **osteomalacia**. Both these conditions are more common in the Asian population of the British Isles, possibly due to a combination of dark skin, lack of exposure to sunlight and dietary deficiencies.

## Calcitonin

Calcitonin, the final hormone involved in the control of calcium and phosphorus metabolism, is secreted from the parafollicular cells of the thyroid gland. It is a peptide containing 32 amino acids. Unlike parathyroid hormone it is secreted in response to a high level of circulating calcium ions and lowers their level by favouring deposition of calcium in bones. It seems to be much less important than parathormone and its role is not yet clear. It does not have to be given to patients who have had their thyroid gland removed.

## Coordinated regulation of body calcium

Levels of calcium ion in the extracellular fluid are normally very precisely regulated. As already indicated, this is maintained mainly by parathyroid hormone and activated vitamin D (1,25-dihydroxycholecalciferol). Parathyroid hormone acts in a simple negative feedback loop whereby a fall in calcium triggers release of the hormone, which restores the calcium level. In parallel to this, an adequate calcium intake in the diet, combined with an appropriate level of activated vitamin D, ensures enough calcium in the bones. This framework is sufficient for the understanding of many disturbances of calcium but in real life things are rarely simple, and these hormones and other active agents have been shown to act at many sites, sometimes in conflicting ways (**Fig. 2.6.19**).

Other hormones are also thought to play a part in calcium metabolism. Corticosteroids appear to lower calcium concentration, whereas growth hormone causes a rise. Cortisol and, to some extent, thyroxine, favour breakdown of protein, including the collagen in bones. This weakens the bones and also causes loss of calcium as a secondary effect.

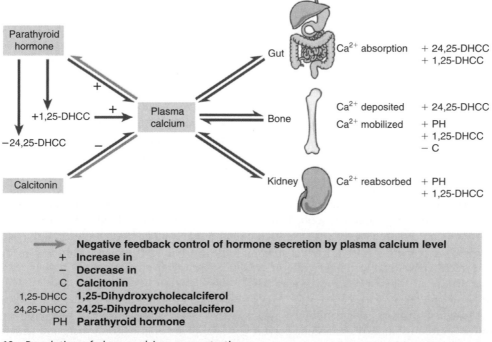

**Negative feedback control of hormone secretion by plasma calcium level**
- **+** **Increase in**
- **−** **Decrease in**
- **C** **Calcitonin**
- **1,25-DHCC** **1,25-Dihydroxycholecalciferol**
- **24,25-DHCC** **24,25-Dihydroxycholecalciferol**
- **PH** **Parathyroid hormone**

**Figure 2.6.19**   Regulation of plasma calcium concentration

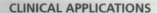

## OSTEOPOROSIS

This term refers to loss of substance in bones. It is often diagnosed on X-ray when the normally bold outlines of major bones become reduced in size and density. Technically, **osteoporosis** refers to loss of collagen; **osteomalacia** refers to loss of the calcium phosphate minerals. However, one condition tends to merge into the other. In practice, the term 'osteoporosis' is commonly used to describe a fall in X-ray density of bones. Such a fall in density accompanies ageing, especially in postmenopausal women. The bones become fragile and liable to fracture, particularly the vertebrae, wrist and neck of femur. Fractures of the femur, often from a minor fall, are a major cause of disability and death in older women and, to a lesser extent, in men.

The risk of osteoporosis is increased by a low bone mass in adolescence. Inadequate dietary calcium and inadequate weight-bearing exercise in the first two to three decades of life seem to be important factors here. In later life, some loss of bone mass seems inevitable but the loss is slowed by maintaining adequate dietary calcium and exercise. Protection against osteoporosis is one of the benefits of hormone replacement therapy after the menopause. Signs and symptoms of osteoporosis due to vertebral collapse include lower back ache and loss of height. Often individuals will be diagnosed as having this condition when they are X-rayed for a fractured wrist or hip following a fall.

## Growth and development

Growth involves an increase in length, size and weight, with the deposition of additional protein and bone mineral. Development involves a highly coordinated pattern of bodily changes through fetal life, childhood and adolescence, culminating in the normally developed adult man or woman.

The normal pattern of rate and extent of growth and development is complex and is influenced by a number of different factors. First, **genetic factors** lay down the basic guidelines for overall height achieved, as indicated by the correlation of adult height between parents and children, and for the pattern and timing of growth spurts. Different norms apply to different races. Disturbed patterns leading to abnormal function are often genetic in origin, as with Down syndrome.

Second, the genetic pattern can be modified by a variety of **adverse circumstances** that can stunt growth and distort development. Striking examples occur in early fetal life at the time that major organs are appearing. Drugs (e.g. heroin, alcohol, smoking, thalidomide) and viruses (e.g. rubella) are well known for adverse effects, from general stunting to severe organ abnormalities. At all stages of development, malnutrition, including vitamin deficiencies, and chronic illness can cause stunting and distortion. Rickets and osteoporosis due to inadequate calcium intake are two examples. A childhood diet inadequate in overall amount or in vitamins or other micronutrients will result in an adult who does not reach his or her genetic potential in terms of height and organ perfection. In the other direction, someone who is 'overnourished' in childhood will not exceed his or her genetically predetermined stature but might suffer from obesity.

On a world scale, long-term poor nutrition leads to reduction in adult size and, in a way, this can be seen as an adaptive response to a bad situation; a smaller adult requires less food than a larger individual. These changes can take some generations to be reversed because smaller women tend to have smaller babies. The increase in population height in the twentieth century in well nourished populations might be related in part to this trend. The onset of reproductive function in young women, as indicated by the menarche (first menstruation), has been shown to move progressively to an earlier age in the same general time span. In general, the menarche is delayed by malnutrition and menstruation can cease when there is severe weight loss.

Third, the normal rate and pattern of growth and development are regulated through the **endocrine** system. In general, endocrine disturbances in childhood, like other chronic illnesses, stunt or distort growth. Particularly dramatic are the rare disturbances of growth hormone secretion (considered below), when too little can result in the individual being a dwarf in adulthood and too much can cause the person to be a giant.

The rate of growth varies considerably during childhood. In proportion to body size it is greatest in early fetal life. The rapid rate of growth during fetal life continues into infancy but significantly decelerates through early childhood. There is a further deceleration before puberty, which is followed by the pubertal growth spurt. The age at which this growth spurt occurs varies considerably between female and male, being around 10.5–13 years in girls, and 12.5–15 years in boys. In general, the younger this growth spurt occurs, the shorter the final height achieved. During this period there is very considerable variation in stature and development between individuals of the same chronological age. However, charts have been produced showing average and usual range of growth for male and female (the yellow line in **Fig. 2.6.20** shows the average trend). It is

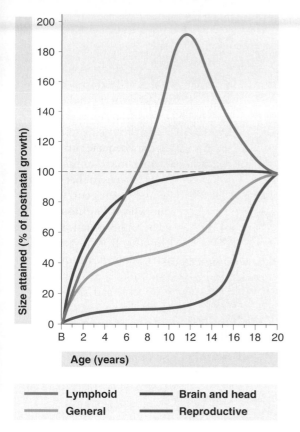

**Figure 2.6.20** Growth curves for different body tissues (adapted from Tanner, 1962)

Lymphoid — Brain and head

General — Reproductive

helpful to plot individual progress in relation to these growth charts, so that sudden deviation from the normal trend can be spotted and investigated.

Different tissues vary in the rate and timing of growth and **Fig. 2.6.20** demonstrates the variation between tissues at different ages as a percentage of the size at age 20. Note that the brain (the brown line) completes its growth relatively early whereas the reproductive system (purple) remains rudimentary until puberty. The role of hormones in maturation of the reproductive system is discussed in Chapter 6.3.

We now look at the hormone that plays a major part in the control of overall body (somatic) growth – growth hormone.

## Growth hormone (somatotrophin)

Growth hormone is a single, large, polypeptide chain of 191 amino acids formed in the anterior pituitary gland. The structure of this hormone is very similar to that of prolactin (also formed in the anterior pituitary gland) and human placental lactogen. As expected, there is some overlap in activity between growth hormone and prolactin.

Growth hormone modifies metabolism in a number of different ways to favour growth. It stimulates

an increase in the length of bones through cellular activity at their growing ends. In addition, it has a general anabolic action by favouring protein synthesis in various tissues. This enables the increase in cell mass required for growth in general.

The effects of growth hormone are complex and it seems to act in two main ways. First, it stimulates cell activity directly through binding to specific receptors on the cell membranes of the target organs. Second, it stimulates the liver and other tissues to produce other factors that help to mediate its effects. These factors are known as somatomedins, one of which resembles insulin in structure and is known as insulin-like growth factor (IGF).

**Figure 2.6.21** summarizes the complex effects of growth hormone, which make all the difference between reaching adulthood with a severely reduced body size and developing normally.

## Other metabolic effects and regulation of growth hormone

If growth hormone were concerned only with growth to adulthood, its secretion might be expected to cease when growth was complete. However, it continues to be secreted throughout life and the rate of secretion is variable, depending on various stimuli. It thus seems that at least some of its actions are important for situations such as exercise and in responding to a lack of glucose. Because it is associated with going to sleep, it is tempting to suggest that growth hormone is involved in tissue repair (anabolism) after the relative catabolism inducted by cortisol during the day. However, it is difficult to draw simple conclusions about a situation with the complexity indicated in **Fig. 2.6.22**. This figure indicates that, like other anterior pituitary hormones, growth hormone secretion is regulated by hypothalamic releasing and inhibiting hormones (or factors). The inhibiting hormone is called **somatostatin**.

Proof of the vital role of growth hormone in normal growth has come from providing it to children whose **impaired growth** is associated with lack of growth hormone. When given the hormone, they start to grow at a normal rate. Because the hormone is specific to the human it was referred to as human growth hormone (hGH) and was initially (some decades ago) obtained post-mortem from human pituitary glands. Risks of infection would preclude such methods nowadays and, fortunately, the hormone can now be produced by recombinant DNA techniques.

In children, as mentioned earlier, excessive secretion of growth hormone leads to the condition known as **gigantism**. In most cases, excessive growth can be identified in childhood using growth charts.

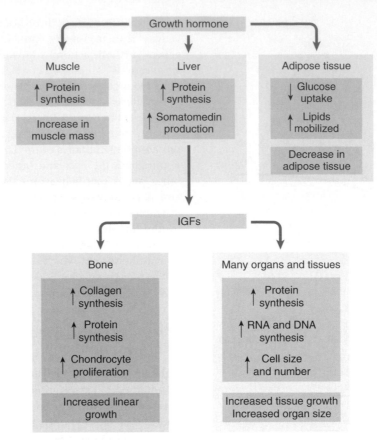

**Figure 2.6.21**   The effects of growth hormone

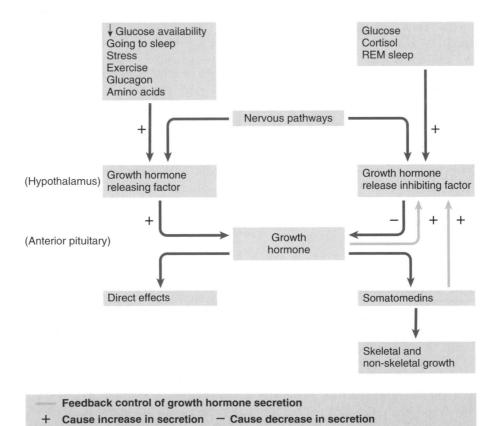

**Figure 2.6.22**   Control of growth hormone secretion

Reduction of the excessive growth hormone level (for example by removing an anterior pituitary tumour of cells that secrete it) terminate the excessive growth so that adult height is nearer normal.

In adults, a surge of growth hormone cannot increase height because the epiphyses of the long bones are fully ossified. In this case, greatly increased secretion of growth hormone, possibly as the result of a pituitary tumour, causes the tissues to grow within the confines of the person's height. Although many organs increase in size, the condition is most noticeable in the extremities, and so is called **acromegaly** (*Acro*, extremities; *megaly*, enlargement). It is most marked in the bones and soft tissues of the hands, feet, face and lower jaw, which become enlarged, with coarsening of the skin (**Fig. 2.6.23**). Compare this figure with **Fig. 2.6.6**, in which the features and skin are fine, and **Fig. 2.6.7**, in which the skin is coarsened but the features not enlarged. The patient is likely to have required progressively larger sizes of shoes. Shaking hands with such a patient conveys the effect of being engulfed in an exceedingly large hand. The changes of acromegaly can take years to develop and so might be attributed to ageing alone. However, the person is likely to be very embarrassed by the changed features and will therefore require very sensitive support from all involved in his or her care. Because growth hormone favours mobilization of glucose and other energy sources, its effects are antagonistic to insulin and the patient is quite likely to have features of diabetes mellitus. As with gigantism in children, treatment is based on bringing growth hormone effects down to normal and, again, the sooner treatment is started, the better the outcome.

## Coordinated control of growth and development

As indicated previously, growth is a complex process, basically determined by genetic makeup, modified by such factors as diet and illness, and requiring the coordinated activity of a number of hormones. Reduction in growth during illness is often followed by a period of 'catch-up' growth when the rate is considerably above normal to allow the child to return to the previous growth curve (Faulkner & Tanner, 1986).

The number of hormones involved in the normal growth and development of an individual is indicated by the range of abnormalities of hormone secretion that can result in disturbed growth and abnormal development. Obviously, growth hormone is involved, but so also are thyroid hormones, parathyroid hormone, vitamin D and calcitonin, glucocorticoids, insulin and the sex hormones, as well as the pituitary hormones regulating the release of many of these.

The importance of different hormones varies at different stages in growth and development. During fetal life those hormones that are central to these processes after birth (growth hormone, thyroid hormone and the sex hormones) are relatively unimportant. The mother at this stage provides much of the hormonal environment. After birth, the child must produce his or her own endocrine environment. Disturbance of any of these is like severe chronic illness in that it distorts the normal smooth following of the growth-chart course. Thyroid hormones are particularly important in that they have a major role in development as well as growth.

As mentioned earlier, hypothyroidism of the new born (**cretinism**) leads to not only dwarfing, but also to infantile bodily proportions, coarse features and, most importantly, mental retardation. Unless treated at an early stage some of the effects, including the mental retardation, will be permanent.

The glucocorticoid hormones (e.g. cortisol) have a regulatory effect on tissue growth and in excess they inhibit growth in height. Children requiring steroid therapy need careful monitoring of growth and their therapy should be adjusted as far as possible to allow normal growth.

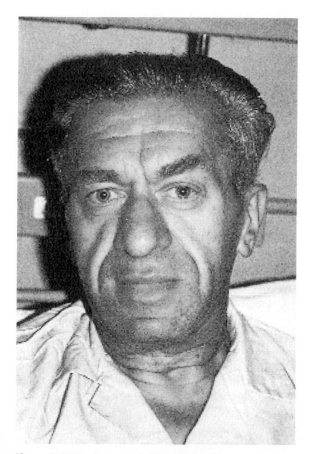

**Figure 2.6.23** A person with acromegaly

The effect of the gonadotrophic and sex hormones on the gonads and the development of secondary sexual characteristics are discussed in Chapter 6.3. However, during puberty a number of other bodily changes also occur. There is a considerable increase in growth rate, resulting in a gain in height of the order of 25 cm, and changes in general body size and shape. This growth spurt comes early in puberty in girls but late in boys. Most of the height increase is in the trunk, in the length of the vertebral column, rather than in the legs. In addition, increased width of shoulders in boys and size of pelvis in girls occurs. The endocrine mechanisms of these changes are not clear.

An increase in androgen secretion from the adrenal cortex occurs between the ages of 5 and 8 years in both boys and girls, and is thought to be a preliminary to changes during puberty. The endocrine control of puberty is not fully understood. The hypothalamus appears to have a major role, with an increase in secretion of gonadotrophic-releasing hormones. It has been suggested that the pineal gland might also be involved. Whatever the initiator, the growth spurt during puberty is due to the activity of both growth hormone and sex hormones. The sex hormones are thought to be mainly responsible for the changes in the vertebral column and shoulders and hips, whereas growth of the legs is due largely to the activity of growth hormone.

In childhood, the distribution of different types of tissue within the body is similar in girls and boys. In adulthood, men have about one and a half times the lean body mass and skeletal mass of women, and women have much more body fat than men (25 versus 15%). The differences in fat distribution and amount between the sexes are thought to be due to the secretion of testosterone preventing the female pattern of fat deposition. The increased body mass in men is due to androgen activity and includes much greater muscle power.

## Response to life-threatening challenge

To survive in adverse environmental conditions, an individual must be able to adapt to change. The nervous system is of major importance in responses requiring thought or planned activity. However, the brain is also involved in immediate unconscious responses. These are mediated largely by the brainstem and adjoining areas. The hypothalamus, in particular, is involved and, not surprisingly, involves the endocrine system in these emergency innate responses.

Situations that can kill a previously healthy person in a short time include contact with deadly infection, encounter with a threatening situation (attacking animal or person, earthquake), extreme heat and cold, and serious injury involving widespread tissue damage and loss of blood. The response to infection relies heavily on the immune system, which in turn is regulated in part by hormones and related chemicals, including cytokines. This system is considered in detail in Chapter 6.2. At this stage we consider the stress response, which is a pattern of bodily activities that, with variations, is involved in survival in the face of all the deadly threats (including infection) mentioned above.

## The stress response

The dangerous situations mentioned above tend to fall into two groups – those where the response must be extremely rapid, with the outcome determined in less than a minute, and those where the response, 'fight for life', must continue for days. In the first situation, described as the 'fright, flight, fight response' by Cannon and de la Paz in 1911, the sympathetic nervous system and the adrenal medulla dominate, whereas in prolonged stress situations (e.g. patient with multiple injuries in intensive care) the adrenal cortex is particularly important. In many situations the two responses overlap and blend. The sympathetic response is known to the general public in terms such as 'getting the adrenaline going', and correctly so, as the hormonal response of the adrenal medulla is about 80% **adrenaline** (epinephrine). The second response is sometimes known as the metabolic response to stress/trauma and relies heavily on the adrenal glucocorticoid **cortisol**. Stress is considered fully in Chapter 2.7.

### The adrenal medulla

Functionally, the adrenal medulla is a part of the sympathetic nervous system. During embryonic life it develops from an outgrowth of nervous tissue that becomes surrounded by what is, in terms of function, a completely separate gland, the adrenal cortex (compare the merging of the anterior and posterior lobes of the pituitary gland). The sympathetic nervous system is discussed in Chapter 2.5.

The neurotransmitter of the postganglionic sympathetic nerve fibres is **noradrenaline** (norepinephrine), and this is also one of the hormones secreted by the adrenal medulla. However, **adrenaline** (epinephrine) is the major hormone of this gland. The two hormones (named catecholamines from their chemistry) are very similar in structure and are formed from the amino acid tyrosine. They are stored in vesicles in the adrenal gland and released in response to signals from sympathetic preganglionic fibres (**Fig. 2.6.24**). Although sympathetic nerves can

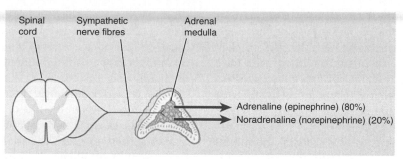

**Figure 2.6.24** Secretions of the adrenal medulla

promote rapid 'fight or flight' by direct communication with the heart and the muscular system, the same system can also produce a slightly slower, but massive and longer-lasting effect through adrenal medullary adrenaline (epinephrine) and noradrenaline (norepinephrine), which are carried round the circulation as hormones to the same target organs.

## Actions of adrenal medullary hormones

In general, these hormones stimulate activity of the neuromuscular system, the cardiovascular and respiratory systems, and have various metabolic effects. These actions prepare the body for immediate activity in response to environmental challenge, and occur rapidly – within the time taken for the blood to circulate around the body. Briefly, alertness is increased, muscular movements become very powerful and their reflex components are quicker than usual. These effects explain how in emergencies and, to some extent, sporting and athletic performance in highly emotionally charged atmospheres, people can do things that are not possible in more mundane situations. Also, the heart rate accelerates rapidly and the heart pumps more vigorously to produce the necessary increase in cardiac output. Airways dilate and glucose is mobilized into the bloodstream.

The actions of these hormones, as of noradrenaline (norepinephrine) released at the postsynaptic endings of the sympathetic nervous system, are mediated through their stimulation of $\alpha$- and $\beta$-receptors on the cell membranes of the target organs:

- **$\alpha$-receptors** mediate the stimulation of circular smooth muscle in blood vessels to cause vasoconstriction. Vasoconstriction in the skin is responsible for the pallor seen in someone who has had a severe shock, and also in a patient who has had severe haemorrhage.
- **$\beta$-receptors** are subdivided into two main types. **$\beta_1$-receptors** mediate cardiac effects, including increase in heart rate and increase in speed and force of contraction of cardiac muscle.

**$\beta_2$-receptors** relax smooth muscle in the blood vessels of skeletal muscle to cause vasodilation and relax smooth muscle in the airways to cause bronchodilation.

These actions have been worked out largely by means of drugs that can selectively block or stimulate a certain type of receptor. These drugs are now widely used for treating disease. For example, $\beta_2$-stimulants relax and dilate the airways in asthma without stimulating $\beta_1$-receptors to make the heart race. A $\beta$-blocking drug can slow the heart rate if this is excessive.

The effects of sympathetic activation are not all helpful. Thus, severe anxiety, which might be experienced by a patient on admission to hospital, can reduce the ability to understand and retain information and to make decisions such as giving permission for surgery. This needs to be borne in mind and adequate time given to explanations and discussion. If information is to be used later, for example when given at an out patient appointment, having it in writing to be read in calmer conditions can be most helpful.

The effects of adrenaline (epinephrine) and noradrenaline vary somewhat, and this can largely be explained by differing affinities for $\alpha$- and $\beta$-receptors. Although both hormones stimulate both receptors, noradrenaline produces relatively more stimulation of $\alpha$-receptors. This results in vasoconstriction, so **noradrenaline** tends to cause **hypertension**, raising both systolic and diastolic arterial blood pressure.

Adrenaline, on the other hand, produces more $\beta$-stimulation. This stimulates the heart to increase its rate and power, so increasing cardiac output. Adrenaline causes vasoconstriction and pallor in the skin because blood vessels there contain many $\alpha$-receptors and few $\beta$-receptors, but it causes vasodilation in other sites well supplied with $\beta$-receptors. This leads to a circulatory state similar to that found in physical exercise, where there is a large cardiac output and a wide pulse pressure (large rise in systolic pressure, only small rise in diastolic). Thus, **adrenaline** tends to cause a **hyperdynamic** circulation – rapid bounding pulse; it also tends to raise the blood glucose level.

When responding to emergencies, the two hormones work together to support prompt and vigorous activity in the threatened healthy person. They also have a role in the injured and those who have lost blood. In this case, the circulation tends to collapse and the hormones help to maintain just enough circulation for the brain and heart, with little being sent to the skin and gut.

The isolated effects of the adrenal hormones are illustrated by the very rare **adrenal tumour** (phaeochromocytoma). Excessive secretion of noradrenaline by the tumour leads to hypertension, with both systolic and diastolic pressures elevated. Excessive secretion of adrenaline leads to tachycardia, a high pulse pressure, hyperglycaemia, tremor and an increased metabolic rate. α- and β-blockers dramatically remove the effects and have to be used very skilfully during surgery for the tumour – handling it can result in wild fluctuations in heart rate and blood pressure, risking serious complications.

## Secretion, metabolism and excretion

The effects of sympathetic activity, including those of the adrenal medullary hormones, are rapid both in onset and in disappearance, thus allowing speedy adaptation to environmental changes. This activity is regulated by the central nervous system from the nuclei in the brainstem, which are the origins of the nerve supply to the sympathetic nervous system.

Activity of the brainstem nuclei is affected by many internal and external factors. Nervous connections from the cerebral cortex, limbic system and hypothalamus allow secretion as a result of emotions. Victims of serious trauma, such as a road traffic accident, who experience widespread tissue damage, have widespread stimulation of pain fibres. This results in a huge input to the thalamus and, even though the patient is unconscious, this can lead to powerful sympathetic stimulation (and also hypothalamic stimulation considered below).

Higher sympathetic fibres descend to the spinal cord, and adrenal medullary secretion is activated by nerve impulses passing from the spinal cord along the sympathetic preganglionic nerve supply to the glands (see Fig. 2.6.24).

Normally, most catecholamines are secreted during daytime activity. Sympathetic fibres maintain the arterial blood pressure by causing vasoconstriction, mainly in skin. During physical exertion, sympathetic activity is marked. Not only are adrenaline and noradrenaline released from the adrenal medullae but the noradrenaline that is released at nerve endings spills over into the circulation. The catecholamine level falls rapidly when we go to bed and remains low, reducing alertness and favouring sleep. Most people have experienced the sudden alerting that can be caused by a sudden noise. Sleep usually takes some time to return, as the catecholamines take a corresponding time to fall to low levels again.

Although adrenaline levels are usually higher than noradrenaline levels in the blood, the ratio seems to vary to some extent with the stimulus. Thus hypoglycaemia appears to cause the secretion of relatively large amounts of adrenaline, which is much more effective in restoring the blood glucose level.

The catecholamines have a very short half-life of about 2 minutes, as befits hormones whose action is best terminated nearly as rapidly as it starts. Catecholamines are rapidly metabolized by enzymes that are widely distributed throughout the body. The products are excreted, mainly in the urine.

The actions of these hormones are invaluable during strenuous exercise and when immediate action is important, but they not uncommonly occur in situations when physical activity is not of benefit, and indeed might be impossible. For example, patients waiting for dental treatment or entering hospital might have a raised blood pressure and pulse rate due to raised anxiety resulting in an increase in catecholamine secretion.

## The adrenal cortex

The other main part of the stress response involves the adrenal cortex. The effects of the adrenal cortical response begin more slowly and last longer than those mediated through the adrenal medulla. These effects correspond quite closely with those of the adrenal cortical hormone cortisol. The adrenal cortex is derived from cells closely related to those that form the ovaries and testes, and these organs synthesize steroid hormones. The adrenal cortical steroids are generally referred to as corticosteroids. There are many of them (see Fig. 2.6.4) and different hormones are formed in different parts of the cortex. The adrenal cortex has three layers. The outer **zona glomerulosa** (looks microscopically rather like renal glomeruli) produces mineralocorticoids, mainly aldosterone (discussed earlier as an important regulator of sodium and potassium). The middle **zona fasciculata** secretes glucocorticoids, mainly cortisol. The inner **zona reticularis** secretes small amounts of sex hormones – androgens – in both males and females. There is some overlap in production, and particularly in the activity of the different groups of hormones. In particular, the glucocorticoids such as cortisol also have mineralocorticoid activity, although much less than aldosterone. In the stress response the activity of the **glucocorticoids** is particularly important.

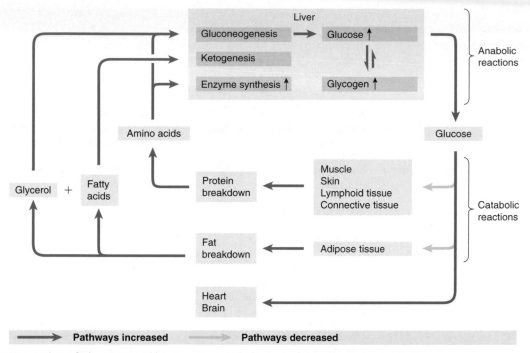

**Figure 2.6.25**   Action of glucocorticoid hormones on carbohydrate, fat and protein metabolism

## Actions of glucocorticoid hormones

Steroid hormones, including the glucocorticoids, cross the cell membrane easily to act on the nucleus and stimulate the formation of mRNA, and thus regulate enzymes that control cell function. In addition to these **direct actions**, glucocorticoids also regulate other actions indirectly. They must be present to allow some other hormones to have their full effects; for instance, the catecholamines influence a number of metabolic pathways only in the presence of glucocorticoids. Such indirect actions are called **permissive effects**.

Glucocorticoids are particularly concerned with modification of the metabolism of carbohydrates, fats and proteins in a way (**Fig. 2.6.25**) that mobilizes energy for the many extra activities needed to survive serious physical stress. Such effects are the opposite to those of insulin, which favours storage of these metabolites. Thus, whereas insulin is an anabolic hormone, the glucocorticoids are catabolic, particularly with respect to body protein. By favouring conversion of amino acids into glucose, the glucocorticoids reduce the amino acid pool, impairing the maintenance of skeletal muscle protein and reducing the synthesis of new protein in antibody and inflammatory responses.

Although the glucocorticoids are generally catabolic, some of the extra glucose generated is stored temporarily in the liver as glycogen, an anabolic effect. Some of the fatty acids released will be converted into ketones in the liver and used as an energy source by other tissues, as happens in starvation. When there is an inappropriately high level of glucocorticoids in Cushing's syndrome (see below and **Table 2.6.6**), some of the excess energy sources are converted into fat deposits, another anabolic action.

### CLINICAL APPLICATIONS

**Steroid therapy** has been widely used with good effect for many years. It involves artificial steroid drugs that are closely related to cortisol but have less mineralocorticoid effect. Although these drugs are widely referred to as 'steroids', they are in fact synthetic glucocorticoids, used mainly for their **anti-inflammatory effect**. Rheumatoid arthritis and asthma are two common distressing conditions whose effects are produced by inflammation – leading to painful joints and narrowed airways, respectively. Synthetic steroids such as prednisone can be injected into joints or inhaled into the airways to excellent effect. In some cases they are given by mouth in high doses but here there is an increased risk of serious side-effects (see later under Cushing's syndrome, in which a tumour can produce excessive amounts of corticosteroids). However, inflammation is an essential stage in the process of wound healing (see Chapter 6.1) and if this inflammation is prevented or reduced by corticosteroid therapy, wound healing will be slow because the initial fibrous tissue is not laid down normally.

**Table 2.6.6**  Disturbances in Cushing's syndrome

| | | |
|---|---|---|
| Protein catabolism ↑ → protein depletion | Thinning of skin and subcutaneous tissue<br>Muscles poorly developed<br>Reduced protein replacement | Skin easily damaged → bruises, lacerations<br>Lacking in strength<br>Poor wound healing |
| Changed fat distribution | Moves from periphery<br>Collections in face, upper back, abdominal wall | Thin limbs<br>'Hump' between shoulders<br>Stretching → striae |
| Altered glucose metabolism | Hyperglycaemia, ↓ bd in glucose utilization | Diabetes mellitus in susceptible people |
| Altered fluid and electrolyte balance | Sodium and water retained<br><br>Potassium depletion | Moon-face, hypertension (85% of patients)<br>Muscle weakness |
| Effects on bone metabolism | Loss of collagen matrix<br>Anti-vitamin D effect<br>Increased calcium excretion | Osteoporosis – softening and demineralization of bone |
| Response to infection | ↓ Fibrosis and inflammation<br>↓ Systemic effects of infection<br>↓ Antibody formation | Infection spreads readily<br>No obvious effects of spread<br>Reduced ability to combat infection |
| Effect on nervous system | Acceleration in basic EEG rhythms → mental aberrations | Increased appetite, insomnia, euphoria<br>Toxic psychoses |

Corticosteroids also cause a **reduction in the immune response** because this response depends heavily on protein synthesis. They are thus of value in treating serious allergic reactions, including severe blood transfusion reactions. They are also used to reduce the risk of organ transplant rejection and in the treatment of autoimmune diseases, in which the body makes antibodies against some of its own tissues. However, suppression of antibody formation inevitably impairs the body's response to serious infection (see Chapter 6.2).

Excessive glucocorticoids hinder the inflammatory activities associated with healing and this can play a part in their increasing the risk of peptic ulcer. As they keep the body in a state of hypermetabolism, it is not surprising that glucocorticoids can cause a degree of psychological tension and, indeed, cause personality changes.

As the glucocorticoid hormones have mineralocorticoid activity, high levels can cause excessive retention of salt and water, with increased risk of oedema and hypertension.

The effects of excessive inappropriate levels of glucocorticoids are seen in **Cushing's syndrome**. Various causes exist (**Table 2.6.7**) but tumours of

**Table 2.6.7**  Causes of Cushing's syndrome

| |
|---|
| Cushing's disease due to excess secretion of ACTH from the pituitary gland |
| Adrenocortical tumours – adenoma or carcinoma |
| Ectopic ACTH syndrome – secretion of ACTH by malignant or benign tumours of non-endocrine tissue |
| Iatrogenic:<br>• corticosteroid administration<br>• ACTH administration |

the pituitary gland are the most common 'internal' or 'endogenous' cause, and corticosteroid therapy is a common 'external' or 'exogenous' cause. The widespread effects of Cushing's syndrome are summarized in **Table 2.6.6**. Osteoporosis is a relatively common problem and can affect the vertebrae, causing them to collapse with painful effects. Some rise in glucocorticoid levels occurs with severe mental stress but the levels are much below those of Cushing's syndrome.

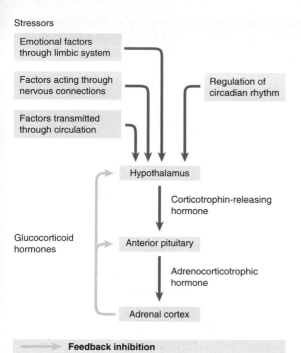

Stressors

Emotional factors through limbic system

Factors acting through nervous connections

Factors transmitted through circulation

Regulation of circadian rhythm

Hypothalamus

Corticotrophin-releasing hormone

Glucocorticoid hormones

Anterior pituitary

Adrenocorticotrophic hormone

Adrenal cortex

Feedback inhibition

**Figure 2.6.26**   Regulation of glucocorticoid secretion

The glucocorticoids are transported in the plasma bound to a globulin protein, **transcortin** or **corticosteroid-binding globulin** and, to a lesser extent, to albumin.

Steroid hormones are converted in the liver to a number of other mainly, but not entirely, inactive steroids, which are largely excreted in the urine. In disease of the liver, degradation of glucocorticoids is depressed and inappropriate levels of steroid hormones accumulate and contribute to the metabolic disorders of liver failure.

## Regulation of glucocorticoid secretion

There is considerable variation in the rate of glucocorticoid secretion at different times during each 24-hour cycle, with a minimum around midnight, a sharp rise prior to normal waking and relatively high levels during the day. This is an important **circadian rhythm.** Circadian rhythms are bodily changes with a cycle length of about (*circa*) a day. This circadian rhythm is maintained by a hypothalamic 'clock'.

The circadian rhythm is overridden, again via the hypothalamus, in severe physical stress to produce much higher levels, which can persist for days. This cortisol response is essential for **survival after trauma.** Patients who cannot produce it are at risk of collapsing and dying with even moderate injuries that would not normally be life-threatening.

Glucocorticoid regulation is summarized in Fig. 2.6.26. Many aspects of glucocorticoid regulation

via hypothalamus (**corticotrophin-releasing hormone; CRH**) and pituitary (**adrenocorticotrophic hormone; ACTH or corticotrophin**) are similar to regulation of thyroid hormones via thyrotrophin-releasing hormone and thyroid-stimulating hormone (**see Fig. 2.6.8**). Again, hormonal negative feedback on the pituitary gland is important and has a major implication for **long-term glucocorticoid (steroid) therapy.** At high levels of therapy, the feedback suppression is complete and the unstimulated pituitary cells and unstimulated adrenal cortical cells eventually atrophy so that the patient can no longer produce the life-saving cortisol surge if a major injury occurs. Such patients are advised to carry documentation, such as a Medic Alert bracelet. Then, if they are admitted to casualty unconscious from an injury, they will need supplementary cortisol injections, as would a patient with Addison's disease (below).

### CLINICAL APPLICATIONS

If the level of cortisol drops (as in **chronic adrenal insufficiency – Addison's disease**), the patient is unable to meet the quite considerable 'stress' of daytime living – maintaining the circulation in the upright posture and taking muscular exercise from time to time. Low blood pressure, very poor energy and nausea result and the patient is in serious danger of succumbing to even moderate injury or infection. Release of adrenocorticotrophic hormone is not inhibited and the levels rise. **Melanocyte-stimulating hormone** release is increased concurrently and causes the increased pigmentation found in this condition. Replacement therapy with glucocorticoids is required. Mineralocorticoids are usually also deficient and the patient must have a fairly high salt intake and possibly also a mineralocorticoid. If these patients sustain moderate to severe injury, or are seriously ill for any other reason, they are likely to require extra doses of cortisol. This treatment must be maintained until recovery is well under way. Blood pressure is carefully monitored, as a fall below normal suggests that not enough cortisol is being given.

Adrenocorticotrophic hormone is a peptide containing 39 amino acids. Interestingly, it is synthesized as a part of a large precursor molecule, which is also the precursor for melanocyte-stimulating hormone and the analgesic endorphins and enkephalins (endogenous opiates).

Adrenocorticotrophic hormone acts by binding to membrane receptors on adrenal cortical cells and stimulates the conversion of cholesterol to the steroid hormones. It also stimulates the release of glucocorticoids from the cell, but has only a small effect on the output of mineralocorticoid hormones.

At first sight it might seem strange that glucocorticoids have a **vital role in survival** after major trauma including surgery, as they can hinder healing and response to infection. However, it seems that the responses produced by the surge of cortisol and other hormones and nervous influences in this situation are absolutely essential for survival. In this situation, healing and response to infection do not seem to be seriously impaired. A clue to the key role of cortisol is that, in its absence, patients tend to collapse, with low blood pressure that fails to respond to blood and fluid transfusions but does respond to cortisol. This could be regarded as the ultimate permissive role of cortisol – permission to avoid fatal circulatory collapse!

## Conclusion

The endocrine system and the nervous system interact closely in the control of the body. The endocrine system is generally responsible for the range of metabolic functions that ensure that the general, unconscious activities of all the cells of the body occur in a coordinated way and body function continues, not only from day to day but at times of unusual physical stress. Knowing about the effects of the different hormones and the processes that regulate their activity should help nurses to understand the signs and symptoms, and the medical treatment given to patients with disorders of the endocrine system. This can help nurses to predict the problems likely to be met by such patients and to plan and provide the most appropriate nursing care.

---

## Clinical review

In addition to the Learning Objectives at the beginning of this chapter, the reader should be able to:

- Describe the body's hormonal response to environmental stressors and the importance of this in adaptation
- Apply knowledge of the function of the different hormones when assessing needs and planning care for patients with alteration in endocrine function

---

## Review questions

1. How do hypothalamic hormones reach the anterior lobe of the pituitary?
2. Which part of the pituitary has nervous communication with the hypothalamus?
3. What are the two main biochemical groups of hormones?
4. How can the activity of a cell be regulated by hormones?
5. What determines the blood levels of a hormone?
6. Which organs are mainly responsible for the metabolism and excretion of hormones?
7. What are catabolism and anabolism?
8. How do the thyroid hormones act at the cellular level?
9. What hormones are synthesized by the thyroid gland?
10. What is the role of iodine in the thyroid gland?
11. What action does thyroid stimulating hormone have on the thyroid gland?
12. Which organ is particularly vulnerable to a sudden drop in blood glucose?
13. How effective is glycolysis in generating ATP?
14. How effective is the Krebs' cycle in generating ATP?
15. What effects do insulin and glucagon respectively have on blood glucose levels?
16. Where is insulin synthesized?
17. Where does ADH act and what is its action?
18. What is the action of aldosterone?
19. What is angiotensinogen and why is it important?
20. What is the action and the effect of parathyroid hormone (PTH)?
21. What is the effect of calcitonin?
22. What are the main $\alpha$ and $\beta$ effects of catecholamines?

23  Where do the glucocorticoid hormones work and what action do they have?
24  How do the glucocorticoids help patients to survive major surgery and trauma?
25  How do the effects of hormones compare and contrast with the effects of nerves?
26  How do the controlling mechanisms for different hormones differ with respect to involvement of the brain?

## Suggestions for further reading

Boore, J.R.P. (1978) *Prescription for Recovery*. London: Royal College of Nursing. (Reprinted as Hayward, J. & Boore, J.R.P. (1994) *Research Classics from the Royal College of Nursing*. London: Scutari Press).
*This monograph reports an experimental study on the effect of preoperative preparation on postoperative recovery. The results indicate that preoperative preparation of patients to reduce anxiety can reduce corticosteroid hormone secretion and the risk of postoperative infection.*

Ganong, W.F. (2003) *Review of Medical Physiology*, 21st edn. New York: McGraw Hill.
*This is a concise textbook packed with facts, strong on endocrinology. For those who want to check-out the finer details.*

Greenspan, F.S. & Gardner, D.G. (2001) *Basic and Clinical Endocrinology*, 6th edn. East Norwalk, CT: Lange Medical.
*This textbook covers the physiology of the endocrine system and also the causes and effects of the various disorders and their treatment.*

Groër, M.W. & Shekleton, M.E. (1989) *Basic Pathophysiology: A Holistic Approach*, 3rd edn. St Louis: Mosby.

*This book examines the physiological disturbances of disease within a systems theory approach but with a strong emphasis on coping and adaptation.*

Pestana, C. (2000) *Fluids and Electrolytes in the Surgical Patient*, 5th edn. Philadelphia: Lippincott, Williams and Wilkins.
*This book is written for nurses and examines in detail the fluid and electrolyte disturbances to which surgical patients are prone, and the effects of such problems on their physiological functioning.*

Price, S.A. & Wilson, L.M. (2003) *Pathophysiology: Clinical Concepts of Disease Processes*, 6th edn. St Louis: Mosby.
*This book examines the causes and effects of disordered bodily functioning. It provides the necessary information for developing a good understanding of the physiological aspects of disease.*

Tanner, J.M. (1990) *Foetus into Man: Physical Growth from Conception to Maturity*, 2nd edn. Cambridge, MA: Harvard University Press.
*This book examines in detail the stages and control of human growth.*

## References

Cannon, W.B. & de la Paz, D. (1911) Emotional stimulation of adrenal secretion. *American Journal of Physiology*, **28**; 64–70.

Conn, J.W. (1977) Primary aldosteronism. In: Genest, J. et al. (eds) *Hypertension*. New York: McGraw-Hill, pp. 768–780.

Faulkner, F. & Tanner, J.M. (1986) *Human Growth: a Comprehensive Treatise*, vols 1–3. New York: Plenum Press.

Passmore, R. & Robson, J.S. (1976) *A Companion to Medical Studies. Vol 1. Anatomy, Biochemistry, Physiology and Related Subjects*, 2nd edn. Oxford: Blackwell Scientific, p. 27.10.

Tanner, J.M. (1962) *Growth at Adolescence*, 2nd edn. Oxford: Blackwell.

## Acknowledgement

I wish to acknowledge the contribution of Professor Jennifer R.P. Boore in laying the foundation of this chapter in previous editions.

# Stress

*Benita Wilson*

## LEARNING OBJECTIVES

After studying this chapter the reader should be able to:

- Give three reasons why an understanding of stress is important for nurses

- Identify and briefly describe the three major models of stress, including the changes associated with the general adaptation syndrome

- Describe the physiological changes associated with the sympatho-adrenomedullary (SAM) axis the hypothalamic–pituitary–adrenal (HPA) axis

- Identify the importance of the stress response for adaptation

- Identify the importance of stress as a causative factor in disease and list

  ten diseases in which stress is implicated

- Describe in detail how stress can contribute to the development of atheroma and identify the manifestations of this in four organs of the body

- Describe the effects of stress on the integrity of the gut and skin, the immune system and glucose metabolism

- Identify the types of circumstances associated with illness and treatment that can result in stress, and give an example of each type

- Describe the nursing interventions to minimize stress in patients

## INTRODUCTION

It is particularly important that nurses understand the concept of stress because stress influences the health and welfare of both patients and healthcare staff.

Stress has been implicated in the aetiology of a number of different diseases and in the severity or recurrence of symptoms in established disease. Furthermore, the degree of stress perceived by a patient can influence that person's recovery from illness or surgery; there is also evidence to suggest that nursing interventions to minimize stress can enhance postoperative recovery (Broome & Llewelyn, 1995).

Equally important for nurses to understand is the part that stress plays in their own lives. There is considerable evidence to demonstrate that high levels of stress are associated with the nursing role and can result in burnout, a state whereby nurses fail to interact effectively with patients and carry out their work automatically (McGrath, Reid & Boore, 1989).

Stress and those factors that are considered stressful have been studied in many professional groups, including student nurses (Lindop, 1991), trained nurses (Lees & Ellis, 1990) and nurse managers (Baglioni, Cooper & Hingley, 1990). Whereas some situations are stressful for only one group, such as a student nurse's lack of confidence in carrying out procedures (Parkes, 1985), other situations result in stress for nurses at any grade; dealing with death and bereavement proves difficult for many nurses. In addition, nurses move house, have rows with their boyfriend or girlfriend, have babies and experience the range of life events and daily hassles that have been identified as stressful (Evans & Johnson, 2000; Holmes & Rahe, 1967).

This chapter introduces different models of stress so that the patient's physiological responses to stressful situations and circumstances can be understood. These responses are then explained and explored in some detail. The role of stress in the aetiology of disease is discussed with reference to its influence on existing disease and illness. Finally, the role of illness and treatment in causing stress is considered in relation to the approaches that nurses can utilize to help patients minimize the effects of stress in their lives.

## What is stress?

Traditionally, stress has been difficult to define effectively, and it can in fact be described in three different ways: as a stimulus, as a response and as a transaction. Although the third description would now be recognized as the most valuable approach, it is important to understand the nature of all three models to be able to avoid confusion and identify when patients are experiencing stress.

## Stress as a stimulus

In this model, stress is seen purely as an external force that acts upon the individual. This view of stress as a stimulus originated in the field of engineering and considers stress in terms of forces applied to structures. When such stress occurs, it creates strain, which can result in fractures; if the stress is allowed to continue or increase, the structure will eventually break. It follows, then, that stress in humans is usually seen as an aversive or noxious stimulus within the individual's environment that produces a strain reaction, which is often treatable but that can be damaging. Early researchers claimed that stress was what happened *to* the individual, not what happened *within* them; that is, that stress was a situation or set of circumstances in the external environment rather than symptoms exhibited by the individual (Gross, 1998). Although this approach accepts that stress thresholds can vary due to individual differences, it fails to explain why the 'load' necessary to cause the strain within the individual cannot be quantified or defined. Unlike the predictable weight-bearing capacity of a wooden lintel or metal beam, the necessary load can reduce or

increase in response to situations and experiences encountered by an individual. For further explanation, see Bailey and Clarke (1989), who describe and critically review this model.

## Stress as a response

This model identifies stress as an endogenous response to stressors or factors within the environment (internal and external). The work supporting this approach focuses on biological changes; in essence, stress is the non-specific effect of any demand on the body (Ursin & Olff, 1993). Hans Selye (1976) was the first major researcher in this area. He described stress as 'a state manifested by a specific syndrome, which consists of all the non-specific changes within the biological system'. That is, the changes occur as a result of any stressor, yet they form a clearly differentiated syndrome; so the changes are the same for everyone and are the response to all stressors. In his early work, Selye found that different rats exposed to different acute noxious agents (such as cold, surgical injury and excessive exercise) responded by displaying a group of very similar negative symptoms.

Selye confirmed these findings with human subjects in his observations of hospital patients experiencing various injuries and illnesses. He was interested in the 'just being ill' syndrome – the group of symptoms that include the general aches and pains, raised temperature, malaise, furred tongue, etc. that are common to many illnesses. Seyle claimed that these characteristics were not just attributable to the illness but were also symptomatic of the stress response. He argued that this response could make a significant contribution to the physical pathology, that is to say that illness is a stressor that causes the stress response, which in turn exacerbates the existing illness and pathological changes. Although others have added to and refined the original description of the changes in stress, Selye's version of the stress response still stands. He called this response the triphasic **general adaptation syndrome**, comprising of the **alarm reaction, stage of resistance** and **stage of exhaustion**. **Figure 2.7.1** demonstrates the variation in resistance throughout these stages. The changes identified by Seyle are associated with increased secretion of corticosteroid hormones from the adrenal cortex.

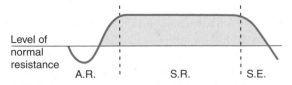

**Figure 2.7.1**  The general adaptation syndrome (see text for phases). A.R., alarm reaction; S.R., stage of resistance; S.E., stage of exhaustion

The alarm reaction is triggered by the encounter of a stressor, which activates the hypothalamic–pituitary–adrenal (HPA) system. During the initial shock phase, blood pressure and muscle tension drop briefly before the countershock phase, which alerts the subject to possible threat. If the stressor subsides, nervous and endocrine system activity rapidly return to normal levels. However, if the stressor persists, the body attempts to adapt to the demands of the environment and the stage of resistance is reached. Although endocrine and sympathetic activity might drop slightly in this stage compared with the alarm phase, they are still maintained at a higher than normal level. There might be few outward signs of stress but the body's ability to resist additional stressors could be impaired. In this stage, the body has a finite ability to cope with the physiological demands made upon it and, in time, resources might become so depleted that the final stage is reached.

The stage of exhaustion occurs when the individual's physiological ability to resist the stressor is exceeded. There is a depletion of bodily resources and the symptoms of the alarm stage reappear, making the individual more vulnerable to what Selye terms 'diseases of adaptation' – peptic ulcers, enlargement of the lymph and thymus glands, shrinkage of the adrenal cortex, hypertension and illnesses that result from an impaired immune system. If this stage is allowed to continue, the body becomes exhausted.

Despite Seyle's work providing a good basis for understanding the physiological effects of stress, his early work failed to consider the variations in individual perceptions of stressors (Ur, 1991). Mason (1975) illustrated how the same stressors produced different patterns in the secretion of adrenaline (epinephrine) and noradrenaline (norepinephrine) in different individuals. In addition, Mason highlighted how stressors do not always bring about the same response in the same individual (Mason et al., 1976). He explained that the body is not passive when reacting to stressors, suggesting that judgements are made that then influence the physiological response. Although Selye's later work accepted the role of conditioning factors in modifying the way in which an individual might respond to stressors, it did not go far enough in explaining how or why this occurs.

## Stress as a transaction

The key to understanding this third model is the suggestion that the word 'transaction' refers to the interaction between the individual and the environment. This concept of transaction adds an important dimension in that it reinforces the individual as an active participant. The emphasis is on whether individuals recognize an imbalance between the perceived demands of the situation and their perception of their resources to cope. This includes an appraisal of biological, psychological and social assets. The evaluation of whether the resources will meet the demand is based on the individual's subjective judgement and does not necessarily reflect reality as seen by others. Yet this estimation will determine the outcome of whether the stress response will occur. It is the subjective nature of stress that makes it so elusive and difficult to define. **Figure 2.7.2** shows the elements of this approach as described by Cox (1978).

Three types of cognitive appraisal are used when an individual is confronted with stressors (Lazarus & Folkman, 1984). **Primary appraisal** refers to the initial assessment of whether the demand threatens the person's well-being and whether any resources are available. **Secondary appraisal** is the estimation of the perceived resources to meet the demand. If an imbalance exists between demand and capability, the person feels unable to cope and a stress response will occur. However, if he or she feels able to cope with the demand, then the stress will not occur. The sequence of these two mental processes can change depending on the individual and the situation encountered. The third type of appraisal is **reappraisal**, when the individual assesses the effectiveness or otherwise of the coping behaviour.

### CLINICAL APPLICATIONS

Of the three approaches to considering stress, this model is the most useful for nursing and the most comprehensive in explanation. It is this model that provides the rationale for Lazarus & Folkman's (1984) widely accepted definition of stress:

*...a pattern of negative physiological states and psychological responses occurring in situations where people perceive threats to their well-being which they may be unable to meet.*

The crucial element is that it is the individual's *perceptions* of both the threat and the available resources that dictate the physiological responses. Consequently, the experience of stress will not occur if the individual perceives that he or she can master the situation (Karasek & Theorell, 1990). This scope for adaptation to demand highlights the nurse's role in working with patients to enhance their coping abilities and thus minimize stress.

The stress as a transaction model illustrates how the psychological aspects of stress are as important as the physiological. However this chapter will now focus on an explanation and discussion of the physiological aspects of stress.

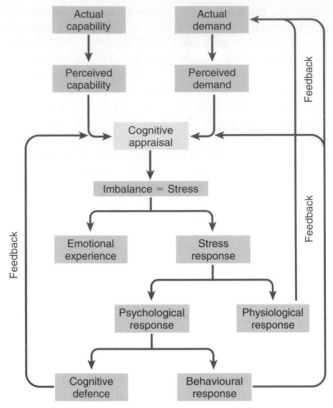

**Figure 2.7.2**   The transactional model of stress

## The physiological changes of stress

Although Selye described the changes associated with increased levels of corticosteroid hormones, it is now clear that the secretion of the majority of hormones is altered by stress.

The hypothalamus, a neuroendocrine gland, plays a central role in stress because it regulates the secretion of the majority of hormones in the human body, as discussed in Chapter 2.6. The hypothalamus receives impulses from the cerebral cortex via the limbic system. The perception by the cerebral cortex is influenced by the emotional impact provided by the interpretations of the limbic system (Myers, 1998), which in turn influences the activity of the hypothalamus. Thus, the secretion of all the hormones whose activity is regulated by the hypothalamus is modified in stress. As some of these hormones influence the activity of other hormones not directly regulated by the hypothalamus, the physiological changes in stress might be even wider than is at first apparent.

Selye's description of the stress response dealt with only one aspect of the phenomenon, that which occurs relatively slowly. However, there are two aspects of the stress response: (i) the acute, short-lasting response is initiated by sympathetic nervous activity and the secretion of catecholamines from the adrenal medulla; and (ii) the slower, longer-lasting response is caused mainly by the action of glucocorticoid hormones from the adrenal cortex gland instigated by the HPA.

## The sympatho-adrenomedullary (SAM) axis (the fast stress response)

This rapid reaction is also known as the **flight or fight** response (Cannon, 1927). It occurs very rapidly, in parallel with the HPA, as catecholamines, stored in vesicles in the cells ready for release, are secreted rapidly from the sympathetic nervous system and the adrenal medulla in response to hypothalamic influence (Martini, 2001). The adrenal medulla enlarges, secreting catecholamines such as adrenaline (epinephrine) and noradrenaline (norepinephrine), which, as sympathomimetics, mimic sympathetic branch activity and help to maintain the increased physiological activity characteristic of this response. Detailed information about the actions of these hormones is provided in Chapter 2.6.

It is important to realize that the changes that occur in the SAM help prepare the body to respond rapidly and effectively to real or imagined threat (Clow, 2001). The supply of oxygen to the tissues is increased as the heart rate is increased, the blood pressure raised and respiration rate increased. More nutrients are made available to the tissues by increased release of glucose and fatty acids into the

**Table 2.7.1** Physical signs (including common clinical measurements) and symptoms which may occur in acute stress (from Boore et al., 1987)

| Site | Physiological basis | Physical signs and common clinical measurements | Physical symptoms |
|---|---|---|---|
| Cardiovascular system | Increased cardiac rate and output | Tachycardia<br>Pulse of full volume<br>Raised blood pressure | Pounding heart<br>Palpitations<br>Chest pain<br>Headache |
| Respiratory system | CNS arousal<br><br>If the hyperventilation is not in response to physiological need, low ppCO$_2$ results and leads to vasodilatation, fall in blood pressure and, in extreme cases, tetany | Increased rate and depth of ventilation<br>Tetany in extreme cases | Dizziness, faintness, panic (in extreme cases)<br>Tingling in the extremities<br>Muscle spasm (in extreme cases) |
| Gastrointestinal system | Reduced blood supply to and reduced secretion in gastrointestinal tract<br>Decreased or increased mobility of tract | <br><br><br>Vomiting<br>Diarrhoea<br>Constipation<br>Anorexia or overeating | Dry mouth indigestion/dyspepsia<br><br><br>Nausea<br>Diarrhoea (often frequent)<br>Constipation<br>Anorexia or overeating |
| Skin | Contraction of pilomotor muscles<br>Cholinergic sweating<br>Reduced blood supply | Erection of hair<br><br>Sweating<br>Pallor | <br><br>Clammy palms |
| Eye | Contraction of radial muscle | Dilated pupils | Blurred vision |
| Muscle | CNS arousal | Muscle tension, tremor<br>Muscle spasm in severe cases<br>Lack of coordination | Headache<br>Muscle tension, tremor, twitching<br>Lack of coordination<br>Back pain |
| General | CNS arousal<br><br>Increased metabolic rate | Insomnia<br>Restlessness<br><br>Low grade pyrexia | Insomnia<br>Restlessness<br>Fatigue/weakness<br>Feeling hot or cold |

CNS, central nervous system; ppCO$_2$, partial pressure of carbon dioxide.

bloodstream. The body is prepared for injury by increasing the coagulability of the blood so that loss of blood will be minimized. The increased arousal of the nervous system will ensure a rapid response. The signs and symptoms of acute stress are detailed in **Table 2.7.1**. These physiological and biochemical changes are extremely valuable when a physical threat is present. However, if a physical response is not appropriate, the enhanced physiological and nervous arousal is tiring and can often be counterproductive.

## The hypothalamic–pituitary–adrenal (HPA) axis (the slow stress response)

Physiological stress is characterized by the activation of both the SAM and the HPA axes (Moynihan et al., 1994). During stressful situations, the hypothalamus is influenced by impulses from the cerebral cortex and the limbic system. The emotional content of the limbic impulses is important because the magnitude of the stress response is related to the level of an individual's emotional arousal (Biondi & Pancheri, 1995). The hypothalamus initiates the flow of corticotrophic releasing hormone (CRH) via the infundibulum, which is linked to the anterior pituitary gland. In turn, the anterior pituitary gland secretes adrenocorticotrophic hormone (ACTH) into the bloodstream. This targets the adrenal cortex, which in response secretes various corticosteroids, including glucocorticoids such as corticosterone, cortisone and hydrocortisone. High blood glucocorticoid concentrations lead to increases in:

- the mobilization of fats and tissue protein
- liver gluconeogenesis (the creation of new glucose)
- fat catabolism (Thibodeau & Patton, 1992).

These characteristics of the stress response are important in enhancing the body's ability to cope with additional and/or continued physical demands. The additional nutrients released into the bloodstream are directed to the tissues where they are most required. Increased breakdown of protein releases amino acids into the bloodstream for any necessary tissue repair. Increased retention of water and sodium leads to increased fluid volume, making the body more able to cope with blood loss, and at the same time the blood's coagulability is increased. Inflammation is reduced in stress and this can increase the body's ability to cope with physical demand. The physiological effects of glucocorticoids secreted in stress are shown in **Table 2.7.2**.

The response resulting from the activity of glucocorticoids is much slower to develop for two reasons. First, the increased amounts of the hormones have to be synthesized within the cells of the adrenal cortex before they can be secreted into the circulation. Second, the effects of these hormones often occur through the stimulation of the formation of enzymes in the target cells of the body; both of these activities take time. Similarly, the effects last longer because the enzymes thus produced remain functioning for a prolonged period. Detailed information on the actions of these hormones is given in Chapter 2.6.

## Other hormone changes in stress

The secretion of nearly every hormone is altered in stress (Carola, Harley & Noback, 1992) and the changes that occur are summarized in **Table 2.7.3**. The major effects result in increased catabolism, which increases the availability of nutrients for energy, and an increase in the extracellular fluid volume, thus enhancing the body's ability to cope with trauma and haemorrhage.

## Stress as a causative factor in disease

Although stress is essentially an adaptive response and is necessary for continued life and health, it can also play a part in the aetiology of disease (Sternberg, 2001). The major concern of normal physiology is to maintain homeostasis and in stress homeostasis is disrupted. In the normal stress response, the homeostatic disturbances are fairly rapidly returned to normal when the person affected no longer perceives the situation as threatening and recognizes his or her ability to cope.

A number of deleterious effects can occur as a result of prolonged periods of raised hormone levels (see **Table 2.7.2**) and these are the same if the high levels result from stress or another cause. Prolonged stress has been implicated in the development of a number of diseases, examples of which are shown in **Table 2.7.4**. In some circumstances, even though stress might not have played a role in the initial aetiology of a condition, it could play a part in initiating an exacerbation of a chronic disease. The mechanisms by which stress results in the development of some important and relatively common disorders is explained below.

## Disturbances to the circulation

One of the major causes of disease in developed countries in the twentieth century was the development of atheroma, a thick porridge-like substance that is laid down in the major arteries of the body (Tortora & Grabowski, 2000) and is a major cause of death in Western civilization (Ross, 1988). By causing reduced circulation to the organs of the body, atheroma can result in a number of different conditions depending on the part of the body affected, for example:

- angina and myocardial infarction affecting the heart
- transient ischaemic attacks and cerebrovascular accidents affecting the brain
- peripheral vascular disease causing intermittent claudication and, later, gangrene of the legs
- blockage of the mesenteric arteries supplying the gut leading to loss of function of the intestinal muscle and thus resulting in intestinal obstruction.

Stress plays a major role in the development of atheroma, although other factors such as smoking (which might itself be a behavioural response to stress), diet, high blood pressure (discussed below) and genetic factors are also important. A number of

**Table 2.7.2** Physiological effects of glucocorticoid secretion in stress (from Boore et al., 1987)

| Body function or site | Glucocorticoid effect | Short-term physiological effects | Additional long-term physiological effects |
|---|---|---|---|
| Carbohydrate metabolism | Stimulates hepatic gluconeogenesis<br>Enhances elevation of blood glucose produced by other hormones e.g. adrenaline, glucagon<br>Inhibits uptake of glucose by most tissues (not brain) by antagonizing peripheral effects of insulin<br>Inhibits activity of glycolytic enzyme hexokinase | Increased plasma glucose<br><br><br><br>*Glycosuria (if renal threshold exceeded)<br><br>(Steroid diabetes) | |
| Protein metabolism | Stimulates breakdown of body protein and depresses protein synthesis<br>Stimulates hepatic deamination of amino acids | Increased plasma levels of amino acids<br>Increased nitrogen content of urine<br>Negative nitrogen balance | *Muscle wasting<br>*Thinning of the skin<br>*Loss of hair<br>*Depression of the immune response |
| Lipid metabolism | Promotes lipolysis | Increased plasma levels of fatty acids and cholesterol<br>Increased ketone body production and ketonuria | *Redistribution of adipose tissue from periphery to head and trunk |
| Calcium metabolism | *Antagonizes vitamin D metabolites and so reduces calcium absorption from gut<br>Increases renal excretion of calcium | | *Osteoporosis<br><br><br>Kidney stones |
| Vascular reactivity | Permissive for noradrenaline to induce vasoconstriction<br>Reduces capillary permeability | *Prevents stress-induced hypotension | |
| Inflammatory response | *Stabilizes membranes of cellular lysosomes (inhibiting their rupture)<br>*Suppresses phagocytosis<br>*Reduces multiplication of fibroblasts in connective tissue and hence decreases production of collagen fibres<br>*Inhibits formation and release of histamine and bradykinin | *Inhibition of inflammation<br><br><br><br>*Decreased formation of granulation tissue<br><br><br>*Reduced allergic response | *Gastric ulceration<br><br><br><br>*Reduced rate of wound healing |
| Immune response | *Reduced immunoglobulin synthesis<br>*Decreased levels of lymphocytes, basophils and eosinophils<br><br>*Atrophy of lymphoid tissue | *Decreased white blood cell count<br>*Immunosuppression and decreased resistance to infection | |

*(Contd)*

**Table 2.7.2**  (*Contd*)

| Body function or site | Glucocorticoid effect | Short-term physiological effects | Additional long-term physiological effects |
|---|---|---|---|
| Water and electrolyte balance | Enhances sodium ion and water reabsorption in distal tubules and collecting ducts of renal nephrons<br>Reciprocal potassium and hydrogen ion excretion (mineralocorticoid effect) | Increased extracellular fluid volume | |
| Blood | *Enhances coagulability<br>*Reduces levels of lymphocytes basophils and eosinophils<br>*Increases levels of erythrocytes, platelets and neutrophils | *Reduced blood clotting time<br>*Decreased white blood cell count<br>*Haemoconcentration (increased viscosity) | |
| Central nervous system | *Emotional changes (in excess or deficiency)<br>May facilitate learning and memory (ACTH may, independently facilitate learning and memory) | *Emotional changes<br><br>Increased rate of learning<br>Enhanced learning | |

*These physiological effects occur only when high plasma levels of glucocorticoids, similar to those found during steroid therapy, are present.

**Table 2.7.3**  The secretion and effects of other hormones in stress (from Boore et al., 1987)

| Hormone | Endocrine gland of origin | Physiological functions | Effect of stressor on secretion | Physiological effects in stress |
|---|---|---|---|---|
| Somatostatin | Hypothalamus | Inhibits secretion of growth hormone and thyroid stimulating hormone<br><br>Suppresses output of insulin and glucagon | Inhibited | Secretion of growth hormone and thyroid stimulating hormone facilitated<br>Secretion of insulin and glucagon increased |
| Antidiuretic hormone | Hypothalamus and posterior pituitary | Increased water reabsorption from the distal tubule and collecting duct of renal nephrons<br>May also influence learning by direct action on the brain | Increased | Increased extracellular fluid volume<br><br>Enhanced learning |
| Growth hormone | Anterior pituitary | Reinforces carbohydrate and lipid mobilizing effects and insulin antagonism of catecholamines and cortisol | Increased in acute stress | Promotes gluconeogenesis and elevation in blood glucose |

*(Contd)*

**Table 2.7.3** (*Contd*)

| Hormone | Endocrine gland of origin | Physiological functions | Effect of stressor on secretion | Physiological effects in stress |
|---|---|---|---|---|
| | | May stimulate uptake of amino acids by injured tissue, but unable to counteract catabolic effect of cortisol on body protein | Cortisol suppresses release, so decreased in chronic stress | Facilitates tissue growth and repair<br>Retarded growth in chronic stress |
| Thyroid stimulating hormone<br>Thyroxine and Tri-iodothyronine | Anterior pituitary<br><br>Thyroid | Raised metabolic rate acts synergistically with catecholamines | Increased in acute stress but secretion suppressed by cortisol in chronic stress | Potentiation of catecholamine effects in acute stress |
| Aldosterone | Adrenal cortex | Increased sodium ion reabsorption from distal tubule and collecting duct of nephron | Increased | Increased extracellular fluid volume |
| Glucagon | Pancreas (α-cells) | Promotes glycolysis and gluconeogenesis<br>Presence of cortisol permissive for these actions | Hypoglycaemia is major stimulus for secretion but large increases in secretion also occur in response to other stressors, such as cold exposure, exercise and acute anxiety | Raised plasma glucose |
| Insulin | Pancreas (β-cells) | Promotes entry of glucose into most body cells<br>Anabolic effect on lipid and protein metabolism | Catecholamines suppress release<br><br>Cortisol and Growth hormone antagonize peripheral effects | Actions inhibited |
| Gonadotrophins (Follicle stimulating and luteinizing hormones) | Anterior pituitary | Secretion of gonadal steroids reduced | Inhibited | Irregularity or cessation of menstrual cycle<br>Failure of ovulation<br>Infertility |

the effects of stress contribute to the development of these disorders:

1. Both catecholamine and corticosteroid hormones stimulate the breakdown of adipose tissue, and the levels of free fatty acids in the blood are raised (O'Hara, 1996). These are then available to be incorporated into **atheroma**. The blood vessels are thus narrowed and have roughened linings.

2. The narrowed arteries reduce the supply of oxygen to the tissues. This results in **angina** when the heart's demand for oxygen is greater than the supply, **transient ischaemic attacks** when the brain's demand is greater than the supply, or **intermittent claudication** when the leg's demand is greater than the supply.

3. Catecholamines increase tissue metabolism and heart rate and thus increase the heart's demand

**Table 2.7.4** Some diseases in which stress is or might be an aetiological factor

| | |
|---|---|
| Coronary heart disease | Cerebrovascular accident |
| Hypertension | Migraine |
| Bronchial asthma | Peptic ulceration |
| Ulcerative colitis | Spastic colon |
| Diabetes mellitus | Hyperthyroidism |
| Reproductive disorders | Growth retardation |
| Rheumatoid arthritis | Multiple sclerosis |
| Eczema and dermatitis | Cancer |
| Autoimmune disease | Allergies |
| Infections | |

for oxygen, which cannot be supplied (Bohus & Koolhaas, 1993), leading to **angina**.

4. The viscosity of the blood is increased and clotting time reduced, thus **blood clots** are more likely to form against the rough linings of the arteries (Tortora & Grabowski, 2000) and block them partially or completely. Complete obstruction of an artery will lead to death and loss of function of the tissue supplied by that artery, e.g. **intestinal obstruction, myocardial infarction, gangrene** of the leg, **cerebrovascular accident**.

5. Corticosteroids increase potassium and magnesium loss and sodium retention in the body, and thus alter the electrolyte balance at the cardiac cell membranes. The resulting abnormal function is thought to result in **myocardial infarction** when there is reduced oxygen availability (Bohus & Koolhaas, 1993).

6. Sustained high levels of catecholamines may deplete high-energy phosphates (the energy stores) in cells and, thus, be toxic to cardiac muscle (Ramsey, 1982).

7. Catecholamines increase the blood pressure and, in susceptible individuals, frequent release of catecholamines because of stress can result in **hypertension** (Groër & Shekleton, 1989). This increases the risk of atheroma formation and the risk of a **cerebrovascular accident**. Hypertension can also result in cardiac hypertrophy, aortic aneurysm, cerebral ischaemia and nephrosclerosis, which can lead to renal failure (Martini, 2001).

8. Elevated levels of glucocorticoids can lead to memory impairment by damaging some hippocampal neurons involved in the consolidation of memory (Sapolsky, 1994).

## Endocrine disorders

A number of disorders result from disturbed interaction of the different hormones secreted in the body, and some of these are identified in Chapter 2.6. Because stress alters the secretion of so many of the hormones, it is reasonable to expect a variety of endocrine disturbances to be associated with stress.

Diabetes mellitus is a condition with a very complex aetiology and it has been hypothesized that stress plays a part in the development of non-insulin dependent diabetes (Vander, Sherman & Luciano, 2000). In animal experimentation, stress, although not the primary cause, has been shown to be a factor in precipitating the development of the disease (Carter et al., 1987; Mazelis et al., 1987). However, much of the evidence for this in humans is based on anecdotal and retrospective reports, and it has not been proved that stress is a factor in the development of this disease (Wilkinson, 1991). Nevertheless, there are various ways in which stress could influence the development or presentation of diabetes mellitus (see Chapter 2.6):

1. Catecholamines stimulate the release of glucose from the liver and, as the blood glucose rises, this excess will stimulate the pancreas to release more insulin. If this is not adequate then hyperglycaemia develops.

2. Corticosteroids counteract the effect of insulin. Thus, in prolonged stress, glucose does not enter the cells normally and the blood glucose level rises. Some people predisposed to develop diabetes mellitus have a lower than normal amount of insulin in the pancreatic cells. The high blood glucose levels stimulate the release of insulin and might exhaust the insulin-secreting pancreatic cells; the person develops diabetes mellitus.

3. A number of other hormones also antagonize insulin and can result in diabetes mellitus. People with acromegaly due to excessive amounts of growth hormone secretion, or with thyrotoxicosis, have a higher incidence of diabetes mellitus than the general population (Alberti & Hockaday, 1983).

4. There is evidence that psychological stress and poor diabetic control often coexist but evidence to support a relationship is inconclusive (Pickup & Williams, 1991). However, stress might result in modifications to behaviour that reduce compliance with dietary advice or insulin administration leading to loss of metabolic stability.

Growth retardation is another example of an endocrine disorder that occurs due to the inhibition of the hypothalamic hormone, which stimulates growth hormone release (Gardener, 1972).

## The immune system and inflammatory response

Prolonged high levels of glucocorticoid secretion, as can occur in stress, will reduce the immune and inflammatory responses of the body. Those affected are more prone to infection and to cancer because increased corticosteroid levels:

1. Suppress the inflammatory response and formation of new granulation tissue (Likar et al., 1963) and lead to a reduction in phagocytosis (Greendyke, Bradley & Swisher, 1965). Infection is not localized and can spread more readily throughout the body.
2. Decrease levels of lymphocytes and other white blood cells, which will reduce the body's ability to combat infection.
3. Result in reduced immunoglobulin formation (Groër & Shekleton, 1989) due to increased protein breakdown and depressed protein synthesis.
4. Depress cellular immunity (Ursin & Olff, 1993), resulting in impaired surveillance for abnormal cells that should no longer be recognized as 'self'. Thus, cells that have become malignant are less likely to be destroyed by the normal immune mechanisms and the malignant cells are able to multiply and spread.

## Influence on protein structures

One of the actions of glucocorticoids is to increase protein breakdown, with many of the amino acids released being used in gluconeogenesis (to form new glucose). This increase in protein breakdown is linked with a reduction in the formation of new protein with deleterious results, including:

- thinning of the skin
- muscle wasting
- loss of hair
- slowing of wound healing.

In addition, this change in protein synthesis is often associated with other changes of stress to cause or aggravate disease associated with the integrity of the gut lining or the skin.

Peptic ulceration is a relatively common condition frequently associated with stress (Guyton, 1992). Normally, a balance is achieved between the gastric juices and other potential causes of damage and the resistance of the gut wall to these substances; the integrity of the lining of the stomach and duodenum (the sites of peptic ulceration) is maintained. The minor damage continually occurring to the gut wall is repaired very rapidly through cell division. The potentially damaging effects of the hydrochloric acid produced in the stomach is prevented by a number of mechanisms, including the secretion of a slightly alkaline layer of mucus that acts as a barrier over the gastric mucosa and the regulation of secretion of gastric hydrochloric acid by negative feedback mechanisms. Stress interrupts the normal situation in several ways (Groër & Shekleton, 1989):

1. Increasing the levels of substances that can damage the gut lining by stimulating an increase in hydrochloric acid and pepsinogen secretion.
2. Reducing the ability of the gut lining to resist the action of the gastric juices by:
   - slowing wound healing, and thus minor damage to the mucosa remains open to the action of the gastric acid and can develop into an ulcer
   - causing a decrease in mucosal blood flow, which results in cellular hypoxia and tissue damage
   - inhibiting the normal protective inflammatory response of the gut mucosa and thus allowing attack by the gastric juices.
3. Increasing the frequency of behavioural responses to stress, some of which can reduce the resistance of the gut lining; these include smoking, drinking alcohol, or taking certain drugs (such as aspirin).

## The role of illness and treatment in causing stress

Discussion so far has concentrated on ways in which stress can influence the development or presentation of disease, but equally it is necessary to consider how illness and resulting treatments can be the cause of stress.

### CLINICAL APPLICATIONS

Lazarus (1966) identified six events that can induce the stress response, many of which are experienced by patients:

- uncertainly about physical survival
- uncertainty about maintaining one's identity
- inability to control the immediate environment

- pain and privation
- loss of loved ones
- disruption of community life.

Mishel (1984) identified four types of circumstance that are associated with uncertainty in patients. He established a strong relationship between uncertainty and stress as a consequence of a patient's perception of the situation and his or her ability to cope with the demands of:

- discomfort, incapacitation and other symptoms of illness
- management of special treatment procedures and their side-effects
- technical environments, including relating with medical and other healthcare providers
- assessment of the future and reassessing independence.

This relationship between uncertainty and stress was reinforced by the work of Volicer and Bohannon (1975), who developed a Hospital Stress Rating Scale consisting of 49 items. The items causing the most stress were ranked in order of severity:

1. Thinking you might lose your sight.
2. Thinking you might have cancer.
3. Thinking you might lose a kidney or some other organ.
4. Knowing you have a serious illness.
5. Thinking you might lose your hearing.
6. Not being told what your diagnosis is.
7. Not knowing for sure what illness you have.
8. Not getting pain medication when you need it.
9. Not knowing the results of or reasons for your treatments.

These studies all seem to indicate that the traditional role of being a patient can be stressful in itself. While experiencing illness, patients might feel powerless, helpless and passive, as all responsibility and decision making regarding their care is taken, on their behalf, by health professionals. Nichols (1995) argues that typical general hospital entry involves patients adopting a role of required helplessness for the benefit of the institution. He claims that patients can feel excluded from the process of caring for themselves and that this experience takes away their personal status, dignity and control.

## Approaches to helping patients minimize stress

This chapter has concentrated on the physio-logical effects of stress but has also acknowledged the importance of psychological aspects. Awareness of these psychological factors can help nurses minimize the physiological aspects of the stress response.

## CLINICAL APPLICATIONS

The transactional model predicts that the perception of control can mediate the effects of stressors (Krause & Shaw, 2000). Stress will not be experienced if individuals perceive that they can master the situation (Karasek & Theorell, 1990). This is demonstrated in cross-cultural studies that have shown how workers with little or no control over their work environment are more likely to suffer heart disease than workers with a high degree of control over their work environment (Cheng et al., 2000).

Studies have demonstrated how 'informational control' can be used in healthcare settings to help reduce postoperative pain, improve the rate of wound healing and increase general well-being (Haywood, 1975), and reduce distress for children in the emergency room (Chamberlain, 2000). Informational control includes exploring how patients perceive the situation and providing information to enable them to understand the environment and what is happening. This control enables patients to evaluate the demand on them and make appropriate decisions about their resources and ability to cope. It is therefore important to ensure that they receive clear, honest and frequent information about their condition and treatment. This could involve spending time with patients after they have received bad news and providing an environment to allow them to express their feelings, organize their reactions, recognize their own strengths and begin to identify coping mechanisms (Rusk, 1971).

Cognitive control requires individuals to think about the situation they are in so as to alter the way that they perceive the threat. Such control can be implemented in two ways, either problem focused or emotion focused.

Problem-focused strategies reduce the demands of the stressor by exploring the resources available to deal with the situation. Examples of this strategy could include using cognitive processes (thinking) to define the problem, seek alternative solutions and evaluate their pros and cons before finally implementing the best course of action. To alter the problem causing the stress could be as simple as requesting medical help for a condition, seeking-out treatments or securing money to pay a bill. For the strategy to reduce the demands of the stressor and ameliorate the effects of stress, it is vital that individuals perceives that change can be effected by their efforts.

Emotion-focused strategies attempt to prevent negative emotions becoming so overwhelming that the individual perceives them as uncontrollable (Atkinson et al., 2000). Moos (1988) divided emotion-focused coping into two types of strategy, behavioural and cognitive. Behavioural strategies include physical exercise and activity, the use of alcohol and drugs, and seeking social support from family and friends.

Cognitive control usually involves a reappraisal of the stressor. Attempts are made to restructure the thought patterns and redefine the meaning of the stressor e.g. 'I know it is painful but this operation will put an end to the pain I feel on a daily basis'. The perception of the threat and the individual's ability to cope is restructured. Taylor (1983) utilized this strategy to help female breast cancer sufferers come to terms with the effects of their surgery.

The use of control strategies, informational and cognitive, will not eliminate stressors but will help individuals perceive them in a less negative manner, thus making them less disruptive (Antoni et al., 2000).

Other patient-centred strategies that nurses can use to help minimize stress in their patients include:

1. Encouraging patients to identify the questions that they need to ask (Coles, 1990), refer them to counselling services if necessary.
2. Providing information that allows patients to play an active role in their own treatment and recovery (Bailey & Clarke, 1989).
3. Involving patients and their families in the planning of care, and helping them to carry out the plan of care (Nichols, 1993).
4. Managing pain (Sofaer, 1998).
5. Providing clear information about what patients should do and how they will feel after discharge from hospital, and making adequate arrangements for appropriate community care (Wilson-Barnett & Fordham, 1982).

Nursing care to minimize stress includes both physical and psychological interventions. Some of the approaches that can be used are relatively straightforward and can be utilized by all nurses. However, some of the psychological approaches to the management of stress require specialist skills and knowledge that comes from additional training. Bailey & Clarke (1989) discuss a number of these in detail and their book is recommended for further study.

## Conclusion

This chapter introduced the models of stress so that the physiological effects of stress could be considered and discussed in some detail. Understanding the models highlights how approaches to care can minimize the stress response. The recognition that nurses can use their interpersonal skills to help patients re-evaluate their perceptions of a situation is crucial in the management of stress.

---

## Clinical review

In addition to the Learning Objectives at the beginning of this chapter, the reader should be able to:

- Identify situations associated with illness or treatment that often cause stress

- Describe the approaches that nurses can use to minimize the stress experienced by patients

---

## Review questions

1 What are the stages and major changes in the general adaptation syndrome?
2 What leads to stress in the transactional model?
3 How does the emotional impact of stress alter hormone levels in the body?
4 Describe the effects of the 'fight or flight' reaction on the cardiovascular and respiratory systems.
5 Which hormones are responsible, respectively, for the SAM and HPA systems?
6 What physiological changes result from the HPA axis due to glucocorticoid secretion?

7   Why might stress lead to atheroma?
8   Why might stress lead to increased susceptibility to infection?
9   Why might stress lead to peptic ulceration?
10  Distinguish between informational and cognitive control as stress reduction strategies.

## Suggestions for further reading

Bailey, R. & Clarke, M. (1989) *Stress and Coping in Nursing*. London: Chapman and Hall.
*This is an excellent book for developing a broad understanding of stress. It reviews the theory and research on stress and coping and gives considerably more psychological detail than could be included in this chapter. It will help nurses to understand and cope with their own stress and to help patients cope with stress.*

Boore, J.R.P. (1978) *Prescription for Recovery*. London: Royal College of Nursing. Reprinted in Hayward, J. & Boore, J.R.P. (1994) *Research Classics from the Royal College of Nursing, Vol. 1*. London: Scutari Press.
*This monograph reports an experimental study on the effect of preoperative preparation on postoperative recovery. The results indicate that preoperative preparation of patients to minimize anxiety can reduce corticosteroid hormone secretion and the rate of postoperative infection.*

Broome, A. & Llewelyn, S. (1995) *Health Psychology: Processes and Applications*. London: Chapman and Hall.
*Unusually, this book provides an introduction to health psychology from a British perspective. The chapter by Nichols highlights some of the problems and issues in using client-centred care to reduce stress in institutional settings.*

Burnard, P. (1991) *Coping with Stress in the Health Professions: A Practical Guide*. London: Chapman and Hall.
*This accessible handbook deals with the issues of stress in relation to health professionals. It provides clear advice on the effects of stress and some instructional activities to help combat such effects. It also suggests how support systems for individuals and groups could be structured.*

Conduct and Utilization of Research Project (CURN) (1981) *Distress Reduction through Sensory Preparation*. New York: Grune and Stratton.
*This book is based on Jean Johnson's work on the value of giving information about the sensations to be experienced*

by patients during various procedures. It gives guidelines on the translation of her research findings into nursing practice.

Conduct and Utilization of Research Project (CURN) (1981) *Mutual Goal Setting in Patient Care*. New York: Grune and Stratton.
*This book is one of a series that provides guidelines on the translation of research findings into nursing practice. It contains several research papers relevant to the topic and then examines approaches to implementation.*

Cox, T. (1978) *Stress*. London: Macmillan.
*This book covers both the nature of stress and its effects, as well as its experience and management. It draws upon a wide range of disciplines and gives a broad view of the subject.*

Grossman, A. (ed) (1987) *Neuroendocrinology of Stress. Baillière's Clinical Endocrinology and Metabolism, 1 (2)*. London: Baillière Tindall.
*This volume consists of eleven chapters, each of which discusses in depth one aspect of stress. It includes causation, regulation and detail about some of the physiological results of the stress response.*

Jones, F. & Bright, J. (2001) *Stress: Myth, Theory and Research*. Harlow: Prentice Hall.
*An interesting and approachable book that gives a comprehensive insight into all areas of stress. It includes chapters on the measurement of stress, its physiology, individual differences in reactions to stress, stress at home and work, and a selection of strategies for stress reduction.*

Selye, H. (1976) *The Stress of Life*, 2nd edn. New York: McGraw-Hill.
*This is the classic text on stress, slightly updated since the first edition in 1956. Some of the English is a bit old fashioned but it gives an interesting account of the development of the stress concept by Selye.*

## References

Alberti, K.G.M.M. & Hockaday, T.D.R. (1983) Diabetes mellitus. In: Weatherall, D.J., Ledingham, J.G.G. & Warrell, D.A. (eds) *Oxford Textbook of Medicine*. Oxford: Oxford University Press.

Antoni, M.A., Gruess, D.G., Gruess, S. et al. (2000) Cognitive-behavioural stress management intervention effects on anxiety, 24 hour urinary norepimepherine output and t-cytotoxic/suppressor cells over time

among symptomatic HIV-infected gay men. *Journal of Consulting and Clinical Psychology*, **68**; 31–45.

Atkinson, R.L., Atkinson, R.C., Smith, E.E. et al. (2000) *Hilgard's Introduction to Psychology*, 13th edn. Fort Worth: Harcourt College Publishers.

Baglioni, A.J., Cooper, C.L. & Hingley, P. (1990) Job stress, mental health and job satisfaction among UK senior nurses. *Stress Medicine*, **6**; 9–20.

Bailey, R. & Clarke, M. (1989) *Stress and Coping in Nursing*. London: Chapman and Hall.

Biondi, M. & Pancheri, P. (1995) Clinical research strategies in psychoimmunology: A review of 46 human research studies (1972–1992). In: Leonard, B.E. & Miller, K. (eds) *Stress, the Immune System and Psychiatry*. Chichester: John Wiley and Sons.

Bohus, B. & Koolhaas, J.M. (1993) Stress and the cardiovascular system: central and peripheral physiological mechanisms. In: Stanford, S.C., Salmon, P. & Gray, J.A. (eds) *Stress: From Synapse to Syndrome*. London: Academic Press.

Boore, J.R.P., Champion, R. & Ferguson, M. (1987) *Nursing the Physically Ill Adult*. Edinburgh: Churchill Livingstone.

Broome, A. & Llewelyn, S. (1995) *Health Psychology Processes and Applications,* 2nd edn. London: Chapman and Hall.

Cannon, W.B. (1927) The James–Lange Theory of Emotions: A critical re-examination and an alternative theory. *American Journal of Psychology, 39;* 106–124.

Carola, R., Harley, J. & Noback, C.R. (1992) *Human Anatomy and Physiology, 2nd edn. New York: McGraw Hill.

Carter, W.R., Herman, J., Stokes, K. & Cox, D.J. (1987) Promotion of diabetes onset by stress in the BB rat. *Diabetologia, 30;* 674–675.

Chamberlain, J. (2000) Easing children's psychological distress in the emergency room. *Monitor on Psychology, 31;* 40–42.

Cheng, Y., Kawachi, I., Coakley, E.H. et al. (2000) association between psychosocial work characteristics and health functioning in American women: Prospective study. *British Medical Journal, 32;* 1432–1436.

Clow, A. (2001) The physiology of stress. In: Jones, F. & Bright, J. (eds) *Stress: Myth, Theory and Research*. Harlow, UK: Prentice Hall.

Coles, C. (1990) Diabetes education: Letting the patient into the picture. *Practical Diabetes, 7*(3); 110–112.

Cox, T. (1978) *Stress*. London: Macmillan.

Evans, G.W. & Johnson, D. (2000) Stress and open office noise. *Journal of Applied Psychology, 85;* 779–783.

Gardener, L.I. (1972) Deprivation dwarfism. In *Readings from the Scientific American* (1972) *Human Physiology and the Environment in Health and Disease,* Part IV, *Responses to Psychosocial Stress*. San Francisco: W.H. Freeman.

Greendyke, R.M., Bradley, E.M. & Swisher, S.N. (1965) Studies on the effects of administration of ACTH and adrenal corticosteroids on erythrophagocytosis. *Journal of Clinical Investigation, 44;* 746–753.

Groër, M.W. & Shekleton, M.E. (1989) *Basic Pathophysiology: A Holistic Approach*. St Louis: Mosby.

Gross, R.D. (1998) *Psychology: The Science of Mind and Behaviour,* 3rd edn. London: Hodder & Stoughton.

Guyton, A.C. (1992) *Human Physiology and Mechanisms of Disease,* 5th edn. Philadelphia: W.B. Saunders Company.

Holmes, T.H. & Rahe, R.H. (1967) The social adjustment rating scale. *Journal of Psychosomatic Research, 11;* 213–218.

Karasek, R. & Theorell, T. (1990) *Healthy Work. Stress, Productivity and the Reconstruction of Working Life.* New York: Basic Books.

Krause, N. & Shaw, B.A. (2000) Role specific findings of control and mortality. *Psychology and Aging, 15;* 617–626.

Lazarus, R.S. (1966) *Psychological Stress and the Coping Process*. New York: McGraw-Hill.

Lazarus, R.S. & Folkman, S. (1984) *Stress, Appraisal and Coping*. New York: Springer.

Lees, S. & Ellis, N. (1990) The design of a stress management programme for nursing personnel. *Journal of Advanced Nursing, 15;* 946–961.

Likar, L.J., Mason, M.M. & Rosenkrantz, H. (1963) Response of the level of acid mucopolysaccharide in rat granulation tissue to cortisol. *Endocrinology, 72;* 393–396.

Lindop, E. (1991) Individual stress among nurses in training: Why some leave whilst others stay. *Nurse Education Today, 11*(2); 110–120.

McGrath, A., Reid, N. & Boore, J. (1989) Occupational stress in nursing. *International Journal of Nursing Studies, 16*(4); 343–358.

Martini, F.H. (2001) *Fundamentals of Anatomy and Physiology,* 5th edn. New Jersey: Prentice Hall.

Mason, J.W. (1975) A historical view of the stress field. *Journal of Human Stress, 1;* 22–36.

Mason, J.W., Maher, J.J., Hartley, L.H. et al. (1976) Selectivity of corticosteroid and catecholamine responses to various natural stimuli. In: Serban, G. (ed) *Psychopathology of Human Adaptation*. New York: Plenum.

Mazelis, G., Albert, D., Crisa, C. et al. (1987) Relationship of stressful housing conditions to the onset of diabetes mellitus induced by multiple, sub-diabetogenic doses of streptozotocin in mice. *Diabetes Research, 6;* 195–200.

Mishel, M.H. (1984) Perceived uncertainty and stress in illness. *Research in Nursing and Health, 7;* 163–171.

Moos, R.H. (1988) *Coping Responses Inventory Manual.* Palo Alto, CA: Social Ecology Laboratory, Department of Psychiatry, Stanford University and Veterans Administration Medical Centers.

Moynihan, J.A., Brenner, G.J., Cocke, R. et al. (1994) Stress induced modulation of immune function in mice. In: Glaser, R. & Kiecolt-Glaser, J. (eds) *Handbook of Human Stress and Immunity*. San Diego: Academic Press.

Myers, D.G. (1998) *Psychology,* 5th edn. New York: Worth.

Nichols, K.A. (1993) *Psychological Care in Physical Illness*. London: Chapman and Hall.

Nichols, K.A. (1995) Institutional versus client-centred care. In: Broome, A. & Llewelyn, S. (eds) *Health*

*Psychology Processes and Applications,* 2nd edn. London: Chapman and Hall.

O'Hara, P. (1996) *Pain Management for Health Professionals.* London: Chapman and Hall.

Parkes, K. (1985) Stressful episodes reported by first-year student nurses: A descriptive account. *Social Science and Medicine,* **20**(9); 945–953.

Pickup, J.C. & Williams, G. (1991) *Textbook of Diabetes.* Oxford: Blackwell, pp. 784–791.

Ramsey, J.M. (1982) *Basic Pathophysiology, Modern Stress and the Disease Process.* London: Addison-Wesley.

Ross, R. (1988) The pathogenesis of atherosclerosis. In: Braunwald, E. (ed) *Heart Disease: A Textbook of Cardiovascular Medicine.* Philadelphia: W.B. Saunders.

Rusk, T.N. (1971) Opportunity and technique in crisis psychiatry. *Comprehensive Psychiatry,* **12**; 249–263.

Sapolsky, R.M. (1994) *Why Zebras don't get Ulcers.* New York: Freeman.

Selye, H. (1976) *The Stress of Life,* 2nd edn. New York: McGraw-Hill.

Sofaer, B. (1998) *Pain: Principles, Practice and Patients,* 3rd edn. Cheltenham: Stanley Thornes (Publishers) Ltd.

Sternberg, R.J. (2001) Neuroendocrine regulation of autoimmune/inflammatory disease. *Journal of Endocrinology,* **169**; 429–435.

Taylor, S.E. (1983) Adjustment to threatening events: A theory of cognitive adaptation. *American Psychologist,* **38**; 1161–1173.

Thibodeau, G.A. & Patton, K.T. (1992) *The Human Body in Health and Disease.* St Louis: Mosby Year Book.

Tortora, G.J. & Grabowski, S.R. (2000) *Principles of Anatomy and Physiology,* 9th edn. New York: Wiley.

Ur, E. (1991) Psychological aspects of hypothalamo–pituitary–adrenal activity. In: Grossman, A. (ed) *Psychoendocrinology. Baillière's Clinical Endocrinology and Metabolism,* **5**(1); 79–96. London: Baillière Tindall.

Ursin, H. & Olff, M. (1993) The stress response. In: Stanford, S.C., Salmon, P. & Gray, J, A. (eds) *Stress: From Synapse to Syndrome.* London: Academic Press.

Vander, A.J., Sherman, J.H. & Luciano, D.S. (2000) *Human Physiology: The Mechanisms of Body Function,* 5th edn. New York: McGraw Hill.

Volicer, J.V. & Bohannon, M.M. (1975) A hospital stress rating scale. *Nursing Research,* **24**; 352–359.

Wilkinson, G. (1991) Psychological problems and psychiatric disorders in diabetes mellitus. In: Pickup, J.C. & Williams, G. (eds) *Textbook of Diabetes,* pp. 784–791. Oxford: Blackwell.

Wilson-Barnett, J. & Fordham, M. (1982) Recovery of fitness. In *Recovery from Illness.* Chichester: Wiley.

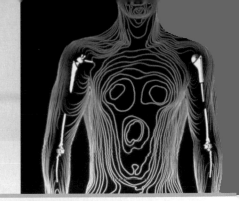

# Section 3

# Mobility and support

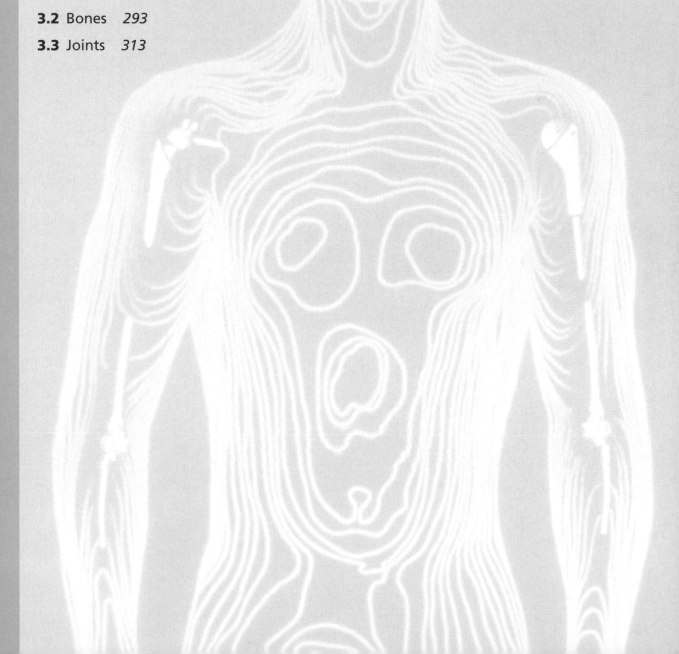

# Chapter 3.1

# Skeletal muscles

*Susan M. McLaren*

## LEARNING OBJECTIVES

After studying this chapter the reader should be able to:

- List the functions of skeletal muscle

- Describe the different levels of organization of skeletal muscle in fasciculi, individual fibres and at the molecular level

- Discuss the events leading to muscle contraction, i.e. stimulation of motor nerves, neuromuscular transmission and excitation-contraction coupling

- Explain how each of these events can be allayed or prevented by pathological disorders, electrolyte disturbances and drugs, citing relevant clinical examples

- Demonstrate an understanding of the 'sliding filament hypothesis' of muscle contraction

## INTRODUCTION

The primary function of skeletal muscle is to allow movement, not only of the whole body but of parts of the body relative to each other, so that an individual can move and explore the physical environment. Muscle is a tissue that is structurally specialized for contraction, a property that enables it to transform chemical energy into the mechanical work that causes movements of bones at a joint. Movements are not only generated at joints but also in soft tissues, for contractions of skeletal muscle also bring about movements of the eyeball, palate, tongue and voluntary sphincters. In addition, muscles play an important role in maintaining body posture; it is the sustained partial contractions of muscles that allow us to remain in one body position for long periods of time, as when sitting or standing.

Another important function of skeletal muscle is to assist body heat production. It has been estimated that only 25% of the chemical energy generated in skeletal muscle is actually used to do mechanical work, the rest is dissipated as heat. Heat production in muscle can be adjusted when a person is exposed to extremes of environmental temperature. In cold conditions, for example, shivering occurs. This process of involuntary muscle tremor increases heat production in muscle, so that body temperature is maintained when the environmental temperature fails (see Chapter 6.1). In health, approximately 33–50% of total body protein is found in skeletal muscle; during starvation this reserve can be substantially reduced for metabolic utilization.

## Gross anatomy

The skeletal muscle mass forms 40–50% of the body weight in an adult. It is divided into more than 600 individual muscles that vary in size, shape and arrangement of cells. Elongated muscle cells, which are also known as **fibres**, are bound together by connective

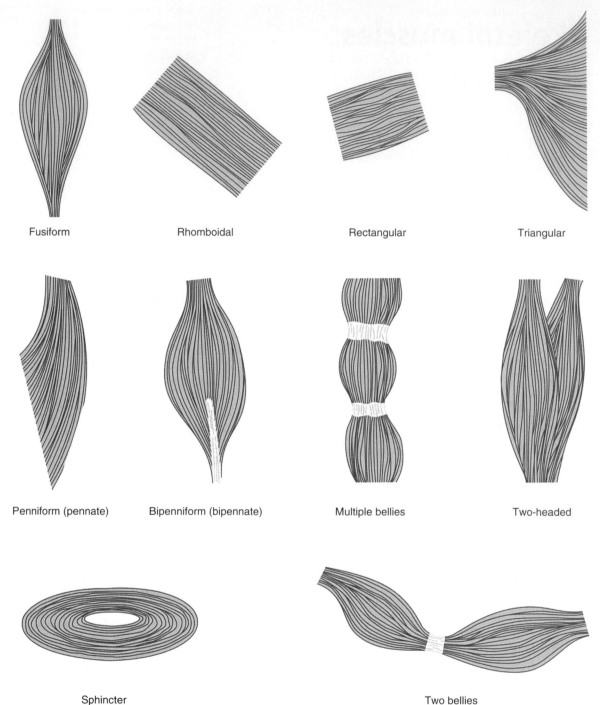

Figure 3.1.1 The variety of muscle shapes based on the arrangement of fasciculi

tissue in bundles, or **fasciculi**. Some of the most common arrangements of fasciculi found within muscles are shown in **Fig. 3.1.1**.

Fibre length is crucial in determining the range of movements that can be performed by a muscle, whereas the strength of contraction depends on fibre numbers and size. If the mean length of fibres is increased, then so too is the range of movement, and vice versa. However, in a muscle with an oblique arrangement of fibres, although the fibres are short, giving a limited range of movement, the fibre numbers are increased, giving the muscle greater strength.

## Fibre classification

In recent years, skeletal muscle fibres have been classified on the basis of morphological, physiological and biochemical characteristics into different types. On the basis of the form of the contractile protein myosin present (which determines mechanical characteristics), three types are currently distinguished in humans: the type 1, type 2A and type 2X fibres (Berchtold et al., 2000). Type 1 fibres have a small diameter, are enervated by small motor neurones, have a slow contractile speed, possess a high oxidative and low glycolytic capacity, are high in myoglobin and contain myosin in a heavy chain isoform known as MHC-1 (see p. 274). By contrast, type 2A fibres are of intermediate diameter, are enervated by large motor neurones, have fast contractile speed and contain intermediate quantities of myoglobin and the heavy chain isoform of myosin MHC-2A. Finally, type 2X fibres have a large diameter, are enervated by large motor neurones, have a fast contractile speed, possess a low oxidative and high glycolytic capacity are low in myoglobin and the myosin heavy chain isoform MHC-3.

In addition to the major fibre types summarized above, a number of intermediate subtypes have been identified. These contain two or more of the myosin isoforms in a single fibre. Skeletal muscle possesses a remarkable 'plasticity', or adaptive potential, which allows fibres to change in size and content of muscle protein isoforms. Factors that bring these changes about include growth factors (e.g. insulin-like growth factor), hormones (e.g. growth hormone, thyroid hormones), ageing, neuronal inputs and physical exercise.

## CLINICAL APPLICATIONS

In health, a factor that influences fibre length and mass is the stress generated when a muscle is put through its full range of movement. If the workload of muscle is increased during athletic training, the fibres increase in size (hypertrophy) and muscle strength is greatly increased. Endurance training increases the slow type 1 fibres (MHC-1), whereas weight training and rapid sprinting increase fast type 2 fibres (MHC-2 and MHC-3). Thus, the nature of exercise, and probably the training status of the muscle, can affect the type of response (Bruton, 2002).

Lack of exercise, when muscles are not exercised due to limb pain, prolonged bedrest, joint immobilization or the flaccid paralysis that follows a cerebrovascular accident, produces marked effects on fibre length and mass. In these circumstances, muscles are not exercised through their full range of movement and, as a consequence, the fibres atrophy, shorten and the joint may become stiff and immobile. Inevitably, the range of movement becomes limited and the strength of muscle contraction is diminished, leading to weakness. Unless physiotherapy is instituted at an early stage, muscles can become permanently fixed, shortened and resist stretching, causing a **contracture deformity** that is difficult to treat. Atrophy is a common pathological change found in diseased muscles. It can follow protein–energy malnutrition when body protein reserves in muscle are severely reduced. Anthropometric assessment of the protein reserve can be extrapolated from measurements of midarm muscle circumference. Such measurements, which comprise part of the process of nutritional assessment, can be used to monitor an individual's response to nutritional repletion, as muscle mass is restored (Taylor & Goodinson-McLaren, 1991). Anthropometric measurements assume that the mass of a muscle group in the limbs (arm, calf or thigh) is proportional to its protein content and that it is also a reflection of total body muscle mass. Both of these assumptions can be challenged. More sophisticated techniques used in the measurement of body composition, for example magnetic resonance imaging (MRI) and dual X-ray absorptiometry (DEXA), can be used to provide more precise quantification of tissue-system level components such as muscle (Ellis, 2000; Pietrobelli et al., 1998).

## Prime movers, antagonists and synergists

Muscles do not act in isolation: more than one muscle supplies a joint and their action is integrated. Furthermore, muscles can cross more than one joint so that when they contract, movement occurs at all joints crossed. Unfortunately, this can present problems, because, unless action at some of the joints is prevented, a purposeful movement cannot be made. This difficulty is overcome by utilizing the combined actions of muscles as prime movers, antagonists and synergists. Muscles that initiate and maintain a desired movement are known as **prime movers**, whereas those that resist the actions of prime movers and are capable of producing the opposite movement are known as **antagonists**. When the prime movers shorten and contract, the antagonists relax and lengthen but their structural and physical properties offer resistance to the prime movers. Towards the end of the movement, a brief contraction of the antagonists opposes the prime movers to bring about 'braking' deceleration. For example, when the forearm is flexed the biceps brachii muscle is the prime mover. The triceps brachii, which is the antagonist, relaxes but is also capable of constructing and extending the forearm **(Fig. 3.1.2)**. In certain circumstances, prime movers

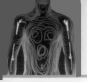

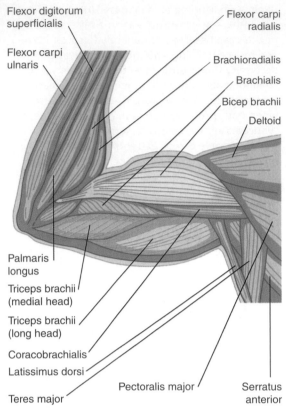

Figure 3.1.2 Muscles of the medial aspect of the arm and forearm

Labels for Figure 3.1.2:
- Flexor digitorum superficialis
- Flexor carpi ulnaris
- Palmaris longus
- Triceps brachii (medial head)
- Triceps brachii (long head)
- Coracobrachialis
- Latissimus dorsi
- Teres major
- Pectoralis major
- Flexor carpi radialis
- Brachioradialis
- Brachialis
- Bicep brachii
- Deltoid
- Serratus anterior

and antagonists contract in unison to stabilize movements at a joint, most commonly when some part of the body must be held rigid and immobile, for example the knee joint in the standing position.

If a muscle crosses more than one joint, or if it produces more than one type of movement at a single joint, it is essential that unwanted movements that are generated during contraction are removed. **Synergistic muscles** are muscles that cancel out such unwanted movements, helping the prime movers to produce the desired effect.

## Muscle attachment

Muscles are attached to the periosteum, a dense layer of connective tissue on the surface of a bone, by tendons. Two types of attachment, known as **the origin** and **the insertion**, are made here. During muscle contraction the site of origin remains relatively fixed and the insertion moves. Contraction of a muscle therefore brings the sites of origin and insertion closer together.

In addition to providing muscle with firm attachments, **tendons** must transmit the forces generated during muscle contraction to bone. To perform these functions effectively, tendons consist of white fibrous connective tissue containing parallel bundles of collagen fibres. This enables them to retain flexibility but resist stretching when a pulling force is applied. Fibrocartilage is present and gives added strength to the areas where tendons merge with bone.

## Connective tissue

Muscles are enclosed by a very extensive network of fibrous connective tissue, which is penetrated by blood vessels, nerves and lymphatics. Surrounding the entire muscle is a smooth layer of connective tissue – the **epimysium** – which allows the muscles to slide over adjacent structures during movement (**Fig. 3.1.3**). A finer septum of connective tissue, the **perimysium**, subdivides the muscle into bundles of fibres, and finally each fibre or muscle cell is surrounded by a very fine layer of connective tissue, the **endomysium**. In addition to providing muscle with a supporting framework, the connective tissue matrix condenses into the tendons, which provide muscles with their origin and insertion on bone. Furthermore, the physical properties (viscosity, elasticity) of the connective tissue matrix allow relaxed antagonists to offer resistance to prime movers during movement. Elasticity is an important property of both the connective tissue matrix and the tendons. It is these structures that act like a spring during muscle contraction, transmitting the forces generated in muscle to bone.

## Nerve supply

Each skeletal muscle is supplied by one or more nerves containing both sensory and motor fibres. Three types of motor nerve are present: **myelinated $\alpha$ efferent nerves**, which relay from the anterior horn cells of the spinal cord to muscle fibres; **myelinated $\gamma$ efferents**, which supply the muscle spindles; and **non-myelinated autonomic efferents**, which supply smooth muscle in the walls of arterioles. A number of **sensory afferent fibres** are present, some of which terminate in proprioceptors in the muscle spindles, tendons and connective tissue. **Proprioceptors** are concerned with the detection and signalling of information on movement and body position to the central nervous system; their action is essential to coordinate and grade muscle contraction. They are stimulated by the mechanical deformation or vibration created when muscles and joints move, and also

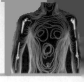

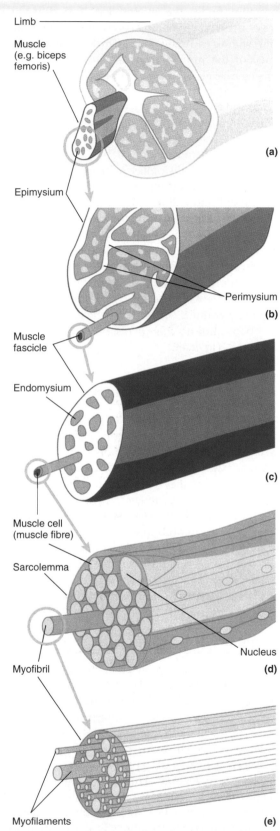

Limb

Muscle
(e.g. biceps
femoris)

Epimysium

**(a)**

Perimysium

**(b)**

Muscle
fascicle

Endomysium

**(c)**

Muscle cell
(muscle fibre)

Sarcolemma

Nucleus

Myofibril

**(d)**

Myofilaments

**(e)**

**Figure 3.1.3** Cross-section of entire thigh muscle
(a) dissected into increasingly smaller parts showing
(b) a single muscle, (c) and (d) microscopic views of
the muscle and (e) the ultrastructural arrangement of
contractile filaments

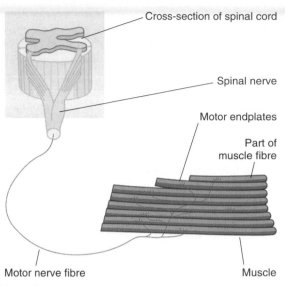

Cross-section of spinal cord

Spinal nerve

Motor endplates

Part of
muscle fibre

Motor nerve fibre

Muscle

**Figure 3.1.4** A motor unit showing the spinal nerve,
the motor nerve fibre and muscle fibres served by
the fibre

by changes in body position. Muscle spindles relay
information on length and on speed of contraction
in muscle fibres. A fuller discussion on sensory receptors is given in Chapter 2.2, and on muscle spindles
in Chapter 2.1.

Some of the sensory afferent nerves terminate as
free-nerve endings in the endomysium and tendons,
responding to the stimuli created by compression,
inflammation, ischaemia and necrosis of muscle
fibres. These nerves are concerned with the signalling
of painful stimuli, although it is perhaps misleading
to call one fibre a 'pain fibre' because pain appears to
be detected by an imbalance in fibre activities (see
gate control mechanism, Chapter 2.3).

Contraction of skeletal muscle is voluntarily controlled. The areas of the brain that control voluntary
movement are the cerebral cortex, cerebellum, basal
ganglia and brainstem nuclei. Motor tracts descend
from these areas to synapse, in the anterior horn of
the spinal cord, with the lower motor neurones that
supply skeletal muscles (**Fig. 3.1.4**). Motor nerves
can originate from one or all of the cervical, thoracic,
lumbar or sacral segments of the spinal cord, ultimately terminating at the **motor endplate** or **neuromuscular junction**.

On entering a skeletal muscle, the axon of a motor
neurone divides into a number of unmyelinated
branches that supply groups of muscle fibres. Each
muscle fibre is innervated by one of these branches.
A **motor unit** consists of one motor neurone and
the muscle fibres supplied by its branches, which
can range in number from as few as ten to several
hundred. Very precise movements of the fingers or
the eye are brought about by stimulation of the
motor units containing smaller numbers of fibres.

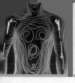
## Blood supply

Skeletal muscles have a very extensive blood supply, receiving in total 1 litre (L) of blood each minute, which is 20% of the resting cardiac output. The capillary network is vast, consisting of 300–400 capillaries/$mm^3$ of muscle tissue. Autoregulation of blood flow to skeletal muscle is mediated by the vasodilator nitric oxide, produced by the vascular endothelium (Stamler & Meissner, 2001).

In healthy subjects performing maximum exercise at a steady level, the total muscle blood flow increases up to 15–20 L/min to meet the additional oxygen requirements of muscle cells. However, in athletes, muscle blood flow during exercise can reach an astounding 30 L/min! This increase in the blood supply to muscle during exercise is known as **exercise hyperaemia** and is brought about by the relaxation of precapillary sphincters.

### CLINICAL APPLICATIONS

The blood supply to skeletal muscle can be impaired in a number of disorders, including arterial thrombosis, polyarteritis, trauma and bone fractures. Prolonged ischaemia of muscle can lead to fibre necrosis and contracture deformities such as Volkmann's ischaemic contracture (see also p. 289).

## Microanatomy

Approximately 10–100 μm in diameter, skeletal muscle cells or fibres are elongated, cylindrical and taper at the ends (**Fig. 3.1.5**). Fibre length is variable, ranging from a few millimetres in short muscles to 30 cm in the long sartorius muscle of the upper leg.

The terminology used to describe some of the structural components of muscle cells differs from that used for other kinds of cell. The **sarcolemma** forms the plasma membrane, the **sarcoplasm** the cytoplasm and the **sarcoplasmic reticulum** is similar to the endoplasmic reticulum of other cells. Whereas all body cells have one nucleus, skeletal muscle cells contain several nuclei distributed around the periphery of the sarcoplasm (**Fig. 3.1.5**). The term used to describe this feature, peculiar to the skeletal muscle cell, is **syncytium**. It is formed from the fusion of uninucleate myoblast cells during embryological development.

Inside the cell, the sarcoplasm is filled with **myofibrils** – longitudinally-running fibres 1–2 μm in diameter. Myofibrils possess a banded structure that gives skeletal muscle its characteristic 'striped'

appearance under the microscope. Two different types of filament containing contractile proteins are found within each myofibril. Thick filaments are formed of the protein **myosin**, whereas thin filaments consist of three different proteins, **actin**, **troponin** and **tropomyosin**. Thick and thin filaments are arranged alternately in the myofibril, as shown in **Fig. 3.1.5b**. Structurally, myosin is composed of two heavy (MHC) and two light chains (MLC). Three myosin heavy chain isoforms, MHC-1, MHC-2A and MHC-2X are genetically expressed in humans and provide a basis for classifying muscle fibres (Berchtold et al., 2000; Bruton, 2002). Because of the overlap of thick and thin filaments, the banded structure showing A, H, M, I and Z bands is visible on electron microscopy. The area between two Z lines is known as a **sarcomere**. Several sarcomeres are arranged along each myofibril. During contraction, the thick and thin filaments slide against one another, shortening the myofibrils. This reduces the width of the I and H bands but no change occurs in the width of the A-band (**Fig. 3.1.6**).

## Intracellular tubular systems

Two tubular systems penetrate each muscle cell. One of these is known as the **transverse tubular system** or **T-system**, which consists of tubules, lined by sarcolemma, extending from the cell exterior into the sarcoplasm where they branch and terminate near the A–I band of the sarcomere.

The other, wholly internal, system is formed by fine tubules – **sarcotubules** – of the sarcoplasmic reticulum. These end in closed sacs, the terminal cisterns, near the A–I-band of each sarcomere. Both tubular systems play an important role in the events that precede and follow muscle contraction.

## Myoglobin

Myoglobin is a haem-protein, abundantly distributed throughout the sarcoplasm. Like haemoglobin, it combines reversibly with oxygen and is capable of providing a temporary store for oxygen. It performs this function when the capillary supply to muscle is transiently decreased during contraction, and when the oxygen demands of cells are increased during exercise. The myoglobin content of muscle fibres increases in response to endurance training.

An interesting property of myoglobin is that it combines with oxygen far more effectively than does haemoglobin at lower oxygen tensions. For example, at an arterial $PO_2$ of only 4 kPa (30 mmHg), myoglobin is 95% saturated with oxygen, whereas haemoglobin is only 50% saturated.

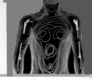

## CLINICAL APPLICATIONS

Myoglobin can escape into the circulation following crush injuries to muscle, or any other insult that brings about severe necrosis of muscle, e.g. pressure ulcer necrosis, drug toxicity and in some of the disorders known collectively as the **muscular myopathies**. In these circumstances, myoglobin is excreted in the urine but might form casts in the nephron and lead to acute renal failure.

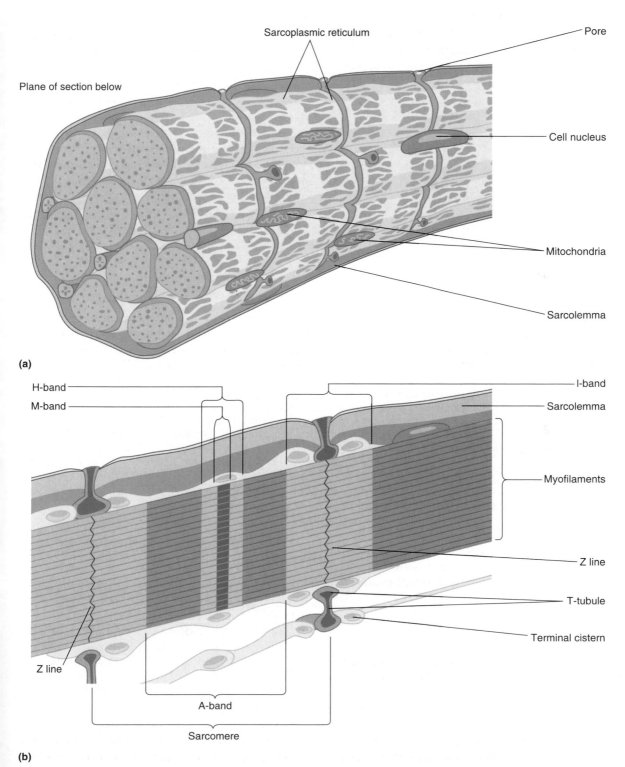

**(a)**

**(b)**

**Figure 3.1.5**  The structure of (a) a skeletal muscle cell showing the nuclei just under the sarcolemma and (b) a longitudinal section of a myofibril

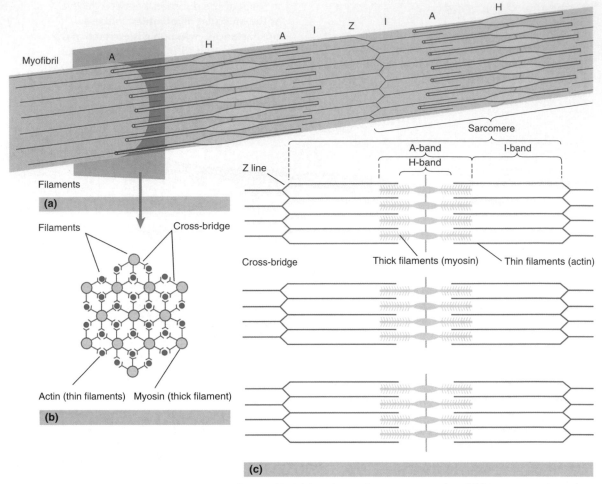

**Figure 3.1.6** Diagrammatic representation of a myofibril (a) with sarcolemma removed and (b) in cross-section. The Z-lines mark the ends of the sarcomeres. (c) Shows the components of the sarcomere. The thick filaments run the width of the A-band and the thin filaments run the length of the I-band and overlap with the thick filament in the A-band. The H-band is composed solely of thick filaments. During contraction, the filaments overlap to a greater extent and the sarcomere shortens

## Molecular structure of the thick and thin filaments

To understand how contraction is brought about in skeletal muscle, it is essential to visualize the arrangement of actin and myosin within the thin and thick filaments.

### Thick filaments

More than 100 myosin molecules are found in a single thick filament. If it were possible to examine one thick filament in isolation, we would see a structure very much like that shown in **Fig. 3.1.7**. Each myosin molecule possesses a double, club-shaped head, followed by a double-stranded 'tail' that is coiled in a helix. All myosin molecules are assembled together in the thick filament so that the heads protrude at the surface and the tails form a cylindrical rod.

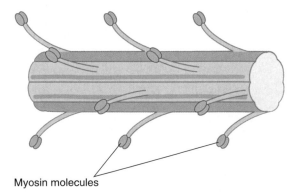

Myosin molecules

**Figure 3.1.7** Structure of a thick filament of skeletal muscle

According to the **sliding filament hypothesis**, during contraction the globular myosin heads form cross-bridges, which attach to binding sites on the thin actin filaments. Repeated attachments of the myosin heads slide the thin filaments towards

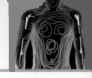

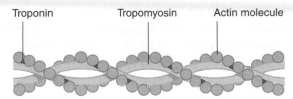

**Figure 3.1.8** Structure of thin filament of skeletal muscle

the centre of the thick filaments, shortening the myofibril. It is this concerted shortening of myofibrils that brings about contraction of the muscle cells.

## Thin filaments

Actin, troponin and tropomyosin are the proteins that form the thin filaments. The actin molecules are arranged in two helical strands, which are intertwined with a third strand of tropomyosin, as shown in **Fig. 3.1.8**. Another protein, troponin, is interspersed at regular intervals along the thin filament.

In resting muscle, the orientation of tropomyosin blocks the binding sites on actin, preventing the formation of cross-bridges. However, during muscle contraction, this inhibition is removed by calcium ions, allowing cross-bridges to form between actin and myosin.

## Muscle contraction

Before muscle contraction can occur, the following sequence of events must take place.

1. **Stimulation of the motor nerves.** This leads to the arrival of an electrical impulse, the action potential, at a motor nerve terminal.
2. **Neuromuscular transmission.** The transfer of a chemical signal from the nerve terminal to the sarcolemma brings about a change in electrical potential, known as 'depolarization', of the membrane. Following this, an action potential is fired in the muscle cell.
3. **Excitation–contraction coupling.** The generation of an action potential in the muscle cell is followed by activation of the contractile filaments. Shortening of the myofilaments inside the muscle cell, mediated by calcium ions, brings about muscle contraction.

A number of disorders affecting nerve or muscle can disrupt these events, leading to problems of muscle weakness, impaired mobility or even paralysis. In the following pages, stimulation of motor nerves, neuromuscular transmission and excitation–contraction

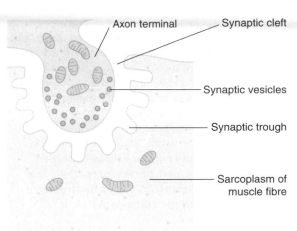

**Figure 3.1.9** The neuromuscular junction

coupling are discussed individually, together with some of the disorders that might impair them.

## Stimulation of motor nerves

Muscle contraction is brought about by stimulation of motor nerves controlled by areas of the brain such as the cerebral cortex, cerebellum, brainstem nuclei and basal ganglia. Upper motor neurones descend from these higher centres to synapse in the anterior horn of the spinal cord with the lower motor neurones that supply skeletal muscles. An electrical signal, the action potential, is transmitted along myelinated motor nerves by saltatory conduction, (this process is described in Chapter 2.1).

Inside the muscle, a motor neurone branches to form a number of unmyelinated terminals, each of which supplies an individual muscle cell at the motor endplate or neuromuscular junction. The action potential finally arrives at this specialized junction between nerve and muscle, also known as the neuromuscular synapse (**Fig. 3.1.9**). Here, the nerve terminal is separated from the muscle cell sarcolemma by a cleft approximately 30–50 μm wide. Transmission of the signal from nerve to muscle is accomplished by release into the synapse of a chemical transmitter, acetylcholine.

### CLINICAL APPLICATIONS

Disorders affecting the relay of impulses by motor neurones are broadly classified as either upper or lower motor neurone lesions. If the nerves are damaged, then, clearly, muscle contraction will be impaired in some way. **Upper motor neurone lesions** are those that affect the centres in the brain concerned with the control of voluntary movement. Such lesions include Parkinson's disease, multiple sclerosis and cerebrovascular accidents. Typically, upper motor neurone disorders create problems of muscle weakness and paralysis. In addition, abnormalities in muscle tone might be present, such as spasticity or rigidity. Abnormalities of movement including ataxia, intention tremor, poor muscle coordination, jerky movements (chorea) or writhing movements (athetosis) can also feature in some disorders, depending on the nature and site of the lesion.

By contrast, **lower motor neurone disorders**, which include the peripheral neuropathies, lead to muscle weakness accompanied by atrophy of muscle fibres, and sometimes sensation is impaired.

## Neuromuscular transmission

Acetylcholine is stored in a number of vesicles inside the axon terminal. Arrival of an action potential depolarizes the nerve terminal, triggering an influx of calcium ions from the extracellular fluid. Following this, the vesicles move towards the terminal membrane, fuse with it and discharge at least 1 million molecules of acetylcholine into the synaptic cleft. Acetylcholine diffuses across the cleft, binding to specific protein molecules in the sarcolemma, which are known as receptors. Following this, an electrical signal (the action potential) is fired, which spreads longitudinally along the muscle cell and is conducted down the T-system. Contraction of the muscle cell follows a few milliseconds later.

Acetylcholine then diffuses away from the receptors in the sarcolemma and is broken down (hydrolysed) by the enzyme acetylcholinesterase, which is also present in the synaptic cleft. One of the products of this hydrolysis is choline, which is transported back into the nerve axon and used to resynthesize acetylcholine.

## Electrical events

The muscle cell has a negative resting potential that is created by a separation of electrical charge across the plasma membrane (the sarcolemma). In effect, the inside of the membrane is negatively charged (−90 mV) with respect to the outside. The reason for this negative potential, which is caused by an unequal distribution of ions across the cell membrane, is discussed in Chapter 2.1.

## Depolarization

Both muscle and nerve are 'excitable' cells, which means that it is possible to change their negative resting potential. A decrease in the membrane potential towards 0 mV (i.e. *less* negative), which increases excitability, is known as **depolarization**, whereas an

*increase* in the negative potential, which decreases excitability, is termed **hyperpolarization**. These changes are brought about by a phased selective increase in the permeability of the cell membrane to positively charged sodium and potassium ions, a process that generates the action potential in nerve and muscle cells.

### The action potential

The combination of acetylcholine with receptors in the sarcolemma of the muscle cell generates a small depolarization known as the endplate potential. Channels open in the sarcolemma, allowing positively charged sodium ions to enter the muscle cell, which decreases the negative membrane (sarcolemma) potential towards 0 mV (**Fig. 3.1.10**). Within 0.5 ms, this small depolarization moves the membrane towards a **critical threshold**, at which point a massive depolarization occurs and an action potential is fired. Other channels open in the sarcolemma, increasing its permeability to both sodium and potassium ions, although the permeability change initially favours the sodium ions. Positively charged sodium ions enter the muscle cell, reversing the membrane potential, which at the peak of the action potential is +30 mV. At this point **inactivation** occurs, the sodium channels close and potassium channels, which have been opening slowly, reach a maximum. Potassium ions move out of the muscle cell, **repolarizing** the membrane back towards the negative resting potential. In fact, it is repolarized to a value slightly below the resting potential so that, technically speaking, at this point

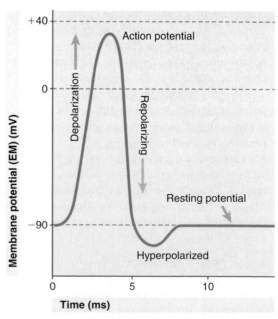

**Figure 3.1.10** Phases of the action potential in muscle

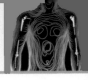

the cell is hyperpolarized. The sequence of electrical events from the initial depolarization of the endplate to the conclusion of the action potential takes only 5–8 ms. From the generation of the action potential, the muscle cell has gained a small quantity of sodium ions and lost potassium ions. The intracellular resting concentrations of these two ions are restored by the action of the sodium/potassium ATPase pump, returning the membrane potential to its resting value of −90 mV.

## CLINICAL APPLICATIONS

### IMPAIRED NEUROMUSCULAR TRANSMISSION

There are several circumstances in which the depolarization of the sarcolemma can be impaired or prevented. Some of the most common are:

- a decrease in the release of acetylcholine due to toxins or electrolyte imbalances
- a blockade of acetylcholine receptors by drugs, or by antibodies in the case of myasthenia gravis
- a change in excitability of the sarcolemma caused by drugs or electrolyte imbalances.

### DECREASED ACETYLCHOLINE RELEASE

Acetylcholine release can be abolished by a number of toxins, which are fortunately rare! One of the best known examples is the botulinum exotoxin, which is produced following food poisoning with *Clostridium botulinum* bacteria. The exotoxin produced by the bacteria abolishes acetylcholine release at the skeletal neuromuscular junction and in the parasympathetic nervous system. This leads to skeletal muscle paralysis with involvement of the respiratory muscles. Effects of parasympathetic blockade include decreased gut motility and retention of urine. Death can be caused by respiratory failure unless the individual is admitted to an intensive care unit and mechanically ventilated.

Calcium ions play a vital role in mediating the release of acetylcholine from vesicles inside the nerve terminal – actions that are opposed by magnesium ions. If the extracellular concentration of magnesium ions is raised then calcium-mediated acetylcholine release is blocked, leading to weakness or paralysis of skeletal muscle with respiratory embarrassment. Magnesium excess occurs if excretion is impaired by severe dehydration or by renal failure and in situations in which magnesium replacement therapy is

excessive. The treatment consists of using dialysis to promote magnesium excretion in patients with renal failure and, in the case of severe dehydration, promoting urinary excretion by fluid replacement therapy. The effects of excess magnesium ions on calcium-mediated acetylcholine release can be reversed by administering intravenous calcium gluconate solution.

If the concentration of free calcium ions in the extracellular fluid is reduced (normal 2.00–2.55 mmol/L), the excitability of skeletal muscle is increased, thus leading to tetany. This is not what we would expect from a knowledge of the role of calcium ions on acetylcholine release! The explanation is that initial reductions in the calcium concentration are directed at muscle excitability, and it is only when the calcium concentration in extracellular fluid is reduced well below 1 mmol/L that neuromuscular blockade is observed.

### ACETYLCHOLINE RECEPTOR BLOCKADE

Drugs such as tubocurarine and pancuronium are used therapeutically to block neuromuscular transmission. They act by competing with acetylcholine for receptor sites on the muscle cell sarcolemma. These drugs can be displaced from the receptors and their effects reversed by increasing the local concentration of acetylcholine at the synapse. This is achieved by the administration of anticholinesterase drugs, such as neostigmine and pyridostigmine. Tubocurarine and pancuronium are both used to achieve muscle relaxation during surgery; to facilitate intermittent positive pressure ventilation (IPPV) and to control the severe muscle spasms caused by tetanus infection. As these drugs paralyse the respiratory muscles, IPPV is always employed whenever they are used.

### MYASTHENIA GRAVIS

Myasthenia gravis is an uncommon disorder, affecting 1 in 18 000 individuals. It can occur at any age but is most common after 30 years (Drachman, 1978). Although the cause of this disorder is not fully understood, 75% of myasthenic patients have an abnormality of the thymus gland. More than 85% have raised anti-acetylcholine receptor antibodies present in their serum. These antibodies, which are produced by the thymus, bind to acetylcholine receptors, reducing the numbers available to combine with released acetylcholine. As a result, when endplate potentials are generated they might be inadequate to trigger an action potential in the skeletal muscle cell. Muscle weakness and fatigue result (**see Table 3.1.1**).

**Table 3.1.1** Effects of muscle disorders on activities of daily living

| Muscle group affected | Disorder | Activities affected problems |
|---|---|---|
| Neck muscles | Duchenne dystrophy<br>Myotonia dystrophica<br>Polymyositis | Inability to support head leading to difficulties during eating, restriction of vision, communication, reading |
| Respiratory muscles | Myasthenia gravis<br>Duchenne dystrophy<br>Polymyositis<br>Hypokalaemic paralysis | Breathing impaired, leading to dyspnoea |
| Extraocular muscles | Myasthenia gravis<br>Hypokalaemic paralysis<br>Hyperthyroid myopathy | Impaired vision<br>Diplopia<br>Paresis of eye muscles |
| Jaw muscles | Myasthenia gravis<br>Polymyositis<br>Myotubular myopathy | Difficulty with chewing food |
| Facial muscles | Myasthenia gravis<br>Myotonia dystrophica | Altered facial expression<br>Ptosis impairing visual field |
| Muscles of palate, pharynx, larynx, tongue | Myasthenia gravis<br>Polymyositis | Dysphagia, dysarthria, difficulty in coughing |
| Proximal muscles of the arms and legs | All primary myopathies | Restricted movement<br>Difficulties meeting hygiene needs, dressing, walking on the flat and up stairs |
| Distal muscles of the arms and legs | Myotonia dystrophica<br>Rarely, in the later stages of some other primary myopathies | Effects on hands and fingers lead to impaired fine movements, sewing, fastening buttons, writing, etc.<br>Effects on leg muscles cause tripping, high-stepping gait |
| Quadriceps muscles at the knee | Many primary myopathies | Difficulties in standing, walking |

It is a characteristic feature of this disorder that the muscle weakness becomes progressively worse as muscles are repeatedly used, probably because it takes time to resynthesize acetylcholine and repeated use decreases the supply available to produce an effective depolarization. Rest therefore improves this progressive weakness in some muscles.

The severity of the disorder can fluctuate through periods of mild and severe exacerbation, with remissions in some individuals, or pursue an extreme course that ends in death due to respiratory paralysis.

Neuromuscular transmission can be improved by increasing the concentration of acetylcholine at the motor endplate. Anticholinesterase drugs such as neostigmine (Prostigmin) and pyridostigmine bromide (Mestinon) achieve this by inhibiting the enzyme acetylcholinesterase, which hydrolyses acetylcholine.

Immunosuppressive drugs such as prednisone, azathioprine and cyclophosphamide reduce the production of anti-acetylcholine receptor antibodies. These drugs are the treatment of choice for elderly patients or those with a poor response to removal of the thymus. In severe cases, immunosuppressive drugs can be used in conjunction with plasma exchange (see below).

Although surgical removal of the thymus is effective in some cases, it is not usually successful in patients aged over 50 years.

Plasma exchange involves the removal of large volumes of plasma from the circulation and its replacement by fresh plasma, or a plasma equivalent, so that hypovolaemia is prevented. In the management of myasthenia gravis, the aim of plasma exchange is to deplete the patient's serum of anti-acetylcholine receptor antibodies. At present, plasma exchange is restricted to the management of myasthenia

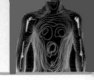

gravis in patients with a severe form of the disease. Great improvements in the condition of these patients have been reported following its use (Glassman, 1979).

As the degree of muscle weakness and immobility caused by this disorder varies, the nurse should make individual assessments of the patient's capacity to perform the activities of daily living, and care should be planned accordingly. Bearing in mind that the muscle weakness of myasthenia gravis is increased by repeated activity and alleviated by rest, nursing care is aimed at planning the activity of the patient's day to avoid muscle fatigue by supervising periods of rest and activity and setting small goals that are easily achieved. Maximum use should be made where necessary of physiotherapy aids, such as frames and tripods to assist walking, and the maintenance of good posture. The nursing management of other problems associated with this disorder are discussed at the end of this chapter.

## ALTERED EXCITABILITY OF THE MUSCLE CELL

As described earlier, calcium ions play a vital role in mediating both acetylcholine release and excitation–contraction coupling.

If the concentration of calcium ions is decreased in plasma, the permeability of the muscle cell sarcolemma to sodium ions is increased. As a result, the excitability of the membrane is increased, bringing it nearer the critical threshold at which an action potential is fired. As the plasma calcium concentration falls, this increased excitability can precipitate a condition known as **hypocalcaemic tetany**. Features of this include numbness and tingling of the extremities, muscle cramps, carpopedal spasms, dysphasia and, in severe cases, laryngeal spasms and convulsions. A positive Chvostek's sign might be present, i.e. contraction of the facial muscles occurs when the facial nerve is tapped.

Hypocalcaemia can be caused by hypoparathyroidism, excessive urinary losses of calcium ions in chronic renal diseases and through the gut due to fistulae, diarrhoea, or prolonged nasogastric aspiration. Hypocalcaemic tetany is treated by administering either oral or intravenous calcium gluconate replacements.

Disturbances in potassium balance can also have repercussions on the depolarization of the sarcolemma. Remember that the resting potential of muscle cells is approximately −90 mV. If the plasma potassium concentration falls, more potassium ions are lost from the cell. As a result, the negative resting potential increases in value above −90 mV, hyperpolarizing the membrane and moving it further from the threshold at which an action potential is fired. The result is muscle weakness and, in severe depletion states, paralysis. Potassium depletion can occur when excessive losses from the gut of potassium-rich fluid occur in prolonged vomiting, diarrhoea and in patients receiving nasogastric aspiration for intestinal obstruction. Hyperaldosteronism, Cushing's disease, respiratory and metabolic alkalosis and prolonged therapy with diuretics such as furosemide can also lead to potassium depletion. The treatment consists of careful oral or intravenous potassium replacement therapy.

Hyperkalaemia, which can occur in acute renal failure and in adrenocortical deficiency states, has complex effects on the membranes of nerve and muscle. Excitability is increased in slight to moderate hyperkalaemia but it is reduced in severe hyperkalaemia, where it leads to weakness and paralysis of skeletal muscle. However, the effects on the heart usually lead to cardiac arrest before any signs of paralysis have set in.

Alterations in the potassium concentrations in plasma and muscle cells are features of the hypo- and hyperkalaemic metabolic myopathies. Altered excitability of the cell membrane leads to intermittent attacks of muscle weakness and paralysis. A number of drugs prevent cholinergic receptors responding to acetylcholine by maintaining the sarcolemma in a constant state of depolarization. This **depolarizing blockade** causes an immediate flaccid paralysis of skeletal muscle. Suxamethonium, which is used in the same circumstances as pancuronium, is an example of this type of drug.

## Excitation–contraction coupling

The generation of an action potential in the muscle cell must be followed by activation of the contractile machinery in the myofibrils if contraction is to occur. This process is known as excitation–contraction coupling. As described earlier, contraction is brought about by shortening of the myofibrils when the thin actin filaments slide inwards against the thick myosin filaments, propelled by the myosin cross-bridges.

In the resting muscle cell, sliding of the filaments is prevented by the configuration of tropomyosin on the thin filament, which conceals crucial binding sites to which the cross-bridges attach. Therefore, an essential step in activating the contractile machinery of the muscle cell is to expose these actin-binding sites.

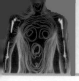

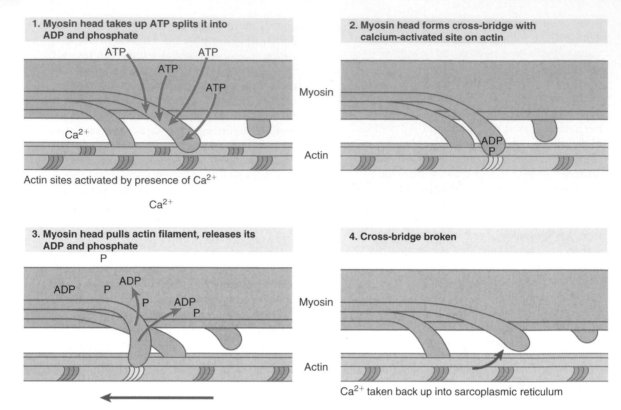

**1. Myosin head takes up ATP splits it into ADP and phosphate**

Actin sites activated by presence of $Ca^{2+}$

$Ca^{2+}$

**2. Myosin head forms cross-bridge with calcium-activated site on actin**

Myosin

Actin

**3. Myosin head pulls actin filament, releases its ADP and phosphate**

Myosin

Actin

**4. Cross-bridge broken**

Myosin

Actin

$Ca^{2+}$ taken back up into sarcoplasmic reticulum

**Figure 3.1.11** Diagrammatic representation of the sliding filament theory showing how the thick filaments of skeletal muscle move relative to one another as cross-bridges are formed and broken

When an action potential is fired, it is transmitted longitudinally along the cell and down into the T-tubular system, which is lined by sarcolemma. Depolarization of the sarcolemma lining the T-tubules triggers the release of calcium ions into the sarcoplasm from terminal sacs of the sarcotubular system (sarcoplasmic reticulum). More specifically, it is currently suggested that depolarization of the sarcolemma lining the T-tubules brings about changes in the structure of the dihydropyridine receptor (DHPR) within the membrane. Subsequently, signal transmission from DHPR to the ryanodine receptor (RyR), which is the major channel for calcium release from the sarcoplasmic reticulum, brings about an increase in the concentration of the calcium concentration in the sarcoplasm by about 100fold (Berchtold et al., 2000).

Calcium ions then bind to troponin on the thin filaments and allow the tropomyosin strand to alter position, exposing the binding sites on actin that are essential for cross-bridge formation. Myosin heads on the thick filaments then attach to the actin binding sites and form a series of cross-bridges.

For the cross-bridges to propel the thin filaments inwards, energy must be supplied by the conversion of the energy-rich compound adenosine triphosphate (ATP) to adenosine diphosphate (ADP) plus inorganic phosphate. This chemical reaction is accomplished by the enzyme adenosine triphosphatase, which is present in the myosin head. Release of energy from ATP allows the myosin heads to move to a different angle (**Fig. 3.1.11**), pushing the thin filaments inwards towards the centre of the thick filaments.

As action potentials continue to arrive, this process is repeated many times. Cross-bridges form, break and reattach along the thin filaments, sliding them inwards. In this way, concerted shortening of the myofibrils inside the muscle cells brings about contraction of the muscle as calcium ions are repeatedly released.

To enable relaxation to take place, calcium ions dissociate from troponin and are pumped back into the sarcoplasmic reticulum by an ATP-powered pump. Inside the sarcoplasmic reticulum, calcium ions are stored bound to the protein calsequestrin.

Removal of the calcium ions allows tropomyosin to block the active sites on the actin filaments again, breaking the cross-bridges. **Figure 3.1.12** summarizes the events occurring before, during and after muscle contraction. For further information on excitation–contraction coupling, see Berchtold et al. (2000).

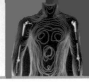

delay in returning calcium ions to the sarcoplasmic reticulum after muscle contraction.

In Duchenne muscular dystrophy, which is a genetically determined (X-linked, recessive) *non*-myotonic dystrophy affecting 1 in 3500 boys, the protein dystrophin, which spans the muscle fibre sarcolemma, is absent. This leads to membrane destabilization and the initiation of complex processes resulting in alterations in intracellular calcium handling (Blake et al., 2002). Increased entry of calcium ions into the cell, leading to hypercontraction of myofibrils followed by fibre degeneration and necrosis, are pathophysiological features.

A number of drugs can inhibit excitation–contraction coupling. Dantrolene sulphate is used to prevent the spastic movements that often follow spinal cord injury, cerebrovascular accidents, cerebral palsy and multiple sclerosis. In many of the disorders affecting skeletal muscle, including muscular dystrophies, degenerative changes are seen in the structure of the muscle cells. In many of the congenital disorders, abnormal myofibrils are present. If the contractile machinery of the cell is damaged, muscle cells cannot contract effectively. It is not surprising, then, to find that muscle weakness is one of the major problems associated with these disorders.

## Types of contraction

Contraction is the process of generating force in a muscle; it does not necessarily lead to shortening of the muscle. In the preceding section, the process whereby force (tension) is developed in the contractile filaments of the muscle fibres was described. Tension is transmitted by the muscle tendon to bone at the point of insertion. Tension developed by the muscle is applied to a load, which is the object to be moved or supported. The load consists of the bone, the part of the body to be moved and any external object that is being supported or lifted. Resisting the tension exerted by the muscle is the force, which is produced by the weight of the load. To lift a load, the tension generated by the muscle must be greater than that exerted by the load (see also lever systems, Chapter 3.3).

During an **isotonic contraction**, the tension developed in the muscle remains constant and the muscle shortens, lifting the load. Mechanical work is done, and movement is produced by the contraction. In contrast, during an **isometric contraction**, tension is increased in the muscle but this is insufficient to lift the load and shortening does not occur. In this case, mechanical work is not done, and movement is not produced. Isometric contractions are

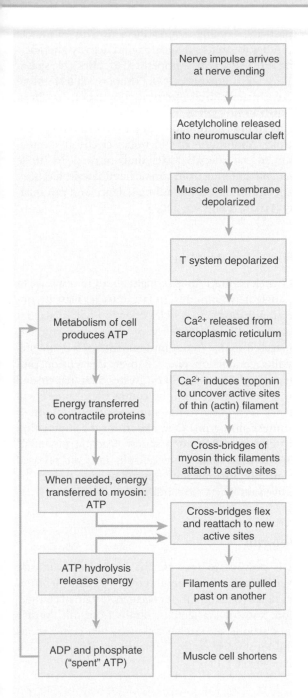

**Figure 3.1.12** Summary of the sequence of events involved in muscle contraction

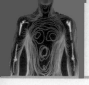
performed when supporting a load in a fixed position or when pushing against a flat immovable surface. Isometric exercises, which develop tension in muscles without bringing about movement, are frequently used as part of a physiotherapy programme to prevent weakness, atrophy and contractures in patients who are immobilized. They are particularly useful in situations where, for a variety of reasons, isotonic movements cannot be performed, for example, in patients with joint disease when isotonic, active or passive movements can precipitate painful spasms.

> ### CLINICAL APPLICATIONS
>
> External low-level electrical stimulation of muscle, which produces only a small fraction of a maximum voluntary contraction, can be used to achieve therapeutic benefits. A study by Levine et al. (1990) has shown that electrical stimulation of the gluteus maximus in seated individuals can produce changes in the shape, configuration and undulation of tissue, altering the seating interface pressure distribution beneficially. This technique could have future valuable applications in the prevention of pressure ulcers.

## Muscle tonus

**Muscle tone** is defined as the resistance offered to passive stretch of the muscle. It is determined by the muscle nerve supply and its control, and also by the elastic and contractile properties of muscle.

**Tonic contractions** are the sustained partial contractions of muscle that are so important for maintaining posture. They are brought about by the asynchronous contraction of small numbers of muscle fibres producing tautness rather than movement.

**Flaccidity** (flabbiness) is the term used to describe a decrease in muscle tone (decreased resistance to passive stretch). It is a feature of disorders that directly affect muscle (myopathies) or its lower motor neurone supply (peripheral neuropathies). A flaccid paralysis is an early feature of cerebrovascular accidents or spinal cord injuries.

By contrast, **spasticity** is the increased muscle tone that accompanies higher neural lesions such as stroke and Parkinson's disease. It is caused by a decreased transmission of nerve impulses down inhibitory pyramidal paths (see Chapter 2.3). Excitatory impulses relayed to the anterior horn cells then predominate to a greater extent than normal, increasing muscle tone and causing either spasticity or rigidity. A rigid muscle has a very great resistance to passive stretch due to its sustained suntraction. The local application of cold is of considerable benefit in treating spasticity. Cooling reduces the sensitivity of muscle spindles to stretch, reducing reflex activity and altering its viscoelastic properties to alleviate spasm (Price & Lehmann, 1990; Thomas, 2000). More recently, functional electrical stimulation has been shown to strengthen muscle power and reduce spasticity in the rehabilitation of patients suffering from stroke. Application of functional electrical stimulation to the affected lower limb muscles in stroke patients suffering from spastic hemiparesis, has been reported to improve standing balance and gait quality (Isakov & Bowker, 2002).

## Twitch contraction

A twitch contraction is brought about in response to a single nerve stimulus. In fact, muscles usually contract in response to a series of action potentials, not just one. If the frequency of nerve stimulation is increased so that one stimulus arrives before the preceding contraction phase is over, the tension produced in the muscle will be greater than that created by a single twitch and the contractile response will increase. In other words, **summation** or addition of contractions occurs. One reason for the summation in tension is that, as a series of action potentials arrives, more and more calcium ions are released from the sarcoplasmic reticulum, increasing the active sites where cross-bridges can form.

## Tetanus

It is possible to increase the frequency of muscle stimulation to a maximum point where further summation of tension cannot occur. A sustained contraction, known as a tetanus, results from this. Muscle contractions are rarely single twitches; summations and incomplete tetanic contractions play the greater part (**Fig. 3.1.13**).

## Recruitment

One way of increasing the tension (force) developed in the muscle is to increase the number of fibres that contract by a process known as recruitment. This is accomplished when more motor neurones are activated by higher control centres so as to increase the number of active motor units. This is one means by which muscle contractions are graded to match the demands of a particular task. As described earlier, muscle tension must exceed the force generated by a load if that load is to be lifted.

The force of muscle contraction is also increased if the resting length of the muscle fibres is increased.

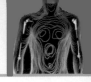

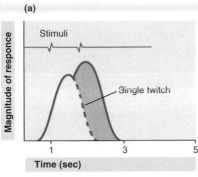
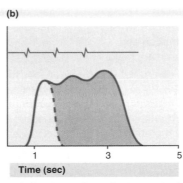
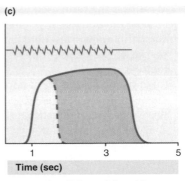

**Figure 3.1.13** The development of tetany in skeletal muscle under increasingly frequent stimuli from (a) to (c)

## Energy supply

The energy for contractions is provided by ATP. Energy is released when ATP is converted to ADP plus inorganic phosphate by the action of adenosine triphosphatase. It is vital that ATP is rapidly reconstituted to replenish the energy supply. This can be accomplished by using another high-energy phosphate compound as a 'back-up' energy source; such a back-up is **creatine phosphate**. The following chemical reaction replenishes the ATP supply, catalysed by the enzyme creatine phosphokinase (CPK):

$$\text{creatine phosphate} + \text{ADP} \xrightarrow{\text{CPK}} \text{ATP} + \text{creatine}$$

    ↑                                  ↓

energy for          used to regenerate creatine
contraction         phosphate energy store

Although creatine phosphate provides an immediate reserve energy supply at the start of contraction, additional ATP sources must be mobilized. Oxidative phosphorylation in the muscle cell supplies most of the ATP required during moderate activity. However, during intense exercise the oxygen delivery to muscle is transiently impaired by the contractions, which impede arterial blood flow. This reduces the ATP supply from oxidative phosphorylation. In such circumstances the ATP is provided by glycolysis, a process that can occur in the absence of oxygen, using glycogen stores in the muscle cell as an energy substrate. Lactic acid is the end-product of this process.

## Effects of exercise on muscle strength

Muscle strength is defined as the maximum voluntary resultant force of short duration that an individual can bring to bear on the environment. It is crucial to the performance of functional abilities and can be influenced by training intensity, frequency and duration (Bohannon, 1990).

Strength training is characterized by increased muscle activity in response to high resistance and low numbers of repetitions. To increase strength, a muscle must be subjected to a load that is greater than normal; this load needs to be progressively increased to produce incremental gains in strength. In strength training, the 'training zone' can be defined as loads ranging from 60 to 80% of maximal voluntary performance for normal individuals and from 80 to 100% for athletes (Komi & Hakkinen, 1998). Greater frequency of training, in terms of numbers of sessions and their content, increase strength proportionally. Subjects training once a week achieve only one-third the rate of improvement of those training daily.

Increasing the duration of individual isometric contractions does not affect the amount of strength but benefits the rate at which increases in strength are obtained. Longer duration of exercise (days, weeks, months) is required to build up strength to a plateau, or 'limiting strength'. The length of time an individual must train to build up muscle strength depends on the regimen, but benefits can be reported in healthy individuals within 4–6 weeks. However, longer periods of time might be necessary to demonstrate improvements in non-healthy individuals undergoing rehabilitation. Strength training leads to morphological adaptations, including hypertrophy (see below), in muscle. For a detailed review of the impact of strength and endurance training/detraining on muscle see Bruton (2002).

### CLINICAL APPLICATIONS

#### DISORDERS AND MORPHOLOGICAL CHANGES AFFECTING SKELETAL MUSCLE

All those disorders that primarily impair skeletal muscle are collectively known as **myopathies**. **Primary myopathies** are caused by intrinsic defects within the muscle fibre, for example the genetically determined myotonic and non-myotonic muscular dystrophies. **Secondary myopathies** arise as a sequel to endocrine, metabolic or vascular disorders; they are not caused by intrinsic defects in the muscle fibre.

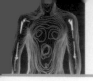

**Myositis** is the term used to describe an inflammatory myopathy, for example polymyositis and dermatomyositis. Here, inflammation and fibrosis of the muscle connective tissue are major features.

For many disorders, but particularly the muscular dystrophies and congenital myopathies, there is as yet no effective medical treatment to allay the progression of muscle degeneration. However, the physiotherapy and nursing measures outlined on the following pages can do much to attenuate or delay disabilities. Genetic counselling is essential for individuals suffering from many of the muscular dystrophies and the periodic paralyses to provide information on the risks of transmitting hereditary disorders to offspring.

## DEGENERATIVE CHANGES IN MUSCLE

Muscle disorders are characterized by a number of degenerative changes that decrease the size of fibres and impair their intracellular structure and the integrity of surrounding connective tissue. If fibres are damaged, they cannot contract effectively, if at all. It is not surprising to find that in severely affected muscles these degenerative changes lead to pain, with decreased muscle strength, tone and mass, impairing voluntary movement.

### Atrophy

Atrophy is a decrease in muscle fibre mass that can follow damage to the nerve supply or prolonged immobility (e.g. bed-rest or limb fixation), athletic detraining or weightlessness experienced during space travel. Atrophy is also a common feature of many diseases (e.g. cachexia, diabetes mellitus, hyperthyroidism and fasting). Protein synthesis declines, individual muscle fibres shorten and decrease in diameter and, as a result, muscle force and power decline (Fitts et al., 2000). Exactly what the cellular basis for atrophy is remains to be fully explained but, in addition to decreased protein synthesis, enhanced breakdown (proteolysis) might account for it. Recent reviews of research evaluating different models of muscle wasting in animal studies have suggested that accelerated muscle proteolysis via the ubiquitin–proteasome pathway is responsible for atrophy resulting from disuse, fasting, denervation and that induced by some disease states (Jagoe & Goldberg, 2001). An interesting feature of muscle fibres undergoing atrophy is that a segmental elimination of fibres occurs, that is, only part of the fibre (myonuclei and cell organelles) is removed without affecting its viability. It has been suggested that apoptotic cell death affecting only part of the fibre underlies this feature of atrophy (Sandri, 2002).

### Hypertrophy

In healthy individuals, strength training increases muscle mass, marked by increases in the cross-sectional area of type 1 and type 2 fibres, with the changes in type 2 taking place more rapidly. An increase in the expression of myosin isoform MHC-2A occurs, together with reduction in MHC-2X. Type 2A fibres possess higher fatigue resistance and oxidative capacity than type 2X.

Hypertrophy is also found in a number of pathological conditions, for example the form of dystrophy known as myotonia congenita; both muscle fibre size and numbers are increased here.

As the increased muscle mass in Duchenne dystrophy is mainly due to fatty infiltration with only minor increases in fibre numbers, it is more correctly described as **pseudohypertrophy**; it predominantly affects the calf muscles.

### Necrosis (fibre death)

Fibre necrosis is a common feature of many muscle disorders. It is present in the muscular dystrophies and metabolic myopathies and can follow trauma, ischaemia, inflammation and infection of muscle. Necrosis can also be caused by toxic injury when drugs such as pentazocine are administered, via the intramuscular route, for prolonged periods.

### Defects in the sarcolemma and sarcoplasmic reticulum

In muscle fibres, the sarcolemma (or cell membrane) consists of two areas: a basement lamina of glycoproteins inside which is the lipoprotein plasma membrane. If the basement lamina and the endomysium of connective tissue outside it are extensively damaged, no 'scaffolding structure' exists to assist the regeneration of a new fibre. Traumatic and ischaemic injuries most commonly cause this type of 'non-selective' damage and this limits regeneration.

### Myofibrillar abnormalities

Alterations in the structure of myofibrils are seen in many muscle diseases in which fibres are undergoing necrotic changes. Myofibrils can become hypercontracted, 'clumped' and disassembled due to the action of phagocytes.

### Congenital abnormalities

Abnormal structures in the myofibrils are found in the congenital myopathies. In central core disease, for example, cores of disorganized myofibrils are found in the centre of the fibre.

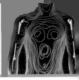

## Other changes

In a healthy muscle fibre, several nuclei are distributed around the periphery of the sarcoplasm. In a diseased muscle fibre, the nuclei increase in number and move towards the centre of the sarcoplasm. This might be a feature of regeneration. Fatty infiltration and fibrosis of muscle are found in the muscular dystrophies. Inflammation and fibrosis of muscle connective tissue occurs in inflammatory myopathies such as polymyositis.

## REGENERATION OF SKELETAL MUSCLE

The full complement of skeletal muscle fibres appears to be established by birth or in the early postnatal period. Subsequent increases in muscle size are achieved by increasing the length and diameter of existing fibres.

Exactly how regeneration of skeletal muscle takes place following injury has not been fully explained. It has been suggested that primitive satellite cells, which retain their powers of division, persist in skeletal muscle. Following injury, they move towards areas of damage in the fibre. The satellite cells then divide, giving rise to immediate myoblast cells that fuse together to form a multinucleate muscle fibre. A healthy muscle will regenerate after necrosis if the blood and nerve supplies are intact and the cause of injury is removed.

To what extent regeneration takes place depends on the degree of damage to the fibre and adjacent tissues, and whether or not any pathological activity decreases. Non-selective necrosis of the entire fibre with its basement lamina and the surrounding endomysium can result in less effective regeneration because vital 'scaffolding' structures are damaged. Trauma and ischaemia are causes of this type of injury. Regeneration is more effective if the basement lamina and endomysium are left intact, despite necrosis of the remainder of the fibre.

## INVESTIGATIONS OF MUSCLE DISEASE

### Electromyography

Electromyography is an invaluable technique in the diagnosis of muscle and nerve disorders. A needle electrode is inserted through the skin into the muscle to make an extracellular recording of motor unit action potentials. In healthy muscle, motor unit action potentials are usually 1–2 mV in amplitude, last for 2–8 ms and have two or three distinct phases. In muscle disease, degeneration of fibres leads to low-amplitude, short-duration motor unit action potentials, which might also be polyphasic.

## Enzyme tests

Enzymes are released into the circulation from muscle fibres that degenerate. Enzyme measurements are therefore useful in the diagnosis of skeletal muscle disease. Those most commonly used include:

- **creatine phosphokinase (CPK)**: the most sensitive; levels are increased during mild and severe degeneration.
- **aldolase, aspartate aminotransferase (AST)** and **lactate dehydrogenase (LDH)**: levels are all increased in serum during rapid degeneration of muscle.

## Blood and urinary creatine

Creatine is vital to muscle energy metabolism. Muscle diseases or trauma that cause severe fibre necrosis will result in an increase in the concentration of blood and urinary creatine.

## Muscle biopsy

This is another useful technique in the diagnosis of muscle disease. Samples are taken for histopathological examination from an affected muscle.

## SIGNS OF PRIMARY MUSCLE DISORDERS

Some of the most common signs of muscle disorders are:

- decreased muscle strength
- decreased muscle mass (atrophy)
- decreased muscle tone (flaccidity).

Clinical manifestations resulting from muscle disorders include:

- muscle weakness
- fatigue
- delayed relaxation (myotonia)
- intermittent paralysis
- pain.

## MEDICAL ASSESSMENT

A full medical assessment of the patient is carried out by the physician. This involves taking a medical history in which the family history and onset and duration of symptoms are noted. Body muscle groups are assessed individually by asking the patient to perform a range of motion exercises and noting alterations in tone and muscle strength. Patterns of weakness are noted, together with the extent of atrophy. Tendon reflexes are also tested; they are reduced in muscle disease. A full examination of the nervous system is necessary if coordination is impaired and tremor or abnormal movements such as chorea,

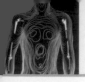

athetosis and dystonia are present. These are the signs of upper motor neurone lesions.

## PLANNING CARE

A full nursing history should be taken and an assessment made to identify the problems that exist for the patient. Observations of muscle strength, range of movement, mobility and posture should be made to establish to what extent the patient is able to carry out the activities of daily living. Some of the most common problems for patients with muscle disorders are discussed below, and the effects of muscle disorders on activities of daily living are summarized in **Table 3.1.1**.

### Weakness and fatigue

Muscle weakness, wasting and fatigue are common problems resulting from muscle disorders. Weakness might be restricted to one group of muscles, for example, the pelvic girdle in corticosteroid myopathy, or it might become progressively more widespread involving the limbs and pelvic and shoulder girdles, as is the case in many muscular dystrophies and in congenital and secondary myopathies (proximal muscles, nearer the trunk, are usually affected to a greater extent).

Depending on the extent and severity of weakness, mobility might be impaired. Weakness can affect the respiratory and pharyngeal muscles, leading to difficulties in breathing and swallowing for those afflicted with myasthenia gravis, polymyositis and hypokalaemic periodic paralysis.

Fatigue occurs in healthy muscle after intense exercise but in diseased muscle it can occur readily following any activity. Affected individuals complain of tiring easily and might be exhausted by tasks that they finished with ease before the onset of illness. This is most noticeable in patients suffering from myasthenia gravis, where muscle weakness and fatigue increase excessively with repeated use and are improved by rest.

Bearing this in mind, nursing care is aimed at planning the activities of the patient's day to avoid exacerbating muscle weakness or precipitating fatigue and exhaustion by supervising periods of rest and activity. Initially, small, easily achieved goals should be set, to foster independence and boost morale. Activities can be increased gradually as muscle strength is regained. Rapid regression of muscle weakness occurs when the underlying adrenal or thyroid disorders are treated in the endocrine myopathies. Anticholinesterase drugs such as neostigmine and physostigmine are used to alleviate muscle weakness in patients suffering from myasthenia gravis.

### Stiffness

Delayed relaxation of muscles (myotonia) can result in slow, stiff movements in patients suffering from the myotonic muscular dystrophies. In myotonia congenita, delayed relaxation of muscles is most severe after rest and is exacerbated by cold; warmth and exercise improve the condition. In this disorder, muscles are hypertrophied so the atrophy and weakness do not cause problems. Administration of drugs such as procainamide, phenytoin or quinine sulphate can improve delayed relaxation of voluntary muscle in the myotonic muscular dystrophies.

### Intermittent paralysis

Attacks of intermittent muscle weakness and paralysis are features of the metabolic myopathies. In the hypokalaemic form of periodic paralysis, the attacks of muscle weakness tend to occur in the evening, often following a heavy, carbohydrate-rich meal or after heavy exercise. A fall in the plasma potassium ion concentration and a rise in the concentration inside the muscle cell occur, altering its excitability. Potassium chloride is given orally to treat the attacks and as a preventive measure in the evenings; acetazolamide is also used to treat the disorder. Patients should restrict their dietary intake in the evenings and reduce the carbohydrate content, as well as avoiding heavy exercise.

### Immobility

The extent of immobility experienced by individuals with muscle weakness and wasting depends on the progressive nature of the disorder. Duchenne muscular dystrophy is so relentlessly progressive that walking can be impossible by the age of 10 years and many of those afflicted die in young adulthood. By contrast, the non-progressive nature of some of the congenital myopathies, e.g. central core disease, allows some of these individuals to remain active throughout life. Most patients afflicted with myotonia dystrophica are unable to walk by 35 years of age.

As described earlier, muscle fibre length is crucial in deciding the range of movement possible, whereas fibre numbers and size influence muscle strength. Longer fibres give a greater range of movement, and increased size and greater numbers impart greater strength to muscle. A major influence on fibre size is the stress and strain imposed by daily use. If the workload of a muscle is increased then healthy fibres increase in size (hypertrophy), giving the muscle greater strength. If muscles are not used, they undergo atrophy; the fibres shorten and

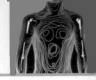

decrease in diameter. Atrophy, leading to muscle weakness, wasting and impaired mobility, is a pathological feature in muscle disorders. It can also occur if the nerve supply to a muscle is impaired, or due to disuse if mobility is restricted.

A major problem is that muscles can atrophy and shorten, leading to a **contracture** at the joint, which severely limits movement; a permanent deformity can result. Therefore, it is vital that any individual afflicted with a muscle disorder receives regular physiotherapy exercises during the course of the day, which will attenuate atrophy and build up muscle bulk in healthy fibres, thereby promoting strength and preventing disabling contractures. Active and passive exercises must be instituted to maintain range of movement, and maximum use must be made of all aids to ambulation – tripods, walking frames, etc. Immobile limbs must not be left in flexed positions, which can cause flexion contractures, and other deformities such as foot or wrist drop must be prevented by the use of bed footboards and splints.

Contractures can also develop when prolonged ischaemia results in necrosis of muscle. This usually occurs in association with bony factures involving the humerus, femur or tibia, although it can also follow thrombosis of the arterial supply to the muscle as a result of atherosclerotic disease.

Following fracture reduction, the formation of a haematoma and oedema can lead to obstruction of the muscle arterial supply. If the ischaemia is not relieved within 4 hours, serious muscle necrosis will take place. Subsequent fibrosis and scar tissue formation then lead to shortening of the muscle, causing a contracture deformity. A classic example of this is seen in **Volkmann's ischaemic contracture**, which can follow a supracondylar fracture of the humerus at the elbow. Ischaemia of the arterial supply to the flexor muscles of the forearm leads to a flexion deformity of the forearm, wrist and fingers. To prevent this, nurses must be able to recognize and report the signs of 'muscle' ischaemia, which in this case include the absence of a radial pulse, severe pain with pallor and coolness of the extremities. Postoperative elevation of the arm will reduce oedema formation. Immediate treatment of this condition includes the removal of tight bandages or splints to improve the circulation, and surgical relief of the cause of ischaemia, if necessary.

## Pain

Muscle pain can occur in healthy muscles as a result of severe exercise. Most people are familiar with **cramps**, the short, painful, involuntary tetanic contractions of muscle that can follow sudden exercise, especially in those unaccustomed to taking it! Exercise-related pain in healthy muscle usually disappears within a few days.

However, pain can also follow traumatic injury, infection, inflammation and ischaemia of muscle. It can be diffuse or localized, depending on the nature of the disorder. In patients with peripheral vascular disease, an ischaemic muscle pain develops in the calf muscles on walking – **intermittent claudication**. Muscle spasms are sustained muscle contractions that can be reflexly induced by pain, ischaemia and mechanical damage. Persistent muscle pain that is not related to exercise or injury and is associated with decreased muscle tone, strength and atrophy suggests that an underlying muscle disease is present. Nurses should attempt to locate the source of the pain and assess its quality; any precipitating causes, such as exercise, should be identified. Analgesia and rest should then be provided together with immobilization and elevation of a painful limb. Pain associated with severe inflammatory disorders such as polymyositis is alleviated when corticosteroid drugs are administered to reduce the inflammation. Ischaemic pain is treated by alleviating the underlying causes. Drugs such as Praxilene (naftidofuryl oxalate) can be useful in relieving muscle pain in patients suffering from peripheral vascular disease.

## Dyspnoea

Dyspnoea can sometimes occur in disorders that directly affect the muscles of respiration (e.g. myasthenia gravis, polymyositis) and in those that impair the nerve supply to the respiratory muscles (e.g. Guillain–Barré syndrome).

Resulting weakness of the respiratory muscles decreases the vital capacity of the lungs, and the patient might be unable to expectorate pulmonary secretions effectively; pooling of secretions then leads to dyspnoea. If dysphagia is also present, saliva or food debris might be inhaled into the trachea, resulting in airway obstruction. Chest physiotherapy, pharyngotracheal suction and nursing the patient in an upright position (which allows maximal lung expansion) are some essential preventive measures.

Respiratory weakness might be so severe in some patients that respiratory failure develops. Intermittent positive pressure ventilation (IPPV) is then necessary.

## Dysphagia

Weakness can affect the muscles of the pharynx and jaw in patients suffering from myasthenia gravis or polymyositis, leading to difficulties in swallowing and chewing food. Following assessment of dysphagia and dietetic referral, a softer diet with smaller, more frequent meals might be recommended instead of large meals and bulky foods, which require extensive chewing and swallowing. Prostigmin 1 mg may be given subcutaneously before meals to myasthenic patients, to assist chewing and swallowing. In severely dysphagic patients, in whom oral ingestion of food is unsafe and has been contraindicated following assessment, nutritional needs can be met either by nasogastric feeding or by parenteral nutrition.

Further details on the use of modified food textures in swallowing disorders and on screening for dysphagia can be found in Penman & Thompson (1998) and guidelines published by the Royal College of Speech and Language Therapists (1998).

Many other problems arise for patients suffering from muscle disorders. Weak, immobile patients are vulnerable to all the complications of immobility, including pressure ulcers, deep vein thrombosis, chest infections and disuse osteoporosis. Implementing all the physiotherapy and nursing measures that keep the patient as mobile as possible will do much to prevent these complications and other disabilities, as will the prophylactic use of sheepskins, air mattresses and at least 2-hourly changes of position for immobile patients. Depression and disturbances of body image can result from the physical changes brought about by muscle disease.

## DEVELOPMENTAL ISSUES

### EMBRYOLOGICAL DEVELOPMENT

During the first 4 weeks of embryological development, the segmentally arranged somites derived from mesoderm give rise to the myotomes from which skeletal muscle originates. It is unusual for muscle to arise from single myotomes, most are formed by fusion of adjacent somites. Muscle primordia developing from myotomes can migrate to form distant attachments and layers of muscle can arise by splitting of primordia. Two distinct cords of muscle on the dorsal and ventral surfaces of the spinal column form the extensor muscle of the spine (dorsal) and the prevertebral musculature of the abdominal and thoracic walls.

## EFFECTS OF AGEING

Muscle constitutes 40% of body cell mass, the largest reserve of protein in the body. It is affected not only by disease (see below) but also by ageing. Between the middle years extending up to the age of 80 years, approximately 30% of muscle mass is lost, a process called sarcopenia. Histologically, this is evident in loss of myofibrillar proteins and a relative increase in connective tissue and fat components. The decline in muscle area, mass and, as a consequence, strength, is particularly evident. Muscle strength and fibre number decline by similar proportions, although loss of type II fast twitch fibres can be particularly noted (Beaufrere & Boirie, 1998; Hyatt et al., 1990). A number of factors might be responsible for the effects of ageing on muscle including inactivity, inadequate dietary intakes due to anorexia, and changes in the regulation of protein turnover and mass by decreased secretion of growth hormone and insulin-like growth factor-1. Other hormonal deficits associated with muscle changes in ageing are testosterone and thyroid hormone.

The diminution in muscle mass and strength can result in a loss in functional capacity, together with an increased risk of falls, injuries and reduced physical work capacity in elderly subjects. However, there is encouraging evidence to suggest that gentle exercise programmes to increase muscle strength, volume and other dimensions of performance can have beneficial effects on physical function and levels of dependency (Fisher et al., 1991; Frontera et al., 1988). More specifically, progressive resistance exercise training has proved effective in attenuating the effects of ageing, bringing about an increase in muscle protein synthesis, muscle protein mass, strength and power (Parise & Yarasheski, 2000). Improvements in maximal oxygen consumption have also been reported (Coudert & Van Praagh, 2000). Increasing dietary intakes of amino acids via use of supplements have been reported to increase muscle protein synthesis in older adults (Volpi et al., 1999).

## Clinical review

In addition to the Learning Objectives at the begining of this chapter, the reader should be able to:

• Define the terms 'prime mover', 'antagonist', and 'synergist', and explain how the actions of these muscle groups are coordinated during movement

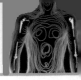

- Describe the microstructure of a single skeletal muscle fibre
- Describe the molecular structure of the thick and thin filaments within a myofibril
- Discuss the process of neuromuscular transmission and briefly explain how this process can be impaired or prevented
- Discuss the aetiology of myasthenia gravis; describe the medical treatment and nursing care that should be given to individuals afflicted with this disorder
- Explain the ionic events that form the basis of the action potential in a skeletal muscle cell
- Define the terms 'resting potential', 'depolarization', 'repolarization' and 'hyperpolarization'
- Discuss how muscle tone is altered in primary myopathies and upper motor neurone lesions
- Describe the common signs and clinical manifestations of muscles disorders
- Review the major problems that can arise in individuals afflicted with myotonia dystrophica, Duchenne dystrophy and polymyositis, and outline what nursing care is indicated
- Explain how a contracture deformity can be allayed or prevented
- Differentiate between an isotonic and an isometric muscle contraction

## Review questions

1. How much of your body is made up of skeletal muscle?
2. Which actions do prime movers perform?
3. Which connective tissue surrounds the individual muscle fibres?
4. Describe a motor unit.
5. How much of the cardiac output goes to skeletal muscles at rest?
6. Which contractile proteins do myofibrils contain?
7. Which protein are the thick filaments made of?
8. Which ion is involved in excitation–contraction coupling?
9. Which neurotransmitter is released into the skeleton neuromuscular junction?
10. What does acetylcholine bind to on the sarcolemma?
11. Describe the process of depolarization.
12. What does botulinum toxin do and what is its effect on skeletal muscle?
13. What happens when the concentration of calcium ions is decreased in extracellular fluid?
14. In addition to calcium ions and contractile proteins, what else is required for contraction of skeletal muscle to take place?
15. Describe what happens in skeletal muscle contraction.
16. Which enzyme measurements are used in the diagnosis of skeletal muscle disease?

## Suggestions for further reading

Dos Remedios, C.G., Chabra, D., Kekic, M. et al. (2003) Actin-binding proteins: Regulation of cytoskeletal filaments. *Physiology Reviews*, **83**; 433–473.
*Excellent contemporary review on the function of actin in the cell skeleton – for enthusiasts.*

Grimley Evans, J. & Franklin Williams, T. (1992) *Oxford Textbook of Geriatric Medicine*. Oxford: Oxford University Press.
*A classic test. Excellent reviews on human ageing and associated disorders, including muscle.*

Lieber, R. (2002) *Skeletal Muscle Structure and Function: The Physiological Basis of Rehabilitation*. Philadelphia: Lippincott, Williams and Wilkins.
*Detailed applications of muscle physiology to rehabilitation.*

Palastanga, N., Field, D. & Soames, R. (2002) *Anatomy and Human Movement*. Oxford: Butterworth-Heinemann.
*Well-illustrated sections on muscle and their related structures.*

Sobczak, J. (2002) *Alive and Kicking: The Carer's Guide To Exercise For Older People*. London: Age Concern.
*Of interest to those working in care homes who wish to facilitate chair-based exercise for older people.*

Walton, J. (2001) *Disorders of Voluntary Muscle*. Cambridge: Cambridge University Press.
*An authoritative, classic text recently updated.*

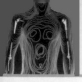

## References

Beaufrere, B. & Boirie, Y. (1998) Aging and protein metabolism. *Current Opinion in Clinical Nutrition and Metabolic Care,* **1**(1); 85–89.

Berchtold, M.W., Brinkmeier, H. & Muntener, M. (2000) Calcium ion in skeletal muscle: Its crucial role for muscle function, plasticity and disease. *Physiological Reviews,* **80**(3); 1215–1275.

Blake, D.J., Weir, A., Newey, S.E. & Davies, K.E. (2002) Function and genetics of dystrophin and dystrophin-related proteins in muscle. *Physiological Reviews,* **82**; 291–329.

Bohannon, R.W. (1990) Exercise training variables influencing the enhancement of voluntary muscle strength. *Clinical Rehabilitation,* **51**; 449–462.

Bruton, A. (2002) Muscle plasticity: Response to training and detraining. *Physiotherapy,* **88**(7); 398–408.

Coudert, J. & Van Praagh, E. (2000) Endurance exercise training in the elderly: Effects on cardiovascular function. *Current Opinion in Clinical Nutrition and Metabolic Care,* **3**(6); 479–483.

Drachman, D. (1978) Myasthenia gravis. *New England Journal of Medicine,* **298**(3); 136–186.

Ellis, K.J. (2000) Human body composition: In-vivo methods. *Physiological Reviews,* **80**(2); 649–680.

Fisher, N., Pendergast, D. & Calkins, E. (1991) Muscle rehabilitation in impaired elderly nursing home residents. *Archives of Physical and Medical Rehabilitation,* **72**; 181–185.

Fitts, R.H., Riley, D.R. & Widrick, J.J. (2000) Micro-gravity and skeletal muscle. *Journal of Applied Physiology,* **89**; 823–839.

Frontera, W., Meredith, C.N. & O'Reilly, K. (1988) Muscle strength conditioning in older man: Skeletal muscle hypertrophy and improved function. *Journal of Applied Physiology,* **64**; 1038–1044.

Glassman, A. (1979) Immune responses: the rationale for plasmaphoresis. *Plasma Therapy,* **1**(1); 13.

Hyatt, R., Whitelaw, M., Bhat, A. et al. (1990) Association of muscle strength with functional status of elderly people. *Age and Ageing,* **19**; 330–336.

Isakov, E. & Bowker, B. (2002) Influence of a single FES treatment on hemiparetic legs. *Physiotherapy,* **88**(5); 269–272.

Jagoe, R.T. & Goldberg, A.L. (2001) What do we really know about the ubiquitin–proteasome pathway in muscle atrophy? *Current Opinion in Clinical Nutrition and Metabolic Care,* **4**(3); 183–190.

Komi, P.V. & Hakkinen, K. (1998) Strength and power. In: Knuttgen, H.G. & Tittel, K. (eds) *The Olympic Book of Sports Medicine.* Oxford: Blackwell Scientific Publications, pp. 181–193.

Levine, S.P., Kett, R.L., Cedarna, P.S. & Brooks, S.V. (1990) Electrical muscle stimulation for pressure sore prevention: Tissue shape variation. *Archives of Physical and Medical Rehabilitation,* **71**; 210–214.

Parise, G. & Yarasheski, K.E. (2000) The utility of resistance exercise training and amino-acid supplementation for reversing age-associated decrements in muscle protein mass and function. *Current Opinion in Clinical Nutrition and Metabolic Care,* **3**(6); 489–495.

Penman, J.P. & Thompson, M. (1998) A review of the textured diets developed for the management of dysphagia. *Human Nutrition and Dietetics,* **11**; 51–60.

Pietrobelli, A., Wang, M. & Heymsfield, S.B. (1998) Techniques used in measuring human body composition. *Current Opinion in Clinical Nutrition and Metabolic Care,* **1**; 439–448.

Price, R. & Lehmann, J.F. (1990) Influence of muscle cooling on the viscoelastic response of the human ankle to sinusoidal displacements. *Archives of Physical and Medical Rehabilitation,* **71**; 745–748.

Royal College of Speech and Language Therapists (RCST) (1998) Clinical guidelines by consensus for Speech and Language Therapists. London: RCST Publications.

Sandri, M. (2002) Apoptotic signaling in skeletal muscle fibres during atrophy. *Current Opinion in Clinical Nutrition and Metabolic Care,* **5**(3); 249–253.

Stamler, J.S. & Meissner, G. (2001) Physiology of nitric oxide in skeletal muscle. *Physiological Reviews,* **81**(1); 209–240.

Taylor, S. & Goodinson-McLaren, S.M. (1991) *Nutritional Support: A Team Approach.* London: Wolfe Publishing.

Thomas, M.A. (2000) Modalities used in the treatment of fractures. In: Hoppenfield, S. & Murthy, V.L. (eds) *Treatment and Rehabilitation of Fractures.* Philadelphia: Lippincott, Williams and Wilkins, pp. 27–30.

Volpi, E., Mittendorfer, B., Wolf, S.E. & Wolfe, R.R. (1999) Oral amino acids stimulate muscle protein anabolism in the elderly despite higher first-pass splanchnic extraction. *American Journal of Physiology, Endocrinology and Metabolism,* **277**; E513–E520.

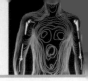

# Bones

*Susan M. McLaren*

---

## LEARNING OBJECTIVES

After studying this chapter the reader should be able to:

- List the functions of bone

- Describe the architecture, composition and vascular supply of bone

- Discuss the origin and function of osteoblasts, osteocytes and osteoclasts

- Describe the processes of endochondral and intramembranous bone ossification

- Explain how growth in length and diameter of bone is achieved

- Identify the pathophysiological features of common bone disorders, together with the rationale for treatment

---

## INTRODUCTION

Current knowledge of the microstructure and physiological functions of bones is far from complete and, in many instances, there is controversy. Outward appearances can be misleading, for bone is far from being the structurally inert, reinforced concrete so frequently envisaged. Instead, it is a dynamic tissue with a high metabolic activity, which is continuously undergoing complex, structural alterations under the influences of mechanical stressors and hormones.

Bone is considered to have a dual role, providing mechanical support and mineral homeostasis. Four major functions are ascribed to it:

1. Provision of a structural support for body tissues and an attachment for muscles, tendons and ligaments.
2. Formation of the lever systems that permit body movement (see Chapter 3.3).
3. A major role in mineral homeostasis by providing a reservoir of body calcium, phosphorus and magnesium salts (see Chapter 2.6).
4. Formation and protection of haemopoietic tissue in the bone marrow (see Chapter 4.1).

Bone is a specialized form of connective tissue that is made durable by the deposition of minerals such as calcium and phosphate within its infrastructure. It is well fitted to withstand the deforming forces generated during body movement: its ultimate tensile stress and compressive strength compares favourably with other structural materials such as granite and cast iron (**Table 3.2.1**). In addition, its elastic properties confer flexibility and a diminished likelihood of fracturing under stress, and protection against the impact of a deforming force is afforded by its soft tissue covering. In an adult, skeletal bone forms one of the largest tissue masses in the body, weighing 10–12 kg.

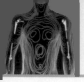

**Table 3.2.1** Physical characteristics of bone (adapted from Passmore and Robson, 1976)

|  | Ultimate tensile strength (kg/mm²) | Ultimate compressive strength (kg/mm²) |
| --- | --- | --- |
| Cortical bone | 7–10 | 14–21 |
| Cast iron | 7–21 | 42–100 |
| Granite | 10–20 | 9–26 |

## Composition of bone

Three major components are found in bone:

1. an organic matrix of collagen, which imparts tensile strength
2. a mineral matrix of calcium and phosphate, which imparts compressive strength and rigidity
3. bone cells, including osteoblasts, osteoclasts, osteocytes and fibroblasts.

The organic matrix of bone comprises 25% of its total weight and is known as **osteoid**. By far its greatest component is collagen (95%), with hyaluronic acid and chondroitin sulphate constituting the remainder of the matrix. By contrast, the mineral matrix of bone consists of amorphous calcium phosphate and a crystalline structure similar to hydroxyapatite.

The mechanisms underlying the process of bone mineralization are poorly understood. Amorphous calcium phosphate is transformed into apatite crystals, which become oriented along the collagen molecules of the organic matrix. The physical properties of the collagen fibres and, in particular, their banded structure, favour formation of the hydroxyapatite crystals $3Ca_3(PO_4)_2Ca(OH)_2$. Surface ions of the hydroxyapatite crystals are hydrated, forming a shell through which exchange of ions with the body fluids occurs; this provides a basis for the modelling and remodelling of bone throughout an individual's lifetime. The process of mineralization is initially very rapid, with 70% mineralization occurring within a few days, although completion can take up to 6 weeks.

## Architecture of bone

Two forms of architecture are distinguished, woven and lamellar bone. **Woven bone** is a transitional, relatively fragile form most commonly seen during phases of rapid bone formation in embryonic life or at zones of **endochondral ossification** (see p. 298).

It is also found during fracture repair, and some persists in the adult near sites of tendon insertion and ligament attachment.

Lamellar bone is of greater durability, manifest in its structure, which consists of layers in each of which the collagen fibres have a different orientation. Two forms of lamellar bone are distinguished: compact, **cortical bone** and spongy, cancellous, **trabecular bone**.

## Compact bone

Compact, cortical bone forms the outer area of all bones. It is found in the shafts of long bones where it encloses the marrow cavity, and in the outer and inner parts of flat bones. The functional units of compact bone are the **Haversian systems** or **osteons**, which are 0.2–0.5 mm in diameter. These consist of a central canal oriented parallel to the long axis of the bone, through which pass an arteriole, capillary, venule and nerve. Each Haversian canal is surrounded by concentric lamellae (**as shown in Fig. 3.2.1**), which contain **osteocytes** within grooves known as **canaliculi**. Adjacent osteocytes communicate via a system of microcanaliculi, which permeate the bone, facilitating the exchange of nutrients and movement of waste products. This is particularly important because osteocytes are not in direct contact with blood vessels. Around each Haversian system is a 'cement line', which the canaliculi do not cross. Due to the constant remodelling of bone, great variation in the mineralization of osteons and the diameter of Haversian canals occurs. Some canals appear irregular and enlarged due to the removal of mineral and matrix that might be occurring. Remains of earlier systems are also found, forming the interstitial lamellae shown in **Fig. 3.2.1**. Finally, circumferential lamellae are found beneath the periosteum and endosteum.

## Trabecular bone

Unlike the regular structure found in compact bone, this form contains fewer Haversian systems and is organized into a lattice of trabeculae in which red or fatty marrow fills the cavities. Bone remodelling occurs on the surface of the trabeculae and the lacunae containing osteocytes are scattered throughout the matrix. Spongy, cancellous, trabecular bone is found in vertebrae, flat bones and at the end of long bones (**Fig. 3.2.2**).

### Epiphysis and diaphysis

**Figure 3.2.2** shows the typical anatomical features of a long bone. The central shaft, or **diaphysis**, is formed of compact bone, and at each end is the **epiphysis**. The latter extends from beneath the articular cartilage

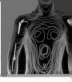

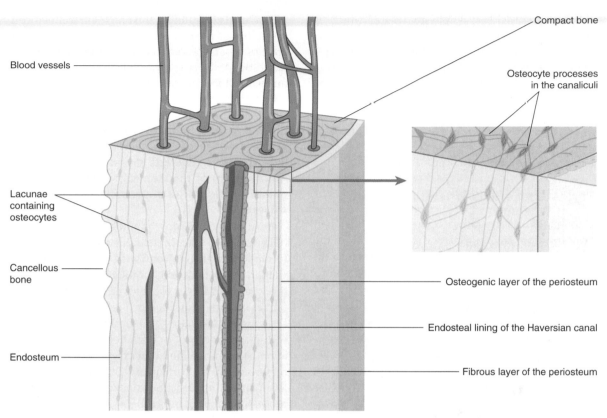

**Figure 3.2.1** The longitudinal and cross-sectional appearance of compact cortical bone

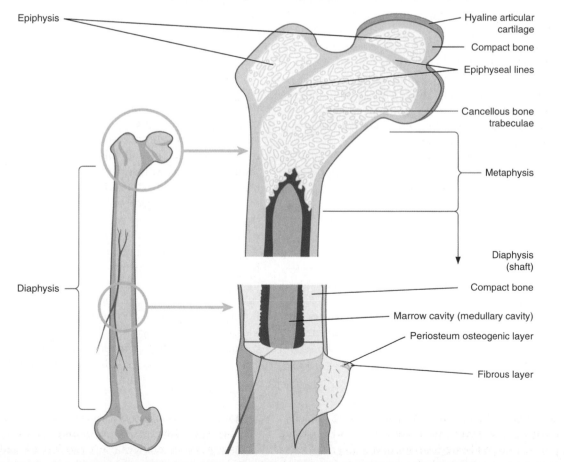

**Figure 3.2.2** Structural components of the femur showing the epiphysis, metaphysis and diaphysis

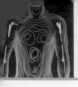

inwards towards the epiphyseal plate, which is formed of cancellous bone. The joint capsule is attached around the synovial joint formed at the epiphysis, as shown in Chapter 3.3. Adjacent to the growth plate is the growing end of the diaphysis, called the **metaphysis**. During growth, the epiphyses are separated from the diaphyses by this growth plate of cartilage. However, once growth is completed in adult life, the plate becomes fully calcified and remains as the epiphyseal line.

## Periosteum and endosteum

Contiguous over the surface of most bones is a tough layer of fibrous connective tissue known as the **periosteum**. This does not cover the articular cartilage surfaces of the synovial joint. The outer, fibrous layer of the periosteum transmits blood vessels and provides a site of attachment for ligaments and muscles. Beneath this is a layer of **osteoblasts**, cells that contribute to the increased growth in diameter of bone in this region. Until growth is complete, the periosteum is not firmly attached to the underlying bone except at the epiphyseal plate. The periosteum is abundantly supplied with myelinated and unmyelinated nerve fibres. These comprise sensory fibres (which detect pain, pressure changes and vibration) and some autonomic vasomotor fibres.

### CLINICAL APPLICATIONS

Stimulation of the sensory fibres due to traumatic injury accompanied by tearing of the periosteum or due to the increased pressure generated by a tumour can result in bone pain, which is always severe and continuous in nature.

A fine, inner layer of tissue, known as the **endosteum**, lines the marrow cavity of the bone. This contains osteoblasts, osteoclasts and the cells that are their precursors.

## Bone cells

The origin of bone cells remains controversial. One major theory proposes that precursor cells originate in bone marrow and that osteoblasts and osteocytes differentiate from haemopoietic stem cells, whereas osteoclasts differentiate separately, from mononuclear phagocytic cells.

### Osteoblasts

Osteoblasts are present on all bone surfaces, in single layers adjacent to the unmineralized osteoid of newly forming bone. They are uniform in size and are linked to adjacent osteoblasts by fine cytoplasmic processes.

A characteristic feature is their high intracellular concentration of the enzyme alkaline phosphatase. This appears to play a key role in the mineralization of bone by destroying pyrophosphate, which is an inhibitor of this process.

Functions of the osteoblast include the synthesis and secretion of the constituents of the organic matrix, including collagen and protein–polysaccharides (glycoproteins and proteoglycans). In addition, osteoblasts promote mineralization (calcification) of the matrix, controlling the rapid phases of this process in the initial stages (the first 4 days).

In summary, during physiological growth and bone turnover, osteoblasts fulfil a vital role in bone formation, which is controlled by 1,25-dihydroxy vitamin D3, parathyroid hormone, diverse growth factors, cytokines and eicosanoids (Hughes et al., 1998). Phases of bone resorption by osteoclasts (see below) are coupled to phases of deposition by osteoblasts within the process of calcium homeostasis. Combination of hormonal and other regulatory factors with receptors on the osteoblast generate signals that affect osteoclast function, underpinning this cyclic process. Signalling mechanisms relayed from osteocytes to osteoblasts and osteoclasts are also influential in bone remodelling.

### Osteocytes

Osteocytes are derived from osteoblasts that have become trapped in lacunae by the matrix they have secreted. Fine cytoplasmic processes extend through the microcanaliculi of lacunae, linking adjacent osteocytes. At present, the precise role of these cells is uncertain but it is thought they might detect microdamage in the bone matrix and initiate bone remodelling through signal transmission relayed to osteoblasts and osteoclasts (Qiu et al., 2002). Bone adjacent to the wall of the osteocyte (perilacunar bone) contains fewer collagen fibres and is more soluble in terms of mineral content. Furthermore, the size of the lacunae appears to increase following either vitamin D or parathyroid hormone administration. It has been suggested that the osteocyte might also act as a 'bone pump', releasing calcium from perilacunar bone in response to these hormones (**osteocytic osteolysis**). Other functions ascribed to the osteocytes include synthesis of some collagen and control of matrix mineralization, long-term calcium exchange and plasma protein uptake.

### Osteoclasts

These cells are responsible for the resorption of bone and are abundant on or near surfaces undergoing erosion. They show a great variation in size and are highly mobile: some are small and contain one

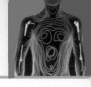

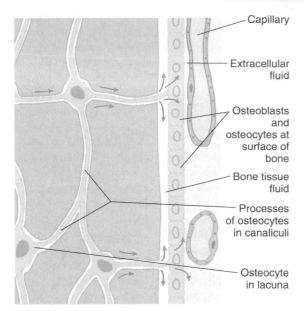

Figure 3.2.3 Exchange of tissue fluid between bone and blood circulation

nucleus, others are multinucleate giant cells. At their site of contact with bone is a brush border of microvilli, which infiltrates the disintegrating bone surface. To facilitate bone resorption, osteoclasts contain a large number of enzymes for lysis of the mineral and organic matrix. They also contain high levels of the enzyme acid phosphatase. A number of hormones are known to control the activities of the osteoclasts, notably parathyroid hormone, thyroxine, calcitonin, oestrogens and metabolites of vitamins A and D. To make calcium available for physiological requirements, osteoclast activity is enhanced by parathyroid hormone and thyroxine. This action is opposed by calcitonin when the opposite conditions apply (see Chapter 2.6).

## Bone tissue fluid

Bone surfaces are covered by a layer of osteoblasts and osteocytes, which separate the bone tissue fluid from the extracellular fluid and the blood capillary supply. Metabolites must cross this barrier to reach bone. In the bone, movement of ions and other metabolites then occurs via the bone fluid in the lacunae and canaliculi. The distribution of bone fluid is shown in **Fig. 3.2.3**. Bone fluid differs from extracellular fluid in both mineral and protein content: the potassium concentration is higher than that of plasma but the calcium, magnesium, sodium and albumin concentrations are all markedly lower.

## Blood supply

Long bones are supplied by three major vessel types: the nutrient artery, the periosteal arteries and the

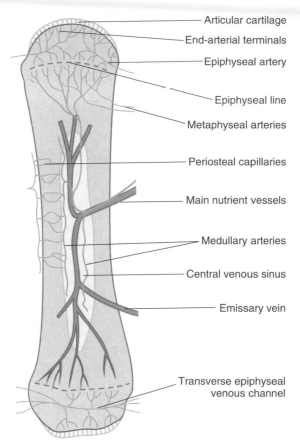

Figure 3.2.4 Blood supply to long bones

metaphyseal and epiphyseal arteries (**as shown in Fig. 3.2.4**). The nutrient artery arises from a systemic artery, pierces the diaphysis through a foramen and gives rise to ascending and descending medullary arteries within the marrow cavity. In turn, these give rise to arteries supplying the endosteum and diaphysis.

The periosteal blood supply passes from the periosteal network via Volkmann's canals to the lamellae of compact bone. Approximately one-third of cortical bone and a large proportion of epiphyseal and metaphyseal bone are supplied by periosteal vessels. The periosteal blood supply is increased when growth is complete and the periosteum becomes firmly attached to the underlying bone.

### DEVELOPMENTAL ISSUES

The metaphyseal and epiphyseal supply of long bones changes with age. During growth, a special circulation to each epiphyseal growth plate exists but, once growth is complete, this changes. Metaphyseal and epiphyseal arteries arise from systemic arteries, entering the bone foramina as shown in **Fig. 3.2.4**. Note that they are separated by the growth plate. Nutrients are supplied to the epiphyseal ossification centres by the epiphyseal

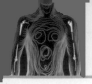

arteries and to newly formed bone by the metaphyseal arteries. Once growth is complete, the two groups of arteries anastomose freely.

At rest, the arterial flow rate to the skeleton is approximately 12% of the cardiac output, or (2–3 mL/100 g/min) (Brookes, 1971). With regard to the mechanisms controlling the osseous circulation, the vasculature has been shown to be responsive to the majority of vasodilator and vasoconstrictor substances (McCarthy, 1998). Vascular endothelial cells secrete a number of factors that could potentially influence the activity of bone, notably nitric oxide, interleukins and growth factors. Blood flow is greatly increased in the presence of inflammation, infection and following fracture. Local production of nitric oxide, which is a potent vasodilator and angiogenic stimulus, might account for the high blood flow following fracture. The flow rate to the marrow is increased in hypoxaemia, when red cell production is increased to raise the oxygen transport capacity.

## EMBRYOLOGICAL DEVELOPMENT OF BONE

By the fourth week of embryological development, structures that give rise to the musculoskeletal system are apparent. Paired blocks of segmentally arranged mesoderm present on either side of the spinal cord and form somites. These show a characteristic regional distribution: 4 occipital, 8 cervical, 12 thoracic, 5 lumbar, 5 sacral and 8–9 coccygeal somites. Subsequently, a cavity develops in each somite demarcating three distinct areas: the dermatome, myotome and sclerotome. Skeletal muscle develops from the myotome, a proportion of the dermis and connective tissue of the skin from the dermatome and vertebral centra, neural arches and costae from the sclerotome. In contrast, the skeleton and muscle of the jaws develop from mesoderm of the pharyngeal arches of the embryo.

Limb buds also become marked in the fourth week of embryological development. Initially out-growths from the trunk, the forelimbs develop first. Each bud comprises a core of mesenchyme enclosed by ectodermal epithelium, the precursor of the epidermis. From the mesenchymal core subsequently develop the skeletal axis of limb bones, periosteum, joints and their associated structures. The latter include tendons, ligaments, periosteum, muscles, dermis, connective tissue, blood vessels and lymphatics. Nerves develop by axomic sprouting from the spinal cord, invading the limb bud.

The earliest skeletal framework on the developing embryo arises from mesenchyme cells, which lay down membranes of fibrous connective tissue. During fetal growth, the fibrous tissue is almost completely replaced by hyaline cartilage templates. Subsequently, bone can develop by ossification of cartilage (endochondral) or replacement of fibrous connective tissue (membranous) ossification. Ossification is begun in early fetal life but is not completed until the third decade of adult life.

### Endochondral ossification (Fig. 3.2.5)

This is the process by which pre-existing cartilage templates are replaced by bone. A signal that ossification is about to occur is the appearance of centres of ossification within the shaft of the bone. Chondrocytes in this region hypertrophy and the surrounding lacunae expand to form cavities within the matrix. The result is that the cartilage matrix degenerates rapidly to form irregular spicules. Subsequent calcification of the cartilage matrix cuts off the nutrient supply to the chondrocytes, which eventually die. While this is occurring, perichondral osteogenic cells are stimulated to form a circumferential periosteal collar of bone around the mid-region of the shaft. As blood vessels grow inwards from the periosteum, they carry with them periosteal cells that give rise to marrow cells, osteoblasts and osteoclasts. The osteoblasts deposit bone matrix around the scaffolding of calcified cartilage spicules, forming trabecular bars. Within the shaft, spaces invaded by marrow cells become confluent, eventually forming a true marrow cavity. From the centre of the shaft, ossification extends towards the bone ends by the same sequence of events, and the central endochondral bone rapidly converges with the periosteal collar. Initial sites of bone formation in the shaft and periosteal collar are known as **primary centres of ossification**. They first appear in long bones during the first 7–8 months of intrauterine life. At birth, the ends of most long bones still consist of cartilage but **secondary ossification centres** in the epiphyses appear during the first 5 years of childhood.

### Intramembranous bone formation (Fig. 3.2.6)

In this form of ossification, direct replacement of fibrous connective tissue by bone occurs. Intramembranous bone formation occurs in bones of the cranium, lower jaw and clavicle. The imminent ossification of the tissue is signalled by its increase in vascularity. Following this, mesenchyme cells proliferate, hypertrophy and differentiate into osteoblasts, which synthesize the collagen fibres and proteoglycans of the osteoid matrix. Under the influence of the osteoblasts, mineralization follows rapidly. Spicules of developing bone gradually enlarge, forming trabeculae in a closely interwoven

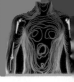

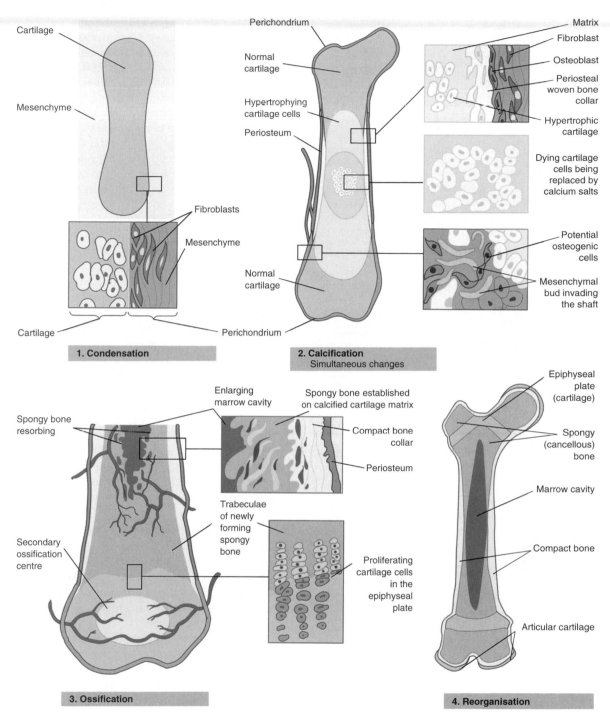

**Figure 3.2.5** Schematic representation of the events occurring during endochondral bone formation in the femur. This type of bone formation involves the replacement of a cartilaginous model of the bone by bone itself

network. Osteoblasts are eventually trapped within lacunae in the matrix that they synthesize. Here, they gradually lose the potential for proliferation and differentiate into osteocytes. In the final stages of intramembranous ossification, the trabeculae are remodelled and replaced by cancellous or compact bone. However, if the bone remains spongy, the labyrinth is rapidly filled by mesenchyme cells, which develop into marrow.

## GROWTH OF BONE

### Growth in length

Growth in the length of a bone is achieved by endochondral ossification and growth in diameter by apposition on existing bone surfaces.

Longitudinal growth of bone takes place by endochondral ossification at the bone ends, a process that depends on the production of

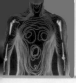

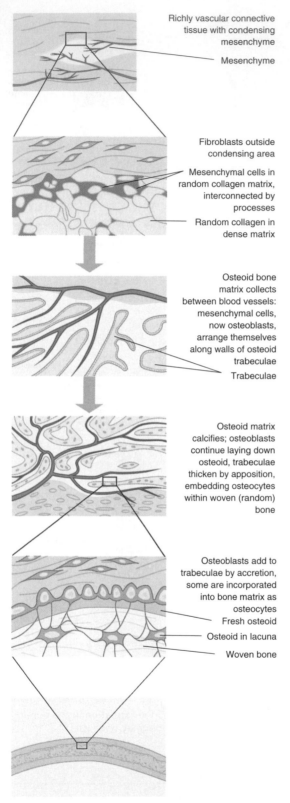

Richly vascular connective tissue with condensing mesenchyme

Mesenchyme

Fibroblasts outside condensing area

Mesenchymal cells in random collagen matrix, interconnected by processes

Random collagen in dense matrix

Osteoid bone matrix collects between blood vessels: mesenchymal cells, now osteoblasts, arrange themselves along walls of osteoid trabeculae

Trabeculae

Osteoid matrix calcifies; osteoblasts continue laying down osteoid, trabeculae thicken by apposition, embedding osteocytes within woven (random) bone

Osteoblasts add to trabeculae by accretion, some are incorporated into bone matrix as osteocytes

Fresh osteoid

Osteoid in lacuna

Woven bone

**Figure 3.2.6**  The process of intramembranous bone formation (e.g. in flat bone growth)

cartilage at the epiphyseal plate. At the epiphyseal growth plate, cartilage cells known as **chondrocytes** are arrayed in columns extending from the epiphysis inwards towards the shaft.

Four zones are distinguished within the columns of chondrocytes. The outer zone is one of proliferation, where chondrocytes are actively dividing, and this is located furthest from the shaft. Beneath this lie zones of maturation and hypertrophy where chondrocytes are gradually enlarging, becoming vacuolated and degenerating. The innermost zone is one of calcification, where osteogenic cells encroach on the lacunae left by the chondrocytes, differentiate into osteoblasts and lay down endochondral bone, as described earlier. Thus, at one end of the epiphyseal plate, cartilage is produced, and at the other end it is degenerating, so growth in the length of bone is dependent on the proliferation of new cartilage cells. As this process continues, bone trabeculae in the diaphysis are eroded by osteoclasts to ensure that the marrow cavity lengthens as growth proceeds.

At the end of the growth period, under the influence of growth hormone and gonadal hormones, the epiphyseal plate is entirely replaced by bone, unifying the epiphysis and diaphysis, a process known as **synostosis**. In most individuals, the epiphyseal plates are fused and no further lengthwise growth is possible by the late teens/early twenties. Premature arrest of bone growth can occur if the epiphyseal plate is fractured. Although growth in length of most bones is completed by 20 years of age, the clavicle is the last bone to ossify completely in the third decade of life.

### Growth in diameter

Growth in diameter of the bone shaft is achieved by deposition of new membranous bone under the periosteum. This is rapidly ossified to keep pace with the growth in length attained by endochondral ossification.

One vestige of the original cartilaginous template of the long bone persists throughout adult life: this is the articular cartilage covering the surface of the epiphysis, which remains as an integral structure in the synovial joint (Chapter 3.3).

### Remodelling of bone (Fig. 3.2.7)

The process of bone remodelling continues through-out life, long after growth has ceased. Remodelling comprises phases of bone formation in which new matrix is secreted and calcified, followed by resorp-tion of mineralized bone. Younger bone has a more rapid turnover, and there is an increase in skeletal mass until the age of 50 years, followed by a slow decline. With the exception of growing

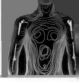

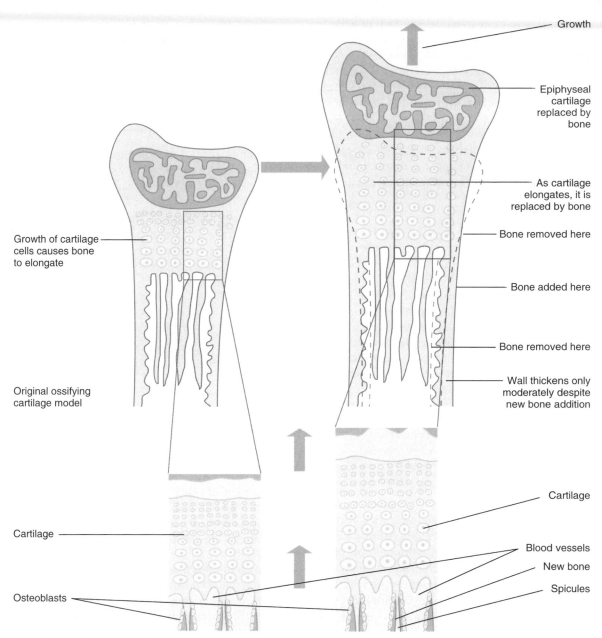

**Figure 3.2.7** The process of bone remodelling that takes place during bone growth

bones, rates of deposition and resorption are equal, so the total bone mass remains the same in young adults. At any one time, 3–5% of the adult skeletal mass is being actively remodelled by osteoblasts, which continually deposit bone on the outer surface and cavities, and osteoclasts which resorb bone. Remodelling of bone occurs in cycles of activity in which resorption precedes formation. The process is initiated by activation of a group of osteoclasts over a period of a few hours or days. This is followed by a period of resorption, extending from 1 to 3 weeks, in which osteoclasts erode tunnels 1 mm in diameter through the bone. Resorption is succeeded by bone formation for a period of 3 months: osteoblasts

deposit bone inside the tunnels around blood vessels. In this manner, new osteons are formed and the Haversian canal is all that remains of the original cavity created by the osteoclasts. In the new mineralized bone, the osteoblasts form osteocytes.

The value of remodelling is that it allows bone to adapt to external stressors, adjusting its formation to increase strength when necessary. In addition, the shape of bones can be rearranged to support mechanical forces more effectively. A number of internal factors also control bone remodelling, for example vitamin D, calcitonin and parathyroid hormone, all of which are concerned with calcium and phosphate homeostasis.

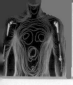

In summary, bone remodelling can provide a means of increasing or decreasing the concentration of minerals released into plasma to regulate mineral balances; it also allows the skeleton to adapt to mechanical loading and finally to repair microdamage caused by cyclic loading. Currently, the mechanisms underpinning what appears to be targeted and non-targeted remodelling in bone are not fully understood. It has been hypothesized that osteocyte apoptosis signals remodelling in response to microdamage that results in cracking across canalicular connections (Burr, 2002).

## Mechanical stress and pressure

### CLINICAL APPLICATIONS

Bone is deposited in proportion to the load it must carry; the converse also applies, for an immobilized bone rapidly decalcifies, a phenomenon known as **disuse osteoporosis**. Very rapid losses of calcium from weight-bearing bones have been observed in healthy individuals confined to bed for a period of 12 weeks (Zerwekh et al., 1998). Increased bone *resorption* underpinned this, reflected by an increase in urinary hydoxyproline excretion and hypercalciuria. These effects were reversed once normal activity was resumed.

Similar effects have been observed in astronauts, who are subjected to recumbency and weightlessness for prolonged periods. In the Gemini series of flights between 1965 and 1970, some individuals lost up to 20% of their bone mass. The problem was alleviated on later flights by instituting a planned exercise programme (Pace, 1977). A review of the research relating to the impact of extended duration space flight, for example on the Mir space station, has confirmed rates of bone calcium loss of around 250 mg per day. Changes in the endocrine regulation of bone metabolism during longer space flights are not fully understood. However, increased bone resorption might result in decreases in circulating parathyroid hormone and 1,25-dihydroxy vitamin D and, in turn, reduced calcium absorption from the gut (Smith & Lane, 1999).

Since the work of Bassett (1971), the possible role that biophysical events play in controlling bone remodelling has been acknowledged but remains enigmatic. It has been suggested that a stimulus for bone formation and destruction in remodelling could be mainly electrical. A deforming force might generate mechanical stress in bone, producing an electric signal. In turn, this could alert the bone mesenchymal cells to adjust the bone's mechanical properties to meet the need that has arisen by activating the formation of osteoblasts or osteoclasts (see also Fracture healing, p. 305). This contrasts with the suggestion that osteocyte signalling in response to microdamage is the stimulus for remodelling (Burr, 2002).

## Hormones and mineral homeostasis

The maintenance of blood calcium and phosphate concentrations is, to a significant degree, dependent on the resorption and mineralization of bone. These processes are regulated by vitamin D, parathyroid hormone and calcitonin. If the plasma calcium concentration falls, release of parathyroid hormone is evoked and this in turn stimulates the formation of $1,25(OH)_2$ vitamin D in the kidney. This acts to increase the resorption of bone, and the intestinal and renal reabsorption of calcium, raising the plasma calcium concentration. In contrast, if the plasma calcium concentration rises, calcitonin is released, which inhibits bone resorption, achieving a reduction in the plasma calcium concentration. Controversy has surrounded the extent to which bone contributes to mineral homeostasis but its contribution to short-term regulation cannot be denied. It also provides a reservoir for the long-term buffering of plasma calcium over a period of months and years. The endocrine control of calcium homeostasis is described in Chapter 2.5.

A number of other hormones and vitamins also exert effects on calcium and phosphate homeostasis, as these are primarily directed towards skeletal homeostasis, they will be considered here:

- **Growth hormone** is essential for healthy bone growth, particularly in the epiphysis. A deficiency of the hormone causes dwarfism whereas an excess produces gigantism and, after fusion of the epiphyses, **acromegaly**. In acromegaly, the size of the skeleton is increased but this is accompanied by reduced bone density with osteoporotic changes.
- **Thyroxine** in excess produces marked skeletal changes. An increased bone turnover occurs, in which resorption predominates, resulting in increased plasma calcium and phosphate concentrations with hypercalciuria. In contrast, a deficiency of the hormone (hypothyroidism) in childhood (**cretinism**) causes growth retardation with a delay in the appearance of the epiphyseal centres; in adults, bone turnover is decreased.
- **Oestrogen and testosterone** deficiency contributes to osteoporosis. In females, oestrogen deficiency contributes to **postmenopausal osteoporosis**, probably by enhancing the sensitivity of bone cells to parathyroid hormone.

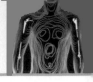

A progressive decrease in height with age has been attributed to changes in the vertebral column, together with postural effects caused by generalized osteoporosis. Height decreases by 1–3 cm/20 years postmaturity, although this is dependent on race and sex (Heymsfield et al., 1984). Together with growth hormone, the sex hormones bring about the increased growth of bone, which leads to fusion of the epiphyses in young adults.

- **Insulin** promotes the uptake of amino acids into bone and enhances their incorporation in components of the organic matrix.
- **Glucagon** can inhibit bone resorption and possibly bone formation in certain circumstances, but its role in bone metabolism is still unclear.
- **Cortisol**, in excess (as occurs in individuals with Cushing's syndrome and during steroid therapy) causes a decrease in bone formation accompanied by increased resorption. High doses suppress bone resorption and low doses stimulate it. The changes produced by corticosteroids on bone can lead to osteoporosis and pathological fracture.
- **Prostaglandins** are 20-carbon, short-chain fatty acids with potent systemic effects. The E series prostaglandins comprises stimulators of bone resorption in vitro and these might be involved in mediating the effects of neoplasms on bone structure.

A number of **vitamins** are required for the healthy growth of bone, notably vitamins A and C:

- **Vitamin A** is essential for the synthesis of matrix components, such as collagen and glycosaminoglycans, and also promotes the activity of osteoclasts and their production from progenitor cells. Deficiency of vitamin A causes remodelling failure associated with bony overgrowth, while an excess increases demineralization and vulnerability to fracture.
- **Vitamin C** is also essential for the synthesis of collagen. In deficiency states, bone formation is impaired and healing is delayed.

## DEVELOPMENTAL ISSUES

### THE EFFECTS OF AGEING

Age is the most important determinant of bone mass, which decreases with age in both sexes after a plateau at about 35–40 years. Maximal bone mass is attained at 25–30 years. Bone loss with age incorporates two phases: slow, involving losses of cortical and trabecular bone in both sexes, and the more rapid accelerated loss of trabecular bone that occurs after the menopause in females. The

underlying physiological changes that result in bone loss include decreased production of systemic or local growth factors that regulate osteoblast function (secretion of insulin and growth hormone is reduced by up to 45% with advanced age), and decreased sensitivity of intestinal calcium transport mechanisms to the active metabolite of vitamin D. Reduced production of the enzyme responsible for the formation of this metabolite of vitamin D in the kidney also occurs with ageing, which also exerts a negative effect on calcium absorption. For the effects of hormones and menopause, see p. 755.

Changes in the biomechanical properties of bone which occur with ageing have been investigated and age-related osteoporotic fractures have been attributed to a diminution in bone mineral or mass. Adverse changes in the collagen network have also been demonstrated, which could lead to a decreased toughness of bone (Wang et al., 2002). Low bone mineral density has been associated with an increased mortality risk. Many factors could influence this, notably oestrogen, body mass index, smoking or comorbidity (van der Klift et al., 2002). See also osteoporosis, p. 304.

## CLINICAL APPLICATIONS

### DISORDERS AFFECTING BONE STRUCTURE

#### Paget's disease: osteitis deformans

A recent survey in the UK established a prevalence in Paget's disease of about 2% over the age of 55 years (Cooper et al., 1999). This disorder is marked by increased bone turnover in focal areas of the skeleton, leading to changes in bone architecture. An uncontrolled, intense increase in the activity of both osteoblasts and osteoclasts is present and the cortical and cancellous bone is replaced by coarse trabeculae. This new bone is soft, inadequately mineralized and, as it invades the medullary cavity, the dimensions of the bones increase. Eventually the bone marrow is displaced by a highly vascular, fibrous tissue. Bones of the axial skeleton are most commonly affected (the skull, vertebral column, pelvis). The problems that result can be formidable, including severe disability due to deformity, bone pain related to arthritic changes, microfissuring and fractures and pressure generated by encroachment of nerves. Nerve compression can result in deafness and other neurological complications can set in because of bone distortion and overgrowth. Cardiac failure can occur, related to the increased blood flow through the affected bones.

The treatment of Paget's disease is aimed at reducing symptoms, preventing complications and

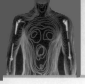

using drug therapy to suppress the excessive bone turnover. A recent review providing evidence-based guidelines, supports a range of symptomatic and specific treatments (Selby et al., 2002). Biphosphonate drugs (e.g. tiludronate, risedronate, pamidronate), which bind to the hydroxyapatite crystals in bone inhibiting osteoclast activity at sites of resorption, provide the primary treatment. Calcitonin, which inhibits bone resorption by a direct action on osteoclasts, is recommended for possible use in patients in whom biphosphonates are not tolerated or ineffective. It is not a first line treatment because of its side-effects and weaker activity.

### Osteitis fibrosa: hyperparathyroidism

The primary cause of hyperparathyroidism is an adenoma of the parathyroid, which secretes excessive amounts of parathyroid hormone (PTH). However, the disorder is also found in chronic renal failure accompanied by hypocalcaemia, which stimulates excessive parathyroid hormone secretion. The pathological features include an increase in the activity of the osteoclasts, leading to excessive bone resorption. As a compensatory response, an increase in the production of woven bone occurs in which mineralization is slowed. The resulting major problems for the affected individual include skeletal pain, tenderness and fractures. As calcium ions are lost from bone, the plasma calcium level rises, leading to weakness and lethargy, polyuria and thirst. Renal stones can form as a consequence of hypercalciuria, and an acute arthritis might be precipitated. The treatment comprises surgical removal of the adenoma, together with short-term replacement of calcium reserves by an increased dietary intake. Postoperative hypocalcaemia can be a problem where the bone disease has been extensive; this can be prevented by the administration of high-dose vitamin D.

### Osteomalacia

This disorder is the adult form of rickets, a disorder of bone in which defective mineralization of the organic matrix is present. Excess osteoid is the characteristic feature, leading to problems of bone pain, persistent tenderness, deformity, fracture and delayed healing. Muscle weakness may be triggered by a related myopathy, causing immobility and abnormal gait or posture. The disorder is caused by vitamin D deficiency, which might be due to a poor intake in the diet, defective synthesis due to lack of exposure to sunlight or to malabsorption syndromes. It might also be associated with chronic hepatic or renal failure, in which vitamin D cannot be metabolically activated. The treatment of osteomalacia is focused on providing oral vitamin D supplements (25–125 mg daily) and correcting the dietary intake if malnutrition is a contributing cause. In children, rickets can result from inadequate exposure to ultraviolet light or from dietary deficiency of vitamin D.

### Osteoporosis

Osteoporosis has been defined as 'a systemic skeletal disease characterised by low bone mineral density and microarchitectural deterioration of bone tissue, leading to bone fragility and increased risk for fracture' (Pachucki-Hyde, 2001). Osteoporotic bone is normal in composition but reduced in quantity due to an excess of bone resorption over formation. Risk factors for osteoporosis include genetic factors, which exert a negative impact on the achievement of peak bone mass (the amount of bone accumulated at the end of skeletal growth): as a consequence females, Caucasians and Asians have a greater risk than males and other races. In children, variables that adversely affect normal growth can attenuate peak bone mass and contribute to the development of osteoporosis (Lappe, 2001).

Other risk factors are those that influence bone loss, that is, ageing, nutrition, lifestyle and medical conditions. Insufficient oestrogen secretion during the menopause can result in osteoporosis, or it might occur as a result of the predominance of bone resorption over secretion, which is a feature of old age. In both sexes the latter might be related to hormonal deficiencies or to a poor dietary intake of calcium and phosphate. Calcium and vitamin D deficiency increase age-related bone loss due to secondary hyperparathyroidism (Sahota & Hosking, 2001).

Lifestyle factors that increase the risk are smoking, a sedentary lifestyle associated with a decreased bone mineral density and excessive alcohol consumption (Pachucki-Hyde, 2001). Medical conditions associated with osteoporosis include Cushing's disease, in which increased cortisol secretion accelerates renal calcium loss, reduces gut calcium absorption, increases bone resorption and reduces bone formation. Acromegaly, hyperthyroidism, malabsorption syndromes and neurological disorders such as stroke, where immobility results from paralysis, have also been associated with osteoporosis.

Any immobile patient is at risk of developing disuse osteoporosis. It is an alarming fact that the plasma calcium rises, as does urinary excretion, after only 1–2 days bedrest. Over a period of 4–6 weeks this can amount to losses of 10–14 g calcium, serious enough to complicate recovery following bone fracture. In addition, hypercalciuria can lead to the deposition of

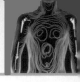

stones in the renal tract; a complication that can be prevented by increasing fluid intake sufficiently to raise the flow rate of urine. Thus, early ambulation and physiotherapy are essential if disuse osteoporosis is to be prevented in patients confined to bed. In limbs immobilized by a plaster cast, isometric exercises might be sufficient to prevent the problem.

Whatever the aetiology, the pathological features of osteoporosis include thinning of cortical bone by resorption, enlargement of the Haversian canals and loss of trabeculae from cancellous bone. The bone appears fragile and porous and can fracture spontaneously. The problems experienced by the affected individual include pain related to fractures and deformity, disability and shortening of limbs if fractures become compressed. Remedial measures include the maintenance of regular physical activity in the elderly, ensuring an adequate dietary intake of calcium, and the use of oestrogen replacement therapy in menopausal women who are affected. Hormone replacement therapy (HRT) has been shown to exert a protective effect against postmenopausal bone loss (Johnell et al., 2001). Physical exercise training programmes alone or in combination with HRT, can benefit bone mass and strength (Cheng et al., 2002). In established osteoporosis, biphosphonate drugs are the preferred treatment (McClung & McClung, 2001; Rizzoli et al., 2001).

## FRACTURES

Bone will fracture or break when its capacity to absorb energy is exceeded, most commonly following traumatic injury. Fractures are classified on the basis of location or complexity, as shown in **Fig. 3.2.8**.

### Fracture healing (Fig. 3.2.9)

A number of stages are distinguished in fracture healing: the inflammatory, reparative and remodelling stages. The **inflammatory stage** is the first stage after the fracture, when extensive disruption of the blood vessels, endosteum, periosteum and muscles might have occurred. Haemorrhage is followed by clot formation, during which the fibrin network enmeshes bone and muscle debris, erythrocytes, leucocytes and marrow cells. Within 12 hours, blood vessels dilate, allowing neutrophils to infiltrate the site. After 24 hours has elapsed, monocytes infiltrate, phagocytosing the tissue debris and fibrin, assisted by the neutrophils, which lyse fibrin and tissue fragments. The extensive invasion of blood capillaries at 72 hours concludes the inflammatory stage. Fibroblasts originating from the periosteal connective tissue, marrow and endosteum also infiltrate the site at this stage, proliferating to form chondroblasts or osteoblasts.

In the subsequent **reparative stage**, the chondroblasts synthesize collagen and proteoglycans, uniting the bone ends in a fibrous connective tissue known as **callus**. Within 14–17 days, the callus has calcified and, as hydroxyapatite, becomes deposited in the connective tissue matrix; ossification is gradually completed. Osteoblasts lay down trabeculae of cancellous bone at the fracture ends and osteoclasts destroy dead bone, keeping the marrow cavity patent.

**Remodelling** of bone by osteoblasts and osteoclasts concludes the healing, a process that takes several months to complete and involves replacement of cancellous by compact bone.

### Factors affecting fracture healing

A number of factors can impair the healing of a fracture. Some of the most important are loss of the blood supply, displacement of bone fragments, loss of the blood clot in open fractures and infection. Less commonly, the administration of corticosteroids, lack of vitamin D and protein–energy malnutrition can all hinder healing. The principles of fracture treatment are therefore to minimize all the factors listed above, to correct any displacement that has occurred and to facilitate healing in a position that will ensure the maximum retention of function.

Correction of displacement is achieved by performing either an open or closed surgical reduction, depending on the nature of the fracture, under local or general anaesthetic. In revision joint surgery, spinal fusion and following trauma, tissue-typed bone allografts can be used to support bone growth and healing (Kropp et al., 2003). Immobilization can be achieved in three ways: splinting in a plaster of Paris cast, applying traction via a metal pin inserted in the bone or using internal fixation with a pin and plate. Traction might initially be applied to correct displacement, disengage the bone ends and overcome excessive muscle spasm, which enhances displacement.

In fracture non-union characterized by the presence of soft tissues in the gap and by the failure of mineralization, vascularization and bone formation, healing can be promoted using pulsed electromagnetic fields. Beneficial cellular effects include the promotion of angiogenesis, increased mineralization, matrix synthesis and endochondral ossification (Bassett, 1993; Darendeliler et al., 1997, cited by van Nguyen & Marks, 2002). After a fracture has healed, electrical stimulation can be used to reduce muscle spasm. Therapeutic heat, which increases

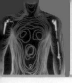

### (a) On the basis of severity

| Type of fracture | Features |
|---|---|
| Closed (simple) | Skin intact<br>No communication<br>with surface |
| Open (compound) | Skin broken<br>Communication from<br>bone to surface<br>Open wound |
| Complicated | Fractured bone penetrates<br>adjacent organs, blood<br>vessels, nerves, etc. |
| Complete | Fracture extends<br>completely through the bone |
| Incomplete<br>'Greenstick' | Fracture extends only<br>partially through bone;<br>occurs only in pliable<br>bones of child |
| Comminuted | Bone broken in two or<br>more places<br>Fragmented |
| Displaced | Bone fragments<br>separated |

### (b) Direction of fracture

| Type of fracture | Features |
|---|---|
| Transverse | Across the bone |
| Oblique | At an oblique angle to<br>the longitudinal axis<br>of the bone |
| Spiral | Fracture forms spiral<br>'twist' encircling bone;<br>produced by rotatory<br>force |
| Linear | Parallel to the longitudinal<br>axis of the bone |

### (c) According to deforming force

| Type of fracture | Features |
|---|---|
| Compression | Adjacent cancellous<br>bones compacted;<br>usually heals rapidly<br>due to minimal soft<br>tissue injury caused<br>by deforming force |
| Avulsion | Bone pulled apart;<br>ligaments remain intact |
| Stress | Undisplaced microfracture<br>caused by repetitive<br>stress, e.g. athletic<br>training may summate<br>to macrofracture |

### (d) According to anatomical location

| Type of fracture | Features |
|---|---|
| Osteochondrial | Involves articular<br>cartilage at a joint and<br>underlying bone |
| Extra- or<br>intracapsular | Without or with capsular<br>involvement at the joint |
| According to the<br>major bone and<br>area involved | i.e. Supracondylar fractures<br>of the humerus |

This classification is not comprehensive.
Pathological fractures occur in bone which
is weakened by disease, e.g. in Paget's
disease and in osteoporosis.
Some fractures are still characteristically
named, e.g. Colles' fracture of the
distal radius and Pott's fracture of the
distal fibula.

**Figure 3.2.8**　Classification of fractures

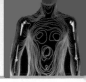

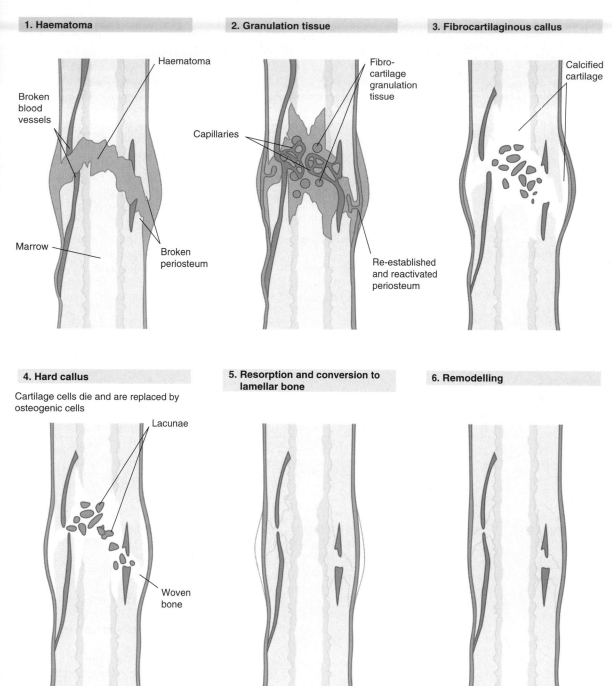

**1. Haematoma**

Haematoma

Broken blood vessels

Marrow

Broken periosteum

**2. Granulation tissue**

Fibro-cartilage granulation tissue

Capillaries

Re-established and reactivated periosteum

**3. Fibrocartilaginous callus**

Calcified cartilage

**4. Hard callus**

Cartilage cells die and are replaced by osteogenic cells

Lacunae

Woven bone

**5. Resorption and conversion to lamellar bone**

**6. Remodelling**

**Figure 3.2.9** The process of healing of a bone fracture

bloodflow, can be applied using hot packs or ultrasound during fracture rehabilitation, to reduce pain and muscle tension (Thomas, 2000).

The complications that can follow bone fractures, and the nursing care that can prevent them, are summarized in **Table 3.2.2**.

Ensuring an adequate nutritional intake of energy, protein, vitamins A, B, C and D, calcium and phosphate is essential to promote the healing of fractures. Following traumatic injury, a metabolic injury response occurs that significantly

increases requirements for energy, nitrogen and micronutrients (Frayn et al., 1984). Dietary provision must take account of this if it is to be effective. In a survey by Dickerson et al. (1986), the postoperative food intake of elderly female patients who had undergone surgery for fractured neck of the femur was measured. In many, the nutritional intake of protein, energy, calcium, thiamine, vitamins C, A, D and iron was found to be inadequate despite the adequate provision of food. A later study by

**Table 3.2.2** Complications following fractures: prevention and treatment

| Complication | Cause | Prevention/treatment |
| --- | --- | --- |
| Avascular necrosis of bone which delays union | Bone and soft tissue damage resulting in diminished accessibility of fracture site to blood vessels<br>May be caused by initial trauma or surgical intervention, e.g. pin and plates, insertion of metal medullary rods<br>Extensive necrosis may occur, e.g. head of femur following subcapital fracture of neck | Avoidance of weight bearing until healing adequate to provide support without risk<br>Prosthetic replacement of necrotic head of femur<br>Surgical arthrodesis (fixation of a joint) advised in certain cases |
| Joint stiffness and contractures | Prolonged immobility following fracture<br>Formation of scar tissues, fibrosis, ischaemic contracture of muscles<br>Local oedema following fracture (e.g. hand injury) | Maintain maximum activity during immobilization with appropriate active/passive physiotherapy exercises<br>Isometric exercises may be sufficient to prevent muscle wasting in an immobilized limb<br>Volkmann's ischaemic contracture may require surgical release<br>Elevate limb following injury, to decrease oedema |
| Fat embolism | Embolism caused by flocculation of fat chylomicrons in plasma<br>Triggered by release of kinins and thromboplastins from damaged tissue<br>May lead to cerebral, pulmonary, or renal infarction | Early recognition of signs vital: cyanosis, haemoptysis, hypoxaemia, tachycardia, pyrexia, convulsions, confusion, coma<br>Full supportive measures including IPPV in ITU<br>Low dose heparin therapy to clear lipaemia<br>Intravenous dextran to improve circulation to ischaemic tissue |
| Deep vein thrombosis | Venous stasis due to immobility<br>Clotting cascade triggered by release of kinins and thromboplastins released from damaged tissue | Early detection of signs vital: calf pain on dorsiflexion of the foot, pyrexia, local swelling and tenderness<br>Prophylactic or therapeutic heparin administration<br>Intravenous dextrans to prevent circulatory sludging<br>Deep breathing exercises and limb exercises to prevent venous stasis<br>Application of Tubigrip stockings<br>Early remobilization and resumption of physical activities |
| Local oedema | Following removal of splints from limbs<br>Cause uncertain<br>? Temporary disequilibration of Starling forces | Apply firm bandage<br>Elevate limb intermittently<br>Initiate exercises as advised by physiotherapist |
| Infection | Following common compound fracture or open reduction | Early recognition of signs – pyrexia, pain, swelling, discharge of pus through sinus – not always visible if splint in situ<br>Antibiotics following identification of organism<br>Strict asepsis during wound excision and dressing procedures |

*(Contd)*

| Table 3.2.2 (Contd) | | |
| --- | --- | --- |
| **Complication** | **Cause** | **Prevention/treatment** |
| | | High protein/energy diet with adequate vitamin C to promote healing |
| Pressure ulcers | Immobility: prolonged pressure on bony prominences<br>May arise under splints and plaster due to local friction<br>Prolonged pressure due to incorrect splinting can lead to nerve palsy | Alleviation of local pressure by 2-hourly or more frequent turning, use of ripple mattresses, sheepskins<br>Scrupulous attention to skin hygiene<br>Early remobilization<br>Careful padding of splints and plaster over bony prominences<br>Maintain nutritional status: ensure diet contains adequate protein, energy, vitamins to meet individual needs<br>Avoid heavy night sedation, which decreases spontaneous movements during sleep<br>Established ulcers: implement above, with other specific treatments, e.g. aseptic technique during application of sterile dressings, antibiotics if infection occurs, application of 'opsite' dressing, treatment with ultraviolet light |

IPPV, intermittent positive pressure ventilation; ICU, intensive care unit.

Jallut et al. (1990) demonstrated that elderly patients with a femoral neck fracture did not adequately adjust their spontaneous food intake to meet energy and protein needs. The results supported the view that these patients would benefit from oral supplementation above their spontaneous food intakes, providing an extra 200–300 kcal/day containing 20 g protein. Reasons why elderly patients who have sustained fractures cannot increase their food intakes postoperatively remain speculative, but probably include the high prevalence of post-traumatic confusion in these patients, linked to general frailty, weakness and anorexia. The benefits of supplemented tube feeding in this group have been demonstrated by Bastow et al. (1983) and included a positive impact on recovery, reducing the risk of morbid complications (wound and non-wound related) and mortality. More recent studies by Hartgrink et al. (1998) in older adults recovering from hip fracture have shown that overnight enteral tube feeding can increase energy and protein intakes, resulting in significant improvements in nutritional status in comparison with a control group who were not enterally fed. In a randomized, controlled clinical trial, Porter & Johnson (1998) evaluated the use of protein supplements (20 g/day, 5 days a week) for 6 months in older adults recovering from femoral fracture. Outcomes included improvements in biochemical indicators of nutritional status, minimization of bone loss and decreased length of stay in a rehabilitation setting.

Given these findings, it is vital that nurses supervise patients at meal times and alert the nutritional support team if, for any reason, food intake is impaired. Failure to provide nutritional support could lead to delayed healing, slower remobilization and an increased risk of complications.

## Clinical review

In addition to the Learning Objectives at the beginning of this chapter, the reader should be able to:

- List the major functions ascribed to bone
- Describe the three major components of bone

- Write short notes on each of the following: woven bone, compact bone, trabecular bone, Haversian systems
- Draw a diagrammatic section through a named long bone, labelling the major anatomical features including the vascular supply
- Discuss the origin and functions of osteoblasts, osteoclasts and osteocytes
- Briefly explain how bone tissue fluid differs in composition from extracellular fluid
- Compare and contrast the processes of endochondral and intramembranous ossification
- Explain how growth in length and diameter of bone is achieved

## Review questions

1  What is the major constituent of the organic matrix of bone?
2  What passes through the central canal of the Haversian system?
3  What is the metaphysis?
4  What are the different bone cells called?
5  What is the effect of parathyroid hormone and thyroxine on bone?
6  How do long bones receive their blood supply?
7  What is ossification?
8  How is endochondral ossification distinguished from intramembranous ossification?
9  What effect does vitamin D have on bone?
10  What is the essential difference between osteomalacia and rickets?
11  Which factors can lead to osteoporosis?

## Suggestions for further reading

Bassey, J. & Dinan, S. (2001) *Exercise for Strong Bones*. London: National Osteoporosis Society.
*A step-by-step programme to prevent osteoporosis, aimed at the general public. This text would be helpful to nurses working in primary prevention.*

Burkhardt, P., Dawson-Hughes, B. & Heaney, R.P. (2001) *Nutritional Aspects of Osteoporosis*. San Diego: Academic Press.
*A comprehensive look across the lifespan at nutritional factors influencing the development of osteoporosis and a review of dietary aspects of management.*

Canalis, E. (2000) *Skeletal Growth Factors*. Philadelphia: Lippincott, Williams and Wilkins.
*Excellent review of a highly specialized area.*

Cowin, S.C. (2001) *Bone Mechanics Handbook*. London: CRC Press.
*Good reference text for enthusiasts.*

Dreschner, J., Hofman, C.R., Piesco, N.P. & Agarwal, S. (2003) Signal transduction and mechanical strain in chondrocytes. *Current Opinion in Clinical Nutrition and Metabolic Care*, 6; 289–293.

Hertel, K.L. & Trahiotis, M.G. (2001) Exercise in the prevention and treatment of osteoporosis. *Nursing Clinics of North America*, 36(3); 441–452.

Hoppenfield, S. & Murthy, V.L. (2000) *The Treatment and Rehabilitation of Fractures*. Philadelphia: Lippincott, Williams and Wilkins.
*Comprehensive discourse on the medical, physiotherapy and occupational therapy aspects of management. A great deal of information relevant to nursing.*

Kessenich, C.R. (2001) Diagnostic imaging and biochemical markers of bone turnover. *Nursing Clinics of North America*, 36(3); 409–415.

Papapoulos, S.E. (2001) Catabolic and anabolic signals in bone: Therapeutic implications. *Current Opinion in Clinical Nutrition and Metabolic Care*, 4; 191–196.

Woolf, A.D. (2002) *Bone and Joint Futures*. London: BMJ Books.
*A highly focused, prognostic review of the burden, diagnosis and future management of bone and joint disease.*

# References

Bassett, C.A. (1971) Biophysical principles affecting bone structure. In: Bourne, G.H. (ed) *The Biochemistry and Physiology of Bone*, 2nd edn. London: Academic Press, pp. 1–76.

Bassett, C.A. (1993) Beneficial effects of electromagnetic fields. *Journal of Cellular Biochemistry*, **51**; 387–389.

Bastow, M., Rawlings, J. & Allison, S.P. (1983) Benefits of supplementary tube feeding after a fractured neck of femur. *British Medical Journal*, **287**; 1589–1592.

Brookes, M. (1971) *The Blood Supply of Bone: An Approach to Bone Biology*. London: Butterworths.

Burr, D.B. (2002) Targeted and nontargeted remodeling. *Bone*, **30**; 2–4.

Cheng, S., Sipilä, S., Taaffe, D.R. et al. (2002) Change in bone mass distribution induced by hormone replacement therapy and high-impact physical exercise in post-menopausal women. *Bone*, **31**; 126–135.

Cooper, C., Schafheutle, K., Dennison, E. et al. (1999) The epidemiology of Paget's disease in Britain: Is the prevalence decreasing? *Journal of Bone Mineral Research*, **14**; 192–197.

Darendeliler, M.A., Darendeliler, A. & Sinclair, P.M. (1997) Effects of static magnetic fields and pulsed electromagnetic fields on bone healing. *International Journal of Orthodontics, Orthnographics and Surgery*, **12**; 43–53.

Dickerson, J., Fekkes, J., Goodinson, S.M. & Older, M. (1986) Post-operative food intake of elderly fracture patients. *Proceedings of the Nutrition Society*, **45**; 7a.

Frayn, K.N., Little, R.A. & Stoner, H.B. (1984) Metabolic control in non-septic patients with musculoskeletal injuries. *Injury*, **16**; 73–79.

Hartgrink, H.H., Wille, J., Konig, P. et al. (1998) Pressure sores and tube feeding in patients with a fracture of the hip: a randomised clinical trial. *Clinical Nutrition*, **17**(6); 287–292.

Heymsfield, S., McManus, C., Seitz, S. et al. (1984) Anthropometric assessment of adult protein-energy malnutrition. In: Wright, R. & Heymsfield, S. (eds) *Nutritional Assessment*. Oxford: Blackwell Scientific Publications, pp. 27–77.

Hughes, F.J., Buttery, L.D.K., Hukkanen, M.V.J. & Polak, J. (1998) Nitric oxide and osteoblast function. In: Hukkanen, M.V.J., Polak, J.M. & Hughes, S.P.F. (eds) *Nitric Oxide in Bone and Joint Disease*. Cambridge: Cambridge University Press, pp. 105–120.

Jallut, D., Tappy, L. & Kohut, M. (1990) Energy balance in elderly patients after surgery for a femoral neck fracture. *Journal of Parenteral and Enteral Nutrition*, **14**(6); 563–567.

Johnell, O., Kanis, J.A., Oden, A. et al. (2001) Targeting of hormone replacement therapy immediately after menopause. *Bone*, **28**: 440–445.

Kropp, L., Mann, S., Drain, J. et al. (2003) Setting up a satellite bone harvesting service to supply cancellous bone graft. *Journal of Orthopaedic Nursing*, **7**; 70–72.

Lappe, J.M. (2001) Pathophysiology of osteoporosis and fracture. *Nursing Clinics of North America*, **36**(3); 393–400.

McCarthy, I. (1998) Modulation of bone blood flow by nitric oxide. In: Hukkanen, M.V.J., Polak, J. & Hughes, S.P.F. (eds) *Nitric Oxide in Bone and Joint Disease*. Cambridge: Cambridge University Press, pp. 129–140.

McClung, B. & McClung, M. (2001) Pharmacologic therapy for the treatment and prevention of osteoporosis. *Nursing Clinics of North America*, **36**(3); 433–440.

Pace, N. (1977) Weightlessness: A matter of gravity. *New England Journal of Medicine*, **297**; 32–37.

Pachucki-Hyde, L. (2001) Assessment of risk factors for osteoporosis and fracture. *Nursing Clinics of North America*, **36**(3); 401–408.

Passmore, R. & Robson, J.S. (1976) *Companion to Medical Studies*, 2nd edn. London: Blackwell Scientific.

Porter, K.H. & Johnson, M.A. (1998) Dietary protein supplementation and recovery from femoral fracture. *Nutrition Reviews*, **56**(11); 337–340.

Qui, S., Rao, D.S., Palnitkar, S. & Parfitt, A.M. (2002) Age and distance from the surface but not menopause reduce osteocyte density in human cancellous bone. *Bone*, **31**; 313–318.

Rizzoli, R., Schaad, M.A. & Uebelhart, B. (2001) Osteoporosis in men. *Nursing Clinics of North America*, **36**(3); 467–478.

Sahota, O. & Hosking, D.J. (2001) The contribution of nutritional factors to osteopenia in the elderly. *Current Opinion in Clinical Nutrition and Metabolic Care*, **4**; 15–20.

Selby, P.L., Davie, M.W.J., Ralston, S.H. & Stone, M.D. On behalf of the Bone and Tooth Society of Great Britain and the National Association for the Relief of Paget's Disease (2002) Guidelines on the management of Paget's disease of bone. *Bone*, **31**; 366–373.

Smith, S.M. & Lane, H.W. (1999) Gravity and space flight: effects on nutritional status. *Current Opinion in Clinical Nutrition and Metabolic Care*, **2**; 335–338.

Thomas, M.A. (2000) Modalities used in the treatment of fractures. In: Hoppenfield, S. & Murthy, V.L. (eds) *Treatment and Rehabilitation of Fractures*. Philadelphia: Lippincott, Williams and Wilkins, pp. 28–30.

van der Klift, M., Pols, H.A.P., Geleijnse, J.M. et al. (2002) Bone mineral density and mortality in elderly men and women: The Rotterdam Study. *Bone*, **30**; 643–648.

van Nguyen, J. & Marks, R. (2002) Pulsed electromagnetic fields for treating osteoarthritis. *Physiotherapy*, **88**; 458–470.

Wang, X., Shen, X., Li, X. & Mauli Agrawal, C. (2002) Age-related changes in the collagen network and toughness of bone. *Bone*, **31**; 1–7.

Zerwekh, J.E., Rumi, L.A., Gottschalk, F. & Pak, C.Y.C. (1998) The effects of twelve weeks bed rest on bone histology, biochemical markers of bone turnover, and calcium homeostasis in eleven normal subjects. *Journal of Bone Mineralisation Research*, **13**; 1594–1601.

# Chapter 3.3

# Joints

*Susan M. McLaren*

## LEARNING OBJECTIVES

After studying this chapter the reader should be able to:

- Describe the general functions of joints in the musculoskeletal system

- Explain how movement in humans is brought about by the concerted actions of muscles, bones and joints within lever systems

- Describe how lever systems can be manipulated to gain a mechanical advantage

- Classify joints according to the structure and degree of movement they permit

- List the characteristic features of fibrous, cartilaginous and synovial joints

- Describe the structure, function and anatomical sites of synovial, cartilaginous and fibrous joints

- Discuss the pathophysiological features of joint dysfunction together with the rationale for therapeutic interventions

## INTRODUCTION

Joints, or articulations, are the specialized structures found where two or more bones meet. They have the following functions:

- To facilitate movement of different parts of the body relative to each other. Immovable fibrous joints provide the exception to this.
- To confer stability on movement.
- To assist in the maintenance of body posture.

Preceding chapters have considered aspects of mobility and support in relation to the physiology of muscle and bone. Movement in humans is brought about by lever systems in which the integral components are provided by bones, muscles and joints acting in concert. A fuller discussion of movement is now given and this chapter begins with a necessary, though simple, presentation of lever principles. Understanding the properties of lever systems is both useful and relevant because, as will be shown, they can be manipulated to advantage in clinical nursing practice. However, the physiology of movement, which includes lever mechanics, is a complex subject, and for the enthusiast suggestions for further reading can be found in the bibliography.

The embryological development of joints is discussed in conjunction with that of other skeletal structures on p. 298.

## Lever systems

A lever is best visualized as a rigid bar that rotates about a pivot, or fulcrum (plural: fulcra) when a force is applied to the lever (i.e. the bar). The distance between the fulcrum and the point of application of effort, or applied force, is known as the effort arm. The resistance arm is the distance between the fulcrum and point of application of the load, or resisting force. This resisting force tends to rotate the lever in a direction opposite to that produced by the effort.

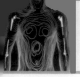

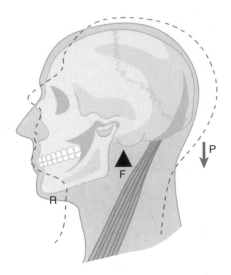

The shorter the effort arm, the greater is the applied force required to balance or lift the load

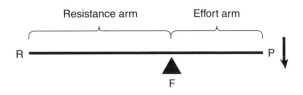

First-class lever

**Figure 3.3.1**  An example of a first-class lever

In the body, the components of a lever system are provided by bones, which act as levers, and joints, which act as fulcra. The position of muscle insertion on bone is the application point of effort and the weight of the bone itself, plus the weight of that part of the body to be moved, forms the load.

## Classification of lever systems

Lever systems are classified according to three arrangements along the lever of its components: the fulcrum, and the application points of effort and load.

### The first-class lever (**Fig. 3.3.1**)

The fulcrum occupies an intermediary position between the points of application of effort and load. An example of a first-class lever system is raising the head; the atlanto-occipital joint is the fulcrum and the weight of the head is the resistance.

### The second-class lever (**Fig. 3.3.2**)

In this system, the point of load application is located between the fulcrum and the point of effort application. Rising on tiptoe utilizes a second-class

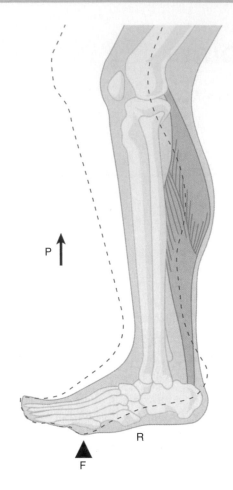

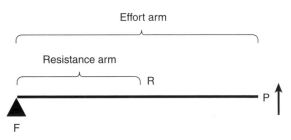

The shorter the resistance arm, the smaller is the applied force required to balance or lift the load.

Second-class lever

**Figure 3.3.2**  An example of a second-class lever

lever, with the joint at the ball of the foot providing a fulcrum. Effort is applied at the insertion point of the flexor muscles of the lower leg and body weight is the load.

### The third-class lever (**Fig. 3.3.3**)

The point of effort application is situated between the fulcrum and the load. Third-class levers are the most commonly found in the body. Unfortunately, this type of lever requires the application of a large effort to produce movement of comparatively small

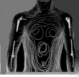

The shorter the resistance arm, the smaller is the applied force required to balance or shift the load

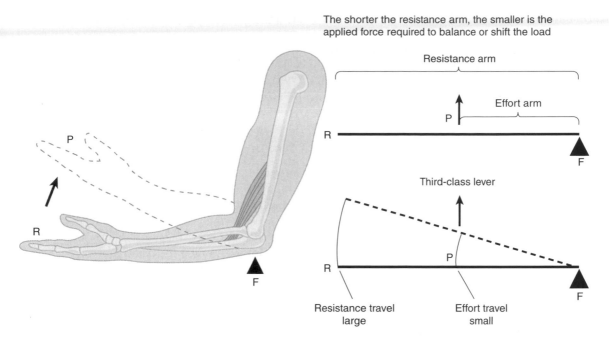

**Figure 3.3.3**  An example of a third-class lever

loads. A classic example is when the biceps muscle flexes the forearm. In this instance, the elbow joint forms the fulcrum, the biceps muscle insertion is the point of effort application and the weight of the arm is the load.

## Manipulation of lever systems

Traumatic injuries to bones, muscles, ligaments and joints can occur when lever systems are overloaded. To explain how this can come about, let us consider to begin with a lever of the first class (**see Fig. 3.3.1**).

A 5 kg weight 20 cm from the fulcrum is just balanced by a 10 kg weight 10 cm from the fulcrum. The mathematical principle involved here is:

> effort × effort arm (length)
> = resistance × resistance arm (length)

The effort needed to keep the lever in balance can be lessened by lengthening the effort arm. If the effort arm was 40 cm in length, the effort required would be only 2.5 kg. If the effort arm was shorter, say 5 cm, 20 kg effort would be required to keep the lever in balance. However, if the effort arm was *very* short, then the effort required to keep the lever in balance might be so great as to bend or break the lever.

Most body lever systems are of the third class, where the effort arm and fulcrum are anatomically fixed, and the effort arm is indeed very small. To gain maximum advantage in these systems, the length of the resistance arm can be altered because effort arm length cannot be altered. Transposing the measurements from **Fig. 3.3.1** to a third-class lever (**Fig. 3.3.3**),

we find that if the resistance arm is shortened to 10 cm, then only 5 kg effort is required to keep the lever in balance; whereas if the resistance arm is longer, say 40 cm, a 20 kg effort will be required.

### CLINICAL APPLICATIONS

The application of such principles is clearly of great importance to nurses when lifting or turning patients, or assisting patients with lifting exercises. By carrying loads as close to the body as possible, the resistance arm is decreased and thus less force needs to be exerted by muscles and less strain is exerted on the body lever systems. For example, lifting a straight limb requires the development of considerably more force by muscle than when the limb is bent at the knee joint. Any action with a short resistance arm is less tiring and is also more economical in terms of energy expenditure.

However, there are situations when moving straight limbs and developing greater forces in muscle are used to advantage. Following meniscectomy (removal of meniscus cartilages in the knee joint), straight-leg raising exercises both strengthen and increase muscle mass, giving the joint greater stability, an essential postoperative requirement.

### Classification of joints

Joints are classified, according to structure and the type of movement they permit, as **fibrous,** cartilaginous or synovial. A number of subclasses are distinguished within each of these categories and a few exceptions are found in which features of more than one class merge.

## Fibrous joints – synarthroses

Two features are characteristic of this class:

1. Either no movement is permitted, or movement is severely limited.
2. Fibrous connective tissue is present between the articulating surfaces, merging into the periosteum on either side.

Bones of the skull are united by short, compact fibrous strands, the sutural ligament, to form an immovable fibrous joint (**Fig. 3.3.4**). This articulation is reduced in adult life as ossification progresses. An equally simple fibrous joint is formed between the tooth and its socket. Although serving to anchor the tooth firmly in the jaw, this type of joint does allow slight movements to take place when food is chewed. Another fibrous joint is formed where the distal end of the fibula articulates with the tibia. At this joint, some slight movement is possible because the fibrous strands uniting the bones are long, forming what is known as the interosseus ligament.

## Cartilaginous joints – amphiarthroses

A limited amount of movement is permitted by the flexible fibrocartilage present between opposing bone ends. Two subclasses are distinguished, the symphyses and the synchondroses; the latter usually ossify in adult life and are thus immovable.

### Symphyses

At symphyses, the fibrocartilage takes the form of a pad or disc inserted between the hyaline plates of the articulating surfaces. Typical examples are found at the pelvic symphysis pubis (**Fig. 3.3.5**) and in the intervertebral joints of the spinal column. Compression of the intervertebral disc permits movements limited to small degrees of flexion, side flexion and extension.

Extensive and complex arrangements of ligaments and muscles act as important stabilizing structures on the joint and, together with the thickness of the disc, they act to limit movement. Resistance to movement is provided by the elastic structure of the disc, which allows bones to recoil to their original position once a compressing force is removed. The elasticity of the intervertebral disc also enables it to act very much like a shock absorber, uniformly redistributing pressures that are generated during movement and lifting heavy loads. It is formidable to think that intervertebral joints can be subjected to stresses equivalent to several hundred kilogrammes weight when the spine is flexed and loads are lifted. Rupture of the disc has occurred when loads of 500–600 kg have been applied, the fracture usually occurring at the weakest spot, the hyaline endplates.

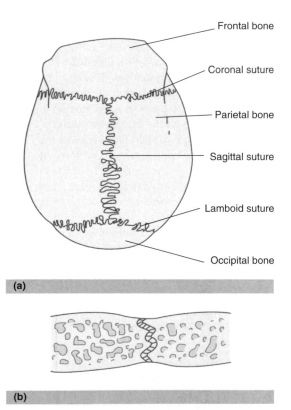

Frontal bone

Coronal suture

Parietal bone

Sagittal suture

Lamboid suture

Occipital bone

**(a)**

**(b)**

**Figure 3.3.4** Fibrous joint (skull) (a) superior aspect of skull; (b) transverse section of fibrous joint

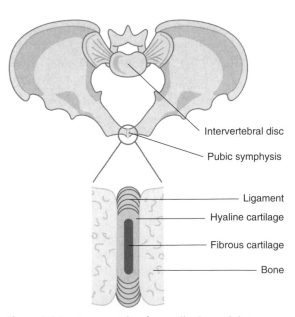

Intervertebral disc

Pubic symphysis

Ligament

Hyaline cartilage

Fibrous cartilage

Bone

**Figure 3.3.5** An example of a cartilaginous joint (the pelvis) showing a transverse section of the pubic symphysis

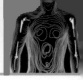

## CLINICAL APPLICATIONS

Intervertebral discs can slip out of place (**prolapse**) as a result of degenerative changes or flexion injuries, which are caused by heavy lifting. Degenerative changes are seen in the structure of the intervertebral disc, usually after the third decade of life, and are probably caused by mechanical stress. Once degeneration has occurred, the disc can no longer function as an effective shock absorber and this increases the load borne by the joints of the vertebral arch, leading to back pain. Degenerative changes might alone be sufficient to lead to prolapse of the disc or this might be triggered by minor trauma caused by, for example, coughing or sneezing, associated with degeneration. A prolapsed disc (**Fig. 3.3.6**) can compress the spinal nerve or its roots and stretch or tear adjacent tissues. In some cases, the prolapse could be severe enough to compress the spinal cord. Such prolapses can occur in any region of the vertebral column but the lumbar vertebrae are most commonly affected.

Major problems for the patient are pain and limited movement. Back pain can radiate to the arm or leg, depending on the site of prolapse, and is aggravated by straight-leg raising, bending or lifting. Numbness and tingling might be present in affected limbs and movement is limited by local muscle spasm around the affected vertebrae. If the spinal cord is compressed, the effects on motor nerve tracts can lead to weakness, uncoordinated movements and abnormal gait. Bladder function might also be impaired.

Treatment includes bedrest on a firm mattress and the provision of anti-inflammatory analgesics, to allow the pain and inflammation to subside. A cervical collar can be worn to support and

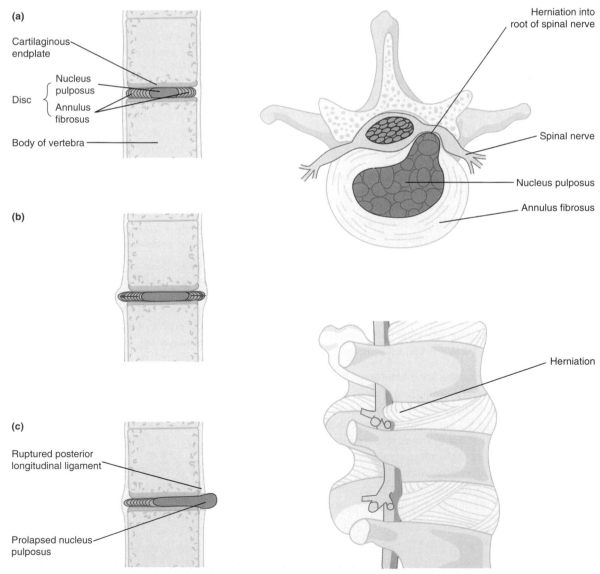

**Figure 3.3.6**   Compression of a vertebral disc leading to herniation – a 'slipped disc'

immobilize the neck following a cervical disc prolapse. In some circumstances, cervical or pelvic traction is applied to increase the distance between adjacent vertebrae, allowing the prolapse to subside and to relieve painful muscle spasms. Surgical excision of the disc might be necessary if these measures fail or if control of bladder function is impaired.

### Synchondroses

Synchondroses are cartilaginous joints that ossify in adult life and thus permit little, if any, movement. Typical synchondroses are found where the epiphysial plate of cartilage is present between the epiphysis and diaphysis of long bones, and where the upper ribs articulate with the sternum at the sternocostal joints.

## Synovial joints – diarthroses

Most of the body joints are synovial, that is to say, they are freely movable in a number of planes. They are classified by anatomical structure and the range and axes of movement they allow.

A classification of synovial joints, together with the range of movement they permit, is presented in **Table 3.3.1**. Definitions of the types of movement permitted are listed and illustrated in **Table 3.3.2**.

---

### CLINICAL APPLICATIONS

The range and types of movement characteristic of a synovial joint can be modified by diseases and, when making a nursing assessment of the patient with limited mobility, the nurse should bear the following points in mind:

- Range of movement at a joint decreases with age. The presence of stiffness or even increased mobility might not be a feature of an underlying disease.
- If impaired movement is present at any joint, the effects on coordinated movements, posture and balance as a whole must be established.

---

A number of structural features are common to all synovial joints, irrespective of classification (**Fig. 3.3.7**). A capsule of fibrous connective tissue surrounds the articulating bones like a sleeve. Lining the capsule is a highly specialized synovial membrane, which secretes a lubricant fluid into the cavity of the joint. Hyaline cartilage covers the opposing bone ends, which are not in direct contact. All of these structural components possess properties that allow movement in a number of planes.

### The joint capsule

A capsule of fibrous connective tissue containing a high percentage of collagen fibres and abundantly supplied with blood capillaries encases the joint. The capsule is attached on either side to the periosteum of the articulating bones. Joint stability is increased if intra- or extracapsular ligaments are present (**Fig. 3.3.8**) and by the mass and tension in surrounding muscles.

Innervation of the capsule is complex: the main supply branches from the nerve supply to those adjacent muscles that produce movement at that joint. Additionally, a number of afferent sensory nerves are found within the capsule and its surrounding ligaments. Myelinated afferent nerves terminate in a number of sensory receptors, known collectively as proprioceptors, and convey information on joint movement to the somatosensory cortex and cerebellum. Together with visual, auditory and vestibular nerve inputs, this information subserves our sense of position and facilitates balanced and coordinated movements.

### The synovial membrane

Beneath the fibrous capsule lies the synovial membrane: a thin, highly vascular membrane that covers all surfaces inside the joint with the exception of the articular cartilages. Its surface is highly folded in some areas to form microscopic projections known as **villi**.

The membrane has two regions: an outer cellular layer 'approximately three cells thick' next to the joint cavity rests on an inner fine meshwork of connective tissue. Within the cellular layer are phagocytic type B cells, which are responsible for the production of synovial fluid components such as hyaluronic acid.

In addition to its rich capillary network, the synovial membrane is abundantly supplied with lymphatic vessels and some sensory nerve fibres.

### Synovial fluid

In composition, synovial fluid resembles a filtrate of plasma and, as such, is similar to the fluid found in the pleural and peritoneal cavities, where body surfaces are also in close apposition. The protein content is low ($<20\,g/L$; plasma $60–80\,g/L$) and most of it is combined with hyaluronic acid. In health, the volume of synovial fluid is small, approximately $0.2–0.4$ mL in the knee joint. It is a highly viscous fluid but, when subjected to the shearing forces produced by movement, its viscosity is lowered. It is, therefore, an ideal joint lubricant. **The very thin film of fluid, dispersed between the articulating cartilages when they move relative to one another, effectively reduces friction.**

It is the presence of the complex of hyaluronic acid and protein that gives synovial fluid its characteristically high viscosity and lubricant properties. Some of this complex appears to be adsorbed directly onto the cartilage, providing added lubrication and protection

## Table 3.3.1 Classification and range of movement in synovial joints

| Synovial joint | Site | Articulating surfaces | Range of movements |
|---|---|---|---|
| 1 Hinge joint | (a) Elbow | Distal humerus with proximal ulna (humeroulnar joint) | Movement is restricted about a single tranverse axis |
| | (b) Tooo Fingers | Between phalanges (interphalangeal joint) | Flexion, extension |
| | (c) Ankle | Distal tibia and fibula with talus (talocrural joint) | Flexion (dorsiflexion) Extension (plantar flexion) |
| | (d) Knee | Femur and tibia | Flexion, extension, slight rotation when leg flexed |
| 2 Pivot joint | (a) Elbow | Radius with ulna (proximal radioulnar joint) The head of the radius forms a pivot which rotates within a ring formed by an ulnar notch | Rotation (pronation, supination) |
| | (b) Vertebral column | First cervical vertebra (atlas) with second cervical vertebra (axis). Here, the atlas (ring) rotates about the odontoid process of the axis (pivot) | Rotation |
| 3 Gliding joint | | Apposed flat bone surfaces glide together. Movement is limited by extensive ligature | |
| | (a) Shoulder girdle | 1 Clavicle with sternum and cartilage of 1st rib (sternoclavicular joint) | Gliding, limited motion in several directions |
| | | 2 Clavicle with scapula (acromioclavicular joint). | Gliding, rotation of scapula on clavicle |
| | (b) Hand | Some articulations between carpals | In concert with radiocarpal joints, describe varying degrees of flexion, extension, adduction, abduction, circumduction |
| | Foot | Articulations between bases of metatarsals (tarsometatarsal joint) | Limited to slight gliding movements |
| | (c) Vertebral column | Facets of articular processes of adjacent vertebrae | Range of movements between adjacent vertebrae is small but extensive in vertebral column as a whole |
| | | Cervical vertebrae 2–7 Thoracic vertebrae | Flexion and extension, side flexion and rotation are limited cervically |
| | | Lumbar vertebrae | Flexion, extension, side flexion, no rotation |
| 4 Ball and socket joint | | One articulating surface is shaped to form a spherical head, which rotates in a cuplike depression in the reciprocal surface | Very extensive range of movements |
| | (a) Hip | Head of the femur with the acetabulum of the pelvis | Flexion, extension, abduction, adduction, internal and external rotation, circumduction |
| | (b) Shoulder | Head of the humerus with the glenoid cavity of the scapula | |
| 5 Saddle (sellar) joint | | Articulating surfaces both saddle shaped, the convex surface of one bone is inserted into the concave surface of the other | Movements permitted in two directions at 90° to each other |
| | Hand Base of thumb | First metacarpal with carpal (trapezium bone) | Flexion, extension, abduction, adduction, opposition |
| 6 Ellipsoid joint | | Both surfaces ellipsoidal, one with a longer radius of curvature | Movements permitted in two directions at 90° to each other |
| | Wrist | Distal radius with 3 carpals; the scaphoid lunate and triquetral bones (radiocarpal joint) | Flexion, extension, radial flexion, moving hand towards thumb Ulnar flexion moving hand towards little finger True rotation is impossible but circling movements may be produced by a combination of wrist and forearm movements |
| | Hand | Metacarpals with phalanges | Flexion, extension, adduction, abduction |
| | Foot | Metatarsals with phalanges | |

**(1) Hinge joint**

**(2) Pivot joint**

**(3) Gliding joint**

**(4) Ball and socket joint**

**(5) Saddle (sellar) joint**

**(6) Ellipsoid joint**

## Table 3.3.2  Types of movement of synovial joints

**Circumduction:**
A combination of movements that makes a body part describe a circle.

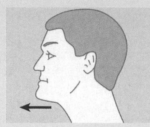

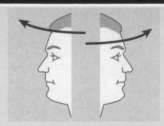

**Rotation:**
The pivoting of a body part around its axis, as in shaking the head. No rotation of any body is complete (i.e. 360 degrees).

**Protraction:**
The protrusion of some body part, e.g. the lower jaw.

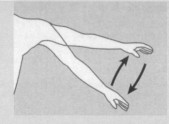

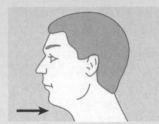

**Retraction:**
The opposite of protraction.

**Abduction:**
A movement of a bone or limb away from the median plane of the body. Abduction in the hands and feet is the movement of a digit away from the central axis of the limb. One abducts the fingers by spreading them apart.

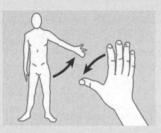

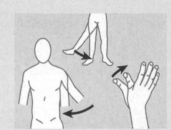

**Adduction:**
The opposite of abduction, involving approach to the median plane of the body or, in the case of the limbs, to the central axis of a limb.

**Inversion:**
An ankle movement that turns the sole of the foot medially. Applies only to the foot.

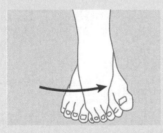

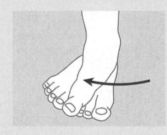

**Eversion:**
The opposite of inversion. It turns the sole of the foot laterally.

**Supination:**
The opposite of pronation. When the forearm is in the extended position, this movement brings the palm of the hand upward.

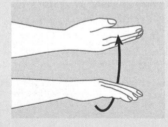

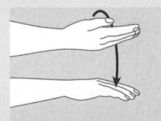

**Pronation:**
A movement of the forearm that in the extended position brings the palm of the hand to a downward position. Applies only to the forearm.

**Extension:**
The opposite of flexion, it increases the angle between two movably articulated bones, usually to a 180-degree maximum. If the angle of extension exceeds 180 degrees (as is possible when throwing back the head), this action is termed hyperextension.

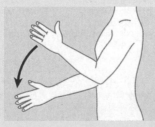

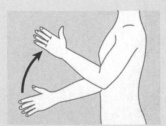

**Flexion:**
The bending of a joint; usually a movement that reduces the angle that two movably activated bones make with each other. When one crouches, the knees are flexed.

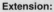

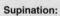

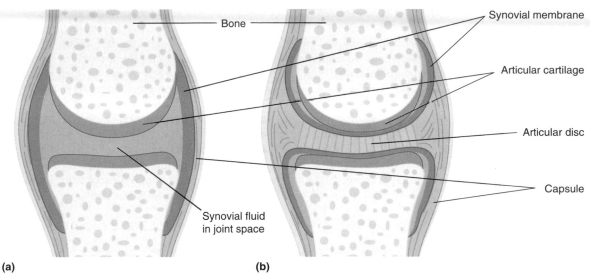

Figure 3.3.7 Diagrammatic representation of a synovial joint with section through (a) a simple synovial joint and (b) a synovial joint that contains articular cartilage

Bone

Synovial membrane

Articular cartilage

Articular disc

Capsule

Synovial fluid in joint space

(a)

(b)

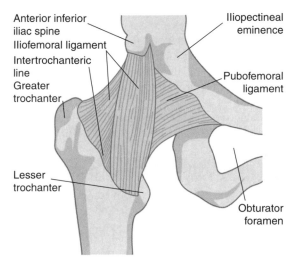

Anterior inferior iliac spine
Iliofemoral ligament
Intertrochanteric line
Greater trochanter

Iliopectineal eminence

Pubofemoral ligament

Lesser trochanter

Obturator foramen

Figure 3.3.8 Posterior aspect of a synovial joint (the hip) showing arrangement of extracapsular ligaments

from erosion. However, the exact mode of action of the synovial fluid as a lubricant is as yet incompletely understood.

A number of cellular components are also present in synovial fluid, mainly leucocytes and synovial cells. In health, their number is very small and most cells are phagocytic, functioning mainly in the removal of debris.

In addition to its function as a lubricant, synovial fluid also fulfils a nutritive role in permitting the free diffusion of nutrients to articular cartilage and other intracapsular structures.

## Articular cartilage

Opposing bone ends are covered by closely moulded hyaline cartilage, which can reach a depth of 2–3 mm

in the hip joint. In composition, the cartilage consists of cells known as chondrocytes embedded in a matrix that they both maintain and secrete. Collagen fibres are present in the matrix together with proteoglycans (protein–polysaccharide complexes), mainly chondroitin and keratin sulphate. Water forms a considerable proportion of the matrix – at least 70% of the wet weight – and is osmotically held in place by the proteoglycans. Deeper zones of the cartilage might be calcified in the adult.

It has been estimated that the articular cartilage on the head of the femur can be subjected to loads of two and a half to five times body weight during walking. How then does cartilage withstand these continual stresses without mechanical failure? Present evidence suggests that when cartilage is subjected to forces generated during joint movement, due to its high proteoglycans–water content, it deforms elastically. Under conditions of sustained pressure, fluid may be squeezed out of the matrix. The ability to deform elastically reduces the forces acting on the cartilage and protects the underlying bone surfaces. In this way, articular cartilage is able to withstand considerable mechanical loading without failure.

### DEVELOPMENTAL ISSUES

### THE EFFECTS OF AGEING ON JOINTS

Ageing is the single most important risk factor for osteoarthritis, which shows a sustained and progressive increase in epidemiological surveys in elderly populations, in whom it is a major cause of pain and disability (Doherty & Lohmander, 2002). Mild degrees of osteoarthritis are evident in almost all X-rays of joints in elderly individuals, and moderate to severe changes are present in

64%. However, despite radiographic evidence of joint degeneration, many individuals remain symptom free. The presence of osteophytes (see p. 296) appear to be a universal age-associated attribute but it is difficult to determine their pathological significance and there is little evidence that they cause symptoms. However, the relationship between osteoarthritis and disability is important because analysis of the global burden of disease has shown that osteoarthritis is ranked fourth in terms of its negative impact on health in women and eighth in men (Murray & Lopez, 1997).

## CLINICAL APPLICATIONS

Women show an interesting increased prevalence and severity of osteoarthritis of the hands, knees and feet, whereas men are affected most frequently and severely in the spine and intervertebral discs. Both sexes are affected equally by osteoarthritis of the hip. Osteoarthritis of the knee and hip are dominant causes of disability and, in addition to increasing age and gender, a number of risk factors that vary in magnitude of effect at each joint site have been implicated in their development (Doherty & Lohmander, 2002; Felson & Zhang, 1998; Lievense et al., 2002). Genetic factors are influential in the disease affecting both joint sites, whereas obesity,

the presence of Heberden's nodes and trauma, and repetitive mechanical loading incurred by specific categories of occupation or athletic use, affect development of osteoarthritis of the knee. In contrast, a history of congenital joint disease affecting the hip, obesity, occupational and athletic loading are more influential than the presence of Heberden's nodes and trauma in osteoarthritis of the hip. Prevalence of hip osteoarthritis is lowest in Asian populations and highest in white Europeans; osteoarthritis affecting the knee does not show a dominant predisposition in racial impact.

## THE PATHOPHYSIOLOGY OF JOINT DYSFUNCTION

A number of disorders can affect the integral components of synovial joints and their related structures – muscles, tendons, ligaments and nerves. Although a detailed consideration of the aetiology and pathology of disease processes is not appropriate here, the pathophysiology of inflammatory, metabolic and degenerative diseases affecting joints will be related to the specific joint components. These pathophysiological effects will in turn be considered in relation to the clinical nursing problems that subsequently arise. A summary of disorders affecting joints is shown in **Table 3.3.3**.

**Table 3.3.3** Common disorders affecting joints

| Classification | Disorder | Aetiology | Joints affected | Joint component affected |
|---|---|---|---|---|
| Degenerative | Osteoarthrosis | Unknown; heredity, trauma, congenital factors, pre-existing diseases are all important | Symmetrical involvement of weight-bearing joints; interphalangeal and metacarpal joints of hand, knee, elbow, shoulder, jaw, and cervical, thoracic and lumbar intervertebral joints | Degeneration of articular cartilage Degeneration of intervertebral discs |
| Inflammatory | Rheumatoid arthritis | Unknown; possibly autoimmune; pre-existing infection or injury, and genetic factors are important HLA-D4 antigen carriers are at risk | Peripheral synovial joints; metacarpophalangeal, metatarsophalangeal and interphalangeal joints of hands and feet; later spread involves the elbow, hip and cervical spine | Synovial membrane Synovial fluid Articular cartilage Capsule Ligaments Tendons |
| | Juvenile arthritis (Still's disease) | Unknown, may be associated with growth disorders | Distal interphalangeal joints, cervical spine, hip and sacroiliac joints | As above |

*(Contd)*

**Table 3.3.3** (Contd)

| Classification | Disorder | Aetiology | Joints affected | Joint component affected |
|---|---|---|---|---|
| | Rheumatic fever | Hypersensitivity reaction to Group A streptococci | Wrists, ankles, knees, elbows | All joint components |
| | Reiter's syndrome | Venereal origin or may follow some forms of dysentery | Peripheral synovial joints, particularly of lower limbs | All joint components |
| | Psoriatic arthritis | Carriers of certain human leucocyte antigens (HLA) are at risk, e.g. HLA-38 | Peripheral, sacroiliac, thoracic and cervical spine | All joint components |
| | Ankylosing spondylitis | HLA-B27 | | |
| Metabolic | Gout | *Primary*: enzyme defect in uric acid metabolism (hypoxanthine-guanine phosphoribosyl transferase) *Secondary*: some form of (thiazide) diuretic therapy causes urate retention (impaired renal clearance of urate) | First metatarsopha-langeal joints; subsequent involvement of joints in hands, knees, feet | Synovial membrane Deposition of monosodium urate crystals triggers synovitis |
| | Pseudogout | Associated with diabetes mellitus, hyperparathyroidism | Knee joint, subsequent spread to hip, pelvis, shoulder | Synovial membrane Deposition of calcium pyrophosphate crystals triggers synovitis Synovial fluid alkaline phosphate decreased |
| Infective | Bacterial arthritis | Systemic spread of gonococci, meningococci staphylococci and streptococci from other sites May complicate traumatic injuries or rheumatoid arthritis | Symmetrical widespread involvement | All joint components involved |
| | Viral arthritis | Associated with viral infections of rubella, chickenpox, hepatitis | As above | All joint components involved |
| | Tuberculous arthritis | Systemic spread from primary focus of mycobacterium TB | Vertebrae, hip joint | All joint components involved |
| Traumatic injuries | Minor trauma | Common in athletes due to overtraining before adequate muscle control gained | Individual joints vary in susceptibility to injury | Synovitis affecting synovial membrane Ligaments torn, effusion of fluid into capsule Ligaments ruptured |
| | Sprain | | | Haemarthrosis may be present |
| | Dislocation | External injury | | Fracture of cartilage surfaces |

## DYSFUNCTION IN THE SYNOVIAL JOINT

### The synovial membrane: inflammatory change

**Synovitis** is a term used to describe inflammatory changes that are localized within the synovial membrane; the term **arthritis** describes the extended inflammation that involves other joint structures. Synovitis can be precipitated by any of the following.

**Injury** can result from minor trauma, e.g. caused by athletic overtraining before adequate muscle control is attained.

**Irritation** can be caused by the synovial deposition of monosodium urate crystals in gout or by bleeding (**haemarthrosis**) into the joint, associated with trauma, haemoglobinopathies and blood dyscrasias. It might also follow primary degenerative osteoarthrotic changes in cartilage. **Osteoarthrosis**, also referred to as **osteoarthritis**, is not a true arthritis because inflammation is not the primary event but follows degenerative changes in cartilage. By contrast, in rheumatoid arthritis the primary event is inflammation of the synovial membrane due to autoimmune events, with degeneration of cartilage and bone occuring as sequelae to this.

**Infection** can be acquired following trauma or precipitated by blood-borne viral or bacterial infections from other foci.

**Immunological reactions** have been extensively investigated in the development of rheumatoid arthritis (Catrina et al., 2002; Katrib et al., 2001; Smith et al., 2001). The inflamed synovial membrane becomes swollen, hyperaemic and infiltrated by lymphocytes and macrophages, predominately from the bloodstream, in response to the local production of chemoattractant proteins. Examples of the latter include monocyte chemoattractant protein-1 (MCP-1) and macrophage inflammatory protein-1$\alpha$ (MIP-1). Lymphocytes and macrophages subsequently generate a cascade of pro-inflammatory cytokines, notably interleukin-1$\alpha$, interleukin-1$\beta$, interleukin-6 and tumour necrosis factor (TNF)$\alpha$, which play a pivotal role in the initiation of inflammation. The cytokines act to release peptidase enzymes, the matrix metalloproteinases (MMPs), which degrade the extracellular matrix of the cartilage underlying the synovial membrane. Other important actions of the cytokines are to stimulate the production of nitric oxide by enzyme activation in macrophages; the enzyme induced is nitric oxide synthase (NOS). In turn, nitric oxide stimulates the production of pro-inflammatory prostaglandins via induction of the enzyme cyclo-oxygenase (COX) (Salvemini, 1998). Overall, the actions of prostaglandins amplify the other inflammatory processes triggered by the cytokines.

In rheumatoid arthritis, the synovial membrane proliferates rapidly to form a pannus of tissue, which infiltrates and reduces the joint space and can bind together opposing articular surfaces. As a result of inflammatory changes, the joint becomes swollen and stiff, and its range of movement can be limited. Although the synovial membrane is not extensively supplied with free nerve endings, pain is often felt, particularly on movement.

### Synovial fluid changes

The appearance and properties of synovial fluid are markedly altered in a number of disorders; thus, aspiration of fluid from the joint is an essential investigation in the early stages of any joint disorder.

Volume increases in fluid within the joint are characteristic of inflammatory disorders. Increased numbers of leucocytes are present ($>2000$/mL) and the fluid might have a turbulent, purulent or blood-stained appearance. Concentrations of matrix metalloproteinases rise significantly in synovial fluid in the early stages of rheumatoid arthritis in comparison with osteoarthritis, where concentrations are lower. Loss of synovial fluid from the joint space can occur during the late stages of degenerative diseases such as osteoarthritis, or inflammatory disorders such as rheumatoid arthritis. In both, surface fissuring of cartilage, together with the increased pressures generated in the joint during movement, can force fluid down into subchondral bone to form cysts. Changes in volume and composition do not necessarily accompany traumatic injuries, although bleeding into the joint and effusions of synovial fluid are common features.

Altered viscosity can occur where synovial fluid is diluted and increased in volume. Loss of viscosity can also be brought about by the release of enzymes, such as hyaluronidases, from synovial cells and leucocytes during the inflammatory changes of rheumatoid arthritis. These enzymes can break down the vital hyaluronic-acid–protein complex in synovial fluid.

If synovial fluid is lost, or its physical properties are impaired, then great pressures are set up in the joint during movement and the loss of lubrication results in stiffness and an impaired range of joint movement. This is compounded by inflammatory changes in the synovial membrane. Pain can arise as a result of pressures exerted on the capsule by an increased volume of synovial fluid and the inflamed, proliferating synovial membrane.

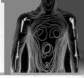

## Articular cartilage and bone: degenerative changes

Release of matrix metalloproteinases by cytokines trigger the degeneration of extracellular matrix in rheumatoid arthritis, despite the production of matrix metalloproteinase enzyme inhibitors by chondrocytes and other cells. Destruction of cartilage and juxta-articular bone can follow and, in some cases, a generalized osteopenia can occur due to bone resorption by osteoclasts, the aetiology of which is not established (Hirayama et al., 2002). Factors that contribute to this process of bone resorption in rheumatoid arthritis include circulating cytokines, corticosteroid treatment, alterations in mineral metabolism and immobilization.

By contrast, primary focal degradation of cartilage occurs in osteoarthritis, together with sclerosis of subchondral bone and formation of **osteophytes** (van der Kraan & van den Berg, 2000). Chondrocytes produce interleukin-1 and tumour necrosis factor $\alpha$, which trigger the production of metalloprotease enzymes (as described above). In addition, interleukin-1 also inhibits the synthesis of structurally important matrix proteoglycans in articular cartilage. Local cytokine production in turn stimulates the synthesis of nitric oxide, which appears to exert two important effects in osteoarthritis. First, it acts as a mediator of interleukin-1 in the inhibition of chondrocyte proteoglycan synthesis and, second, it interferes with the actions of vital growth factors for cartilage, for example insulin-like growth factor (IGF-1). Current views on the pathophysiology of osteoarthritis are that it encompasses changes in both repair and degradation processes. Initially, cartilage repair by anabolic growth factors such as insulin-like growth factor and transforming growth factor (TGF) $\beta$ occurs, stimulating matrix synthesis and inhibiting its breakdown. But this is followed later by dominance in the degradation of the cartilage matrix (chondroitin sulphate, collagen) by cytokine-triggered catabolic metalloprotease enzymes.

As a result of enzyme activity, the healthy, smooth appearance of cartilage is lost and surface fissuring appears. Although regenerating cartilage initially replaces the damaged tissue, this is deposited unevenly at the joint margins and ossifies to form the marginal spurs of bone (**osteophytes**) characteristic of the disease.

Inevitably, all these degenerative changes result in the loss of the compressible properties of hyaline cartilage and extensive shearing forces are generated on bone during movement, a surface that is ill-suited to cope with this. Wearing of the thickened bone surfaces can be followed by fracture and collapse, so that the bone no longer functions as a component of an efficient lever system. Progressive loss in the range of movement at affected joints occurs and this might be accompanied by deformity and instability of the entire joint structure. Bone pain might be present, and is far more severe than that related to elevated intracapsular pressures. Degeneration of vertebral joints can cause nerve root compression, resulting in numbness, pain and sensory impairment, and problems with micturition might arise if the caudae equinae are involved. These problems related to vertebral joints are most likely to present with disorders such as osteoarthritis.

## The joint capsule and its surrounding structures

All the pathophysiological changes that have been described in relation to other joint components can eventually extend to involve the fibrous capsule and the surrounding structures – muscles, tendons, ligaments and nerves – that play a vital role in mobility and stability.

In rheumatoid arthritis, distension of the capsule, which is plentifully supplied by pain fibres, by the increased bulk of synovial fluid and pannus causes pain. The pain can be increased by mechanical changes that produce local ischaemia and muscle spasm, and contractures of the joint can occur if the painful limb is held for a prolonged period in a position that minimizes discomfort.

Deformity can also arise from distension and weakening of the capsule and its surrounding ligaments. The resulting limited movement is further aggravated by muscle spasm and fibrosis and, together with erosion of the capsular structure, the joint can become unstable and dislocate.

**Dislocation** caused by external injury (a direct blow or shearing force) is associated with the rupture of extracapsular ligaments, effusion of fluid into the fibrous capsule and displacement of articulating bones. A **subluxation** is an incomplete dislocation. Treatment consists of reduction of the dislocation, with surgical repair of the capsule and ligaments if necessary. This is followed by immobilization to promote healing. During this period, exercises must be introduced to maintain the range of motion in a synovial joint and prevent contractures. A traumatic injury that injures the highly vascular synovial membrane can cause bleeding into the joint, which in turn causes synovitis. In this situation, aspiration of blood from the joint cavity might be necessary.

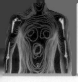

## A SUMMARY OF PROBLEMS: A RATIONALE FOR PLANNING NURSING CARE

The previous section examined pathophysiological changes in the synovial joint brought about by some common disorders. The three major interrelated problems that have emerged – pain, limited movement and deformity – will now be examined in relation to the rationale for planning nursing care. Reference is also made to some aspects of medical treatment, physiotherapy and dietetics.

### Pain

The causes of pain associated with joint disorders can be summarized as follows:

- **Pressure** exerted on the capsule by inflammatory processes within the synovia, and an increased volume of synovial fluid (e.g. inflammatory and infective disorders).
- **Compression** of nerve roots, which follows trauma or degeneration of intervertebral synovial and cartilaginous joints.
- **Collapse** of bone following cartilage erosion (e.g. degenerative disorders such as osteoarthritis, later stages of rheumatoid arthritis).
- **Spasm** in muscle and tendons (any disorder).

Pain caused by inflammation can be relieved in the first instance by the administration of either a non-steroidal anti-inflammatory analgesic drug (NSAID) (e.g. indomethacin or phenylbutazone) or a COX-2 selective agent. Both categories of drug act on biochemical pathways to prevent the synthesis of pro-inflammatory prostaglandins, NSAIDS inhibit the enzyme prostaglandin synthetase and COX-2 inhibit cyclo-oxygenase. Specifically, in rheumatoid arthritis, **second line** drugs that have a slower onset of action (e.g. azathioprine, methotrexate, chloroquine and parenterally administered gold) can retard the progression of tissue damage (van Riel, 2002).

Approaches to drug therapy that target the cytokines responsible for inflammation are in the process of evaluation. For example, anti-tumour necrosis factor α therapy (Etanercept) has been shown to reduce the production ('down regulation') of metalloproteinase enzymes, which cause inflammation and degeneration of extracellular matrix in rheumatoid arthritis (Smith et al., 2001).

Pain resulting from osteoarthritis can respond to simple analgesia with paracetamol (Doherty & Lohmander, 2002). In both rheumatoid and osteoarthritis, corticosteroids, which have immunosupressive and anti-inflammatory actions, can be given either orally or injected into the joint as a medical procedure.

The inflammatory process can be halted by rest, either by resting and immobilizing the affected joint in a splint or by instituting bedrest if several joints are involved in a severe inflammatory disorder such as rheumatoid arthritis. Aspiration of an increased volume of fluid within the joint is a medical procedure that can alleviate pressure on the capsule and thus provide pain relief.

When cartilage erosion and collapse of the underlying bone have occurred the use of anti-inflammatory analgesics, as already described, might be inadequate to control bone pain, which is usually severe, and the use of more potent opiate-related analgesics, e.g. Diconal or Omnopon, may be necessary. Bone pain is exacerbated by loading, therefore the use of walking aids or other devices to prevent loading stresses on joints, together with appropriate lifting techniques, will do much to alleviate pain.

Pain caused by muscle spasm can be alleviated in a number of ways. Splinting the joint with plaster of Paris or moulded fibreglass splints will enable the muscle to relax and thus reduce pain. Muscle relaxation can also be achieved by physiotherapy techniques such as hydrotherapy (see p. 329) and the application of local heat treatments via heating pads or paraffin wax baths. Passive exercises in an acutely inflamed joint can exacerbate or precipitate painful muscle spasm, so isometric exercises (i.e. that develop tension in muscles without moving the joint) are advisable. Although these exercises are initiated on the advice of the physiotherapist, it is important to reinforce them. Constraining the body in one position for a lengthy period can increase the severity of muscle and joint pain, and this is particularly true if movement during sleep is restricted. For this reason, it is unusual for potent hypnotic drugs, which reduce sleep movements, to be prescribed for an individual with joint disease; a combination of sedative and anti-inflammatory drugs is given instead.

Pain produced by compression of a nerve root can be relieved by a combination of traction and local heat treatment, initiated as a medical decision. This is particularly useful in treating joint pain caused by degenerative changes in the cervical spine. Surgical decompression can be considered if these conservative measures fail (traction is considered at greater length in Chapter 3.2).

### Immobility and stiffness

The causes of limitation of movement associated with joint disorders can be summarized as follows:

- **Loss of joint space** due to proliferation of synovial tissue (rheumatoid arthritis).

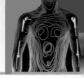

- **Loss of physical properties** of synovial fluid, or loss of fluid *per se* (inflammatory or degenerative disorders).
- **Degenerative changes** in bone and cartilage; loss of the compressive properties of cartilage with subsequent loading of bone (osteoarthrosis, late stages of rheumatoid arthritis).
- **Fibrosis** of the capsule, and ligaments and tendons.
- **Spasm** of muscle.

## Assessment of mobility

Normal movement can be defined as a voluntary and automatic, coordinated skeletal muscle activity essential for carrying out the tasks of daily living. An individual's capacity for movement is determined by the possession of physical abilities, the motivation to move and a free, non-restrictive environment (Hollerbach, 1988). The preceding chapters have examined the integrated operation of muscles and bones at joints that bring about movement, but how can such mobility be assessed? Assessment of mobility is an important component of evaluating the response to rehabilitation in individuals whose physical functions have been impaired by trauma, by inflammatory or degenerative disease affecting muscles, bones and joints and by a variety of central nervous system disorders such as cerebrovascular accident or 'stroke'.

Diverse approaches to the assessment of mobility have been developed, including global assessments of functional abilities in the performance of activities of daily living (ADL) and more specific functional tests investigating particular limbs or range of movement at joints.

One of the most extensively used global methods of assessment is the Barthel Index, which investigates abilities to perform ten self-care activities (feeding, grooming, bowels, bladder, dressing, chair/bed transfer, toilet, mobility, stairs and bathing), at different levels of dependency over a 0–20 point scale (Mahoney & Barthel, 1965). The use of ordinal scales with a summed score has its limitations: they provide a crude level of measurement, lack comparability and independence of the items included, and suffer from 'ceiling effects', where the top score does not imply total recovery. However, the Barthel Scale has demonstrated reliability and validity, and scores obtained from it have been predictive of length of hospital stay, placement on discharge and ability to live in different residential settings (Granger & Dewis, 1979; Wade et al., 1985).

The functional independence measure (FIM) is another example of an approach to quantify the ability to perform activities of daily living (Oczkowski & Barreca, 1993). This utilizes a 7-point scoring system for independence across 18 items of care, providing a motor score for 13 items (feeding, grooming, bathing, dressing upper body, dressing low body, toileting, bladder, bowel, bed transfers, wheelchair transfers, toilet transfers, bath transfers and locomotion). Five items score cognitive abilities and this cognition score can be added to that obtained for motor independence to give a total score.

Several functional motor assessments have focused on the lower limbs. Robinson & Schmidt (1981) devised a simple assessment of walking ability that can be used in hospital setting without the need for the complex, specialized and expensive equipment normally used to assess human gait. This involves patients walking 10 m on the flat over a timed period, on a floor banded in 3 cm distances. As the patient walks, an observer records and measures velocity, stride, step length and step frequency. In contrast, Stewart et al. (1990) have devised a simple timed walking test for use with elderly patients. This involved the subjects walking using 'usual' aids, as far as possible, on a flat vinyl floor, over a 2-minute period, on two consecutive days. This test was able to detect significant improvements in subjects undergoing active rehabilitation, unlike a conventional rating scale, which did not detect improvement.

Assessments of the dynamic behaviour of joints during a range of functional abilities can be helpful in the determination of disease impact and monitoring responses to physiotherapy. Flexible electrogoniometry offers an improvement in comparison with standard techniques of assessing joint range of motion during the performance of functional activities (Rowe et al., 2001). Alternative approaches include the development of scales to evaluate joint damage, for example the mechanical joint score (MJS), which provides a clinical index of joint damage in rheumatoid arthritis (Johnson et al., 2002). This ordinal scale evaluates damage in the metatarsophalangeal and metacarpophalangeal joints, wrists, elbows, shoulders, knees and ankles. The mechanical joint score demonstrated strong correlation with the Larsen X-ray score of hands and feet (Larsen et al., 1977) and moderate correlation with the Stanford Health Assessment Questionnaire (Kirwan & Reeback, 1986). The latter is one of the most widely used indices of joint function and measures the patient's perception of disability, not that of the health professional.

A number of nursing actions can alleviate some of these problems. Immobility caused by increases in intracapsular bulk due to inflammation of the synovial membrane can be alleviated by the correct administration of anti-inflammatory analgesics (i.e. regularly, as prescribed by the medical staff, and after meals to reduce the potential problem of gastrointestinal side-effects) and measures previously described.

Rest of the affected joint, or bedrest if several joints are involved, will help to reduce the great pressures that are generated during movement due to loss of synovial fluid, joint space and cartilage, and which can cause further cartilage erosion. Excessive or abnormal use of the joint will accelerate cartilage fissuring and destruction, therefore loading stresses on weight-bearing joints should be prevented by using walking aids (e.g. tripods, walking frames) and lifting techniques, by supervising exercise periods, and asking the dietician to advise a weight-reducing diet if the individual is obese. Other dietary measures may bring benefit (see p. 329).

Immobility can be reduced by using physiotherapy exercises that maintain the range of movements in unaffected joints, followed by the introduction of active and passive exercises in affected joints as soon as inflammation and pain have subsided. Exercise also increases muscle mass and tension, thereby promoting stability in the affected joint. In a number of instances it might be advisable to institute, as soon as possible, exercises that attempt to maintain normal joint function, e.g. prolonged rest and immobilization can be harmful in ankylosing spondylitis, resulting in further ankylosis and impairment of mobility. Pain relief is an essential prerequisite here.

### Deformity

Joint deformity can be acquired as a result of the following.

- **Distension** of the articular capsule by increased intracapsular pressures, which result in the capsule and ligaments becoming weakened and loose.
- **Collapse** of bone and degeneration of cartilage.
- **Prolonged immobilization** of a joint in an abnormal position, which can cause contracture deformity.

Measures to prevent capsular distension and loading collapse of bone and cartilage are discussed above. Contracture deformities can occur in any immobile patient who holds a limb close to the body with the joint flexed for a prolonged period of time. This is followed by muscle atrophy and shortening. The individual with a painful joint is particularly vulnerable because there might be a tendency to hold

the joint in a position that minimizes pain, and a flexion deformity might result. Vital preventive measures include the effective use of analgesia, frequent changes of position for immobile patients, avoiding flexion position, and putting joints through a normal range of movement as soon as possible. In practice, deformity results from the exposure of the joint to a deforming force. Therefore preventing deformity by maintaining good posture is an important aspect of nursing care. Patients with joint disorders should be nursed on firm mattresses, walking aids should be used to maintain a correct upright posture, table heights should be adjusted to prevent continual stooping and the patient should be positioned with the back straight when sitting up and with one pillow when lying down.

Splinting is used extensively to correct existing joint deformity; serial splinting can be used to overcome a fixed flexion deformity. Splinting is carried out by a skilled technician or physiotherapist on medical advice.

## Surgical intervention

Surgical intervention is indicated when the conservative methods of treatment already described have failed. The aim of surgery is directed at relief of pain and immobility, and correction of deformity. **Synovectomy**, a procedure that excises proliferating synovial tissue, is often successfully employed in rheumatoid disease to reduce pain by preventing capsular distension deformity. **Arthrodesis**, or excision of the joint, can be undertaken where cartilage is degenerating and collapse of bone has occurred. This measure alleviates deformity and instability at the expense of loss of movement.

An important achievement has been the advent of the **replacement arthroplasty**, in which the joint is reconstructed and a prosthetic implant replaces one or more of the articulating bone surfaces, for example, hip joint replacement. Loss of the compressible properties of cartilage, with subsequent erosion and collapse of the underlying bone, is a fundamental cause of immobility in the diseased joint and it is an unfortunate fact that, once lost, cartilage does not regenerate.

## Electromagnetic therapy

Recently, van Nguyen & Marks (2002) have reviewed the evidence for using pulsed electromagnetic fields in the treatment of osteoarthritis and other musculoskeletal conditions. The rationale for this intervention in the treatment of osteoarthritis is that cartilage exposed to an electrical field increases its proteoglycans content, which might reflect elevated chondrocyte synthesis of this vital component of the cartilage matrix. Bone repair, ligament and tendon healing are also reported to benefit from pulsed electromagnetic fields, which could be used in situations where these tissues are involved in osteoarthritic symptomatology. The beneficial outcomes of these tissue-level effects include reductions in joint and muscle pain, stiffness and swelling. Although the research evidence is currently limited and further evaluation is needed, it supports the application of this technique in the attenuation of pain and disability in osteoarthritis.

## Dietary therapy

The use of dietary supplements such as fish and plant oils in the treatment of rheumatoid arthritis has evoked interest and divergent opinion in recent years. Dietary ingestion of fish oils rich in omega-3 fatty acids can lead to the incorporation of these fatty acids into macrophages, which play a pivotal role in the initiation of joint inflammation. Once incorporated, omega-3 fatty acids close-down cytokine production and, thereby, pro-inflammatory responses (Mayer et al., 1998). A review of the evidence relating to therapeutic effects of fish oils in rheumatoid arthritis concluded that a modest benefit can be gained. Further investigation is necessary to confirm these benefits, to establish safe doses and to evaluate potential long-term toxicity (Eerola & Peltonen, 1998). Similar conclusions relate to the therapeutic effects of ingesting oil of evening primrose, which is high in gamma linoleic acid. Metabolism of this oil produces prostaglandins of the E series, which are anti-inflammatory.

## Hydrotherapy interventions

A review of the research evidence relating to the effectiveness of physiotherapeutic hydrotherapy has concluded that high- to moderate-quality evidence supports benefits in a range of inflammatory and degenerative musculoskeletal conditions (Geytenbeek, 2002). Critical appraisal of the research studies reviewed found that physiotherapeutic hydrotherapy benefited joint mobility, strength, pain, functional ability and other selected outcomes. Particular benefits accrued in older adults and those suffering from rheumatic conditions.

## Clinical review

In addition to the Learning Objectives at the beginning of this chapter, the reader should be able to:

* Provide a classification of the common disorders affecting joints
* Relate pathophysiological changes to limitations in movement and other problems that result from common disorders affecting synovial and cartilaginous joints

## Review questions

1 How are joints analogous to lever systems?
2 Which is the most efficient class of lever system?
3 What is the most common type of lever system found in the body?
4 Why is it better to lift loads as close to the body as possible?
5 How do fibrous and cartilaginous joints essentially differ from synovial joints?
6 Why are there sensory receptors in joints?
7 What is the main function of synovial fluid?
8 How do synovitis and arthritis differ?
9 What is the difference between rheumatoid arthritis and osteoarthritis?

## Suggestions for further reading

Burkhardt, P., Dawson-Hughes, B. & Heaney, R.P. (2001) *Nutritional Aspects of Osteoporosis.* San Diego: Academic Press.
*Definitive text on this subject.*

Casimiro, L., Brosseau, L., Milne, S. et al. (2002) Acupuncture and electro-acupuncture for the treatment of osteoarthritis. Online. Available: www.cochrane.org/cochrane/revabstr/ab003788.htm

Edwards, S. (2002) *Neurological Physiotherapy.* Edinburgh: Churchill Livingstone.
*Some excellent information of interest to nurses in the sections on management of acute rehabilitation and complex disability management and splinting.*

Evans, R.C. (2001) *Illustrated Orthopaedic Physical Assessment.* St Louis: Mosby.
*Emphasis on rheumatology in the first two chapters: well illustrated joint range of movement in later sections.*

Goss, G.L. (1998) Orthopaedic nursing. *Nursing Clinics of North America,* **33**(4). Philadelphia: WB Saunders.
*A series of multi-author papers relating to the nursing assessment and management of conditions affecting bones and joints, with integrated pathophysiology.*

Hukkanen, M.V.J., Polak, J.M. & Hughes, S.P.F. (1998) *Nitric Oxide in Bone and Joint Disease.* Cambridge: Cambridge University Press.
*A highly accessible background text reviewing the research relating to the influence of nitric oxide in pathological processes.*

Maddison, P.J., Isenberg, D.A., Woo, P. & Glass, D.N. (1998) *Oxford Textbook of Rheumatology,* 2nd edn. Oxford: Oxford University Press.
*A comprehensive review of the scope of rheumatology and its treatment. Highly recommended reference source.*

Palastanga, N., Field, D. & Soames, R. (2002) *Anatomy and Human Movement: Structure and Function,* 4th edn. Oxford: Butterworth-Heinemann.
*Well illustrated, detailed reference text, combining up to date theoretical information with practical applications.*

Woolf, A.D. (2002) *Bone and Joint Futures.* London: BMJ Books.
*Evaluates the future burden of bone and joint conditions, together with priorities for care.*

## References

Catrina, A.I., Lampa, J., Ernestam, S. et al. (2002) Anti-tumour necrosis factor (TNF) alpha therapy (etanocerpt) down-regulates serum matrix metalloproteinase (MMP)-3 and (MMP)-1 in rheumatoid arthritis. *Rheumatology,* **41**; 484–489.

Doherty, M. & Lohmander, S. (2002) The future diagnosis and management of osteoarthritis. In: Woolf, A.D. (ed) *Bone and Joint Futures.* London: BMJ Books.

Eerola, E. & Peltonen, R. (1998) The gastrointestinal system. In: Maddison, P.J. et al. (eds) *Oxford Textbook of Rheumatology,* 2nd edn. Oxford: Oxford University Press, pp. 255–271.

Felson, D. & Zhang, Y. (1998) An update on the epidemiology of knee and hip osteoarthritis with a view to prevention. *Arthritis and Rheumatology,* **41**; 1343–1355.

Geytenbeek, J. (2002) Evidence for effective hydrotherapy. *Physiotherapy,* **88**(9); 514–529.

Granger, C.V. & Dewis, L.S. (1979) Stroke rehabilitation: analysis of repeated Barthel Index measures. *Archives of Physical and Medical Rehabilitation,* **60**; 14–17.

Hirayama, T., Danks, L., Sabokbar, A. & Athanasou, N.A. (2002) Osteoclast formation and activity in the pathogenesis of osteoporosis in rheumatoid arthritis. *Rheumatology,* **41**; 1232–1239.

Hollerbach, A.D. (1988) Assessment of human mobility. In: *AAANS Neuroscience Nursing. Section 5.* pp. 283–302. New York: Appleton and Lange.

Johnson, A.H., Hassell, P., Jones, P.W. et al. (2002) The mechanical joint score: A new clinical index of joint damage in rheumatoid arthritis. *Rheumatology,* **41**; 189–195.

Katrib, A., Tak, P.P., Bertouch, J.V. et al. (2001) Expression of chemokines and matrix metalloproteinases in early rheumatoid arthritis. *Rheumatology,* **40**; 988–994.

Kirwan, J.R. & Reeback, J.S. (1986) Stanford Health Assessment Questionnaire modified to assess disability in British patients with rheumatoid arthritis. *British Journal of Rheumatology,* **25**; 206–209.

Larsen, A., Dale, K. & Eek, M. (1977) Radiographic evaluation of rheumatoid arthritis and related conditions by standard reference films. *Acta Radiologica Diagnostica,* **18**; 481–491.

Lievense, A.M., Bierma-Zeinstra, A.P., Verhagen, A.P. et al. (2002) Influence of obesity on the development of osteoarthritis of the hip; a systematic review. *Rheumatology,* **41**; 1155–1162.

Mahoney, F.I. & Barthel, D.W. (1965) Functional evaluation: The Barthel Index. *Maryland State Medical Journal,* **14**; 61–65.

Mayer, K., Seeger, W. & Grimminger, F. (1998) Clinical use of lipids to control inflammatory disease. *Current Opinion in Clinical Nutrition and Metabolic Care,* **1**(2); 179–184.

Medical Research Council (1976) *Aids to the Examination of the Peripheral Nervous System.* London: HMSO.

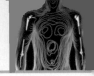

Murray, C.J.L. & Lopez, A.D. (1997) *The Global Burden of Disease.* Geneva: World Health Organization.

Oczkowski, W. & Barreca, S. (1993) The functional independence measure: its use to identify rehabilitation needs in stroke survivors. *Archives of Physical Medicine and Rehabilitation*, **74**; 1291–1294.

Robinson, J.L. & Schmidt, G.L. (1981) Quantitative gait evaluation in the clinic. *Physical Therapy*, **61**; 351–353.

Rowe, P., Myles, C.M., Hillman, S.J. & Hazlewood, M.E. (2001) Validation of flexible electrogoniometry as a measure of joint kinematics. *Physiotherapy*, **87**(9); 479–485.

Salvemini, D. (1998) Nitric oxide and prostaglandin interactions in acute and chronic inflammation. In: Hukkanen, M.V.J., Polak, J.M. & Hughes, S.P.F. (eds) *Nitric Oxide in Bone and Joint Disease.* Cambridge: Cambridge University Press, pp. 70–90.

Smith, M.D., Slavotinek, J., Au, V. et al. (2001) Successful treatment of rheumatoid arthritis is associated with a reduction in synovial membrane cytokines and cell adhesion molecule expression. *Rheumatology*, **40**; 965–977.

Stewart, D.A., Burns, J.M.A., Dunn, S.G. & Roberts, M.A. (1990) The two minute walking test: A sensitive index of mobility in the rehabilitation of elderly patients. *Clinical Rehabilitation*, **4**; 273–276.

van der Kraan, P.M. & van den Berg, W.B. (2000) Anabolic and destructive mediators in osteoarthritis. *Current Opinion in Clinical Nutrition and Metabolic Care*, **3**(3); 205–211.

van Nguyen, J. & Marks, R. (2002) Pulsed electromagnetic fields for treating osteoarthritis. *Physiotherapy*, **88**(8); 458–470.

van Riel, P.L.C.M. (2002) The future diagnosis and management of rheumatoid arthritis. In: Woolf, A.D. (ed) *Bone and Joint Futures.* London: BMJ Books.

Wade, D.T., Langton-Hewer, R., Skilbeck, C.E. & David, R.M. (1985) *Stroke: A Critical Approach to Diagnosis, Treatment and Management.* London: Chapman and Hall.

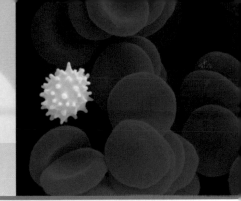

# Section 4

# Internal transport

# Chapter 4.1

# The blood

*Susan E. Montague*

## LEARNING OBJECTIVES

After studying this chapter the reader should be able to:

- Describe the appearance and major constituents of blood

- Outline the major functions of blood

- State the approximate blood volume of a baby, child and adult and give reasons for variations

- Describe the origin of the various constituents of plasma and relate these to the interpretation of biochemical estimations performed clinically

- List the major groups of plasma proteins and explain their functions

- Describe how blood cells are produced and how this process is regulated

- Describe the characteristics and functions of mature red blood cells

- Demonstrate understanding of the structure and functions of haemoglobin A

- Describe the functions of the various types of white blood cell

- State the functions of platelets

- Outline the key stages in the process of haemostasis

- Describe the genetic and physiological bases of the major blood group systems and explain their clinical significance

## INTRODUCTION

An inevitable consequence of the increasing size of organisms and cell specialization that took place during evolution was that cells tended to lose direct contact both with each other and with the external environment. As exchange with their immediate environment became insufficient for these cells to maintain dynamic equilibrium, so a biological need arose for a means of connecting each specialized group of cells – an internal transport system. Indirect exchange

between all cells and the external environment was then made possible by such a system.

In all complex animals, including humans, the function of internal transport is primarily fulfilled by the specialized tissues that comprise the heart and blood vessels – the cardiovascular system (see Chapter 4.2) – and by the fluid transport medium contained within them – the blood, which is the subject of this chapter. Even minor injuries frequently result in the walls of small blood vessels, lying close to the body surface, being breached and blood lost to the exterior. The fact that blood is quite commonly shed gives it an unusual significance, in that it is probably the only internal body tissue that most people have seen and can describe.

Religious and other historical records show that, for thousands of years, in all cultures and societies, people have recognized that blood is a vital fluid, the major loss of which rapidly leads to death. As a result, it has often been assigned magical properties, such as the power of rejuvenation. In many societies it has come to symbolize desirable human qualities such as courage, purity and fertility, as well as to represent strong beliefs about kinship and race. Descriptions of past and present human beliefs and knowledge of blood make fascinating reading, allowing insights into the reasons behind apparently irrational human behaviour in relation to the loss, donation and transfusion of human blood. A fuller discussion of this topic is beyond the scope of this book but the interested reader will find suggestions for further reading on this subject at the end of this chapter.

Blood is circulated throughout the body propelled by the pumping action of the heart. In the capillary beds of the tissues it comes into close proximity with the thin layer of interstitial tissue fluid that directly surrounds the cells of the body. As a transport medium, blood carries a wide variety of substances that are involved in all aspects of cell function. As blood passes through the capillaries its composition changes as components such as oxygen, carbon dioxide, nutrients and waste products are exchanged, across the capillary walls, with components in the tissue fluid. This continuous exchange functions to maintain an optimum internal environment for cell and tissue function and is thus the basis of homeostasis.

## Appearance, composition and major functions of blood

Newly spilled human blood typically appears as a homogeneous, opaque, somewhat syrupy fluid, which is dark red in colour. The fluid solidifies into a sticky clot, which exudes a clear fluid within a few minutes.

If, however, a sample of blood is placed in a glass tube, prevented from clotting (coagulating) by the addition of anticoagulant and allowed to settle, or spun in a centrifuge, it separates into its major components (**Fig. 4.1.1**). These are a pale yellow, slightly opalescent liquid – the **plasma** – which in health constitutes approximately 55% of the total volume, and a lower deposit of formed elements; the latter are the **blood cells** and **platelets**. As can be seen in

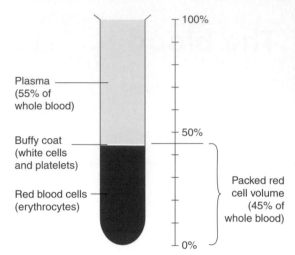

**Figure 4.1.1** The appearance of anticoagulated whole blood when allowed to settle

Fig. 4.1.1, the red cells (erythrocytes) normally constitute nearly all of the cellular deposit. They are topped by a very thin 'buffy coat' that consists of the white cells (leucocytes) and platelets. In health these account for less than 1% of blood volume. So, despite its appearance, blood is not a homogeneous substance but a complex fluid containing a variety of cells and platelets in suspension and chemicals in solution.

## Blood weight and volume

Blood constitutes approximately 6–8% of an adult's body weight. The proportion is lower for the obese adult because fatty tissue contains relatively little blood, and is slightly higher in infancy and childhood. The sum of the red cell volume and the plasma volume gives the total blood volume, because the volume of white cells and platelets is negligible:

red cell volume + plasma volume
= whole blood volume

A newborn baby weighing 3.4 kg would be expected to have a total blood volume of approximately 0.25 litre (L), a 70-kg adult male to have 4.8 L and a 51-kg adult female to have 3.3 L. An appreciation of such volumes is important for an understanding of the amount of blood loss that may be tolerated by an individual and to fluid replacement requirements.

It is also important to appreciate that blood is not evenly distributed throughout the body. Normally, it is contained in the blood vessels of the cardiovascular system (see Chapter 4.2), and some tissues are much more vascular (contain more blood vessels) than others.

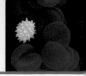

# An outline of the functions of blood

Blood provides a medium for the following physiological processes:

## Internal transport

Blood carries a wide variety of substances to and from the body cells and in so doing supports the following metabolic functions:

- **Respiration**. The respiratory gases oxygen and carbon dioxide are carried on haemoglobin molecules in red cells and in plasma. Exchange of these gases with the external environment takes place in the lungs.
- **Nutrition**. Nutrients, absorbed from the intestine, are carried in the plasma and passed to the external environment, primarily via the kidneys.
- **Maintenance of water, electrolyte and acid–base balance**. Through continuous exchange of its constituents with those of tissue fluid, blood has an essential role in this aspect of homeostasis.
- **Metabolic regulation**. Hormones and enzymes, both of which affect the metabolic activity of cells, are carried in plasma.

## Defence against infection by foreign organisms

Defence against infection is a primary function of white blood cells. Chapters 6.1 and 6.2 describe the protective inflammatory and immune responses, respectively.

## Protection from injury and haemorrhage

The protective inflammatory response is the localized response of tissues to injury.

Prevention of haemorrhage is a function of the platelets and a series of clotting and fibrinolytic factors present in plasma. Haemostasis, the process of stopping bleeding from a damaged blood vessel, is described later in this chapter.

## Maintenance of body temperature

Blood carries heat and because it circulates between body core and periphery it provides the material basis for heat exchange between the tissues and the external environment.

of the blood. As obtaining a specimen of venous blood, by venepuncture, is a relatively straightforward invasive procedure, the results of biological and biochemical analysis of such a specimen frequently provide a major aid to medical diagnosis, a guide to treatment and an important means of monitoring a patient's progress. Changes in the composition of blood, secondary to disease elsewhere in the body, are far more common than those due to primary disorders of blood itself. Nevertheless, as we shall see in this chapter, primary disorders of the blood, or loss of blood from the circulation, have widespread effects on body function and produce diverse health problems.

All personnel involved in handling blood or blood products should take precautions, such as wearing protective gloves and safe disposal of sharps, to avoid inadvertent infection with pathogenic blood-borne organisms, for example hepatitis B and the human immunodeficiency virus (HIV), the virus that causes acquired immune deficiency syndrome (AIDS).

## Plasma

Plasma is a pale yellow, slightly opalescent fluid, comprising approximately 55% of the total blood volume – 2.5–3.0 L in an adult. Its major constituents and properties are summarized in **Table 4.1.1**.

Plasma contains clotting factors and, given an appropriate stimulus such as exposure to air, will form a clot. The clear fluid exuded from clotted whole blood and clotted plasma is called **serum**. The constituents of serum are the same as those of plasma minus the small quantities of clotting factors, such as fibrinogen, that are destroyed during the process of clotting.

**Table 4.1.1** Major constituents and properties of plasma

| Constituent | % |
|---|---|
| Water | 90 |
| Protein | 8 |
| Inorganic ions | 0.9 |
| Organic substances | 1.1 |

| Property | Value |
|---|---|
| Specific gravity (relative to water) | 1.026 |
| Viscosity (relative to water) | 1.5–1.75 |
| pH | 7.35–7.45 |
| $H^+$ concentration | 35–45 nmol/L |

Plasma forms about 20% of the body's total extracellular fluid of about 15 L and its composition is very similar to that of the other major extracellular fluid, the interstitial (tissue) fluid; the main difference is in protein content. Interstitial fluid contains only about 2% protein, whereas plasma contains 8%. This is because most of the plasma protein molecules are too large to pass through the capillary walls into the interstitial fluid. The small amount of protein that does 'leak' through passes eventually into the lymph (see Chapter 6.2) and is returned to the circulation.

### CLINICAL APPLICATIONS

The constituents of plasma reflect overall metabolic function and are frequently the subject of biochemical estimation in chemical pathology laboratories for clinical purposes.

## Plasma proteins

Plasma contains between 60 and 80 g of protein per litre. Plasma proteins are classified into groups according to their molecular size, water solubility and electrophoretic mobility (migration when placed in an electrically charged field). There are three major groups: **albumin**, **fibrinogen** and **globulin**. Further fractions – alpha ($\alpha$), beta ($\beta$) and gamma ($\gamma$) – can be distinguished within the globulin grouping.

Albumin is normally present in larger quantities than either fibrinogen or any of the globulin fractions. In health, albumin accounts for 60% of the plasma protein, globulins 36% and fibrinogen 4%. The relative proportions and amounts of plasma proteins can alter in certain diseases, and electrophoretic tracings indicating such changes can aid medical diagnosis.

### Origin of the plasma proteins

Plasma albumin, fibrinogen, $\beta$ globulins and most of the $\alpha$ globulins are synthesized exclusively by the liver. The remaining plasma proteins are produced by other tissues. The $\gamma$ globulins (immunoglobulins, Ig) are produced by cells of the immune system (see Chapter 6.2). There are many more proteins, present in plasma in very low concentrations, which have important biological functions. These trace proteins include most of the clotting factors (see later), as well as hormones and enzymes.

The albumin molecule (molecular mass 69 000) is the smallest plasma protein molecule and is just too large to pass through the capillary walls. In severe nephritis (kidney disease), however, the damaged glomerular capillaries 'leak' albumin into the nephron and the urine can contain large quantities of this protein. The liver has the reserve capacity to synthesize and replace a daily albumin loss of approximately 25 g, provided adequate nitrogen (protein) is obtained from the diet to sustain this extra synthesis. As a result, large quantities of albumin can be lost from the body without producing symptoms of disease. Following haemorrhage, plasma proteins are restored to normal levels in a few days, provided the body has sufficient amino acids to synthesize them.

With the exception of thromboplastin and calcium ions, all of the clotting factors are proteins and are synthesized by the liver. Vitamin K is essential in the production of some of these, for example prothrombin. In liver disease, the physiological effects of reduced hepatic synthesis of plasma proteins can produce health problems. These are discussed in Chapter 5.2 and include disordered clotting and the formation of ascites.

## Functions of the plasma proteins

### Intravascular osmotic effect

Plasma protein molecules do not diffuse readily across the capillary wall because their diameter is greater than that of the pores in the capillary wall. The small quantities of protein, mainly albumin, that do leak through the wall, pass from the interstitial space into the blind-ended lymph capillaries and are returned to the blood via the lymphatic vessels.

Only substances that cannot pass through the pores of a semi-permeable membrane can exert an osmotic effect, and hence it is the dissolved protein in the plasma and interstitial fluid that is responsible for the osmotic effect occurring at the capillary wall. This is often referred to as colloid **osmotic pressure** or **oncotic pressure**.

The osmotic effect of plasma proteins plays a major role in the formation and re-absorption of tissue fluid and in determining the normal distribution of water between blood and tissue spaces. The mechanics of this important process are described in Chapter 4.2.

The albumin in plasma is the source of 70–80% of the colloid osmotic pressure. This is because the osmotic pressure of a solution is determined by the *number* of dissolved particles unable to pass through the membrane, rather than their weight and size. Not only is there twice as much albumin as globulins in plasma but albumin molecules are also considerably smaller than globulin molecules in weight and size.

When plasma colloid osmotic pressure becomes abnormally low, this affects the distribution of water between blood and tissue spaces, and oedema may result (see Chapter 4.2). The major causes of reduced plasma colloid osmotic pressure are:

- decreased production of plasma protein, as for example, in liver disease or protein malnutrition
- excessive loss of plasma protein from the body, as for example, in nephritis or severe burns
- increased porosity of capillary walls, as for example, in inflammation and allergic reactions.

## Contribution to the viscosity of plasma

Plasma and cells contribute almost equally to the **viscosity** of the blood, which is between two and five times that of water. The viscosity of plasma is mainly due to its protein content. Despite its relatively small quantity, the asymmetrical shape of the fibrinogen molecule means that fibrinogen contributes as much to plasma viscosity as albumin.

## Transport

Many substances that are insoluble in water are carried partially or wholly bound to plasma protein molecules. Substances bound to plasma proteins are unable to enter the cells and take part in metabolism. This is of clinical importance, particularly in the case of drugs, where the bound substance forms a reservoir that must be saturated before the drug can have effect. One substance can also displace another from a binding site, rendering the freed one biologically active. (Further discussion and examples of such interactions can be found in pharmacology texts.) Albumin molecules bind calcium, bilirubin, bile acids and several drugs, for example aspirin, phenylbutazone, thiazide diuretics, digoxin, penicillin, sulphonamides, tolbutamide and tryptophan.

Specific α globulin molecules bind the hormones cortisol and thyroxine. β globulins carry cholesterol and other lipids, vitamins A, D and K, insulin and iron (transferrin), and γ globulins bind circulating antigens and histamine. The carriage of some of these substances can affect the carriage of others, and hence their uptake by the tissues. For example, aspirin and sulphonamides compete with bilirubin for binding sites on albumin molecules. The presence of these drugs thus facilitates the diffusion of bilirubin into the liver and other tissues.

## Protein reserve

Plasma proteins function as a labile **protein store**, forming part of the body's amino acid pool. They can be broken down into their constituent amino acids by the cells of the mononuclear phagocytic system and, as a last resort, can form a source of replacement amino acids for tissue protein in conditions of dietary protein deficiency or intestinal malabsorption. Plasma may be given, intravenously, as a source of protein, but the use of proprietary amino acid preparations for infusion has superseded this practice.

## Clotting and fibrinolysis

**Clotting** and clot breakdown (**fibrinolysis**) are functions of plasma and most of the recognized clotting and fibrinolytic factors are plasma proteins. The processes of clotting and fibrinolysis are described in more detail later in this chapter.

## Inflammatory response

One of the early features of some types of **inflammation** is the walling-off of the area by a mesh of fibrin (fibrin clot). This fibrin mesh functions to delay the spread of bacteria and toxins from the initial area of penetration and forms a framework for repair. Fibrin is formed from the soluble plasma protein, clotting factor fibrinogen.

Plasma **kinins**, for example bradykinin, are polypeptides that contribute to the events of the inflammatory response. They cause contraction of smooth muscle, vasodilation and decreased blood pressure, increased vascular permeability, and they stimulate nerve endings producing pain. In high concentrations they promote the migration of white blood cells into the tissues. **Complement** (see Chapter 6.1) consists of a system of plasma proteins that acts in a complex sequence to augment inflammatory and immune defence mechanisms.

## Protection from infection

The γ globulins (immunoglobulins, Ig) are produced by plasma cells of the B-lymphocyte series of cells and function as **antibodies**. Each antibody is a specific protein capable of binding and inactivating a specific antigen on, for example, a bacterial cell, virus, or pollen, which it recognizes as foreign in the acquired immune response (see Chapter 6.2). Five classes of antibody make up the immunoglobulins: these are IgM, IgG, IgA, IgD and IgE.

## Maintenance of acid–base balance

Some of the amino acid constituents of proteins have free carboxylic acid groups (COOH). Other amino acids have free basic amino groups ($NH_2$/$NH_3OH$).

**Table 4.1.2** Normal ranges of concentration of inorganic ions in plasma

| Ion | Concentration (mmol/L) |
|---|---|
| Sodium (Na$^+$) | 135–146 |
| Potassium (K$^+$) | 3.5–5.2 |
| Calcium (Ca$^{2+}$) | 2.10–2.70 |
| Chloride (Cl$^-$) | 98–108 |
| Hydrogen carbonate (HCO$_3^-$) | 23–31 |
| Phosphate (PO$_4^{2-}$) | 0.7–1.4 |

Proteins can therefore ionize as acids or bases (that is, they are amphoteric molecules) and so can operate in both acidic and basic **buffering** systems.

At the pH of blood (7.35–7.45, hydrogen ion concentration 35–45 nmol/L), plasma proteins ionize as anions and act as hydrogen ion acceptors, 'mopping up' excess hydrogen ions. However, plasma proteins account for less than one-sixth of the buffering power of the blood, the protein (haemoglobin) in the red cell, being a far more potent hydrogen ion acceptor.

## Inorganic ions

The inorganic ions **(electrolytes)** of plasma are almost identical to those found elsewhere in the extracellular fluid. Sodium is the major cation and chloride and hydrogen carbonate (bicarbonate) the major anions. **Table 4.1.2** presents their normal ranges of concentration. Reference ranges vary between laboratories, depending on the characteristics of the population from which they were derived and the precise measurement techniques employed.

### CLINICAL APPLICATIONS

Changes in plasma electrolyte concentration are followed by similar changes in the interstitial fluid. These, in turn, affect cell function. For example, potassium depletion following the increased losses that can occur in severe diarrhoea and vomiting affects tissue excitability, causing muscle weakness and abnormalities in the conduction of the cardiac impulse. Calcium is also necessary for the normal excitability of tissues and the calcium ion deficiency that occurs, for example, in alkalosis, can result in tetany. Sodium deficiency occurs infrequently in temperate climates but arises in severe diarrhoea and vomiting and in some renal and endocrine diseases. It leads to a reduction in the volume of the extracellular fluid. The resultant fall in blood pressure produces weakness, dizziness, mental confusion and fainting. A fuller discussion of electrolyte disturbances is given in Chapter 5.4.

The **osmolality** (see Chapter 1.2 for explanation) of plasma is approximately 285 mosmol/kg of water. Solutions used in **intravenous replacement therapy** must be isotonic with normal body fluids or damage to cells may occur; 0.9% (154 mmol/ 308 mosmol) sodium chloride solution and 5% (278 mmol/278 mosmol) dextrose solution are examples of commonly used isotonic solutions.

## Substances in transit in plasma

Plasma contains a multitude of substances in transit to various tissues. These may be in simple solution or carried bound to plasma protein molecules. Many are present in very small quantities.

### Gases

Inspired **gases** dissolve in plasma to a degree normally dependent only on their solubility in water and their partial pressure at the alveolar membrane.

Oxygen is not very soluble in water, and consequently arterial blood with a partial pressure of $O_2$ of 13 kPa (100 mmHg) only carries 3 mL/L (0.13 mmol/L) of oxygen dissolved in the plasma. This amount is physiologically insignificant. Oxygen is carried mainly in the blood attached to haemoglobin molecules in the red blood cells (see later in this chapter).

Carbon dioxide is more water soluble than oxygen. Approximately 5% of that transported in the blood is carried in simple solution and about 90% as hydrogen carbonate ions in the plasma.

Other gases, such as inhalation anaesthetics, also vary in their solubility. Nitrous oxide, for example, produces a rapid induction because the blood rapidly becomes saturated and the drug quickly becomes able to enter the brain (Galbraith et al., 1999).

### Organic substances

**Table 4.1.3** summarizes reference ranges of various **organic substances** in serum. These might vary from those quoted by other sources because, as pointed out earlier, the ranges given depend on the characteristics of the population from which they were derived and the precise laboratory techniques employed.

### Nutrients

The most abundant **nutrient** in plasma is glucose **(Table 4.1.3)**, the primary source of energy for cellular metabolism. Other nutrients in transit include amino acids, fatty acids, triglycerides, cholesterol and other lipids, and vitamins.

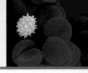

**Table 4.1.3** Normal serum levels of various organic substances

| Organic substance | Concentration |
|---|---|
| Glucose | |
|     fasting | 3.3–5.5 mmol/L |
|     after a meal | <10.0 mmol/L |
|     2 hours after glucose | <5.5 mmol/L |
| Urea | 2.7–8.5 mmol/L |
| Uric acid (urate) | 150–580 μmol/L |
| Creatinine | 40–110 μmol/L |
| Bilirubin | 3–21 μmol/L |
| Aspartate aminotransferase (AST) | 5–30 iu/L |
| Alanine aminotransferase (ALT) | 5–30 iu/L |
| Hydroxybutyrate dehydrogenase (HBD) | 150–325 iu/L |
| Creatine kinase (CK) | <130 iu/L |
| Amylase (AMS) | 150–340 iu/L |
| Alkaline phosphatase (ALP) | 21–100 iu/L |
| Acid phosphatase (ACP) | <8.2 iu/L |

iu = international unit.

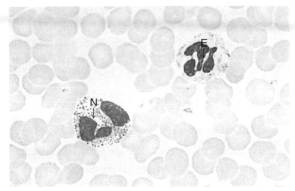

**Figure 4.1.2**   Colour slide of whole blood showing erythrocytes and two leucocytes (labelled). N, neutrophil; E, eosinophil

## Waste products of metabolism

These include urea, uric acid and creatinine, which are excreted by the kidney, and the bile pigment, bilirubin, which is excreted in the bile **(Table 4.1.3)**.

## Hormones

**Hormones**, such as cortisol and thyroxine, are carried in plasma attached to plasma proteins to their target cells from the endocrine gland that secreted them into the blood.

## Enzymes

Except for those enzymes involved in clotting, the removal of intravascular clots and the complement system, most of the **enzymes** found in plasma derive from the normal breakdown of the cells of blood and other tissues and have no metabolic function in the plasma itself.

Monitoring the activity of certain enzymes in plasma can be a useful diagnostic index for specific abnormalities. For example, serum amylase (AMS) is raised in people with acute pancreatitis. However, very few enzymes are produced by only one specific tissue and it is often the pattern, or change, in levels obtained from measuring the serum level of two or three enzymes over time that aids diagnosis, rather than single values. For example, the levels over time of four markers are commonly measured to detect the cell death that occurs in myocardial infarction. These are creatine kinase (CK), its cardiospecific isoenzyme (CK-MB) and the very sensitive cardiospecific proteins troponin T and troponin I (Boon et al., 2002).

## Other substances

Other exogenous chemicals can be absorbed into the blood and transported in the plasma. **Drugs** are probably the major example and these can be the subject of biochemical estimation in cases of poisoning.

## Cellular components of blood

The cellular elements of blood comprise approximately 45 percent of its volume **(see Fig. 4.1.1)**. There are three major types:

- red blood cells, or **erythrocytes**, which are the most numerous and make up nearly all of the cellular deposit
- white blood cells, or **leucocytes**
- platelets, which together with the leucocytes form the thin 'buffy' coat **(see Fig. 4.1.1)**.

A major part of basic haematological investigation (**haematology** is the study of blood and blood-forming tissues) involves counting the number of each type of cell present per unit volume of blood. In health, the numbers of cells in peripheral blood remain constant within quite narrow limits, that is, they are homeostatically regulated. The information given by a full blood count, the most basic of laboratory tests, has increased enormously in the last 20 years and the complex, automated blood cell analysers that provide the information, are now standard equipment in hospitals in the United Kingdom. Blood cell counts are expressed per litre of blood and electronic counters are now capable of measuring the red blood cell count (RBC), the white blood cell count (WBC), the platelet count, the haemoglobin level and the mean volume of red blood cells (MCV). Other red cell indices can then be derived.

**Figure 4.1.2** shows the appearance of a prepared film of normal blood. Of course the cells are not coloured in this way in the body – the colour is due to the dyes used as the blood film is prepared for study. Microscopy allows further assessment of blood cell morphology and is necessary to identify red cell inclusions, for example, the malarial parasite.

## DEVELOPMENTAL ISSUES

### HAEMOPOIESIS (THE FORMATION OF BLOOD CELLS)

Haemopoietic cells first appear in the yolk sac of the 2-week embryo. By 6 weeks, haemopoiesis has become established in the embryonic liver and by 12–16 weeks the liver has become the major site of blood cell formation. It remains an active haemopoietic site until 2 weeks after birth; the spleen is also active during this period. The bone marrow becomes an active haemopoietic site from about 20 weeks gestation and gradually increases its activity until it becomes the major site of production about 10 weeks later.

At birth, actively haemopoietic (red) marrow occupies the entire capacity of the bones and continues to do so for the first 2–3 years of postnatal life. The red marrow is then very gradually replaced by inactive, fatty, yellow marrow. The latter begins to develop in the shafts of the long bones and continues until, by 20–22 years, red marrow is present only in the upper epiphyses (ends) of the femur and humerus and in the flat bones of the sternum, ribs, cranium, pelvis and vertebrae (Hoffbrand et al., 2001). However, because of the growth in body and bone size that has occurred during this period, the total amount of active red marrow (approximately 1000–1500 g) is nearly identical in the child and the adult. Adult red marrow has a large reserve capacity for cell production and fatty marrow is capable of reversion to haemopoietic marrow in diseases in which blood cell production is increased. In childhood and adulthood it is also possible for haemopoietic sites outside marrow, such as the liver, to become active if there is excessive demand as, for example, in severe haemolytic anaemia or following haemorrhage. In old age, red marrow sites are slowly replaced with yellow, inactive marrow.

Red marrow forms all types of blood cell and is also active in the destruction of red blood cells, brought about by tissue macrophages present in the lining of the marrow blood sinuses. Red marrow is, therefore, one of the largest and most active organs, approaching the size of the liver. About two-thirds of its mass functions in white (myeloid/non-lymphoid) cell production (**leucopoiesis**) and one-third in red (erythroid) cell production (**erythropoiesis**), although there are approximately 700 times as many red cells as

white cells in peripheral blood. This apparent anomaly reflects the shorter life span and hence greater turnover of the white blood cells in comparison with the red blood cells.

## Haemopoietic cells (Fig. 4.1.3)

A common, pluripotent stem cell with the appearance of a small to medium-sized lymphocyte gives rise to a series of progenitor (precursor) cells for the main myeloid and lymphoid cell lines (Hoffbrand et al., 2001). Stem cells also give rise to natural killer cells, dendritic cells and osteoclasts (part of the mononuclear phagocytic system). Each type of cell can be identified by immunological identification of 'cluster differentiation' (CD) molecules on the cell surface.

Stem cells are capable of self-renewal and this characteristic is progressively lost in precursor cells and their descendants as they differentiate and develop. This capacity for self-renewal is significant in that it allows the bone marrow to remain in homeostatic steady-state in terms of the cells that compose it, even though it is a major site of cell production. Another important concept is that the system amplifies itself many times. It has been calculated, for example (Hoffbrand et al., 2001), that a single stem cell can produce one million mature blood cells after just 20 divisions.

Unlike stem cells, differentiated precursor cells are capable of responding to haemopoietic growth factors (see below) to increase production of their particular cell line when necessary. Stem cells either from bone marrow or, more recently, from umbilical cord blood can be transplanted in circumstances where there are major abnormalities or deficiencies in blood cell lines (see below).

The specific development of erythrocytes, granulocytes, platelets and lymphocytes from the pluripotent stem cell through committed precursor cells is described within the section in this chapter on that cell type. **Figure 4.1.3** summarizes diagrammatically the major stages of haemopoiesis.

## *Haemopoietic growth factors*

Haemopoietic growth factors are glycoprotein hormones that regulate the production of haemopoietic cells and the function of mature blood cells. They may act locally at the site they were produced or circulate in plasma. Lymphocytes, monocytes, endothelial cells and fibroblasts are the major cell sources except for erythropoietin (epo; see later), most of which is synthesized in the kidney and thrombopoietin (tpo), which is synthesized in the liver. The biological effects of growth factors are mediated through specific receptors on the target cells.

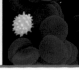

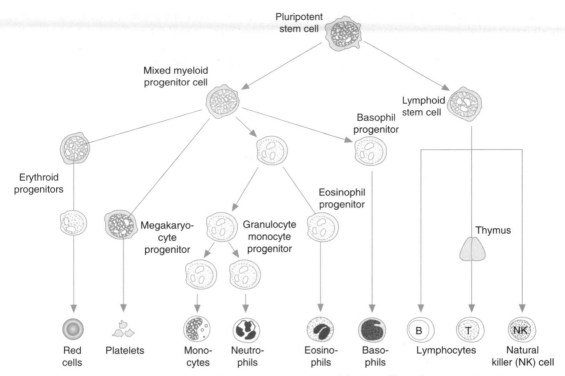

Figure 4.1.3    A summary of the major stages of haemopoiesis. Adapted from Hoffbrand, A.V., Pettit, J.E. & Moss, P.A.H. (2001) *Essential Haematology*, 4th edn. Oxford: Blackwell Science, Figure 1.4, p. 3

## CLINICAL APPLICATIONS

### BONE MARROW BIOPSY (ASPIRATION)

Bone marrow aspiration or trephine biopsy is performed in order to confirm a diagnosis suggested by clinical examination of the patient and investigation of the peripheral blood cells. These tests provide information about the normality of haemopoiesis, the relative numbers of different types of cell present and can also demonstrate the presence of foreign cells, for example in metastatic cancer and Hodgkin's disease.

In aspiration, a needle is inserted into the marrow and a liquid sample of marrow withdrawn. In biopsy, a solid core of bone is removed, using a bone-biopsy trephine needle to reach the marrow. Suitable sites require red marrow to be present under a relatively thin layer of bone. The tibia is frequently used in young children and the sternum and posterior iliac crest in adults. The area is first infiltrated with local anaesthetic and the needle, which is fitted with a guard, is pushed through the bony cortex into the medullary cavity and marrow fragments are aspirated using a syringe. The procedure is carried out, aseptically. As well as assisting with the procedure, nursing responsibilities include explanation to the patient, skin preparation and assessing for pain and bleeding at the site following the aspiration. Haemorrhage can be a particular risk if the patient's clotting mechanism is abnormal due to illness, as in leukaemia.

## BONE MARROW (BMT) AND STEM CELL TRANSPLANTATION

Until recently, allogenic BMT has been the only potentially curative treatment for people with severe aplastic anaemia, leukaemias and severe, congenital immune deficiency and haemopoietic disorders. The treatment is most effective in young patients (under 20 years), although older patients can also be transplanted. Complications, such as infection and graft-versus-host disease (GVHD) are common and can be severe. Stem cells from other sources, such as umbilical cord blood, are now also being used in transplants.

Healthy marrow or stem cells for transplantation are collected from a normal histocompatible donor (often a sibling). In the United Kingdom there has been debate and publicity around the ethical basis of the creation and subsequent genetic selection of human embryos ('designer babies') to provide a perfect immunological match for a stem cell transplant for a sick sibling. Although this procedure is accepted in the United States, it was only in 2003 that a British couple won permission in the Court of Appeal in the United Kingdom to undergo this procedure (see www.news.bbc.co.uk/2/hi/health/3002610.stm). Marrow or stem cells from umbilical cord blood are then administered intravenously to the recipient, who has previously been immunosuppressed with chemotherapy and irradiation. The stem cells of the donor marrow settle in the recipient's marrow cavity and, if the graft is successful, begin to release cells into the blood after about a fortnight, producing enough cells to meet the patient's needs in about 3–4 weeks.

It is also possible for the patient's own marrow or stem cells to be collected, frozen and treated intensively before it is re-infused. This is **autologous bone marrow transplantation/stem cell transplantation** and is used to rescue the patient following the effects of radical chemotherapy and/or irradiation (Craig et al., 2002).

## Red blood cells (erythrocytes)

### Erythropoiesis (the production of red blood cells)

Mature red blood cells develop from committed precursor cells **(see Fig. 4.1.3)**. The maturation process for erythrocytes is characterized by the following:

- gradual appearance of haemoglobin and disappearance of ribonucleic acid (RNA) in the cell
- progressive degeneration of the cell's nucleus, which is eventually extruded from the cell
- gradual loss of cytoplasmic organelles, for example mitochondria
- gradual reduction in cell size.

The young red cell is called a **reticulocyte** because of the reticular network (reticulum) present in its cytoplasm. This reticulum is composed of ribonucleic acid. As the red cell matures the reticulum disappears. A reticulocyte normally takes about 4 days to mature into an erythrocyte, spending about 1–2 days in the bone marrow and 1–2 days in the liver or spleen or circulation.

Between 2 and 6% of a newborn baby's circulating red cells are reticulocytes; this reduces to less than 2% in a healthy adult. However, the reticulocyte count increases considerably in conditions in which rapid erythropoiesis occurs, for example following haemorrhage or acute haemolysis of red cells.

### Regulation of erythropoiesis

In health, erythropoiesis is regulated so that the number of circulating erythrocytes is maintained within a narrow range. Normally, a little less than 1% ($2 \times 10^{11}$) of these cells are produced per day and these replace an equivalent number that have reached the end of their life span.

Erythropoiesis is stimulated by hypoxia. However, oxygen lack does not act directly on the haemopoietic tissues but instead stimulates the production of a hormone, **erythropoietin**. This hormone then stimulates haemopoietic tissues to produce red cells. Erythropoietin is a glycoprotein with a molecular weight of 34 000. Approximately 90% of erythropoietin is formed in the peritubular complex of the kidney. It is inactivated by the liver and excreted in the urine. Various factors can affect the rate of erythropoiesis by influencing erythropoietin production.

### Endocrine factors

Thyroid hormones, thyroid-stimulating hormone, adrenal cortical steroids, adrenocorticotrophic hormone and human growth hormone (hGH) all promote erythropoietin formation and so enhance erythropoiesis. In thyroid deficiency and anterior pituitary deficiency, anaemia may occur due to reduced erythropoiesis. Polycythaemia (see below) is often a feature of Cushing's syndrome. However, very high doses of steroid hormones seem to inhibit erythropoiesis. Androgens stimulate and oestrogens depress the erythropoietic response. In addition to the effects of menstrual blood loss, this effect might explain why women tend to have a lower haemoglobin concentration and red cell count than men.

## CLINICAL APPLICATIONS

Plasma levels of erythropoietin are raised in hypoxic conditions. This produces an **erythrocytosis** (increase in the number of circulating erythrocytes) and the condition is known as **secondary polycythaemia**. A physiological secondary polycythaemia is present in the fetus (and residually in the newborn) and in people living at high altitude because of the relatively low partial pressure of oxygen in their environment. This phenomenon is the physiological basis for athletes training at high altitude to enhance the oxygen-carrying capacity of their blood, for example, prior to the Mexico City Olympic Games, which were staged at high altitude. The practice of 'blood doping' or 'blood boosting', in which athletes are transfused with their own, or a compatible, blood with a high red cell count is a risky and not very effective practice carried out in the hope of improving performance. Secondary polycythaemia occurs as a result of tissue hypoxia in diseases such as chronic bronchitis, emphysema and congenital cardiovascular abnormalities associated with right-to-left shunting of blood through the heart (i.e. bypassing the lungs), for example Fallot's tetralogy. Erythropoietin is also produced by a variety of tumours of both renal and other tissues. Conversely, the severe anaemia associated with end-stage renal failure can be treated with human recombinant erythropoietin.

The oxygen-carrying capacity of the blood is increased in polycythaemia but so is the blood viscosity, and the latter produces circulatory problems such as raised blood pressure and risk of thrombosis.

In **primary polycythaemia** (polycythaemia rubra vera), there are increases in the numbers of all the blood cells and plasma erythropoietin levels are normal. The cause of this condition is a clonal malignancy of a marrow stem cell (Hoffbrand et al., 2001).

The underlying cause of secondary polycythaemia is treated with the aim of eliminating hypoxia. Venesection (blood letting) is sometimes employed to reduce red cell volume to normal levels. Frequently, blood is removed, centrifuged to remove cells and the plasma returned to the patient (**plasmapheresis**).

In **anaemia** there is a reduction in blood haemoglobin concentration due to a decrease in the number of circulating erythrocytes and/or in the amount of haemoglobin they contain. Anaemia occurs when the erythropoietic tissues cannot supply enough normal erythrocytes to the circulation. In anaemias due to abnormal red cell production, increased destruction and when demand exceeds capacity, plasma erythropoietin levels are increased. However, anaemia can also be caused by defective production of erythropoietin as, for example, in renal disease.

Dietary substances that are essential for normal erythropoiesis are summarized in **Table 4.1.4**. Requirements for iron, vitamin B12 and folic acid are further discussed in the section on anaemia on pp. 350–52.

## Characteristics of mature erythrocytes

### Numbers

Erythrocytes are by far the most numerous of the blood cells. The normal **red cell count** (RBC or RCC) is $5.5 \times 10^{12}$ per litre of blood in men and $4.8 \times 10^{12}$ per litre in women (see **Table 4.1.5** for reference ranges for red cell indices).

When blood is allowed to settle, or is centrifuged under standard conditions, the red cells normally make up almost all the volume of the cellular sediment (**see Fig. 4.1.1**). The proportion of the blood sample composed of packed red cells (the **packed cell volume, PCV**) is 0.47 in men and 0.42 in women. This measure is also known as the **haematocrit (Hct)**. The haematocrit indicates red cell mass relative to total blood volume and so values are reduced in anaemia and raised in polycythaemia.

### Morphology

Mature circulating erythrocytes are biconcave disc-shaped cells with a mean diameter of 7.2 μm and a thickness of 2.2 μm (**Fig. 4.1.4**). They have a mean cell volume (MCV) of approximately 85 fl (femtolitres; see Chapter 1.1). Their relative excess of surface area over volume maximizes exchange of nutrients and respiratory gases with their environment and also makes them very deformable, which allows them to pass through the capillaries even though these have a diameter of approximately 6 μm.

Erythrocytes have a complex protein–lipid membrane, the surface of which is the site of various antigens which determine the different blood groups (see later). Many of the cell's enzyme systems are

| **Table 4.1.4** | Dietary substances that are essential for normal erythropoiesis |
|---|---|
| **Substance** | **Utilization** |
| **Protein** | Synthesis of globin part of haemoglobin and cellular proteins<br>Very low protein intake retards haemoglobin synthesis |
| **Metals**<br>Iron<br>Trace metals: manganese and cobalt | <br>Contained in haem portion of haemoglobin<br>There is no evidence that these substances are essential for erythropoiesis in humans. Cobalt is essential for vitamin B12 synthesis in ruminants since these animals manufacture this vitamin |
| **Vitamins**<br>Vitamin B12 (hydroxocobalamin) and folic acid<br>Vitamin C (ascorbic acid)<br><br><br><br>Vitamin B6 (pyridoxine), riboflavin and vitamin E | <br>Involved in DNA synthesis and hence essential to the maturation of red cells<br>Necessary for normal folate metabolism<br>Facilitates absorption of iron by reducing ferric iron to ferrous iron<br>Very low levels required before effect seen and the anaemia of vitamin C deficiency (scurvy) is usually the result of blood loss<br>Deficiency of these substances has been associated, occasionally, with anaemia |

**Table 4.1.5**  Reference ranges for red cell indices

| Index | Normal range |
|---|---|
| Red cell count (RBC or RCC)<br>Males<br>Females | <br>$4.5–6.5 \times 10^{12}$/L<br>$3.9–5.6 \times 10^{12}$/L |
| Reticulocyte count | 0.2–2.0% of RBC |
| Haematocrit (Hct)/Packed<br>red cell volume (PCV)<br>Males<br>Females<br>Mean cell volume (MCV) | <br><br>40–52%<br>36–48%<br>80–95 fl |
| Haemoglobin concentration (Hb)<br>Males<br>Females | <br>135–175 g/L<br>115–155 g/L |
| Mean cell haemoglobin (MCH) | 27–34 pg |
| Mean cell haemoglobin<br>concentration (MCHC) | 20–35 g/dL |
| Erythrocyte sedimentation<br>rate (ESR)<br>Males<br>Females | <br><br>1–5 mm/h<br>5–15 mm/h |

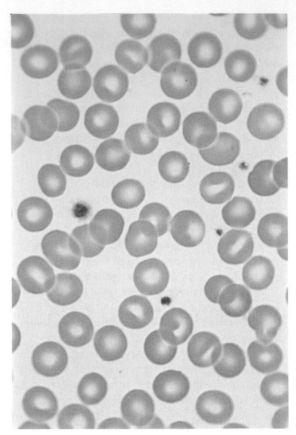

**Figure 4.1.4**  Mature erythrocytes. Reproduced with permission from Hoffbrand, A.V. & Pettit, J.E. (2002) Color Atlas of Hematology, 3rd edn. St Louis: Mosby

located in the membrane, including those that function in the transport of glucose (which is the red cell's sole source of energy) across the membrane. The fragility of red cell membranes varies slightly between normal cells and changes in some abnormal states. This fragility is related to cell shape, the basic principle being that 'slender' cells rupture less easily than 'plump' cells. The membranes of red cells in people with hereditary spherocytosis, for example, show increased fragility. Very defective red cells such as these might haemolyse in the circulation.

Mature erythrocytes lack nuclei and so are unable to divide or to synthesize new proteins. This means that they have a limited life span of 100–120 days. They also lack certain cytoplasmic organelles, for example mitochondria.

The major constituents of a red cell are the protein pigment haemoglobin and a variety of enzymes and other substances that are the products of red cell metabolism. These enzymes and intermediary metabolites are essential to the optimum functioning of haemoglobin and to intracellular stability. Interestingly, although the red cell has evolved to carry oxygen, it obtains its energy predominantly through the anaerobic process of glycolysis. The constituents of red cells are surrounded by intracellular fluid and by a cytoplasmic stroma, or framework, which provides a structural basis for the cell's metabolic function.

## Haemoglobin (Hb)

Haemoglobin is a red-coloured protein pigment found within red blood cells. The normal concentration of haemoglobin in blood is 155 g/L (2.28 mmol/L) in males and 140 g/L (2.06 mmol/L) in females.

Each red cell contains 30 pg (picograms; see Chapter 1.1) of haemoglobin – **mean cell haemoglobin (MCH)**. This represents about 640 million haemoglobin molecules. The **mean cell concentration of haemoglobin (MCHC)** in an erythrocyte is 320 g/L.

### Functions of haemoglobin

The main function of haemoglobin is oxygen uptake in the lungs, carriage in the blood and release in the tissues. This function is dependent on the partial pressure of oxygen at these sites. Haemoglobin also carries carbon dioxide as carbaminohaemoglobin (at sites different from its oxygen carriage sites). This carriage of carbon dioxide should not be confused with that of carbon monoxide. The latter poisonous gas displaces oxygen from its molecular carriage sites (see later). Haemoglobin is a powerful buffer in the maintenance of blood pH. All these functions are described further in Chapter 5.3.

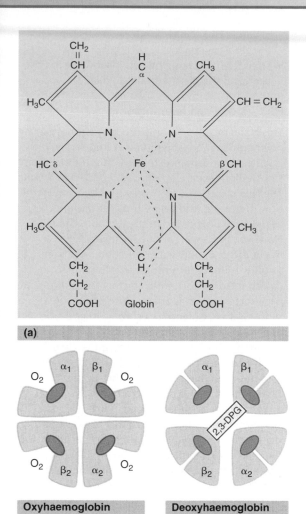

**(a)**

Oxyhaemoglobin　　　　Deoxyhaemoglobin

● Haem

**(b)**

**Figure 4.1.5** (a) The molecular structure of the haem molecule and (b) a diagram of oxygenated and deoxygenated haemoglobin. 2,3-DPG, 2,3-diphosphoglycerate. Adapted from Hoffbrand, A.V., Pettit, J.E. & Moss, P.A.H. (2001) *Essential Haematology*, 4th edn. Oxford: Blackwell Science, Figures 2.7 and 2.8, p. 17

## Synthesis

Haemoglobin synthesis takes place during erythropoiesis. Mature red cells are unable to perform this function.

## Molecular structure

Haemoglobin has a molecular mass of 68 000. Each molecule consists of two major portions

- the iron-containing pigment **haem**
- the protein **globin**.

**Haem** is composed of ring-shaped organic molecules called pyrrole rings (**Fig. 4.1.5a**). Four of these are joined by bridges to form a larger ring structure (**Fig. 4.1.5b**). An iron atom in the ferrous ($Fe^{2+}$) form is then taken up and held centrally by the nitrogen atom of each pyrrole ring. About 300 mg of haem are synthesized daily. The great majority of this becomes incorporated in haemoglobin and the remainder becomes part of the muscle pigment, myoglobin and some cellular enzymes.

Abnormalities of haem synthesis can be inherited or acquired. They are caused by disorders of the enzymatic control of the process. Increased porphyrin production can occur in bone marrow and in the liver. The most common condition resulting from disordered synthesis is **acute intermittent porphyria**. This is inherited as a dominant characteristic but can also be provoked by drugs such as steroid hormones, sulphonamides and barbiturates. Symptoms are mainly abdominal (vomiting and pain) and cardiovascular (tachycardia and hypertension), and are due to increased porphyrin synthesis. Large quantities of porphobilinogen and other intermediary metabolites can be detected in the urine.

Like all proteins, **globin** consists of a long chain of amino acids. Four types of globin molecule occur in normal human haemoglobin. These are distinguished by slight differences in the amino acid composition of the globin chain and are called alpha ($\alpha$), beta ($\beta$), delta ($\delta$) and gamma ($\gamma$). Each haemoglobin molecule contains four coiled globin molecules.

There are three important, normal, human haemoglobins.

|  | Globin chain content | |
|---|---|---|
| HbA | | |
| (the major adult haemoglobin) | $2\alpha$ | $2\beta$ |
| HbA$_2$ | | |
| (the minor adult haemoglobin) | $2\alpha$ | $2\delta$ |
| HbF | | |
| (fetal haemoglobin) | $2\alpha$ | $2\gamma$ |

At birth, HbF makes up two-thirds of the haemoglobin content and HbA the remaining third. By 5 years of age, adult haemoglobin proportions have been obtained. These are HbA > 95%, HbA$_2$ < 3.5%, HbF < 1.5%.

## The haemoglobin molecule: its structure and function

Each haemoglobin molecule has four coiled globin chains attached to four haem groups and each haem group contains one ferrous iron atom. This atom has one bond to enter into a loose and reversible combination with a molecule of oxygen, to form **oxyhaemoglobin** ($HbO_2$).

The poisonous gas carbon monoxide (CO) combines with haemoglobin in the same way, but more easily and less reversibly because haemoglobin has about 250 times greater an affinity for carbon monoxide than it has for oxygen. The compound formed is called **carbon monoxyhaemoglobin** (HbCO) and the presence of this substance in the blood blocks the availability of haemoglobin for oxygen transport. Carbon monoxide poisoning therefore produces an anaemic hypoxia.

Each haemoglobin molecule can potentially carry four molecules of oxygen **(see Fig. 4.1.5b)**. At full saturation this means that one mole of haemoglobin is capable of carrying 4 moles of oxygen. The haemoglobin concentration of the blood is, therefore, a sensitive index of the oxygen-carrying capacity of the blood.

Haemoglobin picks up oxygen molecules one at a time. The reversible binding of each oxygen molecule changes the configuration of the globin and so increases the affinity of the haemoglobin molecule for oxygen. As a result, the affinity of the haemoglobin molecule for the fourth oxygen molecule is twenty times greater than for the first. This phenomenon accounts for the sigmoid shape of haemoglobin's oxygen dissociation curve, which is so important physiologically and is described in Chapter 5.3.

Various factors affect the affinity of haemoglobin for oxygen and so shift the oxygen dissociation curve to the right (decreased oxygen affinity), or left (increased oxygen affinity). These factors include pH, temperature and the presence of the substance **2,3-diphosphoglycerate** (2,3-DPG) in the red cell. 2,3-DPG is an intermediary metabolite of glycolysis (glucose breakdown) occurring within the red cell. Increasing temperature, decreasing pH (i.e. increasing acidity) and increasing levels of 2,3-DPG (precisely the conditions found in the tissues), all reduce haemoglobin's affinity for oxygen, shifting the dissociation curve to the right and so facilitating oxygen delivery in the tissues.

The structure of the haemoglobin molecule also affects its oxygen affinity. For example, HbF has a higher oxygen affinity than HbA. This allows the fetus to obtain adequate amounts of oxygen from the partial pressure of oxygen in the placental blood supply (which is lower than that occurring in the mother's lungs).

Genetic mutations producing changes in the globin chains can produce abnormal haemoglobin molecules with either high or low oxygen affinities.

## CLINICAL APPLICATIONS

### ABNORMAL HAEMOGLOBINS (HAEMOGLOBINOPATHIES)

Several abnormal haemoglobins have now been identified and can be distinguished by electrophoresis. The abnormalities always affect the globin part of the molecule and can be divided into two groups:

- There is substitution of an amino acid in a globin chain by another amino acid, for

example HbS, which produces sickle-cell anaemia (see below).
- The rate of globin synthesis is subnormal; this produces the disease thalassaemia.

### HbS – sickle-cell haemoglobin

This is the most commonly occurring abnormal haemoglobin and is found most frequently in people of African ancestry, but also in those from the Mediterranean region, Saudi Arabia and India. The HbS molecule differs only slightly from HbA in that the amino acid valine replaces glutamic acid as the sixth amino acid in the β globin chains. However, this small change in structure has a major effect on molecular function. HbS is less soluble in the reduced form and the molecules link to form crystals, which distort the red cell into a characteristic sickle shape. Such cells have a reduced life span and so a chronic haemolytic anaemia occurs in people with HbS (**sickle-cell anaemia**). Sickle cells also increase the viscosity of the blood, resulting in reduced blood flow and sometimes complete vascular obstruction.

An individual will suffer from sickle-cell anaemia if he or she is homozygous for the sickle-cell gene, that is, the sickle-cell gene has been inherited from both parents. About 1 in 400 people of African descent suffer from this disease. The anaemia is severe and typically punctuated by crises of a variety of types, for example a vaso-occlusive, 'painful' crisis. In tropical countries, mortality rate in childhood is high but in Western countries, where sophisticated treatment is possible, more than half of patients live beyond 40 years of age (Sergeant, 2001).

A heterozygous individual who has inherited one normal and one sickle-cell gene has the **sickle-cell trait**. Heterozygotes are usually completely well because their red cells do not contain sufficient HbS to produce sickling at normal partial pressures of oxygen. However, they might be at some risk when subjected to hypoxic conditions, for example at altitude and during and following administration of certain anaesthetic gas mixtures. For this reason, all patients of African descent should be screened routinely for HbS before being given a general anaesthetic.

Sickle-cell trait offers some protection against malaria, probably because the malarial parasite is less successful in establishing itself in red cells containing HbS. The result is an increased survival of heterozygotes over HbA homozygotes in areas where malaria is endemic and the mortality rate, from malaria, relatively high, for example, tropical Africa. This occurrence is called 'heterozygote advantage'. This has led to the HbS gene occuring at higher frequencies than would be expected from its mutation rate alone.

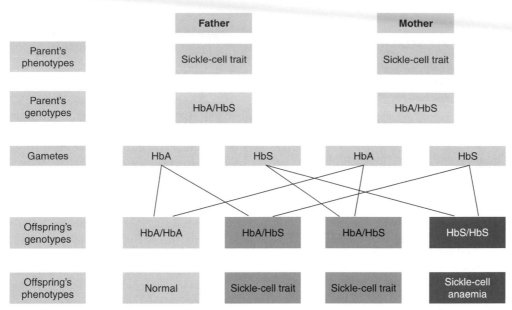

**Figure 4.1.6**  The inheritance of sickle-cell anaemia

**Figure 4.1.6** illustrates that heterozygous parents who carry the sickle-cell gene have a 1 in 2 chance of producing a child with sickle-cell trait, and a 1 in 4 chance of producing an offspring who is homozygous for either the normal HbA gene or the HbS gene for sickle-cell anaemia.

## Thalassaemia

In **thalassaemia** there is a genetically determined deficiency in the production of either the α or the β chain of normal adult haemoglobin (HbA). A wide variety of conditions occurs, ranging from some that are so severe that they result in death in utero, to others that are detectable only on laboratory investigation (Weatherall & Clegg, 2001).

All living cases of **thalassaemia major** are due to abnormalities of β globin synthesis, because α deficiencies lead to death in utero. β thalassaemia occurs mainly in people from Mediterranean countries and the Middle and Far East. In Britain most affected patients are Greek, Greek Cypriot or Indian. These individuals suffer from severe anaemia, due to their reduced levels of normal haemoglobin. Additionally, their abnormal haemoglobin has a reduced ability to release oxygen and its presence decreases the life span of the red cells. Treatment consists of:

- blood transfusions to raise haemoglobin concentration
- splenectomy in cases where red cell destruction by the spleen exceeds red cell production
- drugs – iron chelators, such as desferrioxamine, to reduce iron load
- folic acid administration because the huge haemopoiesis that occurs greatly increases folate requirements

- bone marrow transplant in young patients from a human leucocyte antigen (HLA)-compatible sibling or parent
- stem cell tranplantation.

The carrier state can be detected for both sickle-cell anaemia and thalassaemia major, so affected individuals can be offered genetic counselling. It is also possible to discover, antenatally, if a fetus has the disease and some parents choose to terminate a pregnancy when it is known that the fetus is affected.

## The function of red cells

The haemoglobin content and morphology of mature erythrocytes, described in preceding paragraphs, enable them to function efficiently as oxygen and carbon dioxide transporters. Haemoglobin also functions as a powerful buffer.

In addition, red cells contain the enzyme carbonic anhydrase, which catalyses the reaction:

$$CO_2 + H_2O \underset{\text{carbonic anhydrase}}{\rightleftharpoons} H_2CO_3$$

carbon   water        carbonic
dioxide                acid

$$\rightleftharpoons H^+ + HCO_3^-$$

hydrogen   hydrogen
ion           carbonate
               ion

This enzyme has an important function in facilitating carbon dioxide carriage, as hydrogen carbonate ions ($HCO_3^-$), in plasma. The function of the red cell in respiration is fully described in Chapter 5.3.

## CLINICAL APPLICATIONS

### THE ERYTHROCYTE SEDIMENTATION RATE (ESR)

If diluted blood containing an anticoagulant is allowed to stand in a narrow vertical tube, the red cells slowly settle because their density is greater than that of plasma. The erythrocyte sedimentation rate (ESR) is determined by measuring the length of the column of clear plasma, above the cells, after 1 hour. The normal range is 1–5 mm/h in men and 5–15 mm/h in women, and there is a progressive increase with age (Hoffbrand et al., 2001).

Red cells tend to sediment more rapidly when they can pile on top of one another to form columns (like piles of plates), which are called **rouleaux**. The ESR is primarily a measure of the tendency of the red cells to form rouleaux. This tendency is dependent on the concentration of plasma proteins, particularly fibrinogen and globulins, and hence is directly related to plasma viscosity. Plasma viscosity measurements replace ESRs in some centres. Rouleaux formation is also enhanced by the presence in plasma of proteins that are the by-products of inflammatory and neoplastic disease.

The ESR is raised in a wide range of systemic inflammatory and neoplastic diseases, and in pregnancy. The highest values (> 100 mm/h) are found in chronic infections such as tuberculosis. It is often used as a screening test when diagnosis is uncertain and to monitor the course of a chronic illness. It is generally viewed as a useful indicator of 'wellness'. An ESR of greater than 12 mm/h is usually considered indicative of disease.

### ANAEMIA

Anaemia occurs when the haemoglobin concentration of the blood falls below 135 g/L in adult males and 115 g/L in adult females. From the age of 3 months to puberty, less than 110 g/L indicates anaemia, whereas 150 g/L is the lower normal limit at birth. This happens when, for whatever reason, the erythropoietic tissues cannot supply enough normal erythrocytes to the circulation. Anaemia is therefore not a disease in itself but a sign of disease. Its general effects on a person are the direct result of a reduction in the oxygen-carrying capacity of the blood. The severity of symptoms is related both to the haemoglobin concentration of the blood and to the length of time over which the anaemia developed.

Many young adults with chronic anaemia do not experience health problems until their haemoglobin has fallen below 80 g/L, but older people may have unpleasant symptoms at 110 g/L. The major problems that occur are:

- shortness of breath on exertion
- palpitations (awareness of the heart beat)
- feelings of tiredness and weakness
- loss of appetite and dysphagia (difficulty in swallowing)
- sore mouth and tongue (glossitis)
- pins and needles (paraesthesiae)
- intermittent claudication (shooting pains in the legs), particularly on exertion
- chest pain – angina pectoris
- oedema (swelling) of the ankles at the end of the day (may be due to mild heart failure induced by the anaemia)
- in severe anaemia, central nervous system symptoms appear and these include: faintness and giddiness, tinnitus (ringing in the ears), headache and spots before the eyes due to retinal haemorrhages.

An anaemic person appears pale because of the lack of the pigment haemoglobin in the blood. This pallor is evident in the skin and mucous membrane of the conjunctiva, mouth and tongue and in the nail beds.

### Classification of anaemia

Anaemia can be usefully classified according to its pathophysiology. There are three major types of disturbance which result in anaemia:

- decreased production of red cells
- increased loss of red cells
- increased destruction of red cells.

Anaemia is also described in terms of the size and colour (which reflects haemoglobin concentration) of the circulating red blood cells. Red cells can be **microcytic** (of small size), **normocytic** (of normal size) or **macrocytic** (of large size). They can also be **hypochromic** (pale in colour) or **normochromic** (normal in colour). For example, a microcytic, hypochromic anaemia is characteristic of iron deficiency, and a macrocytic, normochromic anaemia is typical of vitamin B12 deficiency.

It is important that the underlying cause of the anaemia is identified and treated, if this is possible. The only treatment in severe anaemia is blood transfusion but this procedure is especially hazardous for people with anaemia (unless the condition is due to acute haemorrhage) because of the possibility of fluid overload. If transfusion is essential, packed cells are preferable to whole blood and units should be given slowly, to minimize the above risk.

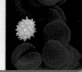

## Iron-deficiency metabolism and iron-deficiency anaemia

The body of an adult normally contains 4–5 g (75–90 mmol) of iron. The majority of this is in haemoglobin (2.5 g, 45 mmol) and a further 1.5 g (27 mmol) is in storage in the tissues. Small quantities are found in the muscle pigment, myoglobin and in some intracellular enzymes, such as cytochrome oxidase.

Iron requirements are obtained from dietary sources. Foods vary both in their iron content and in the availability of iron for absorption. Iron is mainly obtained from meat, liver, eggs, green vegetables and fruit. A mixed Western daily diet typically contains 10–15 mg, of which only 5–10% is absorbed, and this is enough to meet normal requirements.

In the stomach, gastric acid causes the bound iron to be released and converted to the ferrous form. Ferrous iron is then absorbed in the duodenum and jejunum. Normally only about 5–10% of the daily intake is absorbed, although a greater amount might be absorbed if body stores of iron are deficient. Absorption of 0.5–1.0 mg (9–18 µmol) of iron is sufficient for the requirements of a healthy man.

The amount of iron required each day to compensate for losses from the body and growth varies with age and sex. It is highest in pregnancy and in adolescent and menstruating females. The need for iron is greater for women of reproductive age than for men because of the blood loss that occurs during menstruation. Pregnancy increases iron requirements considerably, particularly in the last 2 months when the fetus and placenta are growing rapidly. Growing children also require more iron than a healthy adult man. These groups are therefore most likely to develop anaemia due to iron deficiency (Hoffbrand et al., 2001).

Iron is carried in the plasma bound to the protein, **transferrin**. It is stored in the tissues (liver, spleen, bone marrow and cells of the mononuclear phagocytic system) in two forms. About two-thirds of storage iron are attached to the tissue protein **apoferritin** and is stored as **ferritin**. The remaining third is stored as **haemosiderin**, which is a conglomerate of ferritin molecules. Trace amounts of ferritin occur in plasma and the quantity indicates the magnitude of body iron stores. Serum iron concentration is normally 13–32 µmol/L (70–175 µg/dL). If iron deficiency develops, iron stores are depleted first, followed by haemoglobin and then myoglobin and enzymes. During pregnancy, fetal iron requirements take precedence over those of the mother.

Although red cells and their constituent haemoglobin are continually being broken down, the vast majority of the iron released is retained for reutilization in the body. Only small amounts of iron are excreted: in urine and bile, desquamated cells of the skin and gut mucosa, and in menstrual fluid. In healthy adults, this amount balances that absorbed from the diet.

**Iron poisoning** can occur when storage of iron is greatly increased (**siderosis**). The main causes of iron overload are increased intestinal absorption and excessive parenteral administration, as, for example, in multiple blood transfusions. The former can be due to failure to control iron absorption, as in **haemochromatosis**, an inherited condition associated with cirrhosis of the liver. Increased absorption might also be due to regular high iron intake. This is usually the result of regularly ingesting large quantities of cheap wine and cider, which contain high levels of iron. Acute iron poisoning is a significant cause of death in young children and the result of accidentally ingesting attractively coloured iron tablets.

Excessive parenteral administration of iron usually occurs in the form of multiple blood transfusions as, for example, in the treatment of the haemolytic anaemia of thalassaemia.

Iron poisoning, whether acute or chronic, is treated by administration of the chelating agent, desferrioxamine, which both reduces iron absorption from the gut and increases iron excretion in the urine.

The causes of iron deficiency (see below) follow from the physiology described in the preceding paragraphs.

- poor diet
- excessive requirements
- lack of gastric acid
- malabsorption
- blood loss.

The history of a person with iron deficiency anaemia might contain features that reflect the cause of the iron deficiency, and it is important that this cause is found and treated whenever possible.

In most cases of iron deficiency anaemia, the amount of iron required to restore normal amounts of haemoglobin and replenish iron stores cannot be supplied in the diet and so additional iron preparations are required. Whenever possible, these are given orally, for example as ferrous sulphate. Gastrointestinal upsets of various kinds can occur as side-effects. Intramuscular and parenteral iron preparations are available but their use is associated with unpleasant side-effects, such as skin staining and anaphylactic reactions, and so they are given only when it is necessary to replace iron stores rapidly.

## VITAMIN B12 AND ITS DEFICIENCY

**Vitamin B12** (hydroxocobalamin) is synthesized by bacteria and occurs in significant amounts only in foods of animal origin, that is, meat, liver, eggs, milk and cheese. Humans obtain all their vitamin B12 from their diet: a mixed diet contains 5–30 μg per day and the daily adult requirement is 2–3 μg. This requirement balances the daily loss from the body, largely in urine and faeces.

Vitamin B12 is absorbed in the ileum, mainly in combination with **intrinsic factor (IF)**, a glycoprotein secreted by the main gastric glands into the gastric juice (see Chapter 5.1). During absorption, IF is split from the vitamin B12.

Vitamin B12 is transported in plasma bound to plasma protein. It is rapidly taken up by the tissues, especially the liver, and liver stores may last for several years, even if no further vitamin B12 is absorbed.

Deficiency of this vitamin causes anaemia because the vitamin is necessary for the synthesis of a precursor of thymine. Thymine is a constituent of deoxyribonucleic acid (DNA) and so DNA formation is limited in vitamin B12 deficiency; this causes increased size of red cell precursors and megaloblastosis.

The major causes of vitamin B12 deficiency are as follows.

- Lack of gastric intrinsic factor. The most common reason for this is autoimmune gastric atrophy, and it is this condition that produces the classical Addisonian **pernicious anaemia** of vitamin B12 deficiency. Total and partial gastrectomy result in loss of IF.
- Malabsorption of the IF/B12 complex.
- Strict vegetarian (vegan) diet, containing no animal products.

Vitamin B12 deficiency is treated by intramuscular injections of hydroxocobalamin, administered monthly or even less frequently. Typically, the patient feels significantly better within 48 hours of commencing treatment.

## FOLIC ACID (FOLATE) AND ITS DEFICIENCY

**Folic acid** is present in foods of animal and vegetable origin but is destroyed by heat. The major dietary sources are liver, green vegetables and oranges. A typical Western diet contains 500–800 μg per day and the daily adult requirement is 100–200 μg. This excess of intake over requirement compensates for the poor absorption of some forms of the vitamin and for losses through cooking.

Folates are absorbed in the duodenum and jejunum and liver stores are sufficient to last a few weeks if intake ceases. Small amounts are excreted in urine and faeces. Like vitamin B12, folates promote thymine synthesis and hence DNA synthesis. As a result, folate **deficiency** causes a megaloblastic anaemia with essentially the same features as vitamin B12 deficiency anaemia, except that neurological deficiency does not occur, and intrinsic factor activity and gastric acid are normal.

The major causes of folic acid deficiency are:

- poor diet
- increased requirements
- malabsorption
- the presence of folic acid antagonists, for example the antimitotic drug methotrexate.

Treatment is with oral folic acid preparations and the response is usually rapid.

## The life span and breakdown of red cells

The life span of normal red cells in a normal circulation is approximately 120 days. As they have no nucleus, red cells are unable to replace structural proteins and enzymes needed for normal function. As red cells circulate in the blood, the plasma membrane becomes progressively damaged in the microcirculation (the minimum diameter of which is 3.5 μm) until it eventually ruptures.

Old red cells are ingested and destroyed by the macrophage cells of the mononuclear phagocytic system (phagocytic cells found in bone marrow, liver, lymph nodes, spleen and subcutaneous tissues). The spleen, in particular, functions in the removal of abnormal red cells, and splenomegaly (enlargement of the spleen) is often a clinical feature of conditions in which abnormalities of red cells occur. Very defective red cells, such as those in sickle-cell disease or spherocytosis, haemolyse in the circulation.

### Haemoglobin breakdown

Within the macrophage cells, the ring of the haem in each haemoglobin molecule is opened by oxidation, so that the haem ring becomes a straight chain. This causes the haem to split from the globin portion of the molecule. The globin is catabolized (broken down) to its constituent amino acids and these enter the general metabolic pool to be reutilized in the synthesis of new protein.

Iron is removed from the opened haem ring and the majority is reutilized in the synthesis of new iron-containing compounds, mainly haemoglobin. The remainder is retained in storage forms in the tissues. Only a minute amount is lost from the body.

The remainder of the haem molecule is converted into the pigment bilirubin and transported to the liver, bound to plasma albumin. In the liver it is conjugated with glucuronic acid to form a water-soluble

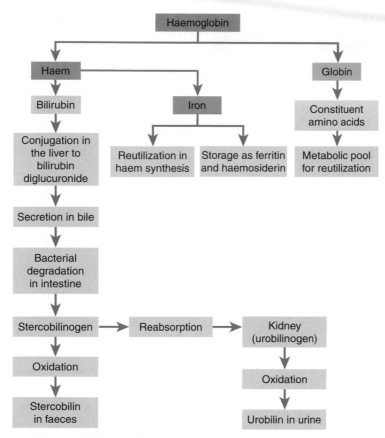

**Figure 4.1.7** A summary of haemoglobin breakdown

compound that is excreted in the bile. The excretion of bilirubin is described fully in Chapter 5.2. **Figure 4.1.7** summarizes the breakdown of the haemoglobin molecule.

Specific mechanisms exist to prevent the loss from the body of haem, and the iron it contains, during red cell destruction. Normally, this process occurs within macrophage cells so that haemoglobin is contained. However, if haemolysis occurs in the circulation, haemoglobin is released into the blood. The molecular mass of haemoglobin (68 000) is such that the molecule will pass into the glomerular filtrate and be excreted in the urine.

Excretion of haemoglobin is prevented by the presence of the plasma proteins **haptoglobins** and **haemopexin** in the plasma. These bind to free haemoglobin and haem, respectively, forming molecular complexes that are too large to be excreted and are instead taken up by the mononuclear phagocytic system. Only when both these mechanisms for iron conservation are saturated will free haemoglobin be excreted in the urine (haemoglobinuria).

## White blood cells (leucocytes)

The blood of a healthy adult contains $4–11 \times 10^9$ white blood cells per litre (there are 1000 erythrocytes in the blood for every leucocyte). This is the **white cell count (WCC** or **WBC)**, which, unlike the red cell count, represents only a small proportion of the total number of white cells in the body because the majority are in the tissues. Within these limits, quite large variations can occur in an individual, from hour to hour, as various physiological factors (such as exercise and emotion) influence white cells to enter or leave the circulation. The white cell count of a newborn baby is normally approximately double that of an adult and gradually decreases to reach adult values at between 5 and 10 years of age.

Several types of white cell can be distinguished on examination of a stained blood film. Cells are classified into groups on the basis of various morphological characteristics, such as the presence or absence of a granular cytoplasm, the staining reaction of the cytoplasm and the shape of the nucleus. A **differential white cell count** is obtained by classifying and counting the first 100 white blood cells observed on examining a blood film and expressing the result as a percentage of the total. Reference ranges for the different types of white blood cell are given in **Table 4.1.6**.

An increase in the white cell count above the normal range (i.e. greater than $11 \times 10^9$/L) is called a **leucocytosis**, and a decrease below the normal range (i.e. less than $4 \times 10^9$/L) a **leucopenia**. If a specific

**Table 4.1.6** Reference ranges for the white blood cell count

| White cell type | Count per litre of blood |
|---|---|
| All white cells (WBC or WCC) | $4-11 \times 10^9$ |
| Differential white cell count, in absolute numbers and as percentage of total count (parentheses): | |
| neutrophils | $2.0-7.5 \times 10^9$ (40–75) |
| eosinophils | $0.04-0.4 \times 10^9$ (1–6) |
| basophils | $0.0-0.1 \times 10^9$ (0–1) |
| monocytes | $0.2-0.8 \times 10^9$ (2–10) |
| lymphocytes | $1.5-4.0 \times 10^9$ (20–45) |

type of white cell is causing the abnormal count it is described accordingly, for example a neutrophil leucocytosis or a lymphocytosis.

## Types of white blood cell

### Granulocytes (polymorphonuclear leucocytes)

These cells are characterized by the presence of granules in the cytoplasm and a lobed nucleus, hence their names. They are 10–14 μm in diameter. Within the group, three cell types can be distinguished from the staining reaction and size of their cytoplasmic granules. They, too, have been named accordingly:

- **Neutrophils** contain cytoplasmic granules of varying size that stain violet with a neutral dye. As they are by far the most numerous of the granulocytes (see Table 4.1.6) and have the most lobular nucleus, neutrophils often monopolize the term polymorphonuclear leucocyte (PML) (Fig. 4.1.8a).
- The cytoplasm of **eosinophils** contains large, distinctive granules which take up an acidic dye and stain red. The nucleus typically has two lobes (Fig. 4.1.8b).
- **Basophils** have large, basophilic cytoplasmic granules that take up a basic dye and stain blue/black. The nucleus typically has two to three lobes (Fig. 4.1.8c).

### The production of granulocytes (granulopoiesis)

Granulocytes arise from bone marrow stem cells. Precursor cells develop from pluripotential stem cells under the influence of interleukin growth factors. A mixed myeloid precursor cell type then gives rise to new cells, which are increasingly committed to red

cell, platelet granulocyte and monocyte production (Hoffbrand et al., 2001) (see Fig. 4.1.3). As can be seen from **Fig. 4.1.3**, neutrophils and monocytes arise from a single progenitor type.

Postnatally, production of granulocytes normally occurs only in red marrow. **Granulopoiesis** is characterized by progressive condensation and lobulation of the nucleus, a reduction in the amount of cytoplasmic organelles, for example mitochondria, and the development of an abundance of cytoplasmic granules in the cells involved.

The development of a polymorphonuclear leucocyte can take a fortnight but this time can be considerably reduced when there is increased demand, as, for example, in bacterial infection. The red marrow also contains a large reserve pool of mature granulocytes so that for every circulating cell there might be 50–100 cells in the marrow.

Mature cells pass actively through the endothelial lining of the marrow sinusoid into the circulation. In the circulation, about half the granulocytes adhere closely to the internal surface of the blood vessels. These are called **marginating cells** and are not normally included in the white cell count. The other half circulate in the blood and exchange with the marginating population.

Within 7 hours, half the granulocytes will have left the circulation in response to specific requirements for these cells in the tissues. Once a granulocyte has left the blood it does not return. It can survive in the tissues for 4 or 5 days, or less, depending on the conditions it meets.

The turnover of granulocytes is, therefore, very high. Dead cells are eliminated from the body in faeces and respiratory secretions, and are also destroyed by tissue macrophages (monocytes).

### Functions of granulocytes

**Neutrophils** are actively mobile, phagocytic cells and their shape is constantly changing due to amoeboid movement. The granules in their cytoplasm are enzymes that have a digestive, or lytic, action.

The major **function** of neutrophils is in inflammation of bacterial origin. The vascular endothelium becomes sticky at the site of the inflammation. Neutrophils adhere to this sticky endothelium and to each other, forming clumps. They then actively move into the tissues, probably passing between the junctions of the endothelial cells. This process is known as **diapedesis**.

In the tissues, neutrophils are attracted to the site of inflammation by various substances produced there, for example bacterial toxins and components of the inflammatory and immune responses. This process is known as **chemotaxis**. When a neutrophil

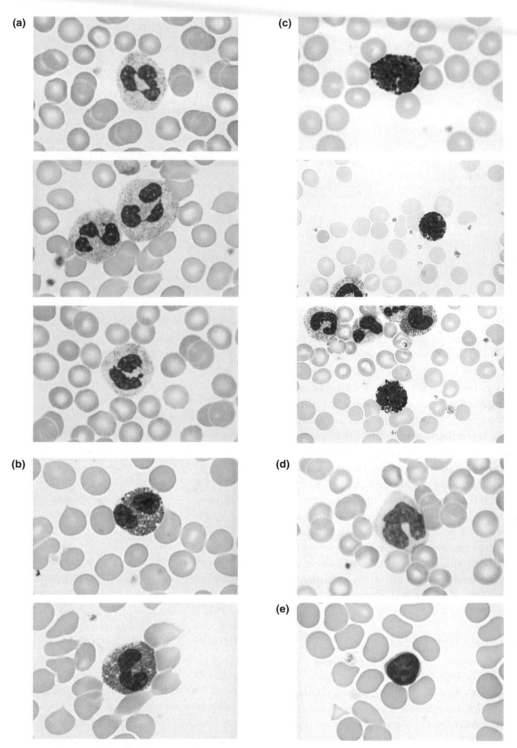

**Figure 4.1.8** Leucocytes: (a) neutrophils, (b) eosinophils, (c) basophils, (d) monocyte and (e) lymphocyte. Reproduced with permission from Hoffbrand, A.V. & Pettit, J.E. (2002) Color Atlas of Hematology, 3rd edn. St Louis: Mosby

comes into contact with a bacterium, **phagocytosis** (cell eating) occurs **(Fig. 4.1.9)**. The cell membrane of the neutrophil becomes invaginated until the bacterium is completely engulfed in a digestive vacuole. Phagocytosis occurs much more easily if the bacterium is coated with immunoglobulin or complement, a process called **opsonization**.

Once the bacterium is completely engulfed, the lytic enzymes of the granules are released into the digestive pouch where they digest and kill the bacterium.

Neutrophils also act as scavengers in the tissues, removing small inanimate particles such as antigen-antibody complexes. For this reason they are

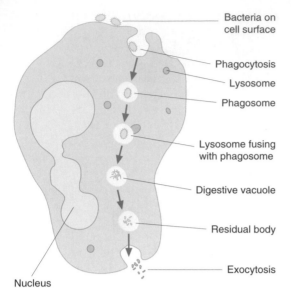

Bacteria on
cell surface

Phagocytosis

Lysosome

Phagosome

Lysosome fusing
with phagosome

Digestive vacuole

Residual body

Exocytosis

Nucleus

**Figure 4.1.9**   Phagocytosis by a neutrophil

sometimes called **tissue microphages** (Greek: *micro* = small, *phage* = swallow), whereas monocytes are tissue macrophages. The ability of neutrophils to metabolize without oxygen is crucial to their function of removing bacteria and cell debris in necrotic tissue.

Large numbers of neutrophils can be destroyed during an acute inflammatory response to a bacterial infection. The contents and cell debris of dead neutrophils form the **pus** that occurs at such a site, for example a boil, abscess or infected cut.

Some bacteria produce toxins that act as pyrogens (fever-producing substances). It is likely that these induce fever by interacting with neutrophils to produce a polypeptide called **leucocyte** (or **endogenous**) **pyrogen**. This polypeptide is able to cross the blood–brain barrier and affect the temperature-regulating centre in the hypothalamus.

The secretion of adrenaline (epinephrine) in acute stress produces a transient increase in the number of circulating neutrophils. Increased levels of adrenocorticotrophic hormone and glucocorticoids, for example hydrocortisone, which occur in stress and steroid therapy, also increase the number of circulating neutrophils. However, the action of these hormones impairs the ability of neutrophils to migrate into the tissues and so resistance to infection is impaired despite their increased numbers.

**Eosinophils (see Table 4.1.6 and Fig. 4.1.8b)** are mobile, phagocytic cells. They destroy animate and inanimate particles, but less actively than neutrophils and monocytes. Their cytoplasmic granules contain most of the lytic enzymes found in neutrophil granules.

Eosinophils enter inflammatory exudates and have a special role in defence against parasites, in allergic responses and in the removal of fibrin formed during inflammation.

**Basophils (see Table 4.1.6 and Fig. 4.1.8c)** are the circulating counterparts of **tissue mast cells** (i.e. they become mast cells on entering the tissues). The cytoplasmic granules of basophils contain histamine and heparin. Mast cells are widely distributed in the body and are commonly found in close proximity to the walls of small blood vessels. They are able to bind specific IgE antibody to their surface and subsequent exposure of a basophil that has done this to the antigen for which the bound IgE is specific, leads to rapid breakdown and loss of the basophil's histamine granules.

Basophils are involved in **anaphylactic reactions**, which are mainly due to the effects of the release of **histamine**. In humans, histamine produces vasodilation and hence a fall in blood pressure and rise in heart rate. It increases the tone of most types of smooth muscle and stimulates exocrine secretion. It also produces itching or, in high concentrations, pain. Antihistamine drugs, for example promethazine (Phenergan) and loratadine (Clarytyn) are very effective against anaphylactic conditions. **Heparin** is a powerful anticoagulant. In anaphylaxis, blood clotting is inhibited due to the release of heparin.

## Agranulocytes

These white blood cells are so called because of the non-granular appearance of their cytoplasm when viewed with a light microscope, although very small granules are in fact present. Two types of cell are distinguished, monocytes and lymphocytes.

Monocytes (see Table 4.1.6 and Fig. 4.1.8d) are large cells with a diameter of 10–18 μm. They have a large oval or indented nucleus which is pale staining and positioned non-centrally. The cytoplasm appears clear and stains pale blue. It contains many mitochondria and other cytoplasmic organelles, and may contain very fine granules, known as azurophilic granules. Monocytes are produced in the bone marrow, developing from precursors in common with granulocyte neutrophils (see Fig. 4.1.3).

Mature cells spend only a short time in marrow and after about 30 hours leave the blood to enter the tissues where they mature and carry out their principal functions.

Monocytes are actively phagocytic and, in the tissues, they mature into larger cells called **macrophages** (Greek: *macro* = big, *phage* = eat), which can survive in the tissues for periods of months or even years. These cells form the mononuclear phagocytic cells of the mononuclear phagocytic system (reticuloendothelial system) in bone marrow, liver, spleen and lymph nodes. Tissue macrophages (sometimes called **histiocytes**) respond more slowly than neutrophils to chemotactic stimuli. They engulf and destroy bacteria, protozoa, dead cells and foreign matter. They also facilitate the immune response by processing antigen structure and presenting antigen at the lymphocyte's surface. This is essential if full antigenic stimulation of both T and B lymphocytes is to take place.

Lymphocytes (see Table 4.1.6 and Fig. 4.1.8e) are round cells containing large round nuclei. The cytoplasm stains pale blue and appears non-granular under light microscopy. However, some cytoplasmic granules and organelles are present.

Morphologically, lymphocytes can be divided into two groups: the more numerous **small lymphocytes**, with a diameter of 7–10 μm; and **large lymphocytes**, which have a diameter of 10–14 μm. Lymphocytes are produced in bone marrow (see Fig. 4.1.3) from primitive precursors, the lymphoblasts and prolymphocytes. Immature cells migrate to the thymus and other lymphoid tissues, including that found in bone marrow, and undergo further division, processing and maturation.

Functionally, there are two main types of lymphocyte: **T (thymus processed or dependent) lymphocytes**, which are involved in cell-mediated immune responses, for example against intracellular organisms including bacteria, viruses, protozoa and fungi, and also against transplanted organs. T lymphocytes account for 80% of lymphocytes in blood. **B (bursa or bone marrow dependent) lymphocytes** produce plasma cells, which secrete antibodies (immunoglobulins) and so produce humoral immunity. T and B lymphocytes are morphologically indistinguishable, and their identification is dependent on the detection of surface markers. B lymphocytes have membrane-bound surface immunoglobulins and T cells do not; 60–80% of lymphocytes circulating in the blood are T cells. During the first 2 years of life lymphocytes are the most numerous of white blood cells, constituting approximately 50% of the white cell count. This falls to normal adult levels (20–40%) at between 5 and 10 years of age.

Lymphocytes spend a very small proportion of their life cycle in the blood and most of it in the lymphoid tissues. At any one time there are many more lymphocytes in the tissues than in blood. However, unlike granulocytes, lymphocytes recirculate between the blood and lymphatic tissues, returning to the blood via the thoracic duct. Both T and B lymphocytes can have a short or long life span. However, T cells are generally long lived (2–4 years) and B cells typically have a shorter life span, measured in days or weeks.

As circulating lymphocytes represent only a tiny proportion of the cells in the body's lymphoid tissue, even major abnormalities of lymphoid function might not be apparent from the white cell count.

## CLINICAL APPLICATIONS

The major causes of an abnormally raised lymphocyte count (**lymphocytosis**) include lymphoid malignancy and viral infection, particularly that caused by the Epstein–Barr virus, the causative agent of infectious mononucleosis (glandular fever). A decreased lymphocyte count mainly reflects reduced numbers of T lymphocytes. It might be due to immune deficiency disease or be the result of high levels of circulating glucocorticoids (steroids), cytoxic therapy, or malignant disease, for example Hodgkin's disease.

Chapter 6.2 on acquired immune defences discusses the functions of these cells in much more detail.

**Leukaemia** is produced by a malignant proliferation of leucopoietic tissue. The disease is classified according to its course and duration and the predominant affected white cell type, for example acute lymphoblastic leukaemia and chronic myeloid leukaemia. The former is mainly a disease of childhood and the latter usually affects middle-aged adults.

Characteristically there is a leucocytosis consisting mainly of immature and abnormal white cells of the type affected. The malignant leucopoietic tissue also infiltrates and displaces other haemopoietic tissues and may infiltrate the liver and spleen.

People who have leukaemia are prone to infection because a large proportion of their white cells are not fully functional due to cellular immaturity. They might also be anaemic because of depressed erythropoiesis and prone to bleed because of reduced platelet production. The major clinical features of leukaemia are due to these three factors.

Leukaemia is usually diagnosed from an examination of the person's blood count and the results of a bone marrow biopsy. The most effective therapy includes intensive cytotoxic chemotherapy and supportive measures such as the use of broad-spectrum antibiotics to prevent infection, and blood transfusion to increase levels of red cells, mature white cells and platelets. Bone marrow and/or stem cell transplant might also be considered.

## White cell antigens

**Antigens** on the surface of white blood cells can be either specific to the cell type or also present on other cells of the body. Of the latter type, the most important clinically is the **human leucocyte antigen** (HLA) system. This genetically determined set of antigens occurs on the surface of most body cells and forms the basis of tissue typing for the purposes of matching prior to organ transplantation. For this reason the HLA system is sometimes called the **major histocompatibility complex** (MHC).

The major clinical application of HLA typing is in the selection of compatible donor/recipient pairs for organ transplantation. It is also worth noting the interesting association of certain HLA antigens with the occurrence of certain diseases. Over 100 diseases, including ankylosing spondylitis and diabetes mellitus, are associated with the presence of specific HLA antigens. However, the precise mechanism by which the presence of certain antigens affects susceptibility to a particular disease remains unclear.

## Platelets

Platelets are the smallest cellular elements in blood. They are colourless, non-nucleated, discoid bodies, with a diameter of 2–4 μm, a volume of 7 fl and a life span of 7–10 days. The number of platelets in a normal adult's blood ranges from 150 to $400 \times 10^9$ per litre. This is the **platelet count**. Children have similar levels of circulating platelets. In animal physiology, platelets are sometimes called thrombocytes and the prefix 'thrombo', which relates to the function of platelets in clot (thrombus) formation, is used in human physiology in terms relating to platelet production and under- and overproduction (see below).

### Production (thrombopoiesis)

Platelets are produced in bone marrow. They are formed in the cytoplasm of a very large cell, the **megakaryocyte**, derived in bone marrow from a megakaryoblast that has differentiated from the

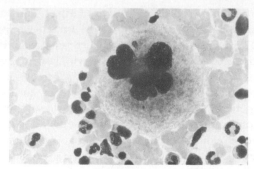

**Figure 4.1.10** Megakaryocyte. Reproduced with permission from Hoffbrand, A.V. & Pettit, J.E. (2002) Color Atlas of Hematology, 3rd edn. St Louis: Mosby

pluripotential stem cell (**see Fig. 4.1.3**). The megakaryocytes enlarge by a number of mitotic replications, which take place inside the cell, and the cytoplasm then becomes granular and fragments at the edge of the cell (**Fig. 4.1.10**). This process is called **platelet budding**. Each megakaryocyte produces about 4000 platelets and the whole process from stem cell to platelet budding takes about 10 days.

Platelet production is under the control of a humoral growth agent, **thrombopoietin**, which is produced in the liver and kidney.

At any one time, about two-thirds of the body's platelets are circulating in the blood and one-third is pooled in the spleen. There is constant exchange between the two populations. They are destroyed by platelet plug formation and by macrophages in the spleen and the liver.

## Structure of platelets

Under the light microscope, platelets are normally disc shaped and their structure appears relatively simple, with a transparent cytoplasm and a central, more darkly staining, granular area. Electron microscopy and biochemical analysis reveal a far more complex structure.

The platelet plasma membrane has the dimensions of, and contains the usual components of, a cell membrane. It is the site of many enzymes and also contains glycoprotein receptors (GP) for numerous substances, such as collagen, adrenaline (epinephrine) and serotonin (5-hydroxytryptamine; 5-HT). These glycoproteins are crucial to the platelet functions of adhesion and aggregation (see below), which are the initial steps of platelet plug formation. The platelet plasma membrane also contains phospholipids that provide a surface for the important conversion of clotting factor X to Xa and in the activation of prothrombin (II to IIa). The platelet plasma membrane dips in and out of the cytoplasm providing a very large surface area, like an open series of canals, onto which clotting factors can be adsorbed.

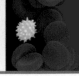

The platelet cytoplasm contains microtubules and microfilaments composed of a contractile protein called **thombosthenin**, which functions in clot retraction. The cytoplasm also contains numerous dense granules, which are composed of the nucleotides adenosine diphosphate (ADP) and adenosine triphosphate (ATP), serotonin and calcium. Other specific granules occur frequently and are collectively known as α granules. These contain certain clotting factors and growth factors. Lysosomes and peroxisomes are also present. When the platelets release their granules these are discharged into the open cytoplasmic canal system.

## Functions of platelets

The major functions of platelets are in haemostasis (the arrest of bleeding). Through **adhesion** to the damaged endothelium of a blood vessel, **release** of cytoplasmic granules and **aggregation** (interaction with each other so that they stick together), they form a **platelet plug**, which can stop blood flow. Haemostasis is initially dependent on the formation of this plug, which occurs very rapidly. The plug is normally stabilized later by the formation of a fibrin clot.

Platelets also function in blood clotting, providing essential coagulation factors various stages in the formation of a clot and in clot retraction and a phospholipid surface on which the process of clotting occurs. These important functions of platelets are described in more detail in the next section on haemostasis.

Platelets store and transport histamine and serotonin, both of which are released when platelets are destroyed and function in the early response to injury, affecting the tone of smooth muscle in blood vessel walls.

Normal platelets probably have a nutritional function, supplying the endothelial cells of blood vessels with nutrients, because these cells atrophy in platelet deficiency. They secrete a growth factor (platelet-derived growth factor; PDGF), which stimulates proliferation of smooth muscle cells in artery walls and can hasten vascular healing following injury.

### CLINICAL APPLICATIONS

Abnormalities of platelet production and/or function are one of the most common causes of defects in haemostasis. The latter is usually normal until the platelet count falls to $40 \times 10^9$/L (normal range is 150–400 $\times 10^9$/L). When the count falls below $20 \times 10^9$/L, spontaneous bleeding is likely to occur. An abnormally low platelet count is called **thrombocytopenia**. An abnormally high platelet count (**thrombocytosis**) occurs in several diseases, for example myeloid leukaemia, and immediately after splenectomy.

## Haemostasis: The physiological arrest of bleeding

Haemostasis is a fundamental homeostatic process that functions to prevent the loss of blood from the vascular system and to ensure the patency of the blood vessels. Normally, it is very effective in controlling bleeding from breached capillaries, arterioles and venules, and even small arteries and veins, but it is insufficient to halt haemorrhage from large vessels. In the last-mentioned situation, non-physiological intervention, first aid, medical and surgical measures are required to control blood loss.

Natural haemostasis stops blood loss because constituents of the blood and damaged blood vessel wall react together to form a solid mass that blocks the hole in the vessel. Bleeding will also slow, or cease, if the blood pressure within the vessel approaches or becomes equal to the external hydrostatic pressure. This can occur either if there is a local or general fall in blood pressure or if inflammation and the accumulation of blood in the surrounding tissues raise the external pressure.

For clarity of description, haemostasis can be divided into four phases. However, it should be recognized that the events of these phases interact and are synergistic; they do not occur in a straightforward sequence. The four phases of haemostasis are as follows.

1. Contraction of the smooth muscle cells in the wall of the breached vessel, with resultant vasocontriction – the myogenic reflex.
2. Formation of a platelet plug.
3. Formation of a fibrin clot (blood clotting or coagulation) and retraction of the fibrin clot.
4. Fibrinolysis – the breakdown of a fibrin clot.

Haemostasis is outlined in **Fig. 4.1.11**, and the events of each of the above phases are described below.

### Phase 1: vasoconstriction (the myogenic reflex)

Immediately after injury, reflex vasoconstriction and retraction of the severed ends of injured blood vessels occurs and spreads to adjacent small vessels. The reduced blood flow allows contact activation of platelets and clotting factors and reduces the likelihood of the platelet plug (Phase 2) being washed away. Serotonin and thromboxane $A_2$, released from platelets, potentiate this reflex vasoconstriction, which lasts approximately 20 minutes.

Capillary walls contain no smooth muscle and so are not stimulated to constrict. In capillary bleeding, blood flow through the capillary bed can be reduced by reflex contraction of precapillary sphincters.

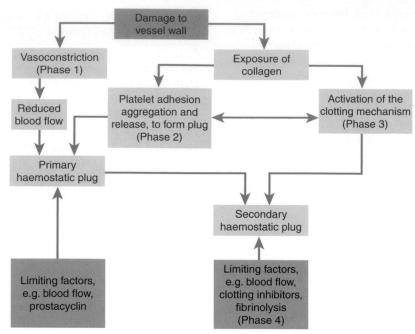

Figure 4.1.11   An outline of the main events in haemostasis

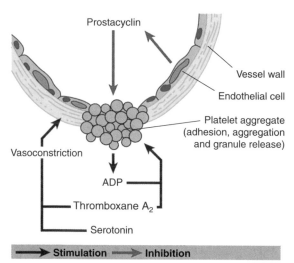

Figure 4.1.12   Summary of events in the formation of a platelet plug

Additionally, adhesion of the endothelial (intimal) surfaces of capillaries and small blood vessels may occur following vasoconstriction, and this may seal the hole.

## Phase 2: the formation of a platelet plug (Fig. 4.1.12)

### Platelet adhesion

Damage to a blood vessel wall that exposes collagen and elastin microfilaments in the subendothelium causes passing platelets to adhere to the site, because platelets have membrane-based collagen receptors. Adhesion to collagen is facilitated by membrane

glycoproteins and by von Willebrand factor. This is a very large molecule that also carries clotting factor VIII (see later).

Platelet adherence causes the release of adenosine diphosphate (ADP) from the platelet, red cells and vessel wall. The ADP triggers platelet membrane changes that lead to the platelets assuming a spherical shape with pseudopodia, instead of their more characteristic disc shape. These membrane changes promote platelet aggregation (interaction with one another so that they stick together). Platelet aggregation is also promoted by many other substances, such as serotonin and certain clotting (coagulation) factors.

### Platelet release

The process of platelet adhesion and aggregation is reversible until the platelets discharge or 'release' their granules. Granule contents include ADP, serotonin, lysosomal enzymes and a heparin antagonist. After platelet release has occurred, white blood cells begin to adhere to the degranulated platelets and clotting or coagulation (Phase 3) occurs.

During aggregation, the unstable substance **thromboxane $A_2$ (TXA$_2$)** is produced by the platelets from prostaglandin precursors and is a powerful inducer of both aggregation and vasoconstriction.

### CLINICAL APPLICATIONS

The production of thromboxane $A_2$ is inhibited by non-steroidal anti-inflammatory drugs, for example aspirin and phenylbutazone. This action

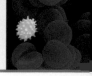

partially explains the antithrombotic effect of these drugs and their ability to prolong the bleeding time. The antithrombotic drug sulphinpyrazone (Anturan) also inhibits platelet prostaglandin synthesis and hence adhesion and aggregation.

Within the endothelial cells of the vessel wall, prostaglandin endoperoxides are converted into **prostacyclin**, a substance that powerfully inhibits aggregation and produces vasodilation. Prostacyclin has now been synthesized and is a potential antithrombotic agent for clinical use. The drug dipyridamole (Persantin) exerts its antithrombotic effect by enhancing the action of prostacyclin.

## Platelet aggregation

Thromboxane $A_2$ and ADP released from platelets cause additional platelets to aggregate at the site of the blood vessel injury. ADP causes the platelets to swell and encourages adherence of adjacent platelets. This adherence stimulates further release of cytoplasmic granules, promoting further aggregation. This positive feedback process leads to the formation of a platelet plug large enough to seal the area of endothelial injury (Hoffbrand et al., 2001).

Platelet aggregation also activates platelet phospholipid in the platelet plasma membrane (also known as platelet factor 3). This functions as a surface on to which various blood clotting factors bind and react as a result of their physical proximity; the formation of the complex that activates prothrombin occurs in this way. Once thrombin has been formed from activated prothrombin, it also acts as a powerful stimulus to further platelet aggregation.

In summary, three distinct mechanisms act to produce platelet aggregation and the formation of a platelet plug.

1. granule release following platelet adhesion
2. thromboxane $A_2$ generation and ADP release
3. the formation of thrombin in the clotting sequence.

The early stages of haemostasis are dependent on constriction of the damaged vessel wall and the formation of a platelet plug. The platelet plug is formed within a few seconds of injury and can withstand a blood pressure of up to 100 mmHg (13.3 kPa), and so might be sufficient to stop bleeding from small vessels. However, if the plug is not stabilized by fibrin fibres around the aggregated platelets, it is likely that it will break down and bleeding will restart after about 20 minutes. This phenomenon can occur after relatively minor injury, such as a dental extraction, in untreated people with a clotting disorder but normal platelet function, for example those with haemophilia.

The normal formation of the platelet plug is as important for haemostasis as blood clotting.

## Phase 3: the formation of a fibrin clot (blood clotting or coagulation)

It is important to understand that the process of blood coagulation is a massively amplifying system in which a sequence of reactions form a cascade that culminates in the production of a fibrin clot. The cascade sequence is amplifying in that minute amounts of the earlier factors result in the conversion of large amounts of fibrinogen into fibrin. The entire sequence takes 3–8 minutes (the bleeding time). Surface contact initiates a sequence of reactions in which an inactive proenzyme is converted into an active enzyme (identified by the suffix 'a'). The active enzyme then catalyses the activation of the second proenzyme in the sequence, and so on until the formation of the proteolytic enzyme thrombin, which catalyses the conversion of the soluble plasma protein fibrinogen to the insoluble fibrin clot. The initiation of this enzyme cascade, or 'waterfall', needs a concentration of circulating coagulation factors at the site of injury, and this is achieved on the platelet phospholipid surface (described above) and on exposed collagen fibres and tissue factor.

The essential endpoint of the process of coagulation is the formation of the insoluble protein **fibrin** from the soluble plasma protein **fibrinogen**. Thrombin splits off two peptides (fibrinopeptides A and B) from fibrinogen to form fibrin monomers. These monomers then polymerize to form a fibrin clot, which, in the presence of calcium ions and clotting factor XIII **(Table 4.1.7)**, stabilizes by cross-linking into a more permanent clot **(Fig. 4.1.13)**. Insoluble fibrin is laid down as a network of fine white threads that stick to each other and to tissue cells, and which entangle blood cells and platelets. (White fibrin threads can be seen if a blood clot is washed in water.) A new clot is a soft, jelly-like mass. This gradually retracts by more than a half, squeezing out serum. Clot retraction is dependent on normal platelet function, requiring the contractile platelet protein, **thrombosthenin**. A retracted clot is more solid and elastic and forms a tougher, more efficient haemostatic plug.

The coagulation factors involved in blood clotting were discovered mainly during the 1940s and 1950s. In 1961, an International Convention agreed that they should be designated Roman numerals for identification purposes. The numbers designated indicate the historical sequence of their discovery. The coagulation factors used currently are shown in **Table 4.1.7**.

In the circulation (in vivo) the process of coagulation is initiated by tissue damage. This damage generates tissue factor (coagulation factor III), sometimes known as thromboplastin. As tissue factor is extrinsic to blood, this activation mechanism has been called the **extrinsic system** and is the usual way

## Table 4.1.7 Coagulation factors

| Factor number | Factor name |
|---|---|
| I | Fibrinogen |
| II | Prothrombin |
| III | Tissue factor* (thromboplastin) |
| V | Labile factor* |
| VII | Proconvertin (stable factor) |
| VIII | Antihaemophilic factor A* (antihaemophilic globulin (AHG)) |
| IX | Christmas factor (antihaemophilic factor B) |
| X | Stuart–Prower factor |
| XI | Plasma thromboplastin antecedent (antihaemophilic factor C) |
| XII | Hageman contact |
| XIII | Fibrin stabilizing factor |
| | Prekallikrein (Fletcher factor) |
| | High-molecular-weight kininogen* (HMWK) (Fitzgerald factor) |

In their active form, most coagulation factors are proteolytic enzymes. Those marked with an asterisk act as cofactors to enzymic reactions.

of initiating coagulation in the body. In the presence of calcium ions, factor III forms a complex with factor VII, activating factor VII. This complex activates factors IX and X. The process is then amplified as factor Xa generates small amounts of thrombin, which activates cofactors V and VIII **(Fig. 4.1.14)**. The extrinsic system is rapid, the endproduct of a fibrin clot being produced in 10–14 seconds – the prothrombin time (PT). The amount of thrombin generated by this rapid route is too small to produce sustained clotting. However, it is large enough to trigger thrombin's positive feedback effects by activating factor IX. The classic 'intrinsic' pathway (see below) then produces the large amounts of thrombin required. Thus, the classic view of two parallel pathways has been replaced with an interactive cross-over process in which the extrinsic system provides the means for recruiting the more potent classic pathway.

The second 'classic' or 'intrinsic' pathway for blood coagulation is thought not to take place naturally in vivo but instead explains results obtained in coagulation testing 'in vitro'. It has been called the 'intrinsic' mechanism because only constituents of blood take part in the reactions. It is initiated by contact with a negatively charged surface between factor XII, kallikrein and high-molecular-weight kininogen (HMWK). Such surface contact activates factor XII, which then activates factor XI. Activated factor XI activates factor IX. Activated factor IX then forms a molecular complex with factor VIII and platelet phospholipid (platelet factor 3). This complex activates factor X. Once activated, factor Xa reacts with its cofactor Va, in the presence of platelet phospholipid (platelet factor 3), which provides a surface on which the reagents are concentrated. This complex is termed **prothrombin activator**. Once factor X is activated, clotting occurs in seconds, due to the rapid formation and action of thrombin. In other words, in normal clotting the first appearance of fibrin can take several minutes but, once fibrin has been formed, its production is complete within seconds. The intrinsic pathway normally takes 30–40 seconds and is measured by the activated partial thromboplastin time (APTT).

The extrinsic in vivo mechanism of blood clotting is summarized in **Fig. 4.1.14**, which includes indication of where the main inhibitors of the process have their effect. This level of detail is included here to illustrate the interactive nature and complexity of the system, and the control mechanisms that exist. Although they appear complex, the mechanisms described here are, in fact, an oversimplification of actual events. It is not expected that students (other than those particularly interested in this subject) will necessarily remember the detail. Understanding the overall concepts of amplification, cascade reaction

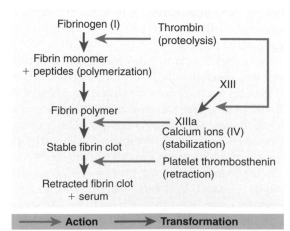

**Figure 4.1.13** Events in the formation of a fibrin clot from fibrinogen

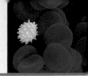

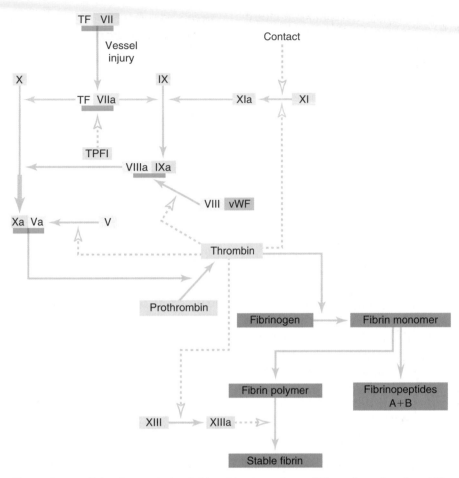

**Figure 4.1.14**   The pathway of blood coagulation initiated by tissue factor (TF) on the cell surface. When plasma comes into contact with TF, factor VII binds to TF. The complex of TF and activated VII (VIIa) activates X and IX. TF pathway inhibitor (TFPI) is an important inhibitor of TF/VIIIa. VIIIa–IXa complex greatly amplifies Xa production from X. The generation of thrombin from prothrombin by the action of Xa–Va complex leads to fibrin formation. Thrombin also activates XI (dashed line). V and XIII. Thrombin cleaves VIII from its carrier von Willebrand factor (vWF) greatly increasing the formation of VIIIa–IXa and hence of Xa–Va. Pale green, serine proteases; yellow, cofactors. Reproduced with permission from Hoffbrand, Pettit, Moss. *Essential Haematology* 4e. © 2001 Blackwell Science.'

and control systems is important. **Figure 4.1.15** summarizes the process and shows that the essential endpoints of both the intrinsic and extrinsic systems are common from the point of activation of factor X.

## Physiological inhibition of coagulation

The process of coagulation is tightly regulated (Norris, 2003). Blood almost certainly contains natural inhibitors of all the clotting factors and their presence forms a crucial protective mechanism against widespread coagulation. These inhibitors regulate the generation and destruction of the active enzymes so that clotting does not spread from the site of blood loss and widespread intravascular coagulation is prevented. Several natural clotting inhibitors (anticoagulants) have been identified. Probably the most important of these is antithrombin.

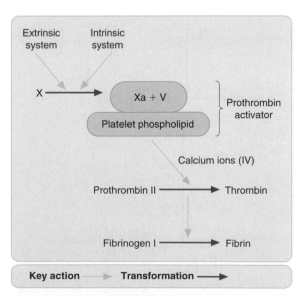

**Figure 4.1.15**   The essential reactions of the coagulation sequence

Antithrombin (AT) inhibits thrombin and several other coagulation factors. Deficiency of this plasma protein is inherited as a dominant condition. Low levels are associated with an increased tendency to intravascular clotting (thrombosis), particularly during pregnancy. Oral contraceptives containing oestrogen also depress the level of antithrombin.

The first inhibitor to have an effect is tissue factor pathway inhibitor (tFPI), present in platelets and plasma, which prevents the action of factors Xa and VIIa, as well as the action of tissue factor. Protein C and protein S combine to inactivate coagulation cofactors V and VIII, preventing further thrombin production.

## Phase 4: fibrinolysis (the dissolution of a fibrin clot) (Fig. 4.1.16)

Fibrinolysis is the normal process by which fibrin is degraded into soluble products that are then removed by cells of the mononuclear phagocytic system. Fibrinolysis takes place much more slowly than clotting. In health, the body maintains a homeostatic balance between the continual deposition of small amounts of fibrin and fibrin breakdown. The gradual removal of a blood clot by fibrinolysis is the final part of the normal process of healing, occurring after the breach has been healed. The fibrinolytic system also prevents excess fibrin deposition.

Fibrin is broken down by the proteolytic enzyme plasmin. Like thrombin, this enzyme is not present in plasma but is produced by the activation of the soluble plasma protein, plasminogen. Plasminogen is synthesized in the liver and is present in body fluids as well as in plasma. It has an affinity for fibrin and becomes absorbed on to a fibrin clot as the latter forms.

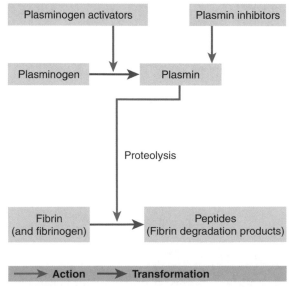

**Figure 4.1.16** Fibrinolysis

### Tissue plasminogen activator and fibrinolytic agents

Tissue plasminogen activator (tPA) is produced by endothelial cells. It binds to fibrin and in so doing enhances the conversion of plasminogen to plasmin. In its turn, tissue plasminogen activator is inactivated by plasminogen activator inhibitor (PAI) and circulating plasmin is inactivated by antiplasmin and macroglobulin. They inactivate plasmin by forming a complex with the molecule. This prevents widespread destruction of fibrin.

Activated protein C destroys inhibitors of tissue plasminogen activator and so stimulates fibrinolysis. However, thrombin inhibits fibrinolysis by activating thrombin activated fibrinolysis inhibitor (TAFI) (Hoffbrand et al., 2001).

## Role of endothelial cells in haemostasis

The endothelial cells lining blood vessels play an active role both in the maintenance of the patency of the blood vessel wall and in the haemostatic response. These cells produce the basement membrane that separates the protein fibres (collagen, elastin) of the connective tissue (subendothelial) supporting the blood vessel from the blood. Damage to the endothelium leads to blood loss and activation of the haemostatic mechanism (Hoffbrand et al., 2001). The endothelial cells synthesize a number of factors, some of which enhance and some of which inhibit haemostasis. Tissue factor, prostacyclin, von Willebrand factor (vWF), plasminogen activator, antithrombin (AT), thrombomodulin (TM – the surface protein receptor that binds thrombin and activates protein C) are all synthesized. Tissue factor pathway inhibitor (tFPI) and nitric oxide (NO) cause vasodilatation and so inhibit platelet aggregation and the initiation of haemostasis.

## Tests of haemostasis

Tests of haemostasis can be divided into two groups: screening tests and specific tests that identify the disorder. The latter, which include, for example, specific clotting factor assays, are performed in specialized laboratories. Screening tests assess the function of each of the components of haemostasis, that is:

- vascular function (bleeding time)
- platelet number (platelet count and bleeding time)
- platelet aggregation (platelet aggregometry)
- coagulation (clotting time, activated partial thromboplastin time, prothrombin time and thrombin time)
- fibrinolysis (fibrin degradation products).

Details of the conduct of the above tests can be found in haematology texts (e.g. Hoffbrand et al., 2001).

## Defects of haemostasis

### CLINICAL APPLICATIONS

#### INCREASED FRAGILITY OF CAPILLARY WALLS AND PLATELET DISORDERS

Increased fragility of capillary walls and disordered platelet function prolong the bleeding time. Bleeding from capillary beds occurs after only minor injury or even apparently spontaneously. Normally, such bleeding would be arrested quickly by vessel contraction and platelet plugging. Capillary bleeding shows itself as bruising and as haemorrhagic areas under the skin. Blood loss from nose bleeds and at menstruation is also greater than normal.

The major causes of increased capillary fragility are a reduced platelet count (thrombocytopenia), autoimmune disorder and the effect of drugs, for example penicillin, oxytetracycline, aspirin and thiazide diuretics. Old age and Cushing's syndrome produce atrophy of the supporting connective tissue of capillaries and bleeding, combined with lack of white cell phagocytic activity, leaves brown areas of haemosiderin under the skin (age spots). Typically, these appear on the backs of the hands because of the frequency of minor injury at these sites.

Wherever possible, the cause of the bleeding disorder is treated. Other therapeutic measures include the administration of anti-inflammatory and immunosuppressive agents, splenectomy and platelet transfusion.

### CLOTTING DEFECTS

Significant deficiencies of functional forms of clotting factors arise from rare inherited defects in their synthesis. Almost always, deficiency of a clotting factor leads to a bleeding disorder in which clotting time is prolonged but bleeding time remains normal.

### The haemophilias

The haemophilias are the most common of the hereditary clotting disorders, with an incidence of $30–100/10^6$ population. **Haemophilia A (classical haemophilia)** is due to deficiency of clotting factor VIII. It is transmitted as a sex-linked recessive disorder (that is, the gene is on the X chromosome), so the disease occurs only in men, who inherit an abnormal X chromosome from their unaffected, carrier mothers. However, 33% of patients have no family history and in them the disease presumably results from spontaneous mutation. **Figure 4.1.17** illustrates the inheritance of haemophilia in a family with a carrier mother and normal father. Theoretically, the chances are that half of the children will be normal and, of the other half, the males will have haemophilia and the females will be carriers of the disease.

Where there is evidence that a woman might be a carrier of haemophilia, either through her family history or because she has borne an affected son, assessment of her clotting factor activity can confirm this and genetic counselling should be made available to her.

**Haemophilia B** occurs about six times less frequently than classical haemophilia. It is caused by a deficiency of clotting factor IX and is also inherited as a sex-linked recessive gene. It is clinically identical to haemophilia A and it was not until factor IX was discovered that the two conditions were distinguished. Factor IX deficiency

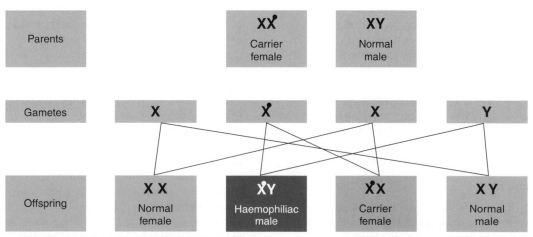

**Figure 4.1.17**    The inheritance of haemophilia

is commonly called **Christmas disease**, after the first sufferer identified.

In both haemophilia A and Christmas disease the severity of the bleeding disorder depends on the level of active clotting factor present in the plasma. Spontaneous bleeding occurs at very low levels (<5%).

**von Willebrand disease is** the most common inherited bleeding disorder. The mechanism is autosomal dominant with variable expression so that the severity of the bleeding disorder varies. There is a deficiency in von Willebrand factor (vWF), a protein synthesized by endothelial cells. vWF has two major roles: promoting platelet adhesion to damaged endothelium and functioning as a carrier molecule for factor VIII.

People with coagulation factor deficiencies are usually cared for as outpatients at specialist centres. Therapy now consists of the intravenous administration of a concentrated preparation of the relevant active clotting factor, obtained from normal human plasma, although plasma of UK origin is no longer used because of the risk of contamination and the potential of infection with variant Creutzfeldt–Jakob disease (vCJD), although it is not known whether this disease is transmissible between humans from blood products (McClelland, 2001). The aim is to raise the patient's plasma level to about 30% of the normal activity of that factor. Through this treatment, it is possible to arrest serious bleeding and hence prevent the development of chronic deformities. Clotting factor therapy also allows people with haemophilia to undergo surgery with far less risk of life-threatening haemorrhage. In most cases, following education, the patient, or a member of his family, is able to administer the clotting factor preparation at home.

It is important to remember that people with disorders of haemostasis and those on antithrombotic therapy have an increased tendency to bleed. Special care should therefore be taken when administering injections to such people. Those with severe haemophilia are not given intramuscular injections because of the risk of bleeding into the muscle. Instead, when necessary, drugs are given via careful subcutaneous or intravenous injections. People at risk of excessive bleeding should be advised not to participate in activities that carry a substantial risk of accidental injury, such as contact sports. They should also avoid ingesting irritant substances, such as aspirin, because these can cause internal bleeding.

### Thrombosis

Thrombosis is the process of clot formation within the cardiovascular system of a living person. A **thrombus** (plural: thrombi) is an intravascular blood clot, that is a clot that forms within the blood vessels. Venous thrombi consist of a fibrin web enmeshed with platelets and red blood cells. Arterial thrombi are composed mainly of platelets with little fibrin.

Blood does not normally clot unless it is shed from the vascular system. Its intravascular fluidity is dependent on the properties of the normal endothelial lining of the blood vessels, the rate of blood flow and the presence of natural clotting inhibitors. In 1846, Rudolf Virchow described a triad of situations that predispose to intravascular clotting:

* damaged vessel endothelium
* slow blood flow
* hypercoagulable blood.

Virchow's triad remains valid and thrombi are most likely to form when these conditions exist.

Nearly 50% of British adults die as a result of one of the three major types of thrombosis and many more suffer the chronic disabling results of non-fatal occurrences. The three major types of life-threatening thrombosis are:

* **coronary thrombosis**: arterial thrombosis leading to myocardial infarction (a heart attack)
* **cerebral thrombosis**: arterial thrombosis leading to cerebral infarction (this type of cerebrovascular accident is the most common form of stroke)
* **pulmonary embolism**, embolus from a venous thrombosis, usually in the deep veins of the calf, leading to pulmonary infarction (see below).

Risk factors for arterial thrombosis relate to the development of atherosclerosis and research has led to the development of coronary artery thrombosis risk profiles based on age, sex, blood pressure, serum cholesterol, cigarette smoking, glucose intolerance and electrocardiogram abnormalities (see Chapter 4.2).

Inherited conditions associated with increased risk of venous thrombosis are at least as common as the hereditary bleeding disorders. Activated protein C resistance (factor V Leiden gene mutation) and antithrombin deficiency (an autosomal dominant condition) are two examples of these conditions, of which there are several (Norris, 2003). Acquired risk factors for venous thrombosis include venous stasis and immobility, malignancy, oestrogen therapy (the contraceptive pill or hormone replacement therapy) and various blood disorders, especially those that increase blood viscosity such as polycythaemia.

**Deep vein thrombosis** (DVT) accounts for the formation of over 90% of venous thrombi. These thrombi usually form in the pocket-like valves of the deep veins of the calf during prolonged periods of immobility, especially when lying supine, for example either during or following an abdominal operation. Lying supine increases the pressure in the leg veins and produces venous stasis. The sustained pressure can also damage the venous endothelium. In recent years there has been publicity surrounding certain instances of DVT and subsequent pulmonary embolism occurring in people following long haul air travel. The risk of venous thrombosis in these circumstances is apparently increased by the immobility associated by long periods of sitting in relatively cramped conditions in an aeroplane cabin. The risk is exacerbated by the presence of other risk factors for venous thrombosis (see above). Prevention of DVT is the same as in any other circumstances (see below) and mainly involves ensuring that the leg muscles are regularly exercised and leg veins supported.

Deep vein thrombosis might not become clinically apparent. The inflammation associated with its occurrence sometimes produces pain in the calf, especially on dorsiflexion of the foot (**Homans' sign**) and flushing, heat and swelling in the affected area. Superficial leg veins can act as a collateral circulation, enabling blood to bypass the thrombus.

Deep vein thrombi are not a major health hazard in themselves. However, in a small proportion a fragment of the thrombus breaks away. This fragment (an embolus) is transported through the venous system to the right side of the heart and passes into the pulmonary arterial tree where it can block one of the vessels. The size and severity of effect of the pulmonary infarction thus produced depend on the size of the embolus and the vessel it has blocked. Pulmonary embolism has a mortality rate of 50% and is one of the main causes of sudden death.

It is therefore important to prevent the occurrence of deep vein thrombosis. This can be done by taking action to prevent venous stasis in the leg veins. Teaching a preoperative or bedridden patient the importance of, and how to do, deep breathing exercises (which aid the respiratory pump) and leg exercises (which increase the muscular pump effect) is probably helpful. Prophylactic leg exercises should be performed passively on unconscious and uncooperative patients. Pressure on the leg veins is also reduced by regular changes in position and by the use of bed cradles. Other important preventive measures include the application of elastic stockings. These support the calf muscles and aid venous tone. Intermittent pneumatic compression of the calves, using electrical apparatus, has also been shown to be beneficial. Low-dose anticoagulant therapy, for example

aspirin in low daily doses can be prescribed for some high-risk patients.

People with a previous history of thrombosis, or who are known to be at particular risk of its development, can be maintained prophylactically on long-term antithrombotic therapy (see below).

## Antithrombotic therapy

The treatment and prevention of thrombosis involves three classes of drug:

- anticoagulants
- antiplatelet drugs
- fibrinolytics.

### Anticoagulants

**Anticoagulants** prevent blood from clotting either by inhibiting the normal function of coagulation factors, or by inhibiting their production. The main use of anticoagulant drugs is to prevent thrombus formation or the extension of an existing thrombus in the slower moving venous side of the circulation. They are less useful in preventing thrombus formation in arteries, where thrombi are formed mostly of platelets, with little fibrin. However, because of the many links between platelet activation and the coagulation cascade, it is not surprising that anticoagulants can also have a beneficial effect in preventing coronary artery disease, or that platelets have some effect on venous thrombosis. Anticoagulants inhibit thrombogenesis and either inhibit thrombin or prevent thrombin being produced.

### Heparin

**Heparin** is a powerful anticoagulant both in vivo and in vitro. It is ineffective if given orally, being broken down by digestive enzymes, and so is given either intravenously, or subcutaneously.

Heparin is secreted by mast cells in the tissues. It is extracted for clinical use from the lungs and gut of slaughtered cattle. Natural heparin can help maintain the normal fluidity of the blood but its precise physiological role has not been established. Heparin acts by inhibiting the action of thrombin. It does so by combining with antithrombin to produce an even more powerful thrombin inhibitor. As a result, the time taken for blood to clot is greatly increased. Protamine sulphate neutralizes the activity of heparin. Standard or unfractionated heparin (UFH) consists of a mixture of heparin polymers, from which can be extracted **low-molecular-weight heparins (LMWH)**, for example, dalteparin (Fragmin) and enoxaparin (Clexane), which appear to be equally effective, have a longer duration of action and a more predictable anticoagulant response.

## Vitamin K

**Vitamin K** deficiency is characterized by prolonged blood clotting time and severe bleeding. The vitamin is present in both plant and animal food sources and is also synthesized by bacteria in the large intestine. Deficiency is usually the result of reduced absorption rather than low levels in the gastrointestinal tract, except in circumstances of prolonged anorexia and when prolonged antibiotic therapy destroys the normal bacterial flora of the gut.

Vitamin K is fat soluble and therefore its absorption from the gut is dependent on the absorption of fats and on the normal function of bile salts and lipase enzymes in the gut. Deficiency of the vitamin can occur in any condition in which the flow of bile is decreased, in pancreatic disease and in chronic diarrhoea. The body stores very little vitamin K, so the effects of deficiency become apparent in about a month. Vitamin K is required for the synthesis of clotting factors II (prothrombin), VII, IX and X in the liver. Deficiency of the vitamin therefore leads to abnormal synthesis of these factors and hence a prolonged blood clotting time. Liver disease is one of the most common causes of an acquired defect in blood clotting and so the prothrombin time test for clotting is often used as a test of liver function.

At birth, vitamin K and hence prothrombin levels are low. This is due to deficiency in the mother's vitamin K stores and to the baby's initial lack of intestinal bacteria to synthesize the vitamin. Prothrombin levels are usually normal by 2 weeks after birth. If the baby is born prematurely, levels are even lower because of deficient liver cell function due to immaturity. If prothrombin levels are low, there is a greatly increased risk of haemorrhage and so vitamin K is given to the baby, usually intramuscularly. Administration of the vitamin usually produces a rise in prothrombin to normal levels in about 48 hours.

**Vitamin K antagonists**, such as the **coumarins (e.g. warfarin)** and the **indanediones (e.g. phenindione)** prolong clotting time by blocking the action of vitamin K and so reducing the synthesis of prothrombin and clotting factors VII, IX and X. They are effective when administered orally.

The first vitamin K antagonist to be discovered was dicoumarol. **Dicoumarol** is a product of sweet clover fermentation and was discovered after it caused an epidemic of haemorrhaging in cattle in Alberta, Canada, in 1921. It has a similar molecular structure to vitamin K and acts as an antagonist by replacing the vitamin at its normal site of action. As a result, inert clotting factors are produced.

Other vitamin K antagonists are derived from dicoumarol. They differ mainly in their speed of onset of effect and duration of action. Warfarin and other vitamin K antagonists were first used as rat and mouse poisons. Vitamin K antagonists are widely used for people at risk from thrombosis, and the prothrombin time test is used to assess their therapeutic effect. This should be two to three times normal, reflecting a 5–15% clotting factor activity. Individual response varies widely and so regular monitoring is essential.

### Antiplatelet drugs

**Antiplatelet drugs** were mentioned in the section on platelet function. They have different modes of action:

- **Enzyme inhibitors**: for example aspirin, which inhibits the enzyme cyclo-oxygenase (COX), which is needed for the manufacture of prostaglandins including thromboxane. Dipyradimole is a phoshodiesterase inhibitor that antagonizes the uptake of adenosine into platelets.
- **Platelet ADP receptor antagonists**: for example, clopidrogel and ticlodipine. These block ADP receptors on the platelet surface.
- **Glycoprotein IIb/IIIa antagonists**: for example, Abciximab and Tirofiban. These compete with fibrinogen to occupy the glycoprotein IIb/IIIa receptor on the platelet surface and so block platelet aggregation.

### Fibrinolytic agents

**Fibrinolytic agents** are widely used in clinical practice as 'clot-busting' drugs. Tissue plasminogen activator has been synthesized using recombinant DNA technology (rtPA Alteplase). Haemolytic streptococci produce streptokinase (SK), which is able to combine with plasminogen and convert other plasminogen molecules to plasmin. Tenecteplase is the first fibrinolytic agent to match the efficacy of tissue plasminogen activator with a single dose, making it a significant drug in prehospital emergency care. It is produced from snake and bat venom models (Blann et al., 2002).

The substances **epsilon-aminocaproic acid (EACA)** and **tranexamic acid (AMCA)** inhibit fibrinolysis and are used clinically to reduce bleeding at sites where active fibrinolysis occurs, for example the uterus or following dental extraction. They are also used as antidotes to the therapeutic fibrinolytic agents such as streptokinase.

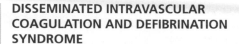

## DISSEMINATED INTRAVASCULAR COAGULATION AND DEFIBRINATION SYNDROME

In disseminated intravascular coagulation (DIC), widespread clotting occurs throughout the circulatory system. This condition can arise in a variety of usually serious illnesses, for example major trauma and surgery, septicaemia, widespread malignancy and mismatched transfusion. Activation of intravascular clotting is precipitated by entry of tissue fluid into the blood or by widespread damage to the vessel endothelium.

Paradoxically, bleeding is the major feature of DIC because clotting factors have been used up intravascularly (defibrination syndrome). Other problems are the result of microthrombi lodging in the arterial blood supply and producing infarctions, in tissues such as brain, lung and kidney. Haemolytic anaemia also occurs as a result of red cells being damaged by intravascular fibrin strands. Treatment is primarily directed at the usually severe cause of the DIC. Antithrombotic drugs and transfusion of platelets and clotting factor preparations may also be given, alongside other supportive therapies (Collins, 1998).

## Blood groups

Over 400 different, genetically determined, antigens can be identified on the surface of human red blood cells. An **antigen** is a substance that stimulates antibody formation and combines, specifically, with the antibody produced. Some of these antigens are specific to red cells and others are also present on white cells, platelets and on the cells of other tissues. People can be divided into groups (blood groups) according to the presence or absence of particular antigens on the surface of their red cells.

## The major blood group systems

More than 12 different blood group systems and subdivisions of these have now been identified. Some of these have been designated letters and others are named after the individual in whom they were first identified. They include the ABO, Rhesus (Rh; CDE/cde), MNS, P, Lutheran (Lu), Kell (K), Lewis (Le), Duffy (Fy) and Kidd (Jk) blood group systems.

### CLINICAL APPLICATIONS

#### SIGNIFICANCE

Blood groups become clinically significant when blood transfusion is performed and when a pregnant woman is carrying a fetus that has inherited (from its father) a blood group different from that of its mother. In both these situations the clinical importance of a particular red-cell antigen depends on three factors:

* frequency of occurrence in the plasma of the corresponding antibody
* the ability of this antibody to produce haemolysis of red cells following combination with the antigen
* in pregnancy, the ability of the antibody to cross the placenta.

On this basis, the ABO and Rhesus blood group systems are by far the most important. Usually, the other systems cause clinical problems only in cases of repeated blood transfusion and in second and subsequent incompatible pregnancies.

## The ABO blood group system: The classical blood groups

The ABO blood groups were discovered in 1900, when Landsteiner demonstrated that blood from two individuals could be mixed successfully only if their blood groups matched. This discovery marked the beginning of safe blood transfusion.

The **ABO antigens** occur on the red cell membrane and on most other cells, including white blood cells and platelets. They are glycoproteins, which differ only in one carbohydrate molecular residue and appear on the red cells by about the sixth week of fetal life. At birth they have reached about one-fifth of the adult level.

In 80% of the population who possess secretor genes, the ABO agglutinogens (antigens) are also found in soluble form in body fluids and secretions, e.g. plasma, saliva, semen and sweat. The stability of the antigens allows their detection in dried fluids and this is of great importance in forensic medicine.

### Inheritance of ABO blood groups

The locus (site) that determines the ABO blood groups is on chromosome nine and three alleles – A, B and O – can occur at this site. Each parent transfers one of his/her two genes to their baby. **Table 4.1.8** illustrates how a person's ABO blood group is genetically determined. There are four possible phenotypes – A, B, AB and O – because the A and B genes are codominant and dominant over O (which is amorphic), so that AO and BO react like AA and BB, respectively.

### The frequency of occurrence of the ABO blood groups

The frequency of occurrence of each of the four ABO blood groups varies widely within different

**Table 4.1.8** The inheritance of the ABO blood groups

| If a baby receives | O + O | A + O | A + A | B + O | B + B | A + B |
|---|---|---|---|---|---|---|
| His or her genotype is | OO | AO | AA | BO | BB | AB |
| His or her phenotype (blood group) is | O | A | A | B | B | AB |

**Table 4.1.9** The frequency of occurrence of the ABO blood groups in the populations of the United Kingdom and Western Europe

| Group | Percentage occurrence |
|---|---|
| O | 46 |
| A | 42 |
| B | 9 |
| AB | 3 |
| All groups | 100 |

populations. **Table 4.1.9** shows the frequency of occurrence of each group in the United Kingdom and Western Europe; groups O and A are by far the most common. However, the percentages of the four blood groups vary considerably in different parts of the United Kingdom and even wider variations exist between the populations of Western Europe and those of other countries and continents.

## Antigens and agglutination

The A and B blood group antigens are sometimes called **agglutinogens** because, in the presence of their specific antibody (an agglutinin), agglutination of the red cells occurs. In **agglutination**, the red cells lose their outline and become massed in clumps. These clumps are sometimes described as having the appearance of paprika pepper. The size of the red cell clumps depends on the strength of the antibody. Agglutination is then usually followed by haemolysis. Agglutination is a quite different process to blood coagulation (clotting) and should not be confused with the latter. O antigen does not normally act as an agglutinogen as it does not usually evoke production of a corresponding antibody.

## Antibodies (agglutinins)

The antibodies (or agglutinins) that correspond to the A and B antigens are called anti-A or alpha, and anti-B or beta. Unusually these antibodies are present in the absence of their corresponding antigen and without any immunizing stimulus such as incompatable blood transfusion or pregnancy.

Antibodies are produced by the plasma cells of the immune system (see Chapter 6.2). They are IgM immunoglobulins and are found in plasma and in other body fluids. Certain bacteria and viruses contain antigens so similar to A and B that they trigger production of anti-A and anti-B. Normally, people make antibodies against the A and B antigens that are **not** expressed on their own cells. Natural exposure probably occurs via the gastrointestinal tract. About 50% of newborn babies have some anti-A and/or anti-B antibodies in their blood from placental transfer. Actively produced anti-A and anti-B are measurable at about 3 months of age and reach adult levels by about 10 years. There are marked variations in antibody titre between individuals at all ages (McClelland, 2001).

If an antigen is present on the red cells of an individual the corresponding antibody must be absent from the plasma because if it was present agglutination would occur. If the serum of the four ABO blood groups is examined, it is usually found that:

- group A blood serum contains anti-B
- group B blood serum contains anti-A
- group O blood serum contains both anti-A and anti-B
- group AB blood serum contains neither anti-A nor anti-B.

## Determination of ABO group

To determine the ABO group of a blood sample, two test sera, one containing anti-A and one containing anti-B, are used. A variety of techniques is available for ABO grouping. In the slide technique, a small volume of each antiserum is placed on a slide and labelled, and then an equal volume of the diluted blood sample is added to each serum. After 10 minutes the slides are observed for agglutination. **Figure 4.1.18** illustrates the results for a blood sample of each ABO group.

## The Rh (Rhesus) blood group system

After Landsteiner's discovery of the ABO blood group system, the majority of blood transfusions were successful. However, sometimes patients receiving a transfusion of ABO-compatible blood would suffer a transfusion reaction. In addition, some mothers were delivered of an ABO-compatible baby

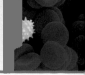

| Blood group (antigen on cells) | Serum containing | |
|---|---|---|
| | anti-A | anti-B |

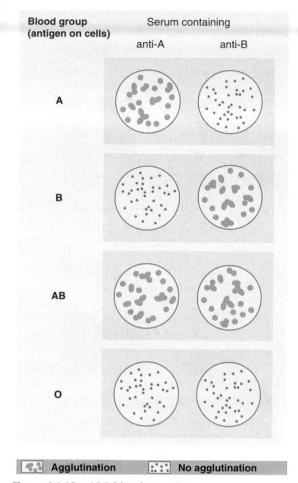

| Agglutination | No agglutination |
|---|---|

**Figure 4.1.18** ABO blood grouping

who had severe haemolytic anaemia (haemolytic disease of the newborn). It was believed that this anaemia was caused by incompatible blood group antibodies (agglutinins) present in the mother's plasma, crossing the placenta and destroying her baby's red cells.

These clinical problems were not clearly understood until Landsteiner joined forces with the American immunologist, Alexander Wiener. In 1939 they discovered the Rhesus (Rh) blood group system, and went on to discover other blood group systems.

The Rh system is so called because the antigens were discovered on the red cells of Rhesus monkeys. Red cells from a Rhesus monkey were injected into a rabbit and, as a result, the rabbit's immune system formed an antibody that agglutinated the Rhesus red cells. It was then found that if Caucasian human red cells were mixed with serum from the immunized rabbit, agglutination occurred in 85% of cases. The occurrence of agglutination indicated the presence of Rh antigen on the human red cells. Individuals with Rh antigen on their red cells are termed **Rh positive**; those with no Rh antigen on their red cells are termed **Rh negative**.

## Rh Antigens and their inheritance

Rh antigens are specific to red cells and three closely linked genes on chromosome 1 are responsible for their production or non-production. Each of the three genes has two alleles, called CDE/cde. Alleles C, D and E are dominant over c, d and e. Of these three genes, D is by far the most important clinically (Nairn & Helbert, 2002). The presence of the D allele gives rise to the Rh antigen, D. The d allele is amorphic and so produces no antigen. The term **Rh positive**, then, refers to the presence of antigen D on the red cell surface.

Two examples of the inheritance of the D and d Rh blood group antigens are shown in **Fig. 4.1.19**. One gene is received from each parent. As D is dominant over d, the genotypes DD and Dd both give rise to Rh-positive red cells and the dd genotype produces Rh-negative red cells.

## Frequency of Rh blood groups

The frequency of the Rh antigens varies in different parts of the world. For example, in the United Kingdom and Western Europe, 83% of people are Rh positive (DD and Dd) and 17% Rh negative (dd); in Japan, 99.7% of the population are Rh positive and only 0.3% Rh negative.

## Rh (anti-D) antibody

Unlike the ABO system's anti-A and anti-B, anti-D antibody does not occur naturally in the plasma of Rh-negative individuals. However, immune production of anti-D can be stimulated by contact of an Rh-negative individual's immune cells with the Rh-positive (D) antigen. This **alloimmunization** (immunization against antigens that the individual lacks) can occur in two ways:

- Following transfusion with Rh-positive blood.
- The red cells of an Rh-positive fetus enter the circulation of its Rh-negative mother. Such escape of fetal red cells happens most often at delivery but can also occur in therapeutic, threatened and spontaneous abortion, ectopic pregnancy, antepartum haemorrhage and during invasive prenatal procedures. The mother's titre of anti-D is unlikely to be high enough to cross the placenta and destroy her Rh-positive fetus' red cells during a first pregnancy.

As antigen d is amorphic, there is no corresponding anti-d antibody and so transfusion of an Rh-positive person with Rh-negative blood does not give rise to antibody production.

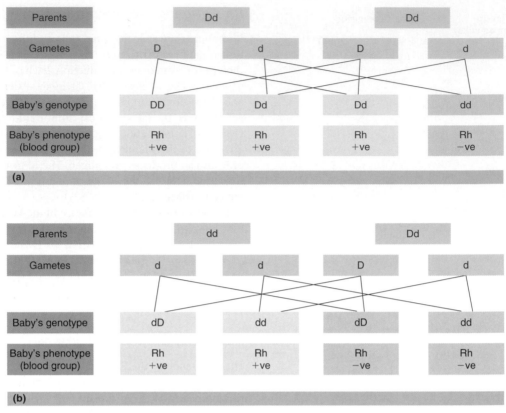

**Figure 4.1.19** The inheritance of the D and d Rh blood groups when (a) both parents are Rh-positive heterozygotes and (b) when the mother is Rh-negative and the father is an Rh-positive heterozygote

## Blood transfusion

### CLINICAL APPLICATIONS

Blood for transfusion has always been and still is a limited and expensive resource. Over the years, techniques have been developed that enable blood to be separated into its various components. These techniques allow modern transfusion practice to aim to give patients only the blood component they lack and therefore need, for example factor VIII in classical haemophilia. Not only does **blood component therapy** represent a more economical use of blood, it also removes many of the health risks associated with whole blood transfusion when this is not required.

Outside the body (in vitro), blood can be prevented from clotting by the addition of sodium citrate, sodium oxalate or sodium edetate (EDTA: ethylenediamine-tetra-acetic acid). These precipitate calcium ions (factor IV) and the clotting sequence is therefore inhibited. For example:

Calcium + sodium → calcium citrate + sodium
ion        citrate      (insoluble            ion
                         precipitate)

These substances cannot be used as anticoagulants within the body (in vivo) as the resultant severe reduction in plasma calcium ions would produce clinical problems, such as severe tetany. Blood collected for transfusion and for laboratory analysis of blood cells or clotting factors is usually anticoagulated with citrate phosphate dextrose with adenine. Use of this anticoagulant and preservative solution increases the storage period of red cells from 21 to 35 days.

### BLOOD GROUPS AND BLOOD TRANSFUSION

When blood from one individual is transfused into another, it is essential to avoid red cells being agglutinated. Agglutination will occur if the antigens present on the red cells come into contact with their corresponding antibodies.

Usually, it is unnecessary to consider the antigens on the cells of the transfusion recipient because the antibodies in the donor's plasma are diluted to such a degree by the much larger volume of the recipient's plasma. This dilution ensures that the donor's antibodies do not cause agglutination of the recipient's red cells. Normally, therefore, it is only *necessary to exclude incompatibility between the antigens on the donor's cells and the antibodies in the recipient's plasma*.

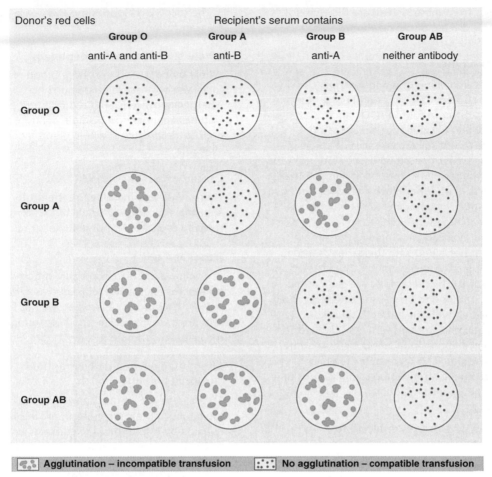

Donor's red cells

Recipient's serum contains

| | Group O<br>anti-A and anti-B | Group A<br>anti-B | Group B<br>anti-A | Group AB<br>neither antibody |

Group O

Group A

Group B

Group AB

🔴 **Agglutination – incompatible transfusion**   ⦙⦙⦙ **No agglutination – compatible transfusion**

**Figure 4.1.20**   The results of transfusing blood of each of the four ABO blood groups into recipients of each group. Group O is known as the 'universal donor' type and group AB is known as the 'universal recipient' type

## The ABO blood group system

**Figure 4.1.20** shows the results of transfusing blood of each of the four ABO groups into recipients of each group. The occurrence of agglutination indicates an incompatible transfusion. It can be seen that intra-group transfusion is always compatible. A recipient of group AB can receive blood from any of the four ABO groups without agglutination occurring. Similarly, group O blood can be given to recipients of all four groups. For this reason, group AB individuals have been termed 'universal recipients' and group O individuals 'universal donors'. However, these terms are not valid because they ignore the effect of other blood group systems, in particular the Rh system, in blood transfusion. Consequently they should no longer be used.

## The Rh blood group system

As described earlier, Rh antibodies do not occur naturally but a person who is Rh negative will produce anti-D if immunized with Rh-positive blood. If an immunized Rh-negative person subsequently comes into contact with Rh-positive

red cells, agglutination and haemolysis of these red cells will occur. This could occur on further transfusion of incompatible Rh-positive blood and when an immunized Rh-negative woman is pregnant with an Rh-positive fetus.

It is therefore essential that no Rh-negative person is transfused with Rh-positive blood, except in extreme emergency when no Rh-negative blood is available. This is particularly important for female patients prior to the menopause, as their sensitization to antigen D could adversely affect their subsequent ability to bear a child.

## Other blood group systems

Other blood group systems are of relatively minor clinical significance as antibodies do not occur naturally in the plasma and it is unusual for the antigens of these systems to evoke antibody formation, even after incompatible blood transfusion. However, with repeated transfusions of incompatible blood, antibody formation sometimes occurs and can produce agglutination on subsequent transfusion. Occasionally, too, antibodies from these systems are the cause of haemolytic disease of the newborn.

### Cross-matching

Direct cross-matching of blood for transfusion with the recipient's blood is routinely performed prior to transfusion for the ABO and Rh systems. It has now also become routine laboratory procedure to test for the presence of atypical antibodies from other blood group systems in the serum of the recipient. This is done prior to cross-matching so that donor blood that does not have the corresponding antigens can be selected.

Cross-matching for the ABO and Rh systems is performed by mixing a sample of the already grouped donor blood with the patient's serum and observing for agglutination. The latter does not occur if the blood samples are compatible. Each unit of blood to be transfused is individually cross-matched with the patient's serum. Additionally, the patient's serum is screened for the presence of abnormal antibodies. Accurate direct cross-matching represents the only safeguard against transfusion complications due to blood group incompatibility.

### The effect of storage on blood for transfusion

Donated whole blood can be stored at 2–6°C for up to 35 days without excessive loss of viability. Red cell metabolism is significantly decreased at 4°C and, as a result, the red cells swell and their fragility is increased. The amount of spontaneous haemolysis that takes place increases with the length of storage. Following transfusion, stored red cells become normal within 48 hours.

Leucocytes and platelets are destroyed within a few days of donation and so these cells cannot be obtained from stored blood. Plasma can be stored, in liquid form, for many months. It can also be frozen successfully. Dried plasma can be preserved for years at a wide range of temperatures. It is reconstituted with sterile water prior to transfusion. However, UK donations have white cells removed as a precaution against variant Creutzfeldt–Jacob disease (vCJD) (**leucocyte depleted blood**) and for the same reason plasma is not utilized (McClelland, 2001).

### Blood component therapy

The objective of blood component therapy is either to give the patient the particular component of blood that is lacking, for example platelets, or to substitute a normal for an abnormal component, for example exchange of normal red cells for sickle cells in sickle-cell anaemia.

The following blood components are available for transfusion:

### Whole blood (leucocyte depleted)

**Whole blood** is used to restore blood volume following acute, severe haemorrhage. In an emergency, concentrated red cells and a plasma volume expander, for example dextran, can be used as a substitute if whole blood is not available.

### Concentrated (packed) red cells

These constitute the ideal treatment for severe anaemia in which additional blood oxygen carrying capacity but not volume is required.

### Frozen red cells

Red cells can be frozen in liquid nitrogen (−196°C) for several years. Glycerol is used as a protective agent. This procedure is expensive but **frozen red cells** are a very useful method of storing selected red cells, for example those of a rare blood group.

### Alternative oxygen delivering fluids ('artificial blood')

Several types of synthetic oxygen carrying substitutes, for example, perfluorocarbons and haemoglobin solutions, are currently undergoing research trials. As yet, however, none of these **red cell substitutes** is considered safe for widespread clinical use (McClelland, 2001).

#### Platelets

**Platelets** must be transfused within 5 days of preparation because of their short survival time. They are mainly required to arrest bleeding due to thrombocytopenia. Platelets from ABO- and Rh-compatible donors are usually given because of the presence of the ABO antigens on platelets and red cell contamination of the platelet preparation.

#### Granulocytes

Methods of producing **granulocyte** preparations for transfusion are as yet experimental. Granulocytes can be obtained in sufficient quantities only by leucopheresis from a single donor. Occasionally, patients with chronic granulocytic leukaemia volunteer as donors because they have high levels of circulating granulocytes. Granulocyte preparations are used fresh because the cells have a short survival time. They are contaminated with red cells and so must be compatible with the recipient's ABO and Rh groups. They are mainly used when antibiotic therapy is unable to control severe infection in patients with neutropenia due to marrow suppression. Currently, white cells are not utilized from UK donors, for the reasons discussed previously.

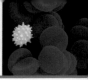

### Plasma

Currently, plasma of UK origin is not utilized in blood donation as a precaution against variant Creutzfeldt–Jacob disease (vCJD) (McClelland, 2001).

Plasma is transfused to increase blood volume and to replace plasma that has been lost from the circulation, for example following burns. As in whole blood transfusion, relatively small volumes of plasma can be transfused without considering the effects of the antibodies present. This is because the antibodies are diluted to harmless levels by the recipient's plasma. However, if large volumes of plasma are to be transfused, agglutination might occur. To avoid such agglutination, **conditioned plasma** is used. Conditioned plasma is a preparation from which the antibodies have been previously removed by contact with red cells.

**Plasma substitutes**, such as a solution of the polysaccharide dextran, are sometimes used in an emergency and to avoid the risk of transmitting serum-carried diseases. The large dextran molecules are retained in the circulation and so exert an osmotic effect similar to that of the plasma proteins. This osmotic effect draws fluid into the blood, increasing its volume and hence blood pressure. Plasma components available for clinical use are summarized in **Table 4.1.10**.

The risk of transmitting serum-carried infections diseases in plasma transfusing varies according to the precise component used. Most methods of preparation destroy microorganisms.

## ADVERSE EFFECTS OF TRANSFUSION

Blood transfusion is a common occurrence in hospital wards. As well as being potentially lifesaving, it is also a potentially hazardous procedure for the recipient as a variety of complications can occur. To avoid such problems, the National Blood Service takes stringent precautions to ensure that each unit of blood released is suitable for transfusion, and strict safety measures are followed by the hospital blood bank and ward staff involved in administering the transfusion. As a direct result of these safety measures, blood transfusion is usually a relatively safe procedure, although severe and even fatal reactions do occur occasionally. The large majority of these are due either to administrative errors, for example misidentification of the patient or a blood sample, or to maltreatment of the blood between the time it leaves the blood bank and is transfused.

**Table 4.1.10** Plasma components for clinical use

| Plasma component | Major uses |
| --- | --- |
| Plasma protein fraction (PPF) | Plasma replacement |
| | Blood volume expansion |
| Human albumin | Albumin replacement in hypoalbuminaemia, e.g. in nephrosis |
| Fresh frozen plasma (FFP) | Clotting factor deficiencies, e.g. DIC, anticoagulant overdose, liver disease |
| Cryoprecipitate (factor VIII, fibrinogen) | Classical haemophilia<br>von Willebrand disease<br>Fibrinogen deficiency |
| Factor VIII concentrate and freeze-dried factor VIII | Classical haemophilia |
| Factor IX concentrate | Christmas disease |
| Human immunoglobulin (Ig) (γ globulin) | Hypogammaglobulinaemia<br>To produce passive immunity to common viral diseases such as rubella (German measles), measles and chickenpox |
| Human specific globulin (specific antibodies) | Rh anti-D for prevention of Rh immunization<br>To produce passive immunity to rare, life-threatening diseases, e.g. tetanus |

DIC, disseminated intravascular coagulation.

## Types of transfusion reaction

Acute, life-threatening complications of transfusion are very rare and include:

- acute, haemolytic transfusion reaction
- infusion of an infected unit of blood
- severe allergic reaction or anaphylaxis
- transfusion-associated lung injury (TRALI).

In all situations, new signs and symptoms that occur during a transfusion must be monitored carefully and taken very seriously because they could herald the onset of a serious reaction.

Immunization can occur against the antigens the patient lacks (**alloimmunization**). Recipients of multiple transfusions can develop antibodies to antigens in the donor blood that have not been grouped and cross-matched. Antigens that trigger alloimmunization are present on red cells, white cells, platelets and plasma proteins. Alloimmunization of the recipient is not in itself a problem but on subsequent transfusion the antibodies formed might produce an incompatible transfusion reaction (see below).

A transfusion reaction due to **ABO incompatibility** is one of the most serious complications of blood transfusion. The clinical problems associated with this reaction are due to the effects of the acute intravascular agglutination and haemolysis that occur. The antigen–antibody reaction probably also triggers the complement and clotting cascades and so may initiate disseminated intravascular coagulation (DIC).

When an ABO-incompatible transfusion is commenced, the recipient often experiences a burning sensation radiating up the arm along the track of the vein from the transfusion site. Within a few minutes he or she might complain of severe pain in the lumbar region, tightness in the chest and difficulty in breathing. These symptoms are probably due to agglutinated red blood cells blocking small blood vessels in the kidneys and lungs. The patient's temperature and pulse rate rise and the blood pressure falls; febrile rigors might be experienced.

The occurrence of such a reaction is an acute emergency and prompt diagnosis and treatment are often life saving. For this reason, it is important that a nurse caring for a patient undergoing transfusion observes him or her particularly carefully during the first 15 minutes of transfusion. Frequent monitoring of how the patient is feeling, as well as of the temperature, blood pressure and pulse rate, is essential throughout the transfusion. An early symptom is often the patient's perception that something is amiss. If an ABO-incompatible reaction is suspected, the transfusion should be stopped immediately but the intravenous infusion is maintained for use in treatment. The remaining blood is retained for analysis. The reaction is unlikely to be fatal if less than 50 mL of blood has been transfused.

ABO-incompatible reactions also produce urticarial rashes and diarrhoea and vomiting. The glomerular filtration rate (GFR) decreases due to the fall in blood pressure and to the deposition of thrombi in the renal blood vessels. Free haemoglobin colours the plasma red and is filtered into the renal nephrons, where it can be precipitated as acid haematin, obstructing the tubule lumen. Haemoglobin is also excreted in the urine (haemoglobinuria). The fall in glomerular filtration rate and obstruction of the renal tubules lead to a decrease in the volume of urine produced and, in severe cases, to anuria. If renal failure occurs, blood levels of potassium, urea and other nitrogenous compounds increase, with serious metabolic consequences. To monitor renal function, it is important that all urine produced by the patient is measured and retained for analysis.

A patient who is anaesthetized or unconscious is particularly at risk of a severe reaction because he or she is unable to complain of the early warning symptoms. The oozing of blood from a surgical wound (due to defibrination syndrome) is sometimes the first sign of a major transfusion reaction in an anaesthetized patient.

Treatment aims to maintain blood pressure and renal perfusion. Anaemia can be corrected by transfusion of compatible packed red cells. If disseminated intravascular coagulation and defibrination syndrome occur, transfusion of platelets and clotting factors might also be required.

## Other incompatibilities

Transfusion reactions due to **other antibodies** can occur in patients who have received multiple transfusions. The reactions are usually relatively mild, involving fever and anaphylactic responses such as urticarial rash. Purpura can follow transfusion when platelet antibodies exist. The presence of antibodies reduces the survival of the transfused target cells.

### Allergic reactions

**Allergic reactions** to blood transfusion are quite common. They vary in severity from a minor rise in temperature, itching urticarial rash, through to acute laryngeal and periorbital (around the eyes) oedema and anaphylaxis. The latter conditions occur only rarely and require urgent treatment.

### Pyrogenic reactions

**Pyrogenic reactions** produce a rise in temperature, as their name suggests. Pyrogenic reactions, usually of unknown origin, used to be one of the most common types of transfusion reaction, but are now much more rare. This is partly due to the introduction of plastic transfusion packs and partly because of greater understanding of the causes of transfusion reactions, which allow the reactions to be more accurately identified. The severity of a pyrogenic reaction is usually related to the speed of the transfusion. The patient rarely becomes shocked, so although a rise in temperature is unpleasant, these reactions are not usually dangerous. Pyrogens might be present in the donor blood as a result of bacterial growth in the transfusion medium prior to sterilization.

## Metabolic reactions

**Metabolic reactions** usually occur only when large volumes of blood (5 units or more) are transfused rapidly.

Stored blood contains citrate anticoagulant and increased levels of potassium. The latter can produce **hyperkalaemia** until the transfused red cells regain their normal state (usually within 48 hours). Hyperkalaemia can cause cardiac irregularities and, in severe cases, ventricular fibrillation. The citrate anticoagulant precipitates calcium ions. Normally, citrate is converted to hydrogen carbonate in the liver but this process can be delayed in massive transfusion and **hypocalcaemia** resulting in severe muscle spasm (tetany) can occur. Hypocalcaemia can be prevented by giving calcium gluconate to a patient receiving a massive transfusion.

## The temperature of and the maltreatment of blood

Blood is stored at 2–6°C. Large volumes that are transfused rapidly can significantly lower body temperature and might produce cardiac irregularities. Blood transfusion should be commenced within half an hour of removal from the blood bank and transfusion completed within 5 hours of its removal from controlled storage. During this time the unit should be stored at room temperature. **Blood for transfusion should never be frozen, stored in the ward refrigerator (the temperature of these is often unreliable), heated, or have anything (e.g. drugs), added to it.** All these procedures can severely damage and haemolyse red cells. If large volumes of blood are to be given rapidly, the blood can be passed through a commercial blood-warming apparatus or the blood bag can be warmed in water at 37°C. The temperature of the water must be measured using a reliable thermometer.

## Thrombophlebitis

**Thrombophlebitis** is inflammation of a vein, often accompanied by thrombus formation. It occurs most commonly as a result of trauma to the vessel wall. The incidence of thrombophlebitis as a complication of blood transfusion has greatly decreased since the introduction of plastic giving sets. If thrombophlebitis occurs, the transfusion will probably need to be resited.

## Microvascular obstruction

Microaggregates of platelets and fibrin occur in stored blood. These can **obstruct** small pulmonary blood vessels and so special filters are often used when large volumes of blood are to be transfused rapidly.

## Circulatory overload

**Circulatory overload** occurs most commonly when anaemic patients are transfused with whole blood. This is because they need only the additional oxygen-carrying capacity of the red cells and not the additional volume. Anaemic patients with existing cardiac disease are particularly at risk. The increased blood volume produced by the transfusion can precipitate cardiac failure and pulmonary oedema.

## Abnormal haemostasis

Platelets and some clotting factors do not survive storage. Therefore, massive transfusion with stored blood might significantly reduce the recipient's platelet count and clotting factor titres and thus produce **abnormal haemostasis**. To prevent this, a unit of fresh frozen plasma may be given for every four or five units of blood transfused.

## Infected blood

It is extremely rare for blood for transfusion to become **contaminated** with microorganisms. Although blood is an ideal culture medium, the low temperature at which it is stored limits bacterial growth. Gram-negative *Pseudomonas* and coliform bacilli, capable of reproducing at 4°C, are the most common contaminants.

Occasionally, bacteria are introduced into the blood during the transfusion. These can multiply and reach dangerous levels if the transfusion is slow.

Transfusion of infected blood produces fever, rigors, pains in the chest and abdomen, and hypotension (septicaemic shock). The condition is frequently fatal. If infected blood is suspected, the transfusion is stopped immediately but the intravenous infusion is maintained. The blood is retained for culture. Treatment includes antibiotic therapy and supportive measures for shock.

### Transmission of infectious disease

The selection of blood donors is intended to exclude anyone whose blood might be harmful to the recipient. In the United Kingdom, every donation is screened for evidence of syphilis, hepatitis B, hepatitis C, HIV1 and HIV2. Currently, plasma of UK origin is not utilized in blood donation and leucocytes are removed from blood as a precaution against variant Creutzfeldt–Jacob disease (vCJD) (McClelland, 2001).

In other countries, criteria for donor selection can be different from those used in the United Kingdom. Despite the screening of donors for hepatitis B surface antigen, viral hepatitis remains a serious complication of blood transfusion. Transmission of other **bloodborne diseases**, such as malaria, syphilis and brucellosis, via transfused blood is extremely rare because of donor screening. Universal donor screening (which has operated since 1985) for the human immunodeficiency virus (HIV), which causes acquired immune deficiency syndrome (AIDS), and requests to those at high risk of carrying the virus not to donate their blood now mean that people requiring blood transfusion run practically no risk of HIV infection as a result of undergoing treatment. All blood units taken are tested for anti-HIV as a further precaution.

### Iron overload (haemosiderosis)

Haemosiderosis occurs when repeated transfusions of red cells are given in the absence of haemorrhage, for example in the treatment of thalassaemia major. Excess iron, as haemosiderin, is deposited in the cells of the mononuclear phagocytic system and this eventually damages the liver, heart muscle and endocrine glands. Iron chelation therapy with desferrioxamine is given to reduce the problem of iron overload.

### Fetomaternal incompatibility

Fetal blood cells can carry antigens, inherited from the father, that are not present on the mother's blood cells. If these fetal blood cells enter the mother's circulation across the placenta, her immune system will be stimulated to produce IgG antibodies to the foreign antigens. Fetal blood cells most commonly enter the mother's blood during parturition. This alloimmunization of the mother has no harmful effects, in itself, but predisposes her to immune problems if she should subsequently require blood transfusion or tissue transplantation. If an alloimmunized woman becomes pregnant with another fetus whose blood cells carry the same incompatible antigens, her antibodies might cross the placenta and enter the fetal circulation. The clinical effects on the fetus vary according to the specificity and potency of the maternal antibodies.

### Rh Haemolytic disease of the newborn

The most severe form of **haemolytic disease of the newborn** is caused by maternal Rh anti-D antibodies. Before the prophylactic use of IgG anti-D was introduced in 1967, Rhesus haemolytic disease of the newborn was responsible for about 800 stillbirths and neonatal deaths annually in the United Kingdom.

#### Effects on the fetus

The effects on the fetus are due to agglutination and haemolysis of its Rh-positive red cells by maternal anti-D. The most severe damage occurs when maternal anti-D levels are high throughout the pregnancy. In this situation the fetus develops severe haemolytic anaemia, an enlarged liver, spleen and heart and gross oedema (**hydrops fetalis**). It dies either in utero or soon after birth.

In less severe cases, the baby develops jaundice (**icterus gravis neonatorum**) within 24 hours of birth because its liver is unable to conjugate the large amounts of bilirubin produced from haemoglobin breakdown following the haemolysis of its red cells. In utero, excess bilirubin is transferred across the placenta and excreted by the mother's liver. The baby's liver might be so severely damaged that death occurs from liver failure. If the baby's serum bilirubin reaches very high levels (over 270 μmol/L), this stains the basal ganglia in the brainstem yellow and damages them. This condition is called **kernicterus** and produces changes in muscle tone and athetoid cerebral palsy.

The newborn baby might not be anaemic because of its very high rate of erythropoiesis. Its blood contains raised levels of immature red cells (**erythroblastosis fetalis**). As the rate of red cell haemolysis is highest at birth, anaemia might develop within days.

#### Prevention

Since the late 1960s it has been possible to prevent anti-D haemolytic disease of the newborn by preventing Rh-negative women developing anti-D. This can be done in the following ways.

- By ensuring that an Rh-negative woman does not receive a transfusion of Rh-positive blood.

• By administering anti-D to every Rh-negative mother who might have been sensitized with the D antigen, provided she has not been exposed previously. As discussed earlier (see p. 371), there are a number of circumstances in which this sensitization might occur but the most likely is at parturition. The dose of anti-D destroys the leaked fetal red cells before the mother's immune system is stimulated to produce the antibody. For this reason it must be given as soon as is possible, and certainly within 72 hours of sensitization (usually delivery).

### Treatment

The titre of anti-D in the mother's blood is monitored in known affected pregnancies. Intensive plasmapheresis to reduce the anti-D titre can reduce the severity of fetal disease.

The fetus can also be monitored: amniocentesis allows assessment of the bilirubin content of the amniotic fluid and it is also possible, via fetoscopy, to obtain fetal blood samples for analysis.

**Treatment** for severe fetal disease is exchange transfusion with Rh-negative blood. Intrauterine exchange transfusion can be performed but the procedure is more frequently carried out after birth. The exchange transfusion is given via the umbilical vein. Approximately 10 mL of the baby's blood is removed first and then an equal volume of Rh-negative blood is transfused. The procedure is then repeated. In this way, the baby's Rh-positive blood is progressively removed so that it does not have to metabolize the degradation products of its own blood cells. The transfused Rh-negative cells correct the baby's anaemia. These cells have a normal life span, of approximately 120 days, by which time the maternal anti-D has disappeared.

### ABO haemolytic disease of the newborn

Several factors protect the fetus from the effects of ABO fetomaternal incompatibility so that ABO haemolytic disease of the newborn is uncommon even though ABO incompatibility between mother and fetus occurs in 20% of births. These factors include:

• the relative weakness of fetal A and B antigens
• the occurrence of A and B glycoproteins on other tissues and in body fluids; this diverts maternal anti-A and anti-B, which cross the placenta, away from the fetus' red blood cells.

ABO haemolytic disease can occur in a first pregnancy because anti-A and anti-B are naturally present in the plasma. Group A and group B babies of group O mothers are most frequently at risk. Although this situation occurs in about 25% of pregnancies, only about 1% of babies show a degree of haemolysis and jaundice and the condition is usually mild.

## The blood in ageing

### DEVELOPMENTAL ISSUES

There is no significant change in either the rate of red blood cell formation or in red cell indices, such as the haematocrit and mean cell haemoglobin concentration, in elderly human beings. White cell and platelet counts and indices, and clotting time also show no age associated alterations.

Plasma levels of triglyceride lipids (fats) and cholesterol begin to increase as early as 20 years of age and this continues steadily with increasing age. The evidence for causal connection between the lipid and cholesterol content of a person's diet and the occurrence of atheromatous disease of the coronary (and other) arteries (coronary heart disease) is extremely complex (LaRosa et al., 1999). Heredity, smoking and diet are all factors involved in the changes in the heart and blood vessels that occur with age.

## Conclusion

Blood is the fluid that is normally contained within the heart and blood vessels. It is composed of red cells, white cells, platelets and plasma. Its major function is the carriage of organic and inorganic substances, which are continuously exchanged with those contained in the interstitial fluid surrounding the cells. This exchange maintains the composition of the internal environment.

Certain components of blood have a vital function in producing the inflammatory and immune responses and in maintaining the patency of the blood vessels.

The widespread involvement of blood in homeostasis underlies the finding that pathological processes almost always affect its composition. For the same reason, a wide variety of health problems are produced if blood is lost from the circulation and if the blood cells, or the constituents of plasma, are abnormal.

## Clinical review

In addition to the Learning Objectives at the beginning of this chapter, the reader should be able to:

- Give examples of other normal and abnormal human haemoglobins and their effects
- Define the term 'anaemia' and explain the occurrence of the health problems associated with this state
- Outline the metabolism of iron, vitamin B12 and folic acid, and the features of the anaemias produced by deficiency of these substances
- Relate the functions of white blood cells to changes in white cell counts and morphology in illness
- Outline the major health problems associated with platelet deficiency
- Relate the process of haemostasis to the major defects of bleeding and clotting, the occurrence of thrombosis and types of antithrombotic therapy
- Enumerate and discuss clinical problems associated with the transfusion of blood and apply this knowledge to nursing responsibilities in the care of people undergoing blood transfusion
- Describe and explain the occurrence of the major types of fetomaternal blood incompatibility and discuss the prevention of these
- Recognize the importance of policies and procedures relating to the safe handling of blood and blood products

## Review questions

1  Describe the appearance and major constituents of blood and outline its major functions.
2  List the various constituents of plasma and relate these to the interpretation of biochemical estimations performed clinically.
3  Name the major groups of plasma proteins and explain their functions.
4  Describe how and where blood cells are produced and how this process is regulated.
5  Describe the structure and function of mature red blood cells.
6  Outline the structure and functions of haemoglobin A and give examples of other normal and abnormal human haemoglobins and their effects.
7  Define the term 'anaemia' and explain the occurrence of the health problems associated with this state.
8  Describe the functions of the various types of white blood cell and relate the functions of white blood cells to changes in white cell counts and morphology in illness.
9  List the functions of platelets and outline the major health problems associated with platelet deficiency.
10  Outline the key stages in the process of haemostasis and relate the process of haemostasis to three major defects of bleeding and clotting.
11  List risk factors for the occurrence of thrombosis and outline the mode of action of major types of antithrombotic therapy.
12  Explain the genetic and physiological bases of the major blood group systems and explain their clinical significance.

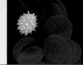
## Suggestions for further reading

BMJ (2002) ABC of antithrombotic therapy. *British Medical Journal*, **325**.
*This volume of the* British Medical Journal *contains several papers on the topic of antithrombotic therapy.*

Hoffbrand, A.V., Pettit, J.E. & Moss, P.A.H. (2001) *Essential Haematology*, 4th edn. Oxford: Blackwell Science.
*Authoritative, clearly presented text. A useful handbook in wards and clinics dealing with people with diseases of the blood.*

McClelland, D.B.L. (ed) (2001) *Handbook of Transfusion Medicine. Blood Transfusion Services of the United Kingdom*, 3rd edn. London: The Stationery Office.

*Intended for all involved in prescribing, supplying and administering blood products.*

Miller, J. (1978) *The Body in Question*. London: Jonathan Cape.
*Fascinating classical text in which Dr Miller considers varieties of pathological experience, and the physical foundations of 'dis – ease'*

The Donor
*News and Information from the National Blood Service. Available from: The National Blood Service, West Derby Street, Liverpool, L7 8TW. A quarterly seasonal free magazine giving news of the service for blood donors.*

## Useful websites and addresses

National Blood Service: www.blood.co.uk
*The National Blood Service is run by the National Blood Authority, which is a special Health Authority within the National Health Service. This website contains information about the service and blood and bone marrow donation.*

www.transfusionguidelines.org.uk
*This website contains the UK Transfusion Services'*

*handbook of transfusion medicine as well as links to other relevant websites.*

www.bcshguidelines.com
*British Committee for Standards in Haematology guidelines.*

www.doh.gov.uk
*A whole series of documents, some of which are concerned with blood and blood precautions.*

## References

BBC News (2003) *Designer baby born to UK couple*. Online. Available: www.news.bbc.co.uk/2/hi/health/3002610.stm

Blann, A.D., Landray, M.J. & Lip, G.Y.H. (2002) An overview of antithrombotic therapy. ABC of antithrombotic therapy. *British Medical Journal*, **325**; 762–765.

Boon, N.A., Fox, K.A.A., Bloomfield, P. & Bradbury, A. (2002) Cardiovascular disease. In: Haslett, C. et al., (eds) *Davidson's Principles and Practice of Medicine*. Edinburgh: Churchill Livingstone, pp. 357–481.

Collins, P.W. (1998) Disseminated intravascular coagulation. *CME Bulletins in Hematology*, **1**; 86–88.

Craig, J.I.O., Haynes, A.P., McClelland, D.B.L. & Ludlam, C.A. (2002) Blood disorders. In: Haslett, C. et al., (eds) *Davidson's Principles and Practice of Medicine*. Edinburgh: Churchill Livingstone, pp. 889–956.

Galbraith, A., Bullock, S., Richards, A. & Hunt, B. (1999) *Fundamentals of Pharmacology: A Text for Nurses and Health Professionals*. Harlow: Prentice Hall.

Hoffbrand, A.V., Pettit, J.E. & Moss, J.A.H. (2001) *Essential Haematology*, 4th edn. Oxford: Blackwell Science Ltd.

LaRosa, J.C., He, J. & Vupputuri, S. (1999) Effect of statins on risk of coronary disease: a meta-analysis of randomized controlled trials. *Journal of the American Medical Association*, **282**; 2340–2346.

McClelland, D.B.L. (ed) (2001) *Handbook of Transfusion Medicine. Blood Transfusion Services of the United Kingdom*, 3rd edn. London: The Stationery Office.

Nairn, R. & Helbert, M. (2002) *Immunology for Medical Students*. St Louis: Mosby.

Norris, L.A. (2003) Blood coagulation. *Best Practice and Research Clinical Obstetrics and Gynaecology*, **17**(3); 369–383.

Sergeant, G.R. (2001) *Sickle Cell Anaemia*, 3rd edn. Oxford: Oxford University Press.

Weatherall, D.J. & Clegg, J.B. (2001) *The Thallassaemia Syndromes*, 4th edn. Oxford: Blackwell Science.

# Chapter 4.2

# Cardiovascular function

*Rosamund A. Herbert    Mandy Sheppard*

## LEARNING OBJECTIVES

After studying this chapter the reader should be able to:

- Discuss the vital significance of maintaining an adequate circulation of blood to the tissues at all times

- Describe the normal structure and function of the heart and vascular system

- Demonstrate how disruption of normal function in any part of the cardiovascular system can lead to abnormal states or disease and interferes with tissue nutrition

- Discuss the common forms of treatment used in cardiac and vascular disease, e.g. rest, surgery, drug therapy, and relate them to the abnormal physiology

- Discuss ways of maintaining a healthy cardiovascular system and ways of reducing the risks of developing cardiovascular disease

- Base your assessment, planning, delivery and evaluation of nursing care of patients with cardiovascular problems on sound physiological principles

- Discuss the various ways of assessing the cardiovascular system and be aware of the significance of parameters being monitored

- Give adequate and comprehensive explanations of normal and abnormal conditions to patients and other colleagues

## INTRODUCTION

The functioning of the human body as a whole depends on the individual and collective functioning of all the cells. For optimal function, each cell depends on being in a stable internal environment with a constant supply of nutrients and removal of unwanted substances; it is the role of the circulatory and lymphatic systems to perform these functions. Blood, the fluid within the circulatory system, is considered in Chapter 4.1, and the lymphatic system is discussed in Chapter 6.2. However, as more is discovered about the cardiovascular system it is becoming apparent that this system is much more than a simple transport system: many aspects of its function are intimately controlled with homeostasis, for example some parts perform endocrine functions.

As maintaining an adequate circulation is vital to health, many of the nurse's observations are concerned with assessing, either directly or indirectly, the state of an individual's circulatory system, e.g. taking the pulse rate, recording blood pressure and assessing the pallor of the skin. Pressure area care can even be included: pressure ulcers develop because pressure (usually the individual's own weight) occludes the circulation to tissues, which become ischaemic. Without adequate perfusion the integrity of the tissue is destroyed and the tissue breaks down (see Chapter 6.1).

## General description of the cardiovascular system

The major function of the cardiovascular system is to ensure an adequate circulation of blood to the tissues of the body at all times and thus to transport substances to and from the individual cells as required. The cardiovascular system is made up of the heart functioning as a pump, with the blood vessels as conveyors of blood and the capillaries as permeable exchange beds. The components of the cardiovascular system need to maintain an adequate flow of blood to the tissues and, at the same time, the correct conditions for an appropriate rate of exchange of materials between the blood and the tissues, i.e. producing a suitable gradient for material diffusing out at the arterial end and back into the blood vessels at the venular end.

The cardiovascular system is dynamic and is capable of maintaining an adequate flow to the tissues under varying circumstances, for example at rest, when exercising, even standing on one's head and when compromised by disease states. As there is a finite volume of blood, this flexibility is achieved by directing blood to where it is most needed and away from less active areas. Conflicts can, and do, arise; for instance, if strenuous exercise is undertaken shortly after eating a large meal, both the gastrointestinal system and the muscles require an increased blood flow, which might not be feasible; it is not possible to supply both systems with large blood flows at the same time. After a meal and during digestion, the gut has priority and strenuous exercise cannot usually be maintained.

However, at all times, maintaining an adequate blood flow to vital organs such as the brain and heart has priority. The cardiovascular system as a whole is controlled and coordinated by centres in the brain, although local influences and reflexes are also very important. Tissues that do not have an adequate blood flow, i.e. are **ischaemic**, show signs of adverse effects quickly.

The main role of the cardiovascular system is that of general transport and can be subdivided into the following.

- **Delivery** of substances to all body tissues to maintain their nutrition and metabolic function, i.e. oxygen, nutrients and other substances manufactured in the body such as hormones, amino acids, defence cells.
- **Removal** of carbon dioxide and metabolic endproducts from tissues and delivery to the appropriate organs for breakdown and elimination, e.g. lungs, liver, kidneys.
- **Dissipation** of heat away from active tissues and its redistribution around the body to maintain normal body temperature.

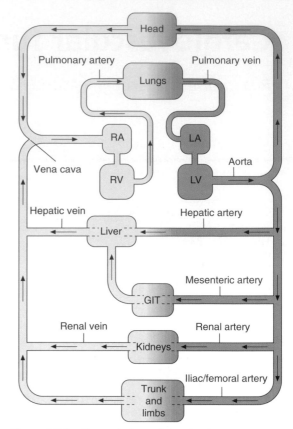

**Figure 4.2.1** General plans of the circulatory system showing (a) diagramatic view

In humans, as in all mammals, there are two distinct circuits within the cardiovascular system, known as the systemic and pulmonary circulations **(Fig. 4.2.1)**. Both circulations originate and terminate in the heart, which is itself functionally divided into two pumps.

The **systemic circulation** supplies all the body tissues and is where exchange of nutrients and products of metabolism occurs; all the blood for the systemic circulation leaves the left side of the heart via the aorta. This large artery then divides into smaller arteries, which deliver blood to all the tissues and organs of the body. These arteries divide into smaller and smaller vessels **(Fig. 4.2.2)**, each with its own characteristic structure and function. The smallest branches are called **arterioles**. The arterioles themselves branch into a number of very small thin vessels, the **capillaries**, and it is here that the exchange of gases, nutrients and waste products occurs. Exchange occurs by diffusion of substances down concentration and pressure gradients. The capillaries then unite to form larger vessels, **venules**, which in turn unite to form fewer and larger vessels, known as **veins**. The veins from different organs and tissues unite to form two large veins, the **inferior vena cava** (from the lower portion of the body) and the **superior vena cava** (from the head and arms), which

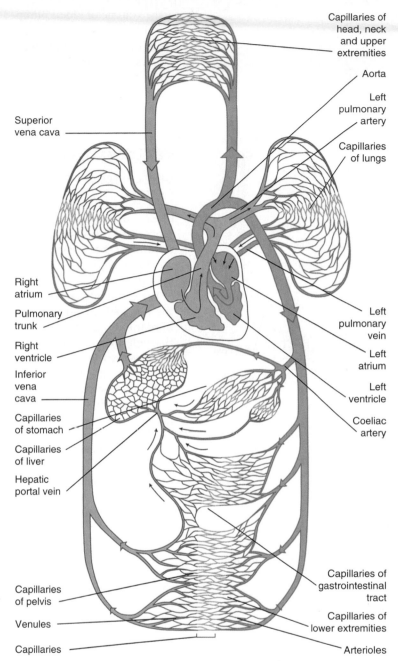

**Figure 4.2.1** (*Contd*)   (b) some of the capillary beds. LA, left atrium; LV, left ventricle; RA, right atrium; RV, right ventricle. Adapted from Watson, R. (1999) *Essential Science for Nursing Students*. London: Ballière Tindall

return blood to the right side of the heart. Thus there are a number of parallel circuits within the systemic circulation **(see Fig. 4.2.1)**.

The **pulmonary circulation** is where oxygen and carbon dioxide exchange between the blood and alveolar air occurs. The blood leaves the right side of the heart through a single artery, the **pulmonary artery**, which divides into two – one branch supplying each lung. Within the lungs, the arteries divide, ultimately forming arterioles and capillaries; venules and veins return blood to the left side of the heart.

All arteries carry blood away from the heart and all arteries, except the pulmonary artery, carry blood with a high oxygen content and deliver this to the tissues. Veins carry blood back to the heart. **Figure 4.2.3** shows the major arteries and veins in the body.

Normally, there is only one capillary bed for each branch of a circuit; however, there are a few instances where there are two capillary beds, one after each other, in series. These are known as **portal systems** or portal circulations. One example of this is in the liver. Part of the blood supply to the liver is venous blood

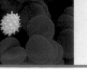

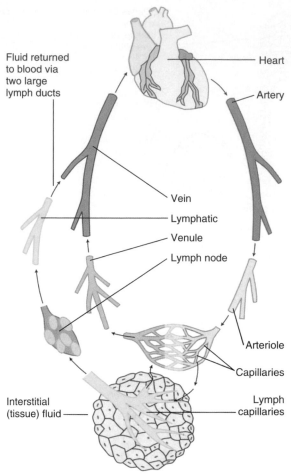

Fluid returned to blood via two large lymph ducts

Heart

Artery

Vein

Lymphatic

Venule

Lymph node

Arteriole

Capillaries

Interstitial (tissue) fluid

Lymph capillaries

**Figure 4.2.2** Relationship between the blood vessels in the circulatory system

coming directly from the gastrointestinal tract and spleen via the hepatic portal vein. This arrangement enables the digested and absorbed substances from the gut to be transported directly to the liver, where many of the body's metabolic requirements are synthesized. Thus there are two microcirculations in series, one in the gut and the other in the liver (for fuller details, see Chapter 5.2).

The force required to move the blood through the blood vessels in the pulmonary and systemic circulations is provided by the heart, which functions as two pumps: the left side of the heart supplying the systemic circulation and the right side the pulmonary circulation. The systemic circulation is much larger than the pulmonary circulation and thus the force generated by the left side of the heart is much greater than that of the right side of the heart. However, as the circulatory system is a closed system, the volume of blood pumped through the pulmonary circulation in a given period of time must equal the volume pumped through the systemic circulation – that is, the right and left sides of the heart must pump the same amount of blood. In a normal resting adult, the

average volume of blood pumped simultaneously is approximately 5 L/min. As there are approximately 5 litres of blood in an adult, this means that the blood circulates around the body approximately once every minute. During heavy work or exercise, the volume of blood pumped by the heart can increase up to 25 L/min (or even 35 L/min in elite athletes).

## DEVELOPMENTAL ISSUES

### DEVELOPMENT OF THE CARDIOVASCULAR SYSTEM

Before considering the detailed structure and function of the heart and circulation it is helpful to consider the development of these structures during fetal growth and the changes that occur at birth.

The embryo obtains its nourishment during the very early stages of development via diffusion of nutrients from the maternal blood flow through the syncitiotrophoblast in the placenta. Blood vessels develop towards the end of the third week and join to form a continuous system of vessels. The primitive heart forms during the fourth and fifth weeks of development and pulsatile movements begin around this time, too. The heart arises from an enlarged blood vessel with a large lumen and a muscular wall. The middle part of the vessel begins to grow faster than the ends and this causes the tube to bulge and twist **(Fig. 4.2.4)**. The vessel at the cranial end of the embryo divides and becomes the aorta and pulmonary artery, whereas part of the vessel at the caudal end becomes the superior and inferior venae cavae.

Inside the developing heart, complex changes occur that result in the eventual development of the four chambers of the heart and the atrioventricular and pulmonary valves. Atrial and ventricular septa divide the tubular heart into separate right and left sides. During the formation of the atrial septum, an opening called the **foramen ovale** develops to establish a communicating channel between the two upper chambers of the heart. If parts of the septa that form the boundaries to the chambers do not develop correctly congenital heart defects can arise (see later). By the seventh or eighth week the normal structures should have been formed.

Throughout fetal life, the placenta transfers maternal oxygen and nutrients to the fetus and transfers waste products out of the fetal circulation. The fetal circulation is different from the normal circulation of extrauterine life. **Figure 4.2.5** shows the normal fetal circulation. Fetal blood is oxygenated via the placenta and

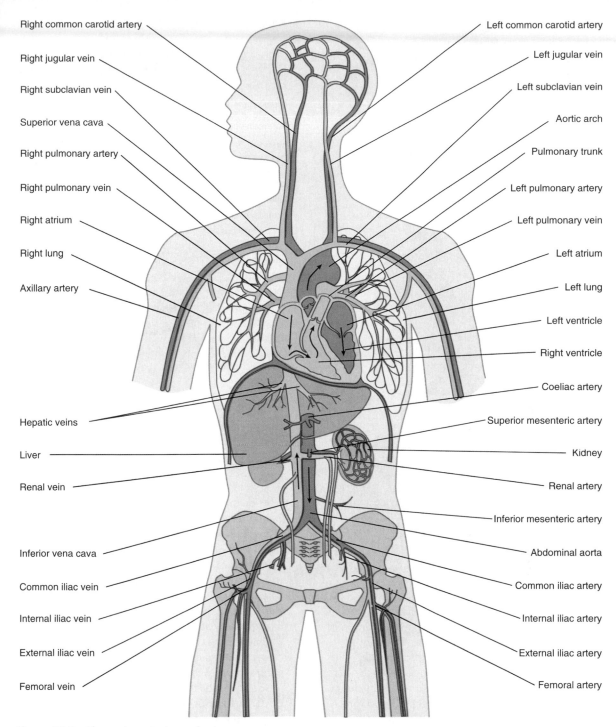

Right common carotid artery

Right jugular vein

Right subclavian vein

Superior vena cava

Right pulmonary artery

Right pulmonary vein

Right atrium

Right lung

Axillary artery

Hepatic veins

Liver

Renal vein

Inferior vena cava

Common iliac vein

Internal iliac vein

External iliac vein

Femoral vein

Left common carotid artery

Left jugular vein

Left subclavian vein

Aortic arch

Pulmonary trunk

Left pulmonary artery

Left pulmonary vein

Left atrium

Left lung

Left ventricle

Right ventricle

Coeliac artery

Superior mesenteric artery

Kidney

Renal artery

Inferior mesenteric artery

Abdominal aorta

Common iliac artery

Internal iliac artery

External iliac artery

Femoral artery

**Figure 4.2.3** The major arteries and veins

returns to the fetus in the umbilical vein. So the umbilical vein carries oxygenated blood and nutrients from the placenta to the fetus. The umbilical vein enters the navel of the fetus and travels towards the liver. About half the blood enters the liver and the rest flows through the **ductus venosus** (a connecting vessel from the hepatic vessels to the vena cava) directly into the inferior vena cava; this facilitates mixing of blood from the lower parts of the fetus. From the inferior vena cava, all the blood flows into the right atrium; most of the blood flows directly through the **foramen ovale** (the opening between the right and left atria), through the left ventricle and is pumped primarily to the heart and brain – this ensures that the heart and brain receive well-oxygenated blood.

Blood from the upper body of the fetus collects in the superior vena cava and will be mixed with the blood from the inferior vena cava in the

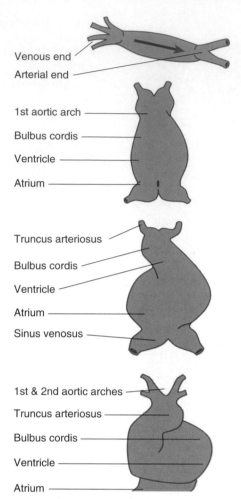

Figure 4.2.4 The embryonic development of the heart showing the external appearance of the fetal heart (adapted from Moore, K.L. (1993) *The Developing Human*, 5th edn, Philadelphia: W.B. Saunders)

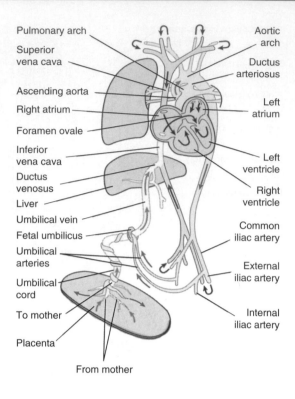

→ **Oxygenated blood from the placenta**
→ **Deoxygenated blood**
→ **Mixture of oxygenated/deoxygenated blood**

Figure 4.2.5 Fetal circulation

right atrium. A small amount of right atrial blood enters the right ventricle and is pumped into the pulmonary artery. Once in the pulmonary artery most of the blood bypasses the lungs by flowing directly into the aorta through the **ductus arteriosus**. A small amount of blood does flow to the lungs; during fetal life the lungs are not expanded and so only need blood for their own tissue development: the placenta provides the gas exchange until the time of birth. The blood from the lungs returns to the left atrium and will leave the heart via the left ventricle in the aorta. The aorta divides to form the common iliac arteries and then branches into the external and internal iliac arteries. The blood in the internal iliac arteries passes into the two umbilical arteries and flows back to the placenta for exchange of gases and nutrients; the external iliac arteries supply the lower part of the fetal body with the blood returning via the inferior vena cava.

At birth, the infant inhales for the first time: the pulmonary vascular resistance falls dramatically and thus a greater volume of blood flows through the lungs and more blood returns to the left atrium. This causes the pressure in the left atrium to increase and the flap of the foramen ovale closes **(Fig. 4.2.5)**. The closure of the foramen ovale is further aided by the fall in pressure that occurs in the right atrium as umbilical flow ceases. So the foramen ovale closes functionally at birth and anatomically several months later.

Soon after birth the smooth muscle of the ductus arteriosus constricts in response to an increased $PO_2$ and also in response to other substances released at birth such as bradykinin, serotonin and prostaglandin inhibitors. The ductus arteriosus closes functionally 15–18 hours after birth and anatomically within 10–21 days. The umbilical arteries constrict at birth to prevent loss of the baby's blood. The umbilical vein remains patent for some time and can be used for exchange transfusion in the newborn baby.

Once the lungs and other systems in the infant's body become established, the special features of the fetal circulation are no longer required. The placenta is expelled by the mother, the umbilical arteries atrophy and become the lateral umbilical ligaments, the umbilical vein becomes the round ligament of the liver and the ductus venosus becomes the ligamentum venosum, which is a fibrous cord in the liver. The flap on the foramen ovale usually closes and becomes a depression in the interatrial septum and the ductus arteriosus atrophies.

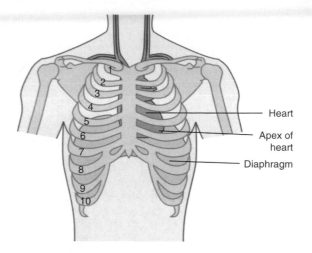

## The heart

### Location and structure (Fig. 4.2.6)

The heart lies in the **mediastinum**, which is the central part of the thorax. It lies between the two pleural sacs that contain the lungs. The mediastinum extends from the sternum to the vertebral column and contains all the thoracic organs except the lungs.

The heart is shaped like a blunt cone and lies with its base towards the head. Approximately two-thirds of its mass lies to the left of the body's midline. The heart is enclosed in a fibrous sac, the **pericardium**, which provides a tough protective membrane around it and anchors it in the mediastinum by its attachments to the large blood vessels entering and leaving the heart, to the diaphragm and to the sternal wall of the chest. Between the pericardium and the heart is a potential space called the **pericardial cavity**. This cavity contains watery fluid, known as **pericardial fluid**, which prevents friction as the heart moves. Inflammation of the pericardium is called **pericarditis** and is often associated with a pericardial friction rub, which can be heard on auscultation of the pericardial area.

### The walls

The walls of the heart consist mainly of muscle called the **myocardium**. It is this muscle that is responsible for pumping the blood (cardiac muscle will be discussed in more detail later). The myocardium is lined on its internal surface by a layer of epithelium, which covers the valves of the heart and the tendons that hold them. This is called the **endocardium**. On the outer surface of the myocardium is an external layer called the **epicardium**. Inflammation of the various layers is referred to as myocarditis, endocarditis and epicarditis, respectively.

### Chambers

The interior of the heart is divided into four hollow chambers, which receive the circulating blood (**Fig. 4.2.7**). The two upper chambers are called the right and left **atria**; they are separated by the **interatrial**

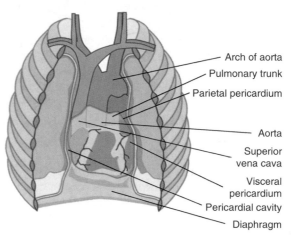

**Figure 4.2.6** Location of the heart and associated blood vessels in the thorax

**septum**. The two lower chambers are called the right and left **ventricles**, and these are separated by the **interventricular** septum. Each atrium is separated from its respective ventricle by a valve. Therefore it is the septa and the valves which divide the heart into four chambers.

### DEVELOPMENTAL ISSUES

As discussed earlier, formation of the heart during early fetal development is a complex process and congenital heart defects are not uncommon. Most of the cardiovascular defects will have developed by the eighth week of gestation. Many causes of congenital heart defects have been identified: environmental risk factors tend to be maternal conditions, for instance viral infections, diabetes, drugs, alcohol and increased maternal age. Genetic factors have also been implicated as there is an increased incidence of defects in the siblings of affected children, although the precise cause is often unknown. Chromosomal abnormalities can

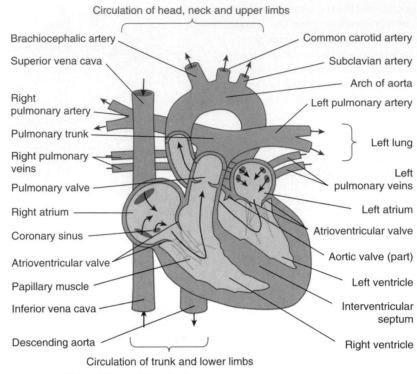

Circulation of head, neck and upper limbs

Brachiocephalic artery
Superior vena cava
Right pulmonary artery
Pulmonary trunk
Right pulmonary veins
Pulmonary valve
Right atrium
Coronary sinus
Atrioventricular valve
Papillary muscle
Inferior vena cava
Descending aorta

Common carotid artery
Subclavian artery
Arch of aorta
Left pulmonary artery
Left lung
Left pulmonary veins
Left atrium
Atrioventricular valve
Aortic valve (part)
Left ventricle
Interventricular septum
Right ventricle

Circulation of trunk and lower limbs

**Figure 4.2.7** The direction of blood flow within the heart

also lead to congenital heart defects, e.g. in Down syndrome and Turner's syndrome.

Abnormalities can occur in the septa that divide the chambers. Such abnormalities most often consist of a hole in the septum (septal defect) that allows a communication either between the atria or between the ventricles. Atrial septal defects usually occur because of failure of the foramen ovale (the opening in the interatrial septum of the fetal heart) to close after birth. Because the pressure in the left atrium is higher than in the right, blood flows from the left atrium into the right. This overloads the pulmonary circulation and decreases the flow in the systemic circulation, which can result in inhibition of body growth. Ventricular septal defects allow mixing of oxygenated and deoxygenated blood so that the oxygenation of the blood pumped into the systemic circulation is decreased. The individual becomes cyanosed (a bluish discoloration of the skin). Septal defects can correct themselves over time but if they do not they can be corrected surgically, either by sewing them together or by covering them with synthetic patches.

Another congenital defect results from the ductus arteriosus remaining open or patent. This is known as patent ductus arteriosus (PDA). If necessary the defect can be treated by ligation of the patent ductus arteriosus. For a fuller discussion of the pathophysiology of alterations in cardiovascular function in children, see MacGregor (2000).

## Valves

The valves that lie between the atria and their ventricles are called the **atrioventricular (AV) valves**. The atrioventricular valve between the right atrium and the right ventricle is called the **tricuspid valve** because it consists of three cusps, or flaps. The atrioventricular valve between the left atrium and the left ventricle is called the **mitral** or **bicuspid valve** because it has two cusps. When the ventricles contract, the pressure exerted on these valves by the blood forces them to close, thus preventing backflow of blood into the atria. To stop the valves themselves being forced backwards into the atria, they are attached to muscular projections of the ventricular wall (**papillary muscles**) by fibrous strands called **chordae tendineae**.

The valves that lie between the ventricles and the major arteries that leave the heart are called the **semilunar valves**, so named because of their half-moon or crescent shape (**Fig. 4.2.8**). The **pulmonary semilunar valve** lies where the pulmonary trunk leaves the right ventricle; the **aortic semilunar valve** lies where the aorta leaves the left ventricle. The semilunar valves are forced open when the ventricles contract, allowing blood to be ejected into the aorta and pulmonary artery. As soon as the ventricles relax, there is a back pressure of blood from the aorta and pulmonary artery that closes the valves. This prevents backflow of blood into the ventricles. Thus the valves ensure one-way flow of blood through the heart.

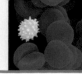
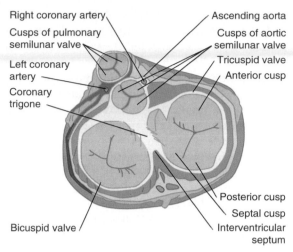

Right coronary artery
Cusps of pulmonary
semilunar valve
Left coronary
artery
Coronary
trigone
Ascending aorta
Cusps of aortic
semilunar valve
Tricuspid valve
Anterior cusp
Posterior cusp
Septal cusp
Interventricular
septum
Bicuspid valve

**Figure 4.2.8**   The valves of the heart (superior aspect)

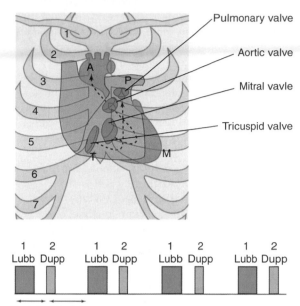

Pulmonary valve
Aortic valve
Mitral vavle
Tricuspid valve

| 1 | 2 | 1 | 2 | 1 | 2 | 1 | 2 |
|---|---|---|---|---|---|---|---|
| Lubb | Dupp | Lubb | Dupp | Lubb | Dupp | Lubb | Dupp |

Systole  Diastole

**Figure 4.2.9**   External anatomical locations of valve sounds A, P, T and M (aortic, pulmonary, tricuspid and mitral valves respectively) of the heart. Note that the sounds are not located directly above the valves. The lower part of the figure shows a phonetic representation of the heart sounds

The closure of the valves defines the period of ventricular contraction because the atrioventricular valves close when the ventricles start contracting and the semilunar valves close when the ventricles stop contracting (i.e. relax). Thus, during each cardiac cycle two **heart sounds** can be heard through a stethoscope applied to the chest wall. The **first heart sound**, which can be described as a 'lubb' sound (long and booming), is associated with the closure of the atrioventricular valves at the beginning of ventricular contraction. The **second heart sound**, which can be described as a 'dupp' sound (short and sharp), is associated with the closure of the semilunar valves at the beginning of ventricular relaxation. The sounds result primarily from turbulence in the blood flow created by the closure of the valves. They can be represented phonetically as in **Fig. 4.2.9**.

Although heart sounds are associated with the closure of the valves, the sounds produced by each valve tend to be heard more clearly in a slightly different position from the anatomical surface projections of the valves. **Figure 4.2.9** shows the surface projections of the valves and the letters, A, P, T, and M (aortic, pulmonary, tricuspid and mitral) indicate where the sounds they produce are best heard. Occasionally, sounds additional to these two heart sounds are heard over a normal healthy heart. For example, in children with thin chest walls, a third heart sound can sometimes be heard during early diastole; this is believed to originate from vibrations of the ventricular walls due to changes in blood flow.

As well as auscultation of the chest for heart sounds, the heart rate is often counted by listening to the **apex beat**. The apex of the heart lies close to the anterior chest wall, usually in the fifth intercostal space in the mid-clavicular line. It produces a pulsation against the chest wall with each ventricular contraction. This pulsation can often be seen and felt in thin individuals and can be heard by auscultation.

## CLINICAL APPLICATIONS

Damage to the heart valves can disrupt the flow of blood through the heart: rheumatic fever and bacterial endocarditis are the most common causes of valvular damage. Rheumatic fever is an autoimmune or allergic disease that can affect many different tissues of the body but especially the heart valves. Damage to the valves can cause the cusps of the valve to stick together, thus narrowing the opening. This is called valvular **stenosis**. At the same time, damage to the edges of the cusps means that they cannot close completely and there is backflow, or regurgitation, of blood through the valve. The valve is said to be **incompetent**. Stenosis and incompetence often coexist but usually one predominates, so the valve is said to be either stenosed or incompetent.

Stenosed or incompetent valves cause sound additional to the normal heart sounds. Normally, when blood flows smoothly in a streamlined manner it makes no sound, but turbulent flow produced either by blood flowing rapidly in the usual direction through an abnormally narrowed (stenosed) valve or backwards through a leaky (incompetent) valve produces a **murmur** or sloshing sound. (Murmur might also be heard if blood is able to move between the two atria or the two ventricles via a septal defect.)

Damaged valves decrease the efficiency of the heart as a pump as more work has to be done either to pump blood through a stenosed valve or to pump the extra blood that flows back through an incompetent valve. In the long term, the effects of valvular damage can result in failure of the pump.

Heart valves can be replaced surgically with either mechanical or tissue valves. Mechanical valves are longer lasting and might be recommended for younger patients. The main disadvantage of mechanical valves is the requirement for anticoagulant therapy. Tissue valves can be animal in origin (porcine) or a preserved human valve (homograph). Tissue valves do not last as long as mechanical valves but there is no need for anticoagulant therapy.

## Direction of blood flow

As already stated, valves ensure one-way flow of blood through the heart **(see Fig. 4.2.7)**. Blood enters the right atrium from the **superior vena cava**, which brings venous blood from the upper portion of the body (i.e. head and arms), and from the **inferior vena cava**, which brings blood from the lower portions of the body (i.e. trunk and legs). This blood passes from the right atrium through the tricuspid valve into the right ventricle, from where it is pumped through the pulmonary valve into the **pulmonary trunk**. The pulmonary trunk divides into the **right** and **left pulmonary arteries**, which carry the blood to the right and left lung, respectively, where gaseous exchange takes place. These are the only arteries to carry deoxygenated blood. This blood returns to the left atrium via four **pulmonary veins**. This is the only place in the body where veins carry highly oxygenated blood. The blood passes from the left atrium into the left ventricle. The left ventricle pumps blood through the aortic valve into the aorta. Arteries branch from the aorta and carry blood to all parts of the body.

## Cardiac muscle

Cardiac muscle combines certain properties of skeletal and smooth muscle. Like skeletal muscle, it is striated and its myofibrils contain actin and myosin filaments (see Chapter 3.1). However, cardiac muscle differs from skeletal muscle in that the cell membranes that separate individual muscle cells have a very low electrical resistance. These membranes are called **intercalated discs (Fig. 4.2.10)**. The action potentials travel from one cardiac muscle cell to another through the intercalated discs without significant hindrance. In this respect, cardiac muscle is similar to smooth muscle. The ability of the action potential to spread to all cells if one cell becomes excited means that cardiac muscle acts as a functional whole. This ability is further enhanced by the shape of the action potential. After an initial spike, the membrane has a plateau of depolarization that lasts for 0.15–0.3 seconds **(Fig. 4.2.11)**. This long duration of the action potential (relative to the velocity of conduction) ensures that the impulse has time to travel over the whole atrial or ventricular muscle mass, causing complete contraction of each muscle mass as a unit, before any portion of the muscle can repolarize and relax. This is essential for efficient pumping.

The action potential is followed by a period in which the muscle is refractory to restimulation. This prevents tetanic contractions and fatigue and ensures that the muscle relaxes between action potentials, permitting it to fill with blood. If there were no relaxation phase, i.e. if tetanic stimulation were possible, no blood would enter the heart and thus the heart's action as a pump would be defunct.

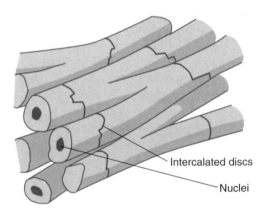

**Figure 4.2.10** The structure of cardiac muscle showing the intercalated discs

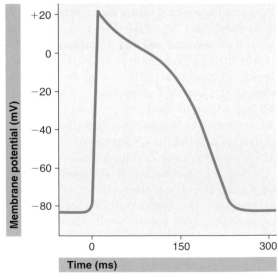

**Figure 4.2.11** The action potential in cardiac muscle

Therefore, three factors affect the way cardiac muscle contracts: (i) the intercalated discs; (ii) the long duration of the action potential and (iii) the long refractory period. These factors, combined with sequential depolarization of the muscle due to the organization of the conducting system (see later), ensure that the heart muscle contracts in a coordinated and effective manner.

The way the actual excitation of the cardiac muscle cell results in contraction (i.e. excitation–contraction coupling) is similar to that of skeletal muscle (see Chapter 3.1). However, in cardiac muscle more of the calcium required for muscle contraction comes from the transverse tubules (T-tubules) rather than from the sarcoplasmic reticulum as in skeletal muscle. The importance of this is that the T-tubules are filled with extracellular fluid, and so the concentration of calcium in the extracellular fluid can alter the strength of cardiac muscle contraction.

As in skeletal muscle, the strength of contraction or tension that a cardiac muscle fibre can generate is related to its length at rest. This is known as the **length–tension relationship** and is discussed in Chapter 3.1 in regard to skeletal muscle. The more the cardiac muscle fibre is stretched before contraction, the greater will be the force of contraction or energy output. This is true up to a critical point, beyond which further increases in muscle length result in a decrease in the strength of contraction because the muscle is stretched beyond its physiological limits.

The length of cardiac muscle fibres is affected by the amount of blood in the chambers of the heart before contraction. Normally, during sedentary activities, the resting length of cardiac muscle (i.e. the length of the muscle fibres during the relaxation phase of the cardiac cycle) does not yield maximum force of contraction, thus leaving a margin for coping with increasing amounts of blood returning to the heart. When venous return to the heart increases, as during exercise, there is a consequent increase in the amount of blood in the ventricles, termed the ventricular end-diastolic volume (VEDV). This stretches the muscle fibres and results in a greater force of contraction and more blood is expelled.

This is the basis of **Starling's law of the heart**, which basically states that the force of contraction of cardiac muscle is proportional to the resting length of the muscle fibres. Therefore, within physiological limits, the more the heart is filled with blood during its relaxation phase, the greater will be the force of contraction, and hence the quantity of blood pumped out during contraction will increase. Other factors affecting the quantity of blood ejected by each ventricle with each contraction (stroke volume) will be discussed later.

## Blood supply – the coronary circulation

When the body is at rest, the oxygen consumption of the heart muscle is approximately 8 mL/100 g/min, which is greater than that of any other tissue.

Oxygenated blood is carried to the cardiac muscle by the right and left **coronary arteries** and their branches **(Fig. 4.2.12)**. The coronary arteries originate from the aorta just beyond the aortic valve. The right coronary artery supplies the right atrium and ventricle and portions of the left ventricle. The left coronary artery divides near its origin into the left anterior descending branch and the circumflex branch. The former supplies blood to the anterior part of the left ventricle and a small part of the anterior and posterior of the right ventricle. The circumflex branch supplies the left atrium and upper front and rear of the left ventricle. The major coronary

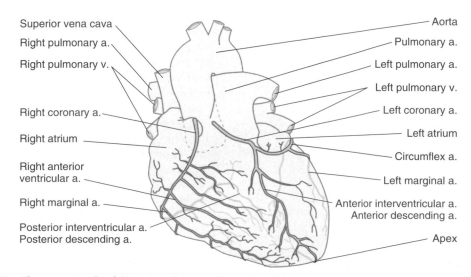

Superior vena cava
Right pulmonary a.
Right pulmonary v.
Right coronary a.
Right atrium
Right anterior ventricular a.
Right marginal a.
Posterior interventricular a.
Posterior descending a.

Aorta
Pulmonary a.
Left pulmonary a.
Left pulmonary v.
Left coronary a.
Left atrium
Circumflex a.
Left marginal a.
Anterior interventricular a.
Anterior descending a.
Apex

**Figure 4.2.12**   The coronary circulation. a, artery; v, vein

arteries lie on the surface of the heart and the branches penetrate deep into the cardiac muscle.

Most of the venous blood from the left ventricular muscle returns to the right atrium through the **coronary sinus**, which is a thin-walled vein without any smooth muscle to alter its diameter. Most of the venous blood from the right ventricular muscle flows through the small anterior cardiac veins into the right atrium.

## Factors that influence coronary blood flow

The coronary blood flow shows the property of **autoregulation** or automatic self-regulation. This enables individual vessels to regulate blood flow by altering their own arteriolar resistance. This is not a unique property of the coronary vessels, but it ensures a constant blood flow at perfusion pressures (mean arterial pressure) between 60 and 180 mmHg provided that other influencing factors are held constant. At this point it might be helpful to refer to the section 'Blood vessel diameter' (p. 427) before considering the specific factors affecting the coronary circulation.

### Aortic pressure

The primary factor responsible for maintaining blood flow to the cardiac muscle is the **aortic pressure**, which is generated by the heart itself. Generally, an increase in aortic pressure will result in an increase in coronary blood flow, and vice versa. However, under normal conditions blood pressure is kept within relatively narrow limits by the baroreceptor mechanism (see later) so that changes in coronary blood flow are primarily caused by changes in the resistance of the coronary vessels.

### Demand for oxygen

The major factor affecting the resistance of the coronary vessels is the **demand for oxygen** of the myocardium. At rest, oxygen extraction from the coronary circulation is almost three times greater than in the normal circulation. Therefore, when the demand for oxygen is increased, little additional oxygen can be removed from the blood unless the flow is increased. Blood flow increases almost directly in proportion to oxygen need due to dilation of the blood vessels. It is believed that oxygen lack causes this dilation of the coronary arterioles indirectly, by inducing the release of a vasodilator substance from the myocardium into the interstitial fluid where it can relax the coronary arterioles. Examples of vasodilator substances are nitric oxide, adenosine, rising concentrations of potassium and hydrogen ions, generation of lactic acid and elevated local temperatures. Some possible mechanisms are discussed

more fully under control and coordination of the cardiovascular system.

### Nervous control

The **autonomic nervous system** has an indirect effect on coronary blood flow. Sympathetic stimulation increases heart rate and contractility, and this increases the demand for oxygen. The primary action of sympathetic nerve fibres on the coronary arterioles is to cause vasoconstriction, but this response is overruled by the metabolic demands for oxygen in the tissue. So the net result of stimulation of sympathetic nerves to the heart is to elicit a marked increase in coronary blood flow. Conversely, parasympathetic stimulation slows the heart rate and has a slight depressive effect on contractility, which results in a decreased cardiac oxygen consumption and therefore coronary blood flow decreases.

### Compression of vessels during systole

Unlike other arteries in the body, the majority of blood flow in the coronary arteries occurs during diastole rather than in systole because when ventricular cardiac muscle contracts (systole) it compresses the vessels within it, thus reducing blood flow. As higher pressures are generated in the left ventricle than the right, this **compression effect** is more marked in this area. During diastole, the cardiac muscle relaxes and no longer obstructs blood flow. **Figure 4.2.13** shows the effects of systole and diastole on coronary blood flow.

---

### CLINICAL APPLICATIONS

#### CORONARY HEART DISEASE

Myocardial cells rely on the coronary arteries for a supply of oxygenated blood and if this is compromised then heart function is also compromised. In coronary heart disease (CHD), the coronary arteries become narrowed due to the presence of atheromatous plaques, and this affects blood flow to the myocardial cells beyond the plaques. (How these plaques form and factors that predispose an individual to develop such plaques are considered in detail later in the chapter because the atherogenic process affects all blood vessels, not just those in the coronary circulation; see p. 431.)

Coronary heart disease is a continuum that clinically commences with angina, in which the oxygen requirements of the myocardial cells are greater than the supply of oxygenated blood. This results in myocardial ischaemia ('blood starvation'). At the other end of the continuum is myocardial infarction, in which the supply of oxygenated blood falls below the level required

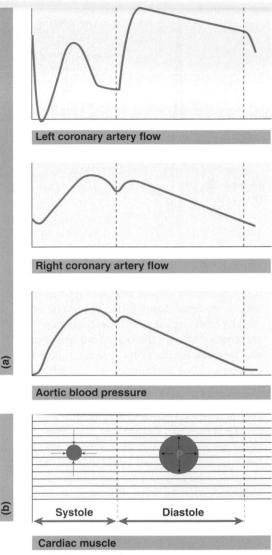

Left coronary artery flow

Right coronary artery flow

Aortic blood pressure

(a)

(b)

Systole | Diastole

Cardiac muscle

**Figure 4.2.13** (a) Schematic representation of the blood flow in the left and right coronary arteries and aortic blood pressure respectively, showing (b) the compression of a blood vessel in the myocardium during systole and diastole (based on Gregg, 1965)

Coronary heart disease (also known as coronary artery disease or ischaemic heart disease) is one of the major causes of death in industrialized societies. In the United Kingdom, approximately 300 000 people suffer a myocardial infarction each year and this leads to approximately 140 000 dying as a result (Peterson et al., 1999).

When trying to understand the aetiology, risk factors and potential treatments for coronary heart disease, it is important to remember that it results from two different processes – atherosclerosis and thrombosis. Some factors influence only one of these processes but some influence both. The classic risk factors for coronary heart disease are smoking, high blood cholesterol and high blood pressure, but the aetiology of these disease processes is much more complex than this; many factors are known to be involved and many of the risk factors themselves are interlinked.

Risk factors for coronary heart disease can be divided into those that are modifiable (i.e. that can be influenced by treatment and lifestyle changes) and those that are non-modifiable. Some risk factors that are not modifiable by an individual include increasing age, male gender, race and genetic predisposition. However, other risk factors can be modified, including raised serum cholesterol, hypertension, smoking, obesity, high alcohol intake, sedentary lifestyle, diabetes and psychosocial factors such as anxiety and stress: it is these factors that should form the focus of health promotion activities either with those known to be at risk or with the general population at large. Much can be gained from increasing exercise levels for those who do not undertake much exercise (see later) and from eating a healthy diet with a lower fat intake and at least five portions of fruit and vegetables a day: diets high in fruit and vegetables do seem to help prevent heart disease. Lowering elevated cholesterol levels has repeatedly been shown to be beneficial (see also the section on atherosclerosis, p. 432). However, some high cholesterol levels can be familial in origin (familial hypercholesterolaemia); one study (Marks et al., 2002) found that it was cost-advantageous to screen family members with familial hypercholesterolaemia rather than to treat the eventual coronary artery disease. The American Heart Association recommends that cholesterol levels should be measured at about 5 years of age, as a way of promoting cardiovascular health early in life (Tanne, 2002). Other potential influences for coronary heart disease include chronic infection, fetal malnutrition and psychosocial factors (Haines et al., 2001; Walker, 1999).

to maintain cell viability, resulting in infarction and necrosis (death) of the myocardial cells. Coronary artery spasm can also cause intermittent narrowing of coronary arteries and has the same effect resulting in myocardial ischaemia. Over time, if the constrictions of the coronary arteries occurs over many years, collateral vessels (small communications between arteries) can develop. These help to maintain a level of oxygenated blood supply to the myocardium beyond the narrowing, and this will influence the degree of clinical signs and symptoms. The symptoms of coronary heart disease depend on the degree of obstruction of the vessels and range from ischaemic pain due to moderate obstruction to death in some instances of complete obstruction.

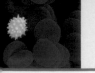
Epidemiological studies (Barker, 1992) suggest that coronary heart disease, along with stroke, hypertension and other diseases, might originate through impaired growth and development during fetal life and infancy.

Further details and issues will be considered in the sections on hypertension, atherosclerosis, and the effects of exercise. For a further discussion of coronary heart disease, see British Heart Foundation (2002), Department of Health (2000), Hubbard (2002) and Walker (1999).

## ANGINA PECTORIS

Often, the first sign that the obstruction of the coronary arteries is great enough to cause ischaemia of the heart muscle is when activities that increase the oxygen demand of the heart cause pain. This pain is called **angina pectoris**. It is usually felt beneath the upper sternum and is often referred to the left arm and shoulder and neck, or even to the opposite arm and shoulder. This distribution of pain is due to the fact that the heart and arms originate during embryonic life in the neck, therefore both these structures receive pain nerve fibres from the same spinal cord segments.

Generally, the pain occurs on exercise or exertion when the increased demand of the cardiac muscle for oxygen cannot be met due to the narrowing of the coronary arteries. The pain usually causes the person to stop the activity. It disappears a few minutes after the cessation of activity when blood flow can again match the oxygen requirements of the muscle. People who suffer from angina pectoris can also feel the pain when they experience emotions that increase the metabolism of the heart.

An exercise tolerance test (ETT) can be performed. This is a 12-lead electrocardiogram (ECG) taken during aerobic exercise, either by using a treadmill or a bicycle. The procedure is carried out to a set protocol using a standardized time/speed and gradient. This is usually known as the Bruce or modified Bruce protocol. Typically, the ST segment becomes depressed during ischaemia **(Fig. 4.2.14)**.

Unstable angina can be a progression from stable angina or it can occur in an individual who has experienced no previous symptoms. It generally lasts more than 20 minutes and is regarded as a medical emergency because the likely progression to myocardial infarction is high.

Treatment for angina pectoris is aimed at decreasing the workload of the heart so that the oxygen requirement of the cardiac muscle is less, thus preventing ischaemic episodes. **Nitrates**, e.g. **glyceryl trinitrate**, taken before activity that is known to cause angina can often prevent it or, if

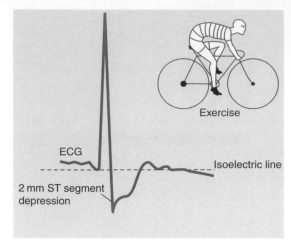

**Figure 4.2.14** ST segment depression on the ECG due to ischaemia of the cardiac muscle during exercise

taken during an angina attack, will often give immediate relief. Some forms of glyceryl trinitrate are given sublingually as this allows rapid absorption through the buccal mucosa. It can also be given via pads on the skin to allow for continuous slow absorption.

Nitrates dilate blood vessels everywhere in the body. Dilation of the arterioles lowers blood pressure, which reduces the resistance that the heart has to pump against and therefore decreases the cardiac work. Consequently, the requirement for oxygen by the cardiac muscle is decreased and hence symptoms are reduced. Venous dilation increases the capacity of the venous circulation and therefore reduces venous return to the heart. The lowered blood volume in the heart decreases the stretch on the ventricular muscle fibres in diastole, resulting in a reduced force of contraction. This again lowers the cardiac work and decreases oxygen consumption. The decreased diastolic stretch on the ventricles allows a greater diastolic coronary blood flow and this also improves oxygenation of the myocardium. Because of their action as vasodilators, one side-effect of nitrates is headaches.

Another group of drugs, the **β-adrenergic sympathetic blocking drugs (β-blockers)**, is also used in the management of angina pectoris to decrease the workload of the heart. Sympathetic nervous activity increases heart rate and contractility, thus increasing cardiac oxygen consumption. Therefore, blocking the sympathetic stimulation of the heart by β-adrenergic blocking drugs, e.g. atenolol or propranolol, reduces oxygen consumption and thus relieves angina. Calcium-channel blocking drugs (sometimes known as calcium antagonists), such as nifedipine or verapamil, are also used in the treatment of angina (as well as for arrhythmias and hypertension). The therapeutic effect of the calcium antagonists results from coronary and peripheral dilatation and decreased myocardial metabolism associated with the decrease in myocardial contractility.

Advice can be given to angina sufferers on ways of adapting their lifestyle to reduce the incidence of attacks. People who smoke should be encouraged to stop smoking as nicotine has a vasoconstrictor effect and so opposes the action of some drugs used in the treatment of angina (it also contributes to atherosclerosis development). Health education and information on diet, stress management and other factors that are known to be implicated in the development of coronary artery disease and atherosclerosis forms an important part of the care of such patients.

## MYOCARDIAL INFARCTION

If there is complete occlusion of a coronary artery, the blood flow to the muscle beyond the blockage ceases and the muscle dies. The wedge-shaped area of dead cardiac muscle is termed an **infarct** and the overall process is called a **myocardial infarction**. Often the person is said to have had a 'coronary occlusion' or a 'heart attack'.

Complete blockage of an artery can be caused by a local blood clot, called a **thrombus**, which develops on an atherosclerotic plaque and grows so large that it completely blocks the lumen of the artery. Alternatively, a clot forming on an atherosclerotic plaque elsewhere can break away (i.e. embolize) and flow downstream until it wedges in a more peripheral branch of the artery causing a blockage at that point.

Sometimes a sudden increase in myocardial oxygen consumption, e.g. during strenuous exercise, in the presence of severely atherosclerotic arteries can have the same effect as complete occlusion of the artery. When a reasonably large coronary artery is occluded, various changes take place within the area of ischaemic muscle. The muscle fibres in the very centre of the area die and this usually causes severe, continuous, crushing retrosternal chest pain, which radiates to the arms, neck and jaw. Unlike angina pectoris, this pain is not relieved by rest and is often associated with nausea, dyspnoea and sweating accompanied by fear, shock and weakness. However, not all people having a myocardial infarction experience chest pain; McNulty (2003) suggests from one study that as many as 25% of individuals might not experience pain.

Around the area of dead muscle is a non-functional area that does not contract, called a zone of injury. Next to this is an area that is mildly ischaemic and therefore contracts only weakly **(Fig. 4.2.15)**. This area is supplied by small collateral arteries (i.e. small branches from other

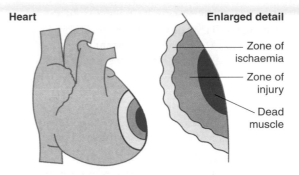

Heart           Enlarged detail

- Zone of ischaemia
- Zone of injury
- Dead muscle

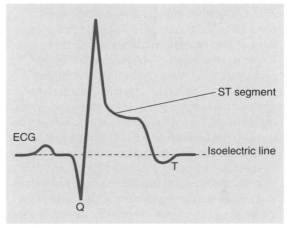

ECG

- ST segment
- Isoelectric line

Q

T

**Figure 4.2.15** Grades of muscle damage following a myocardial infarction and related ECG changes, namely enlarged Q wave, ST segment elevation and T wave inversion

arteries), which are sufficient to provide enough blood to the muscle at rest but not during exercise. Therefore, to prevent an increase in the size of the infarct, i.e. to stop this part of the muscle dying, the patient should be kept at rest and all nursing care should be planned with this in mind.

In the days following myocardial infarction, more of the muscle fibres immediately around the dead area die because of prolonged ischaemia. At the same time, the non-functional area becomes smaller because the size of the collateral vessels increases. Eventually, the dead muscle is replaced by fibrous tissue, which forms a scar that becomes smaller over a period of years.

Although the diagnosis of a myocardial infarction can often be made on the basis of clinical features alone, ECG changes and abnormal serum cardiac enzyme levels are used to formally confirm the diagnosis. Alterations in the ECG result from the changes that are occurring within the muscle of the infarcted area. In approximately 80% of people, the ECG changes will reveal ST segment elevation of 1 mm or more in two neighbouring leads **(see Fig. 4.2.15)**.

Another test for myocardial infarction looks at cardiac enzyme levels in the blood; muscle cells that die release enzymes into the serum and so raised levels of these indicate muscle death. Unequivocal changes in enzyme levels (that are specific to cardiac muscle damage) are an initial rise, then fall, of the iso-enzyme creatine kinase MB and troponin 1.

## Management of patients with an acute myocardial infarction

The key aims of management are to:

- promote healing of the myocardium
- prevent or early detection of complication.

Thrombolytic therapy (such as streptokinase) can be used to restore myocardial perfusion by breaking up or dissolving any thrombi present. It also has the effect of minimizing the area of infarction. Aspirin also has a role in inhibiting platelet aggregation and thrombin formation. The oxygen requirements of the damaged myocardium should be minimized and this can be achieved by bed rest and by alleviating any causes of tachycardia, including pain, nausea and anxiety. Administration of oxygen is also important. The risk of sudden death, usually due to a dysrhythmia such as ventricular fibrillation, is high in the first 24–48 hours after an acute myocardial infarction. When the ventricles fibrillate they do not pump blood, there is no cardiac output and the person dies within 2–3 minutes. Ventricular fibrillation can develop for a number of different reasons, all related to the changes that occur as a result of the muscle damage.

As well as supplying blood to the cardiac muscle, the coronary arteries also supply the tissue of the specialized conducting system (see later). For example, the atrioventricular node is supplied by the right coronary artery in 90% of individuals. Therefore, following coronary occlusion the conducting system is sometimes damaged by ischaemia and oedema, which can lead to arrhythmias such as heart block (see later). Continuous ECG monitoring is standard to detect dysrhythmias. **Table 4.2.1** shows the interventions for patients following an acute myocardial infarction taken from the National Service Framework (NSF) for Coronary Heart Disease (Department of Health, 2000).

Coronary angiography can be undertaken to identify the degree of coronary artery narrowing and which coronary arteries are affected. Coronary angiography can also provide information relating to intracardiac pressures and valve function.

## INTERVENTIONS FOR CORONARY ARTERY DISEASE

The purpose of any intervention or treatment for coronary artery disease is to try to increase the

**Table 4.2.1**  Interventions for patients following an acute myocardial infarction, taken from the National Service Framework (NSF) for Coronary Heart Disease (Department of Health, 2000)

**Before hospital:**
- CPR and defibrillation in the event of a cardiac arrest
- High concentration of oxygen
- Pain relief (2.5–5 mg intravenous diamorphine with an anti-emetic)
- At least 300 mg aspirin orally
- Immediate transfer to hospital

**In hospital:**
- Aspirin 300 mg orally, if not already been given
- Pain relief (as before) if still in pain
- Thrombolytic therapy
- β-blockers, to be continued for at least 1 year
- Consider insulin/glucose infusion for diabetics

**Continuing care:**
- Risk-factor advice and smoking cessation, physical activity and diet
- Low-dose aspirin (75 mg daily)
- β-blockers (for at least 1 year)
- Advice and treatment to keep blood pressure below 140/85 mmHg
- Statins to lower cholesterol concentration either to less than 5 mmol/L or by 30% (whichever is greater)
- Angiotensin-converting enzyme (ACE) inhibitors if symptomatic heart failure
- Control glucose levels and blood pressure in diabetics
- Arrange individualized rehabilitation and secondary prevention

blood flow to the myocardium. However, before any intervention is possible, the degree and specific sites of coronary artery disease, along with cardiac function, must be assessed; a number of investigations that can be employed.

One commonly used investigation is cardiac catheterization, where a dye is instilled into the coronary arteries (coronary angiogram) via a catheter introduced from the femoral artery. The dye enables visualization of the blood vessels. **Figure 4.2.16** shows a typical picture of obstruction of the left anterior descending artery. Dye can also be injected into the left ventricle (a process known as a **ventriculogram**) to assess left ventricular function by looking for areas of uncoordinated contraction due to scarring from previous infarction **(Fig. 4.2.17)**. Cardiac catheterization also provides information about valvular function and intracardiac pressures.

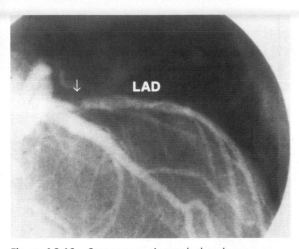

**Figure 4.2.16** Coronary angiograph showing obstruction of the proximal part of the left anterior descending (LAD) artery (courtesy Hallstrom Institute of Cardiology, Sydney, Australia)

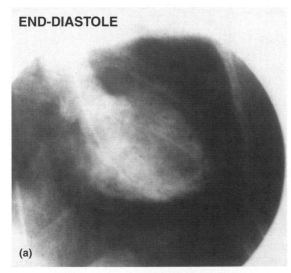

END-DIASTOLE

(a)

END-SYSTOLE

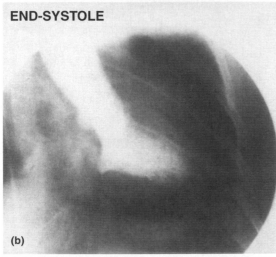

(b)

**Figure 4.2.17** Ventriculogram showing a normal left ventricle (a) at end-diastole and (b) vigorous contraction at end-systole (courtesy Hallstrom Institute of Cardiology, Sydney, Australia)

Other possible investigations are:

- Transthoracic and transoesophageal echocardiography, which can be used to show cardiac anatomy and movement, blood flow, cardiac lesions and valvular function.
- Nuclear cardiology, which can be used to assess myocardial perfusion and left ventricular function (PET and MUGA scanning).
- Cardiac magnetic resonance imaging (MRI), which can provide information about aortic disease, pericardial disease, coronary artery disease and valvular disease.

The two main interventions for revascularization in coronary artery disease are percutaneous transluminal coronary angioplasty (PTCA) and coronary artery bypass grafting (CABG). Percutaneous transluminal coronary angioplasty is generally used when only one or two vessels are affected by the disease. The procedure involves the insertion of a catheter into the coronary artery, usually via a femoral artery approach. Under imaging, the balloon is inflated, widening the narrowed coronary artery. A stent can also be inserted, and left in place, to maintain the lumen of the artery. Coronary artery bypass grafting involves bypassing the narrowed part of the coronary artery using either arteries or veins.

## CARDIOGENIC SHOCK

About 15% of patients who suffer an acute myocardial infarction have such massive ischaemic damage to the heart that the muscle cannot pump effectively. The cardiac output is reduced, resulting in a decreased blood flow to all the organs of the body, and subsequently to a reduction in their functions. This is known as **cardiogenic shock**. It can also occur after cardiac surgery, massive pulmonary embolism and pericardial tamponade (where effusion of fluid into the pericardium causes severe compression of the heart).

## The conducting system

The heart muscle must contract in an orderly and coordinated fashion to ensure efficient pump action. This is achieved by the conducting system of the heart, which is a network of specialized muscle fibres concerned with the initiation and propagation of the wave of excitation that results in cardiac muscle contraction.

The conducting system consists of the sinoatrial (SA) node, the atrioventricular (AV) node, the atrioventricular (AV) bundle (also called the bundle of His), the left and right bundle branches, and the Purkinje fibres (**Fig. 4.2.18**).

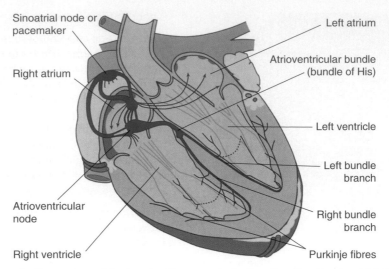

**Figure 4.2.18** The conducting system of the heart with arrows indicating the direction in which the impulse travels

The wave of excitation (impulse) is initiated in the sinoatrial node, which lies in the right atrium near the superior vena cava. It spreads through the muscle mass of both atria causing them to depolarize and contract. It then enters the atrioventricular node, which lies at the base of the right atrium. This node, and atrioventricular bundle, provide the only conduction link between the atria and the ventricles, all other areas being separated by non-conducting connective tissue. This means that malfunction of the atrioventricular node or bundle can cause complete dissociation of atrial and ventricular contractions. Conduction of the impulse through the atrioventricular node is delayed for approximately 0.1 seconds because these nodal fibres have a low conduction velocity. This allows time for the atria to finish contracting and empty their contents into the ventricles before ventricular contraction begins. Once through the atrioventricular node the impulse travels rapidly through the remainder of the conducting system. It enters the atrioventricular bundle and then travels along the left and right bundle branches that lie on either side of the interventricular septum. These branches spread downward towards the apex of the respective ventricles. They then divide into small branches, the Purkinje fibres, which carry the impulse to the many unspecialized ventricular muscle fibres. The impulse then spreads to the remaining muscle fibres via the intercalated discs, resulting in contraction of the ventricular muscle.

The rapid conduction of the impulse once it leaves the atrioventricular node means that depolarization of the whole right and left ventricular muscle mass occurs more or less simultaneously, thus ensuring a coordinated contraction (for a full discussion of the general concept of depolarization, see Chapter 2.2).

The conduction of these electrical impulses in the heart that cause the cardiac muscle to contract produces weak electrical currents that spread throughout the body. By placing electrodes in various positions on the body surface, this electrical activity can be recorded; the recording is called an **electrocardiogram (ECG)** (**Fig. 4.2.23** shows a typical ECG). The P wave represents the depolarization of the atria that results in atrial contraction. The QRS waves together represent the depolarization of the ventricles, which results in ventricular contraction. The ECG will be examined in more detail later on p. 407.

## Automaticity

The sinoatrial node can generate an impulse (that results in the contraction of the cardiac muscle) without any external stimulus. This ability is called **automaticity** or **autorhythmicity** and is due to spontaneous changes in the permeability of the cell membrane to potassium and sodium. There is a gradual decrease in the permeability of the membrane to potassium ions and a natural leakiness of the membrane to sodium ions. This causes a gradual depolarization of the membrane towards threshold, at which point an action potential occurs (**Fig. 4.2.19**). This action potential is transmitted through the conducting system and results in contraction of the cardiac muscle, i.e. the electrical changes precede the muscular contraction. Following the action potential, the membrane potential in cells of the sinoatrial node returns to the initial resting value and gradual depolarization begins again. Thus, rhythmical, repetitive, self-excitation of the cells occurs and causes rhythmical and repetitive cardiac muscle contraction. The sinoatrial node discharges at a rhythmical rate of about 70–100/min. When both divisions of the ANS are blocked (complete autonomic blockade), the heart rate of young adults averages approximately 100 beats/min; this is the **intrinsic heart rate**.

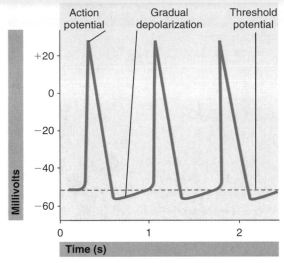

**Figure 4.2.19** Spontaneous rhythmical discharge of the sinoatrial (SA) node

Other areas of the heart also exhibit autorhythmicity, particularly the atrioventricular node and the remainder of the conducting system. The atrioventricular node discharges at a rhythmical rate of 40–60/min and the remainder of the conducting system discharges at a rate somewhere between 15 and 40/min. Normally, these tissues do not have the opportunity to initiate an action potential because they are depolarized by the impulse from the sinoatrial node before they reach their own threshold of self-excitation. The sinoatrial node therefore controls the pace of the heart because its rate of rhythmical discharge is greater than that of any other part of the heart; thus it is known as the normal **pacemaker** of the heart. If for some reason the sinoatrial node were inactive then the tissue with the next fastest autorhythmical rate would take over the pacing of the heart.

## CLINICAL APPLICATIONS

### ABNORMALITIES IN CONDUCTION

Abnormalities in conduction resulting in variations from the normal rhythm, i.e. **arrhythmias** (sometimes called dysrhythmias), can affect the pumping ability of the heart (these are summarized in **Table 4.2.2**). Drugs are often the first line of treatment: for example, digoxin increases the force of myocardial contraction and reduces conductivity within the atrioventricular node. Amiodarone works on all conducting tissues and influences all phases of the action potential; it is generally accepted as the most effective antiarrhythmic (Landowski et al., 2002).

## HEART BLOCK

Occasionally the transmission of the impulse through the heart is blocked at a critical point in the conduction system. Such a phenomenon is called **heart block**. The most common heart block is **atrioventricular block**, in which a disturbance in the conducting tissue of the atrioventricular node, the bundle of His (atrioventricular bundle) or the bundle branches delays or completely prevents transmission of the impulse from the atria into the ventricles. This can occur as a result of damage or destruction of the conducting tissue by ischaemia or as a result of depression of conduction caused by various drugs, e.g. digoxin toxicity.

If transmission of the impulse is completely blocked, as in **third-degree heart block** **(Table 4.2.2)**, atrial and ventricular contractions become totally dissociated. The atria continue to contract at their normal rate, stimulated by the sinoatrial node, but the impulse now cannot be transmitted to the ventricles. Therefore the site in the conducting tissue in the ventricles with the fastest rate of autorhythmicity begins to act as the ventricular pacemaker. Usually, the ventricular rate is less than 40 beats/min as this is the highest autorhythmical rate of the conducting tissue within the ventricles. This is usually insufficient to maintain an adequate blood flow from the heart and results in poor cerebral, coronary and renal perfusion.

Occasionally, complete heart block can occur intermittently. There is normal atrioventricular conduction followed by no conduction at all through the atrioventricular tissue. It can take 5–10 seconds for the ventricles to start contracting at their own inherent rate of 20–40 beats/min. During this time the brain is without a blood supply and the person faints. This is known as **Stokes–Adams syndrome**.

In complete heart block, an adequate heart rate can be maintained by the insertion of an artificial pacemaker, which is an electronic device that delivers an electrical stimulus to the heart via a pacing wire electrode **(Fig. 4.2.20)**. Most pacemakers inserted for complete heart block are known as dual-chamber pacemakers and have one atrial and one ventricular wire. The pacemakers will operate on 'demand', which means that the patient's own heart rate is detected and, if it falls below a present rate, the pacemaker will intervene.

Biventricular pacemakers, where there is a wire to both ventricles, can be inserted to optimize the haemodynamics in patients with heart failure.

The procedure to insert a pacemaker is a simple operation, often performed under local anaesthetic. The pacemaker is usually implanted

## Table 4.2.2a Cardiac arrhythmias

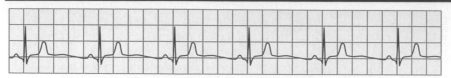

### 1 Normal sinus rhythm (included for reference)

**Description**
Each P wave is followed by a QRS complex
Rate 60–100 beats/min – in this example
the rate is 63 beats/min

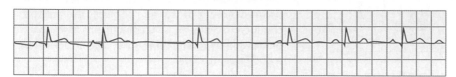

### 2 Sinus arrhythmia

**Description**
Normal variation of sinus rhythm
Heart rate increases with inspiration
and decreases with expiration

**Treatment**
None

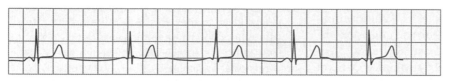

### 3 Sinus bradycardia

**Description**
Sinus rhythm (i.e. each P wave is
followed by a QRS complex);
however, the heart rate at rest is less
than 60 beats/min – in this example
the rate is 50 beats/min

**Causes**
May be normal in athletes
Hypothermia
Increased vagal tone due to bowel
straining, vomiting, intubation,
mechanical ventilation, pain
β-blocking drugs

**Treatment**
Atropine, isoprenaline
If unresponsive to these, may require
temporary ventricular pacemaker

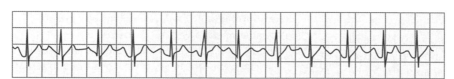

### 4 Sinus tachycardia

**Description**
Sinus rhythm (i.e. each P wave is
followed by a QRS complex); however,
the heart rate at rest is greater than
100 beats/min – in this example the
rate is 125 beats/min

**Causes**
Physiological response to fever,
exercise, anxiety, pain
May accompany shock, left
ventricular failure, cardiac tamponade,
hyperthyroidism, pulmonary embolus
Sympathetic stimulating drugs

**Treatment**
Correction of the underlying cause

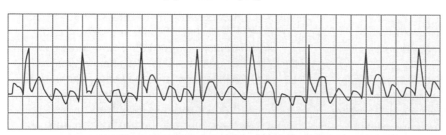

### 5 Atrial flutter

**Description**
Characteristic atrial 'saw tooth' waves
that occur at a regular interval and at a
rate of 250–400 min
Only every 2nd, 3rd or 4th atrial impulse
reaches the ventricles; in this example
every 2nd atrial impulse is followed by a
QRS complex (2:1 block)

**Causes**
Heart failure, pulmonary embolis,
valvular heart disease, digoxin toxicity

**Treatment**
Propranolol; quinidine or digoxin
(unless flutter is due to digoxin toxicity)
Direct current shock (i.e. cardioversion)

## Table 4.2.2b

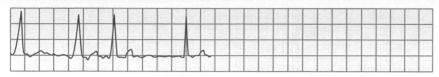

### 6 Atrial fibrillation

**Description**
Atrial activity is seen as rapid, small, irregular waves
Ventricular rate is completely irregular

**Causes**
Congestive cardiac failure, chronic obstructive lung disease, pulmonary embolus, hyperthyroidism, mitral stenosis, post-coronary artery bypass or valve replacement surgery

**Treatment**
Amiodarone,
Digoxin to slow ventricular rate
May require elective direct current cardioversion

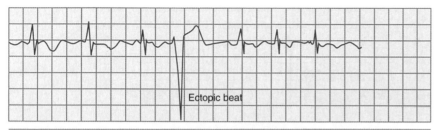

Ectopic beat

### 7 Premature ventricular contraction (ventricular ectopic beat)

**Description**
Beat occurs prematurely
The QRS complex is wide and distorted

**Causes**
Myocardial infarction, heart failure, stimulants (e.g. nicotine, caffeine), drug toxicity (e.g. digoxin, aminophylline), electrolyte imbalance (especially hypokalaemia), anxiety, catheterization of ventricle (e.g. as in a pacemaker)

**Treatment**
None if benign
Lidocaine, procainamide
Stop digoxin if induced by this drug
Potassium chloride if cause is hypokalaemia

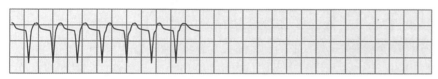

### 8 Ventricular tachycardia

**Description**
QRS complexes are wide and bizarre
No visible P waves
Ventricular rate 140–220 beats/min – in this example ventricular rate is 166 beats/min

**Causes**
Myocardial infarction, drug toxicity (e.g. digoxin, quinidine), hypokalaemia, hypercalcaemia

**Treatment**
Lidocaine,
Amiodarone
If no effect, direct current cardioversion

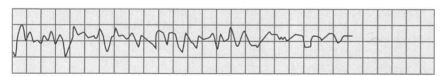

### 9 Ventricular fibrillation

**Description**
Ventricular rhythm is rapid and chaotic
QRS complexes are wide and irregular
No visible P waves

**Causes**
Myocardial ischaemia or infarction, hypo- or hyperkalaemia, congestive cardiac failure, untreated ventricular tachycardia, drug toxicity (e.g. digoxin), electrocution, hypothermia

**Treatment**
Cardiopulmonary resuscitation
Direct current shock 200–400 joules
Antiarrhythmic drugs after resuscitation

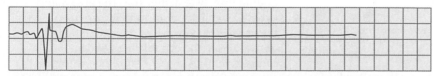

### 10 Asystole

**Description**
Ventricular standstill
No QRS complexes

**Causes**
Myocardial ischaemia or infarction, acute respiratory failure, aortic valve disease, hyperkalaemia

**Treatment**
Cardiopulmonary resuscitation
Calcium chloride
Isoprenaline
Epinephrine

**Table 4.2.2c**

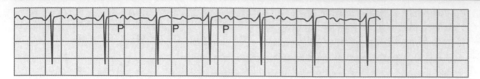

**11 Heart block** 1 First-degree atrioventricular block

Description
PR interval is prolonged
QRS complex normal

Causes
Inferior myocardial ischaemia or
infarction (i.e. right coronary artery
disease), potassium imbalance,
digoxin toxicity, hypothyroidism

Treatment
Correct underlying causes
Discontinue digoxin

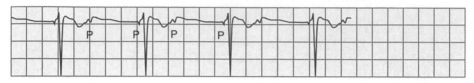

**12 Heart block** 2 Second-degree atrioventricular block

Description
Atrial rate regular but only every 2nd,
3rd or 4th atrial impulse results in a
ventricular contraction – in this example
every 2nd atrial impulse is followed by
a QRS complex (2:1 block)

Causes
Inferior myocardial infarction,
digoxin toxicity, vagal stimulation

Treatment
Atropine
Discontinue digoxin
May require temporary pacemaker

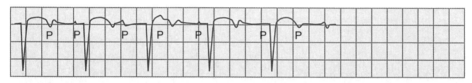

**13 Heart block** 3 Third-degree atrioventricular block

Description
Atrial rate is regular
The ventricular rate is slow and
irregular; however there is no
relationship between the atrial (P)
waves and the ventricular QRS
complexes

Causes
Myocardial ischaemia or
infarction, digoxin toxicity,
complication of mitral valve
replacement

Treatment
Pacemaker

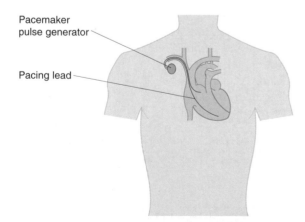

Pacemaker
pulse generator

Pacing lead

**Figure 4.2.20** An artificial pacemaker implanted under
the skin in the upper chest with leads into the heart

under the skin in the upper chest and the leads
to the heart are inserted via the subclavian vein.
Often this procedure is performed as a day
case; in some patients an overnight stay in
hospital is required.

The pacemaker batteries have a life span
of approximately 5 to 6 years. Checks are
performed on the battery yearly, but this might
progress to 6 monthly as the battery life nears
the 6-year point.

## PREMATURE BEATS

Sometimes a small area of cardiac muscle becomes
much more excitable than normal, possibly due to
a local area of ischaemia, overuse of stimulants
such as caffeine or nicotine, electrolyte imbalance
or drug toxicity (e.g. digoxin). The area might
initiate an impulse prior to that from the
sinoatrial node. A wave of depolarization spreads
outward from the irritable area and initiates a
contraction of the heart before one would be
expected from the normal rhythm of the sinoatrial
node. This is called **premature contraction** or
**beat**. The focus at which the abnormal impulse
is generated is called an **ectopic focus** and
might be in the atria or ventricles. The premature

contraction that it initiates is often called an **ectopic beat** (Greek: *ektopos* = displaced). If an ectopic focus becomes so irritable that it establishes rhythmical impulses of its own at a more rapid rate than that of the sinoatrial node, this ectopic focus becomes the pacemaker of the heart.

The output of blood from a premature contraction is decreased because the ventricles have not had normal filling time. Therefore the pulse wave passing to the periphery might be so weak that it cannot be felt at the radial artery. Thus, when the apex beat is counted simultaneously with the radial pulse rate, there is a deficit in the number of pulses felt in relation to the number of beats counted. This is known as **pulse deficit**.

Ventricular premature beats can be treated by giving lidocaine, which reduces the autorhythmicity of the cells and their responsiveness to excitation. If the ectopic beats are caused by digoxin toxicity, then this drug is stopped. Premature beats induced by hypokalaemia are treated by giving intravenous potassium chloride.

## FIBRILLATION

In normal conduction, once the impulses leave the specialized conducting tissue they travel around the heart stimulating the cardiac muscle to contract. The impulses eventually die away because when they return to the originally stimulated muscle this muscle is still in a refractory state.

However, if the length of the pathway along which the impulse travels is lengthened (as might occur in a dilated heart due to congestive cardiac failure), by the time the impulse returns to the starting position the originally stimulated muscle might be out of the refractory state and able to be restimulated. A similar situation occurs if conduction is prolonged, as might happen if there is a blockage in the conduction system, ischaemia of the muscle, or hypo- or hyperkalaemia. Restimulation can also occur if the refractory period is shortened, as in response to various drugs, e.g. epinephrine or in electrocution. Therefore, if an impulse constantly meets an area that is no longer refractory, it keeps travelling around and around the heart in a so-called circus movement. This leads to continuous and completely disorganized contractions called **fibrillation**.

If the ventricles fibrillate, different parts of the ventricle no longer contract simultaneously and therefore no blood is pumped. The person dies within 2–3 minutes if no action is taken. An ECG tracing of ventricular fibrillation is shown in **Table 4.2.2(a)**. The electrical activity in the ventricles is

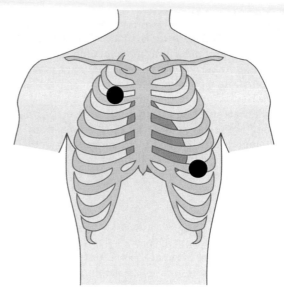

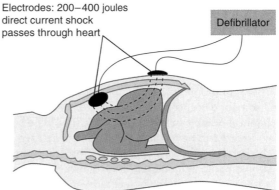

Electrodes: 200–400 joules direct current shock passes through heart

Defibrillator

**Figure 4.2.21**  Electrical defibrillation (a) the circles show the position of the large electrodes ('paddles') across the long axis of the heart, (b) when the defibrillator discharges, a direct current shock passes through the heart

completely disorganized so there are no distinctive wave patterns.

In an attempt to stop the ventricles fibrillating, a very strong direct current can be passed through them, which throws all the ventricular muscle into a refractory period simultaneously. This is called **electrical defibrillation** or **direct current cardioversion**. It is done by placing two large electrodes ('paddles') on the chest, one just to the right of the sternum below the clavicle and the other just to the left of the apex of the heart or the left nipple **(Fig. 4.2.21)**. The direct current (commonly 200–360 joules) passes through the heart causing all impulses to stop for 3–5 seconds, after which it is hoped that the sinoatrial node fires and resumes the pacing of the heart.

When a patient is being defibrillated it is important that nobody is touching either the patient or the bed, otherwise they too will receive the shock.

## CARDIAC ARREST

A fibrillating ventricle is totally inefficient as a pump and therefore fails to maintain an adequate cardiac output. This failure of the heart to maintain an adequate circulation, particularly to the brain, is called **cardiac arrest**, a state that can also result from ventricular tachycardia and asystole **(see Table 4.2.2)**. At normal body temperatures, irreversible changes occur in the brain if circulation fails for more than 2–3 minutes.

The two primary signs of cardiac arrest are:

- unconsciousness
- absent pulses.

Other signs are:

- convulsion, often at the onset of cardiac arrest
- absence of respiration or gasping respiration – this occurs within 20–30 seconds from the onset of cardiac arrest
- dilation of the pupils – this occurs within 30–60 seconds
- no audible heart sounds
- cyanosed pallor.

There is no time to wait for an absolute diagnosis. If someone is unconscious and no carotid or femoral pulse is palpable, he or she should be considered to have had a cardiac arrest. To save the person's life, cardiopulmonary resuscitation should begin immediately. If circulation is restored within 2–3 minutes, complete recovery is possible.

## CARDIOPULMONARY RESUSCITATION

**Cardiopulmonary resuscitation** (CPR) consists of ventilating the patient, to ensure that the blood is oxygenated, and external cardiac massage to circulate this oxygenated blood. The details given below are based on the UK Resuscitation Council (2001) guidelines for basic and advanced life support. The ABC of cardiopulmonary resuscitation is as follows:

- **A: the Airway.** This must be opened by tilting the head back and lifting the chin to stop the tongue falling back. Any debris in the mouth should be cleared out quickly although false teeth should be removed only if poorly fitting.
- **B: Breathing.** If the person is breathing spontaneously, artificial ventilation might not be required. However, in most instances breathing ceases within 20–30 seconds of the onset of cardiac arrest. The person should be artifically ventilated by:
  - mouth-to-mouth or mouth-to-nose ventilation; or
  - mask and bag with oxygen-enriched air; or
  - endotracheal intubation and ventilation with oxygen-enriched air.

Two slow initial breaths should be given. The person should be ventilated approximately 15 times a minute. The efficacy of ventilation is checked by observing if there is adequate chest expansion.

- **C: Circulate.** As the heart is no longer pumping blood efficiently, its action is taken over by external cardiac massage in which the heart is rhythmically compressed between the sternum and the spine to cause blood to be ejected. To perform external cardiac massage, the heel of one hand is placed on the lower half of the sternum and the other hand over the first (avoiding the xiphisternum). The sternum is depressed approximately 4–5 cm by using the operator's body weight through straight arms **(Fig. 4.2.22)**. This compresses the heart between the sternum and the spine and causes blood to be expelled. The sternum should be depressed at a rate of approximately 80–100 compressions a minute. For effective

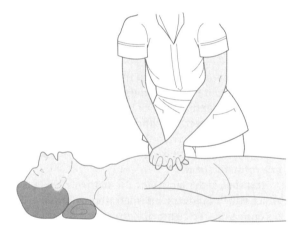

(a)

Sternum

(b)

**Figure 4.2.22** External cardiac massage: (a) position of the operator (b) position of the hands on the lower half of the sternum

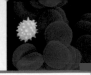

compression the patient should be lying on a firm surface. The efficacy of the compression should be checked by an assistant feeling the femoral pulses.

If the person has been seen to collapse and is reached within 15–30 seconds, a **precordial thump** can be given, i.e. the lower part of the sternum is given a firm thump, once, with the ulnar border of a clenched fist (starting no more than 30 cm from the chest). This manoeuvre is only of value when blood is still circulating in the heart and might be enough to 'shock' the heart into beating again. *This should be performed only if the arrest is witnessed.*

For cardiopulmonary resuscitation, two breaths should be given to every 15 compressions of the heart.

Once cardiopulmonary resuscitation is established, further action can be taken to get the heart pumping effectively by itself again. If facilities are available an ECG should be recorded, remembering that artificial ventilation and cardiac massage must be continued throughout. If ventricular fibrillation is present, electrical defibrillation should be performed. If there is no defibrillator available, intravenous lidocaine as a bolus might be given. If asystole is present, it is vital to get some electrical activity in the heart. Epinephrine and atropine are given. Epinephrine is given, every 3 minutes through an arrest situation.

During cardiac arrest, poor perfusion of tissue induces metabolic acidosis. The acidosis depresses myocardial contractility, induces intracellular loss of potassium (which depresses cardiac response to catecholamines), reduces the threshold for ventricular fibrillation and induces asystole. If the acidosis is not corrected, resuscitation will not be successful.

In the past, sodium bicarbonate was used to correct the acidosis: now, however, the respiratory acidosis should be corrected before administration of sodium bicarbonate. The acidosis is normally corrected by good ventilation, circulation, defibrillation, etc., and sodium bicarbonate is used only during prolonged resuscitation attempts or according to blood gas results. Sodium bicarbonate might also be considered when the cardiac arrest is associated with either a tricyclic overdose or hyperkalaemia.

### Cardiopulmonary resuscitation in children

The procedure just described relates specifically to adults or larger children. The procedure for infants (0–1 year old) and children (1–8 years) is similar and uses the same **ABC** sequence. There are some differences, though; the cause of arrests is commonly prolonged hypoxaemia secondary to inadequate oxygenation caused by respiratory or circulatory failure (only rarely cardiac in origin). Major events necessitating cardiopulmonary resuscitation (CPR) might be injuries, suffocation, aspiration of foreign body (food, toys), smoke inhalation, sudden infant death syndrome or infections, especially respiratory tract infections. The outcome from cardiac arrest is poor in infants and children, and neurological brain damage is not uncommon following cardiac arrests. Therefore the emphasis with children needs to be on prevention and early detection of respiratory difficulties and circulatory impairment. Speed and skill are crucial.

A similar head-tilt, chin-lift manoeuvre is used as with adults, although if there is suspected head or neck trauma care must be taken to prevent injury to the spinal cord. Children seem to find the best position in which to keep their partially obstructed airway open, and so they should be allowed to maintain this. Hyperextension of an infant's neck should be avoided, as should pressure on the soft tissues under the chin as this will cause obstruction of the airway. For infants it is necessary to use mouth to mouth-and-nose, but with larger infants and children mouth to mouth is possible. Two initial slow breaths are given (1–1.5 seconds per breath). As the size of children varies so much, it is not possible to make recommendations on the volume of breath, so the operator should just ventilate until the chest rises. When checking to see if there is a pulse, the brachial or femoral arteries can be used for an infant, and the carotid for a child. If there is a pulse present but no spontaneous breathing, ventilation is continued at the rate of 20–30 breaths per minute for an infant and 15–20 for a child. The ratio of breaths to compressions are 1:5 for an infant and for children aged over 8 it is the same as for an adult, i.e. two breaths for every 15 compressions. Chest compressions in an infant are made using two fingers on the sternum just below an imaginary line between the two nipples moving the sternum just 1–2 cm. For children the heel of one hand is used on the sternum above the xiphoid process with a compression of 2–4 cm.

For further details of both adult and paediatric CPR, see American Heart Association (2000) and Resuscitation Council (2001a, b, c, d) UK guidelines.

## The electrocardiogram

The electrical impulses that precede cardiac muscle contraction arise in the conducting system of the heart. These impulses excite the muscle fibres of the heart and cause them to contract, and it is this coordinated contraction of cardiac muscle that

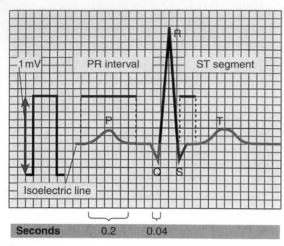

**Figure 4.2.23**   A normal ECG complex

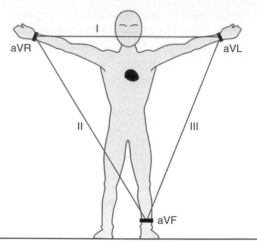

**Figure 4.2.24**   Position of the three limb electrodes in the recording of a six-lead ECG

pumps the blood into the pulmonary and systemic circulations.

The impulse formation and condition produce weak electrical currents that spread through the entire body. By applying electrodes to various positions on the body and connecting these electrodes to an electrocardiograph, an electrocardiogram is recorded. Therefore the electrocardiogram (ECG) is a graphic recording of the electrical processes that initiate the contraction of the cardiac muscle. A typical ECG wave pattern is seen in **Fig. 4.2.23**.

The value of such recordings is that abnormalities in the conduction system or abnormalities in the cardiac muscle itself will result in changes on the ECG and so can be diagnosed. A 12-lead ECG is used for diagnostic purposes as this looks at the heart from 12 different angles.

Sometimes it is necessary to monitor the cardiac rhythm of patients with cardiac abnormalities continuously so that any untoward changes can be observed immediately. For this the ECG signal from just one lead is used.

## ECG leads

The 12-lead ECG includes six recordings from the extremities and six recordings from the chest. Each of the 12 leads looks at the same phenomenon (i.e. the conduction of the electrical impulse through the heart) from a different point. As the electrical currents picked up at each point of recording are slightly different, the waveform patterns will vary between leads. However, for each lead there is a normal waveform pattern.

The six extremity leads are as follows:

Three **bipolar leads**, I, II and III (known as **standard leads**), that record the difference in electrical potential between two points electrically equidistant from the heart.

- lead I records the difference in potential between the left arm and right arm
- lead II records the difference in potential between the left leg and right arm
- lead III records the difference in potential between the left leg and the left arm.

These three leads form an Einthoven triangle whose apices are the two arms and the left leg. The heart is considered to lie in the centre of this triangle (**Fig. 4.2.24**).

Three **unipolar leads** aVR, aVL, aVF (a = augmented; because deflections are small the recordings are augmented 1.5 times). These three leads record the difference in electrical potential between a zero reference electrode and the limb potential:

- aVR records the difference between the zero potential and the right arm
- aVL records the difference between the zero potential and the left arm
- aVF records the difference between the zero potential and the left leg (**Fig. 4.2.24**).

The above six leads can be thought of as 'looking' at the heart in a vertical plane. Leads I and aVL look at the left lateral surface of the heart; leads II, III and aVF look at the inferior surfaces; and lead aVR looks at the atria.

The six **chest leads** are unipolar leads and are recorded from the following positions (**Fig. 4.2.25**):

- $V_1$ 4th right intercostal space at the sternal border
- $V_2$ 4th left intercostal space at the sternal border
- $V_3$ midway between $V_2$ and $V_4$
- $V_4$ 5th left intercostal space in the midclavicular line
- $V_5$ left anterior axillary line at the same horizontal level as $V_4$
- $V_6$ left midaxillary line at the same horizontal level as $V_4$

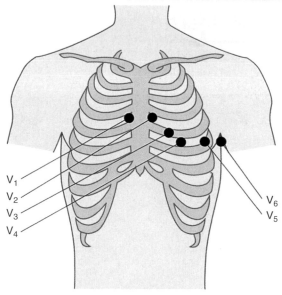

**Figure 4.2.25** Position of the six chest electrodes in the recording of an ECG. When these are combined with the limb leads a 12-lead ECG can be recorded

$V_1$
$V_2$
$V_3$
$V_4$
$V_6$
$V_5$

These leads look directly at the heart in a horizontal plane. Leads $V_1$ and $V_2$ look mostly at the right ventricle; leads $V_3$ and $V_4$ look at the septum between the ventricles and the anterior wall of the left ventricle; leads $V_5$ and $V_6$ look at the anterior and lateral walls of the left ventricle. However, a unipolar chest lead not only records the electrical potential from a small area of the underlying myocardium, it records all the electrical events that occur with each heart beat as viewed from the selected lead site.

For diagnostic purposes it is necessary to look at the heart from these 12 different positions as abnormalities in certain parts of the heart will be more clearly visible (i.e. will cause greater changes in the waveform pattern) in the leads that look most directly at this area of the heart.

**Figure 4.2.26** shows the normal waveform pattern for each lead of the 12-lead ECG.

## Components of the ECG

**Figure 4.2.23** shows a typical ECG complex. The first wave seen is the **P wave**, which represents atrial depolarization that precedes atrial contraction. It is normally in a positive (upwards) direction. After a slight pause, the next three waves, Q, R, S, appear very close to each other. These waves together are called the **QRS complex** and represent depolarization of the ventricles that precedes ventricular contraction. Within the QRS complex, the **Q wave** is the first downward deflection, the **R wave** is the first upward deflection and the **S wave** is the first downward deflection following the R wave. There is a pause after the QRS complex and the next positive wave is the T

**wave**, which represents ventricular repolarization. Occasionally there is a small positive wave after the T wave known as the U wave.

The distance from the beginning of the P wave to the beginning of the QRS complex is known as the **P–R interval**. This represents the time taken for the impulse to travel from the sinoatrial node through the atria to the ventricular fibres. It includes the normal delay of excitation in the atrioventricular node. The **QRS interval** is measured from the onset of the Q wave to the termination of the S wave and represents the total time for ventricular depolarization.

The **ST segment** is the period between the S and T waves, and is part of ventricular repolarization.

The connections of the electrodes to the electrographic apparatus are such that if the wave of depolarization is moving towards the active electrode, the resultant deflection on the ECG will be in an upward direction; if the wave of depolarization is moving away from the electrode, the resultant deflection will be in a downward direction. **Figure 4.2.26** shows the major direction of a normal wave of depolarization. If leads aVR and $V_5$ are taken as an example, in lead aVR the wave of depolarization is mostly travelling away from the electrodes so that most of the deflections are downward; in lead $V_5$ the wave of depolarization is mostly travelling towards the electrode so that most of the deflections are upward. To clarify this further, the genesis of a lead II ECG is followed in more detail in **Fig. 4.2.27**.

The ECG is recorded on graph paper in which horizontal and vertical lines are present at 1 mm intervals. A heavier line occurs every 5 mm. The vertical lines show the time interval (1 mm = 0.04 s, 5 mm = 0.2 s). The horizontal lines show the amplitude (10 mm = 1 mV) **(see Fig. 4.2.23)**. In routine electrocardiograph practice, the recording speed is 25 mm/s.

### CLINICAL APPLICATIONS

#### CALCULATION OF HEART RATE

The **heart rate** is the number of times the heart beats each minute and is represented on the ECG by the number of atrial depolarizations (P waves) or ventricular depolarizations (QRS complexes) that occur each minute. Heart rate can also be measured indirectly by counting the pulse rate. The normal adult heart rate is between 60 and 100 beats/min. It is fastest at birth (130–150 beats/min) and decreases with age until adult values are attained. It is also slightly faster in females than in males. Heart rate diminishes by 10–20 beats/min during sleep. Heart rate increases significantly with exercise: in children this can be up to 200 beats per minute and 180 in adults, although the maximum heart rate attainable does decrease with increasing

**409**

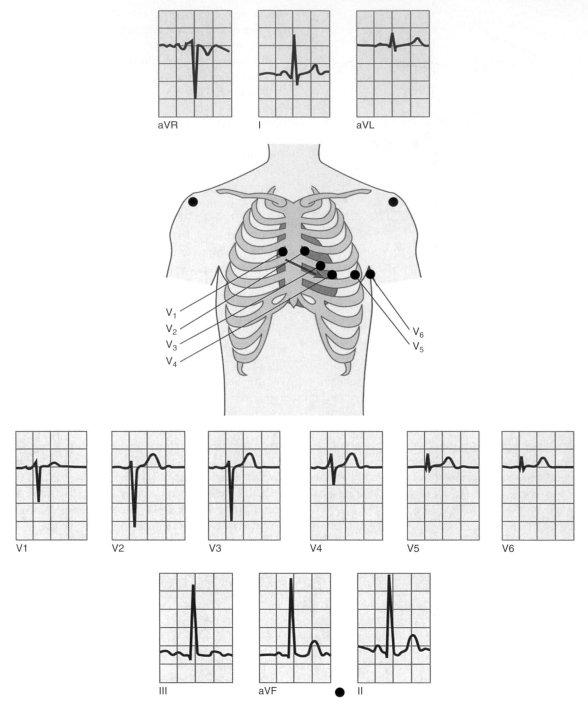

**Figure 4.2.26** Normal complexes for each lead of the 12-lead ECG (with an arrow showing the major direction of the wave of depolarization)

age. Fever also leads to an increase in heart rate. In well conditioned athletes at rest the heart rate is normally 50–60 beats/min.

### RHYTHM (see Table 4.2.1)

The normal rhythm of the heart is called **sinus rhythm**. This denotes that the impulse arises in the sinoatrial node and follows the normal conduction pathway. Thus it implies that a P wave precedes every QRS complex. Variations of sinus rhythm can occur in a normal heart. For example, there may be changes in rate which are related to respiration, the rate increasing with inspiration and decreasing with expiration (see Chapter 5.3). This is known as **sinus arrhythmia** and is more common in children than in adults. These changes in rate can be felt while taking the pulse. Other variations of sinus rhythm are **sinus bradycardia** (Greek: *brady* = slow) in which the heart rate at

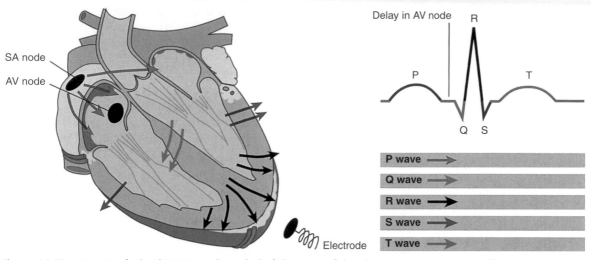

**Figure 4.2.27** Genesis of a lead II ECG, each symbol of the wave of depolarization represents a different waveform on the ECG.
**P wave:** represents atrial depolarization. Wave is in a positive direction because the impulse is travelling towards the electrode.
**Q wave:** represents septal depolarization from left to right. Wave is in a negative direction as the impulse is travelling away from the electrode.
**R wave:** represents depolarization of the apical part of the ventricle and then left ventricular depolarization (because the impulse through the thicker left ventricular muscle mass is stronger than through the right). Wave is in a positive direction as the impulse is travelling towards the electrode.
**S wave:** represents late ventricular depolarization. Wave is in a negative direction as the impulse is moving away from the electrode.
**T wave:** represents late ventricular repolarization. Wave is in a positive direction because repolarization occurs in the opposite direction to depolarization. AV, atrioventricular; SA, sinoatrial

rest is below 60 beats/min, as might occur in well trained athletes or when the body temperature is lowered; and **sinus tachycardia** (Greek: *tachos* = speed) in which the heart rate at rest is above 100 beats/min, as may occur when there is an increased body temperature, e.g. in fever.

## POTASSIUM IMBALANCE

The ECG changes that occur with potassium imbalance are important because the ECG can give a guide to serum potassium levels when direct determination of serum potassium is not possible. The importance of detecting changes in potassium levels is that, in the heart, both hypokalaemia (potassium deficiency) and hyperkalaemia (potassium excess) can diminish excitability and reduce the conduction rate of cardiac muscle. This can lead to cardiac arrest. Therefore the ECG changes indicative of a raised or lowered serum potassium should be reported immediately. The effects of hypokalaemia and hyperkalaemia on the ECG are seen in **Fig. 4.2.28**. In hypokalaemia there is ST segment depression (i.e. the ST segment is below the isoelectric line) and there is a prominent U wave immediately following the T wave. In hyperkalaemia there is peaking of the T wave, the more severe effects including widening of the QRS complex and lengthening of the P–R interval.

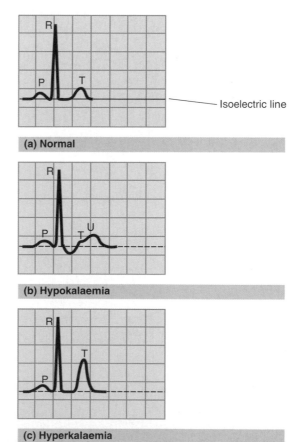

**Figure 4.2.28** ECG complexes in potassium imbalance

## The cardiac cycle

The cardiac cycle is the period from the end of one heart contraction to the end of the next. An understanding of how all the events in the cycle fit together is essential to understanding how the heart acts as an efficient pump.

In a normal cycle, the heart muscle contracts and then relaxes. **Systole** refers to the phase of contraction and **diastole** to the phase of relaxation. As pumping of the blood is achieved mainly by the contraction and relaxation of the ventricles, systole usually refers to the phase of ventricular contraction and diastole to the phase of ventricular relaxation.

First, the events that occur in late diastole will be described. Throughout the description, reference should be made to **Fig. 4.2.29**. It is important to note that the sequences of events in the right and left sides

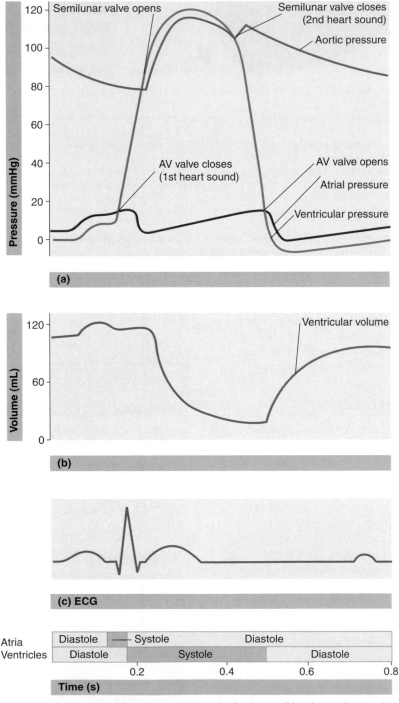

**Figure 4.2.29** The cardiac cycle showing (a) pressure changes in the heart, (b) volume changes in the ventricles and (c) a normal ECG trace relative to time and the phases of the cycle in the atria and the ventricles. AV, atrioventricular.

of the heart are the same. The difference between the right and left side is simply due to the fact that the pressures generated by the right ventricle during systole are considerably lower than those generated by the left ventricle. This is because the total resistance to flow in the pulmonary circulation is less than in the systemic circulation. The difference in the amount of pressure generated by the right and left ventricle is clearly reflected in the size of the muscular ventricular wall, the right ventricular wall being much thinner than the left. Despite the lower pressure, the right ventricle ejects the same amount of blood as the left with each contraction.

### Diastole (late)

In diastole, the atria and ventricles are relaxed. Blood enters the right atrium from the superior and inferior venae cavae, and enters the left atrium from the pulmonary veins. This blood causes the pressure within the atria to be slightly higher than that in the ventricles. This forces the atrioventricular valves to open and blood passes from the atria into the ventricles throughout diastole. For all this time, the pulmonary and aortic valves are closed because the pressures in the pulmonary artery and the aorta are higher than those in the ventricles. This ensures that the blood collects in the ventricles.

Towards the end of diastole the sinoatrial node discharges and the atria depolarize, causing a P wave on the ECG. This depolarization of the atria results in atrial contraction, which pumps any blood remaining in the atria into the ventricles. It is important to note that approximately 80% of ventricular filling occurs before this atrial contraction; atrial contraction merely 'tops up' the ventricles. Therefore atrial dysfunction does not have a great effect on ventricular filling.

The amount of blood in each ventricle at the end of diastole, i.e. just before the ventricles contract, is called the **ventricular end-diastolic volume (VEDV)**. The VEDV determines the **preload**, the pressure generated in the left ventricle at the end of diastole.

Throughout diastole, the pulmonary artery and aortic pressures fall because blood is moving out of arteries into the pulmonary and systemic vasculature.

### Systole

The wave of depolarization initiated by the sinoatrial node passes through the atrioventricular node and into the ventricles, causing them to depolarize. Depolarization of the ventricles is represented on the ECG by the QRS complex. This depolarization triggers contraction of the ventricles, and the pressures within them rises. Almost immediately, the pressures in the ventricles exceed those in the atria, causing the

atrioventricular valves to close and thus preventing backflow of blood into the atria. The turbulence created by the closure of the atrioventricular valves generates the first heart sound.

At the very beginning of ventricular contraction, the pressures in the pulmonary artery and aorta exceed those in the ventricles, therefore the pulmonary and aortic valves remain closed and no blood leaves the ventricles. Each ventricle is contracting but the blood volume within them remains constant. This is known as **isovolumetric ventricular contraction**. This phase of contraction ends when the pressures in the ventricles exceed those in the pulmonary artery and aorta, the semilunar valves open and **ventricular ejection** occurs. The ejection of blood is at first rapid and then tapers off. The amount of blood ejected by each ventricle with each contraction is called the **stroke volume**.

The pulmonary artery and aortic pressures rise as the blood flows in from the ventricles. Peak pressures in the pulmonary artery and aorta occur before the end of ventricular ejection. This is because the rate of ejection of blood from the ventricles during the last part of systole is quite low and is less than the rate at which the blood is leaving the arteries via the arterioles. Therefore the volume of blood, and hence the pressure within the pulmonary artery and aorta, begin to decrease.

Throughout the entire period of ventricular ejection, the atrial pressures rise slowly because of the continued flow of blood from the veins.

### Diastole (early)

Almost as soon as the ventricular muscle relaxes, ventricular pressure falls below the pulmonary artery and aortic pressures, there is a slight backsurge of blood which causes the pulmonary and aortic valves to close. The turbulence created by the closure of these valves generates the second heart sound. For a short time the atrioventricular valves are also closed because the pressure in the ventricles still exceeds that in the atria. Therefore in the early phase of ventricular relaxation the volume of blood in the ventricles remains constant. This is called **isovolumetric ventricular relaxation**. It ends as ventricular pressure falls below atrial pressure, causing the atrioventricular valves to open and ventricular filling to begin. Ventricular filling occurs rapidly at first so that it is almost completed in early diastole.

At a heart rate of 72 beats/min, each cardiac cycle takes 0.8 seconds (s). The period of ventricular diastole (0.5 s) is longer than the period of ventricular systole (0.3 s). During periods of rapid heart rate, as might occur with exercise or emotional stress, there is a marked reduction in the duration of diastole.

However, this does not seriously impair ventricular filling as most filling occurs in early diastole.

## Cardiac output

Cardiac output is the amount of blood pumped by the heart (usually given as a value per minute) and so is the amount of blood available for the transport of nutrients to the tissues. For this reason, cardiac output is central to the function of the circulatory system.

Cardiac output is often defined as the volume of blood pumped out of the left ventricle into the aorta each minute. It is usually expressed in litres per minute (L/min) and can be calculated by multiplying **stroke volume** (the volume of blood pumped out of each ventricle per contraction) by the number of contractions per minute (i.e. the heart rate). Therefore

$$\text{cardiac output (CO)} = \text{stroke volume (SV)} \times \text{heart rate (HR)}$$

For example, if an adult at rest has a heart rate of 72 beats/min and each ventricle ejects about 70 mL of blood with each beat, then

$$\text{cardiac output} = 72\ \text{beats/min} \times 0.07\ \text{L/beat} = 5.0\ \text{L/min}$$

At rest, a normal cardiac output is about 5.0 L/min. This can increase to as much as 25 L/min in a normal person performing strenuous exercise and to as much as 35 L/min in a well-trained athlete. The maximum percentage that the cardiac output can increase above the normal resting cardiac output is called the **cardiac reserve**.

An increased cardiac output, as might be required to supply various tissues and organs with a greater blood flow, e.g. muscles during exercise or the gut during digestion, is achieved by either an increase in heart rate or an increase in stroke volume, or both.

The mechanisms by which heart rates and stroke volume can be altered are as follows.

### Control of heart rate

As was described earlier when discussing the conducting system of the heart, the sinoatrial node, in the absence of any nervous or hormonal influences, discharges spontaneously and rhythmically at about 100 beats/min. If uninfluenced by other factors, this rate set by the sinoatrial node would never vary. However, the rate of the heart does vary to meet the changing requirements of the tissues for oxygen. There are various factors that alter heart rate.

#### Nervous control

By far the most important factor that alters heart rate is the influence of the autonomic nervous system. The heart is supplied by both sympathetic and parasympathetic nerves **(Fig. 4.2.30)**. The sympathetic nerves to the heart originate in the cardiovascular centre, which is a group of neurones within the medulla, innervating the sinoatrial node, the atrioventricular node and portions of the myocardium. Stimulation of these sympathetic nerves causes an increase in heart rate. The parasympathetic nerve to the heart (vagus nerve) originates in the nucleus ambiguus within the medulla. These fibres innervate

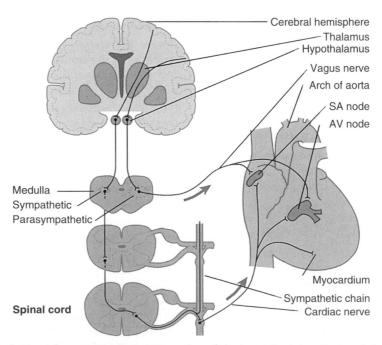

**Figure 4.2.30** Sympathetic and parasympathetic innervation of the heart (based on Tortora & Anagnostakos, 1990). AV, atrioventricular; SA, sinoatrial

the sinoatrial node and the atrioventricular node. Parasympathetic stimulation causes a decrease in heart rate.

At rest a normal adult heart rate is about 60–80 beats/min. This is less than the inherent rate of discharge of the cardiac pacemaker, the sinoatrial node. Therefore, in the resting state, parasympathetic influence is dominant (sometimes known as the **vagal brake**).

Primarily, heart rate is regulated by a balance between the slowing effects of parasympathetic discharge and the accelerating effects of sympathetic discharge.

### Hormonal control

Epinephrine, released from the adrenal medulla, is a sympathetic mediator and therefore causes an increase in heart rate by stimulating the $\beta_1$-receptors in the cardiac muscle conduction system (see Chapter 2.5).

Norepinephrine also influences heart rate. The thyroid hormones enhance sympathetic activity, leading to an increased heart rate and cardiac output. Decreases in either growth hormone or thyroid hormones will result in bradycardia, reduced cardiac output and low blood pressure.

### Stretch

Stretch of the atrial walls by an increased venous return or an increased blood volume can increase the heart rate by as much as 10–15%. This is because there are **stretch receptors** in the wall of the atria that send impulses that stimulate the sympathetic output. This is known as the **Bainbridge reflex**.

Receptors that influence heart rate exist in both atria. They are located mainly at the junctions between the blood vessels and the atria – in the right atrium at its junction with the venae cavae and in the left atrium at its junction with the pulmonary veins. Stretch of these receptors results in impulses going to the brain in the vagus nerve. The efferent discharge back to the heart is via fibres from both divisions of the autonomic nervous system to the sinoatrial node. (The baroreceptor mechanism also responds to changes in blood volume and affects the heart rate, but as its primary response is concerned with control of blood pressure, it is discussed later.)

Atrial stretch receptors are involved with two other mechanisms and, although they are not directly involved with influencing heart rate, a brief consideration will be given here. Stretch of the atrial receptors also causes an increase in urine production; the main mechanism for this response seems to be via antidiuretic hormone (ADH) from the posterior pituitary. An increased blood volume leads to stimulation of the atrial receptors, which leads to a reduction in antidiuretic hormone secretion, and more urine is produced.

The atria themselves also have an endocrine function in that they secrete a hormone known as atrial natriuretic factor (ANF) or atrial natriuretic peptide (ANP) (see also Chapter 5.4). Atrial natriuretic peptide is a peptide hormone released from the atrial cells in response to increased atrial pressure, again as a result of stretching. It has a potent diuretic and natriuretic (excess sodium excretion) effect on the kidneys, and also a vasodilator effect on the arterioles and veins; it is thought to play an important role in the regulation of blood volume and blood pressure. Atrial natriuretic peptide is also produced in the kidneys and walls of blood vessels. Atrial stretch also causes the release of brain natriuretic hormone (BNP), which has similar actions to atrial natriuretic peptide.

---

**CLINICAL APPLICATIONS**

**TEMPERATURE**

A raised body temperature causes an increased heart rate because it increases the rate of discharge of the sinoatrial and atrioventricular nodes. Decreased body temperature, as might occur in exposure to cold or in deliberate cooling of the body during cardiac surgery, decreases heart rate.

**DRUGS**

Administration of certain drugs can alter the heart rate. Such drugs that alter the heart rate are called **chronotropic drugs** (Greek: *chronos* = time). Those that increase the heart rate are called positive chronotropic drugs, e.g. isoprenaline, epinephrine, and those that decrease it are called negative chronotropic drugs, e.g. β-adrenergic blocking drugs such as propranolol.

---

Heart rate is sensitive to other factors, including plasma electrolyte concentrations and hormones other than epinephrine, but these are less important. Generally, heart rate is somewhat faster in females than males and it declines slightly with age.

For a given stroke volume, all the factors that increase heart rate will increase cardiac output and all the factors that decrease heart rate will decrease cardiac output.

### *Control of stroke volume*

#### Venous return and ventricular end-diastolic volume

In a normal heart, the most important factor that controls the amount of blood pumped from a ventricle with each beat (i.e. the stroke volume) is the amount of blood that is in the ventricle immediately before contraction (i.e. the ventricular end-diastolic volume). The more blood in the ventricle before contraction the greater the amount of blood pumped (see p. 393).

As stroke volume is so dependent on ventricular end-diastolic volume, it is important to know what determines ventricular end-diastolic volume. The major determinant is **venous return**. The heart will pump as much blood as is returned to it from the veins, principally due to Starling's law of the heart, which states that the force of contraction is a function of the length of the muscle fibre. The force of contraction adjusts according to the volume of blood in the chambers of the heart, and so the heart is said to **autoregulate**.

As venous return alters ventricular end-diastolic volume, and hence stroke volume, it will also alter cardiac output, as it will be remembered that CO = SV × HR (see p. 414). Hence venous return and the related ventricular end-diastolic volume are crucial determinants of cardiac output. Factors that affect venous return are discussed later in this chapter.

## Nervous regulation

Sympathetic nerves not only supply the sinoatrial node and conducting system, but also innervate the atrial and ventricular myocardium **(see Fig. 4.2.30)**. Sympathetic stimulation causes the release of the sympathetic mediator, norepinephrine, which increases ventricular (and atrial) contractility. **Myocardial contractility** is the strength of contraction at a given degree of stretch (stretch is synonymous with muscle fibre length). It has been shown that muscle fibre length is dependent on ventricular end-diastolic volume, therefore myocardial contractility is the strength of contraction at a given ventricular end-diastolic volume.

Increased contractility results in an increased stroke volume even though ventricular end-diastolic volume does not change. This is possible because, normally, when a ventricle contracts it does not empty completely; the amount of blood that remains after ejection is the **ventricular end-systolic volume (VESV)**. When contractility increases, the ventricle empties more completely, thereby increasing stroke volume. Thus:

SV = VEDV − VESV

where the end-systolic volume is dependent on myocardial contractility. The effect of sympathetic stimulation of the heart on stroke volume is seen in **Fig. 4.2.31**.

Sympathetic stimulation not only causes a more forceful contraction but also a more rapid contraction.

This is important when an increase in heart rate (also the result of increased sympathetic activity) reduces the time available for diastolic filling of the ventricles. If contraction is more rapid, a larger fraction of the cardiac cycle will be available for filling.

Certain drugs can alter myocardial contractility. Drugs that affect contractility are called **inotropic drugs** (Greek: *inos* = fibre). Those that increase contractility are called positive inotropic drugs, e.g. digoxin, epinephrine, and those that decrease contractility are known as negative inotropic drugs, e.g. β-adrenergic blocking drugs such as propranolol.

## Hormonal regulation

Circulating hormones – catecholamine, epinephrine and norepinephrine, released from the adrenal medulla – produce similar changes in myocardial contractility, and hence stroke volume, to those induced by the sympathetic nerves to the heart via the β₁-receptors.

## Arterial blood pressure

An increase in the resistance to the ejection of blood from the ventricles can decrease stroke volume if the force of contraction stays constant. **Resistance to ejection is determined by the distensibility of the large arteries and the total peripheral resistance. This resistance to ejection is called the afterload.**

The arterial blood pressure gives an indication of the degree of afterload. If the arterial blood pressure is raised (i.e. increased afterload) and the force of contraction stays the same, the stroke volume will be reduced. This is because, for the same force of contraction, the muscle fibres are less able to shorten because they are pushing against a greater load. The

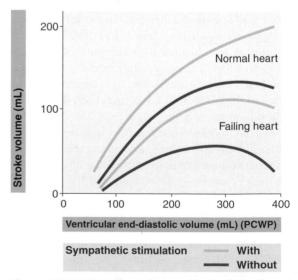

**Figure 4.2.31** The effects of sympathetic stimulation on the normal and failing heart with ventricular end-diastolic volume measured by PCWP (pulmonary capillary wedge pressure) (based on Vander et al., 1990)

ventricle does not empty as much and so stroke volume is decreased.

In a normal heart, changes in blood pressure, up to a certain point, do not affect overall cardiac output. This is due to the self-adjustment of the heart. When the stroke volume falls due to an increased afterload, the ventricular end-systolic volume increases. This end-systolic volume is added to the normal diastolic filling in the next cycle, therefore increasing the volume of blood in the ventricle. This causes a greater stretch on the ventricular muscle which enhances the force of contraction, with a consequent increase in stroke volume. This process continues with each contraction until the original stroke volume is achieved. However, the end-systolic volume and the end-diastolic volume will remain elevated.

Vasodilator drugs, e.g. sodium nitroprusside, phentolamine or nitroglycerine, reduce afterload.

**Figure 4.2.32** summarizes the main factors that can alter cardiac output. A normal functioning heart will pump out all the blood that is returned to it from the veins. Therefore venous return is the primary factor determining cardiac output. Any factors that increase stroke volume or increase heart rate can conceivably increase the cardiac output, and vice versa.

## Measurement of cardiac output

Cardiac output can be assessed indirectly by observing the trends of physiological variables such as heart rate, blood pressure, urine output and peripheral perfusion. In critically ill patients it might be necessary to augment these trends with additional methods of cardiac output measurement.

A long-standing method has been the direct measurement of cardiac output via thermodilution. This involves the placement of a modified pulmonary artery catheter via a central vein, such as the internal jugular or the subclavian vein, into the right side of the heart and then the pulmonary artery. A bolus of cold injectate is introduced via the catheter into the right atrium, which causes a reduction in blood temperature, which is then detected further along the catheter in the pulmonary artery. The temperature reduction has an inverse relationship with the degree that the injectate has been diluted, which in turn has an inverse relationship to the cardiac output.

Cardiac output can also be measured non-invasively by Doppler ultrasound. A probe that emits a continuous wave of ultrasound is placed in the oesophagus, which runs in parallel to the descending aorta. The ultrasound waves produce a signal consisting of a row of triangles, where each triangle shows the variation in blood flow velocity as a bolus of blood is pumped down the descending aorta. From this, the distance travelled by blood down the descending aorta with each cardiac contraction can be calculated. A nomogram derived from weight, height and age takes account of the cross-sectional area of the aorta; the distance travelled by the column of blood multiplied by the cross-sectional area of the aorta provides the stroke volume. Cardiac output is, as would always be the case, calculated by multiplying stroke volume and heart rate.

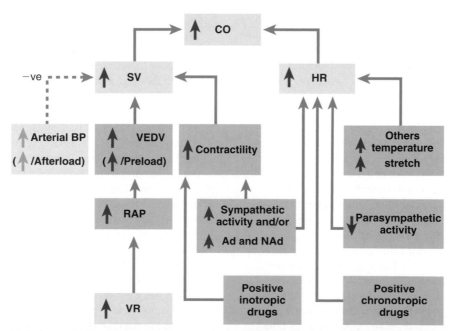

**Figure 4.2.32** Main factors influencing cardiac output (CO). Ad/NAd, epinephrine/norepinephrine respectively; BP, blood pressure; HR, heart rate; RAP, right atrial pressure; SV, stroke volume; VEDV, ventricular end-diastolic volume; VR, venous return

## CLINICAL APPLICATIONS

### HEART FAILURE

It can be seen from the previous discussion that venous return largely determines cardiac output. However, this is only true when the heart is an effective, adjustable pump. If the ability of the heart to pump is impaired, it may not be able to provide an adequate cardiac output to meet the needs of the body, despite a satisfactory venous return. In such a situation the heart is said to have failed. This is known as **heart failure**, **cardiac failure** or **pump failure**. Heart failure is the end stage of all the diseases of the heart and is a major cause or morbidity and mortality. The prevalence of heart failure is increasing as a result of the ageing population and survival from myocardial infarctions (Hobbs, 1999). The Framingham heart study has been the most important longitudinal source of data on the epidemiology of heart failure. Overall prevalence of heart failure is between 3 and 20 people per 1000 population, although this exceeds 100 per 1000 in those aged 65 and over (Davies et al., 2000). There is an approximate doubling in the incidence of heart failure with each decade of ageing, reaching 3% in those aged 85–94.

Causes of heart failure include: coronary artery disease, hypertension, cardiomyopathies, valvular disease, congenital disease, arrhythmias, toxic effects of alcohol (both acute and chronic use), some drugs and some viruses. The most common causes in developed countries are coronary artery disease and hypertension.

Traditionally, heart failure has been regarded as simply a disorder of the heart itself but heart failure is now thought of as a disorder of the circulation as a whole. Many patients have structural cardiac damage that adversely affects cardiac performance, but they do not have heart failure because compensatory mechanisms (both circulatory and neurohormonal) maintain cardiac output and peripheral perfusion. Heart failure develops not when the heart is injured but when compensatory mechanisms are overwhelmed or exhausted.

In the discussion of heart failure we will first consider the pressure and volume changes that occur and then discuss mechanisms that compensate for a decreased cardiac output.

The left and right side of the heart can be considered as two separate pumping systems connected in series. It is possible for one side of the heart to fail independently of the other. For example, myocardial infarction might affect only the left side, or pulmonary disease might affect predominantly the right side. A consideration of the pressure and volume changes that occur when one side of the heart fails independently of the other gives a good understanding of the importance of the integrity of the pumping system.

If the left side of the heart fails, the output of this side is less than the total volume of blood received from the right side. Effects occur in both the vessels behind the pump and beyond the pump. Blood is backlogged behind the left ventricle. This increases the volume and pressure of blood in the left atrium and consequently in the pulmonary veins and the pulmonary capillary bed. The accumulation of blood in the pulmonary capillary bed causes the pulmonary capillary pressure to rise. When it rises about 28 mmHg (3.7 kPa) – the colloid osmotic pressure of plasma – fluid filters out of the capillaries into the interstitial spaces and alveoli of the lungs. Fluid in the interstitial spaces and alveoli is called **pulmonary oedema** and this compromises gas exchange in the lungs (see Chapter 5.3). If severe, pulmonary oedema will be life threatening because the fluid in the alveoli prevents adequate oxygenation of the blood.

The effects beyond the left ventricle are due to the decreased cardiac output. There is a decreased perfusion of the body tissues and effects will depend on how severely impaired the cardiac output is. Renal function especially is depressed, resulting in fluid retention.

Symptoms of left-sided heart failure are related to the high pressures in the pulmonary circulation and the low cardiac output. For example, dyspnoea on exertion (i.e. shortness of breath or difficult breathing during exercise) is due to the low cardiac output failing to provide adequate oxygenation to the tissues plus the increased venous return pooling in the pulmonary circulation, causing pulmonary oedema and consequent reduction in gas exchange.

**Orthopnoea** (difficulty in breathing when lying down) results from the effects of a sudden increase in venous return (which occurs on lying down) not being pumped out by the left side of the heart. Blood accumulates in the pulmonary circulation and so restricts vital capacity. Orthopnoea is relieved by sitting up because this decreases venous return due to the changes in hydrostatic pressure. The nurse should assist the patient into a comfortable, well-supported sitting position that will improve chest expansion and decrease venous return. **Paroxysmal nocturnal dyspnoea** is another symptom of left-sided heart failure, i.e. periods of difficult breathing that occur during the night, probably due to a sudden increase in right ventricular output or in the body's need for oxygen. It is thought that factors such as dreams, nightmares or a full bladder could trigger such occurrences, which may cause the patient typically to rush to breathe out of an open window.

Left-sided heart failure most often results from dysfunction of left ventricular muscle due to myocardial infarction. Other causes may be haemodynamic, such as volume overload that occurs with incompetence of the mitral or aortic valves, or pressure overload as occurs with stenosis of the aortic valve or with systemic hypertension where there is an increased resistance to ventricular ejection (i.e. an increased afterload). In such instances the left ventricle may hypertrophy because of the increased work of pumping extra blood (as occurs with incompetent valves) or of pumping against a resistance (as in hypertension).

If the right side of the heart fails, the output of the right ventricle is less than the total volume of blood being returned to it from the systemic circulation. Blood backlogs behind the right ventricle. This increases the volume and pressure in the systemic venous circulation. (This increased pressure can often be observed because it causes the jugular vein in the neck to be distended or bulging rather than flat.) The systemic capillary pressure is increased and this causes movement of fluid into the interstitial spaces. This fluid is visible as swelling or oedema of the dependent parts of the body where the hydrostatic pressure is greatest, e.g. the ankles, and the sacrum when lying, and this may predispose to the formation of pressure ulcers. The liver and spleen are also distended as they act as reservoirs for the backlogged blood.

The increased venous pressure of right-sided heart failure can be measured by inserting a catheter into the right atrium and connecting it to a pressure transducer. This measurement is called central venous pressure and is described later.

The effects beyond the right ventricle are related to the decreased output. The reduction of blood pumped from the right ventricle means that less blood returns to the left ventricle and subsequently there is a decrease in the cardiac output, which has the same results as a decreased cardiac output from left ventricular failure.

Right-sided heart failure can occur independently of left-sided failure, usually as a result of lung disease when increased resistance to blood flow in the pulmonary circulation eventually causes the right ventricle to fail. When right-sided heart failure is precipitated by lung disease it is called **cor pulmonale**. Most commonly, right-sided heart failure occurs as a result of left-sided failure because the increased back pressure in the pulmonary circulation means that the right ventricle is working against an increased load and eventually fails.

When both sides of the heart fail together, the condition is called **congestive cardiac failure**.

We will now consider the mechanisms that compensate for a decreased cardiac output due to heart failure. Some of these mechanisms are seen to act when the heart failure occurs acutely, others occur when heart failure develops slowly (i.e. chronic heart failure).

When failure is acute, as in myocardial infarction in which the ventricular muscle is damaged, the ventricle cannot pump out all the blood that is returning to it. The cardiac output falls immediately and the blood dams up in the heart, causing the right atrial pressure to rise. The fall in cardiac output leads to a reduction in arterial pressure, which activates the baroreceptor reflex via the carotid and aortic baroreceptors. This results in strong sympathetic stimulation that has two effects:

- It increases myocardial contractility and therefore the efficiency of the heart as a pump.
- At the same time, it causes constriction of the veins, which increases the amount of blood returning to the heart and therefore further increases the right atrial pressure. This increase in right atrial pressure increases the ventricular end-diastolic volume which enhances the ability of the heart to pump (i.e. increases stroke volume) by stretching the muscle fibres.

Both these sympathetic effects help to restore the cardiac output towards normal.

Increased sympathetic activity also causes constriction of the arterioles of less vital organs such as the gut, skin and kidney, and redirects blood to the more immediately essential organs such as the brain and heart.

**Figure 4.2.31** shows the effect of sympathetic stimulation on the failing heart. Pulmonary capillary wedge pressure (see later) is used to measure the left ventricular end-diastolic volume. A raised pulmonary capillary wedge pressure at rest signifies left ventricular dysfunction.

In chronic heart failure a third compensatory mechanism, i.e. expansion of the extracellular fluid volume, occurs. The low cardiac output reduces the blood flow to the kidneys. This is compounded by the effect of the increased sympathetic activity diverting blood flow away from the kidneys. Consequently there is a reduction in the glomerular filtration rate, the renin–angiotensin system is activated and anti-diuretic hormone is secreted, which increases tubular reabsorption of salt and water. This results in expansion of the extracellular fluid volume and therefore increases total blood volume. More blood flows back to the heart causing additional stretch on the muscle fibres which increases the force of contraction, thus helping to return cardiac output towards normal. This is sometimes called **compensated heart failure**.

Atrial natriuretic peptide is also involved in the expansion of extracellular fluid volume. This mechanism can eventually have a detrimental effect if the heart failure becomes more severe. The volume of blood in the ventricles can become so great that the muscle fibres are stretched beyond their physiological limit and cannot produce as much force. More blood remains in the ventricles after ejection, causing the heart to dilate. This is seen on a chest X-ray as an enlarged heart. The effectiveness of the heart as a pump decreases and the cardiac output is again reduced. A vicious circle ensues of further increasing fluid retention, greater stretch of the muscle beyond the physiological limit, still less effective pumping and a further reduction in cardiac output, which eventually leads to death. This is sometimes called **decompensated heart failure**. When this occurs the actions of the sympathetic nervous system become deleterious. The increase in heart rate and contractility further increase the oxygen demands of the heart, cardiac output falls with resultant peripheral vasoconstriction. This in turn increases afterload to the left ventricle, which increases the heart failure. See Gibbs et al. (2000) for a fuller discussion on heart failure.

The diagnosis of heart failure should aim to:

- identify the aetiology
- assess left ventricular function
- exclude other conditions
- estimate the prognosis and risk of mortality (Department of Health, 2000)

Investigations may include:

- 12-lead ECG
- chest X-ray
- echocardiogram
- full blood count, renal, pulmonary and liver function tests
- physical assessment and history
- biochemical marker tests such as B-type natriuretic peptide (BNP). B-type natriuretic peptide is a cardiac neurohormone secreted from the ventricular walls in response to stretching. A level within the normal range (<18.4 picograms (pg)/mL) means that the patient's symptoms are unlikely to be due to heart failure. B-type natriuretic peptide can also be used as a test to rule out heart failure (McDonagh et al., 1998)

Heart failure can range from being asymptomatic (with little or no limitation of physical activity), to mild with slight limitation of physical activity (comfortable at rest but ordinary activity results in fatigue, dyspnoea, palpitations or angina), to moderate (with marked limitation of activity), to severe (the individual is unable to carry out any physical activity without discomfort and symptoms are present even at rest, with increased discomfort with any physical activity).

Diuretics and angiotensin-converting-enzyme inhibitors, combined with non-pharmacological measures, form the basis of treatment in patients with heart failure. Digoxin is used in some instances, too. For a full discussion of the various treatment approaches, see Gibbs et al. (2000).

## Principles of fluid mechanics

### The vascular system

Before discussing the structure and function of blood vessels in detail, it is necessary to consider briefly some of the properties of fluids and the principles that govern the flow of fluids through vessels. The characteristics of the various types of blood vessel will determine the blood flow patterns across the body.

All fluids (when in a confined space) exert a pressure. The term **hydrostatic pressure** refers to the force that a liquid exerts against the walls of its container. The pressure that blood exerts in the vascular system is known as **blood pressure.** Pressure varies with the height of the liquid column and this can be observed in the veins of a person standing up (**Fig. 4.2.33**): the venous pressures in the feet are considerably greater than in the head (this is, of course, related to the effect of gravity). The effect of density on hydrostatic pressure is shown by the fact that 1 mm of mercury (mmHg) exerts the same pressure as 13 mm of water (mmH$_2$O) because mercury is more than 13 times as heavy as water for an equal volume. The SI unit for pressure is the Pascal (Pa) or kilopascal (kPa). However, blood pressure values are usually measured in mmHg. **Table 4.2.3** gives the conversions between kPa and mmHg.

If pressure is exerted on a confined fluid, the pressure will be transmitted equally in all directions – this is known as **Pascal's principle**. If there is a weak point in the container's wall and the pressure exerted is great enough, the container wall may burst. This is what happens when an aneurysm (an abnormal dilatation of an artery) bursts. When an individual is hypertensive, the blood vessels harden or undergo sclerotic changes (**arteriosclerosis**) to prevent the vessels bursting with the elevated blood pressure.

The distensibility of the container also influences the hydrostatic pressure that develops: if the container is distensible, the pressure in the fluid is less than in a rigid container. Haemodynamics is the

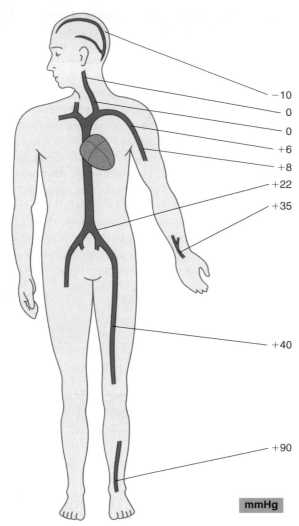

**Figure 4.2.33** Effects of hydrostatic pressure on venous pressure throughout the body in an individual standing still. All figures are approximate in mmHg

| Table 4.2.3 Equivalence of pressure units: approximate conversions between millimetres of mercury (mmHg) and kilopascals (kPa): 1 mmHg equals 0.133 kPa (adapted from Beevers et al., 2001) | |
| --- | --- |
| **mmHg** | **kPa\*** |
| 1 | 0.1 |
| 5 | 0.7 |
| 10 | 1.4 |
| 20 | 2.6 |
| 30 | 4.0 |
| 40 | 5.4 |
| 50 | 6.7 |
| 60 | 8.0 |
| 70 | 9.4 |
| 80 | 10.7 |
| 90 | 12.0 |
| 100 | 13.4 |
| 110 | 14.7 |
| 120 | 16.0 |
| 130 | 17.4 |
| 140 | 18.7 |
| 150 | 20.0 |
| 200 | 26.7 |

*Values in kPa rounded to the nearest decimal place.

study of the movements of the blood and the associated forces.

## Flow of fluids

The flow of a fluid through a vessel is determined by the pressure difference between the two ends of the vessel and also the resistance to flow.

### Pressure difference

For any fluid to flow along a vessel there must be a pressure difference otherwise the fluid will not move. In the cardiovascular system the 'pressure head' or force is generated by the pumping of the heart and there is a continuous drop in pressure from the left ventricle to the tissues and also from the tissues back to the right atrium. Without this drop in blood pressure, no blood would flow around the circulatory system.

### Resistance to flow

Resistance is a measure of the ease with which a fluid will flow through a tube: the easier it is, the less the resistance to flow, and vice versa. In the circulatory system the resistance is usually described as the **vascular resistance**; as it mainly originates in the peripheral blood vessels, it is also known simply as the **peripheral resistance**.

Resistance is essentially a measure of the friction between the molecules of the fluid, and between the tube wall and the fluid. The resistance depends on the viscosity of the fluid and the radius and length of the tube.

### Radius of the tube
The smaller the radius of a vessel, the greater is the resistance to the movement of particles; this increased resistance results from a greater probability of the particles of the fluid colliding with the vessel wall. When a particle collides with the wall, some of the particle's kinetic energy (energy of movement) is lost on impact, resulting in the slowing of the particle. Thus, in a smaller diameter vessel, there will be a greater number of collisions and a reduction in the energy content and speed of the particles moving through the vessel (**Fig. 4.2.34**). This results in a decrease in the hydrostatic pressure.

**421**

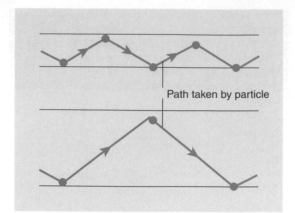

Path taken by particle

**Figure 4.2.34** The effect of the diameter of a vessel on the flow of a fluid. Particles collide more frequently with the wall of the vessel in a narrow vessel and lose energy thus the resistance to particle movement is greater in narrow vessels

Small alterations in the size of the radius of the blood vessels, particularly of the more peripheral vessels, can greatly influence the flow of blood. Atheromatous changes in the walls of large and medium-sized arteries cause narrowing of the lumen of the vessels and result in an increased vascular resistance.

### Length of the tube

The longer the tube, the greater the resistance to the flow of liquid through it. A longer vessel will require a greater pressure to force a given volume of liquid through it than will a shorter vessel. However, the length of the blood vessels in the body is not altered significantly and the overall length is kept to a minimum because of the parallel circuits in the systemic circulation (**see Fig. 4.2.1**).

### Viscosity of the fluid

**Viscosity** is a measure of the intermolecular or internal friction within a fluid or, in other words, of the tendency of a liquid to resist flow. The rate of flow varies inversely with the viscosity: the greater the viscosity of a fluid, the greater is the force required to move that liquid.

Thus, changes in blood viscosity affect flow. Normally the viscosity of blood remains fairly constant but in polycythaemia, in which there is an increased red cell content, the viscosity of the blood can be considerably increased and the blood flow reduced. Severe dehydration, where there is a loss of plasma, can also lead to increased viscosity. Cooling of the blood similarly increases its viscosity: this can occur in the limb extremities in cold weather for example.

The nature of the lining of the tube or vessel also influences the way fluids flow. If the lining of the blood vessel, the endothelium, is smooth, the fluid will flow evenly; this is known as streamline or **laminar flow**.

However, if the lining is rough or uneven or the fluid flows irregularly, **turbulent flow** is set up. Laminar flow is characteristic of most parts of the vascular system and is silent, whereas turbulent flow can be heard, e.g. as happens during blood pressure measurements with a sphygmomanometer and stethoscope.

It is sometimes necessary to measure blood flow in patients and it is usual simply to measure the quantity of blood that passes a given point in the circulation over a given period of time. One method that is used in clinical situations is an **ultrasonic flowmeter** applied to the surface of the skin over a blood vessel. This makes use of the Doppler effect (a shift in the frequency of the ultrasonic waves when they are reflected off the moving blood cells). It is a useful and non-invasive method of assessing the condition of the peripheral arteries, in peripheral vascular disease or after vascular surgery for example.

## The vascular system

To fulfil its role the vascular system must:

- ensure delivery of blood to all tissues
- be flexible and adaptable so that blood flow can be varied according to the metabolic requirements of individual tissues or the body as a whole
- convert a pulsatile blood flow in the arteries into a steady flow in the capillaries to facilitate optimum transfer of substances to and from the cells
- return blood to the heart.

The structure of the vessels in the different parts of the vascular system varies and the differences relate directly to the function of each type of vessel. The walls of all the blood vessels, except the capillaries, have the same basic components (**Fig. 4.2.35**), but the proportion of the components varies with function.

The innermost layer, or **tunica intima** (also known as the tunica interna), is a single layer of extremely flattened epithelial cells, called the endothelium, which is supported by a basement membrane and some connective and elastic tissue. Capillaries are formed from endothelial tissue and do not have the middle and outer layers. The middle layer, or **tunica media**, is predominantly smooth muscle and elastic tissue. The outer layer, or **tunica adventitia (or tunica externa)**, is composed of fibrous connective tissue, collagen and fibroblasts. The tunica media exhibits the greatest variation throughout the vascular tree, for example it is absent in the capillaries but comprises almost the whole mass of the heart. In some larger vessels there is a system known as the vasa vasorum (literally meaning 'vessels of the vessels'),

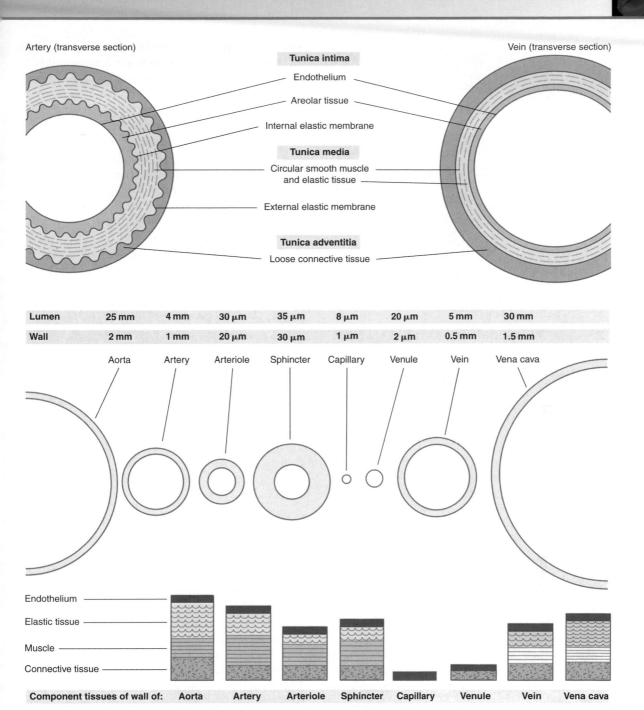

Figure 4.2.35 The structure of blood vessels: arteries, veins and capillaries

which nourishes the more external tissues of the blood vessel walls.

## The arterial system

The **aorta** and **large arteries** are highly elastic and distensible vessels with a relatively large diameter (the lumen of the aorta is approximately 2.5 cm in diameter). As they have relatively wide diameters, they are low-resistance vessels and conduct blood flow through them easily (see above). When the heart contracts and forces blood into the aorta, the elastic fibres are stretched and so the vessel is distended. At the end of ventricular contraction, the force generated by the heart is reduced and so the force stretching the elastic fibres is removed and they tend to return to their initial smaller size. The effect of this elastic recoil in between contractions is to sustain the pressure head: as the arteries return to their original size, the blood in the lumen is forced onwards around the vascular tree. Thus potential energy stored in the elastic fibres during ventricular contraction is converted into kinetic energy moving the blood onwards during the diastolic phase.

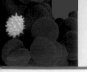
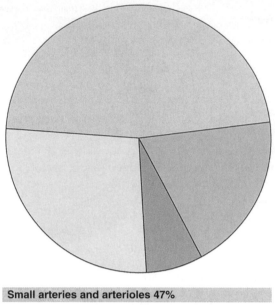

Small arteries and arterioles 47%

Arteries 19%

Veins 7%

Capillaries 27%

**Figure 4.2.36**  Distribution of vascular resistance (based on Despopoulos & Silbernagl, 1991)

This mechanism contributes to the conversion of a pulsatile ejection from the heart to a steady flow through the arterial system.

The **medium-sized arteries** distribute blood to all parts of the body and each has a relatively large diameter (approximately 0.4 cm), which aids blood flow. The walls of these arteries are distensible but, as the vessels become smaller with each further branching or subdivision, the amount of elastic tissue decreases whereas the smooth muscle component increases.

The small arteries, more often referred to as **arterioles**, have a much smaller diameter (20 μm) and a thicker wall with muscle tissue predominating; there can be up to six concentric layers of muscle in some arterioles. The arterioles offer considerable resistance to blood flow because of their very small radius, and are the major site of resistance to flow in the vascular tree (**Fig. 4.2.36**). Thus the total peripheral resistance, that is the total resistance to blood flow, is mainly determined by the radius of the arterioles.

This area of high resistance to blood flow serves several functions: first, together with the elastic arteries, it converts the pulsatile ejection of blood from the heart into a steady flow through the capillaries; second, if no resistance were present and a high pressure persisted into the capillaries, there would be a considerable loss of blood volume into the tissue by transudation of fluid across the capillary

wall. The pulmonary circulation is a *low* pressure circulation partly to prevent this happening; if pulmonary pressures increase for some pathological reason (as discussed earlier), pulmonary oedema may develop.

The arterioles are also important in determining the blood supply to different tissues and regions. There are specialized regions near the junction between the terminal (smallest) arterioles and the capillaries known as **precapillary sphincters**, which consist of a few smooth muscle cells arranged circularly (**see Fig. 4.2.38**). If the sphincters are relaxed and the lumen patent, the capillary beds distal to the sphincter are open and perfused. If the sphincters are partially constricted, blood flow to the capillaries will be reduced and, if fully contracted, no blood will flow through. In active muscle, for instance, many more capillaries are patent due to relaxation of the sphincters and thus blood flow is increased; this has the effect of greatly increasing the surface area available for exchange of substances and at the same time reduces the distance across which substances have to diffuse to reach the cells. The mechanisms that control the arteriolar radius and precapillary sphincters will be considered later. Suffice it to say here that altering the radius is the normal mechanism for controlling the resistance and altering blood flow, and that both the sympathetic nervous system and local factors are involved.

## The capillaries

The capillaries form the part of the circulatory system where the exchange of gases, fluids, nutrients and metabolic waste products occurs between the blood and the individual cells; capillaries are thus sometimes known as the **exchange vessels**. The capillaries form a dense network of narrow, short tubes; they can be as little as 3–4 μm in diameter (i.e. half the diameter of red blood cells) and up to 30–40 μm (these large blood spaces are usually known as *sinusoids*). On average, capillaries have a diameter of 6–8 μm and are approximately 750 μm long (**Fig. 4.2.37**). The total number of capillaries in the body has been estimated to be of the order of 40 000–50 000 million. In the resting state, probably only about 25% of the capillary beds are patent. For exchange of substances to be efficient, it is necessary to have short distances for substances to diffuse, a large surface area (the total cross-sectional area of all the capillaries is about 700 times larger than that of the aorta) and a slow steady flow of blood, about 0.3–0.5 mm/s (the flow velocity is about 700 times lower in the capillaries than in the aorta because of the narrower vessels). This part of the circulatory system is often referred to as the **microcirculation** (**Fig. 4.2.38**).

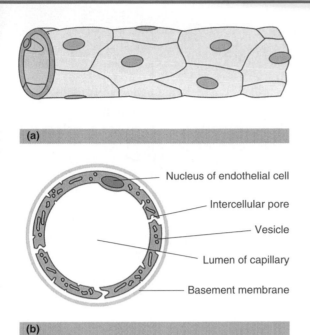

**(a)**

Nucleus of endothelial cell

Intercellular pore

Vesicle

Lumen of capillary

Basement membrane

**(b)**

**Figure 4.2.37** Structure of the capillary showing (a) the surface and (b) a cross-section

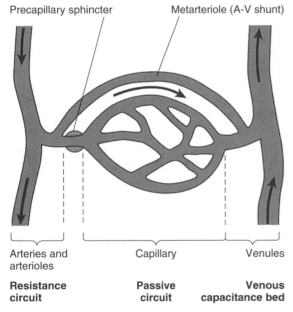

Precapillary sphincter

Metarteriole (A-V shunt)

Arteries and arterioles

Capillary

Venules

**Resistance circuit**

**Passive circuit**

**Venous capacitance bed**

**Figure 4.2.38** Diagrammatic representation of the microcirculation. A-V, ateriovenous

The structure of the microcirculation is modified in different tissues to meet specific functional requirements. Different tissues have varying abundance of capillaries, e.g. dense connective tissue has a poor capillary network as compared to cardiac muscle. Electron microscopy has shown that the nature of the endothelium is not the same in all parts of the circulation. Different kinds of capillary wall have been identified and the terms 'continuous', 'fenestrated' and 'discontinuous' are sometimes used to describe

them, according to the size of the intercellular gaps or pores present in each.

Another modification in the structure of the microcirculation in tissues is the presence of **arteriovenous (A-V) shunts** or **arteriovenous anastomoses**. These are direct connections between the arterial and venous systems that bypass the capillary beds (**Fig. 4.2.38**). If these shunts are patent, blood can flow rapidly through the vessels but does not serve any nutritive purpose. These short connecting vessels have strongly developed muscular control and are under sympathetic nervous control. They are found in many tissues and organs. In the skin, for example, they enable cutaneous blood flow to be increased to allow dissipation of heat from the body surfaces when exercising or in high environmental temperatures (see Chapter 6.1).

The capillary network, whatever its form, drains into a series of vessels of increasing diameter to form venules and veins.

## The venous system

**The venous system acts as a collecting system, returning blood from the capillary networks to the heart passively down a pressure gradient.** The capillaries merge to form venules, which in turn unite to form larger, but fewer, veins that amalgamate finally into the venae cavae. The walls of veins consist of the same three layers as arteries but the elastic muscle components are much less prominent; the walls in general are thinner and more distensible than those of arteries. The vessels have a relatively large diameter (the vena cava is 2–3 cm in diameter) and thus offer low resistance to blood flow. Some veins, especially in the arms and legs, have internal folds of the endothelial lining (**Fig. 4.2.39**) that function as valves and allow blood to flow in one direction only, towards the heart. These valves can be damaged if overstretched by high venous pressures for long periods, for example during pregnancy or in people who stand for extended periods; the valves become incompetent, lose their function and varicose veins develop. As a result of this, oedema and varicose ulcers can develop (**Fig. 4.2.39**).

A major part of the blood volume, approximately 60% (**Fig. 4.2.40**) is contained within the venous system and for this reason veins are sometimes referred to as **capacity vessels**. The capacity of the venous system can be modified by altering the lumen size of the muscular venules and veins; the changes are mediated by altering the **venomotor tone**, that is, the degree of contraction of the smooth muscle in the tunica media. Venomotor tone is mainly under the control of the sympathetic nervous system. Changes in the venomotor tone can increase or

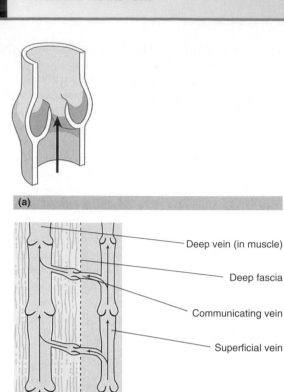

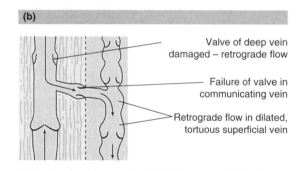

**Figure 4.2.39** Diagram showing (a) a normal venous valve, (b) normally functioning valves in the superficial and deep veins of the leg and (c) the formation of varicose veins when valves in the deep vein become incompetent

decrease the capacity of the venous circulation and therefore can partially compensate for variations in the effective circulating blood volume.

## Venous return

Venous blood flow occurs along relatively small pressure gradients and even small variations in resistance and vessel radius affect the return flow to the heart. As flow can occur only when there is a pressure gradient, the pressure in the venules must at all times be greater than the pressure in the right atrium, and this is normally the situation (**see Fig. 4.2.44**).

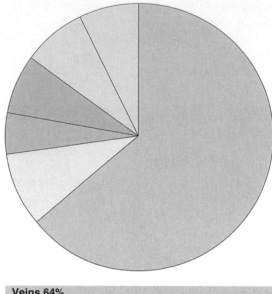

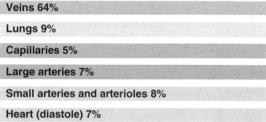

| Veins 64% |
| Lungs 9% |
| Capillaries 5% |
| Large arteries 7% |
| Small arteries and arterioles 8% |
| Heart (diastole) 7% |

**Figure 4.2.40** Percentage distribution of total blood volume in each portion of the circulation

However, the effect of gravity retards venous return: when upright, as the veins are distensible and due to the hydrostatic pressure of a column of blood in the veins below the level of the heart, blood tends to collect or pool in the feet and legs. When vertical, the leg veins take on a circular form which has a greater capacity; when horizontal the veins take on an elliptical shape with a lower capacity. Increased venomotor tone, reducing the diameter and hence capacity of the veins, helps to reduce venous pooling. Venous pooling is a useful term but it suggests stagnation, which does not occur; venous pooling simply indicates that the veins accommodate a greater volume of blood.

One can see the effect of gravity on the veins in the neck: when sitting or standing the neck veins above a level 5–10 cm higher than the heart are not prominent but when lying down the veins distend. This is due to the fact that, in contrast to venous return from the feet, blood from the head returns to the heart aided by gravity when upright. However, the blood supply to the head has to overcome the effect of gravity; failure of this phenomenon can be observed when someone stands up too quickly after bending down and feels dizzy due to a temporary reduction in the effective pressure head delivering blood to the brain.

It is vital that an adequate venous return to the heart is maintained at all times because the cardiac output depends on the venous return – in most instances the cardiac output equals the venous return. Thus, if the venous return falls, cardiac output and blood pressure may also drop. Several mechanisms exist to help maintain the venous return at all times. Increasing the venomotor tone is an important mechanism as it decreases the capacity of the venous system and so aids venous return.

## CLINICAL APPLICATIONS

After a long period of bedrest when the body is not constantly being exposed to the force of gravity and the veins do not have to compensate, venomotor tone is reduced, and this method of reducing the effect of gravity is temporarily less efficient. This should be remembered when helping someone to get up after a period of bedrest. It is essential to move slowly and steadily and to support the person in case he or she becomes dizzy and faint.

Venous return is also assisted by two systems sometimes referred to as the **skeletal muscle pump** and **respiratory pump**. Contraction of the skeletal muscles, especially in the limbs, squeezes the veins and this pushes blood in the extremities towards the heart; backflow is prevented by the presence of numerous valves. There are also many communicating channels that allow emptying of blood from the superficial limb veins into the deep veins when rhythmic muscular contractions occur (**see Fig. 4.2.39**). Consequently, every time a person moves his or her legs or tenses the muscles, a certain amount of blood is pushed towards the heart. The more frequent and powerful such rhythmic contractions are, the more efficient their action. (Sustained continuous muscle contractions, unlike rhythmic contractions, impede blood flow due to the veins being continuously 'blocked'.) The muscle pump mechanism is an efficient system: the venous pressure in the feet of someone walking is of the order of 25 mmHg (3.3 kPa), whereas in the feet of an individual standing absolutely still it is of the order of 90 mmHg (12 kPa; **see Fig. 4.2.33**). So when an individual stands still for long periods of time, the muscle pump cannot operate and venous return is decreased. This can result in people fainting due to an inadequate cerebral blood flow (e.g. soldiers fainting on parade, people fainting in operating theatres after standing still for long periods). Thus it is advisable to contract the muscles of the legs and buttocks voluntarily to aid venous return if standing still for long periods.

Respiration produces cyclical variations in intrapleural and intrathoracic pressure (Chapter 5.3). With each inspiration, the pressure is lowered within the thorax and hence also within the right atrium of the heart; this increases the pressure gradient and aids blood flow back to the heart. Simultaneously, the descent of the diaphragm into the abdomen raises the intra-abdominal pressure and increases the gradient to the thorax, again favouring venous return. With expiration, the pressure gradients are reversed and blood tends to flow in the opposite direction; fortunately this tendency is prevented by the valves in the medium-sized veins.

Thus venous return is maintained by changes in venomotor tone, altering the capacity of the venous system, and by the skeletal muscle and respiratory pumps. Obviously it is also necessary to maintain an adequate circulating blood volume. If the blood volume is depleted for some reason, e.g. dehydration or haemorrhage, in the short term venoconstriction and vasoconstriction in the body's blood reservoirs, such as the skin, liver, lungs and spleen, can increase the effective circulating blood volume. However, the blood volume must be restored eventually by fluid replacement. The pressures in the central regions of the venous system directly reflect the blood volume; thus central venous pressure (CVP), or right atrial pressure, is a good indicator of blood volume, unlike arterial pressures, which are reflexly regulated and controlled (central venous pressure measurements are described later).

## Blood vessel diameter

Blood vessels play an important role in determining local blood flow to tissues and in central reflexes to maintain blood pressure. The diameter of all vessels (except capillaries) is altered by changing the degree of contraction of the smooth muscle in the tunica media of the vessel wall. The muscle is arranged in a circular pattern and, when it contracts, the diameter of the vessel lumen becomes smaller (a process known as **vasoconstriction**); when it relaxes the vessel diameter increases (known as **vasodilation**). Normally, the smooth muscle is in a state of partial contraction all the time, a level of contraction known as the **vasomotor tone**; arteriolar tone refers to the tone of the arterioles and venous or venomotor tone to the tone of the veins. So, by altering the degree of muscle contraction, the radius of the vessel can be increased or decreased.

The smooth muscle of the vessel walls is influenced by both nervous and chemical factors.

### Nervous control of blood vessel diameter

Sympathetic nerves innervate the smooth muscle of all arteries and veins, but the arterioles, precapillary

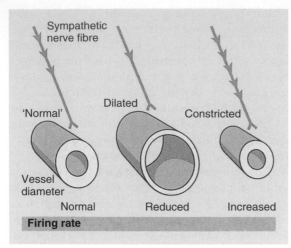

**Figure 4.2.41** Effect of sympathetic nerve firing rate on blood vessel diameter

sphincters and postcapillary venules are more densely supplied with nerve endings than the other vessels. (There are only a few instances of parasympathetic nerve supply to blood vessels, namely the nervi erigentes, which supplies part of the genital tract, and in the salivary glands.) The effect of sympathetic discharge is to cause muscle contraction and hence vasoconstriction. However, due to the fact that the muscle of the vessels is always in a state of partial contraction (the vasomotor tone), the same sympathetic constrictor nerves can also accomplish dilation simply by decreasing the frequency of discharge of impulses along the sympathetic nerve fibres (Fig. 4.2.41). Thus, by increasing the discharge rate, the vessel is constricted, whereas by decreasing the discharge rate the same vessel can dilate. Part of the cardiovascular centre in the medulla oblongata of the brain, described as the vasomotor centre (discussed later), controls the rate of discharge down the sympathetic nerves.

The vasoconstriction that results from increased sympathetic activity causes an increase in the total vascular resistance. An increased sympathetic discharge has other consequences, too. The capillary hydrostatic pressure drops due to the increased arteriolar resistance; this favours the uptake of interstitial fluid from the tissues into the blood and tends to increase the circulating blood volume. Another consequence of the increased sympathetic discharge is to increase the venomotor tone, so the capacity of the venules and veins decreases and venous return increases. These mechanisms are particularly useful in conditions such as haemorrhage when there is a decrease in the circulating blood volume (the opposite effects will occur if the sympathetic discharge is reduced).

The blood vessels in different parts of the body are not all equally affected by the sympathetic output; this is due partly to the variation in distribution of sympathetic nerves to the vessels and also to the varying distribution of $\alpha$- and $\beta$-adrenoreceptors in the smooth muscle (see Chapter 2.5). For example, blood vessels to the skin will vasoconstrict strongly with sympathetic stimulation whereas cerebral vessels show only slight vasoconstriction.

The postganglionic sympathetic fibres normally release norepinephrine and this acts upon the smooth muscle to produce the contraction and vasoconstriction. Epinephrine released from the adrenal medulla causes vasoconstriction in a similar way to the sympathetic nervous discharge (see Chapter 2.5).

The fact that altering blood vessel calibre has several physiological effects is used therapeutically and there are many drugs available that alter blood vessel calibre. For instance, drugs that mimic the action of the sympathetic nervous system (known as sympathomimetics, e.g. dopamine, epinephrine and norepinephrine), cause vasoconstriction; they also have varying effects on the heart. Epinephrine influences both $\alpha$- and $\beta$-receptors and affects both the heart and peripheral vessels, whereas norepinephrine affects mainly $\alpha$-receptors and primarily the vascular system, causing an increase in peripheral resistance. Nicotine increases epinephrine output from the adrenal medulla and so causes vasoconstriction.

## CLINICAL APPLICATIONS

Adrenergic blocking drugs 'block' the activity of epinephrine and norepinephrine at the smooth muscle receptor sites and so cause vasodilation. For example, $\alpha$-receptor blocking drugs are used in the treatment of peripheral vascular disease to increase blood flow to ischaemic tissues; the drugs tend to increase blood flow to the skin rather than to the muscles and so are particularly useful in some instances to assist in the treatment of varicose ulcers. Drugs can also be given that directly affect the smooth muscle in the blood vessel wall, e.g. glyceryl trinitrate (GTN) is a potent vasodilator and is particularly effective in the treatment of angina.

## Chemical control of blood vessel diameter

As well as being affected by sympathetic nervous control, the vascular smooth muscle is also directly influenced by chemical factors such as hormones and locally produced metabolites. The effects of epinephrine and norepinephrine have already been mentioned. A number of other agents have a role, too: for instance, histamine and plasma kinins, released as part of the inflammatory response when tissues are injured, cause vasodilation of the small vessels, whereas angiotensin II, formed by the action of renin on angiotensinogen, is a potent vasoconstrictor. The response of vascular smooth muscle to local metabolites is important and is discussed below.

## Response to local metabolites

The coordination of metabolic needs when tissues are active and require an increased blood supply does not depend on central mechanisms, but is controlled locally. When a tissue is active, there is a local increase of cell metabolic products in the interstitium and these chemicals directly influence the smooth muscle of the precapillary vessels causing vasodilation, and thus increasing the blood flow to the active tissue. This mechanism of increasing blood flow in response to local demand, known as **active hyperaemia**, is highly developed in tissues such as the heart and skeletal muscle, and to a lesser extent in the gastrointestinal tract.

The precise nature of the metabolites that produce this relaxation of the smooth muscle still has to be fully resolved. Many factors have been proposed as vasodilators (e.g. lack of oxygen, high levels of carbon dioxide and lactic acid, decreased pH, hyperosmolarity of the interstitial fluid, adenosine and prostaglandins). The most likely substances are thought to be adenosine (which is also known to be involved in the regulation of coronary blood flow) in skeletal muscle and some prostaglandins, which have been proposed as important vasodilator mediators in some vascular beds.

The smooth muscle of the smaller arterioles and precapillary sphincters shows inherent myogenic activity and the metabolites, whichever they prove to be, suppress this myogenic activity – the sphincters relax and the capillaries governed by them open **(see Fig. 4.2.38)**. With the increased blood flow, the accumulated metabolites are dissipated and the inherent tone can be re-established and the sphincters close again. Thus there is autoregulation of the blood flow in the sense that the increase in blood flow is directly in proportion to the increased activity of the tissue.

Locally mediated vasodilation can be demonstrated easily. If the blood supply to the arm is occluded for a couple of minutes (e.g. using a sphymomanometer cuff inflated to 200 mmHg), the arm goes pale because it is ischaemic. When the cuff is inflated the cells are still metabolizing; the metabolites accumulate as there is no blood flow to remove them. This causes the precapillary vessels to dilate. As the cuff is deflated, once the pressure in the cuff is below systolic pressure,

blood can again flow into the arm. As a result of the vasodilation there is an enlarged capacity in the capillary system and so the arm flushes considerably 'redder' than the other arm due to the increased blood content. In this instance, the ischaemia was responsible for producing the arteriolar dilation and so the process is known as **reactive hyperaemia**.

## Endothelial-mediated regulation

The endothelium, the innermost layer of blood vessels, was originally thought to be a simple passive single layer of cells, however, it is now known that the endothelium plays a key role in controlling cardiovascular function. Doshi et al. (2001) refer to the endothelium as an 'organ' because it is capable of carrying out complex endocrine and paracrine functions and is intimately concerned with controlling vasomotor tone and preventing atherosclerosis and thrombosis. The endothelium is directly sensitive to fluid dynamics and can sense changes in shear stress and responds by switching on genes that leads to synthesis of several substances (Knight, 1999).

The endothelium itself produces a number of potent local vasoactive agents, including the vasodilator molecule, nitric oxide, and the vasoconstrictor peptide, endothelin. So the endothelium is able to produce factors that can cause relaxation or constriction of vascular smooth muscle and so produces vasodilation or vasoconstriction, respectively. The factor that was initially identified to cause vasodilation was named **endothelial-derived relaxing factor (EDRF)** until it was identified as nitric oxide (NO). Stimulation of the endothelial cells by a variety of agents (e.g. acetylcholine, adenosine triphosphate, bradykinin, serotonin, histamine, shear stress of blood flow) results in the production and release of nitric oxide. Nitric oxide has also been found to inhibit platelet aggregation.

The endothelium can also synthesize factors that can cause vasoconstriction, for example endothelin. Endothelin (ET) is a peptide and a very potent vasoconstrictor substance. It has potent effects on smooth muscle cells and fibroblasts and is probably involved in many disease processes. For instance, endothelin has been implicated in the pathogenesis of hypertension, vasospasm and heart failure. Its release is stimulated by angiotensin II, antidiuretic hormone, thrombin, cytokines, oxygen free radicals and shearing forces acting on the endothelium; its release is inhibited by nitric oxide.

The discovery of the role of nitric oxide is revolutionizing many aspects of physiology, and not just in the cardiovascular system. Nitric oxide is a free-radical molecule and is a vital chemical messenger carrying biochemical signals from cell to cell and acting as a trigger in many different physiological

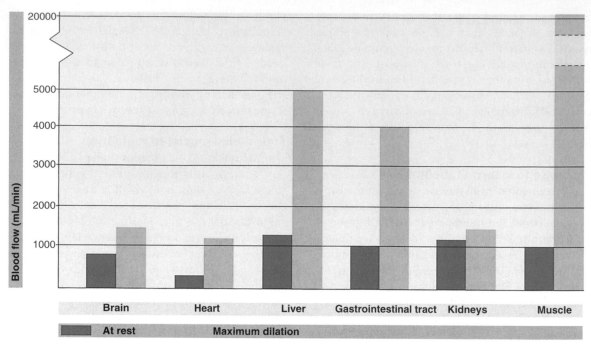

**Figure 4.2.42** Approximate blood flow in selected tissues at rest and at maximal perfusion

processes. The nitric oxide released from the endothelium diffuses into the surrounding layers of muscle in the blood vessel walls: here the nitric oxide triggers events that make the muscles relax and so the blood vessel dilates. Thus blood vessels are kept dilated by a steady release of nitric oxide.

The discovery of the role of nitric oxide has explained aspects not previously understood, for example the role of nitroglycerines in the treatment of angina. It has been known for some time that nitroglycerines dilated blood vessels and reduced blood pressure, but the exact biochemical reason for its efficacy was unknown. We now know that drugs like these work by exploiting the body's natural defence mechanisms for controlling the degree of constriction of blood vessel walls. Endothelial dysfunction may well also have a role in atherosclerosis, septic shock and hypertension, as well as effects on other systems in the body including the central and peripheral nervous systems, immunity and inflammation.

So, by a combination of nervous reflexes and chemical changes, the blood flow to most tissues is regulated according to the metabolic needs (**Fig. 4.2.42** shows the possible extent of the blood flow changes). The chemical control is of overwhelming importance in conditions where there is increased metabolic activity of tissues. For instance, resting skeletal muscle flow is maintained by the influence of sympathetic vasoconstrictor fibres, but when exercising massive vasodilation is achieved by the influence of local metabolites produced by the active tissue.

The control of two of the vital circulations, those of the heart and brain, is predominantly influenced by chemical rather than nervous factors. The coronary vessels are sensitive to oxygen lack and dilate when oxygen levels in the blood drop (for a fuller discussion of control of coronary blood flow, see earlier in this chapter). Blood flow to the brain under normal circumstances varies very little. However, if the chemical composition of the blood or tissue fluid changes markedly, blood flow does alter; the main determinants of the cerebral vascular diameter are the local carbon dioxide, hydrogen ion and adenosine levels along with some endothelial mediated regulation (see Chapter 5.3).

If an individual hyperventilates and expires extra carbon dioxide, the hydrogen ion concentration is reduced and the cerebral vessels constrict; the individual may become dizzy and light-headed due to cerebral hypoxia. Conversely, if the plasma carbon dioxide or hydrogen ion levels increase, the cerebral vessels dilate; this can be observed if an individual breathes air with a high carbon dioxide level, say 7%, when he or she may experience an intense pounding headache due to cerebral vasodilation. A decreased oxygen tension or a rise in body temperature also produces dilation of the cerebral vessels.

The blood flow to the skin, in contrast to the heart and brain, is mainly determined by sympathetic nervous activity and local factors are much less important. Cutaneous blood flow depends not so much on the metabolic activity of the skin itself as on the requirements for maintenance of body temperature, and thus skin blood flow is centrally coordinated. Local reflexes do operate if part of the body is exposed to extremities of temperature (e.g. a hand in

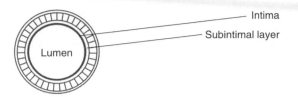

hot water vasodilates). Under maximum heat load, total skin blood flow can be as much as 3–4 L/min, whereas under cold stress the total skin blood flow can be as little as 50 mL/min.

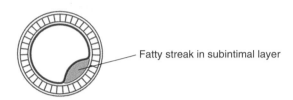

**(a) Transverse section of a normal artery**

## CLINICAL APPLICATIONS

### ARTERIOSCLEROSIS AND ATHEROSCLEROSIS

Structural changes in the walls of blood vessels are very common and lead to changes in the properties and normal functioning of the vessels; but perhaps more seriously, in the long term these changes are also responsible for, or linked with, several of the major diseases prevalent today. **Arteriosclerosis** refers to the hardening of the arteries: muscle and elastic tissue are replaced with fibrous tissue and calcification may occur. Due to the lack of distensibility, arteriosclerotic vessels are less able to change their radius and lumen size. Arteriosclerosis includes atherosclerosis.

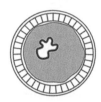

**(b) Early atheromatous plaque**

**Atherosclerosis** refers to hardening and obstruction of the arteries. It is due to the deposition of lipids and other substances, in the form of an atheromatous plaque, in the intima of the medium and large-sized arteries. In affected vessels the intima becomes thickened, smooth muscle cells, collagen and elastic fibres accumulate, and lipids (especially cholesterol) are deposited in the arterial wall **(Fig. 4.2.43)**. The type of artery and where the plaque develops varies with each person. Although much research has been carried out to determine how atherosclerosis develops, the precise mechanisms remain uncertain. The outer part of the plaque is fibrous but the centre is soft and has the consistency of gruel or porridge, hence the use of *athera*, a Greek word meaning gruel. Atherosclerosis is not a simple lesion; a variety of pathological changes occur.

In many cases there is damage to the endothelium of the arteries and endothelial dysfunction probably plays a key part in the pathogenesis and progression of atherosclerosis. Endothelial dysfunction (characterized by an inability to release nitric oxide) occurs early in atherosclerosis, before plaque formation. It also predisposes to thrombosis, leucocyte adhesion and proliferation of smooth muscle in blood vessel walls. Platelets circulating in the blood also adhere to the damaged portions of the endothelium; it is thought that a substance released from platelets, known as platelet growth factor, may promote the proliferation of the smooth muscle cells. Muscle cells, probably from the media, migrate into the intima of the artery wall. The plaque appears above the normal

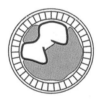

**(c) Advanced atheromatous plaque, narrowing lumen**

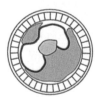

**(d) Ulceration of endothelium**

**(e) Ulceration leading to thrombous formation**

**Figure 4.2.43** Atherosclerotic changes that may occur in arteries. These changes are not, necessarily, sequential

endothelial surface and serum lipids accumulate within it, especially cholesterol and low-density lipoprotein (LDL), which carries cholesterol in the plasma. So the mature plaque is composed of two main constituents: the lipid core is mainly released from necrotic 'foam cells' (monocyte-derived macrophages), which migrate into the tunica intima and ingest lipids. The second part is the connective tissue matrix, which is derived from the migrated smooth muscle cells which proliferate and change to form a fibrous capsule around the lipid core (Grech, 2003).

Clinical problems can ensue from several aspects of plaque formation and atherosclerosis.

The vessels can actually become blocked or stenosed; also, as a result of the endothelial damage and platelet adhesion, an ulcer-like site can develop that can lead to thrombus formation. Sometimes pieces of dead tissue from the damaged arterial wall can break off and lead to an embolus. Stenosis and thrombus and/or embolus formation can occur together. If the process progresses, the intima is 'eaten away' and, especially if the blood pressure is elevated, the vessel can develop an aneurysm.

Atherosclerosis is responsible for most coronary artery and ischaemic heart disease, for much cerebrovascular disease (e.g. strokes), peripheral vascular disease and for most abdominal aortic aneurysms (AAA; about 6000 people per year in the United Kingdom die from a ruptured AAA; Gibson, 2002). The occurrence of atheroma varies in different sites in the body and, as would be expected from the diseases it is associated with, is common in the proximal coronary arteries, the aorta, the iliac, popliteal, femoral and internal carotid arteries and in the circle of Willis in the brain. There is some evidence to suggest that atheroma formation is enhanced in areas where the arteries branch or divide and turbulence in blood flow is increased.

## RISK FACTORS

Many risk factors have been identified as playing a role in the development and progression of atherosclerosis; some of these factors are modifiable and some are not. Some of the risk factors (e.g. smoking and hypertension) may have their own adverse effect by damaging the endothelium. The mechanisms linking smoking and atherosclerosis are complex, but nicotine is thought to increase platelet adhesion and carbon monoxide may increase the permeability of the arterial endothelium, thus enhancing plaque formation. Smokers also have higher fibrinogen levels and a higher blood viscosity, both of which exacerbate atherosclerosis and thrombus formation. Smoking also leads to an increase in many immune cells, which also contribute to the inflammatory responses in atherosclerosis formation. Whatever the precise mechanisms, stopping smoking leads to a significant reduction in cardiovascular disease and reduces atherosclerosis formation. Stopping smoking helps lower cholesterol levels and blood pressure too.

Many studies show a positive relationship between elevated serum cholesterol levels and the incidence of atherosclerosis, especially associated with coronary artery disease. Elevated cholesterol levels may be the result of endogenous (metabolic disease, e.g. diabetes, or genetic) or exogenous (high fat diets, especially saturated fats, and high dietary cholesterol) factors. There is no definitive causal relationship between saturated fat intake in the diet and the serum cholesterol levels but there is evidence that unsaturated fatty acids lower blood cholesterol whereas saturated fats tend to raise it.

There is also convincing evidence that lowering serum cholesterol reduces the risk of subsequent coronary heart disease events and overall mortality. In the past the normal range for cholesterol was 3.6–7.8 mmol/L and levels above 6 regarded as high risk: now the levels regarded as normal are being redefined, with lower ranges being considered. Statins are a group of drugs used for lowering cholesterol levels (e.g. atorvastin and simvastin) and, when they are given to patients who have cardiovascular disease, there is a reduction in further cardiovascular events and improved survival (Hippisley-Cox et al., 2003; Mayor, 2002); fibrates are also used for reducing serum cholesterol levels.

Most researchers believe that the process of atherogenesis begins early in life and that fatty streaks observed in the arterial walls of children may, in some instances, be precursors of atherosclerosis. Some research has also investigated the influence of the very early environment in utero and in infancy, and the effects of maternal nutrition on the expression of coronary heart disease in subsequent adult life (Editorial, 1992). Thus, although there is no proof as to the causal relationship between fats and atherosclerosis, it does seem sensible to reduce the amount of saturated fat in the diet. It is also perhaps important that the body manufactures cholesterol in amounts up to four to six times those found in the diet. There is some evidence to suggest that hypercholesterolaemia itself can alter the normal endothelium.

Many other factors have been associated with the development of arteriosclerosis. It is more common in the industrialized areas of the world. Diabetes and obesity are also known to be causative factors. It has been suggested that atherosclerosis is a result of a more sedentary lifestyle; indeed, regular physical exercise has been found to promote a favourable ratio of lipoproteins in the blood (a higher high-density lipoprotein (HDL) and lower low-density lipoprotein content).

Other dietary factors have been studied; vitamins C and E have antioxidant properties and have been suggested as having a role in preventing free radical damage on lipids in the vessel walls (Shaw et al., 2001). Having a close relative who developed atherosclerosis at an early age also puts a person at risk. There are sex differences too: males are affected more than women until the time of the menopause, when the sex distribution becomes equal. The incidence of atherosclerosis also increases with increasing age.

Atherosclerotic changes can occur in any part of the body. One in five of middle-aged population (65–75 years old) in the United Kingdom have some evidence of peripheral arterial disease (i.e. changes in the vessels in the limbs), although not all of these people will have problematic symptoms (Burns et al., 2003). The most common symptom is muscle pain in the lower limbs when exercising, which is known as intermittent claudication. Peripheral arterial disease is a marker for atherosclerotic changes elsewhere in the body, the risk to the limb affected is low but the risk to life is high because of the possible consequences of changes especially in the coronary and cerebral circulations. 'Best medical practice' (Burns et al., 2003) is to achieve complete and permanent cessation of smoking, antiplatelet agents (usually aspirin) to reduce coagulability, screening for diabetes, reduction of any hypertension, exercise, and lowering cholesterol. Acting on evidence of peripheral arterial disease can significantly reduce general cardiovascular mortality and morbidity.

## Blood pressure in the cardiovascular system

**Blood pressure** refers to the pressure exerted by the blood on the blood vessel walls. All fluids, and blood is no exception, exert pressure on the walls of the vessel that they are held in. The pressure exerted by a liquid against the walls of its container is known as the **hydrostatic pressure** and thus blood pressure is a hydrostatic pressure.

Each blood vessel has its own blood pressure value, for instance arterial blood pressure, capillary blood pressure, venous blood pressure, right atrial pressure, and so on. As can be seen from **Fig. 4.2.44**, the pressure in the blood vessels falls continuously from the aorta to the end of the systemic circulation in the right atrium. The pressures in the pulmonary circulation are considerably lower than in the systemic circulation but there is still a pressure gradient from the right ventricle to the left atrium. The pressure must drop if the blood is to flow. It is also essential for adequate tissue exchange to have a differential blood pressure gradient between the arteriolar and venular ends of the capillary: this ensures that substances can leave the bloodstream at the arteriolar end and returned at the venular end. This is discussed in detail on the section on tissue fluid formation (see p. 444).

When we talk clinically about 'blood pressure' *per se*, we are usually referring to systemic arterial blood pressure. The emphasis on arterial blood pressure is logical and important because it is this pressure that ensures an adequate blood flow to the tissues and to vital organs such as the brain and heart. If the blood pressure falls too far, tissue flow is reduced and so nutrient and gas supplies may become inadequate. A person fainting is an example of this, with a reduced blood supply to the brain.

As we shall see later, there are several reflexes operating to regulate and maintain arterial blood pressure

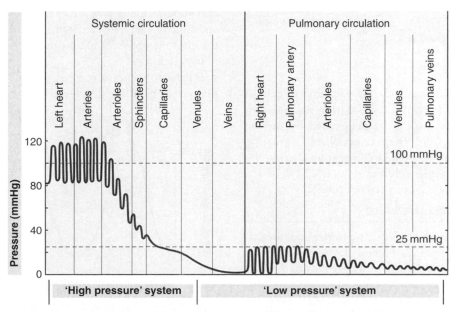

**Figure 4.2.44** Relationship between blood pressure, blood flow and cross-sectional area in the systemic and pulmonary circulation

within normal limits. Blood pressures in other regions of the circulatory system should similarly be kept within normal ranges: for instance, abnormal capillary blood pressures will alter the exchange of fluids to and from the tissues (see later).

Blood pressure is a function of blood flow and vascular resistance. Both moment-to-moment and long-term stability of arterial pressure are necessary for survival. The discussion that follows concentrates mainly on the short-term regulation of blood pressure.

## Blood flow

The circulatory system is a closed system and thus the total flow leaving and returning to the heart will be the same. Thus blood flow is equivalent to cardiac output.

## Pressure difference

This is the difference between the mean pressure in the aorta and the pressure in the vena cava just before the blood enters the heart (this latter value is almost zero). As the blood pressure is essentially the same in the aorta and all *large* arteries, the pressure difference can be said to be equivalent to mean arterial pressure.

## Resistance to flow

This is the *total* resistance to blood flow. As the majority of the resistance is found in the peripheral vessels, especially the arterioles, it is often described as the total peripheral resistance. Thus we have the equation:

$$\text{mean arterial pressure} = \text{cardiac output} \times \text{total peripheral resistance}$$

or

$$BP = CO \times TPR$$

This is one of the fundamental equations of cardiovascular physiology. You can see from the equation that blood pressure can be maintained by altering cardiac output and/or total peripheral resistance. The cardiac output itself is changed by altering the heart rate and stroke volume.

## Arterial blood pressure

Arterial blood pressure fluctuates throughout the cardiac cycle. The contraction of the ventricles ejects blood into the pulmonary and systemic arteries during systole and this additional volume of blood distends the arteries and raises the arterial pressure. When the contraction ends, the stretched elastic arterial walls recoil passively and this continues to drive

blood through the arterioles. As the blood leaves the arteries the pressure falls; the arterial pressure never falls to zero because the next ventricular contraction occurs when there is still an appreciable amount of blood within the arteries (Fig. 4.2.45). Thus the pressure in the major arteries rises and falls as the heart contracts and relaxes. The maximum pressure occurs after ventricular systole and is known as the **systolic pressure**. When the blood pressure in the aorta exceeds that in the ventricle, the aortic valve closes; this accounts for the dicrotic notch (**Fig. 4.2.45**). Once the aortic valve has closed, the blood pressure in the aorta and large arteries falls as blood flows through the arterioles and capillaries to the veins. The level to which the arterial pressure has fallen before the next ventricular systole (i.e. the minimum pressure) is known as the **diastolic pressure**.

The systolic pressure is determined by the amount of blood being forced into the aorta and arteries with each ventricular contraction (i.e. the stroke volume) and also by the force of contraction. An increase in either will increase the systolic pressure. Similarly, if the arterial wall becomes stiffer, as happens in arteriosclerosis, the vessels are not able to distend with the increased blood volume and so the systolic pressure is increased.

Diastolic pressure is also influenced by several factors. The diastolic pressure provides information on the degree of peripheral resistance: if there is increased arteriolar vasoconstriction, this will impede blood flowing out of the arterial system to the capillaries, and the diastolic pressure will rise. Conversely, if the peripheral resistance is reduced by vasodilation, more blood will flow out of the arterial system and thus diastolic pressure will fall. Drugs that modify the degree of arterial vasoconstriction and alter the peripheral resistance will obviously affect the diastolic pressure, and are used for the treatment of hypertension.

The diastolic pressure also depends on the level of the systolic pressure, the elasticity of the arteries and

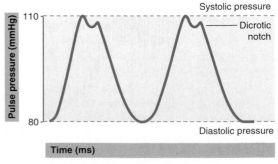

**Figure 4.2.45** Waveform showing variation in blood pressure in main arteries as the heart contracts and relaxes

the viscosity of the blood. Alterations in the heart rate will also affect diastolic pressure: with a slower heart rate, the diastolic pressure will be lower as there is a greater time for blood to flow out of the arteries, and vice versa.

## Pulse pressure and mean arterial pressure

Each ventricular contraction initiates a pulse, or wave, of pressure through the arteries and these pulses can be palpated (felt) wherever an artery passes near the skin and over a bony or firm surface. **Figure 4.2.46** shows the common sites where the pulse is felt. Thus, as there is normally one pulse per heart beat, the pulse rate is used as an easy method for counting the heart rate. The characteristics of the pulse are important: the rate, the pattern of beats and the strength of the pulse all give valuable information on the functioning of the cardiovascular system. Atrial fibrillation can result in a rapid irregular heart

rate; in some instances each ventricular contraction may not be sufficiently strong to transmit an arterial pulse wave through the peripheral artery and can lead to an apex–radial pulse deficit. In these circumstances the heart rate taken at both the apex (with a stethoscope and counting heart rate directly) and radial pulse rate are counted simultaneously.

These palpable pulses represent the difference between the systolic and diastolic pressures and this difference is known as the **pulse pressure**, e.g. the pulse pressure in an individual whose blood pressure is 120/70 mmHg is (120 − 70) = 50 mmHg. Two of the main factors that alter the pulse pressure are the stroke volume and decreased arterial compliance.

It is sometimes useful to have an average, or mean, value for the arterial pressure, rather than maximum and minimum (systolic and diastolic) pressures, as it is the mean pressure that represents the pressure driving blood through the systemic circulation. The **mean arterial pressure** is not a simple arithmetical mean; it is estimated by adding one-third of the pulse pressure to the diastolic pressure. So, for a blood pressure of 120/70 mmHg, mean pressure = 70 + (1/3 × 50) = 87 mmHg.

From the point of view of actual tissue perfusion, it is generally the mean arterial pressure that matters, rather than the precise values of systolic and diastolic pressures. Some automated blood-pressure-measuring machines now give mean arterial blood pressure values.

## Blood pressure values

There is no such value as a 'normal' blood pressure for the population as a whole; there is a usual or 'normal' value for any particular individual, but even that value varies from moment to moment under different circumstances **(Fig. 4.2.47)** and over longer periods of time. Many factors, both physiological and genetic, have an influence on blood pressure and thus it is not surprising that individuals have significantly different, but 'normal', blood pressure values. For these reasons it is more appropriate to refer to a normal range of blood pressure than to a single value: 'normal' adult blood pressures range from approximately 100/60 mmHg to 140/90 mmHg.

Maturation and growth are known to cause predictable increases in blood pressure. In a newborn infant, the blood pressure may be 70/55 mmHg (for a male) or 65/55 mmHg (female), by the age of 5 it may be 95/56 mmHg and at 10 around 100/62 mmHg (MacGregor, 2000) and will increase with growth until the end of adolescence when a value of, say, 120/80 mmHg is reached. Of course, there will be a range of 'normal' values for children as there is for adults. Blood pressure norms have been established

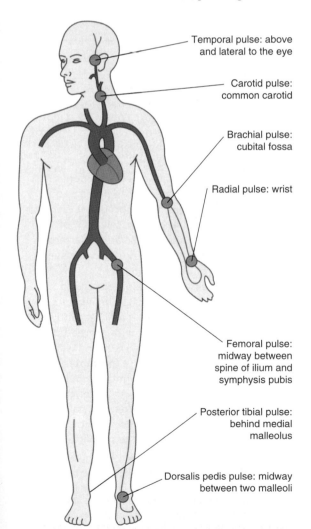

Temporal pulse: above and lateral to the eye

Carotid pulse: common carotid

Brachial pulse: cubital fossa

Radial pulse: wrist

Femoral pulse: midway between spine of ilium and symphysis pubis

Posterior tibial pulse: behind medial malleolus

Dorsalis pedis pulse: midway between two malleoli

**Figure 4.2.46**    Common sites in the body where pulses can be felt

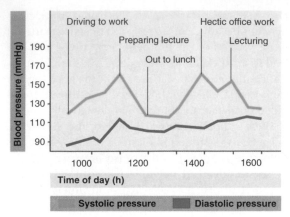

**Figure 4.2.47** Variation in arterial blood pressure over a 'normal' 7-hour period (redrawn from O'Brien & O'Malley, 1981)

using height and specific percentiles identified to help recognition of normal and abnormal values (de Swiet et al., 1989).

Parameters such as age, sex, weight and ethnic origin influence blood pressure values. In Western societies, blood pressure values tend to increase with advancing age, therefore a blood pressure that would be 'normal' for a 70-year-old might be considered 'abnormal' for a 40-year-old. Systolic blood pressure tends to continue rising with advancing age but the rise in the diastolic tends to tail off after about the age of 60. This rise with increasing age is not universal, for example in rural non-Westernized communities the rise in blood pressure with age is minimal (Beevers et al., 2001). The elevation in blood pressure with age is attributed in the main to environmental factors such as sensitivity to salt, increased body mass index and is likely to result from arteriosclerosis (see also the section on Ageing, p. 457). Genetic factors may well be involved in the changes in some individuals.

Men generally have higher blood pressures than women (boys higher than girls, too). Obese people tend to have higher blood pressure values than thin people. There are some racial/ethnic differences but socioeconomic environment is very important, too. Migration studies in Africa have shown that rural people who migrate to urban areas develop a rapid rise in blood pressure within months of arriving (Beevers et al., 2001; Edmunds & Lip, 1999).

The British Hypertension Society recommends that people should have their blood pressure checked every 5 years until the age of 80, because a high blood pressure leads to a significantly increased risk of health problems, especially myocardial infarctions and strokes (Ramsey et al., 1999). The American Heart Association Committee even recommends that blood pressure should be measured from about the age of 3 years (Tanne, 2002). A high or

raised blood pressure is known as hypertension and can be present in one or both of the systolic and diastolic values. There is no evidence of a specific threshold between 'normal' blood pressure and pressures associated with a higher risk (Beevers et al., 2001), which makes decisions about treatment more difficult. Most authorities now agree that a resting systolic value above 140 mmHg and a diastolic pressure persistently exceeding 90 mmHg indicates **hypertension**. Individuals with systolic blood pressure of 120–139 mmHg or a diastolic blood pressure of 80–89 mmHg can be considered possibly to be in a prehypertensive stage (Chobanian et al., 2003); indeed in the United States a blood pressure above 120/80 mmHg would be considered hypertensive. A persistently low blood pressure, **hypotension**, is relatively rare, although temporary or transient hypotension is more common, e.g. in haemorrhage or fainting.

## CLINICAL APPLICATIONS

### HYPERTENSION

Hypertension develops when the long-term control of blood pressure gets out of control; this may occur over many years. Long-term regulation of blood pressure relies on different mechanisms from short-term control; a complex set of interactions concerned with regulation of fluid volume and renal involvement is thought to be in operation for long-term control. Hypertension is one of the most common cardiovascular disorders and can affect people of all ages including children, pregnant women and elderly people. Approximately 50% of people in England aged 65–74 are hypertensive and this percentage increases for people even older (Beevers et al., 2001).

One of the reasons that clinicians are so concerned about the level of an individual's blood pressure is that there is a significantly increased mortality in those with untreated hypertension when compared with individuals with a 'normal' blood pressure (**normotensive**). Many deaths in the United Kingdom could be prevented if blood pressure was better controlled. In the past there was more attention paid to the diastolic pressure value but there is increasing evidence that the height of the systolic blood pressure is a better predictor of both heart attacks and strokes (even when the diastolic value is not raised) (Beevers et al., 2001).

Individuals who are hypertensive usually have few, if any, symptoms and often the hypertension is only diagnosed as part of a routine medical screening, for example for insurance purposes.

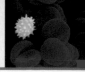

The effects of a raised blood pressure are insidious and develop over many years: the heart (in particular the left ventricle) has to increase in size (detectable by X-ray) and strength to overcome the increased resistance caused by the increased blood pressure. The arteries respond to the increased pressure by hypertrophy of the smooth muscle in their walls, so that they are able to withstand exposure to the higher pressures. Atherosclerosis formation is also potentiated. The blood vessels most commonly affected are the cerebral, coronary and renal vessels; cerebrovascular accidents (strokes) and myocardial ischaemia and infarctions (heart attacks) are the most common clinical manifestations, followed by renal disease. Other complications include heart failure (especially left ventricular failure), atrial fibrillation, peripheral vascular disease, hypercoagulability of the blood and retinopathy.

There has been much research into the causes of hypertension. In a few instances, hypertension is secondary to renal or endocrine disease, but in most cases no clear single identifiable cause is found for **primary** or **essential hypertension**. The aetiology of essential hypertension is almost certainly multifactorial and it is likely to prove to be a combination of genetic and environmental factors. However, what is known is that because arterial blood pressure is the product of cardiac output and total peripheral resistance, all forms of hypertension involve haemodynamic mechanisms – either an increase in cardiac output or total peripheral resistance or both.

Although the cause or causes of primary hypertension are not known, several risk factors have been identified. For instance there is often a positive family history of hypertension: if both parents are hypertensive, there is a significantly greater risk that their children will also develop high blood pressure. Other risk factors include advancing age, high salt intake, obesity, diabetes, a high alcohol intake, elevated cholesterol levels, some drugs (e.g. non-steroidal anti-inflammatory drugs, oral contraceptives, corticosteroids, even liquorice) and acute stress (see the section on atherosclerosis, p. 431). There are also differences in different ethnic groups, with a greater prevalence (and severity) of hypertension in Afro-Caribbean, or black, populations than in their white counterparts (Edmunds & Lip, 1999). There is little convincing evidence, however, that chronic stress causes hypertension (Beevers et al., 2001).

Smoking has a vasoconstrictor effect and so would also exacerbate a raised blood pressure. Events in fetal life and infancy may also predispose to hypertension in adult life (Barker, 1992).

Mechanisms that seem to be involved in the aetiology of hypertension include some that affect the extracellular fluid volume and expand the circulating blood volume. The renin–angiotensin system is likely to be involved, especially the 'local' renin–angiotensin sytems in the kidney, heart and arterial tree, as is increased sympathetic activity, increased vasoconstriction and excessive dietary salt intake, possibly associated with a low potassium intake. Dysfunction of the endothelium has been implicated in essential hypertension, possibly involving endothelin, as has atrial natiuretic peptide secreted by the atria, which could lead to fluid retention and hypertension (for a fuller discussion, see Kornitzer et al. (1999) and Beevers et al. (2001)).

The drug treatments prescribed for hypertension relate to the various mechanisms thought to be involved in the aetiology, i.e. diuretics (e.g. thiazides) to increase sodium and water loss; $\beta$-blockers (e.g. atenolol) and sometimes $\alpha$-blockers too, to reduce sympathetic activity; calcium channel blockers (e.g. amlodipine) reduce peripheral vascular resistance by causing vasodilation. Angiotensin-converting enzyme (ACE) inhibitors are also used; these act on both the local and systemic renin–angiotensin systems and lower peripheral vascular resistance.

The aim of treatment is to reduce the systolic pressure to below 140 mmHg and the diastolic to below 90 mmHg (Chobanian et al. (2003) review the prevention, detection and treatment of high blood pressure). It is usual now for a combination of drugs to be given: most patients will require double or triple therapy, choosing drugs that complement each other. In some hypertensive patients, plasma lipid levels are lowered with the use of statins.

Non-pharmacological treatment or life-style modifications for hypertension are also widely practised, and in most cases should be tried before starting drug regimes. Individuals in the prehypertensive stage should particularly adopt these. Initiatives such as weight reduction, a diet low in salt and fat with an increased intake of potassium from fruit and vegetables (sometimes referred to as the DASH eating plan: Dietary Approaches to Stop Hypertension), moderation of alcohol intake and stopping smoking will all help to reduce hypertension. There is a close positive relationship between alcohol consumption and blood pressure levels.

Increasing exercise levels is also beneficial; this would help in weight loss regimes but physical exercise (e.g. brisk walking, swimming, cycling, etc.) in its own right has positive effects by increasing stroke volume, which in turn would lower heart rate and hence systolic pressure. At least 30 minutes of moderate aerobic exercise per day, most days of the week is recommended (Chobanian et al., 2003). The exercise undertaken should not be of the isometric type because activities such as weight training can raise blood pressure acutely.

Relaxation techniques and biofeedback have been claimed to be successful in reducing blood pressure in some individuals but tend to be used as an adjunct to other treatment approaches.

If hypertension is diagnosed and effectively treated, usually involving drug therapy, much of the cardiovascular-related disease, and the damage to other organs can be prevented.

## Measurement of arterial blood pressure

The first documented measurement of blood pressure dates back to the eighteenth century. In 1773, Stephen Hales, an English theologian and scientist, directly measured mean blood pressure in an unanaesthetized horse by inserting an open-ended tube directly into the animal's neck; the blood entered the tube and rose upwards (to a height of 2.5 m) towards the tube opening until the weight of the column of blood was equal to the pressure in the circulatory system of the horse. This is the basis of a simple pressure manometer, which is still used for measuring blood pressure (see Central venous pressure monitoring). It is also the basis for measuring cerebrospinal fluid pressures during a lumbar puncture.

Catheters can be inserted directly into an artery (the radial artery is often used) to give direct arterial pressure measurements and pressures can be monitored continuously. **Figure 4.2.48** shows an arterial pressure waveform. (For a more comprehensive discussion on direct pressure measurements, see the section on venous pressure, p. 441.)

However, in most instances it is not desirable or practicable to use invasive techniques to measure arterial pressures. In the eighteenth century, an Italian physiologist, Scipione Riva Rocci, invented the **sphygmomanometer** (*sphygmo* = pulse), which enabled a non-invasive measurement of systolic pressure. A rubber inflatable cuff is placed over the brachial artery and the pressure in the cuff is raised until the cuff pressure exceeds that of the blood in the artery. At this point the artery collapses and no radial pulse can be felt as blood is not able to flow through the brachial artery. The pressure in the cuff is then slowly released and the radial pulse reappears. The pressure at which the pulse reappears corresponds to the systolic pressure as it is the point at which the peak pressure (i.e. the systolic) in the brachial artery exceeds the occluding pressure in the cuff.

Traditionally the mercury sphygmomanometer was used as the standard reference for measuring blood pressure (**Fig. 4.2.49a,b**). However, due to hazards associated with mercury (it is toxic), the mercury sphygmomanometer is now being replaced by other automated devices. Most of these devices still operate around the principle of occluding an artery in the arm with an inflation cuff and give blood pressure values by detection of Korotkov sounds (see below) with a microphone or detect arterial blood flow using Doppler, ultrasound or oscillometric techniques. Anaeroid sphygmomanometers work on a bellows system rather than a mercury column. Although automated devices are routinely used, if they are not properly maintained and calibrated against accepted protocols they are liable to give inaccurate readings. O'Brien et al. (2001) review the various blood-pressure-measuring devices available.

Conventionally, blood pressure is measured in millimetres of mercury (written as mmHg); this means that if the blood pressure is 100 mmHg, the

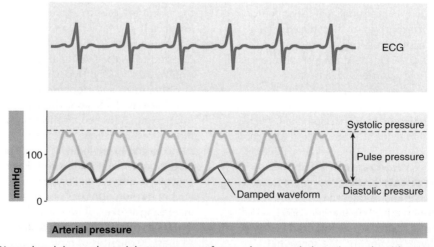

**Figure 4.2.48** Normal and damped arterial pressure waveforms when recorded continuously with a pressure tranducer

pressure exerted by the blood is sufficient to push a column of mercury up to a height of 100 mm. The SI unit for pressure is the pascal (Pa) or kilopascal (kPa) and so sometimes blood pressure may be written as, say, 13.4 kPa instead of 100 mmHg. Often, the automated devices provide the blood pressure readings in both mmHg and kPa (see **Table 4.2.3** for a comparison of mmHg and kPa values).

The original method was developed further a few years after Riva Rocci by a Russian surgeon,

Dr Nicolai Korotkov. Korotkov reported a method for measuring both systolic and diastolic pressures by auscultation, that is, by listening, using a stethoscope placed over the brachial artery and the sphygmomanometer **(Fig. 4.2.49c)**. Various sounds were audible and Korotkov classified the sounds into five phases, which are now known simply as the **Korotkov sounds (Fig. 4.2.50)**. The precise origin of the various Korotkov sounds is not fully understood but they are due primarily to turbulent flow and vibratory phenomena in the brachial artery as it opens and closes with each beat and as the blood flows through the semi-occluded vessel. When the pressure in the blood pressure cuff is greater than that in the artery, the vessel is completely occluded and there is no blood flow and no turbulence, and hence no sound. The systolic pressure value is taken at the point when sounds first start (phase 1) and the diastolic when the sounds disappear (phase 5). Phase 5 correlates well with direct arterial measurement of blood pressure. However in some individuals, especially when the cardiac output is high, the sounds do not disappear (although they do muffle: phase 4), and sometimes persist right down to zero. If sounds do continue to zero, phase 4 should be used; this sometimes occurs in pregnant women, children, anaemic and elderly patients. The fact that phase 4 has been used should be noted.

## CLINICAL APPLICATIONS

Nurses need to ensure that blood pressure measurements are taken under standardized conditions and using the correct technique. Blood pressure values vary according to the situation that the individual is in **(see Fig. 4.2.47)** and many physiological variables influence them.

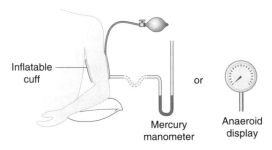

**(a)** Deflated

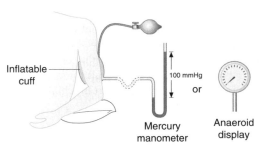

**(b)** Inflated

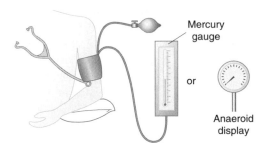

**(c)**

**Figure 4.2.49** Principle of sphygmomanometry; (a) the cuff is deflated; there is no pressure in the cuff, and the mercury levels in the two arms of the U-tube manometer are the same (in actual clinical sphygmomanometers mercury is stored in a reservoir and not in a U-tube as drawn here); (b) the cuff is inflated; pressure in the cuff is equal to the difference in height between the two mercury levels: (c) the auscultatory method for measuring systolic and diastolic pressures. NB: the mercury manometers are being phased out; however they clearly demonstrate the principles behind the technique and so are shown in this diagram

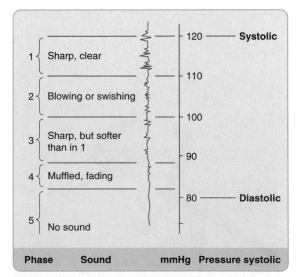

**Figure 4.2.50** The Korotkov sounds

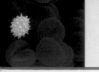
The blood pressure of elderly people varies considerably over time and can be very labile (up and down) in some individuals. For these and other reasons discussed below, one-off or single measurements of blood pressure are notoriously unreliable; automated sphygmomanometry has enabled ambulatory blood pressure measurement, which is useful in some instances.

The individual should rest for at least 5 minutes before measurement and should avoid exertion and not eat or smoke for 30 minutes beforehand. The blood pressure is also influenced by circadian rhythms and is lowest during sleep. Both systolic and diastolic pressures are reported to rise by 10 mmHg or more after a person has eaten a meal. Blood pressure also rises as the bladder fills. Accurate blood pressure measurement in infants and children depends on having the child relaxed and not restless – not easy! Measurements made when a child is eating, sucking or crying will be unrepresentative and usually too high.

The emotional state of the patient, e.g. whether anxious or in pain, will affect blood pressure values but this is often difficult to modify or avoid in clinical situations. Anxiety raises systolic blood pressure, often by as much as 30 mmHg. This defence reaction is a consequence of the fight/flight response; the fact that anxiety influences blood pressure readings should be remembered and noted, especially when intending to use observations taken at the time of admission to hospital as a baseline for subsequent observations or whenever a person is frightened such as before surgery or in an outpatient department. There is also a phenomenon called 'white coat hypertension' where a 'normotensive' person becomes hypertensive during blood pressure measurements (especially taken by a doctor), which then settles to normal levels again afterwards; 24-hour ambulatory blood pressure measurement is useful in cases where this is suspected.

There are also many potential sources for error in the actual measurement technique (Fig. 4.2.51). Posture affects blood pressure, with a tendency to increase from lying to sitting to standing. The ideal position for measurement is sitting comfortably, with the arm supported at heart level or, more specifically, the arm should be horizontal as denoted by the midsternal notch or level with the fourth intercostal space at the sternum. The observer should also support the patient's arm, otherwise the patient will have to perform isometric muscle contractions which can increase both the diastolic and systolic pressures. Raising or lowering the arm away from heart level causes significant changes in blood pressure; the error can be as large as 10 mmHg. The same arm should be used each time, as in some individuals there are differences in the right and left brachial artery pressures.

**State of patient**
Anxiety, pain, fear, recent exercise, full bladder, food, tobacco, alcohol, obesity, arrhythmias

**Nurse**
Training, observer bias, preferred digit, lack of concentration, sight and hearing, distance from sphygmomanometer

**Cuff**
Correct application, dimensions of bladder, positioning of bladder, velcro lost grip

**Patient**
Position, right or left arm, arm supported or not

**Sphygmomanometer**
Not regularly recalibrated

**Surroundings**
Room temperature, noise, other distractions

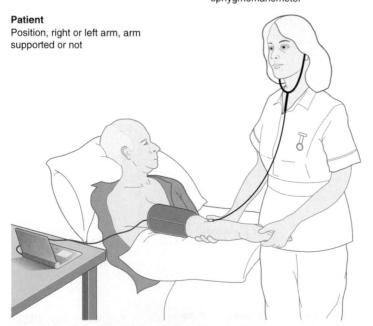

**Figure 4.2.51** Some potential sources of error in blood pressure measurement (based on O'Brien & O'Malley, 1981)

An appropriate size of cuff should also be used; ideally the bladder of the cuff should encircle the arm but if this is not feasible the centre of the bladder must be placed directly over the brachial artery. Miscuffing (i.e. using a cuff the wrong size) is a serious source of error. Recommended bladder dimensions are $4 \times 13$ cm for small children (with a maximum arm circumference of 17 cm), $10 \times 18$ cm for medium-sized children and lean adults (with a maximum arm circumference of 26 cm), $12 \times 26$ cm for the majority of adults (with a maximum arm circumference of 33 cm) and $12 \times 40$ cm for obese adults (with a maximum arm circumference of 50 cm) (Beevers et al., 2001). Tight or constricting sleeves of clothes pushed up to allow application of the cuff will also give false readings.

Equipment must be maintained in good working order; defective control valves should be replaced, as should any cracked or perished tubing. All machines (whatever design) should be recalibrated regularly. Equipment malfunction is a real source of inaccurate blood pressure measurement.

Observer bias, especially by looking at previously charted values and expectations of individuals' values, e.g. older people having higher blood pressures, is also a potential source of inaccuracy with auscultatory methods. For some reason, observers show a strong preference for the terminal digits 0 and 5, e.g. 125/75 mmHg, even though a 5-mmHg mark does not appear on many scales! If using a mercury manometer, the observer should also be at eye level with the scale when reading off the values. Automated devices can give inaccurate readings if the person has severe arrhythmias or tremors, or have weak or low pulses. The oscillometric monitors require adequate puslatile blood flow to the extremities to give an accurate reading.

It is advisable to record an approximate value for systolic pressure by palpation, before auscultation, because in some people the Korotkov sounds appear normally giving the systolic pressure, but then disappear for a short time before returning above the diastolic pressure. This period of silence is known as the **auscultatory gap** and, although nothing can be heard, the pulse can be felt.

On many occasions it is not possible to obtain all the optimum conditions for blood pressure measurement and, if this is the case the qualifying factor(s) should be recorded on the chart, e.g. '150/94 mmHg – patient in severe pain' and the modifying factors taken into consideration when reaching decisions as to the relevance or accuracy of a particular measurement.

If it is not possible to use the arms for blood pressure readings, it is possible, using special large leg cuffs, to record the blood pressure using the Korotkov sounds from the popliteal artery in the popliteal fossa (at the back of the knee). The technique is more cumbersome but is useful in some instances, e.g. for patients with suspected coarctation of the aorta or with arm injuries. Pressure in the arteries of the legs is normally the same as that in the arms.

A crude value for mean arterial pressure can be obtained using the method described earlier to demonstrate reactive hyperaemia. The mean arterial pressure is the pressure level when the arm flushes bright red as blood returns to the arm. This is described as the 'flush method' and is sometimes used in children or in shocked patients when other methods are not possible.

## Measurement of venous pressures

Venous pressures reflect venous return to the heart and cardiac function. As venous pressures are not reflexly maintained at any specific or predetermined level, fluctuations in venous return (especially the circulating fluid volume) and cardiac function are reflected in the venous pressures. Observation of the jugular vein in the neck gives a crude indication of venous pressure: a raised jugular venous pressure (JVP) may indicate cardiac failure, for instance.

The venous pressure most frequently monitored is the **central venous pressure (CVP)**, which is the pressure in the central veins (the superior and inferior venae cavae) as they enter the heart. The central venous pressure is commonly used as a guide to the circulating volume, by reflecting the right atrial filling pressure, which in turn reflects the right ventricular filling pressure (right ventricular end diastolic volume). The assumption is that the right ventricular end-diastolic pressure will reflect the left ventricular end-diastolic pressure.

Central venous pressure measurements can have significant limitations, partly as it is measuring a *pressure* (the right atrial pressure, which acts as a guide to right ventricular end-diastolic volume pressure), which clinically is then used to reflect a *volume* (right ventricular end-diastolic volume).

Right atrial pressures can be affected by a number of factors including: vascular tone, valvular (tricuspid valve) disorders, right ventricular failure and pericardial tamponade. Consequently, the measured pressure may change, although not necessarily as a result of fluid imbalance, and as such it is **the changes**, and not the absolute values of central venous pressure, which are clinically of value.

Access to the right atrium is gained via a central vein, such as the internal jugular or subclavian veins. For insertion of the central venous catheter, the patient is placed in a head-down position to

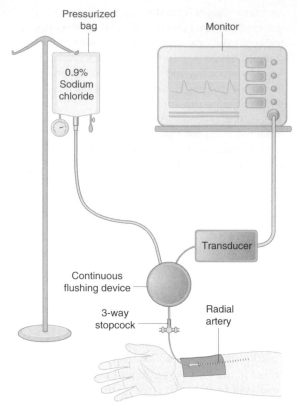

Figure 4.2.52   A direct pressure monitoring system showing the monitoring of central venous pressure

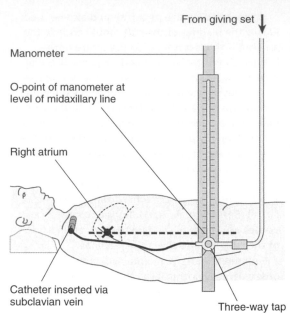

Figure 4.2.53   Measurements of central venous pressure using a fluid manometer system

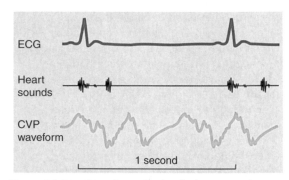

Figure 4.2.54   Waveform obtained when central venous pressure is recorded continuously with a pressure transducer. The electrocardiogram and heart sound recordings are also shown

engorge the veins. After insertion, a chest X-ray is performed to check that the catheter is in the correct position and that a pneumothorax has not been inadvertently caused. The central venous pressure can be measured continuously with a direct pressure monitoring system (transducer; **Fig. 4.2.52**) or intermittently by using a water manometer (**Fig. 4.2.53**). The technique and conditions must be consistent each time a measurement is taken.

## CLINICAL APPLICATIONS

The fluid manometer is usually a branch of a normal giving set linked to a venous catheter via a three-way tap and mounted against a centimetre reference scale. The central line is often used for giving clear parenteral fluids (e.g. saline or dextrose) when not monitoring pressure values. When measurements are being made, the tap is turned so that the pathway between the branch of the giving set and the patient's vein are in direct communication (and the flow of fluid from the intravenous infusion is temporarily stopped). Therefore the fluid level in the manometer directly reflects the central venous pressure. With a simple manometer the central venous pressure is recorded in centimetres of water (strictly this should be centimetres of saline or dextrose). A pressure of 10 cmH$_2$O means a pressure sufficient

to raise a column of water to a height of 10 cm. Central venous pressure pressure is normally in the range of 0–10 cmH$_2$O (1.36 cmH$_2$O is equivalent to 1 mmHg), depending on the zero reference point used (see below).

A transducer is basically a small electronic device that converts one form of energy into another, and in this instance the transducer is converting the physiological variable of venous blood pressure into an electrical signal (it can equally well be used to measure arterial pressures). The electrical signal can then be processed, displayed and recorded at convenience; the values are often displayed on the oscilloscope screen in a waveform (**Fig. 4.2.54**) or as a digital reading. Before use, a transducer must be calibrated against a known pressure source, usually a column of mercury.

The intravascular catheter must remain fully patent for accurate monitoring; thrombus formation or kinking will cause a reduction or damping of the signal (**Fig. 4.2.48** shows a damped arterial waveform). The tendency for thrombus formation is greatest with arterial lines because the relatively high pressure tends to force blood back into the catheter. The likelihood of this happening is reduced by using some form of continuous infusion device between the catheter and the transducer.

All direct blood pressure measurements, whether recorded via a transducer or manometer, must be recorded from a definite zero reference point and the same point must be used in each series of measurements. **Zero referencing** is the technique whereby the effects of both atmospheric and hydrostatic pressures are considered on the ultimate reading. For arterial, central venous and pulmonary wedge pressures (see below), the common reference points are the sternal angle and the midaxillary line in the fourth intercostal space. The midaxillary line is preferred because it is anatomically in line with the right atrium. Placing the transducer or manometer at different levels relative to the patient alters the reading and so it is useless to compare measurements that are made with either the patient or manometer/transducer in different positions. Accurate alignment is achieved by using a spirit level, often attached to a telescopic arm. The zero reference point is often marked on the patient's skin. The patient should ideally be lying flat or, if not flat, at an angle of 45°, and all readings should be taken with the patient in the original position.

The exact position of the zero reference point is not so important when monitoring arterial pressures, which cover a wide range, but is essential with venous pressures, which vary through a small range of values. Measured from the midaxillary line, the normal range of central venous pressure is 5–10 cmH$_2$O (0.5–1.0 KPa); from the sternal angle it is 0–5 cmH$_2$O (0–0.5 kPa). For a transducer, the normal range is 3–8 mmHg (0.4–1.1 kPa). Central venous pressure readings alter during inspiration and expiration as the intrathoracic pressure changes. Intermittent positive pressure ventilation increases the mean thoracic pressure by up to 5 mmHg and this is reflected by a rise in central venous pressure; this must be remembered when interpreting the readings of ventilated patients.

## PULMONARY ARTERY AND CAPILLARY WEDGE PRESSURES

Sometimes it is useful to have more specific information on the function of the left ventricle, as this directly influences blood flow to the systemic circulation. In many clinical cases, right ventricular filling is an accurate reflection of left

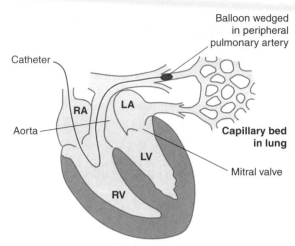

**Figure 4.2.55** Position of a pulmonary artery flotation catheter when 'wedged' in small pulmonary artery

ventricular filling. However, where there is pulmonary hypertension or impaired right ventricular function, as can occur with sepsis or an inferior myocardial infarction, the right heart function and pressures may no longer reflect the left heart function. In such cases the left heart pressures need to be measured directly rather than inferred from central venous pressure readings.

Measurement of left-sided pressures is achieved by inserting a pulmonary artery flotation catheter (PAFC), in the same way as a central venous pressure catheter, accessing the right side of the heart via an internal jugular or subclavian vein. The pulmonary artery flotation catheter continues out of the right heart, following blood flow, into the pulmonary artery. It has a small inflatable balloon near its tip, which when inflated will continue to travel (float) through the pulmonary vasculature until it becomes literally wedged in a small blood vessel (**Fig. 4.2.55**); the balloon blocks or occludes the pressure behind the tip of the catheter. The pulmonary artery flotation catheter is connected to a transducer and monitor, which will display the waveforms and pressures measured. During insertion of the catheter, its correct progression through the right heart and pulmonary circulation is monitored by the changing waveforms. In front of the catheter is the left side of the heart. At the end of ventricular diastole, all cardiac valves between the left ventricle and the pulmonary circulation are open, so that there is a continuous column of blood between the two points. The tip of the catheter can now measure the pressure in the left side of the heart, the left ventricular end diastolic pressure (reflecting the left ventricular end-diastolic volume).

Normally, the balloon is kept deflated (or a section of the lung would become ischaemic due

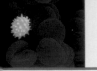

to a lack of blood flow) and the waveform displayed is that of the pulmonary artery **(Fig. 4.2.56)**, which is to where the catheter floats back. When a reading of the pulmonary capillary wedge pressure (PCWP) is required, the balloon is inflated, causing it to move forwards again until it becomes wedged. The normal pulmonary capillary wedge pressure is 4–12 mmHg.

## The formation of tissue fluid

### The capillary wall

In the tissues, blood is contained within the capillaries and is separated from the cells by the capillary wall, which is approximately 0.5 μm in diameter, and the fluid-filled interstitial space. Cells are rarely more than 20 μm away from a capillary. Capillary walls consist of a single layer of endothelial cells, resting on a basement membrane (also known as basal lamina). Electron microscopy has shown the existence of slit-like spaces, with a diameter of 10 nm, between the endothelial cells; these are known as pores. They represent only a very small proportion of the total surface area of the capillary wall. It is through these pores that water and solutes diffuse to and from the blood and interstitial fluid.

Unlike the cell membrane, the capillary wall is not a single semi-permeable membrane. However, if its pores are thought of as the 'pores' in a single membrane, it is possible to examine osmotic effects across the capillary wall.

### Formation and resorption of tissue fluid

Under normal conditions, the volume of the plasma and interstitial fluids changes very little over time, despite very high rates of diffusion of various substances both into and out of capillaries.

At the end of the nineteenth century, the physiologist E.H. Starling pointed out that the mean forces tending to move fluid out through capillary walls are

in near equilibrium with those forces that tend to move fluid from the interstitial spaces into the capillaries. As a result, the volume of fluid passing out of the capillaries, by filtration, almost exactly equals the volume returned. This phenomenon is known as the Starling equilibrium of capillary exchange.

Starling proposed that the direction and rate of transfer between plasma in the capillaries and fluid in the tissue spaces depended on three factors **(Fig. 4.2.57)**:

1. the hydrostatic pressure on each side of the capillary wall
2. the osmotic pressure of protein in the plasma and in the tissue fluid
3. the properties of the capillary wall.

### The capillary blood pressure ($P_{cap}$)

This pressure forces fluid and solutes through the capillary walls into the interstitial spaces. The average pressure in the systemic capillaries is about 25 mmHg (3.3 kPa) but this is a broad generalization, for it represents the midpoint in a capillary where the pressure may be, say, 35 mmHg (4.7 kPa) at the arteriolar end and 15 mmHg (2 kPa) at the venous end. Blood pressure in any capillary is not constant over time; it depends on the arteriolar tone and the resistance offered and, as blood pressure is a hydrostatic pressure, it also depends on the position relative to the heart. The capillary pressure characteristically differs in certain tissues too. For instance, the blood pressure

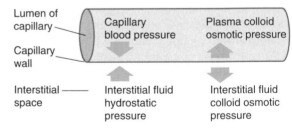

**Figure 4.2.57** Forces affecting fluid movement across the capillary wall

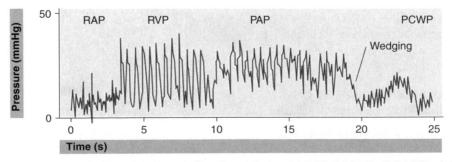

**Figure 4.2.56** Pressure and waveform changes as a flotation catheter passes through the right side of the heart and into the pulmonary artery. PAP, pulmonary artery pressure; PCWP, pulmonary capillary wedge pressure; RAP, right arterial pressure; RVP, right venous pressure

in the renal glomeruli is approximately 70 mmHg (9.4 kPa) and in the lungs 8 mmHg (1.1 kPa).

## The interstitial fluid pressure ($P_{if}$)

Tissue fluid, like any fluid, exerts a hydrostatic pressure. The value for this pressure must be subtracted from the capillary hydrostatic pressure to arrive at the effective transmural pressure, that is, the 'driving' pressure across the wall. The experimental work measuring interstitial fluid pressure gives differing values according to the precise methodology used: some measurements suggest a negative or subatmospheric pressure whereas others indicate pressures between 0 mmHg (atmospheric pressure) and 2 mmHg (0.3 kPa) – the latter figures have been adopted for this text.

## The plasma colloid osmotic pressure ($OP_{cap}$)

This produces fluid movement, by osmosis, into the capillary with a force of approximately 28 mmHg (3.7 kPa).

## The interstitial fluid colloid osmotic pressure ($OP_{if}$)

This produces fluid movement, by osmosis, out of the capillary and has a magnitude of approximately 5 mmHg (0.7 kPa). The process of osmosis is explained in detail in Chapter 1.2 (p. 31).

## *Filtration and absorption of tissue fluid*

As already discussed, the pressures involved vary in different tissues and under different circumstances, therefore hypothetical figures are used to illustrate this example (see also Fig. 4.2.58):

| | | |
|---|---|---|
| $P_{cap}$ (arterial end) | = | 35 mmHg |
| $P_{cap}$ (venous end) | = | 15 mmHg |
| $P_{if}$ | = | 2 mmHg |

| | | |
|---|---|---|
| $OP_{cap}$ (tending to retain fluid in capillary) | = | 28 mmHg |
| $OP_{if}$ (tending to retain fluid in interstitial spaces) | = | 5 mmHg |

### At the arterial end of a capillary

Transmural pressure:

$$P_{cap} - P_{if} = 35 - 2 = 33 \text{ mmHg}$$

Net osmotic pressure:

$$OP_{cap} - OP_{if} = 28 - 5 = 23 \text{ mmHg}$$

Therefore the forces tending to move fluid out of the capillaries exceed those tending to retain fluid by 10 mmHg (1.4 kPa). Thus, at the arterial end, fluid leaves the capillaries.

### At the venous end of a capillary

Transmural pressure:

$$P_{cap} - P_{if} = 15 - 2 = 13 \text{ mmHg}$$

Net osmotic pressure:

$$OP_{cap} - OP_{if} = 28 - 5 = 23 \text{ mmHg}$$

Therefore the forces tending to move fluid into the capillary exceed those tending to move fluid out of the capillary by 10 mmHg (1.4 kPa). Thus, at the venous ends of capillaries, because of the fall in capillary blood pressure that occurs along the length of the capillary, fluid enters the capillaries. Thus a circulation of tissue fluid is established.

As a result of these forces, a small percentage of the plasma volume entering the capillaries is filtered into the interstitial space and flows through the tissues. The vast majority of the volume filtered is reabsorbed at the venous ends of the capillaries. The remaining fluid passes into the lymph capillaries. Lymph drainage plays an important part in maintaining local fluid equilibrium in some tissues.

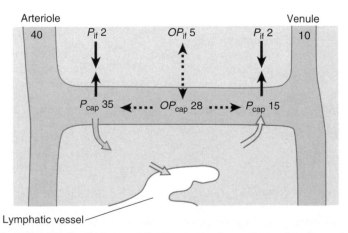

**Figure 4.2.58** Diagram summarizing the forces contributing to the formation and reabsorption of tissue fluid in the systemic circulation. All pressures are in mmHg. $OP_{cap}$, plasma colloid osmotic pressure; $OP_{if}$, interstitial fluid osmotic pressure; $P_{cap}$, capillary blood pressure; $P_{if}$, interstitial fluid pressure. *Note*: Only the magnitude of the $P_{cap}$ alters

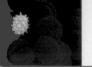
## CLINICAL APPLICATIONS

If these forces become abnormal, the distribution of fluid between the plasma and the interstitial fluid is affected. For example, if mean capillary blood pressure falls considerably, as might occur in severe haemorrhage, the outward forces become less than the inward forces and so more fluid is reabsorbed into the capillary than is filtered. Initially, therefore, following haemorrhage, plasma volume increases at the expense of interstitial fluid volume. Similarly, another example illustrating disturbances in the normal pressures occurs if the plasma protein concentration is increased due to dehydration (for instance by water deprivation, prolonged sweating, severe vomiting and diarrhoea); then water moves by osmotic forces from the tissues to the vascular compartment.

## OEDEMA

More commonly, the imbalance that occurs is such that the outward forces exceed the inward forces and this produces an excessive accumulation of interstitial fluid which is called **oedema**.

Oedema will also develop if there are changes in the permeability of the capillary walls. This can happen due to inflammation or an allergic response. Cytokines are known to mediate increases in vascular permeability (Diskin et al., 1999). If oedema is present for some time, the tissue spaces become stretched and this increases the ease with which further oedema can develop.

Most oedema demonstrates the phenomenon of **pitting**. If the skin over an oedematous area is pressed with the index finger, a pit appears in the tissues and remains for up to 30 seconds after the finger is removed. This is because the oedema has been pushed away through the tissue spaces, by the pressure from the finger, and it takes some time to flow back once the pressure is released.

There are many **causes** of oedema, but there are only four major physiological **mechanisms** underlying its formation; all these result in the outward forces exceeding the inward forces in the affected capillaries. Tissues do not become oedematous until there is quite a large imbalance in these forces acting at the capillary walls. **Table 4.2.4** classifies the causes of

| Table 4.2.4 | Causes of oedema and their physiological mechanisms | |
| --- | --- | --- |
| **Physiological mechanism** | **Cause** | **Examples** |
| Increased mean capillary blood pressure | Increased venous pressure | Back pressure due to reduced cardiac output in cardiac failure |
| | | Venous obstruction due, for example, to pressure from plaster casts/bandages/garters which are too tight |
| | | Fluid overloading with intravenous fluids |
| | Sodium and water retention | Reduced renal blood flow |
| | | Renal failure |
| | Raised aldosterone secretion | Mineralocorticoid effect of corticosteroid therapy |
| | Inability to destroy aldosterone | Liver damage, e.g. cirrhosis |
| Decreased plasma colloid osmotic pressure | Decreased production of plasma protein | Liver damage |
| | Loss of plasma protein from the body | Malnutrition (kwashiorkor) |
| | | Nephrosis, nephrotic syndrome |
| | | Burns, draining wounds and fistulae |
| Increased permeability of capillary walls to protein | Increased porosity of capillary walls | Inflammation, e.g. due to burns and infections |
| | | Allergic reactions, e.g. hives |
| | | Release of cytokines, e.g. tumour necrosis factor, interleukins 1 and 10 |
| Decreased lymphatic removal of protein and tissue fluid (leads to increased interstitial fluid pressure and interstitial fluid colloid osmotic pressure) | Congenital absence of lymphatic vessels | Malignant disease |
| | Blockage of lymphatic vessels | Surgical removal of lymph nodes |
| | | Infestation by parasitic worm, filaria |

oedema according to the four physiological mechanisms involved.

The accumulation of oedema is subject to the force of gravity and so generalized oedema tends to become apparent first in the soft tissues of dependent parts of the body, such as the ankles, wrists and fingers and around the sacrum. **Ascites**, an abnormal accumulation of fluid in the peritoneal cavity, occurs due to physiological mechanisms similar to those of oedema. Localized oedema is most likely to result from an alteration just in one part of the body.

Oedema is treated according to its cause. Diuretics, such as furosemide, are frequently prescribed to promote the excretion of sodium and water. The effectiveness of treatment may be monitored with the help of accurate fluid balance recordings and by recording the weight of the patient, daily, at the same time of day. The skin of an oedematous person requires special care, as waterlogged tissues tend to be deprived of oxygen and nutrients, because of the increased barrier to diffusion, and hence vulnerable to trauma and less able to heal.

In an individual who has varicose veins, the valves in the veins are not functional and the venous and capillary pressures are high. Thus fluid tends to leak out of the capillary and oedema develops. As described above, the normal exchange of gases and nutrients is disrupted; the muscles in the leg can become painful and weak and the skin can become gangrenous and varicose ulcers develop. When a limb is oedematous, as a result of venous stasis, elevation of that limb and the application of an elastic stocking will facilitate venous return (see Diskin et al. (1999) for a fuller review of the pathophysiology and treatment of oedema).

## Interstitial fluid formation and reabsorption in the pulmonary circulation

The mechanics of interstitial fluid formation and reabsorption in the low-pressure pulmonary circulation are essentially the same as for the systemic circulation. The major difference is that the mean blood pressure in pulmonary capillaries is only approximately 8 mmHg (1.1 kPa), much less than the plasma colloid osmotic pressure of 28 mmHg (3.7 kPa).

### CLINICAL APPLICATIONS

**Pulmonary oedema** occurs via the same mechanisms as in the peripheral tissues. The major cause is failure of the left side of the heart to maintain its output of blood. This can result in great increases in pulmonary capillary blood pressure. Pulmonary oedema increases the diffusion barrier between alveoli and blood and, almost invariably, fluid enters the alveoli. It thus interferes with the diffusion of the respiratory gases and this produces hypoxia and breathlessness. In very severe cases, pulmonary oedema can produce death, from asphyxiation, in less than an hour.

As with peripheral oedema, the cause of the condition must be treated. Symptomatic relief can be obtained by nursing the patient sitting up. This maximizes the efficiency of the patient's respiratory effort. Oxygen is usually required to relieve breathlessness and a bronchodilator, such as aminophylline, may also be prescribed. In very severe cases, intermittent positive pressure ventilation may be necessary. Diuretic therapy promotes fluid loss. In acute cases, morphine may be given to allay pain and emotional distress. This drug also produces vasodilation and so helps to reduce blood pressure. Vasodilators, such as sodium nitroprusside, also play a major role in the treatment and prevention of acute pulmonary oedema.

The breathlessness and discomfort produced by pulmonary oedema are extremely frightening and the patient's distress tends to aggravate the condition. The ability of nurses and others in the care team to reassure and calm the patient is therefore also an important aspect of care.

## Control and coordination of the cardiovascular system

The function of the cardiovascular system is to ensure an adequate blood flow to all tissues at all times. All homeostatic mechanisms, and the cardiovascular system is no exception, need an integrating and control centre that receives 'information' from receptors via afferent pathways and coordinates the effector responses.

The coordinating centres that link cardiac and vascular responses are in the medulla and pons of the brain. The major parameter that these centres regulate is the systemic arterial blood pressure, as it is this that ensures blood flow to the tissues, especially to the vital organs of the brain and heart.

As seen earlier, mean arterial pressure can be regulated by altering cardiac output and/or the total peripheral resistance (i.e. $BP = CO \times TPR$). Thus, any factor that influences either cardiac output or peripheral resistance will affect blood pressure, for instance heart rate, stroke volume, radius of arterioles, venomotor tone, circulating blood volume. Many systems are involved in controlling these factors, including

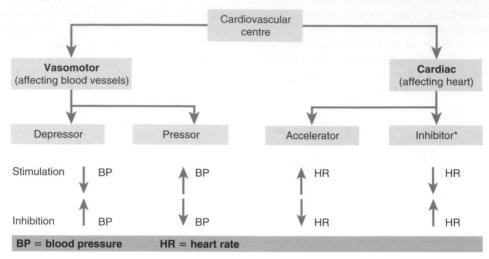

**Figure 4.2.59** Subdivision of cardiovascular control centres. (*The cardiac inhibitory centre corresponds to the nucleus ambiguus)

nervous, hormonal and local factors; some of the systems act rapidly to maintain blood pressure on a short-term basis (e.g. nervous reflexes and local changes) and others operate in the longer term (e.g. hormonal fluid balance mechanisms). Thus the role of the cardiovascular control centres is to integrate the function of the heart and vascular system.

## Medullary cardiovascular centres

In the medulla and pons there is a large diffuse area of interconnected neurones concerned with the regulation of the heart and vascular system. This region, known as the **cardiovascular centre (CVC)**, receives afferent inputs from other parts of the central and peripheral nervous systems and sends out efferents through sympathetic and parasympathetic fibres to the heart and blood vessels. In this way, the cardiovascular centre is able to regulate heart function and blood pressure in accordance with the body's physiological needs.

The cardiovascular centre is sometimes subdivided into discrete units (**Fig. 4.2.59**), e.g. vasomotor centre, cardiac accelerator centre, but there is no clear anatomical separation between these various centres and their function is not always discretely divided up. For instance, the vasomotor centre, the region supposedly exerting control over sympathetic vasoconstrictor activity, also contains neurones that affect the heart and produce positive chronotropic (increase heart rate) and positive inotropic (increase stroke volume) responses. For these reasons, as there are no definite anatomical or functional divisions between the control centres, it is appropriate to use the term **medullary cardiovascular centre**. Thus, for the purposes of this discussion, the controlling centres will be described simply as the cardiovascular

centre. The afferent inputs to the cardiovascular centre are from the baroreceptors and chemoreceptors as well as from the cortex, hypothalamus and other areas of the central nervous system. The efferent pathways are mainly via the sympathetic nerves to the heart (altering the force and rate of contraction) and the blood vessels (altering blood vessel diameter). Sympathetic vasoconstrictor activity in the arterial system increases the peripheral resistance whilst in the venous system it increases the venous return to the heart. The parasympathetic outflow via the vagus nerve arises from the nucleus ambiguus (which corresponds to the centre previously known as the cardiac inhibitory centre). **Figure 4.2.60** summarizes the main afferent and efferent pathways involved.

## The baroreceptor mechanism

The baroreceptor mechanism is the most important of the feedback systems involved in the maintenance of arterial blood pressure on a short-term basis, e.g. during changes in posture, different activity levels. As the parameter being regulated is the arterial pressure, it is appropriate that the major receptors for the feedback loop, i.e. the baroreceptors, are located within the arterial system. The baroreceptors are situated in the tunica adventitia of both the internal carotid artery (especially in the carotid sinus) and the transverse part of the aortic arch (**Fig. 4.2.61**). These areas are linked to the cardiovascular centre by the sinus nerve (part of the glossopharyngeal (IX) cranial nerve) and the aortic nerve (part of vagus (X) cranial nerve), respectively.

The **baroreceptors** are specialized nerve endings that respond to the degree of stretch of the arterial wall, that is, they are stretch receptors. (There are other stretch receptors in other parts of the thorax;

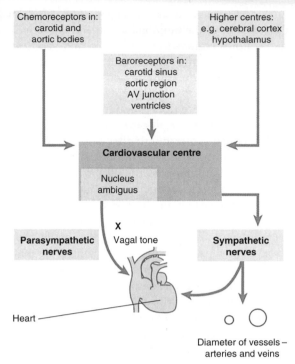

**Figure 4.2.60** Diagrammatic representation of the major afferent and efferent pathways associated with the cardiovascular control centre. (AV, atrioventricular)

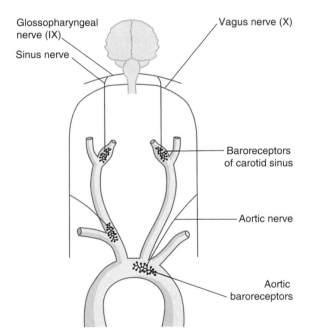

**Figure 4.2.61** Arterial baroreceptor systems

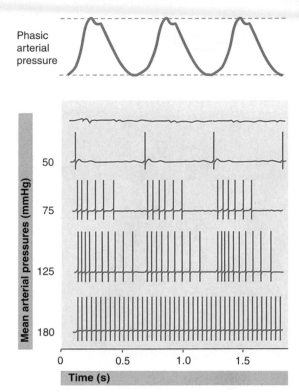

**Figure 4.2.62** Relationship between mean arterial blood pressure and the impulse firing rate in a single afferent nerve fibre from the baroreceptors in the carotid sinus with different levels of a mean arterial pressure. The baroreceptors discharge at a greater frequency as the pressure is increased

see next section). The degree of stretching in the arterial wall is directly related to the blood pressure in the carotid sinus and aortic arch; if there is an increase in the blood pressure, there will be more stretch, and if blood pressure falls, less stretch. The stretching alters the rate of firing of impulses along the nerves to the cardiovascular centre. The baroreceptors are sometimes known as pressoreceptors.

There is always a basal rate of discharge to the cardiovascular centre from the baroreceptors along the afferent nerve fibres. This relates directly to the degree of stretching of the arterial wall; when these endings are stretched there is an increased firing rate in the afferent fibres, which serves to communicate the degree of stretch to the cardiovascular centre in the brain (the region often referred to as the vasomotor centre). So, when the baroreceptors are further stretched, the firing rate increases, and vice versa (**Fig. 4.2.62**). The discharge from the baroreceptors is pulsatile due to the change in the arterial pressure during the cardiac cycle.

The normal action of the cardiovascular centre on this afferent input is *inhibitory* and so an increased blood pressure produces an increased firing rate. This leads to a reduced sympathetic discharge rate to the blood vessels (producing vasodilation) and reduced sympathetic discharge to the heart (producing a decrease in the force and rate of contraction). Simultaneously, there is an increased parasympathetic vagal discharge to the heart, which also reduces the heart rate. The effect of the vasodilation, reducing the total peripheral resistance, and the drop in heart rate and stroke volume, reducing cardiac output, is to cause a drop in the arterial blood pressure. Thus, the

449

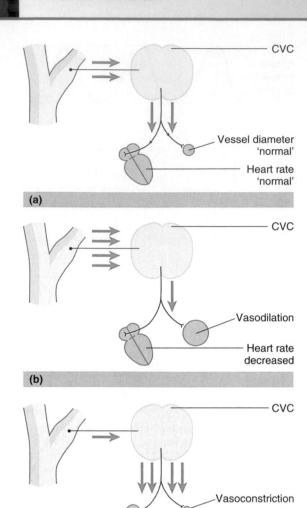

Vessel diameter 'normal'

Heart rate 'normal'

**(a)**

CVC

Vasodilation

Heart rate decreased

**(b)**

CVC

Vasoconstriction

Heart rate increased

**(c)**

**Figure 4.2.63** Representation of the inverse relationship between baroreceptor firing rate and sympathetic outflow to the heart and blood vessels. (a) Pressure 'normal', (b) pressure high, (c) pressure low. (CVC, cardiovascular centre)

initiating stimulus – the increased blood pressure – has been negated, and the blood pressure returned to 'normal':

$$CO \times TPR = BP$$

$$(HR \times SV) \times TPR = BP$$

$$(If \downarrow HR \text{ and } \downarrow SV \text{ and } \downarrow TPR, \text{ then } \downarrow BP)$$

If there is a fall in blood pressure, the firing rate will decrease and, by a reverse of the mechanisms described above, heart rate and force of contraction will increase and vasoconstriction occurs **(Figure 4.2.63)**.

## Other mechanoreceptor reflexes

There are also stretch receptors, similar to baroreceptors, in other parts of the thorax, for instance at the junction between the vena cava and right atrium, at the junction of the pulmonary vein and left atrium, sparse fibres scattered over the atria and ventricles and probably at other sites within the thorax. All the afferent nerve endings are responsive to stretch and mechanical distortion and so are sometimes referred to as **mechanoreceptors**. The impulses from these mechanoreceptors are all carried in the vagus to the cardiovascular centre and so often referred to simply as vagal endings.

The mechanism of action of the cardiac vagal mechanoreceptors is not exactly like the classic baroreceptor system in the systemic arteries; their response is complex. Different receptors seem to have different responses. Some of the receptors seem to play an important role in the control of body sodium and water by acting as blood volume receptors and influence the output of antidiuretic hormone from the posterior pituitary. Atrial natriuretic peptide is also released from the atrial cells (see earlier). Other receptors seem to cause reflex vasodilation, e.g. in the renal circulation.

Activation of some of the fibres from the ventricles seem reflexly to inhibit sympathetic discharge and produce a profound bradycardia. Patients having coronary angiography often show bradycardia when the contrast medium is injected, and it has been suggested that this is due to chemical excitation of these ventricular fibres. The vasovagal syncope and bradycardia of myocardial infarction may also be ascribed to reflexes aroused by an increase in activity of these ventricular fibres.

Stretch of some of the atrial vagal endings causes an increase in heart rate and an increase in the strength of contraction (the Bainbridge reflex). The likely function of this reflex is to help prevent the accumulation of blood in the veins, atria and pulmonary circulation.

Thus the effects of these other mechanoreceptor reflexes are varied, and although they may not be primarily concerned with blood pressure regulation, they play an important role in other cardiovascular reflexes.

## Chemoreceptor input

The chemoreceptors in the carotid and aortic bodies (see Chapter 5.3) can also influence the cardiovascular centre, although they are mainly involved with the regulation of respiration. The chemoreceptors are responsive to oxygen lack, hypercapnia, acidaemia and asphyxia. Under normal circumstances the chemoreceptors only have a small effect on the cardiovascular centre, but under 'emergency' conditions of severe hypoxia or asphyxia they can and do provoke powerful reflex sympathetic effects; for example, a

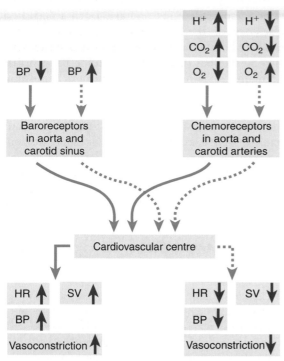

**Figure 4.2.64** Role of the baroreceptors and chemoreceptors in regulating heart function. (BP, blood pressure; HR, heart rate; SV, stroke volume)

decrease in oxygen or increase in carbon dioxide (or hydrogen ion concentration) causes an increase in heart rate and blood pressure (**Fig. 4.2.64**).

## Influence of other areas of the central nervous system

Emotions such as excitement, fear and anxiety can cause an increased heart rate and blood pressure, whereas a sudden shock may induce a bradycardia: the higher centres in the brain are involved in these instances. Stimuli from the hypothalamus influence vasomotor tone and this is one of the mechanisms used to control heat loss and maintain normal body temperature. Pain produces changes in heart rate and blood pressure. The respiratory centres also influence the cardiovascular centre.

## Illustrations of cardiovascular control

The activity of the cardiovascular system is thus coordinated by centres in the brain. As far as the normal control of arterial pressure is concerned, the baroreceptor mechanism is the most important. The baroreceptors respond immediately to a change in arterial pressure and their response is fully active within a minute or so. Besides these direct nervous reflexes, via the cardiovascular centre, there are other moderately rapidly acting (in terms of minutes to

hours) systems that operate for the short-term control of blood pressure, namely hormonal effects, particularly epinephrine and norepinephrine, and intrinsic physical mechanisms altering the shift of fluids from interstitium to plasma.

The baroreceptors are not effective for the long-term control of blood pressure; it seems that the baroreceptor/cardiovascular centre tonic discharge rate becomes reset at a different level when blood pressure is chronically elevated. In the long term, renal and body fluid mechanisms become the dominant pressure-determining factors (see earlier).

A few illustrations of the cardiovascular system 'in action' will now be given. (Most of the separate components of these changes have been discussed earlier in the chapter, so for the details of mechanisms, see the relevant part of the chapter.)

## Changes in posture

When an individual is supine, the arterial and venous pressures are not significantly influenced by the hydrostatic pressure of the blood. However, on standing, due to the effects of gravity, the arterial and venous pressures in the head drop whereas the pressure in the feet and lower parts of the body rises (**see Fig. 4.2.33**). Due to the high compliance of the veins, the limb veins distend and blood tends to pool in the arms and legs. As the venous capacity has increased, the venous return to the heart falls. This is the sequence of events that occurs every time an individual changes from a horizontal to a vertical position. The decreased venous return reduces the stretching of the cardiac muscle fibres and the stroke volume decreases (Starling's law of the heart). As a consequence of the decrease in stroke volume, the cardiac output falls and the arterial blood pressure falls.

This drop in arterial blood pressure is detected by the baroreceptors; the baroreceptors in the carotid sinus are particularly affected. Thus there is decreased baroreceptor activity and the CVC initiates sympathetic activity to increase heart rate, stroke volume and vasoconstriction. The arterial vasoconstriction increases peripheral resistance and the increased venomotor tone enhances venous return to the heart. These changes together correct the blood pressure and compensate for the effect of gravity. The response is complete, in normal healthy individuals, literally within seconds. **Figure 4.2.65** summarizes these changes.

If the body does not correct the blood pressure or if the compensatory mechanisms are sluggish, postural or orthostatic hypotension develops, with dizziness and even fainting if severe. You can observe this mechanism sometimes if you get up too quickly after bending down.

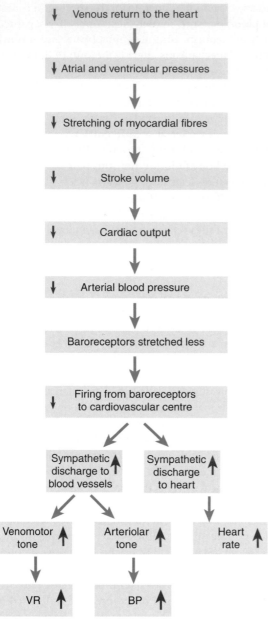

↓ Venous return to the heart

↓ Atrial and ventricular pressures

↓ Stretching of myocardial fibres

↓ Stroke volume

↓ Cardiac output

↓ Arterial blood pressure

Baroreceptors stretched less

↓ Firing from baroreceptors to cardiovascular centre

Sympathetic discharge to blood vessels ↑

Sympathetic discharge to heart ↑

Venomotor tone ↑

Arteriolar tone ↑

Heart rate ↑

VR ↑

BP ↑

**Figure 4.2.65** Sequence of events that occurs immediately after changing posture from lying down to standing up. *Note*: Once venomotor tone has increased and the venous return (VR) to the heart has increased, the heart rate (HR) and blood pressure (BP) return to 'normal'

Patients who are in bed for long periods of time, and thus remain more or less horizontal, do not have to overcome the effects of gravity. (As an aside, this is rather like astronauts in space, in fact much of the work carried out to study the effects of prolonged weightlessness have been done by confining subjects to bed!) Once bed-bound patients start to get up, they often suffer from weakness, dizziness, giddiness or can faint, and this is again often a result of orthostatic hypotension. When confined to bed, patients lose general muscle tone, including that of the blood

vessels, especially veins, and also suffer a decreased efficiency of the cardiovascular reflexes, e.g. the baroreceptor mechanism. The decrease in muscle tone also means that the muscle pump mechanism that normally aids venous return in the vertical position is less efficient.

It has been suggested that bedrest may increase the workload of the heart by increasing the venous return, and hence cardiac output, due to the horizontal position. Certainly there is a decline in general cardiovascular fitness, or a 'detraining effect', due to the reduction in activity levels, which will certainly be deleterious to any patient (see section on exercise).

## CLINICAL APPLICATIONS

### SHOCK AND HAEMORRHAGE

Circulatory shock is not a specific disease but a condition in which the cardiovascular system fails to perfuse all the tissues adequately. There are several ways to classify shock, depending on the origin of the problem, as tissue perfusion can be disrupted in many ways **(Table 4.2.5)**. For instance, failure of the heart to pump properly can lead to cardiogenic shock; insufficient circulating blood volume leads to hypovolaemic shock; septic shock is caused by an overwhelming infection; anaphylactic shock results from an antigen–antibody reaction; and, finally, neurogenic shock results from neural alterations (predominantly a reduced sympathetic control) of vascular smooth muscle tone. Whatever the precipitating cause, shock leads to reduced tissue perfusion, impairment of nutrient delivery to cells and progresses ultimately to organ failure and death unless compensatory mechanisms reverse the process or clinical intervention succeeds. Numerous endogenous substances are released in response to a range of precipitants, including tissue ischaemia, infectious agents and inflammatory disorders. These include eicosanoids, endorphins, cytokines and nitric oxide (also known as endothelium-derived relaxing factor; EDRF). In combination, these substances can cause a range of physiological abnormalities that include vasodilation, increased capillary permeability, and stimulation of neutrophil and platelet activity (Showronski, 1997).

As can be seen from **Table 4.2.5**, there are different sequences of events in shock and so the signs and symptoms will vary. The body attempts to compensate physiologically in the first instance and this will show differing manifestations dependent on the cause. For instance, in hypovolaemic shock the body tries to compensate for the decrease in circulating blood volume by increasing cardiac output and so increases the

**Table 4.2.5** Causes of shock and accompanying features

**Cardiogenic shock**
Failure of the heart to pump effectively (e.g. after myocardial infarction, cardiomyopathy, cardiac arrhythmias, drug toxicity)
Normal or elevated blood volume, with pump failure

**Hypovolaemic shock**
Severe reduction in circulating volume caused, for example, by haemorrhage, gastrointestinal loss, third space losses (i.e. plasma or interstitial fluid)

**Neurogenic or vasogenic shock**
Widespread massive vasodilation (venules, capillaries, and arterioles) resulting from loss of normal sympathetic and parasympathetic control of blood vessels (e.g. after severe head injury, drugs and anaesthetics, trauma to spinal cord or medulla, severe emotional stress and pain)
Fainting due to emotional causes is a transient form of neurogenic shock
No change in blood volume, but drastic decrease in venous return and cardiac output

**Septic shock**
Caused by infections due to bacteria, viruses, fungi or protozoa
Begins with the development of septicaemia, usually from bacterial infections (e.g. *Escherichia coli*) but sometimes viral in origin
Immune and inflammatory response that causes vasodilation and so reduces venous return and cardiac output; fever also leads to increased basal metabolic rate and increased oxygen requirements leading to anaerobic metabolism; release of endotoxins from infection leads to direct cellular damage
Toxic shock syndrome; often follows a localized infection by *Staphylococcus aureus*; is a form of septic shock

**Anaphylactic shock**
Begins as an allergic reaction from allergens (e.g. insect stings, pollens, shellfish, nuts, penicillin)
Hypersensitivity reaction in which histamine and histamine-like substances are released into the blood and cause increased capillary permeability
Often very severe and more acute than other types of shock; progression to death can occur within minutes if emergency treatment not given
Results in vasodilation with resultant hypotension, reduced cardiac output, urticaria, angioedema, rash, tachycardia, bronchospasm and laryngeal oedema

heart rate. Conversely, in the early stages of neurogenic shock because of the low venous return and excessive parasympathetic activity, there is frequently bradycardia. Similarly, in hypovolaemic shock the patient will be pale or an ashen grey colour due to peripheral vasoconstriction and hypoxia, whereas the patient with septic shock will initially present with a warm and flushed skin.

The compensatory mechanisms initially keep tissue perfusion at a sufficient level to prevent cell damage. However, the final common pathway in all types of shock, if no treatment has been instigated, is impairment of cellular metabolism. Once the compensatory mechanisms begin to fail, the hypoxia leads to anaerobic metabolism and an accumulation of lactate. A vicious cycle ensues, leading to cellular damage, release of proteolytic enzymes and histamine production. Changes in the microcirculation follow and an increase in the volume of interstitial fluid results. This then exacerbates the decrease in effective circulating blood volume. In the final stages of shock the changes become irreversible, even if treatment is started, as too much cellular damage has occurred.

Of the various forms of shock, hypovolaemic shock has been the most widely studied; hypovolaemic shock occurs when there is an acute loss of 15–20% of the circulating blood volume. The following section describes the main consequences of haemorrhage.

When an individual suffers a haemorrhage, there is a decrease in the circulating blood volume; this leads to a reduction in the venous return to the heart, and to a reduced stroke volume and cardiac output, and so to a drop in blood pressure. (This sequence of events is the same as when changing from a horizontal to a vertical posture, see p. 452.) In haemorrhage, the drop in blood pressure sets off the baroreceptor mechanism and intense sympathetic activity is established, which causes an increased force and rate of contraction of the heart (so attempting to maintain cardiac output) and the vasoconstriction increases peripheral resistance and venous return. The venoconstriction reduces the size of the blood reservoir in the veins and so increases the effective circulating blood volume.

The intense arteriolar constriction results in a drop in the capillary blood pressure, which has the effect of increasing fluid shifts *from* the tissue spaces *into* the capillaries, and this also increases the effective circulating blood volume.

Under conditions of haemorrhage, the circulation of blood to the vital organs (brain and heart) has priority and so blood is 'shunted' away from less vital areas, i.e. from the skin, skeletal muscle, gut, renal system and spleen, by intense vasoconstriction.

The sympathetic arousal causes the release of epinephrine and norepinephrine from the adrenal medulla, and these hormones augment the effects of the sympathetic nerves. The decreased renal blood flow activates the renin–angiotensin system, which causes more vasoconstriction and also leads to the release of aldosterone to conserve sodium. This in turn leads to increased release of antidiuretic hormone from the posterior pituitary gland, and so tends to conserve water (see Chapter 2.6). The volume receptors in the atria also increase antidiuretic hormone production and release of atrial natriuretic peptide.

Thus there is a wide range of responses to haemorrhage. The above physiological changes explain the common signs and symptoms observed in a shocked patient:

- pale – due to peripheral vasoconstriction
- tachycardia – due to sympathetic arousal
- sweaty – due to sympathetic arousal
- weak pulse – due to low blood volume
- oliguria – due to reduced renal blood flow and fluid-conserving mechanisms.

However, in 'clinical' haemorrhage, if the circulating blood volume is not restored fairly quickly, the tissues deprived of blood, i.e. the ischaemic tissues, will start to necrose. Thus the priority in the treatment of these patients is to replace fluids – often plasma expanders or whole blood are given (see Chapter 4.1).

The blood pressure may well be low; however, it is often the last 'sign' to develop because the cardiovascular reflexes may be 'strong' enough to maintain the arterial blood pressure for some time (this obviously depends on the rate and nature of the haemorrhage). An indication of how effective these compensatory mechanisms are is seen by considering a case of 'controlled haemorrhage' when donating blood: the body is normally easily able to compensate for the loss of 500 mL or so of blood (almost 10% of the total blood volume).

## The effect of exercise on the cardiovascular system

The effects of exercise on the body, and cardiovascular system in particular, need to be considered in two ways – the changes that result during the actual exercise period itself and also the longer-term consequences of undertaking regular exercise. Much has been researched and written on both these areas and this review will consider only the main issues. Health professionals need knowledge in these areas to understand the physiological demands on an individual, perhaps after a myocardial infarction or a period of illness, but also because encouraging people to be active and do more exercise forms an important health promotion message. Although the term 'exercise' is used in this discussion, any form of physical activity or work requires the same physiological responses from the body; thus whether considering walking, cycling, swimming, football, dancing, housework, gardening, the physiological demands are similar. It applies to 'exercise' taken either as part of work or in leisure time.

In a broad sense, physical performance or fitness (the capacity to do physical work) is determined by the individual's capacity for energy output (mainly determined by the cardiovascular and respiratory systems), neuromuscular function, joint mobility and psychological factors, such as motivation. When exercising, as at any other time, the body needs to maintain the chemical and physical equilibrium of the cells. During exercise there is a need to increase the delivery of oxygen and nutrients to the active muscle tissue (this can increase as much as 50 times in an elite athlete) and to also increase the rate of removal of heat, carbon dioxide, water and metabolic waste products. This necessitates a large increase in the exchange of materials between the intra- and extracellular fluids. To prevent the metabolism in the active cells becoming anaerobic (i.e. without oxygen) there needs to be an increase in the cardiac output. The following paragraphs describe the main events to support exercise; as with many activities in the body, the events are coordinated by the autonomic, especially the sympathetic, nervous system.

The 'mental' anticipation of exercise can result in sympathetic arousal and lead to an increase in heart rate even before the exercise starts. Once the exercise is underway, the muscles that are active require an increased blood flow to provide the necessary oxygen and nutrients and to remove waste products. This increased blood flow is achieved by local factors: vasodilation is produced by the accumulation of local metabolites that directly affect the smooth muscle of the arteriolar walls and precapillary sphincters. Thus a greater number of capillary beds are opened up and the distance substances have to diffuse to and from the cells is reduced.

As a consequence of the vasodilation, the peripheral resistance in the muscle drops, and in order to maintain the total peripheral resistance at adequate levels (so that blood pressure does not fall too far), compensatory vasoconstriction occurs, especially in the kidneys and gut. Blood flow to the skin may increase so that the body can lose heat, and arteriovenous anastomoses open up.

For the blood flow to the muscles to increase, the cardiac output must also increase, and this is partly brought about by sympathetic activity. The venous return to the heart is increased by an increased venomotor tone, and especially by the action of the skeletal muscle and respiratory pump mechanisms. The increased venous return (by Starling's law) results in an increased stroke volume. The sympathetic influence also increases the force and rate of cardiac contractions.

The maximum attainable heart rate varies with sex, age and state of physical fitness. As a useful guide, the maximum attainable heart rate is given by the formula 220 – age in years.

The cardiac output increases from the resting value of approximately 5 L/min and can reach 25 L/min (or even 35 L/min in elite athletes).

The systolic blood pressure increases due to the increased stroke volume. The diastolic pressure may increase but, if the total peripheral resistance falls, the diastolic pressure may fall too.

The ability of the cardiovascular system to cope with exercise increases considerably with training. Athletes have a slower heart rate at rest because they have a greater stroke volume – resting heart rates of 40 are not uncommon in very fit people. This increases their reserve when they undertake exercise.

## The effect of exercise on other aspects of body function

To keep exercising, the contractile proteins in the active muscles must have a continuous supply of energy in the form of adenosine triphosphate. The energy comes from the metabolism of foodstuffs, such as carbohydrate in the form of glycogen, and fatty acids in the form of triglycerides. Oxygen is needed for maximum efficiency of the metabolic processes; the aerobic energy output (that is, in the presence of oxygen) is much greater than the anaerobic output: for example glucose can provide 20 times more energy per molecule aerobically than anaerobically.

The purpose of the changes in the cardiovascular system during exercise, described above, is to increase the blood flow and hence the oxygen supply to the active tissues. To saturate the blood fully with oxygen as it flows through the lungs, there also has to be a considerable increase in pulmonary ventilation in order to deliver adequate oxygen into the lungs and to allow removal of carbon dioxide (an endproduct of the metabolism). A typical value for resting gas exchange volume in an adult is around 6 L/min, with a respiratory rate of 10–15 breaths per minute. The volume of gas exchanged during exercise can increase up to around 100 L/min and in elite athletes can even reach 200 L/min, with respiratory rates of 40 or 50 breaths/min.

There is a large reservoir of oxygen carried in red blood cells that is not utilized under normal conditions; that is, not all oxygen is extracted from blood as it flows through tissues. So another way of increasing oxygen delivery to active cells is to increase the extraction of oxygen from the blood. This increased extraction relates to the properties of haemoglobin and is explained by the oxyhaemoglobin dissociation curve (see Chapter 5.3). In active tissues there is a local increase in $PCO_2$ and temperature, and these factors change the properties of haemoglobin and cause the curve to shift to the right; when the curve is shifted to the right, more oxygen is released from the haemoglobin at any given $PO_2$ and so more oxygen is made available to maintain aerobic metabolism.

Muscle tissue is only able to convert a little over 20% of its metabolic energy into mechanical energy, and the remaining energy appears in the form of heat. Thus there is always an increase in local muscle temperature. An increase in the temperature of a tissue increases the rate of metabolism of that tissue and this can be significant. The degree of rise in temperature in a muscle depends on the severity of the exercise, how long the exercise is maintained and environmental conditions. With prolonged exercise the core temperature of the body can increase by several degrees Celsius – this is often observed in marathon runners, for example. Even after the individual stops exercising, the metabolic rate remains high for several hours: this is one of the reasons that exercise helps to keep down the weight of an individual.

The excess heat has to be removed from the body if exercise is to be maintained and temperature homeostasis achieved. Thus heat is removed away from the active muscle via the blood and there is an increase in blood flow to the skin to facilitate heat loss by convection and evaporation (via sweating). This explains why people undertaking exercise appear hot, flushed and sweating. Maintaining thermoregulation in prolonged strenuous exercise can cause conflicting demands on the body's physiology, for example there may be a requirement to increase blood flow to the skin to maximize heat loss and at the same time a requirement for increasing blood flow to active muscles. Excessive sweating can also lead to water and salt loss.

The role of the sympathetic nervous system in coordinating the changes in the cardiovascular system was considered above; the sympathetic nervous system also has a role in aiding gas exchange in the respiratory system by producing bronchodilation and increasing mobilization of nutrients from the liver, which in turn helps to maintain the supply of energy.

There is currently much emphasis on encouraging regular physical activity irrespective of age, ability and state of health: regular exercise makes a major contribution to health and fitness at all ages from childhood to old age. Exercise is beneficial to children in all the same ways that it is for adults. If children are encouraged to enjoy physical activities at an early age, they are more likely to continue exercising regularly throughout their lives. Likewise, undertaking even a minimum amount of low-level activity such as walking can produce substantial health benefits in adults with chronic diseases: physical *inactivity* is associated with an increased risk of death (Martinson et al., 2001). **Table 4.2.6** gives some of the recognized benefits of regular exercise – the list is impressive.

There is convincing research that people who are physically active throughout adult life live longer than those who are sedentary. Early studies showed that those whose work or leisure involved vigorous, regular exercise, were between one-third and one-half as likely to develop or die of coronary heart disease as those whose lives were more sedentary (Jacobson et al., 1991; Morris *et al.*, 1990; Tunstall Pedoe, 1990). Exercise both prevents cardiovascular disease and also plays a key role in recovery and rehabilitation of cardiovascular disease (Miller et al., 1997). Much of the earlier work on exercise and cardiovascular disease considered the positive effects of exercise on men; more recent studies have shown the same positive effects on women (Manson et al., 2002; Stampfer et al., 2000). Manson et al. (2002) conducted a large-scale study in the United States and found that cardiovascular disease in women who exercised and walked the most, occurred at about half the rate of that in those who did not exercise or walk at all.

How much exercise is required? Any level of exercise seems to have some beneficial effects, especially if the individual is unfit to start with (Erikssen et al., 1998). The appropriate amount for an individual will depend on age, current fitness, medical history and so on, but taking at least 30 minutes or so of aerobic activity (such as brisk walking – enough to work up a bit of a sweat), at least five times a week would enable significant effects to be seen (Clark, 2003). Although the benefits of being fitter are acknowledged, the proportion of children and adults taking regular exercise is still relatively low: Baker (2001) reports that about 60% of men and 70% of women get less exercise than they need to ward off ill-health. Some women reported finding it difficult to find the time to exercise – they were too busy (Clark, 2003). Many children in the United Kingdom are also taking too little exercise and, together with increasing levels of obesity amongst children, this is a major cause

**Table 4.2.6** The benefits of regular physical aerobic exercise

Improved cardiovascular function (reduced heart rate at given oxygen consumption; improved efficiency of heart muscle; lower blood pressure)
Inhibition of clotting processes and platelet aggregation
Favourable trend in incidences of cardiac morbidity and mortality
Increased metabolic rate – both during and after exercise
Can reduce obesity due to increased metabolic turnover
Reduced total cholesterol
Favourable increase in ratio of serum high density lipoproteins to low density lipoproteins
Enhanced tolerance to hot environments
Muscle size and strength improve, plus ligament strength (e.g. helps with posture, protects from joint instability and injury, and back pain in pregnancy)
Can help to prevent osteoporosis
Increased capillary density in skeletal muscle
Reduced perceived exertion at given work rate
Can help to maintain normal blood glucose levels, especially in diabetics
Improved functioning of the immune system
Increased rate of endorphin secretion (linked to feelings of well-being, reduced anxiety and stress, and anti-depressant effects)

for concern. Undertaking regular aerobic activity must be incorporated into all healthy lifestyle guidance, along with other aspects such as dietary advice and stopping smoking and, more importantly, somehow translated from guidance into practice.

A discussion on the positive effects of exercise perhaps should not be concluded without an acknowledgement that there are risks associated with some forms of exercise for some people, e.g. eye injuries related to squash, or muscle, tendon and joint injuries associated with running, and there can be consequences from intense training in any activity.

Just as physical exercise and activity have been identified as beneficial to an individual, the converse is also true: lack of activity and exercise leads to a deterioration in physiological functioning of many systems, not least the cardiovascular system. Bedrest (once thought to be a panacea for a wide variety of problems) and low levels of physical activity have been empirically identified as risk factors for a variety of acute and chronic conditions (Topp et al., 2002). The impact of inactivity on the musculoskeletal and cardiovascular systems are marked with atrophy of skeletal muscles, loss in contractility and strength, a general deconditioning of the cardiovascular systems both at rest and when exercise is taken later. The classic study of the effects of bedrest was conducted by Saltin et al. (1968), but Topp et al. (2002) consider the effects, too.

## DEVELOPMENTAL ISSUES

### AGEING AND THE CARDIOVASCULAR SYSTEM

The study of normal changes in the cardiovascular system with ageing is problematic; it is difficult to find a 'coronary-artery-disease-free' population to enable ageing changes, rather than disease-induced changes, to be investigated. It is also particularly important, when comparing the cardiovascular function of young and older people, to ensure that the level of physical fitness is similar in subjects of all ages: as we have already seen, heart rate, blood pressure and cardiac output all vary according to the person's normal level of activity. For some people, ageing can be associated with a general reduction in activity, which tends to produce cardiovascular 'deconditioning'; in other words a loss of fitness. In early work assessing changes in the cardiovascular system with ageing, there was thought to be an inevitable substantial decline in function. However, this is not necessarily the case when care is taken in matching subjects.

Some changes have already been described in this chapter, for example, the maximum heart rate

attainable declines with increasing age and blood pressure tends to increase. Even this change is now known not to be universal, as individuals who live in some isolated societies do not show an increase in blood pressure (see the section on blood pressure, p. 436). It may be that the often-observed age-related increase in blood pressure is more a consequence of environmental factors, including diet and lifestyle.

Nevertheless, there are changes in the structure of the blood vessels. The compliance of the arterial wall declines due to an increase in collagen and its cross-linkages; this, together with atherosclerotic changes, accounts for the increase in blood pressure in many people. The veins lose elastic tissue and become increasingly tortuous, which leads to varicosities in veins subjected to high pressure. There are changes in the heart too; the sinoatrial node becomes invaded by fibrous tissue and shows some loss of cells, which may account for the decline in maximum heart rate. Conversely, there is often an increased heart rate at rest with increasing age. There is enlargement of the left ventricle in some individuals – this is inevitable with less arterial compliance, as there is an increased workload for the heart. There is often thickening of the cardiac valves too.

In some elderly people there is also a decrease in the efficiency of the homeostatic processes and some of the reflexes become less efficient; for instance, there is a decreased baroreceptor sensitivity in some people. Postural or orthostatic hypotension is also more common in elderly people as the postural reflexes are slowed as part of ageing changes. Despite all these changes, the majority of older people who do not have coronary artery disease, show no significant impairment of the cardiovascular system.

'Fit' elderly people also seem to maintain the ability to increase cardiac output when exercising, too. Earlier work showed that there was a decline in the ability of older people to undertake exercise but results from longitudinal studies have shown that the age-related decline in cardiac output is not inevitable. The components of cardiac output can show significant differences with ageing, with a decrease in the heart rate, but exercise stroke volume can increase significantly and to such an extent that elderly people can maintain a cardiac output comparable to that of young subjects who had lower heart rates.

Encouraging older people to be active and take appropriate exercise is very important to maximize cardiovascular function as well as all the other benefits of exercise as shown in **Table 4.2.6**. However, the levels of exercise undertaken must be tailored appropriately to the individual.

## Assessment of the adequacy of the circulatory system

There are many ways of assessing the adequacy of the circulation in the body and of the circulatory system as a whole; some are very simple and others more sophisticated, requiring technical equipment and invasive procedures (Fig. 4.2.66).

For instance, simple observations include assessment of the peripheral circulation by observing the colour and temperature of the skin: with a greater blood flow the skin appears flushed and warmer (e.g. with exercise, cellulitis), and with a decreased blood flow the skin is pale and cold (e.g. peripheral vascular disease, ischaemia, low blood volume). The temperature of the skin in the extremities is often used as an indication of peripheral perfusion in intensive care units. Valuable information can also be gained by observing and touching the patient (Paminter, 2001). Restlessness could be part of the patient's reaction to haemorrhage and confusion could indicate a reduction in cardiac output.

These examples of simple, non-invasive observations are also extremely important and early indicators of physiological deterioration. For example, in haemorrhage, the body compensates, to maintain blood pressure by intense vasoconstriction, mediated by the sympathetic nervous system. Clinical features of sympathetic activation such as tachycardia, tachypnoea, cold peripheries, pallor, and oliguria will alert the practitioner to the possibility of a haemorrhage at a far earlier stage than hypotension. The haemorrhaging patient who is hypotensive is no longer able to compensate, as even with vasoconstriction, the circulating volume is so reduced that blood pressure cannot be maintained.

Many studies have proven the importance of simple patient observations. McQuillan et al. (1998) illustrated that half of the patient admissions to intensive therapy units could have been prevented by closer monitoring of vital signs. Smith & Wood (1998) demonstrated that up to 84% of patients exhibit warning signs in the hours preceding respiratory or cardiac arrest.

Information can also be gained by assessing the symmetry of colour, temperature and pulses on both sides of the body or in both limbs. The development and early signs of pressure sores are indications that the circulation to a particular area is inadequate. The character of the peripheral pulses, e.g. whether weak and thready or bounding, gives qualitative information on the circulation; the pulse obviously gives an easy method of counting heart rate and assessing the regularity of the heartbeat. A strong pulse generally indicates a high stroke volume and a weak pulse a reduction in stroke volume.

The efficiency of the circulatory system as a whole can be assessed by monitoring the function of vital organs, and kidney function is often used. A decreased blood flow to the kidney can lead to oliguria: regular

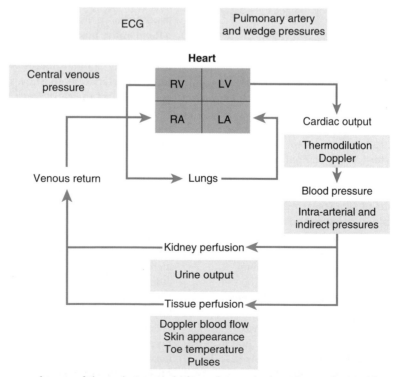

**Figure 4.2.66** Summary of some of the techniques which can be used to monitor and assess the cardiovascular system. LA, left atrium; LV, left ventricle; RA, right atrium; RV, right ventricle

half-hourly or hourly urimeter readings made on catheterized patients who are critically ill are sometimes used to assess renal perfusion which can give information on the fluid volume or progress of, say, shock. Circulating volume can also be assessed by the condition of the skin, where there is hypovolaemia, the skin will be inelastic, i.e. there will be reduced skin turgor. The oral membranes will also look dry in hypovolaemia. Urine will appear more concentrated and the specific gravity will rise. In significant fluid loss, urea may also rise. Arterial blood gas analysis may be useful to indicate a metabolic acidosis that would arise from a significant reduction in tissue perfusion, leading to anaerobic cell respiration with lactic acid production.

Other non-invasive methods, but which require some technical apparatus, are commonly used, for instance sphygmomanometers to measure blood pressure, ECG machines to monitor rate, rhythm and conduction patterns in the heart, or Doppler equipment to monitor blood flow in the peripheral circulation.

Invasive techniques are useful in giving information on venous return to the heart and cardiac function, e.g. central venous pressure measurements, wedge pressures and cardiac output estimations. The circulatory system can also be visualized by injecting radio-opaque substances into the blood and then taking X-rays of the arteries. This technique is called **angiography** or **arteriography,** and the film an arteriogram. Similar procedures can outline the ventricles, e.g. a ventriculogram. Angiography is used in the diagnosis of atherosclerosis. However, invasive procedures do carry some risk to the patients.

These are just some of the numerous possible investigations and ways of monitoring the cardiovascular system. Although the more complex technical investigations are useful, the simple and safe ones should be used first.

## Clinical review

In addition to the Learning Objectives at the beginning of this chapter, the reader should be able to:

- Explain how the structure of the heart is related to its function. In your answer suggest how damage to heart muscle might interfere with its function

- Describe the normal cardiac cycle, linking the electrical and mechanical changes that occur

- Discuss the factors that regulate cardiac output. In your answer define the terms: 'cardiac output', 'stroke volume', 'heart rate', 'Starling's law'

- State Starling's law of the heart and explain why this mechanism is important

- Explain why the maintenance of arterial blood pressure is so important. Discuss the factors that determine blood pressure and explain the changes that occur when a patient gets up after a long period of bedrest

- Discuss the use of central venous pressure monitoring in the critically ill patient

- Discuss the pathophysiology of congestive cardiac failure and explain why oedema formation occurs

- Explain how the circulatory function is altered by atherosclerosis; hypertension; and haemorrhage

## Review questions

1   What functions do the systemic and pulmonary circulations fulfil?
2   Which circulations do the right and left sides of the heart supply?
3   What is the location of the heart?
4   What are the three tissue layers of the heart?
5   Where are the valves of the heart?

6  What function do heart valves serve?

7  What is the origin of the heart sounds?

8  Starting at the venae cavae, describe the direction of blood flow through the heart.

9  What is the consequence of increased venous return to the heart?

10  How does heart muscle receive a blood supply?

11  What is the route of conduction of an electrical impulse from the SA node to the ventricles?

12  Is nervous stimulation necessary to initiate an impulse at the SA node?

13  What does the ABC of cardiopulmonary resuscitation refer to?

14  What do the P-wave, QRS-complex and T-wave of an ECG trace, respectively, represent?

15  If, on an ECG trace, there is one QRS-complex every 25 mm, what heart rate does this show?

16  What are systole and diastole?

17  If cardiac output remains constant and stroke volume increases, what will happen to heart rate?

18  What happens to stroke volume if the ventricular end-systolic volume decreases?

19  What are the three tissue layers of blood vessels and how do veins differ from arteries?

20  Which aspects of the capillary bed enable efficient exchange of substances between blood and peripheral tissues?

21  What function do venous valves serve?

22  What is vasomotor tone?

23  What two factors control blood vessel diameter?

24  If blood pressure is to remain constant, what happens to total peripheral resistance when there is an increase in cardiac output?

25  In which part of the cardiovascular system will an imbalance in osmotic pressure be observed?

26  Why does the production of interstitial fluid not lead to peripheral oedema under normal conditions?

27  What are inotropic and chronotropic effects, respectively, on the heart?

28  What do baroreceptors detect and how do they do this?

## Suggestions for further reading

Astrand, P., Rodahl, K., Dahl, H. & Stromme, S. (2003) *Textbook of Work Physiology: Physiological Base of Exercise*, 4th edn. New York: Human Kinetics Publishers.
*A new edition of the 'Bible' of exercise physiology; a very detailed research-based text covering all aspects of exercise physiology (not for the novice reader!).*

Beevers, G., Lip, G.Y.H. & O'Brien, E. (2001) *ABC of Hypertension*. London: BMJ Books.
*An excellent, readable review of all current aspects concerning the measurement of blood pressure and the aetiology and treatment of hypertension.*

Berne, R.M. & Levy, M.N. (2001) *Cardiovascular Physiology*, 8th edn. St Louis: Mosby Year Book.
*An excellent, comprehensive review of human cardiovascular physiology.*

Chobanian, A.V., Bakris, G.L., Black, H.R. et al. (2003) The seventh report of the joint National Committee on prevention, detection, evaluation and treatment of high blood pressure. *Journal of the American Medical Association*, **289**(19); 2560–2572.
*An excellent article that summarizes the current state of understanding of hypertension management.*

Colquhoun, M.C., Evans, T.R. & Handley, A.J. (1999) *ABC of Resuscitation*, 4th edn. London: BMJ Books.
*Practical concise guide to all major aspects of resuscitation.*

Davies, M.K., Gibbs, C.R. & Lip, G.Y.H. (2000) ABC of heart failure: management, diuretics, ACE inhibitors, and nitrates. *British Medical Journal*, **320**; 428–431.

Diskin, C.J., Stokes, T.J., Dansby, L.M. et al. (1999) Towards an understanding of oedema. *British Medical Journal*, **318**; 1610–1613.
*A useful review of pathophysiology and treatment of oedema.*

Fagan, T. (2002) *Cardiovascular System: A Crash Course*, 2nd edn. London: Mosby.
*Good basic summaries on cardiovascular physiology.*

Gibbs, C.R., Davies, M.K. & Lip, G.Y.H. (eds) (2000) *ABC of Heart Failure*. London: BMJ Publishing. *This book is a compilation of articles taken from the British Medical Journal and is a very useful collection of articles covering all aspects of heart failure.*

Hatchett, R. & Thompson, D. (2002) *Cardiac Nursing: A Comprehensive Guide*. Edinburgh: Churchill Livingstone. *An up-to-date text covering many aspects of cardiac physiology and relevant nursing aspects.*

Iqbal, Z., Chambers, R. & Woodmansey, P. (2001) *Implementing the National Service Framework for Coronary Heart Disease in Primary care*. Abingdon: Radcliffe Medical Press. *An unusual approach, but very readable, incorporating risk factor management with practice.*

Larsen, W.J. (2001) *Human Embryology*, 3rd edn. Edinburgh: Churchill Livingstone. *A readable text, with large, clear diagrams. It addresses the relationship between basic science and embryology, as well as clinical disorders arising out of developmental problems.*

Levick, J.R. (2003) *An Introduction to Cardiovascular Physiology*, 4th edn. London: Arnold. *This new edition of a popular book provides detailed information on all aspects of cardiovascular physiology.*

MacGregor, J. (2000) *Introduction to the Anatomy and Physiology of Children*. London: Routledge. *Includes an informative chapter on the cardiovascular system: very readable and unusual in terms of considering only children's physiology.*

McArdle, W., Katch, F. & Katch, V. (2001) *Exercise Physiology: Energy, Nutrition and Human Performance*, 5th edn. Philadelphia: Lippincott Williams and Wilkins. *A comprehensive and readable review of all aspects of exercise physiology.*

Moore, K.L. & Persaud, T.V.N. (1998) *The Developing Human. Clinically Orientated Embryology*, 6th edn. Philadelphia: WB Saunders. *A detailed and readable text, with nice colour diagrams and case studies.*

Woods, S.L., Sivarajanm Froelicher, E. & Underhill Motzer, S. (2000) *Cardiac Nursing*, 4th edn. Philadelphia: Lippincott Williams and Wilkins. *A useful text with relevant underlying physiology to care of patients with cardiac disease.*

## Useful websites

American Heart Association: www.americanheart.org *Latest information from the United States on all aspects of heart disease in adults and children.*

Blood Pressure Association: www.bpassoc.org.uk *Provides information and support to people with high blood pressure.*

British Heart Foundation: www.bhf.org.uk *A wide range of information for the general public on many individual heart conditions affecting both adults and children, latest statistics and up-to-date information on treatments.*

British Hypertension Society Information Service: www.bhssoc.org *Much information on all aspects of hypertension, and guidance on the latest information on blood pressure measurement.*

Resuscitation Council (UK): www.resus.org.uk *Latest resuscitation guidelines available online.*

## References

American Heart Association in collaboration with the International Committee on Resuscitation (ILCOR). (2000) Guidelines 2000 for Cardiopulmonary Resuscitation and Emergency Cardiovascular Care. An international consensus on science. *Resuscitation*, **46**; 1–448.

Baker, M. (2001) Bodies in motion, minds at rest. *Nursing Times*, **97**(33); 24–25.

Barker, D. (1992) *Fetal and Infant Origins of Adult Disease*. London: British Medical Journal.

Beevers, G., Lip, G.Y.H. & O'Brien, E. (2001) *ABC of Hypertension*. London: BMJ Books.

British Heart Foundation (2002) *Coronary Heart Disease Statistics Database*. London: British Heart Foundation.

Burns, P., Gough, S. & Bradbury, A.W. (2003) Management of Peripheral Arterial Disease in primary care. *British Medical Journal*, **326**; 584–588.

Chobanian, A.V., Bakris, G.L., Black, H.R. et al. (2003) The seventh report of the joint National Committee on prevention, detection, evaluation and treatment of high blood pressure. *Journal of the American Medical Association*, **289**(19); 2560–2572.

Clark, J. (2003) Women too busy to exercise. *British Medical Journal*, **326**; 467.

Davies, R.C., Hobbs, F.D.R. & Lip, G.Y.H. (2000) ABC of heart failure: history and epidemiology. *British Medical Journal*, **320**; 39–42.

Department of Health (2000) *National Service Framework for Coronary Heart Disease*. London: Department of Health.

Despopoulos, A. & Silbernagl, S. (1991) *Color Atlas of Physiology*, 4th edn. New York: Thieme Medical Publishers.

de Swiet, M., Dillon, M.J., Littler, W. et al. (1989) Measurement of blood pressure in children. *British Medical Journal*, **299**; 497.

Diskin, C.J., Stokes, T.J., Dansby, L.M. et al. (1999) Towards an understanding of oedema. *British Medical Journal*, **318**; 1610–1613.

Doshi, S.N., Lewis, M.J. & Goodfellow, J. (2001) Improving endothelial vasomotor function. *British Medical Journal*, **323**; 352–353.

Editorial (1992) Heart disease: in the beginning. *The Lancet*, **339**; 1386–1388.

Edmunds, E. & Lip, G.Y.H. (1999) Hypertension in Afro-Caribbeans. *Modern Hypertension Management*, **1**(2); 14–16.

Erikssen, G., Liestøl, K., Bjørnholt, J. et al. (1998) Changes in physical fitness and changes in mortality. *The Lancet*, **352**; 759–762.

Gibbs, C.R., Davies, M.K. & Lip, G.Y.H. (eds) (2000) *ABC of Heart Failure*. London: BMJ Publishing.

Gibson, J. (2002) Get men's bellies on telly. *Nursing Times*, **97**(2); 13.

Grech, E.D. (2003) ABC of Interventional Cardiology. Pathophysiology and investigation of coronary artery disease. *British Medical Journal*, **326**; 1027–1030.

Gregg, D.E. (1965) In: Buck, T.C. & Patton, H.D. (eds) *Physiology and Biophysics*, 19th edn. Philadelphia: WB Saunders.

Haines, A., Cooper, J., Meade, T.W. (2001) Psychological characteristics and fatal ischaemic heart disease. *Heart*, **85**; 385–389.

Hippisley-Cox, J., Cater, R., Pringle, M. & Coupland, C. (2003) Cross-sectional survey of effectiveness of lipid lowering drugs in reducing serum cholesterol concentrations in patients in 17 general practices. *British Medical Journal*, **326**; 689.

Hobbs, F.D.R. (1999) The scale of heart failure: Diagnosis and management issues for primary care. *Heart*, **82**(supplement IV); IV8–IV10.

Hubbard, J. (2002) The case of the man with myocardial infarction. In: Clancy, J. & McVicar, A.J. (eds) *Physiology and Anatomy: A Homeostatic Approach*. London: Arnold.

Jacobson, B., Smith, A. & Whitehead, M. (1991) *The Nation's Health. A Strategy for the 1990s*. London: King Edward's Hospital Fund.

Knight, J. (1999) Cunning plumbing. *New Scientist*, **6 Feb**; 32–37.

Kornitzer, M., Dramaix, M. & De Backer, G. (1999) Epidemiology of risk factors for hypertension. *Drugs*, **57**(5); 695–712.

Landowski, R., Shulman, R. & Davies, R. (2002) Drugs used in heart disease, Pharmacology 1. *Nursing Times*, **98**(18): 43–46.

MacGregor, J. (2000) *Introduction to the Anatomy and Physiology of Children*. London: Routledge.

Manson, J.E., Greenland, P., LaCroix, A.Z. et al. (2002) Walking compared with vigorous exercise for the prevention of cardiovascular events in women. *New England Journal of Medicine*, **347**; 716–725.

Marks, D. et al. (2002) Cost effectiveness analysis of different approaches of screening for familial hypercholesterolaemia. *British Medical Journal*, **324**(7349); 1303–1306.

Martinson, B.C., O'Connor, P.J. & Pronk, N.P. (2001) Physical inactivity and short-term all cause mortality in adults with chronic disease. *Archives of Internal Medicine*, **161**; 1173–1180.

Mayor, S. (2002) Statins reduce cardiovascular risk. *British Medical Journal*, **325**; 5.

McDonagh, T.A., Robb, S.D., Murdoch, D.R. et al. (1998) Biochemical detection of left ventricular systolic dysfunction. *The Lancet*, **351**; 9–13.

McNulty, P. (2003) Presentation of angina and myocardial infarctions. *American Journal of Cardiology*, **91**(8); 965–968.

McQuillan, P., Pilkington, S., Allan, A. et al. (1998) Confidential enquiry into quality of care before admission to intensive care. *British Medical Journal*, **316**(7148); 1853–1858.

Miller, T. et al. (1997) Exercise and its role in the prevention and rehabilitation of cardiovascular disease. *Annals of Behavioural Medicine*, **3**; 220–229.

Morris, J.N., Clayton, D.G., Everitt, M.G. et al. (1990) Exercise in leisure time: Coronary attack and death rates. *British Heart Journal*, **63**; 325–334.

O'Brien, E. & O'Malley, K. (1981) *Essentials of Blood Pressure Measurement*. Edinburgh: Churchill Livingstone.

O'Brien, E., Weber, B., Parati, J. & Myers, M.G. (2001) Blood pressure measuring devices: Recommendations of the European Society of Hypertension. *British Medical Journal*, **322**; 531–536.

Paminter, S. (2001) Hand-on detection of systemic circulatory deterioration. *Nursing Times*, **97**(27); 40–42.

Peterson, S. et al. (1999) *Coronary Heart Disease Statistics*. London: BHF Statistics Database.

Ramsey, L.E., Williams, B., Johnston, G.D. et al. (1999) British Hypertension Society Guidelines for Hypertension Management 1999: Summary. *British Medical Journal*, **319**; 630–635.

Resuscitation Council (UK) (2001a) *Adult Basic Life Support Resuscitation Guidelines 2000*. London: Resuscitation Council (UK).

Resuscitation Council (UK) (2001b) *Adult Advanced Life Support Resuscitation Guidelines 2000*. London: Resuscitation Council (UK).

Resuscitation Council (UK) (2001c) *Paediatric Basic Life Support Resuscitation Guidelines 2000*. London: Resuscitation Council (UK).

Resuscitation Council (UK) (2001d) *Paediatric Advanced Life Support Resuscitation Guidelines 2000*. London: Resuscitation Council (UK).

Saltin, B. et al. (1968) Response to exercise after bedrest and after training. *Circulation*, **38**(supplement 7); 1–78.

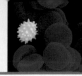

Shaw, K. et al. (2001) Relation between plasma ascorbic acid and mortality in men and women in EPIC-Norfolk prospective study: A prospective population study. *The Lancet*, **357**(9257):657–663.

Showronski, G.A. (1997) Circulatory Shock. In: Oh, T.E. (ed) *Intensive Care Manual.* Oxford: Butterworth-Heinemann, pp. 139–145.

Smith, A.F. & Wood, J. (1998) Can some in-hospital cardiac arrests be prevented? A prospective study. *Resuscitation*, **37**(3); 133–137.

Stampfer, M.J., Hu, F.B., E. Manson, J.E. et al. (2000) Primary Prevention of Coronary Heart Disease in Women through Diet and Lifestyle. *New England Journal of Medicine*, **343**; 16–22.

Tanne, J.H. (2002) Children should have blood pressure and cholesterol checked by age of 5. *British Medical Journal*, **325**; 8.

Topp, R., Ditmyer, M., King, K. et al. (2002) The effect of bed rest and potential of prehabilitation on patients in the intensive care unit. *AACN Clinical Issues*, **13**(2); 263–276.

Tortorta, G.J. & Anagnostakos, N.P. (1990) *Principles of Anatomy and Physiology*, 6th edn. New York: Harper & Row.

Tunstall Pedoe, D. (1990) Exercise and heart disease: Is there still a controversy? *British Heart Journal*, **64**; 293–294.

Vander, A.J., Sherman, J.H. & Luciano, D.S. (1990) *Human Physiology – The Mechanisms of Body Function*, 5th edn. New Dehli: McGraw-Hill.

Walker, J.M. (1999) Coronary heart disease: New epidemiological insights. *Journal of the Royal College of Physicians of London*, **33**(1); 8–12.

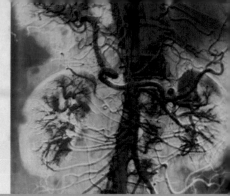

# Section 5

# The acquisition of nutrients and removal of waste

# Chapter 5.1

# The acquisition of nutrients

*Graeme D. Smith*

## LEARNING OBJECTIVES

After studying this chapter the reader should be able to:

- Relate the following oral structures to their function: lips, tongue, taste buds, teeth, salivary glands

- List the constituents of saliva and describe the regulation of its secretion

- Describe how and where peristalsis, segmentation and mass movements occur in the gastrointestinal tract

- Discuss how the generalized structure of the gut wall is adapted throughout its length, according to function

- Describe the neural and hormonal control of gastrointestinal motility and secretion

- List the functions of the stomach and explain fully the mechanism for gastric juice production

- State how the exocrine pancreas contributes to digestion

- Draw a diagram to illustrate the formation, secretion and function of bile

- Describe how the intestinal enzymes complete digestion and summarize the digestion of carbohydrates, proteins and fat

- Describe briefly both the embryological development of the gastrointestinal tract and the changes associated with this system during ageing

## INTRODUCTION

Every day, the average adult consumes approximately 1 kg of solid food and 1.2 kg of fluid. In general, the form in which we eat food is unsuitable for immediate use by the body for growth, repair and the production of energy for the performance of physical work. During its passage though the gastrointestinal tract the food undergoes six processes:

- ingestion
- mastication
- digestion
- absorption
- assimilation of useful components
- elimination of non-usable residues.

The effect of the first three of these – ingestion, mastication and digestion – is to render the food into a state in which it can be absorbed. It is only at the fifth stage, assimilation, that food becomes of use to the body's cells. Substances that are not of use are eliminated at the final stage.

The adult gastrointestinal tract consists of a fibro-muscular tube, approximately 4.5 m long and of variable diameter, that extends from the mouth to the

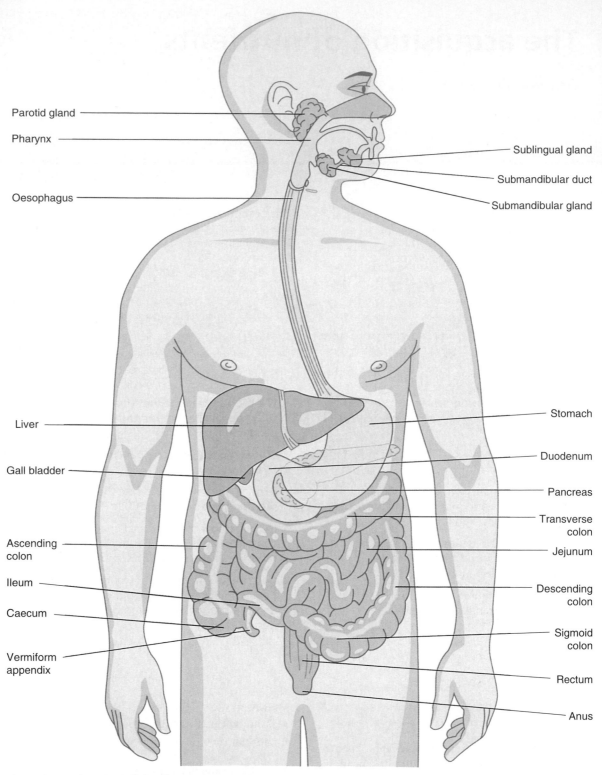

**Figure 5.1.1** Anatomy of the digestive system

anus (**Fig. 5.1.1**). Throughout, the structure of the tract shows variation according to function.

The tract is in contact with the external environment at both ends and, as a result, the potential problem exists of infective agents entering the body via this route. This problem is normally prevented by patches of protective lymphatic tissue throughout the tract and by marked changes in the pH of the medium, which most microorganisms find it difficult to withstand.

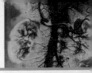

## The mouth

Food is ingested by the mouth, which is the only part of the gastrointestinal tract to have a bony skeleton.

In the mouth, food is mixed with saliva, broken up into small chunks by the teeth, formed into a bolus and propelled backwards into the oesophagus by the tongue.

The mouth is divided into two parts.

- The **vestibule**: that part between the teeth and jaws, and the lips and cheeks. The parotid salivary glands open here.
- The **oral cavity**: this is the inner area, which is bounded by the teeth. The epithelium here is typically 15–20 layers of cells thick and is thus structurally adapted to the amount of friction to which it is subjected during mastication.

## The lips

The lips form a muscular entrance to the mouth. The major muscle of the lips is the orbicularis oris muscle. Lips are necessary for ingestion as they form a muscular passageway for food and fluids and help to grasp particles of food. The act of drinking is accomplished by forming the lips into a tube and simultaneously inhaling – it is, of course, vital to stop the inspiratory process before swallowing fluid to prevent it entering the respiratory tract. During swallowing, the epiglottis blocks the entrance to the trachea and prevents food particles from being inhaled. Once food and fluids are in the mouth, the lips surround and usually close the entrance during chewing and swallowing.

The lips are used in speech, and clear speech in those with injured lips is extremely difficult. A further function of the lips is to convey information about the mood of the person – smiling, grimacing, pursing and kissing. The lips are covered by squamous, keratinized epithelial tissue, which is very vascular and very sensitive. The lips have a large area of the sensory cortex of the brain devoted to receiving sensations from them in relation to actual size of the lips (**see Fig. 2.2.13**).

As there are no sebaceous glands present on the lips, they can quite quickly become chapped and cracked. The lips of individuals who are dehydrated become very dry and the keratinized tissue may peel off; this can lead to bleeding and can be painful. It is for this reason that careful attention must be paid to lubricating the lips in such circumstances (Watson, 1989).

Some individuals carry the herpes simplex virus (type 1) in the cells of the lip area. The virus lies dormant until, for some reason, the individual's resistance is lowered, when the characteristic 'cold sore'

lesion develops. This can cause discomfort and is cosmetically disfiguring. Gloves should be worn when attending to the oral toilet of patients with an herpetic infection of the mouth to prevent the formation of herpetic whitlows on the practitioner's fingers (Holmes & Mountain, 1993).

The inside of the lip is formed from non-keratinized mucous epithelial tissue, and here the profuse blood capillaries lie very close to the surface. It is for this reason that anaemia can be assessed, albeit only roughly, from the colouration of this tissue.

## The teeth

A child has 20 deciduous (milk) teeth and an adult 32 permanent teeth.

The teeth perform several functions during mastication: tearing (the canines), cutting (the incisors) and grinding (the molars and premolars). However, each tooth roughly conforms to the basic structure shown in **Fig. 5.1.2**, with a visible **crown** projecting above the gum and a **root** embedded in the jaw.

**Enamel** covers the crown and the root. This is an extremely hard substance that, when intact, protects the underlying **dentine**, which has a structure similar to bone. Once the enamel is breached, the dentine can be attacked by acids. Bacteria can feed and multiply on sugary residues when the teeth are not properly cleaned. These attacks will eventually result in dental caries and, if untreated, loss of the affected teeth. Proprietary 'fizzy' drinks can be detrimental to teeth because they are both sugary and acidic, some having a pH as low as 3.5.

The **pulp cavity** lies within the dentine and contains nerve fibres. Once the damage caused by dental caries affects this area, intense pain will result when the nerve fibres are stimulated.

### CLINICAL APPLICATIONS

An important nursing function is to attend to the care of the teeth of those unable to do this for themselves. Edentulous individuals (those without teeth) may find eating extremely difficult, and this may be a contributory factor to the nutritional problems of older emaciated or anaemic people. As well as their practical functions, teeth have a cosmetic value and this should be borne in mind when a patient has a dental clearance – a procedure that can have psychological implications. Initially, clear speech may pose problems, in such a person. In older people, the gum tissue covering the jaw tends to shrink and thus dentures that were once well fitting may become loose, making the gums sore and eating difficult. This factor should be

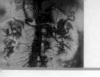
considered when assessing the mouth of an older patient.

*Candida albicans* (thrush) is a fungus that can affect the gums and oral mucosa of those who are very old, very young, debilitated and those on long-term antibiotic therapy in whom the balance of the normal flora of the mouth is disturbed. White, ulcerated plaques form over the affected area. An antifungal substance, such as nystatin in the form of lozenges, mouthwash or tablets, is usually prescribed.

## The tongue

The tongue is formed of striated (voluntary) muscle, which has only one insertion – to the hyoid bone. It is, however, anchored to the anterior floor of the mouth, behind the lower incisor teeth, by a fold of skin called the **frenulum**.

The tongue is very vascular and extremely sensitive, as it is supplied by a large number of nerve endings. We become aware of the tongue's sensory function when it develops a lesion or ulcer. As with the lips, the tongue is represented by a relatively large area of the sensory and motor cortex of the brain in relation to its size (**see Figs 2.2.13 and 2.2.14**). This relatively large cerebral representation in the motor cortex allows innervation of the numerous fine movements of the tongue necessary for speech. If the tongue is injured in any way, then lisping and speech defects can result. Even a tiny lesion on the tongue can cause speech problems.

Apart from its function in speech, the tongue is necessary for swallowing ingested and masticated food. The tongue is very mobile and readily extensible and distensible. It also helps to mix food with saliva.

### CLINICAL APPLICATIONS

Examination of the tongue can give an indication of the health of the individual. Normally, the tongue should be pink, moist and neither smooth nor cracked. It should not appear dry, which indicates a general state of dehydration, nor should it appear furred or brown. A smooth tongue may be seen in pernicious anaemia.

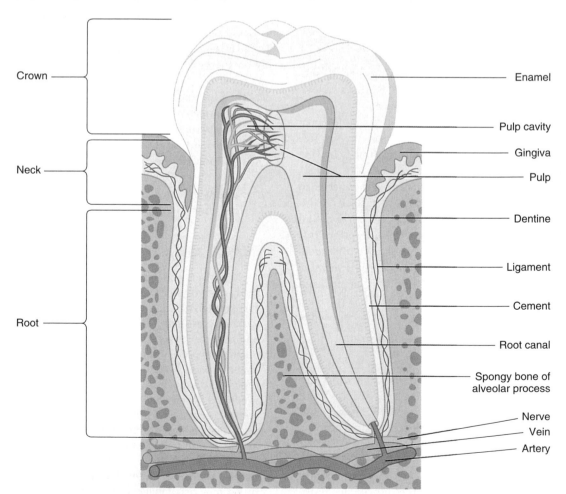

Crown — Enamel

Pulp cavity

Gingiva

Neck — Pulp

Dentine

Ligament

Cement

Root — Root canal

Spongy bone of alveolar process

Nerve

Vein

Artery

**Figure 5.1.2**   Anatomy of a tooth

The tongue and the inside of the mouth should be virtually odourless. A faeculent smell may indicate intestinal obstruction; an ammoniacal, uriniferous smell may indicate liver failure; and a smell of new-mown hay may indicate uncontrolled diabetes mellitus. The mouth may retain for some while odours of food and drink that have recently been ingested, e.g. garlic and alcohol. It is always a good idea to smell the breath of a patient who has been admitted unconscious for clues about the nature of the condition.

An important function of the tongue is that it allows us to taste, and therefore derive enjoyment from food. On the superior surface of the tongue, there are numerous **papillae** – variously called filiform, fungiform, circumvallate and foliate papillae according to their shape (**Fig. 5.1.3**). These areas contain some 10 000 **taste buds**, which allow us to differentiate between the four taste modalities – sweet, sour, salt and bitter. Taste receptor cells (chemoreceptors) lie in these papillae. When chemicals in solution (e.g. dissolved in saliva) stimulate these cells, an impulse is generated. This travels along the nerve fibre supplying each receptor cell, eventually arriving at the sensory cortex of the brain (see Chapter 2.2). Here, the particular taste sensation is distinguished and recognized. It is considered that each of the different types of papillae on the tongue (**see Fig. 5.1.3**) is potentially capable of responding to all types of taste, although each is associated particularly with one modality. Each of the four possible types of taste results in different and distinguishable firing patterns in the nerve fibres, and these are interpreted in the cerebral cortex. Interpretation, which is not always precise, is aided by impulses received from the olfactory nerve, which supplies the olfactory epithelium in the nose (Blank & Mattes, 1990). The fact that taste is potentiated by smell becomes evident when one has a cold: inflammation and hypersecretion of the nasal mucosa impair the ability to smell, and this subsequently impairs the ability to taste food effectively.

## The salivary glands

In terms of their contribution to digestion, these exocrine glands are non-essential; in practical terms, however, they are important as their secretion aids speech, chewing, swallowing and general oral comfort.

There are three main pairs of glands: the parotid glands, submaxillary and sublingual glands. Other smaller glands exist over the surface of the palate, inside the lips and the tongue. These secrete saliva in response to local mechanical stimuli and are not under the control of the parasympathetic nervous system.

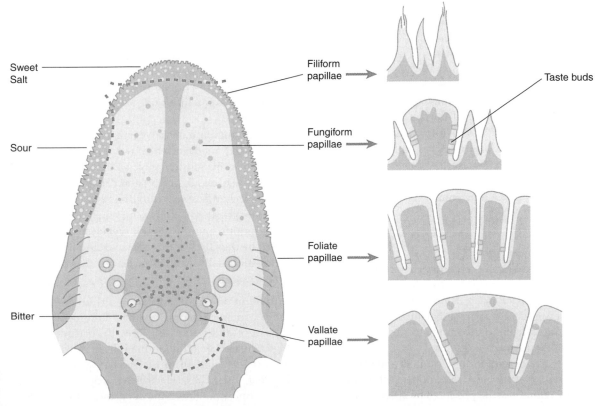

**Figure 5.1.3**   The tongue, showing the papillae

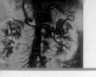

### Parotid glands

These glands are situated by the angle of the jaw, lying posterior to the mandible and inferior to the ear. They are the largest of the three pairs of salivary glands and are supplied by parasympathetic fibres of the glossopharyngeal nerve (the IXth cranial nerve). The parotids produce a watery secretion, which forms 25% of the total daily salivary secretion. This saliva is rich in both enzymes and antibodies (IgA).

---

**CLINICAL APPLICATIONS**

In infectious parotitis (that is, inflammation of the parotids), more commonly called mumps, these glands swell to produce the characteristic appearance of mumps.

---

### Submaxillary glands

This pair of glands lies below the maxilla (i.e. the upper jaw). The submaxillary glands produce a more viscid saliva, which forms 70% of the total daily production. Their nerve supply comes from the facial nerve (the VIIth cranial nerve).

### Sublingual glands

These lie in the floor of the mouth below the tongue and produce a scanty secretion (only 5% of the total produced), which is rich in the protein mucin. This gives saliva its somewhat sticky character. They also are supplied by the facial nerve.

## Saliva

An adult produces approximately 1–1.5 L of saliva a day. Saliva is a mixture of the secretions formed by the salivary glands and is formed mainly of water (99% of total), and normally has a pH of 6.8–7.0. It does, however, become more alkaline as the secretory rate increases during chewing.

Saliva has several functions:

- It cleanses the mouth. There is a constant production of saliva with a backwards flow directed towards the oesophagus. Saliva contains lysozyme, which has an antiseptic action, and also immunoglobulin (IgA), which has a defensive function. In general, a normal flow of saliva helps to prevent dental caries and halitosis. A sudden flush of saliva into the mouth ('water brash') often heralds vomiting.
- Saliva is necessary for oral comfort and the lubrication it provides reduces the friction that would otherwise be produced by speech and chewing. A dry mouth is extremely

uncomfortable, and does not permit easy speech. This condition may occur normally when the subject is nervous, frightened or anxious and when activity of the sympathetic nervous system or the action of drugs inhibits salivary secretion.

---

**CLINICAL APPLICATIONS**

In a patient who is dehydrated, the mouth may be coated with thick secretions. To remove these, frequent, repeated and thorough cleansing of the mouth may be necessary.

Certain drugs, e.g. atropine and hyoscine (scopolamine), block parasympathetic action and therefore cause a dry mouth – that is, they inhibit salivary secretion. It is for this reason that these drugs are often given as part of a premedication prior to surgery. During surgery, it is necessary to reduce the volume of saliva produced. In the absence of the cough reflex, while the patient is anaesthetized, the saliva may be inhaled.

---

- It is necessary for chemicals in food to be in solution (i.e. mixed with saliva) for them to stimulate the taste receptors in the papillae on the tongue. A person who has a dry mouth cannot taste food effectively (and therefore fails to enjoy meals).
- Saliva is necessary for the formation of a **bolus**, that is, a ball of partly broken-up food that is ready to be swallowed. The mucins present in saliva (viscid glycoproteins) help in the moulding and lubrication of the bolus. The role of saliva in swallowing becomes evident if one tries to eat a dry biscuit when anxious or nervous when, consequently, one's salivary secretion is decreased.
- Saliva contains a digestive enzyme, **salivary** or **alpha ($\alpha$) amylase**, which was formerly referred to as ptyalin. Salivary amylase acts upon cooked starch (e.g. bread, pastry) and converts the polysaccharide starch into disaccharides (maltose and dextrins). The longer the starch remains in the mouth, and the more it is chewed, the greater will be the effect of this enzyme. Usually in digestion, salivary amylase plays only a minor and non-essential role.

In addition to the substances already mentioned, saliva contains calcium, sodium, chloride, hydrogen carbonate and potassium ions. If, for some pathological reason (e.g. inflammation, infection or neoplasm) the ducts from the salivary glands become blocked, then these electrolytes may become even more concentrated within the gland, which leads to the formation of salivary stones.

## Control of salivary secretions

The salivary glands are innervated by parasympathetic and sympathetic nerves. Saliva is produced in response to the following:

- **The thought, sight or smell of food.** This is a conditioned reflex. When a substance that is consciously recognized as food is anticipated by thought, sight or smell, impulses travel from the receptor to the cerebral cortex and thence to the medulla in the brainstem. The salivary nuclei are situated in the reticular formation in the floor of the fourth ventricle. Impulses travel from there to the salivary glands and secretion is effected.
- **The presence of food in the mouth.** This produces mechanical stimulation of the salivary glands, and this response represents an unconditioned reflex (i.e. it is not learned). The impulse generated goes straight to the salivary nuclei in the medulla, and does not travel via the cerebral cortex.

Secretion of copious watery saliva occurs as a result of excitation of the parasympathetic nervous system, which also increases blood flow to the salivary glands. The glossopharyngeal and facial nerves (referred to earlier), which supply the salivary glands, form part of the parasympathetic cranial outflow.

**Acetylcholine (Ach)** is the parasympathetic neurotransmitter that brings about salivary secretion; atropine and hyoscine block the receptor sites for acetylcholine and thus inhibit secretion. Conversely, neostigmine inhibits **acetylcholine esterase**, which destroys acetylcholine once it has brought about secretion. The administration of neostigmine therefore increases salivary secretion.

Stimulation of the sympathetic nervous system, such as occurs in stress and extreme anxiety results in vasoconstriction of the blood vessels to the glands, hence only small amounts of concentrated saliva are produced.

### CLINICAL APPLICATIONS

When carrying out a nursing assessment of a patient's mouth, relevant information can be obtained by observing the state of the lips, gums and tongue. It is important to notice the condition of the patient's teeth, and whether or not dental caries is present; the smell of the mouth; any bleeding, thrush (candidiasis) or overt problems such as cracked lips or evidence of herpes simplex.

Before digestion can occur, the ingested and masticated food (now in the form of a bolus) must be swallowed. This process is sometimes referred to as **deglutition**. The food is gathered into a bolus by the tongue and, before swallowing takes place, the mouth is normally closed. To gain an idea of how difficult it is to swallow with the mouth open, think of the problems one experiences in the dentist's chair; under these circumstances, it is possible to swallow only small quantities of saliva. This needs to be remembered when performing mouth care for a patient. The tongue contracts and presses the bolus of food against the hard palate in the roof of the mouth (**Fig. 5.1.4**). It then arches backwards and the bolus is propelled towards the oropharynx.

To ensure that the bolus is not propelled upwards into the nasopharynx, this area is shut off by the soft palate rising. To ensure, too, that the bolus is not propelled into the larynx and respiratory tract, the larynx rises to a position under the base of the tongue and the epiglottis closes over the trachea. Respirations are inhibited so that food and fluids are not inhaled into the trachea during inspiration.

Once the bolus reaches the posterior pharyngeal wall, the musculature there contracts around it. The food, often including up to 100 mL of air, enters the oesophagus and after this point the process becomes involuntary. The earlier stages described are all under voluntary control but, once the bolus touches the posterior pharynx and tonsillar area, impulses are generated that travel to the medulla and trigger off the **swallowing reflex**. This reflex is absent in the deeply unconscious or anaesthetized patient.

## Generalized structure of the gastrointestinal tract

The basic structure of the gastrointestinal tract follows the same pattern from the mouth to the anus, with some functional adaptations throughout (**Fig. 5.1.5**). The digestive tract wall consists of four structural layers.

The **mucosa** is the innermost layer, that is, the layer nearest to the lumen of the tube, and it exhibits a great deal of variation throughout the tract. Mucus-stratified epithelial cells line the lumen (except oesophagus), and it is from this layer that all glands develop. Mucus-secreting cells are situated throughout the epithelium. These cells are subjected to a tremendous amount of frictional wear and tear. The epithelial cells lie on a sheet of connective tissue called the *lamina propria*. Distal to this, there is a thin layer of muscle tissue called **muscularis mucosa**. Patches of lymphoid tissue are found throughout the mucosa; these serve a defensive function.

The **submucosa** lies distal to the mucosa and consists of loose connective tissue, which supports the

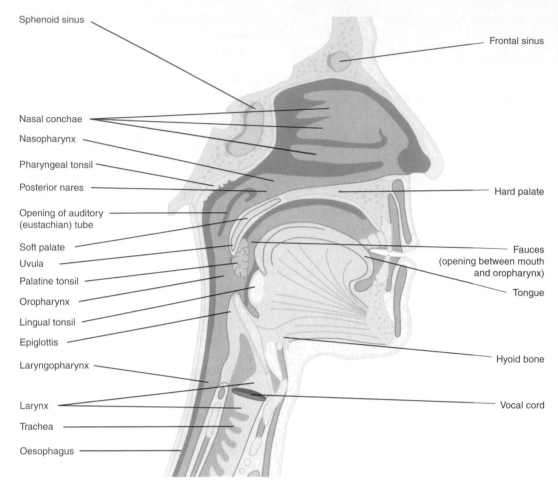

**Figure 5.1.4**   Anatomy of mouth, pharynx and oesophagus (sagittal section)

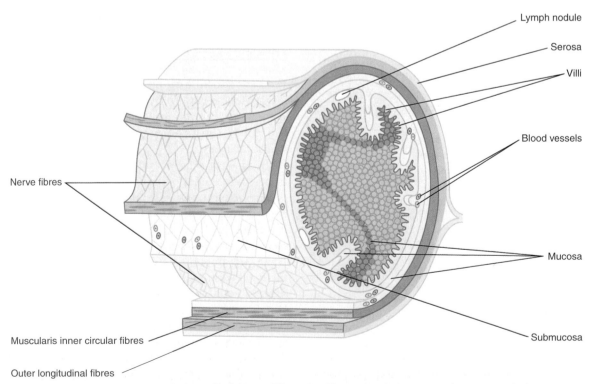

**Figure 5.1.5**   Cross-section through the wall of the small intestine illustrating the mucosa, submucosa and serosa

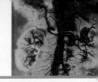

in the abdominal cavity, and carries blood vessels and nerves.

## Blood supply to the gastrointestinal tract

The arteries supplying the abdominal organs of the digestive system are the coeliac and superior and inferior mesenteric arteries. The coeliac artery branches to give rise to the gastric, splenic and hepatic arteries that provide blood to the stomach, pancreas, spleen and liver. The mesenteric arteries supply the intestines.

Venous blood from the stomach, pancreas, spleen and liver is collected together and routed through the liver via the hepatic portal vein. Blood from the remainder of the digestive tract (oesophagus and rectum) escapes the hepatic filter and drains directly into the venous system.

## Motility (movement in the gastrointestinal tract)

Motility refers to contraction and relaxation of the walls and sphincters of the gastrointestinal tract. Motility involves the grinding and mixing of ingested food in preparation for digestion and absorption, it then propels the food along the gastrointestinal tract. Smooth muscle in the gastrointestinal tract enables:

- contractile tone to be maintained even in the absence of food
- activity to be increased and decreased as necessary.

The control of motility and secretion in the gastrointestinal tract is by neural, hormonal and paracrine mechanisms. The neural control is via the extrinsic nerves of the autonomic nervous system. In most instances the mediators of neural or hormonal control are peptides.

### Neural control of the gastrointestinal tract

### Internal nerve plexuses

The gastrointestinal tract receives nerve fibres from the autonomic nervous system. The submucosal and myenteric nerve plexuses form the local internal nervous system of the tract.

In the **submucosal plexus**, parasympathetic nerve fibres synapse with ganglion cells that lie in small clusters within the submucosal tissue. Postganglionic fibres arise from here and travel to the glands and smooth muscle of the tract. Sympathetic fibres also run within this plexus.

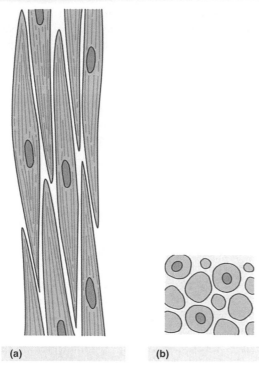

**Figure 5.1.6** The gross structure of smooth muscle (a) surface view and (b) cross-section

blood vessels, lymphatics and nerves carried in this layer. The nerve fibres in this layer form the submucosal or Meissner's plexus.

The **muscularis** layer, as its name suggests, is formed of muscle fibres. The muscle fibres in the gastrointestinal tract are referred to as smooth, involuntary, unstriated or visceral muscle fibres. They exhibit the following characteristics:

- They respond to stimulation by the autonomic nervous system or certain hormones.
- They exhibit continuous rhythmic and inherent contractions that may be modulated by the above stimuli.
- They do not contract as forcefully as striated muscle fibres.
- They do not exhibit the same finely controlled contractions as striated muscles; their contractions bring about rather more diffuse movements of the whole muscle mass.

The fibres consist of elongated spindle-shaped cells with tapered ends (**Fig. 5.1.6**), and with a single centrally located, elongated nucleus; the fibres are bound together in sheets.

The **adventitia** or **serosa** is the outermost, protective layer, formed of connective tissue and squamous serous epithelium. It is continuous with the mesentery

In the **myenteric plexus**, parasympathetic nerve fibres travel to ganglion cells that lie in large clusters within the muscularis layer, between the circular and longitudinal muscle fibres. Postganglionic fibres arise here and innervate the smooth muscle within this layer. This muscle is also supplied with sympathetic fibres from the myenteric plexus.

**Substance P**, a peptide made up of 11 amino acids and found in high concentrations in the gut, is thought to be a chemical mediator, that is, it acts like a neurotransmitter in reflexes at myenteric level. It can therefore be referred to as a **regulatory peptide** or **neuropeptide**. Substance P has been shown to be involved in sending pain impulses along sensory nerve fibres. Indeed, its secretion is decreased by the action of circulating enkephalins (one of the body's natural opiates). For a fuller description of this, see the section on pain in Chapter 2.3. In addition, it brings about vasodilation and contraction of non-vascular smooth muscle.

**Serotonin** (5-hydroxytryptamine, or 5-HT) is also thought to be synthesized within the myenteric plexus and to have a role as an interneuronal transmitter.

Both submucosal and myenteric plexuses run from the oesophagus to the anus, and receive both sympathetic and parasympathetic nerve fibres. There are neuronal connections between the two internal plexuses and activity in one can therefore affect the other. The arrangement of the neurones within the plexuses allows stimulation at the upper end of the tract to be transmitted to distal portions of the tract. Thus, entry of food into the upper oesophagus can lead to gastric and intestinal secretion.

Areas of the gut, for example the stomach, receive direct 'external' autonomic fibres from the vagus nerve (a branch of the parasympathetic nervous system) and the sympathetic nervous system; they also receive autonomic stimulation via the local internal plexuses.

## Autonomic nervous system
(see Chapter 2.5)

Secretion and motility throughout the gastrointestinal tract are under the control of both autonomic nervous and hormonal factors. The effect of the hormonal factors will be discussed later in relation to each relevant area of the tract.

With regard to neural control: in general, parasympathetic activity leads to an increase in both motility and secretion and to relaxation of the gut sphincters. The parasympathetic supply to the oesophagus, stomach, pancreas, bile duct, small intestine and proximal colon is via the **vagus nerve** (Xth cranial nerve). This nerve is very widespread in its connections, supplying areas of the cardiovascular, respiratory and gastrointestinal tracts.

The parasympathetic supply to the salivary glands is via the facial and glossopharyngeal nerves (VIIth and IXth cranial nerves), with the parasympathetic ganglia lying near the glands. The parasympathetic nerve supply to the distal colon is via the *nervi erigentes* in the sacral outflow from the spinal cord.

Activity of the sympathetic nervous system in general leads to a decrease in the blood flow to the gut, and a consequent decrease in secretions and lessening of motility and excitation (i.e. contraction) of the gut sphincters. Within the gastrointestinal tract, as elsewhere in the body, two types of receptor present on the postsynaptic muscle fibres initiate responses to the catecholamines released as a result of sympathetic stimulation. These are termed $\alpha$ and $\beta_2$ ($\beta_1$-receptors are present only in cardiac muscle).

When stimulated, **$\alpha$-receptors** mediate contraction of smooth muscle in the walls of the gastrointestinal tract and the walls of the blood vessels. When stimulated, **$\beta_2$-receptors** bring about relaxation of smooth muscle fibres.

**Table 5.1.1** shows the details of autonomic stimulation of the gastrointestinal tract.

## Regulation of dietary intake

The amount of food we take in daily is regulated only to a certain extent by hunger.

**Hunger** refers to a physiological sensation of emptiness, usually accompanied by contraction of the stomach. There is no direct relationship between the blood sugar level and hunger – diabetic people who are hyperglycaemic often feel hungry. To a large extent, what and how much we eat are dictated by social customs and the pattern of our day; it depends not only on hunger but also on appetite. **Appetite** refers to a pleasant feeling of anticipation of forthcoming food. The two sensations of hunger and appetite are therefore related but quite different. Appetite is affected by one's emotional state, for example someone who is nervous or apprehensive might well lose his or her appetite, that is, become **anorexic**.

The hypothalamus is important in regulating food intake, although the exact mechanism for this is still uncertain. There appear to be two hypothalamic areas that interact in regulating food intake: the **feeding centre** and the **satiety centre**. It is thought that the satiety centre is influenced by the level of glucose utilization in receptor cells in this area of the hypothalamus. These cells are therefore termed **glucostats**.

For details of how to assess a patient's nutritional status, the reader is recommended to consult McLaren & Green (1998) and Shireff (1990). For a fuller discussion of the determinants of food intake, see Kowanko et al. (1999).

**Table 5.1.1** The effects of autonomic stimulation of the gastrointestinal tract

| Area of gastrointestinal tract | Parasympathetic stimulation | Sympathetic stimulation (receptors indicated where appropriate) |
|---|---|---|
| Salivary glands | Profuse watery secretion | α-receptors<br>Sparse viscid secretion |
| Stomach<br>  Motility<br>  Secretion | <br>↑<br>↑ | <br>$\beta_2$-receptors ↓ usually inhibits<br>α-receptors → contraction ↓ |
| Pancreas<br>  (secretion of acinar cells) | ↑ | ↓ |
| Gall bladder and bile ducts | Contraction | Relaxation |
| Small and large intestines<br>  Motility<br>  Secretion<br>  Sphincters | <br>↑<br>↑<br>Relaxation | <br>α- and $\beta_2$-receptors ↓<br>usually inhibits<br>α-receptors → contraction |

↑ increases; ↓ decreases

## The oesophagus

The oesophagus is a thin-walled muscular tube about 25 cm in length. It extends from the pharynx to the stomach and is composed of the same four layers as the bulk of the gastrointestinal tract. The muscular coat of the upper third is composed of skeletal muscle, the lower third smooth muscle with a transitional zone from one to the other between. Both skeletal and smooth muscle fibres are under the control of the vagus nerve.

There are two physiological sphincters in the oesophagus, one at either end:

- upper oesophageal sphincter (crico-pharyngeal sphincter)
- lower oesophageal sphincter (LOS, also known as the cardiac sphincter).

The upper oesophageal sphincter is comprised of skeletal muscle. The lower oesophageal sphincter covers the distal 1–2 cm of the oesophagus; it is not anatomically distinguishable as a sphincter but pressure is normally greater in this region than in the stomach.

## Gastro-oesophageal reflux disease (GORD)

This is a very common gastrointestinal complaint. It is defined as symptoms of mucosal damage (oesophagitis) resulting from exposure to acidic stomach contents. In its simplest form, the symptoms are mild and self-limiting but it can be a chronic disorder with serious consequences. Heartburn, dyspepsia

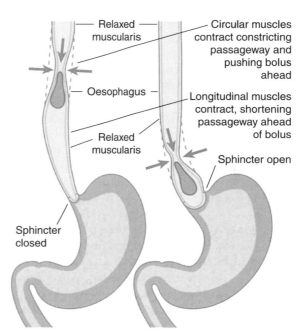

**Figure 5.1.7** The oesophageal stage of swallowing showing peristalsis

and regurgitation are the major symptoms of gastro-oesophageal reflux disease. Gastro-oesophageal reflux disease can respond to simple non-pharmaceutical interventions, including stopping smoking, avoiding problem foods, reducing alcohol and weight reduction. In more severe cases acid-blocking medications ($H_2$-receptor antagonists) or more powerful inhibitors of stomach acid production (proton pump inhibitors) may be required for symptomatic relief.

The movement of food through the oesophagus is by peristalsis (**Fig. 5.1.7**). **Peristalsis** is a coordinated wave of contraction proceeding in an orderly direction from one part of the digestive tract to the next.

In the oesophagus, the wave of contraction is controlled by nerve impulses in the vagus and is coordinated by the swallowing centre in the medulla. The wave takes about 9 seconds to travel the length of the oesophagus.

As the peristaltic waves begin in the oesophagus, the muscle of the lower oesophageal sphincter relaxes, opening the sphincter and allowing the food bolus to enter the stomach. Should any food particles remain in the oesophagus after the first wave of peristalsis, irritation of the mucosa by the food particles evokes a secondary wave of peristalsis that helps to dislodge the remaining food particles and sweeps them into the stomach.

These movements occur progressively throughout the tube in a coordinated manner, and give the appearance of smooth waves of contraction. The process can be initiated by stimulation of the vagus nerve (Xth cranial nerve) and also by stimulation of parasympathetic nerve fibres in the myenteric (Auerbach's) plexus situated in the muscular layer of the tract.

The time taken for food to travel the 20–25 cm of the oesophagus depends on the consistency of the food and the position of the body. Patients who have to eat while flat on their backs may experience some discomfort and difficulty in swallowing – a process that is normally aided by gravity. However, it is possible to swallow when standing on your head! Liquids take only 1–2 seconds to reach the cardiac sphincter but a more solid bolus takes longer, perhaps up to 2–3 minutes. The small amount of air swallowed with the food is usually expelled some time later by belching.

The lower 4 cm of the oesophagus is referred to as the **gastro-oesophageal** or **cardiac sphincter** and is normally in a state of tonic contraction until swallowing occurs, when the circular muscle fibres relax. This is a physiological rather than an anatomical sphincter; the circular muscles in the area act to prevent reflux of the gastric contents into the oesophagus.

**The pressure within the stomach is normally 5–10 mmHg above atmospheric pressure, due to the pressure exerted on the stomach from below by the contents of the abdominal cavity.** Because the pressure within the upper oesophagus is less than this – usually some 5–10 mmHg below atmospheric pressure as the upper oesophagus lies within the thoracic cavity – it can be seen that, without the presence of a functional sphincter, reflux could easily occur. The gastro-oesophageal region lies partly within the abdominal cavity, and this helps to account for the above-atmospheric pressure in this area.

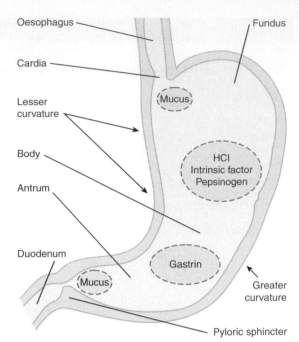

**Figure 5.1.8**   Gross structure of the stomach

## The stomach

### Structure and function

The stomach, continuous with the oesophagus above and the duodenum below, is the most dilated area of the gastrointestinal tract (**Fig. 5.1.8**). It is roughly J-shaped, although the size and shape vary between individuals and with its state of fullness. The stomach is divided into several regions:

- fundus
- cardia
- body
- antrum.

Folds, known as rugae, are present on the inner surface of the stomach. The wall structure of the stomach is similar to the rest of the gastrointestinal tract (**see Fig. 5.1.5**), except that the stomach has an oblique muscular layer in addition to the circular and longitudinal layers in the muscularis. This additional layer

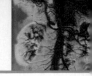

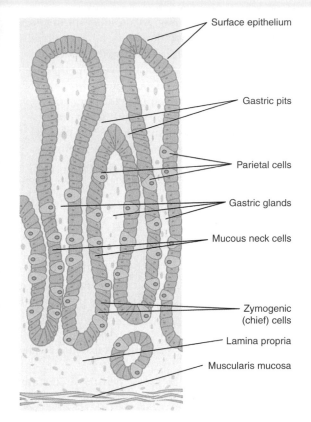

Surface epithelium

Gastric pits

Parietal cells

Gastric glands

Mucous neck cells

Zymogenic
(chief) cells

Lamina propria

Muscularis mucosa

**Figure 5.1.9**  Anatomy of the gastric glands

facilitates distension of the stomach and storage of food.

The epithelium of the body of the stomach (about 75% of the total) is further folded, being composed of **gastric pits** containing microscopic gastric glands (**Fig. 5.1.9**). This arrangement results in a total surface area of some 800 cm$^2$.

Food passes from the stomach to the small intestine via the pyloric canal. This canal is encircled by a band of smooth muscle, the pyloric sphincter.

## Functions of the stomach

### A reservoir for food

This aspect of the stomach's function allows us to eat large meals at quite widely spaced intervals. The importance of this function is demonstrated in patients who have undergone a gastrectomy and who can therefore cope only with small, frequent meals. At rest, the volume of the 'empty' stomach in the adult is approximately 50 mL. However, by **receptive relaxation** of the muscle in the stomach wall as food enters, it can accommodate up to 1.5 L of food and fluids and, under extreme circumstances, can distend to hold nearly 4 L. On the other hand, the stomach of the neonate is only about the size of a hen's egg – something to be remembered when feeding a baby.

This ability of the stomach to store food, together with the presence of the **pyloric sphincter**, allows for the controlled release of gastric contents into the duodenum, and therefore prevents rapid overloading of the small intestine.

### CLINICAL APPLICATIONS

In patients who have had all or a large amount of their stomach resected, this controlled release into the duodenum is not possible. As these patients eat, relatively large, undiluted and therefore highly concentrated amounts of foodstuffs are poured rapidly into the duodenum. This causes distension and stimulates sympathetic nerve fibres in the duodenum and jejunum. Furthermore, because the duodenal contents are hypertonic in relation to plasma and extracellular fluid, fluid moves from the interstitial spaces and from the blood vessels in the gut wall into the lumen of the small intestine to dilute the contents. This results in a quite rapid fall in blood volume and a consequent fall in the cardiac output. As a result, the patient complains of feeling weak, dizzy and faint during or after eating food. This is often referred to as the **dumping syndrome**.

A further problem for these patients may occur when glucose is absorbed very rapidly after a meal. The consequent hyperglycaemia leads to a rapid increase in insulin secretion, and as a result the blood sugar level drops dramatically, causing the patient to become hypoglycaemic.

Not all patients experience these problems after a gastrectomy but for those who do the symptoms are most unpleasant. Such patients may decrease their food intake in an effort to avoid these episodes, with consequent nutritional problems. It is therefore important that patients who have had radical gastric surgery receive dietary advice as part of their care and discharge planning regarding the necessity to take small, frequent meals.

### Intrinsic factor

Intrinsic factor is necessary for the absorption of **vitamin B12 (cyanocobalamin)** in the terminal ileum. Intrinsic factor, a glycoprotein, binds to vitamin B12 in the small intestine to form a complex, which appears to bind to receptors in the ileal wall, allowing vitamin B12 to transfer across the gut wall into the blood. Trypsin is also thought to be necessary for efficient vitamin B12 absorption to occur.

Vitamin B12 is required for healthy functioning of nerve fibres and their myelin sheaths in the spinal cord. It is also necessary for the formation of the red blood cell stroma during erythropoiesis in the red bone marrow.

Lack of vitamin B12 leads to a megaloblastic (pernicious) anaemia and, if untreated, to subacute combined degeneration of the spinal cord (see Chapter 4.1). As a typical human diet normally contains sufficient vitamin B12 to supply our needs, megaloblastic anaemias are usually the result of failure to produce intrinsic factor or of failure to absorb the vitamin in the small intestine. This latter situation may occur following an ileostomy or when chronic diarrhoea exists.

Intrinsic factor is produced by the gastric parietal cells, which also produce gastric acid. Patients who lack intrinsic factor often also lack gastric acid, that is, they have **hypochlorhydria** or **achlorhydria**. Tests used in the diagnosis of megaloblastic anaemia may therefore attempt to elicit gastric acid secretion by, for example, the administration of histamine or, more commonly, pentagastrin. Some patients with megaloblastic anaemia are thought to produce antibodies to their own intrinsic factor, and in these individuals the cause of the disease is autoimmune.

## Gastric absorption

Ingested food is only partly broken down in the stomach and the resulting molecules are still, in general, too large to cross the gastric wall. In addition, carrier systems for the transport of molecules across the gastric wall have not been found. Hence only a small amount of absorption can occur in the stomach. It is possible to absorb the following:

- A small amount of water.
- **Alcohol**: the bulk of alcohol absorption occurs in the small intestine but about 20% may be absorbed in the stomach. If foods containing fat (e.g. milk, cheese) are taken before drinking alcohol, they may help to delay alcohol absorption in the small intestine by slowing down gastric emptying. This will not, however, prevent gastric alcohol absorption.
- **Some drugs**: in particular aspirin. Aspirin (acetylsalicylic acid) is a weak acid and, as such, can cross the stomach wall. In so doing, it increases the hydrogen ion concentration of the cells in the wall, thus lowering their cellular pH. This may cause cell damage. Prolonged aspirin ingestion may therefore lead to gastric irritation (gastritis) and bleeding. As a result, aspirin and other salicylates should never be administered to patients with lesions of the gastric mucosa or dyspepsia, to those on anticoagulant therapy or those with haemophilia. Patients who are prescribed aspirin (e.g. for the treatment of rheumatoid arthritis) are usually given enteric-coated aspirin; the coating on the drug ensures that it is not absorbed in the stomach, and this therefore avoids problems of gastric irritation, bleeding and haematemesis (vomiting of blood).

## The stomach acts as a churn

The stomach converts ingested food to a thick, minestrone-soup-like consistency by mixing it with gastric secretions. This serves to dilute the foodstuffs and thus prevents the entry of a solution into the duodenum that is hypertonic in relation to extracellular fluid. The resulting semi-liquid substance is called **chyme**.

Mixing is achieved by gastric peristalsis. Rhythmic waves of contraction of the three layers of smooth muscle in the stomach wall pass from cardia to pylorus about three times a minute, each wave lasting approximately half a minute. These waves of contraction allow the more liquid contents to leave the pylorus of the stomach quite rapidly and enter the duodenum. As the pyloric muscle contracts, the lumen of the stomach partially closes, and this causes the more solid food in the antrum to pass backwards towards the body of the stomach. This forwards and backwards movement increases the efficiency of gastric mixing. **Motilin** is a regulatory peptide secreted by cells in the duodenum and jejunum in response to acid chyme, which increases gastric motility.

## Secretion of mucus

Mucus consists of a gel, formed of the protein mucin and glycoproteins, which adheres to the gastric mucosa. It is secreted by cells in the necks of the deep gastric glands in both the cardia and the pylorus. **Mucus protects the stomach wall from being digested by the proteolytic enzyme pepsin, which is produced in the stomach (i.e. it prevents auto-digestion).** It also contains some hydrogen carbonate (bicarbonate) and this partially neutralizes gastric acid and so prevents this acid from damaging the gastric cells. It further helps to lubricate the food in the stomach.

To carry out these protective functions, the layer of mucus covering the rugae needs to be at least 1 mm thick.

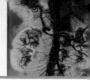

## CLINICAL APPLICATIONS

Mucus hypersecretion occurs in gastric inflammation (gastritis) and as a response to irritant or toxic agents (e.g. alcohol and microorganisms). Additionally, to help patients who have gastric ulcers, mucus secretion can be increased by the administration of carbenoxolone (a liquorice derivative). Protection of the gastric cells does not depend solely on mucus secretion but also on there being intact gastric cell membranes with a low permeability to hydrogen ions and tight junctions between these cells.

Certain substances (e.g. aspirin, alcohol and bile salts) disturb the cellular arrangement of the gastric mucosa and increase the permeability of the cell membranes to hydrogen ions. If the cell membrane is breached, hydrogen ions enter the cell and lower the cellular pH. The subsequent cell damage may lead to hypoxic and eventually necrotic areas of gastric mucosa, and hence to the formation of an ulcer. Healing of such areas is made difficult by the gastric acid in which they are bathed, and by the autodigestive effect of pepsin.

**Histamine** is a substance, produced by circulating mast cells and basophils, which increases gastric acid secretion. It achieves this effect by binding to histamine receptors ($H_2$-receptors) on the gastric parietal cells. $H_2$-receptor blocking agents can therefore be used to decrease gastric acid secretion; such drugs, e.g. cimetidine and ranitidine, are used successfully in the treatment of gastric ulcers. Some peptic ulcers are due to the presence of *Helicobacter pylori* and are treated with bismuth and antibiotics.

## Secretion of gastric juice

Gastric juice consists of a mixture of secretions from two types of cells, both of which are absent from the pylorus:

- **Parietal** or **oxyntic cells**: these secrete hydrochloric acid (HCl), and also the intrinsic factor referred to earlier.
- **Chief** or **zymogen cells**: these secrete enzymes.

Some 2–3 L of juice with a pH of 1.5–3.0 are secreted each day in the adult.

The parietal cells, lying in the gastric pits (**see Fig. 5.1.9**), produce gastric acid and it is thought that these cells have fine channels (canaliculi) leading from the cytoplasm of the cell to the lumen of the gastric pits and through which the acid is discharged into the stomach. There are about 1000 million parietal cells in the healthy adult stomach.

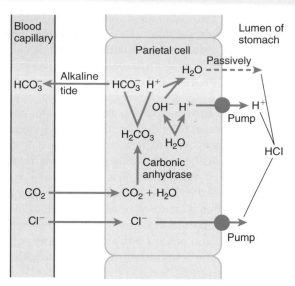

**Figure 5.1.10**   The production of hydrochloric acid within the parietal cells

Hydrogen ions are secreted by the parietal cells *against* a concentration gradient, that is, they are produced by the parietal cells and move into the lumen of the stomach where the hydrogen ion concentration is high, rather than into the blood, which has a low concentration of hydrogen ions. Hydrogen ions are transported actively by a pump mechanism in the cell membrane. Chloride ions, too, are actively secreted against a concentration gradient, and the presence of a similar pump for this action is consequently postulated. The energy for this active transport of both hydrogen and chloride ions is obtained from the aerobic breakdown of glucose.

Blood leaving the stomach via the gastric vein has a lower partial pressure of carbon dioxide than blood arriving at the stomach via the gastric artery. It is therefore postulated that $CO_2$ diffuses into the parietal cells from arterial blood. Within the parietal cell, $CO_2$ combines with water under the influence of the enzyme carbonic anhydrase (CA) to form $H_2CO_3$ (carbonic acid). This dissociates to form hydrogen ions ($H^+$) and hydrogen carbonate ions (bicarbonate, $HCO_3^-$) (**Fig. 5.1.10**). The hydrogen carbonate so produced enters the capillaries and hence the venous blood draining the stomach. This movement of base into the venous blood is referred to as the **alkaline tide**. Thus, in a sense, the parietal cells act as both endocrine and exocrine glands.

## CLINICAL APPLICATIONS

The alkaline tide is of significance in disorders in which there is prolonged vomiting (e.g. hyperemesis gravidarum in pregnancy). In such conditions there is an absolute loss from the body of gastric acid, while the venous blood continues to become more alkaline. This may result in a metabolic alkalosis.

It is thought that within the parietal cell, $H_2O$ dissociates into hydrogen ions ($H^+$) and hydroxyl ions ($OH^-$). The hydrogen ions produced by the dissociation of carbonic acid neutralize the hydroxyl ions produced by the dissociation of water. This leaves the hydrogen ions produced by the dissociation of water to be secreted actively into the lumen of the gastric pits. Equal numbers of chloride ions are similarly secreted actively into the lumen of the gastric pits. Equal numbers of chloride ions are similarly secreted actively into the lumen of the gastric pits; water follows passively to dilute the HCl so formed.

Acid secretion is increased when stimulated by histamine or the hormone gastrin. Pentagastrin, a synthetic gastrin and hence a potent stimulant for acid secretion, can be used clinically to investigate gastric acid secretion.

The **functions of gastric acid** are as follows:

- It inactivates salivary amylase.
- It is bacteriostatic and therefore protective.
- It tenderizes proteins by denaturing them, that is, it alters their molecular structure.
- It curdles milk. The hydrochloric acid acts on casein (a soluble protein in milk) and converts it into paracasein. This combines with calcium ions to form curds preparatory to milk digestion.
- It converts pepsinogen into pepsin.

The chief (or zymogen) cells produce a scanty secretion rich in **pepsinogen**, an enzyme precursor. When gastric pH is below 5.5, this pepsinogen is converted into **pepsin** by hydrochloric acid. Once this conversion has occurred, the pepsin so formed can itself convert pepsinogen into more pepsin. Pepsin is a proteolytic enzyme; that is, it acts on proteins and starts their digestion. It converts proteins into polypeptides (long chains of amino acids) by breaking bonds between specific amino acids. Pepsin is most active when the gastric pH is below 3.5 and it is responsible for between 10% and 15% of all protein digestion. Once chyme leaves the stomach, the activity of pepsin stops due to the change to an alkaline medium.

The secretion of pepsinogen is closely linked to the secretion of gastric acid.

## CLINICAL APPLICATIONS

Stimulation of the vagus nerve leads to the release of acetylcholine at the vagal axon terminations. This stimulates both the chief cells and the parietal cells, and provides the rationale for using agents which block acetylcholine receptors in the treatment of gastric ulcers. Such anticholinergic agents (e.g. propantheline, pirenzepine and metoclopramide, prevent the secretion of both gastric acid and pepsinogen.

### Control of gastric juice secretion

This is both neural and hormonal (humoral) (**Fig. 5.1.11**).

It is usual to describe two phases in the **neural control** of gastric juice secretion, although these two phases are not distinct.

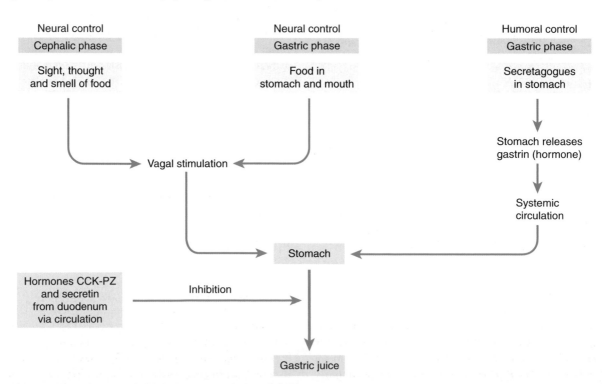

**Figure 5.1.11** Gastric juice secretion. CCK, cholecystokinin

In the **cephalic** or **psychic phase**, secretion is brought about in response to the sight, thought or smell of food. This is a conditioned (i.e. learned) reflex and is mediated by the vagus nerve. Additionally, the presence of food in the mouth leads to gastric secretion. Stimulation of the vagus nerve by such cephalic impulses leads to the release of acetylcholine at the axon terminations. This chemical (as described earlier) stimulates both parietal and chief cells. Surgical section of branches of the vagal nerve (selective vagotomy) will prevent vagal stimulation, resulting in reduced secretion of gastric juice.

The **gastric phase** is not mediated by the vagus nerve. The presence of food in the stomach produces mechanical stimuli, which result in gastric juice secretion. Stretch receptors in the stomach wall respond to distension of the stomach wall and chemoreceptors respond to protein molecules within the stomach. Impulses travel from these stretch and chemoreceptors via afferent nerve fibres to the submucosal plexus. Here, the nerve fibres synapse with parasympathetic neurones and excitatory impulses are conveyed to the parietal cells.

**Hormonal** (humoral) influences also contribute to the gastric (i.e. non-vagal) phase of gastric juice secretion. Throughout the gut there are several such regulatory hormones (or peptides), many of which are also active as transmitters in the central nervous system. For this reason they are sometimes referred to as **neurohormones, neuropeptides** or **neurotransmitters**.

**Gastrin** is a singular term that in fact refers to a group of chemically similar hormones produced by the G cells in the lateral walls of the gastric glands in the antrum of the stomach. There are two main molecular variations of gastrin: G17, with 17 amino acids (present in quite large amounts) and a smaller quantity of G34, with 34 amino acids. It appears that the terminal five amino acids in the molecule (that is, the terminal pentapeptide) form the critical segment for the stimulation of gastric acid secretion. Hence the synthetic gastric acid stimulant is called pentagastrin.

A small amount of gastrin is produced by the duodenal mucosa. This production is sometimes referred to as the **intestinal phase** of the control of gastric juice secretion. Pathologically, gastrin-secreting tumours may occur in the pancreas but it is unlikely that gastrin is normally produced in the pancreas. Such tumours result in a condition termed Zollinger–Ellison syndrome, in which excessive amounts of gastric acid are produced.

Gastrin is secreted in response to the presence in the stomach of certain foodstuffs referred to as **secretagogues**, examples of which are meat, alcohol, tea, coffee and colas, and also in response to the acetylcholine release as a result of vagal stimulation. **Bombesin** – a regulatory peptide – is also called **gastrin-releasing peptide**. It is produced by P cells throughout the gastrointestinal tract and is a potent releaser of most of the regulatory peptides. It is also found in the brain and pancreas.

Once produced, gastrin enters the gastric capillaries and then the systemic circulation. When it reaches the stomach via the bloodstream it:

- stimulates the parietal cells to produce gastric acid by liberating histamine
- has a minor role in stimulating the chief cells to produce pepsinogen
- stimulates the growth of the gastric and intestinal mucosa
- brings about enhanced contraction of the cardiac sphincter, and hence prevents reflux during gastric activity
- stimulates the secretion of insulin and glucagon when it reaches the pancreas via the systemic circulation.

Gastrin secretion is inhibited by the presence of gastric acid in the antrum of the stomach via a negative feedback mechanism. When gastric acid secretion falls, more gastrin is secreted. Thus, when hypochlorhydria or achlorhydria exists, blood gastrin levels are permanently raised.

Circulating secretin from the duodenum similarly inhibits gastrin release (**Table 5.1.2**), as do cholecystokinin, gastric inhibitory peptide, vasoactive intestinal peptide (see later in chapter) and **somatostatin**. Somatostatin is a regulatory peptide that inhibits the release and action of many gut peptides; it is thought to be antagonistic to bombesin. It is found in the gut, thyroid, pancreas and brain. It inhibits the secretion of growth hormone and so is also called growth-hormone-release inhibitory hormone (GHRIH).

## Control of gastric motility and emptying

The time foods remain in the stomach depends upon their consistency and composition. Carbohydrate foodstuffs, together with liquids, leave fastest, then protein-based foods, and finally fatty foods are the slowest to leave the stomach. Hence foods rich in fats, such as fried fish and chips, and cheese, have the highest satiety value and give a feeling of fullness.

When products of protein digestion and acids enter the duodenum, they initiate the **enterogastric reflex** and this results in a slowing of gastric motility. Gastric contents may start to enter the duodenum some 30 minutes after entering the stomach. Gastric emptying is usually complete after 4–5 hours. This, though, will depend on the individual's emotional state; fear

**Table 5.1.2** Factors influencing gastric juice secretion

| Factors stimulating secretion | Factors inhibiting secretion |
| --- | --- |
| Meat products | Catecholamines: |
| Alcohol | adrenaline (epinephrine) and |
| | noradrenaline (norepinephrine) |
| Caffeine-containing drinks | Vagotomy |
| (e.g. coffee and colas) | Fear |
| | Anxiety |
| Vagal stimulation | Depression |
| Anger | Anticholinergics |
| Hostility | Prostaglandins |
| Histamine | Cholecystokinin ⎤ produced when |
| Acetylcholine | Secretin ⎬ chyme enters the |
| Hypoglycaemia | ⎦ duodenum |
| Gastrin | Somatostatin |
| Bombesin | GIP (gastric inhibitory peptide) |
| | VIP (vasoactive intestinal polypeptide) |

and anxiety, and states of generalized sympathetic nervous system stimulation will result in delayed gastric emptying. This explains why, in the operating theatre, it is sometimes found that the stomach still contains food even though the patient has fasted preoperatively.

As already indicated, the structure of the stomach differs from that of the rest of the tract in that the gastric muscle coat consists of three layers and not two, i.e. it contains circular, longitudinal and oblique muscle fibres. It is this arrangement of muscle fibres that facilitates gastric churning. When food enters the stomach, the muscle layer relaxes reflexly – termed **receptive relaxation**. Peristalsis then occurs, which allows mixing of the gastric contents. This peristaltic activity is most marked at the pylorus (from the Greek word for gatekeeper) and indeed may be visible after feeding in a baby with congenital pyloric stenosis or in the adult with secondary pyloric obstruction.

During gastric emptying, the antrum, pylorus and duodenal cap function as one unit. First the antrum contracts, then the pylorus and finally the duodenal cap. This sequence results in squirts of chyme entering the duodenum, and this is sometimes referred to as the **gastric pump mechanism**. Reflux of chyme into the antrum is prevented by the contraction of the pylorus persisting after the relaxation of the duodenal cap.

Once the stomach contents have entered the duodenum, mild contractions occur that persist and increase in intensity over a period of hours. If no food is received, these waves form hunger contractions, each of which can last up to half an hour and may be painful. People who fast for religious reasons, for example, or those who are required to fast preoperatively, may experience these contractions, and become anxious about their origin. It is helpful to warn fasting patients that they may experience such pains and that this is quite normal.

When glucose and fats enter the duodenum, a regulatory peptide called **gastric inhibitory peptide (GIP)** is secreted by the K cells of the duodenal and jejunal mucosa. The GIP decreases gastric secretion and motility and so is considered to be a physiological entergastrone; it also stimulates the secretion of insulin and is thus sometimes referred to as **glucose-dependent insulin releasing peptide**.

**Vasoactive intestinal polypeptide (VIP)** similarly inhibits gastric motility. It is produced by the D cells in the duodenum and colon and is widely distributed throughout the body. It is vasodilatory and acts as a smooth muscle relaxant. In the gut it stimulates the intestinal secretion of electrolytes and water which follows passively by osmosis.

## CLINICAL APPLICATIONS

### NAUSEA

This term refers to the unpleasant sensation which precedes vomiting. It may be accompanied by one or more of the following features:

- pallor
- sweating
- waterbrash (sudden and profuse secretion of saliva into the mouth)
- antiperistalsis (reverse waves of peristalsis from pylorus to cardia).

### VOMITING

This occurs as a result of a reflex and can be defined as the forceful expulsion of gastric and intestinal contents through the mouth. During the process the larynx is closed and the soft palate rises to close off the nasophrynx and so prevent the inhalation of vomitus. The diaphragm and abdominal wall contract strongly, the pylorus closes and this results in a sharp rise in the intragastric pressure, which causes the sudden expulsion of the gastric contents. The muscles of the stomach itself, and of the oesophagus, play a relatively passive role.

The **vomiting centre** is situated in the reticular formation of the medulla oblongata of the hindbrain. Impulses travel from the vomiting centre to the muscles of the abdominal wall and diaphragm via the extrapyramidal tract, and to the stomach via the vagus nerve.

Vomiting may be stimulated by any of the following:

- Irritation of any part of the gastrointestinal tract. Such irritation may be the result of chemical (e.g. alcohol), microbiological (e.g. staphylococci) or mechanical stimuli (e.g. handling of the viscera during surgery); in this respect vomiting can be regarded as an important protective reflex.
- Impulses from the semicircular canals in the ear, for instance in motion sickness.
- Cerebral tumours or a rise in intracranial pressure.
- Higher cerebral centres, as a response to intense anxiety, fear, unpleasant sights or smells, etc.
- Some drugs, for example digoxin, anaesthetic agents, opiates and emetics such as ipecacuanha. Apomorphine is a potent emetic and, as such, can be used in alcohol aversion therapy.

Useful information can be obtained from an examination of the patient's vomitus: if faeculent, this may indicate an intestinal obstruction; if altered blood is present, then a peptic ulcer may be suspected; if undigested food is present, then pyloric obstruction may be a problem.

Vomiting can present the following problems and so care should be directed towards alleviating the effects these problems pose for patients as well as the cause of vomiting:

- Loss of fluid, and also a loss of those electrolytes present in gastric juice, mainly sodium, chloride and potassium.
- Loss of gastric acid, which can result in a metabolic alkalosis. Similar problems can result from long-term nasogastric drainage, when the gastric aspirate is not replaced.
- Exhaustion and soreness of those muscle groups (described earlier) used in vomiting.

- Weight loss and nutritional disturbances if the vomiting is prolonged.
- A sore throat, as a result of a reflux of acid vomitus, together with an unpleasant taste in the mouth.
- If the vomiting is chronic, metabolic acidosis may be more of a problem than the alkalosis just described. Metabolic acidosis will result when the patient starts to utilize body fat as a source of energy once glycogen stores are depleted. Under these circumstances, ketones (e.g. acetoacetic acid) are produced.
- Inhalation of vomitus. This can lead to aspiration pneumonia. Unconscious patients should always be placed carefully in the semi-prone position so that, if they do vomit, the vomitus will drain out of the mouth by gravity and is less likely to be inhaled into the respiratory tract. Inhalation of vomitus can be a cause of death in the unaccustomed drinker who drinks alcohol heavily (for example, at a party), collapses into an unrousable stupor, vomits without waking and inhales the vomitus. A fuller description of the pathophysiology of nausea and vomiting is provided by Hawthorn (1995).

## The small intestine

The small intestine is a convoluted tube extending from the pyloric sphincter to its junction with the large intestine at the ileocaecal valve. It is approximately 6 m long with a 3.5 cm diameter and lies in the central and lower part of the abdominal cavity.

The wall of the small intestine is composed of four layers, consistent with the remainder of the alimentary tract. However, there are three special features in the mucous membrane lining. These are:

1. The surface of the small intestine forms a series of circular folds, which increase surface area available for absorption of nutrients.
2. It has a velvety appearance due to the presence of fine hair-like projections called villi, each containing a lymph vessel (lacteal) and blood vessels.
3. It is supplied with glands of simple, tubular type which secrete intestinal juice.

The mucosa of the small intestine is simple columnar epithelium with four major cell types:

1. Absorptive cells: produce digestive enzymes and absorb digested food.
2. Goblet cells: produce protective mucus.
3. Granular cells: which protect the intestinal epithelium from bacteria.
4. Endocrine cells: produce regulatory hormones.

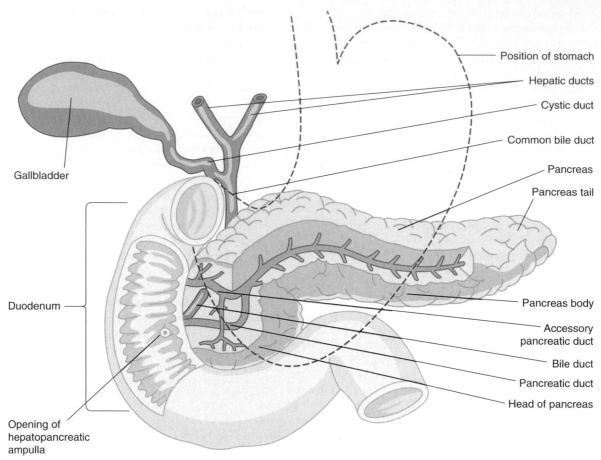

Gallbladder

Duodenum

Opening of
hepatopancreatic
ampulla

Position of stomach

Hepatic ducts

Cystic duct

Common bile duct

Pancreas

Pancreas tail

Pancreas body

Accessory
pancreatic duct

Bile duct

Pancreatic duct

Head of pancreas

**Figure 5.1.12**   Anatomy of the duodenum showing where the gall bladder and pancreas enter

The small intestine consists of three sections (**Fig. 5.1.12**):

- The C-shaped and wider **duodenum**, lying mostly behind the peritoneum. This part is 20–25 cm long. (The name duodenum derives from the Latin word for 12 fingers; in the adult, the length of the duodenum is about equal to the width of 12 fingers.) The loop of this C-shaped area surrounds the pancreas.
- The **jejunum** (meaning empty) forms approximately 40% of the remainder of the small intestine.
- The **ileum** (meaning twisted) is a slightly longer tube making up the final 60%.

The jejunum and ileum are both suspended by mesentery, which carries the blood and nerve supply to these areas. The two areas are, in general, not morphologically distinct. However, some differences are evident between the proximal jejunum and the terminal ileum, for example the jejunum has somewhat thicker walls which are more vascular and folded, whereas the ileum is more sparsely folded on its luminal surface (**Fig. 5.1.13**). Furthermore, in the jejunum there are solitary protective lymph nodes; in

the ileum, however, these are aggregated into groups called **Peyer's patches**.

Most of the small intestine is attached to the posterior abdominal wall by a double fold of serous membrane called peritoneum (**Fig. 5.1.14**). The peritoneum, when folded away from the posterior abdominal wall, looks rather like a fan and supports the blood vessels, lymphatics and nerves that supply the small intestine; this portion of peritoneum is called the **mesentery**. A further fold of peritoneum extends from the liver to the stomach and is called the **lesser omentum**. The **greater omentum** hangs rather like an apron in front of the intestines and is reflected off the stomach. The peritoneum, as well as carrying blood vessels and nerves, serves a protective function and can 'wall off' areas of infection or inflammation, and so prevent the spread of peritonitis.

The major role of the small intestine relates to digestion and absorption. The contractile activity of the intestines mixes and propels the foodstuff towards the ileum.

About 50% of the small intestine can be removed surgically before there is an appreciable effect upon digestion and absorption. Patients who undergo surgery – for whatever reason – that leaves them with

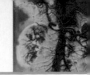

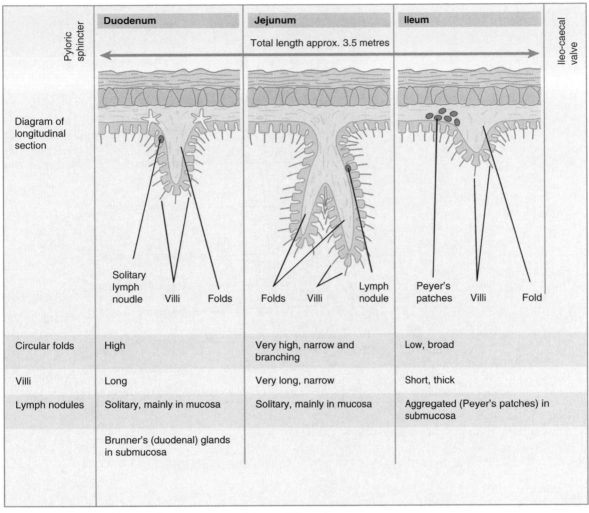

**Figure 5.1.13** The differences between areas of the small intestine

25% or less of their small intestine can survive only with total parenteral feeding, i.e. the infusion into a large vein (usually the superior vena cava) of amino acids, lipids, glucose, vitamins, electrolytes and trace elements in sufficient quantities to meet their full nutritional needs for the rest of their lives (Finlay, 1997).

## The duodenum

By the time the chyme enters the duodenum, salivary amylase has acted upon cooked starch to begin its conversion into maltose and dextrins, and pepsin has acted upon proteins starting their breakdown into polypeptides. The duodenum does not itself secrete digestive enzymes. It does, though, secrete hormones, some of which have already been referred to (e.g. gastric inhibitory peptide, vasoactive intestinal polypeptide, cholecystokinin and motilin).

The duodenum receives the secretions of the pancreatic and common bile duct at a point called the sphincter of Oddi, which lies about 10 cm below the

pylorus at the level of the first to third lumbar vertebrae (L1–3). The secretions produced by both the pancreas and the liver and delivered to the duodenum are alkaline, having a pH in the range 7.8–8.4. There is therefore a sharp change in the pH of the intestinal contents (from the gastric pH of 1.5–3.0) after the addition of bile and pancreatic juice to the duodenal pH of approximately 7.0. The digestive enzymes in the small intestine are, like all enzymes, pH specific, i.e. there is a critical pH for their optimal activity, and act best at a pH of 6.5–7.0. This change in the intestinal pH in the area between the stomach and the duodenum does not favour the reproduction of pathogenic microorganisms.

The first few centimetres of the duodenum (the duodenal cap) receive acid chyme from the stomach and this tissue, therefore (like that of the stomach), must be protected to prevent ulcer formation. In the first part of the duodenum, there are a large number of mucus-secreting glands in the submucosa, called **Brünner's glands**, which are characteristic of the duodenum. The

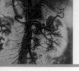
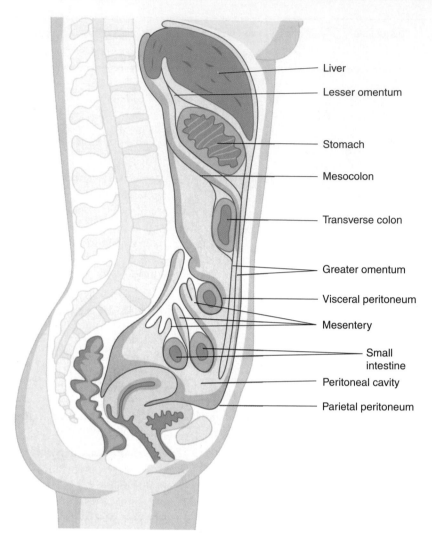

Liver

Lesser omentum

Stomach

Mesocolon

Transverse colon

Greater omentum

Visceral peritoneum

Mesentery

Small intestine

Peritoneal cavity

Parietal peritoneum

**Figure 5.1.14** Sagittal view of the abdomen showing the visceral and parietal peritoneum and the mesentery

mucus is secreted into the bases of the intestinal crypts, that is, into the areas between the mucosal folds.

## The exocrine pancreas

The pancreas is a gland with both endocrine and exocrine functions, and is therefore described as a mixed gland. Only the exocrine function will be described here (see Chapter 2.5 for details of pancreatic endocrine function).

Structurally, the pancreas resembles the salivary glands. It is soft, friable and pink, consisting of a head enclosed within the loop of the duodenum, a body and a tail. The whole lies horizontally below the stomach, the tail extending towards the right of the abdomen (**see Fig. 5.1.12**).

The pancreas has a major role in digestion. Its exocrine digestive function is served by **acinar cells**, which structurally resemble cells of the salivary glands. These cells form and store **zymogen granules**, which consist of protein-based digestive enzymes. These

enzymes are discharged in response to stimulation, mainly hormonal, and are secreted into the pancreatic duct. This duct joins with the common bile duct to form a slightly dilated area called the ampulla of Vater, which then empties into the duodenum via the sphincter of Oddi.

### Pancreatic juice

Between 1.5 and 2 L of juice are secreted daily (most of which is later reabsorbed), with a pH of 8.0–8.4 (it should be remembered that this does not represent the final pH of the duodenal contents, as mixing with acidic chyme will lower the ultimate duodenal pH). The pancreas produces two secretions depending on hormonal stimuli: a copious watery secretion and a scantier one rich in enzymes; a mixture of the two secretions is always released.

### Profuse watery secretion

This contains large amounts of hydrogen carbonate ions, which are manufactured by the cells of the

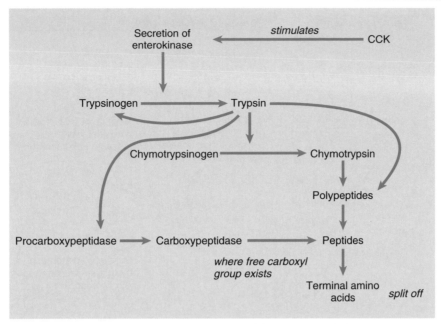

**Figure 5.1.15** Summary of activity of the pancreatic proteolytic enzymes. CCK, cholecystokinin

pancreatic duct in the presence of the enzyme carbonic anhydrase by a process similar to that described earlier for the production of gastric acid. Hydrogen ions are formed in the process and blood leaving the pancreas is therefore more acid than the blood entering it. This is to some extent balanced by the hydrogen carbonate added to the blood during the formation of gastric acid by the stomach. In addition, this watery secretion contains ions of sodium, potassium, calcium, magnesium, chloride, sulphate and phosphate, plus some albumin and globulin.

### Scanty enzyme-rich secretion

Three proteolytic enzymes are produced by the acinar cells of the pancreas. For the reason described earlier in relation to pepsin – namely, to prevent autodigestion – they are secreted in the inactive form. In addition, it is thought that there is a trypsin inhibitor present in the pancreas. **Figure 5.1.15** summarizes the activity of the pancreatic proteolytic enzymes.

**Trypsinogen** is converted into the active form **trypsin** by the enzyme **enterokinase** (also called enteropeptidase) secreted by the duodenal mucosa. The amount of enterokinase produced is increased by the presence of circulating cholecystokinin (CCK).

Trypsin acts on proteins and polypeptides, breaking bonds between the amino acids and thus forming peptides (short sections of amino acid units). Trypsin, once formed, has three further actions:

- It activates trypsinogen to form more trypsin.
- It activates chymotrypsinogen to form chymotrypsin, which has the same proteolytic functions as trypsin.

- In addition, trypsin activates procarboxypeptidase to form active carboxypeptidase.

**Carboxypeptidase** acts on peptides. Whatever their individual molecular structure, all amino acids have an amine group and a carboxyl group. Single amino acids bond together by means of the amine group of one amino acid joining to the carboxyl group of another forming a peptide linkage. Carboxypeptidase splits off the terminal amino acid from the end of a peptide, acting on the free carboxyl group. It thus produces free amino acids.

Pancreatic juice also contains **pancreatic amylase** (sometimes called diastase). This acts on starch and converts it to maltose.

The enzyme **pancreatic lipase** acts on triglycerides, which are neutral dietary fats (triglycerides: molecules made up of three fatty acids and glycerol) and converts them into single fatty acids and glycerol once they have been emulsified by the action of bile salts.

**Ribonuclease** and **deoxyribonuclease (RNAase** and **DNAase)** act on RNA and DNA, respectively, and convert them into free nucleotides.

The secretion of pancreatic juice is primarily under hormonal control, although the vagus nerve has a minor influence (**Fig. 5.1.16**).

### Control of pancreatic juice secretion

**Secretin.** Secretion hormone is produced by S cells deep in the mucosal glands in the wall of the duodenum and upper jejunum in response to acid chyme entering that area. Secretin enters the systemic venous circulation and eventually arrives back at the pancreas

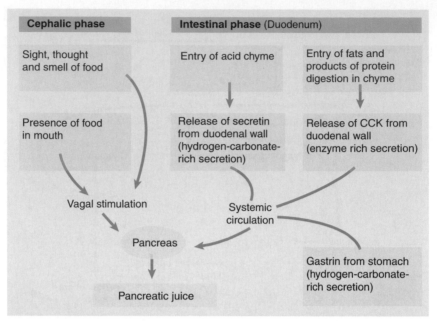

**Figure 5.1.16** Flow chart to illustrate pancreatic juice secretion. CCK, cholecystokinin

via the pancreatic artery, where it brings about the production of a copious watery secretion that is rich in hydrogen carbonate (bicarbonate) ions but low in enzymes. Hydrogen carbonate levels in pancreatic juice may be up to five times greater than in plasma, and the concentration rises as secretion increases.

The actions of secretin can be summarized as follows:

- It increases the secretion of water and hydrogen carbonate by the pancreas.
- It augments the actions of cholecystokinin.
- It decreases gastric secretion and motility.

In molecular terms, secretin is similar to vasoactive intestinal polypeptide, gastric inhibitory peptide and glucagon.

**Cholecystokin**. The molecular structure of cholecystokinin is very similar to that of gastrin. It acts not only in the gut but also as a neurotransmitter in the central nervous system. Cholecystokinin is a hormone. It is secreted by the columnar cells of the duodenal and jejunal mucosal crypts in response to products of protein digestion and fats entering the duodenum. It circulates via the systemic circulation and arrives back at the pancreas, where it stimulates the acinar cells to discharge their zymogen granules; hence it leads to the release of an enzyme-rich secretion. In summary, cholecystokinin:

- stimulates the secretion of an enzyme-rich secretion from the pancreas
- augments the activity of secretin
- slows gastric emptying and inhibits gastric secretion
- increases the secretion of enterokinase

- stimulates glucagon secretion
- stimulates the motility of the small intestine and colon
- causes the gall bladder to contract and therefore to release bile.

The secretion of secretin and cholecystokinin is referred to as the **intestinal phase of pancreatic secretion**.

**Gastrin**. The release of **gastrin** into the circulation by the stomach stimulates the production of a pancreatic secretion rich in bicarbonates. This is sometimes called the **gastric phase of pancreatic secretion**. This is of only minor importance in terms of pancreatic secretion.

**Vagal stimulations**. The **cephalic phase of pancreatic juice secretion** refers to the production of pancreatic juice as a result of **vagal stimulation** brought about by the sight, thought or smell of food, or by the presence of food in the mouth.

Acetylcholine, released as a result of vagal stimulation, acts directly on the acinar cells, bringing about the release of an enzyme-rich secretion similar to that produced in response to stimulation by cholecystokinin. Vagal stimulation is not of major importance in pancreatic secretion.

## The role of bile in digestion

The formation of bile will be further referred to in Chapter 5.2 (on liver physiology); however, the role of bile in digestion will be discussed here.

Bile contains no digestive enzymes; neither does the liver secrete any digestive hormones. The main

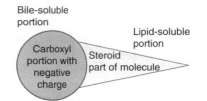

importance of bile in digestion lies in its role in the emulsification of fats and the consequent absorption of lipids and of fat-soluble vitamins and iron.

Bile is a slightly syrupy fluid, with a colour range of greeny-yellow to brown. It consists of water (97%) and bile salts (0.7%). The water contains mucin and hydrogen carbonate. Electrolytically, bile is very similar to pancreatic juice, with a pH of 7.8–8.0. The total volume secreted daily is between 0.5 and 1.0 L.

## Bile salts

The bile salts (see Chapter 5.2) make up 0.7% of the total volume of bile, there being some 2–4 g in total in the body. Bile salts are formed from cholic and deoxycholic acid. Both these acids are steroids manufactured by the liver from cholesterol. In the liver, cholic acid is conjugated with taurine and glycine, which are acid derivatives of the amino acid cystine, to form **taurocholic acid** and **glycocholic acid**. The term 'conjugation' refers to the process during which the substances are joined together chemically with the elimination of water. The bile acids form bile salts with sodium and potassium in solution in the bile, e.g. sodium taurocholate and sodium glycocholate.

Bile salts:

- deodorize faeces
- activate lipase (in the small intestine) and other proteolytic enzymes. (Lipase is water soluble and for its optimal activity fats must be broken down, i.e. emulsified, into small droplets.)
- have a detergent-like action on fats, i.e. they reduce the surface tension of fat droplets and therefore contribute to the emulsification of fats.

The steroid part of the bile salt molecule is lipid soluble and will therefore dissolve in fat droplets. The bile salt molecule also has a water-soluble carboxyl portion, which remains on the surface of the fat droplet and that carries a negative charge. This dissolves in the watery portion of bile. As negative charges repel one another, the charges on the surfaces of the fat droplets cause them to remain separated into small droplets, i.e. they emulsify. Large fat droplets are broken into smaller droplets mechanically as well as chemically due to intestinal activity (**Fig. 5.1.17**).

Bile salts combine with lipids plus lecithin and cholesterol to form **micelles**, which are water-soluble complexes about 1 μm in diameter. Micelles allow fats to be absorbed more easily. If bile salts do not reach the intestine (e.g. in posthepatic jaundice), are lost (e.g. following an ileostomy) or are not produced for some reason, then about 25% of ingested fat may be lost in the stools, which will consequently be bulky and have an offensive odour.

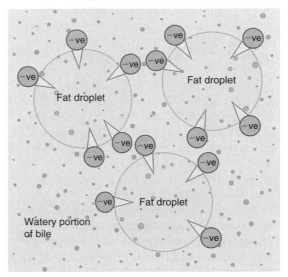

**Figure 5.1.17** Diagrammatic representation of the emulsification of fats

## Bile pigments

These make up 0.2% of the total composition of bile. Bile pigments – mainly **bilirubin** and a small amount of **biliverdin** – are formed from the breakdown of old red blood cells in the reticuloendothelial system – the mononuclear phagocytic system (see Chapter 4.1 for fuller details).

The pigments travel to the liver bound to plasma albumin, where they are conjugated, usually with glucuronic acid, in the presence of the enzyme glucuronyl transferase to form water-soluble bilirubin diglucuronide. This substance enters the bile, giving it its golden colour and, during its passage through the intestine, is subjected to oxidation and acted upon by bacteria. Eventually, **stercobilinogen** is formed, some of which is absorbed into the bloodstream and ultimately excreted by the kidneys, where it is called **urobilinogen**. The remainder within the bowel is converted into **stercobilin** by bacterial action. This is a brown pigment, which colours the faeces.

Bile contains cholesterol, which forms 0.06% of its total composition. Excess cholesterol from the body is excreted in the bile. In addition, bile contains:

- fatty acids
- lecithin
- inorganic salts
- alkaline phosphatase
- excretory products of steroid-based hormones.

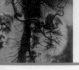

When the normal concentration of cholesterol rises, crystals of cholesterol form within the biliary system and act as nuclei for the deposition of calcium and phosphate salts. This eventually leads to the formation of **gallstones**. About 10% of the middle-aged population of the UK have some gallstones, even though these may not be clinically apparent. Approximately 85% of all gallstones formed are cholesterol based.

If the common bile duct becomes blocked by one of these gallstones, neither bile salts nor bile pigments can enter the duodenum and the build-up of pressure and distension within the gall bladder, as well as the functional spasmodic contractions of the smooth muscle in the bile duct, can result in severe pain (biliary colic). The latter contractions may cause the stone to pass into the duodenum and hence to be eliminated in the faeces. Bile pigments accumulate in the blood and eventually cause the yellow coloration of the skin, which is characteristic of obstructive jaundice. Bile salts, following a similar path, may cause intense itching of the skin. Frequent bathing and the use of a soothing lotion, such as calamine, is sometimes helpful to the patient.

Non-invasive treatment of gallstones is by either gallstone-dissolving drugs, such as methyl tert-butyl ether (MTBE) or chenodeoxycholic acid, or by lithotripsy, whereby shock waves are used to fragment the stones. Surgery is the method of choice only when neither of these non-invasive methods is appropriate to the individual patient. Laparoscopic surgery has markedly reduced postoperative discomfort and shortened hospital stay.

Patients having T-tube drainage of their bile duct after cholecystectomy and exploration of the common bile duct may lose a significant amount of electrolytes, especially sodium, which requires replacement.

## Control of bile secretion and release

The secretion of bile is under the influence of both hormonal and nervous stimuli (**Fig. 5.1.18**). The major stimulus for bile release is cholecystokinin, which is liberated into the circulation in response to fats and products of protein digestion entering the duodenum. It circulates to the gall bladder and there causes contraction of the wall and simultaneously relaxation of the sphincter of Oddi. Substances that bring about contraction of the gall bladder are referred to as **cholagogues**. Once the gall bladder has discharged its contents into the duodenum, further bile will flow directly into the gut from the hepatic cells via the hepatic ducts. This happens continuously in patients who have undergone a cholecystectomy. Stimulation of the vagus nerve during digestion has an action similar to that of cholecystokinin.

The amount of bile secreted by the hepatic cells largely depends upon the blood levels of circulating bile salts. After passage through the intestine in the bile, about 97% of bile salts are reabsorbed in the ileum into the portal circulation, and recycled back to the liver. This is referred to as the **enterohepatic circulation of bile salts (see Fig. 5.2.11)**. The remainder is lost from the body in the faeces. After a meal, therefore, once the products of digestion have reached the ileum, bile salts are reabsorbed into the blood, resulting in a high blood level of bile salts. High blood levels of bile salts stimulate the hepatic cells to increase their own secretion. This is an example of autostimulation. Substances that increase the secretion of bile are referred to as **choleretics**.

A further stimulus to hepatic production of bile salts is thought to be an increase in liver blood flow following a meal.

## Intestinal juice

Juice collected from the intestine contains some digestive enzymes, peptidases and disaccharidases, derived from the break-up of epithelial cells.

The juice is secreted by the jejunum and ileum. The enzymes present in intestinal juice are responsible for the completion of digestion. Up to 3 L of this secretion, with a pH of 7.8–8.0, are normally produced each day by the small intestine in response to local mechanical stimuli and to the chemical stimuli of partially digested food products on the intestinal mucosa. In addition, secretion of intestinal juice is stimulated by circulating vasoactive intestinal polypeptide, and also to some extent by emotional disturbances.

Intestinal juice is rich in mucus, some of which is added by the Brünner's glands in the first few centimetres of the duodenum. The remainder of the watery juice, rich in mucus, is secreted by Lieberkühn's glands in the jejunum and ileum.

The surface area of the small intestine is increased by visible folding of the mucosa into *valvulae conniventes*, and by the presence of finger-like processes, each about 0.5 mm long, called **villi**. These features serve to increase the surface area to 600 times that of a non-folded tube of the same length. The total surface area is further increased by the presence of microvilli on the villous surfaces. This large surface area, of about 200 m$^2$, increases the efficiency of digestion and absorption carried out in the jejunum and ileum. The mucosa of the small intestine is invaginated between adjacent villi to form pits, called the **crypts of Lieberkühn**, where the mucus-secreting glands are located.

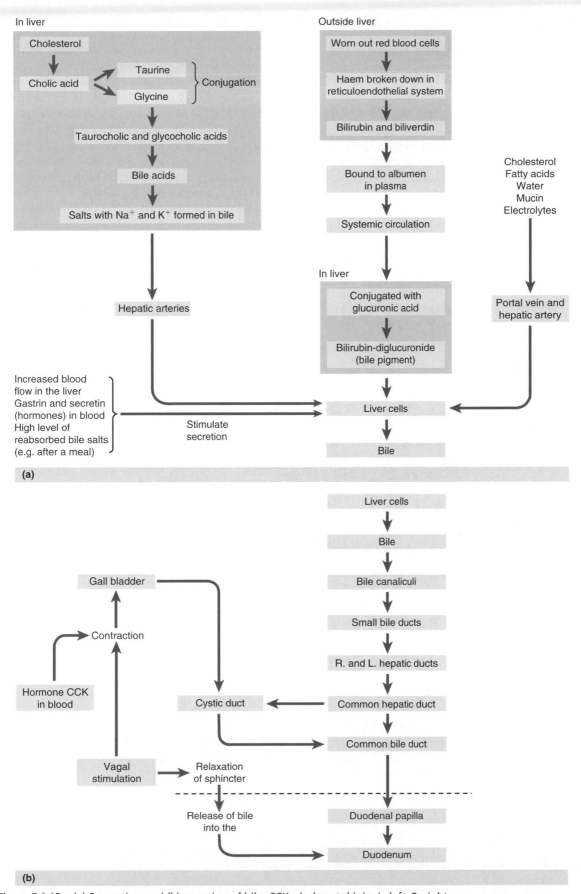

**Figure 5.1.18** (a) Formation and (b) secretion of bile. CCK, cholecystokinin; L, left; R, right

## *Villi* (**Fig. 5.1.19**)

There are 20–40 villi/mm² of the intestinal mucosa. Each villus consists of a finger-like process, the surface of which is covered by simple columnar epithelium continuous with that of the crypts. Within each villus there is a central **lacteal,** which contains lymph and which empties into the local lymphatic circulation; each also has a capillary blood supply, which links with both the hepatic and portal veins. The surface of the villus is usually covered with a layer of mucus that prevents autodigestion by proteolytic enzymes.

Villi contain two main cell types: the **goblet cells,** secreting mucus and situated mainly in the crypts, and the **enterocytes,** which are involved in both digestion and absorption. Enterocytes are tall columnar cells, their nuclei lying towards their bases. Their surfaces are each covered with up to 3000 **microvilli** (microscopic finger-like processes), which increase the villous

surface area. These microvilli give what is known as a brush border to the villus. Enterocytes have many mitochondria to provide for the high-energy demands of enzyme secretion and absorption.

Cell division in the villi is rapid (that is, these cells have a high rate of mitosis) and occurs in the crypts. Cells gradually migrate up from the crypts over a period of about 30 hours to replace those enterocytes being shed from the tips of the villi. There is a very high rate of enterocyte turnover, mainly as a result of the area being subjected to a great deal of friction by the gut contents.

Between enterocytes, at intervals, are situated lymphocytes and plasma cells. These latter secrete IgA, an immunoglobulin that protects the gastrointestinal tract from pathogens. There are also cells in the intestinal wall which secrete serotonin (5-hydroxytryptamine 5-HT). It is known to stimulate the contraction of smooth muscle and may thus have a role in intestinal motility. Identification and characterization of 5-HT receptors has recently led to the development

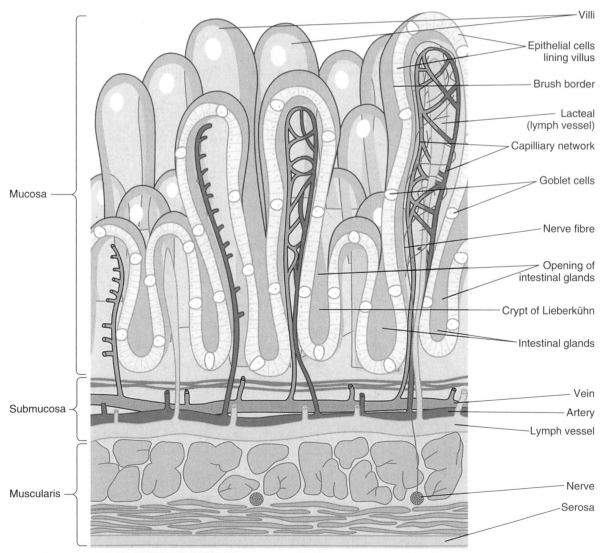

**Figure 5.1.19**   Anatomy (cross-section) of villi

of new pharmaceutical agents that aim to treat gastro-intestinal motility conditions, such as irritable bowel syndrome (Farthing, 1999).

The villi contain a small number of smooth muscle fibres originating from the muscularis coat of the small intestine. Contraction of these muscle fibres assists lymphatic drainage in the central lacteals. The villi also move in response to the mechanical stimulation of food passing along the tract.

### CLINICAL APPLICATIONS

In starvation, the enterocytes shrink, the net result being a decrease in the height of the villi by up to half. The effect of this is to decrease the absorptive powers of the small intestine. Conversely, villi increase in height when actively absorbing nutrients.

## Intestinal enzyme secretion

The outer membrane (i.e. that projects into the lumen of the gut) of the enterocytes contains the remaining enzymes necessary to complete digestion. The juice produced by the glands in the crypts is practically enzyme free, contrary to past theories. Any enzymes present in the actual intestinal juice are probably released from disintegrating shed enterocytes.

### Enzymes present in the enterocyte membrane

- **Aminopeptidases** act on peptides, splitting off amino acids by acting on the amine group at the ends of peptide chains, breaking the peptide bond and thus releasing free terminal amino acids.
- **Dipeptidases** act on dipeptides (i.e. units of two joined amino acids) to break them into single amino acids.
- **Maltase** acts on maltose to convert it into glucose.
- **Lactase** acts on lactose to convert it into glucose and galactose.
- **Sucrase** acts on sucrose to convert it into glucose and fructose.

Digestion is now complete:

- Proteins have been broken down into amino acids.
- Fats have been broken down into fatty acids and glycerol.
- Carbohydrates have been broken down into monosaccharides – glucose, fructose and galactose.

Ingested foodstuffs have been digested and rendered into a form in which they can be absorbed.

## Absorption

Each day, approximately 8–9 L of water and 1 kg of nutrients pass across the wall of the gut from its lumen into its blood supply. This process requires energy, which is derived from the oxidation of glucose and fatty acids. The energy demands of the gastrointestinal tract are extremely high for both secretion and absorption, and also to provide for the rapid rate of mitosis in the epithelial cells lining the tract.

## Transport of nutrients

**Transport of nutrients** across the cell membranes of the gastrointestinal epithelial cells can be either active or passive.

### Active transport

This requires the expenditure of energy. It occurs when the concentration of the substance in the gut is less than the concentration of the substance in the plasma; transport must thus occur against a concentration gradient.

Vitamin B12 and iron are actively absorbed into the bloodstream from the ileum, as are sodium ions, glucose, galactose and amino acids. These substances all require **carrier molecules** to facilitate their absorption. Water follows the passage of these substances passively along an osmotic gradient.

### Passive transport

This requires no energy consumption. Water, lipids, drugs and some electrolytes and vitamins are examples of substances transported passively from the gut into the blood. Passive transport is influenced by concentration and electrical gradients. Some substances require a carrier molecule to assist their passage across the cell membranes of the gut wall. When this carrier-mediated transport occurs passively, it is referred to as **facilitated diffusion**, an example of which is the transport of glucose molecules into cells under the influence of insulin.

## Osmotic transport of water

The 8–9 L of water that are transported daily across the gut wall and reabsorbed into the blood passively follow the passage of actively or passively transported water-soluble substances to restore osmotic balance. If the transport of water required energy, our present average dietary intake would be insufficient to meet this need, and we would have to increase our intake considerably in order to reabsorb water.

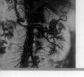

## Absorption of nutrients and minerals

### Monosaccharides (Fig. 5.1.20)

Each day, approximately 500 g of monosaccharides are absorbed; this will vary according to the individual's dietary habits. All such absorption has occurred by the time the terminal ileum is reached.

Monosaccharides pass from the gut lumen across the enterocytes on the villi into the villous capillaries, and thence into the hepatic portal vein. Their active transport is facilitated by a high concentration of sodium ions on the surface of the enterocytes (low sodium levels at this point inhibit transport). Glucose and sodium ions are thought to share the same carrier molecule, which facilitates their transport across the cell membrane of the enterocyte. The concentration of sodium ions *inside* the enterocyte is always low. Sodium moves into the cell along a concentration gradient and

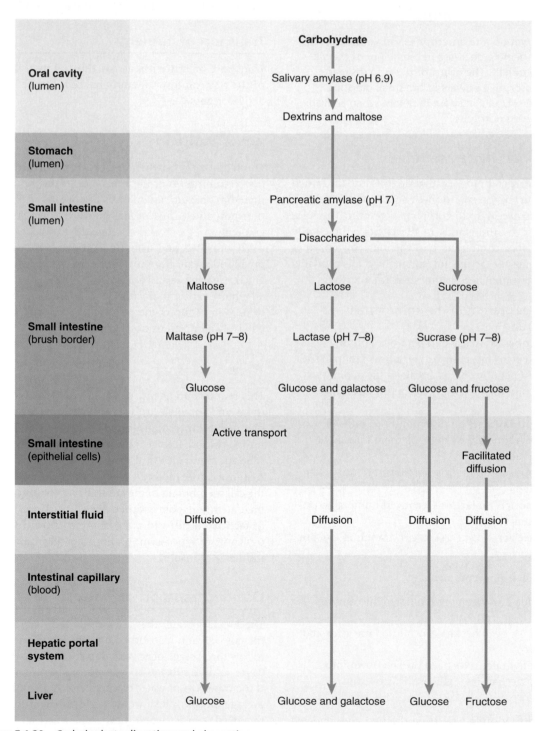

**Figure 5.1.20**  Carbohydrate digestion and absorption

glucose moves with it; sodium is then pumped actively out of the enterocyte into the extracellular spaces of the villi, and glucose moves with it; then both substances pass into the capillary network. The active absorption of sodium ions into the blood is therefore crucial to glucose absorption. Galactose and glucose share a common carrier; fructose, however, requires a different carrier, and its transport is not influenced by sodium.

## Metabolism of monosaccharides

Monosaccharides are transported via the hepatic portal vein to the liver. Here, galactose and fructose are converted into glucose (**Fig. 5.1.21**). Some glucose is converted by the liver under the influence of insulin

into **glycogen**; this is referred to as **glycogenesis**. About 100 g of glycogen (sufficient to maintain blood glucose levels for up to 24 hours) are stored in the liver. Glycogen is also stored within skeletal muscle, and this glycogen, through the action of muscle phosphorylase, can be reconverted to glucose to provide the energy for muscle contraction (see Chapter 3.2).

Glucose surplus to the body's needs for the maintenance of blood glucose levels and glycogen stores is converted by the liver into fat, and stored in fat (adipose) depots throughout the body. Blood glucose is maintained at a resting level of 3.5–5.5 mmol/L by a series of mechanisms described in Chapter 2.6. When the blood glucose level falls, liver glycogen can be

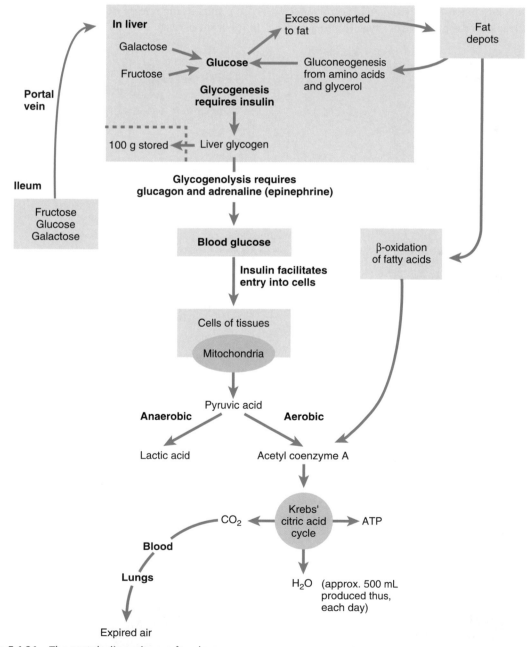

**Figure 5.1.21**   The metabolic pathways for glucose

broken down (**glycogenolysis**) to reform glucose under the influence of glucagon and adrenaline in the presence of the liver enzyme phosphorylase. If glycogen stores are depleted, the liver can manufacture glucose from non-carbohydrate sources (amino acids and glycerol). This process is known as **gluconeogenesis** and occurs only in the liver.

When circulating glucose arrives at the tissues, insulin facilitates its uptake by the cells. This process was referred to earlier as an example of facilitated diffusion. The role of insulin is described fully in Chapter 2.6.

Oxidation of glucose to form energy occurs in the mitochondria of the cells. The glucose is first broken down into pyruvic acid, a process that does not require oxygen (i.e. it is anaerobic). Pyruvic acid is converted aerobically (i.e. in the presence of oxygen) into acetyl

co-enzyme A (acetyl CoA), which then undergoes a series of biochemical changes catalysed by enzymes; these changes are referred to as the **Krebs' citric acid cycle**. They result in the formation of adenosine triphosphate (ATP), water and carbon dioxide. Energy is 'stored' in the adenosine triphosphate molecule. A relatively large amount of energy is released when one of the phosphate bonds in adenosine triphosphate is broken to form adenosine diphosphate (ADP) and free phosphate.

If insufficient oxygen is available for the conversion of pyruvic acid to acetyl co-enzyme A, then lactic acid is formed. Thus, in hypoxic conditions such as shock, blood lactic acid levels may rise and result in a metabolic acidosis. The oxidation of 1 g of glucose results in the release of 16 kj (4 kcal) of energy in the form of heat.

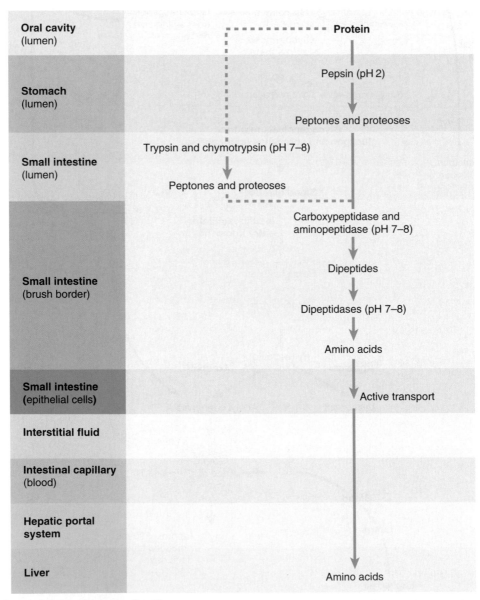

**Figure 5.1.22**  Summary of protein digestion

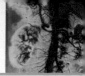

## Amino acids

**Figure 5.1.22** summarizes the digestion of proteins. Each day, approximately 200 g of amino acids are absorbed from the ileum. Absorption of at least 50 g per day is required to remain in positive nitrogen balance and to meet the needs of the adult body for protein for growth and repair of tissues. The amount required to maintain nitrogen balance varies during the life cycle. It is greater, for example, during childhood and in pregnancy.

There appears to be three separate mechanisms for acidic, basic and neutral amino acids involving different carrier molecules. As described earlier for glucose, absorption of amino acids seems to be linked to, and facilitated by, sodium absorption. Sodium on the surface of the enterocyte membrane appears to increase the affinity of the carrier molecules for amino acids. Once the amino acids have entered the enterocyte they appear to move passively into the blood capillaries of the villus and hence pass to the hepatic portal vein.

Most of the absorption of amino acids occurs in the first part of the small intestine. Some amino acids may enter the colon, where they are metabolized by the colonic bacteria.

The 10–20 g of protein present in the faeces is derived from dead bacteria and shed gut epithelial cells.

Proteins, unlike fats and carbohydrates, cannot be stored by the body. Once absorbed into the blood, amino acids enter a common circulating pool (**Fig. 5.1.23**), from where appropriate acids are taken to build up proteins for cell reproduction and growth, the formation of enzymes and hormones, and plasma proteins.

The liver can interconvert amino acids, that is it can use the eight amino acids essential in adults to synthesize other non-essential amino acids. The essential amino acids must be present in the diet for this to occur.

Amino acids can be used to meet energy demands once stores of glycogen are depleted. The oxidation of 1 g of amino acids results in the production of

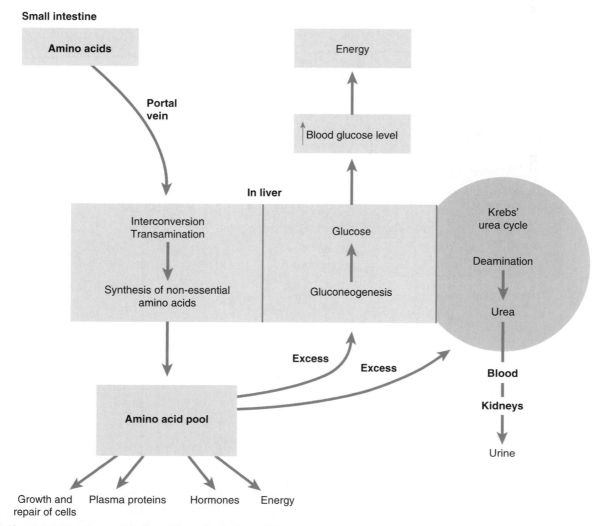

**Figure 5.1.23** The metabolic pathway for amino acids

16 kj (4 kcal) of heat energy. Most amino acids can be converted by the liver into glucose (gluconeogenesis) and any excess amino acids are broken down by the liver by the process of **deamination**. The nitrogen portion of the amino acid is converted into ammonia, which is then converted into urea, via a series of biochemical reactions termed the **Krebs' urea cycle**. Thus the more protein we take in our diet, the more urea will be produced. Urea enters the blood and is excreted in the urine.

## CLINICAL APPLICATIONS

In renal failure, the kidneys are unable to excrete the urea and so blood levels rise, resulting in uraemia. In liver failure, the liver is unable to form urea although it can form ammonia. High levels of this toxic substance build up in the blood, resulting in hepatic coma. In both renal and liver failure, therefore, treatment involves limitation of the dietary intake of protein.

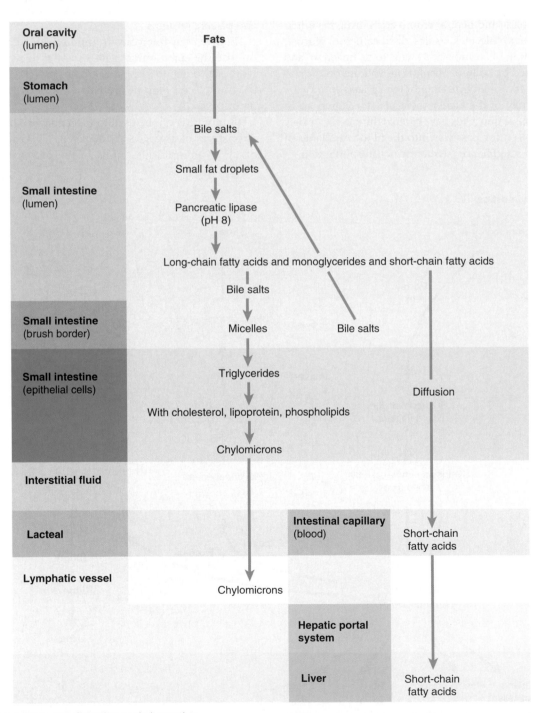

**Figure 5.1.24** Fat digestion and absorption

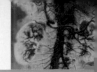

## Fats (**Fig. 5.1.24**)

Each day, about 80 g of fat are absorbed from the small intestine, mostly in the duodenum. Micelles are formed in the duodenum by the action of bile salts on lipids. Micelles are spheres of 3–10 nm in diameter, comprising fatty acids, monoglycerides and cholesterol, which form the transport mechanism for fats. They move to the microvilli on the enterocytes and there they discharge their contents, which enter the enterocytes by passive diffusion. The bile salt portion of the micelle remains within the gut where it is available for further micelle formation.

Short-chain fatty acids (i.e. those with fewer than 10–12 carbon atoms) pass from the enterocyte into the capillary network and thence to the hepatic portal vein, travelling as free fatty acids (**Fig. 5.1.25**). This route accounts for about 20% of fat transport. Longer-chain fatty acids (i.e. those with more than 12 carbon atoms) are resynthesized within the enterocyte

to triglyceride. They become coated with a layer of lipoprotein, cholesterol and phospholipid to form **chylomicrons**. These complexes enter the central lacteals of the villi. The creamy substance so formed in the lacteal is termed **chyle**. This enters the lymphatic circulation and hence, eventually, the bloodstream.

Faeces contain about 5% fat, most of which is derived from bacteria.

### DEVELOPMENTAL ISSUES

Infants lose 10–15% fat in their stools as their ability to absorb fats is not well developed at birth.

Cholesterol is found in the blood, mainly in combination with a protein carrier, as lipoproteins, of which there are three main forms: **high-density lipoproteins (HDLs)**, formed of a large amount of protein combined with a little cholesterol; cholesterol is carried

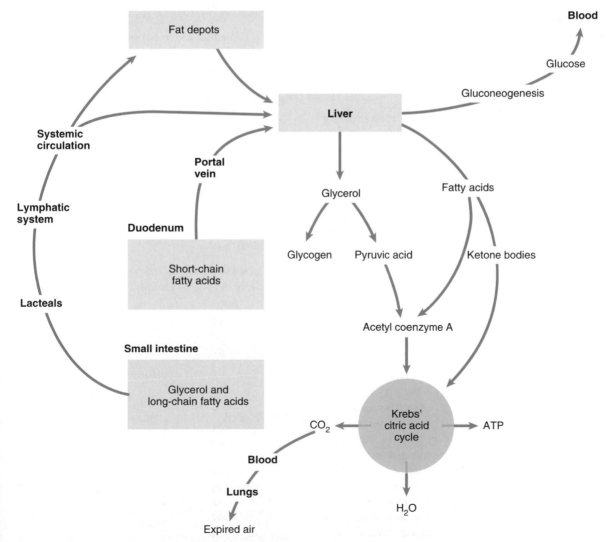

**Figure 5.1.25**　The metabolic pathways for fats

to the liver for excretion in this form, and **low-density lipoproteins (LDLs)** and **very-low-density lipoproteins (VLDLs)**, formed of a little protein combined with a large amount of cholesterol, which represent cholesterol on its way to the tissues, where it is used for the synthesis of bile acids, steroid hormones and cell membranes; 60–70% of the total serum cholesterol is carried in combination with low-density lipoproteins.

### CLINICAL APPLICATIONS

It is thought that it is in the form of low-density lipoproteins and very-low-density lipoproteins that cholesterol is laid down in atheromatous plaques in the arterial wall. The ratio of high-density lipoproteins to low-density and very-low-density lipoproteins has been shown to be increased in the blood of vegetarians, in those whose fat intake is largely polyunsaturated, and in those who take regular exercise to keep fit; this ratio is reduced in those who smoke cigarettes. It is possible that a high ratio of high-density lipoproteins to low-density and very-low-density lipoproteins may afford protection in some way from ischaemic heart disease. For a review of the role of dietary fat see Holmes (1990).

### Fat metabolism (**Fig. 5.1.25**)

The oxidation of 1 g of fat results in the release of 38 kj (9 kcal) of heat energy. Absorbed fat not required for the production of energy is stored in the adipose tissue of fat depots as neutral fat, i.e. triglycerides. These depots are situated in subcutaneous and retroperitoneal tissue.

When fats are required for energy, they are mobilized from the depots under the influence of hormones, e.g. growth hormone or cortisol, and are carried as triglycerides in the blood to the liver. Here they are broken down to fatty acids and glycerol, and released into the bloodstream for use by the cells. The liver can convert glycerol, but not fatty acids, to glucose by gluconeogenesis. Glycerol is converted either to glycogen for storage or pyruvic acid, which enters the Krebs' citric acid cycle (**see Fig. 5.1.25**).

The fatty acids are converted into acetyl co-enzyme A in the presence of oxygen and glucose. This then enters the Krebs' citric acid cycle (mentioned earlier under glucose metabolism). If glucose is not present (as might be the case in starvation or uncontrolled diabetes mellitus), acetyl co-enzyme A metabolism is deranged. In the liver, molecules of acetyl co-enzyme A pair, resulting in the formation of ketone bodies, namely acetoacetic acid and β-hydroxybutyric acid. These can undergo oxidation to release energy; accumulation of these acids in the blood, however, can lead to metabolic acidosis.

## Sodium and water

Each day, depending on thirst and social habits, approximately 2 L of fluid are ingested.

The secretion of digestive juices adds a further 8–9 L of fluid to the gut contents (**Table 5.1.3**). Of this 10–11 L of fluid that daily passes through the gastrointestinal tract, only some 50–200 mL are lost from the body in the faeces; the rest is absorbed, at a rate of 200–400 mL/hour, from the small and large intestines as follows:

- jejunum: 5–6 L reabsorbed in 24 hours
- ileum: 2 L reabsorbed in 24 hours
- colon: 1.5–2 L reabsorbed in 24 hours.

From this, it is possible to estimate the amount of absolute fluid loss from the body if an ileostomy is performed. Sodium irons are actively absorbed in the jejunum, ileum and colon; chloride ions follow passively, as does water.

### CLINICAL APPLICATIONS

Water can either move out of the gut lumen into the blood, or it can move from the blood to dilute the gut contents when these are hypertonic. It is for this reason that hypertonic enema solutions (e.g. magnesium sulphate) result in the production of large watery stools.

Movement of water from the blood into the gastrointestinal tract occurs (as described earlier) in dumping syndrome following major gastric resection or total gastrectomy. The movement of a large volume of water into the gastrointestinal tract can, in some cases, lead to severe shock.

## Potassium

Some potassium is actively secreted into the gut, particularly in mucus. Usually, though, potassium is

**Table 5.1.3** Summary of daily secretion of digestive juices

| Secretion | Volume (mL) | pH |
| --- | --- | --- |
| Saliva | 1000–1500 | 6.8–7.0 |
| Gastric juice | 2000–3000 | 1.5–3.0 |
| Pancreatic juice | 1500–2000 | 8.0–8.4 |
| Bile | 500–1000 | 7.8–8.0 |
| Intestinal juice | 3000 | 7.8–8.0 |

Most of this daily secretion is reabsorbed. If this were not so, 8–9 L would represent an exceedingly high rate of fluid and electrolyte loss. Quite large losses can occur in conditions such as gastroenteritis, cholera and typhoid, and following an ileostomy.

passively absorbed into the blood along a concentration gradient from the ileum and colon.

### CLINICAL APPLICATIONS

In patients suffering from diarrhoea, or in those who have an ileostomy, hypokalaemia can be a potential problem.

## Vitamins

Most water-soluble vitamins (those of the B group, except vitamin B12, and vitamin C) are absorbed passively with water. Vitamins A, D, E and K are fat soluble, and their absorption depends on efficient micelle formation and subsequent entry into the enterocytes. The production of bile salts and the secretion of lipase are thus necessary for the efficient absorption of these vitamins.

Vitamin B12 is absorbed in the terminal ileum. As described earlier, it forms a complex with intrinsic factor from the gastric parietal cells. The complex is thought to bind to receptors on the ileal wall, and vitamin B12 is then able to transfer across the gut wall into the blood.

## Calcium

About 30–80% of ingested calcium is actively absorbed in the upper part of the small intestine under the influence of parathyroid hormone and calcitonin (see Chapter 2.6).

Calcium absorption is facilitated by the active metabolite of vitamin D, formed in the kidney under the influence of parathyroid hormone, called 1,25-dihydroxycholecalciferol. This substance brings about the synthesis of a protein in the gastrointestinal mucosa that binds to calcium ions and is necessary for their transport across the gut wall.

When serum calcium levels fall, more 1,25-dihydroxycholecalciferol is formed and so more calcium can be absorbed from the small intestine. Calcium absorption is facilitated by lactose and proteins, and inhibited by oxalates and phytic acid (found, for example, in cereals and rhubarb) and by phosphate.

## Iron

In the United Kingdom, the average daily intake of iron is 15–20 mg. Only about 5–10% of the total dietary iron intake is absorbed into the blood from the gastrointestinal tract. Each day, about 1 mg of iron is lost from the body through desquamation of skin and via the faeces and urine. In menstruating females there is an additional absolute monthly loss of some 25 mg of iron in an average menstrual flow.

Most of the dietary intake of iron is in the ferric form. However, iron is more readily absorbed in the ferrous form, and reduction from the ferric form to the ferrous form is facilitated by gastric juice and also by vitamin C. Patients who have undergone radical gastric surgery may therefore have problems with iron absorption and may become anaemic.

Iron is actively absorbed in the upper part of the small intestine; thus patients with colostomies and ileostomies should not experience problems with iron absorption. The enterocytes store iron, and more iron is absorbed from the lumen only when these cellular stores are depleted. The enterocytes discharge their iron stores into the blood when serum iron levels fall.

Iron travels in the blood mostly bound to apoferritin, a globular protein, and while in the blood it is referred to as **transferrin**. Once iron binds to apoferritin, **ferritin** is formed. This is the principal storage form of iron, although a small amount is stored as **haemosiderin**. About 70% of the body's iron is in haemoglobin; 3% is in myoglobin, a muscle protein; the rest is stored in the liver as ferritin or haemosiderin.

If the passage of chyme through the small intestine is hastened in any way, there will not be efficient absorption of nutrients. It normally takes about 9 hours from the time of ingestion for nutrients to reach the terminal portion of the small intestine; patients who suffer from chronic conditions resulting in 'intestinal hurry' may well show signs of malabsorption of some nutrients.

## The large intestine

The large intestine, which is divided into several distinct sections, is about 1.5 m long and approximately 6 cm in diameter. It extends from the end of the ileum to the anus. The arrangement of the large intestine and its associated structures is shown in **Fig. 5.1.26**.

The regions of the large intestine include:

- caecum
- ascending colon
- transverse colon
- sigmoid colon
- rectum
- anal canal.

The large intestine has five main functions:

1. storage of food residues prior to their elimination
2. absorption of most of the remaining water, electrolytes and some vitamins
3. synthesis of vitamin K and some B vitamins by colonic bacteria
4. secretion of mucus, which acts as a lubricant for the elimination of faeces
5. elimination of food residues as faeces.

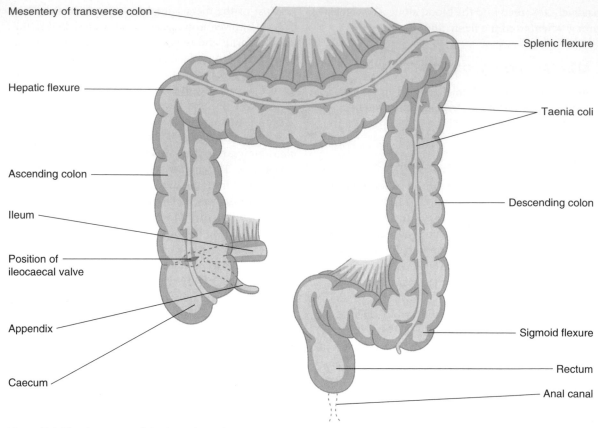

Mesentery of transverse colon

Splenic flexure

Hepatic flexure

Taenia coli

Ascending colon

Descending colon

Ileum

Position of
ileocaecal valve

Appendix

Sigmoid flexure

Caecum

Rectum

Anal canal

**Figure 5.1.26**  Anatomy of the large intestine

Each day, about 1 L of chyme (with a consistency like that of thin porridge) enters the large intestine laterally via the ileocaecal valve. The ileocaecal valve is normally closed, as a result of back pressure from the colonic contents. It has two horizontal folds that project into the caecum and are formed of circular muscle fibres. The valve acts like a sphincter to prevent chyme leaving the small intestine rapidly, i.e. before adequate time has elapsed for full absorption to occur. The ileocaecal valve opens in response to peristaltic waves that bring chyme into contact with it. In addition, when food enters the stomach, a reflex is set up, via the vagus nerve, which stimulates peristalsis in the colon. This causes the caecum to relax and the ileocaecal valve to open. This reflex is called the **gastrocolic reflex**; it is particularly evident after breakfast, when food enters an empty stomach. The consequent colonic peristalsis causes the rectum to fill with faeces, and this results in the urge to defaecate.

Apart from the stomach, the large intestine is the widest part of the gastrointestinal tract and allows the storage of large amounts of food residues, which move slowly through this section of the tract. The large intestine has no villi and hence has a much smaller internal surface area – approximately one-third that of the small intestine.

Throughout the length of the large intestine there are many patches of lymphoid tissue in the muscularis layer of the tube. These have a protective function.

## The caecum

This is a blind-ending pouch about 7 cm long, entered via the ileocaecal valve and leading to the colon. In humans it has no significant function but in herbivorous animals it is concerned with cellulose digestion.

## *The appendix*

This is a vermiform (worm-like) blind-ending sac projecting from the end of the caecum; it is about the size of an adult's little finger. It has no function in humans and there is considerable variation in its position between individuals. It is made up mainly of lymphoid tissue and can enlarge in infection or inflammation. Inflammation (i.e. appendicitis) can occur if the opening of the appendix to the caecum is blocked by a hard mass of faeces (a faecolith) or by swollen lymphoid tissue resulting from inflammation in the area. If this inflammation causes the enlarged appendix to rupture, then faecal material containing bacteria will enter the abdominal cavity and peritonitis is likely to follow.

## The colon

This dilated area of the large intestine is anatomically divided into four main regions (**see Fig. 5.1.26**).

**The ascending colon** (about 50 cm long) turns at the hepatic flexure, or right colic flexure, into the **transverse colon**, which lies slightly 'higher' on the left than the right, transversely below the liver and the stomach.

At the left colic or splenic flexure, the transverse colon turns to form the **descending colon** which is about 25 cm long, on the left of the abdomen. This gives rise to the **sigmoid** (S-shaped) **colon**, about 40 cm long, which empties into the rectum.

The colon differs from the generalized structure of the gastrointestinal tract described earlier in that the longitudinal muscle bands in the muscularis layer are incomplete. As a result, the wall is gathered into three longitudinal flat bands called the **taenia coli**. Because these bands are shorter than the rest of the colon, the wall pouches outwards to form **haustrations** (derived from the Latin word for bucket) between the taeniae when the circular muscle fibres contract. As the haustrations fill and empty, they aid in kneading the colonic contents.

## Functions of the colon

### Storage

The main function of the colon is to **store** unabsorbed and unassimilable food residues. The colon thus acts as a reservoir; 70% of the residue of food is excreted within 72 hours of ingestion and the remaining 30% can stay within the colon for a week or longer. As it does so, progressively more water is **reabsorbed**.

### Absorption of sodium and water

Sodium is actively transported from the colon to the hepatic portal vein, and water and chloride ions follow passively. The amount of water reabsorbed from the colonic contents depends on the length of time the residue remains in the colon. In a constipated person, the food residue remains within the colon for several days and hence most of the water is reabsorbed, resulting in hard pellets of faeces which are difficult to eliminate.

The bulk of the food residue, and hence potential faeces, is made up of cellulose – a substance derived from the cell walls of vegetables and fruits, which humans are unable to digest because they lack the necessary enzyme: cellulase.

Some drugs, for example aspirin, prednisone and some anaesthetics, and also amino acids, can be absorbed by the colonic mucous membrane. Hence steroid retention enemas can be used successfully to reduce inflammation of the colon in patients suffering from ulcerative colitis.

### Secretion of mucus and electrolytes

Mucus contains hydrogen carbonate and hence colonic mucus gives the contents of the colon a pH of 7.5–8.0. In addition, some potassium ions and some hydrogen carbonate ions may be secreted actively into the colon.

### Incubation of bacteria

Many of the bacteria that colonize the large intestine are anaerobic species (i.e. they do not need oxygen for their survival). *Bacteroids fragilis* and *Clostridium perfringens (welchii)* are both anaerobic; *Enterobacter aerogenes* is aerobic, as its name implies, and there are also some streptococci and lactobacilli and *Escherichia coli*. The relatively sluggish movements of the colon are conducive to colonization by bacteria. Many of these bacteria, which compose the gut flora, exhibit a modified symbiotic relationship with humans; that is, each derives mutual benefit from the other and they live together harmoniously. However, these commensals can become pathogenic, especially if introduced into another part of the body, for example, gut bacteria can cause cystitis if introduced into the bladder during catheterization.

The bacteria synthesize vitamin K, thiamine, folic acid and riboflavin in small amounts. The amount produced is not normally nutritionally significant; however, in vitamin deficiency or starvation this contribution may be of some benefit. These bacteria also synthesize a small amount of vitamin B12, but as this vitamin can be absorbed only from the ileum, the amount thus synthesized is normally excreted.

### CLINICAL APPLICATIONS

Patients who are on long-term antibiotic therapy may lose these commensal bacteria, and this loss provides the opportunity for colonization by pathogenic, antibiotic-resistant bacteria, a potential problem that one should be aware of in such patients. The first sign of such a problem is usually diarrhoea.

Bacterial fermentation of food residues produces quite large amounts of gas, called flatus, which consists of nitrogen, carbon dioxide, hydrogen, methane and hydrogen sulphide. Between 500 mL and 700 mL of flatus may be produced each day, although the amount will show considerable variation depending on the food eaten; foods such as baked beans, onions, cauliflower and pulses lead to an increase in flatus production due to fermentation of their residues by the colonic bacteria. The production of flatus may also result from air swallowing in anxiety states (aerophagia). Normal bowel movements allow the expulsion of gases so produced.

In patients who have had abdominal surgery, the smooth muscle activity of the intestine may be inhibited because of trauma resulting from operative handling of the gut. This results in cessation of movements of the small intestine, a condition termed **paralytic ileus**. This may occur not only after abdominal surgery but also as a response to intestinal obstruction. In paralytic ileus, peristalsis stops and thus movement of the gut contents stops; this results in the formation of pockets of gas and fluid. This gas cannot be passed as flatus, and the consequent accumulation of gas and fluid leads to abdominal distension with increase in girth and the production of considerable abdominal discomfort.

If paralytic ileus occurs as a result of abdominal surgery, after a few days the abdominal smooth muscle starts to contract again, peristalsis is once more evident, and flatus can be expelled.

A patient suffering from paralytic ileus should take no food or fluids until flatus is passed – a sign of returning peristalsis. Aspiration of a nasogastric tube helps to remove gases produced and digestive fluids secreted until the paralysis has passed; this may prevent some of the discomfort experienced by the patient.

## The role of dietary fibre in the large intestine

The time taken for food residues to be expelled is directly related to the amount of dietary fibre ingested. Dietary fibre decreases the mouth-to-anus transit time and gives bulk to the diet.

Dietary fibre is made up largely of **cellulose**, the substance found in cell walls. Humans do not produce cellulase, the enzyme found in herbivorous animals such as cows and rabbits, which is necessary to digest and utilize cellulose and, because cellulose cannot therefore be absorbed, it stays in the bowel where it exerts a hygroscopic effect, i.e. it attracts water. Thus, stools high in fibre tend to be bulkier and softer in consistency, and this makes them easier to expel.

Diverticular disease is a condition more prevalent in omnivores (meat and vegetable eaters) than vegetarians, whose diet is always high in fibre; and there is a higher incidence of the condition (about 10% of men and women over the age of 40) in the Western world than in developing countries, where less meat and refined food and more vegetable fibre are eaten.

Diverticula are pouches or sacs that occur in the walls of the intestine as a result of weakness of the muscle layer at that point. They may be congenital. Eating a diet high in fibre does not prevent such diverticula forming (**diverticulosis**); it will, however, help

to prevent **diverticulitis** (inflammation of the diverticula). The latter condition results when hard masses of faeces collect in the diverticula and cause inflammation. This results in increased peristalsis accompanied by discomfort and diarrhoea. Stools high in fibre are softer and pass through the bowel at a speed that is not conducive to pockets of faeces being trapped within the diverticula (Southgate, 1990).

It is estimated that vegetarians eat approximately 41.5 g of fibre daily, whereas omnivores eat only 21.4 g of fibre daily; 33% of a sample of omnivores were found to be suffering from diverticular disease, compared to only 12% of the vegetarian sample.

The longer mouth–anus transit times found in people consuming a low-fibre (refined) diet allow bacterial toxins and metabolites to remain in contact with the gut wall for a longer period of time; this may be linked to the higher incidence of carcinoma of the large intestine and rectum in the Western world compared to developing countries. In addition, the faeces of omnivores contain a higher proportion of *Bacteroides* than do those of herbivores. It is now thought that these bacteria act on bile acids to form carcinogenic products. The slower the bowel transit time, the longer such carcinogens have to exert their effects on the intestinal wall.

A further benefit of a high-fibre diet is that the softer stool produced is easier to expel; thus the necessity to strain at defaecation is eliminated, and this may reduce the incidence of haemorrhoids.

The report of the National Advisory Committee on Nutrition Education (1983) recommended that fibre intake should be increased by 33%, to 30 g per head per day – mainly by increasing consumption of wholegrain cereals.

It should be remembered that an excess of fibre could potentially be harmful (Holmes, 1990). Where high-fibre diets contain high levels of phytate, absorption of both iron and calcium from the gut can be decreased. However, the pattern of eating found in the United Kingdom is such that it is unlikely to contain significantly high levels of phytate (Heaton, 1990).

## Movements of the colon

Although the colon has only incomplete bands of longitudinal muscle fibres, it does have complete bands of circular muscle fibres. When these latter bands contract, segmentation results. Segmentation allows mixing of the colonic contents and facilitates colonic absorption. When the circular muscle bands contract, they divide the colon into segments. Contractions occur about once every half-hour, after which the circular muscle fibres relax and adjacent bands of muscle contract, thus breaking up the first segment of faeces (**Fig. 5.1.27**).

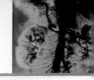

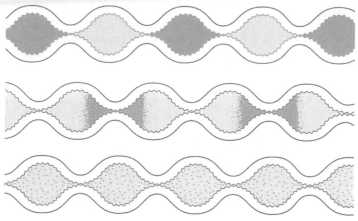

**Figure 5.1.27** Segmentation in the colon

**Segmentation** is a non-propulsive movement and, in the constipated person, it is the main movement that occurs in the large bowel. Peristalsis (described earlier) also occurs in the colon, propelling faeces towards the rectum.

Two or three times a day, usually after meals, an increase in activity occurs in the colon. After meals, especially after breakfast (which is eaten when the stomach is empty), the gastrocolic reflex occurs; this brings about increasing contractions of the terminal ileum, relaxation of the ileocaecal valve and colonic peristalsis. The gastrocolic reflex therefore allows filling of the colon.

Associated with the gastrocolic reflex, the phenomenon of **mass movement** occurs in the colon. Mass movement propels the faeces in the mid-colon towards the rectum; the haustrations in the mid-colon disappear, the tube becomes shortened and flattened by waves of rapidly advancing powerful contractions and the colonic contents are moved at speed, within a few seconds, into the sigmoid colon. The subject only becomes aware of mass movements when faeces enter the rectum.

CLINICAL APPLICATIONS

Analgesics such as morphine, codeine and pethidine decrease these movements in the colon; ganglion-blocking agents and aluminium-based antacids have a similar effect. People taking these drugs therefore may become constipated.

## The rectum

The rectum is a muscular tube about 12–15 cm long, capable of great distension. It is usually empty until just before defaecation. Mass movement of the colon leads to sudden distension of the rectal walls, which brings about what is often termed the 'call to stool',

when the subject becomes aware of the need to defaecate.

The rectum opens to the exterior via the anal canal, which has both internal and external anal sphincters. The **internal anal sphincter** is composed of smooth muscle fibres, and is not under voluntary control. Fibres from the sympathetic nervous system to the internal sphincter are excitatory, i.e. when active they bring about contraction; fibres from the parasympathetic system are inhibitory, and stimulation of these causes relaxation of the sphincter.

The **external anal sphincter** is composed of striated muscle fibres and is under the control of the will from about the age of 18 months.

### DEVELOPMENTAL ISSUES

This control, or continence, is learned, and is not present in the baby and young infant.

### CLINICAL APPLICATIONS

The external sphincter is supplied by the pudendal nerve and is maintained in a state of tonic contraction. This voluntary sphincter control may be lost in people with damage to their pudendal nerve or spinal cord or after a cerebrovascular accident.

## Defaecation

When faeces enter the rectum, afferent impulses travel to the sacral spinal cord. If it is convenient to defaecate, the sacral spinal cord will reflexly initiate defaecation. Impulses travel from the sacral spinal cord not only to the terminal colon and anal sphincter, but also to the cerebral cortex, which can inhibit spinal cord activity if defaecation is not convenient.

## CLINICAL APPLICATIONS

In patients who have had a cerebrovascular accident or who have senile deterioration of their cerebral functions, such inhibition may not be possible and faecal incontinence results. Similarly, in babies or young infants, or in patients with sacral spinal cord lesions, reflex efferent impulses from the sacral spinal cord immediately cause contraction of the terminal colon and relaxation of the sphincters.

Defaecation is thus a reflex response to faeces entering the rectum.

Defaecation is accompanied by some measure of straining. The degree of effort necessary will depend upon the consistency of the faeces. A deep breath is taken and expired against a closed glottis (sometimes called **Valsalva's manoeuvre**). This forced expiration is aided by contraction of the muscles of the abdominal wall, which further serves to raise the intra-abdominal pressure. This, together with contraction of the levator ani muscles, causes the pressure in the rectum to rise to about 26 kPa in the adult. This increase in pressure, together with relaxation of the anal sphincters, leads to the expulsion of the rectal contents. During straining, there is a sharp rise in blood pressure followed by a sudden fall. For this reason, defaecation can sometimes precipitate cerebrovascular accidents.

## Faeces

Approximately 100–150 g of faeces are usually eliminated every day, consisting of 30–50 g of solids and 70–100 g of water. The solid portion is made up largely of cellulose, epithelial cells shed from the lining of the gastrointestinal tract, bacteria, some salts and the brown pigment stercobilin. A small amount of potassium is actually secreted into the faeces in the colon – a fact that becomes significant in diarrhoea, when quite large amounts of potassium may be lost. Indole and skatole are two products of amine breakdown, arising from bacterial decomposition, which give faeces their characteristic odour.

## CLINICAL APPLICATIONS

### DIARRHOEA

This results when movements of the intestine occur too rapidly for water to be absorbed in the colon. Stools are therefore produced in large amounts, and may range from being loose to being entirely liquid, such as the 'rice water' stools associated with cholera. Diarrhoea,

depending on its severity and duration, can be a mere nuisance or fatal. If diarrhoea is severe, large amounts of water (consisting of ingested fluids and digestive juices, together with sodium and potassium) are lost in the stools. This rapidly results in dehydration and electrolyte imbalance. In chronic diarrhoea, hypokalaemia is often found, and loss of alkaline digestive juices may cause a metabolic acidosis. Infants with diarrhoea and vomiting can quickly become severely dehydrated.

The problems that the sufferer is aware of are exhaustion and abdominal pain, possibly embarrassment, anxiety or fear and excoriation of the perineum. While urgent medical management of the condition is essential, nursing activities should in addition be directed towards the relief of these problems.

Causes of diarrhoea are the following:

- **Diet.** Certain foods, notably fruits such as prunes, rhubarb and gooseberries, and highly seasoned dishes can result in diarrhoea. Similarly, diarrhoea may be the result of a high intake of alcohol or of allergies to some foods.
- **Diverticulosis.** This has been discussed in some detail in the section on the role of dietary fibre.
- **Drugs.** Certain drugs, for example antibiotics and iron preparations, cause diarrhoea in some people. Laxatives, by definition, result in the passage of a large, loose stool.
- **Infections.** Organisms such as *Salmonella*, *Shigella* and staphylococci all produce an inflammatory enteritis when present in sufficient numbers. Such intestinal infections are commonly accompanied by nausea and abdominal pain, and usually follow the ingestion of contaminated food.
- **Inflammatory conditions of the gastrointestinal tract.** These include, for example, ulcerative colitis, irritable bowel syndrome and regional ileitis (Crohn's disease). The inflammation leads to an increase in peristalsis and also excess mucus production; intestinal contents are therefore moved rapidly through the large bowel.
- **Malabsorption syndrome.** Bulky, offensive stools are produced in conditions in which, for example, gluten, lactose or fats are not absorbed from the ileum.
- **Neoplasms.** Malignant growths in the bowel may result in a change of bowel habits, such as alternating periods of diarrhoea and constipation.
- **Stress.** Diarrhoea may be a physiological response to stress.

• **Thyrotoxicosis.** In this condition, there is a general speeding up of body activities, and intestinal hurry commonly occurs.

In treating diarrhoea, the predisposing cause must be sought and treated and dehydration and electrolyte imbalances must be corrected. Concurrently, provision must be made for symptomatic relief of the problems presented to the patient by the condition, for example the position of an inpatient's bed in the ward must be carefully considered. If the patient is ambulant, it is helpful to situate the bed not too far from the lavatory. If the patient is on bedrest, then provision must be made for adequate ventilation of the bed area and for deodorant sprays. Soft lavatory paper or tissues are more comfortable for the patient and sometimes a barrier cream for the perineal area is helpful to prevent excoriation. Diarrhoea is an unpleasant condition that causes many patients embarrassment and worry, and reassurance that they are not a nuisance is frequently necessary.

## CONSTIPATION

This term refers to the difficult passage of hard stools. Many people wrongly regard themselves as being constipated if they do not defaecate every day. However, it may be normal for one person to have two bowel actions every day whereas for another it is normal to defaecate only two or three times each week. In this latter case, so long as the stools are of normal consistency and are not difficult to pass, such a person could not be regarded as being constipated.

Constipation is the opposite of diarrhoea in that the food residues become hard, due to the reabsorption of most of the water when they remain in the colon for a long time. They thus become difficult and often painful to eliminate. Constipation frequently occurs when the diet contains insufficient fibre. Food residues tend to remain in the colon until eventually both the colon and the rectum are full of faecal material. This results in the sufferer complaining of a feeling of fullness or of feeling 'bloated'. Abdominal distension may well be evident, and this may lead to a feeling of nausea. In addition, halitosis, a furred tongue, headache, irritability and flatulence may also occur.

When constipated stools are passed, they may be so hard that an anal fissure (a tear in the anal mucosa) occurs with consequent bleeding and pain. The degree of straining necessary to pass such hard stools may result over a period of time in the development of varicosed rectal veins, that is, haemorrhoids or piles. These varicosities occur as a result of the rise in pressure in the rectal veins which accompanies prolonged straining, and this leads to incompetence of the rectal venous valves. Venous return along the rectal veins becomes sluggish, and the veins become distended. The degree of distension may be such that the veins assume a grape-like appearance and, in severe cases, the varicosed rectal veins may prolapse through the anal sphincter. Haemorrhoids further serve to aggravate the problem of constipation as the sufferer tends to delay defaecation in an attempt to avoid the consequent pain.

Causes of constipation are the following:

• **Avoidance of defaecation.** Some examples of conditions in which this may occur have already been described. In addition, embarrassment at having to use a bedpan or commode in the close vicinity of other patients can lead to constipation in any patient in hospital. A patient is required to delay defaecation as a result of a commode, lavatory or bedpan not being available at the time when it is required and might suffer extra discomfort by adding constipation to the existing problems (Wright, 1974).

At home, a patient who is too weak or who is in too much pain (for example, from arthritis) to move to the lavatory may avoid defaecation.

• **Dehydration.** A decrease in fluid intake, or an increase in fluid loss, can cause constipation.

• **Depression and dementia.** Both of these conditions result in a general slowing down of both physical and mental activities. This would include the slowing down of colonic movements and constipation may result. Antidepressant drug therapy may further serve to worsen the condition.

• **Drugs.** Certain analgesics, notably codeine, all narcotics (e.g. morphine and diamorphine), some antihypertensive agents (e.g. methyldopa), anticholinergics (e.g. the antispasmodic propantheline), aluminium antacids (e.g. Aludrox) and iron preparations can all cause constipation.

• **Haemorrhoids.** Varicosities and prolapse of rectal veins can be exceedingly painful and sufferers may attempt to avoid the passage of stools.

• **Hypothyroidism (myxoedema).** Patients suffering from this condition tend to have general depression of all their body activities. Faeces therefore pass through the colon slowly and constipation results.

• **Inactivity.** Exercise tends to stimulate peristalsis and thus defaecation. Patients who are on prolonged bedrest may therefore suffer from constipation. In addition, such patients may suffer from loss of appetite and may therefore decrease their dietary intake. For many reasons, too, they may be reluctant to ask for a bedpan or commode and may therefore delay defaecation.

- **Insufficient dietary fibre.** Dietary fibre is hygroscopic, i.e. attracts water. It therefore provides bulk to the stool and aids elimination. Older patients without their own teeth or with badly fitting dentures may tend to eat a soft, low-fibre diet and thus aggravate the problems arising due to weak musculature of the pelvic floor.
- **Neoplasms.** Change in bowel habits brought about by intestinal growths can lead to alternating bouts of diarrhoea and constipation.
- **Weak musculature of the pelvic floor.** (i.e. the levator ani muscles). In older people, or in multiparous women (i.e. those who have had several babies), the muscles of the pelvic floor tend to become weak and therefore less able to contract efficiently during defaecation, which therefore becomes inefficient.

## Complications of constipation

To initiate the call to stool, a faecal mass of 100–150 g is necessary. If the faecal mass is less than this then straining is necessary to eliminate it. During straining, momentary circulatory stasis occurs, with a sharp increase in the thoracic, intra-abdominal and blood pressures. This can lead to the propagation of thrombi as emboli, which may occlude either the cerebral or pulmonary circulation, depending on their site of origin. The increase in blood pressure can result in the rupture of an existing aneurysm in the cerebral circulation or aorta.

It should be possible to prevent constipation by increasing the intake of dietary fibre to 30 g a day and by encouraging an adequate amount of exercise. People eating a high-fibre diet should increase their fluid intake to prevent its hygroscopic action leading to dehydration.

## Management of constipation

Once constipation has occurred, the following measures, in addition to the above, may be helpful.

The **position** adopted for defaecation affects the efficiency of the mechanism. A comfortable squatting position is more efficient than an upright one. Sitting on a bedpan is uncomfortable and therefore does not aid defaecation; it may in fact increase the amount of straining required. For patients who have suffered a myocardial

infarction, the use of a commode probably causes less overall stress than that associated with the use of a bedpan. Additionally, the assurance of privacy is a psychological help.

The administration of oral or rectal **lubricants**, such as liquid paraffin orally, or glycerine suppositories rectally, serves to soften the faeces. Such lubricants are not absorbed. However, if taken frequently, they may interfere with the absorption of fat-soluble vitamins A, D, E and K.

The most common **bowel stimulants (aperients)** in this group are the senna derivatives, bisacodyl, Senokot and cascara. It is thought that these substances irritate the colonic mucosa and thus aid defaecation. The now seldom-used soap and water enema is an example of an irritant administered rectally.

Examples of **osmotic aperients** are magnesium sulphate (Epsom salts), which can be given either orally or as an enema, oral milk of magnesia, lactulose and phosphate enemas. These substances are hygroscopic, that is, they draw water into the lumen of the gut from the surrounding blood capillaries. A large watery stool will therefore follow their administration.

**Bulking agents** are methylcellulose derivatives, examples of which are dietary fibre, Isogel, Normacol and Celevac. They reduce mouth-to-anus transit time by attracting water to the gut contents and thus providing a bulky but relatively soft stool.

If the above methods fail to manage the problem of constipation, then in extreme circumstances it may be necessary to carry out a manual removal of faeces. This is a painful and embarrassing procedure and should be attempted only by a doctor or trained nurse experienced in the technique. The patient will usually need analgesia or sedation before this procedure. Ross (1998) provides an extensive overview of the causes and control of constipation in the acute hospital setting.

## DEVELOPMENTAL ISSUES

### CHANGES IN THE GASTROINTESTINAL TRACT ASSOCIATED WITH AGEING

The main changes associated with ageing in the gastrointestinal tract occur in the mouth and have been discussed in that section:

- The secretion of saliva decreases and hence a drier mouth (xerostomia) results in potential problems with tasting food, enunciating clearly and swallowing.
- Shrinkage of the maxillary and mandibular bones together with periodontal (gum) tissue may result in loss of teeth. Any previous

neglect of dental hygiene and general wear and tear will have the same effect. Loss of teeth and the need to wear dentures may affect the person's ability to chew food properly (Pettigrew, 1989). This, in itself, is likely to influence the amount of dietary fibre consumed, which in turn may cause an alteration in bowel habits.

- Digestive secretions decrease with age, in particular the secretion of gastric juice. Hypochlorhydria, with consequent decrease in intrinsic factor production, may result in some degree of pernicious, (macrocytic) anaemia (Green, 1985).
- Villous height decreases with age with a concomitant decrease in the surface area available for absorption, especially of folic acid, iron, calcium and vitamins B12 and D.
- Motility throughout the tract decreases, especially in the colon; constipation may be a problem, especially in those whose diet is low in fibre and in whom exercise is restricted.
- Pathologies associated with ageing include carcinomas of the stomach, colon and rectum, gastritis, gall bladder and diverticular disease and haemorrhoids.

## CLINICAL APPLICATIONS

### NURSING ASSESSMENT OF A PATIENT'S BOWEL HABITS

Whether an individual is admitted to hospital or cared for in the community, it is important to assess his or her bowel function. Bowel problems may not be central to the patient's need for care but they can aggravate the primary problems if allowed to develop. In addition, the area in general is one in which the nurse may, with effect, attempt some health education.

Assessment of a patient's bowel habits links with the assessment of his or her state of hydration, the condition of the tongue, the smell of the breath, assessment of food and fluid intake and activity levels.

The following points relating to bowel habits should be assessed by the nurse, either from direct observation or by questioning:

- Frequency of the bowel actions.
- Quantity of stool produced and variation from normal: stools will be increased in volume in patients taking large quantities of fruit and vegetables or in those on a vegetarian diet.
- Consistency of the stool passed: the stool will be softer and larger in those on a high-fibre diet and should float in the lavatory.

- Inexplicable changes in bowel habits in terms of amount, frequency or consistency.
- Presence of mucus in the stool: this may indicate an inflammatory condition in the bowel.
- Presence of blood: according to whether it is fresh or altered, blood may give clues about where in the gastrointestinal tract bleeding is occurring.
- Presence of undigested food: this will occur in conditions of intestinal hurry.
- Colour of the stool: dark stools may result from oral iron preparations; tarry stools may indicate melaena (i.e. bleeding from the gastric or upper intestinal region); pale stools may be the result of obstructive jaundice.
- Offensive odour of stool: this may occur with malabsorption states.
- If the stool is a response to an enema or to aperients, is it an adequate response?
- Pain on defaecation: this may indicate the presence of haemorrhoids, anal fissure, a perineal lesion or constipation.

### GASTROINTESTINAL PAIN

Pain experienced as a response to gastrointestinal (i.e. visceral) stimuli is different in kind from that experienced as a response to cutaneous stimuli. The nerves in the viscera are not able to convey discrete sensations of touch, temperature, etc. to the cerebral cortex; instead, they convey impulses that result from distension of the gastrointestinal wall, and the pattern of these impulses is interpreted in the cerebral cortex. The effect on the individual of pain resulting from gastrointestinal stimuli will vary with, among other factors, that individual's pain threshold, degree of preparation for, or anticipation of, pain and the duration of the pain.

Areas of the gastrointestinal tract will be considered in anatomical order:

#### Mouth

Oral pain can range from that of an inflamed tongue or gums to toothache. With toothache, the nerve endings in the pulp cavity are stimulated and pain impulses travel in the trigeminal nerve to the sensory cortex. Toothache is an example of a pain that can be acute or chronic in nature.

#### Oesophagus

Pain here is often referred to by the sufferer as 'heartburn'. It usually results from reflux of acid gastric contents into the oesophagus, causing irritation of the epithelial tissue. Impulses so produced travel in the lateral spinothalamic tract to the thalamus and thence to the sensory cortex.

### Stomach

Pain here may result from hunger contractions of the stomach; from distension when the stomach is overfull after a heavy meal; and from the formation of a gastric ulcer. This last example results in what sufferers often term a 'gnawing' pain. The inflammation produced around the ulcerated region leads to oedema and an increase in tension in the area. Pain impulses travel to the central nervous system from the stomach along the gastric sympathetic fibres.

### Intestine

Intestinal pain is usually referred to as **colic**, i.e. it results from prolonged contraction (spasm) of smooth muscle. Mechanical obstruction is one condition that can result in colic pain; this occurs when the area of intestine above the obstruction dilates due to the accumulation of gas and fluid. Biliary colic occurs when gallstones obstruct the common bile duct. This leads to an increase in tension in that area, and also to a degree of local ischaemia. Most nerve fibres carrying painful stimuli pass from the intestine to the spinal cord in the region of T11–L2, via sympathetic nerves. Impulses then pass to the thalamus via the lateral spinothalamic tract of the spinal cord, and hence to the sensory cortex.

### Appendix

When this organ becomes inflamed and oedematous, pain is initially felt in the periumbilical region. The explanation for this apparent anomaly is that embryologically the appendix develops from the midgut, lying in the periumbilical area, and its nerve supply reflects this development. A few hours after the pain is first felt, it commonly localizes over the appendix itself. The pain of appendicitis is usually severe.

### Peritoneum

The pain of peritonitis is similarly severe and the patient typically lies very still with a rigid abdominal wall 'guarding' the underlying inflammation. When the visceral (inner) layer of peritoneum is stimulated, a diffuse sensation of pain results that is poorly localized. This diffuse sensation occurs because the peritoneum is insensitive to local mechanical stimuli and contains relatively few pain receptors. In contrast, stimulation of the parietal (outer) layer of the peritoneum by inflammation results in a well-localized sensation of pain.

### Rectum and large intestine

Pain fibres from the rectum accompany the pelvic parasympathetic nerve fibres. Pain from the proximal part of the large intestine is typically experienced as periumbilical; pain from the distal end of the large intestine is experienced as hypogastric.

---

## Clinical review

In addition to the Learning Objectives at the beginning of this chapter, the reader should be able to:

- Teach a student nurse how nutrients are absorbed from the small intestine
- Discuss the importance of the colon and relate this to stoma formation
- Describe how defaecation occurs and relate this to diarrhoea and constipation
- Assess a patient's bowel habits
- Relate types of gastrointestinal pain to their source

---

## Review questions

1 Why does the epithelium of the mouth have so many layers of cells?
2 Why do we not breathe while we are swallowing?
3 Of what type of muscle is the tongue comprised?
4 What are the four taste modalities?

5   What are the functions of saliva?

6   When is saliva produced?

7   What is deglutition?

8   What normally happens when a bolus of food reaches the pharynx?

9   What are the four tissue layers common to the whole of the digestive tract?

10  Which parasympathetic nerve supplies the gastrointestinal tract?

11  How is food propelled down the oesophagus?

12  What are the functions of the stomach?

13  Where is hydrochloric acid produced in the stomach?

14  What is pepsinogen?

15  What are the phases which control gastric juice secretion?

16  What is gastrin?

17  How fast do different foodstuffs leave the stomach?

18  What functions do the mesenteries serve?

19  What secretions are received by the duodenum?

20  Which enzymes are contained in pancreatic juice?

21  How do the actions of cholecystokinin and secretin differ in the control of pancreatic juice secretion?

22  What function does bile perform?

23  What function do villi perform?

24  Why is the rate of cell division in the villi rapid?

25  What is the essential difference between active and passive transport?

26  What happens to most of the water that enters the small intestine?

27  How does glycolysis differ in the presence and the absence of oxygen?

28  How does the body get rid of the excess nitrogen produced in deamination?

29  What are chylomicrons?

30  What is the fate of the acetyl co-enzyme A produced by glycolysis and β-oxidation of fats?

31  Which structure controls the entry of chyme into the large intestine?

32  What function do the taenia coli perform?

33  Which movements occur in the large intestine?

## Suggestions for further reading

Note that most of the further reading suggested here focuses on the way in which a knowledge of the gastrointestinal tract impinges on nursing practice, rather than on physiology *per se*.

Brown, K. (1991) Improving intakes. *Nursing Times*, 87(20); 64–68.
*The report of a survey highlighting the potential problem of the inadequacy of hospital diets.*

Committee on Medical Aspects of Food Policy (1991) *Report on Health and Social Subjects* 41; *dietary reference values for food, energy and nutrients for the UK.* London: HMSO.
*The second report from the CMA panel recommends further cuts in fat and sugar consumption.*

Department of Health (1992) *The Health of the Nation.* London: HMSO.

*This White Paper presents a health strategy for the nation which suggests targets for nutrition to be achieved by 2005, including that at least 60% of people should derive less than 15% of energy from saturated fat, at least 50% of people should derive less than 35% of energy from total fat.*

Holmes, S. (1989) Nutrition and the elderly. *Nursing*, (37); 18–21.
*Sue Holmes considers what can be done by nurses to overcome some of the nutritional problems of ageing.*

Holmes, S. (1990) *Nutrition in Physiological Insights.* London: Distance Learning Centre, South Bank University.
*This forms part of a package of distance learning material, originally designed for students on the Diploma in Professional Studies in Nursing. It reviews the fundamentals of nutrition, patterns of eating behaviour,*

*alterations in need throughout the lifespan and current dietary recommendations.*

Hunter, M. (1989) Nutrition and the elderly. *Nursing Standard*, 4(21); 38–40.
*A clear review of the dietary problems facing older people.*

Krause, M., Mahan, K. & Arlin, M. (1991) *Food Nutrition and Diet Therapy*. London: Baillière Tindall.
*This text gives a good background in the basic theory of nutrition, together with aspects of applied nutrition throughout the lifespan. It should be remembered though that the text is American and hence recommended daily allowances (RDAs) of vitamins, etc. differ from those recommended in the United Kingdom.*

Taylor, M. (1988) Food, glorious food. *Nursing Times*, 84(13); 28–30.
*This article focuses on the need by nurses to improve the nutritional intake of patients in their care to avoid the problem of malnutrition.*

Wade, B. (1989) *A Stoma is for Life*. London: Scutari Press.
*Useful reading for those who care for patients having stoma surgery, looking, as it does, at problems faced by such people in the year following their surgery.*

Waston, R. (1989) Care of the mouth. *Nursing*, 3(44); 20–24.
*A review of the nurse's role in ensuring oral comfort for patients. The article includes some useful references.*

## References

Blank, D. & Mattes, R. (1990) Sugar and spice: similarities and sensory attribute. *Nursing Research*, 39(5); 290–292.

Caddow, P. (1989) *Applied Microbiology*. London: Scutari Press.

Farthing, M. (1999) Irritable bowel syndrome: New pharmaceutical approaches to treatment. *Clinical Gastroenterology*, 13(3); 461–471.

Finlay, T. (1997) Making sense of parenteral nutrition in adult patients. *Nursing Times*, 92(2); 35–36.

Green, R. (1985) Old age. In: Case, R. (ed) *Variation in Human Physiology*. Manchester: Manchester University Press.

Hawthorn, J. (1995) Understanding and management of nausea and vomiting. Oxford: Blackwell Science.

Heaton, K. (1990) Dietary fibre. *British Medical Journal*, 300; 1479–1480.

Holmes, S. (1986) Determinants of food intake. *Nursing*, 3(7); 260–264.

Holmes, S. (1990) Nutrition. In: Gould, D., Hinchliff, S. & Holmes, S. (eds) *Physiological Insights*. London: Distance Learning Centre, South Bank Polytechnic.

Holmes, S. & Mountain, E. (1993) Assessment of oral status: Evaluation of three oral assessment guides. *Journal of Clinical Nursing*, 2(1); 35–40.

Kowanko, I., Simon, S. & Wood, J. (1999) Nutritional care of the patient: Nurses' knowledge and attitudes in an acute care setting. *Journal of Clinical Nursing*, 8(2); 217–224.

McLaren, S. & Green, S. (1998) Nutritional screening and assessment. *Nursing Standard*, 12(48); 26–29.

Moore, K. (1988) *The Developing Human; Clinically Orientated Embryology*, 4th edn. Philadelphia: WB Saunders.

National Advisory Committee on Nutrition Education (1983) *Proposals for Nutritional Guidance for Health Education in Britain*. London: HMSO.

Pettigrew, D. (1989) Investing in mouth care. *Geriatric Nursing*, 10(1); 22–24.

Ross, H. (1998) Constipation: cause and control in an acute hospital setting. *British Journal of Nursing*, 7(15); 907–913.

Shireff, A. (1990) Preoperative nutritional assessment. *Nursing Times*, 86(8); 68–75.

Southgate, D. (1990) The role of dietary fibre in the diet. *Journal of the Royal Society of Health*, 110(5); 174–178.

Watson, R. (1989) Care of the mouth. *Nursing*, 3(44); 20–24.

Wright, L. (1974) *Bowel Function in Hospital Patients*. Royal College of Nursing Research Project, Series 1, No. 4. London: Royal College of Nursing.

# The liver

*Graeme D. Smith*

## LEARNING OBJECTIVES

After studying this chapter the reader should be able to:

- Describe the role of bile salts in the digestion and absorption of fats

- Discuss the significance of the enterohepatic circulation

- Explain the metabolism of bilirubin and the causes of jaundice

- Name the constituents of bile and list their functions

- Describe how bile is secreted from the liver cells to the intestine

## INTRODUCTION

The liver is vital to life. It is an organ that is metabolically active in the synthesis and catabolism (breakdown) of fats, proteins, carbohydrates and vitamins. It also metabolizes and detoxifies hormones, steroids and exogenous substances, such as drugs and alcohol, and secretes bile. This continuous biochemical activity results in the production of a considerable amount of heat, in fact, the amount of heat produced is second only to that of muscular activity. Under basal conditions, the liver is responsible for most of the body heat. The wide variety of reactions taking place in the liver allows for integration and regulation of its various functions. Other body tissues do not demonstrate such a wide functional ability. Although liver tissue has a considerable regenerative capacity, it can malfunction under certain conditions. The diversity of reactions taking place within the organ is then made apparent in the widespread bodily effects of abnormal liver function.

## Structure

The liver is the largest gland in the body, weighing, on average 1.5 kg in men and 1.3 kg in women. It is described as a gland because of its secretory function: it produces bile, which is stored in the gall bladder and subsequently released into the duodenum, where it has the function of emulsifying fat – breaking it down physically, as opposed to chemically – to prepare it for digestion by lipases secreted by the pancreas and the small intestine.

The liver consists of four anatomical lobes, the largest being the right, which lies under the right dome of the diaphragm; the smaller left lobe lies under the left dome. Two lesser segments of the right lobe, the caudate and the quadrate lobes, are located on the under-surface (**Fig. 5.2.1**). The liver is encased by the rib cage so that the organ is not normally palpable (**Fig. 5.2.2**). During a deep inspiration, the lower edge moves 1–3 cm downwards and may be palpated at 'two fingers depth' below the ribs on the right side of the abdomen.

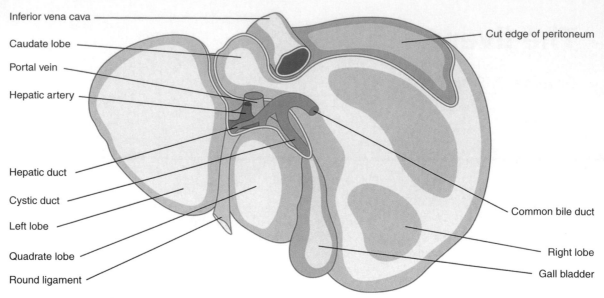

Inferior vena cava

Caudate lobe

Portal vein

Hepatic artery

Hepatic duct

Cystic duct

Left lobe

Quadrate lobe

Round ligament

Cut edge of peritoneum

Common bile duct

Right lobe

Gall bladder

**Figure 5.2.1**   The inferior surface of the liver showing the four lobes

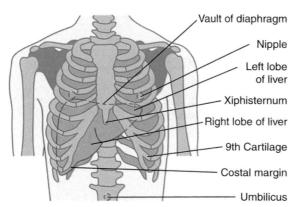

Vault of diaphragm

Nipple

Left lobe of liver

Xiphisternum

Right lobe of liver

9th Cartilage

Costal margin

Umbilicus

**Figure 5.2.2**   The position of the liver in relation to the rib cage

The peritoneum covering the liver forms several ligaments, which attach the organ to the diaphragm and the abdominal wall. The ligament attaching the liver to the abdominal wall is known as the **falciform ligament**.

## Blood supply

The blood supply to the liver is from two sources. The **hepatic artery**, a branch of the coeliac artery, carries arterial blood from the systemic circulation. The **portal vein**, supplied by the splenic and superior mesenteric veins, carries blood drained from the stomach and upper intestine (**Fig. 5.2.3**). These vessels enter the liver on the undersurface (**see Fig. 5.2.1**) at the **porta hepatis**, and divide immediately into right and left branches, which subdivide further through the hepatic tissue. Blood leaves the liver in the left, right and central **hepatic veins,** which open

directly into the inferior vena cava as they leave the liver. Sphincters in all the vascular compartments of the liver regulate the local supply from the hepatic artery and portal vein, as well as the total liver blood flow and capacity of the portal venous bed.

### CLINICAL APPLICATIONS

In certain conditions, for example in cardiac failure, the liver can accommodate up to one-third of the total body blood volume; thus the splanchnic vessels (i.e. those to the viscera) play a major part in the regulation of the general circulation. The vascularity of the liver is responsible for the problems of trauma to the organ caused by stabbing, gunshot wounds or, more frequently, car accidents. A considerable volume of blood may be lost, necessitating rapid repair and supportive measures.

## Histology

Microscopically, liver tissue is divided into **lobules**, 1–2 mm in diameter (**Fig. 5.2.4**). These constitute the functional units of the liver. The approximately hexagonal lobules consist of a central vein from which single columns of **hepatocytes** (liver cells) radiate towards the surrounding thin layer of connective tissue. Within the connective tissue are situated portal canals, each containing a branch of the hepatic artery and portal vein and an interlobular bile duct. Between the layers of cells lie sinusoids, which receive blood from both artery and vein and drain into the central vein. The system of veins runs approximately perpendicular to the portal canals.

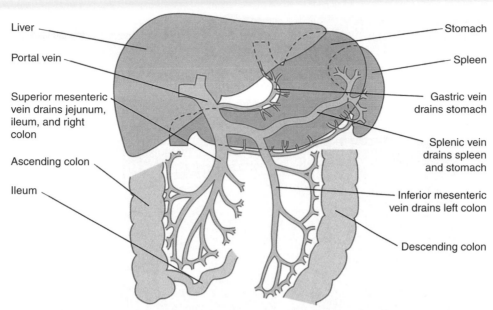

**Figure 5.2.3** The hepatic portal system

Labels (clockwise from top left): Liver · Portal vein · Superior mesenteric vein drains jejunum, ileum, and right colon · Ascending colon · Ileum · Stomach · Spleen · Gastric vein drains stomach · Splenic vein drains spleen and stomach · Inferior mesenteric vein drains left colon · Descending colon

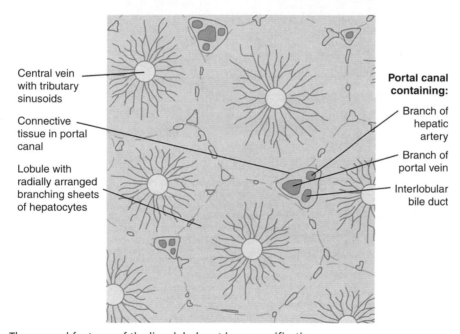

**Figure 5.2.4** The general features of the liver lobules at low magnification

Labels (left): Central vein with tributary sinusoids · Connective tissue in portal canal · Lobule with radially arranged branching sheets of hepatocytes

Labels (right): **Portal canal containing:** Branch of hepatic artery · Branch of portal vein · Interlobular bile duct

Surrounding the liver cells, and in direct contact with them, is a network of minute tubules called the **bile canaliculi**, which carry bile produced in the liver cells. The canaliculi drain into larger ductules and terminate in the interlobular bile ducts of the portal canals. The flow of blood and bile is shown schematically in **Fig. 5.2.5**.

The sinusoids are lined with flat phagocytic cells of the mononuclear phagocytic system (reticuloendothelial system), called **Kupffer cells**. These are important in phagocytosis and also in the production of antibodies. Behind these cells is the space of Disse (**Fig. 5.2.6**), which contains tissue fluid bathing the microvillous border of the hepatocytes. The sinusoidal lining is apparently freely permeable to nutrients and other molecules contained in the plasma. The microvilli maximize the area of liver cells available for absorption of these substances and fluids from the plasma. The area of hepatocytes adjacent to the bile canaliculus also has microvilli projecting into the lumen.

## Biliary drainage

The biliary drainage of the liver is completed as the interlobular ducts join with one another until the left

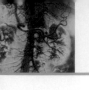

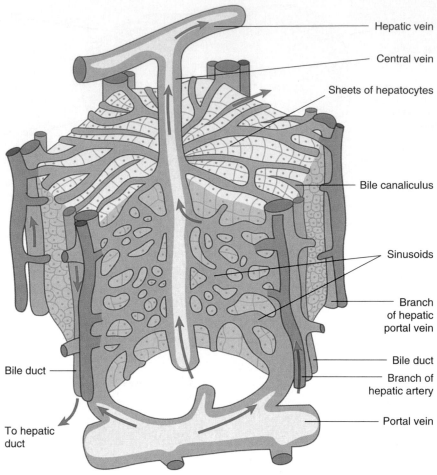

**Figure 5.2.5**   Diagram showing the flow of blood and bile within the liver lobules

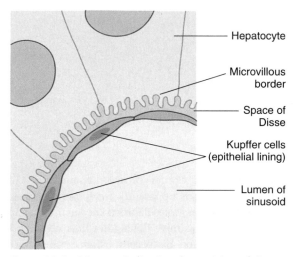

**Figure 5.2.6**   Diagram indicating the position of the space of Disse

and right hepatic ducts emerge from their respective lobes at the prota hepatis and unite to form the common hepatic duct (**Fig. 5.2.7**). This is joined by the cystic duct from the gall bladder, forming the common bile duct. The total length of the common bile duct is 7–8 cm and it opens, in common with the pancreatic duct, via the ampulla of Vater, a spindle-shaped dilation, into the second part of the duodenum 10 cm from the pylorus (**Fig. 5.2.8**). This common opening of the ducts is surrounded by a circular muscle called the **sphincter of Oddi**, which controls the flow of bile into the duodenum. Each duct also possesses its own sphincter so that bile and pancreatic juice may be discharged independently.

## The gall bladder

The gall bladder is a pear-shaped sac with a capacity of about 50 mL. It lies under the right liver lobe, to which it is bound by connective tissue and small blood vessels. The walls consist of a network of elastic and non-striated muscular tissue. The mucous membrane is thrown into folds, producing a honeycomb appearance in the body of the gall bladder, and is lined with columnar epithelium. There are no glands within the gall bladder. The cystic duct joins the gall bladder to the common bile duct.

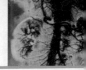

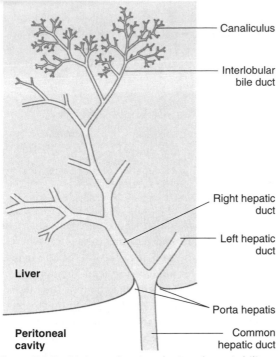

Figure 5.2.7 Diagram showing the intrahepatic biliary drainage (the biliary tree)

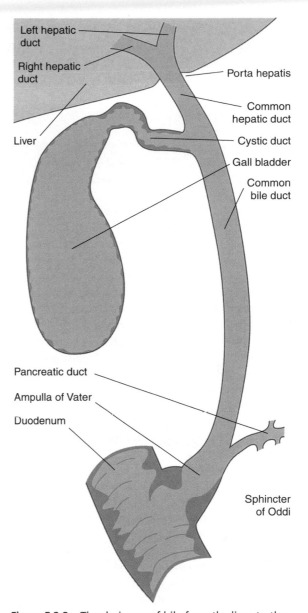

Figure 5.2.8 The drainage of bile from the liver to the intestine (the biliary tract)

## DEVELOPMENTAL ISSUES

The liver and biliary system develop from the hepatic diverticulum (bud). This is derived, during the fourth week of gestation, from endodermal cells in the ventral part of the foregut. The diverticulum enlarges rapidly, separating into two parts: the larger (cranial) part consists of cords of liver cells extending into the septum transversum from which fibrous tissue and Kupffer cells are derived, whereas the smaller (caudal) part expands to form the gall bladder. Haemopoiesis begins during the sixth week but subsides by the end of the pregnancy (see Chapter 4.1). At about 9 weeks gestation, the liver accounts for 10% of the total fetal weight; however, this reduces to about 5% at term. Bile pigments form during weeks 13–16 and enter the duodenum, giving the meconium its characteristic dark green colour (Moore & Persaud, 1993).

The umbilical vein supplies oxygenated blood from the placenta to the portal vein of the developing fetus. Following birth it normally becomes redundant. However, if portal hypertension occurs in adulthood, the remnants can be utilized for colateral circulation.

## Bile

The production of bile is the main exocrine function of the liver, providing an excretory route for several substances.

Bile is a yellowish-green viscous fluid, slightly alkaline in reaction (pH 7–8) and with a bitter taste. About 500–1000 mL are produced daily by the liver and pass into the common bile duct. There is a diurnal rhythm of secretion, more being produced during the day. In the common hepatic duct, above the cystic duct, the bile is 97–98% water and contains 2–3% solids. The main constituents of bile contribute to its functions.

## Bile acids (salts)

Bile acids constitute approximately half the solid matter of bile. In solution, they form salts, usually with sodium. They are important in promoting the absorption of fats and fat-soluble substances from

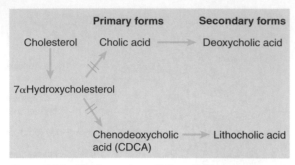

**Figure 5.2.9** The formation of bile acids from cholesterol

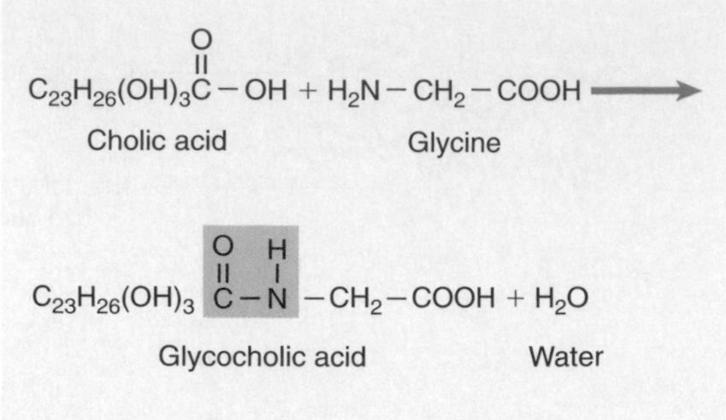

$$C_{23}H_{26}(OH)_3 \overset{O}{\underset{||}{C}} - OH + H_2N - CH_2 - COOH \longrightarrow$$

Cholic acid          Glycine

$$C_{23}H_{26}(OH)_3 \boxed{\overset{O}{\underset{||}{C}} - \overset{H}{\underset{|}{N}}} - CH_2 - COOH + H_2O$$

Glycocholic acid       Water

**Figure 5.2.10** The conjugation of cholic acid with glycine occurring in the liver cells

the intestine. There are 2–4 g of bile salts in the body pool and approximately 0.3–0.6 g are lost in the faeces per day. As the pool remains constant, the liver synthesizes 0.3–0.6 g bile salts per day.

The two primary acid forms, cholic acid and chenodeoxycholic acid (CDCA), are synthesized in the liver from cholesterol (**Fig. 5.2.9**). The secondary forms, deoxycholic and lithocholic acids, are produced in the intestine as a result of bacterial action. Only small quantities of the latter are produced, which are excreted in the faeces. The deoxycholic acid is absorbed with the remaining cholic and chenodeoxycholic acid by the terminal ileum and proximal colon. The synthesis of bile acids is controlled by a feedback mechanism operating at the first reaction (see A in **Fig. 5.2.9**).

Within the liver cells, the bile acids are conjugated with the amino acid glycine or taurine to form glycocholic or taurocholic acid. A **conjugation reaction** involves the formation of an amide linkage (similar to that of amino acid linkages to form proteins) with the elimination of water (**Fig. 5.2.10**). The salts (usually sodium) of these conjugated acids are secreted from the liver cells into the canaliculi. A carrier-mediated mechanism involving active transport against a concentration gradient occurs.

In the bile, the salts form **micelles** – aggregates of molecules having both polar and non-polar characteristics. Micelles keep non-polar, insoluble substances such as cholesterol in solution (**see Fig. 5.1.17**).

The micelles are disrupted in the intestine, allowing the cholesterol to be released and excreted in the faeces; at the same time, the bile salts are operative in the absorption of fat molecules from the lumen (see also Chapter 5.1). Some of the cholate is deconjugated by bacterial action. Unconjugated bile salts diffuse passively into the intestinal cells at all levels of the small intestine, whereas the conjugated ones are reabsorbed into the cells of the lumen by an active transport mechanism in the terminal ileum; a total of 97% is reabsorbed in this way. The remainder continues to the colon where further bacterial degradation occurs followed by passive reabsorption or excretion in the faeces. The reabsorbed bile salts enter the portal venous system draining the intestine. Most are bound to serum proteins and returned to the liver where, at the sinusoids, the salts are taken up by the hepatocytes via a carrier-mediated system. Thus only small amounts enter the systemic circulation. The bile salts taken up by the liver are available for further secretion from the hepatocytes into the bile canaliculi. This cycle is called the **enterohepatic circulation**. It provides a mechanism for the conservation and reutilization of the bile acids and also of other compounds secreted in the bile, such as oestrogenic hormones, progesterone, the thyroid hormones, vitamin A and its metabolites, as well as various drugs (**Fig. 5.2.11**).

The total bile salt pool may circulate between the liver and intestine two to three times during each meal, so that 15–30 g bile salts per day are secreted by the hepatocytes into the canaliculi. Various factors affect the enterohepatic circulation of compounds. These include the extent and rate of secretion of the compound into the bile; the activity of the gall bladder; the fate of the substance in the intestine, particularly the consequences of bacterial deconjugation reactions; and the fate of the substance after reabsorption.

The importance of bile acids is threefold (see Chapter 5.1). First, they activate enzymes involved in the absorption of nutrients such as pancreatic lipase. Second, as emulsifiers they are involved in the digestion and absorption of fats. And finally, high blood levels of bile acids themselves stimulate further bile and bile acid production. They also stimulate a variety of hepatic secretory functions such as phospholipid and cholesterol secretion.

## CLINICAL APPLICATIONS

### ABNORMALITIES OF BILE SALT METABOLISM

Abnormalities of bile salt metabolism and turnover may occur in two ways. Obstruction of the biliary tree results in a decreased quantity of bile salts reaching the intestine and an increased proportion within the liver and serum. As the bile

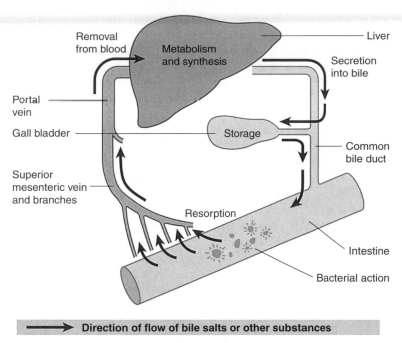

**Figure 5.2.11** Diagrammatic representation of the enterohepatic circulation

salts are required for the digestion and absorption of fat from the intestine, this process is impaired, resulting in an increased excretion of fat within the faeces, known as **steatorrhoea**. In conditions of hepatocellular damage, such as cirrhosis, there is a significant decrease in the total bile acid pool due to a decreased synthesis of bile acids, especially cholic acid in the liver, and an absence of deoxycholic acid due to changes in the colonic flora or intestinal contents, such that the normal production of deoxycholic acid from cholic acid does not occur. This also results in steatorrhoea due to poor digestion and absorption of fats.

## Bile pigments

These are the excretory products of haem and are responsible for the colours of bile and faeces (see also Chapter 4.1). About 260–300 mg of bilirubin are produced in adults per day, although the liver has the reserve capacity to excrete five to ten times this amount. About 75% is derived from the haemoglobin of mature red cells, the breakdown of which takes place in the mononuclear phagocytic (reticuloendothelial) cells of the liver and spleen. The remainder is released in the liver from tissue cytochromes and other haem products. The breakdown of haemoglobin can be summarized as shown in **Fig. 5.2.12**.

### Bilirubin

Bilirubin, the predominant pigment in bile, is yellow in colour, weakly acid, soluble in lipid and sparingly

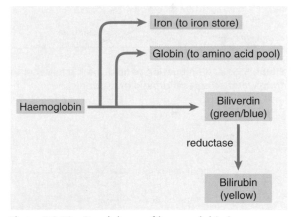

**Figure 5.2.12** Breakdown of haemoglobin in mononuclear phagocytes of the liver

soluble in water. Within cells it interferes with vital metabolic functions. Unconjugated bilirubin is transported in the plasma tightly bound to albumin.

---

### CLINICAL APPLICATIONS

Drugs such as sulphonamides or salicylates compete for binding and so facilitate the diffusion of bilirubin into the liver and other tissues. In neonates, such drug administration would facilitate the entry of unconjugated bilirubin to the brain, increasing the risk of kernicterus.

---

Unbound (lipid-soluble) bilirubin is taken up by the liver cells with ease, whereas the bound complex utilizes a carrier mechanism in the cell membrane.

521

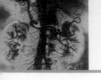

Within the cell, bilirubin is bound to one of two soluble proteins of low molecular weight, called the Y and Z carrier proteins. Competition with other substances may occur. At the smooth endoplasmic reticulum the lipid-soluble unconjugated bilirubin is rendered water soluble, and thus easily excreted, by conjugation to form bilirubin diglucuronide. The reaction is catalysed by the microsomal enzyme bilirubin uridine diphosphate (UDP) glucuronyl transferase (**Fig. 5.2.13**). This reaction can be induced (increased) by drugs such as phenobarbitone or inhibited (decreased) by others – novobiocin, for example.

The secretion of the conjugated bilirubin into the bile canaliculi is poorly understood. It occurs against a large concentration gradient and is probably carrier mediated. The conjugated bilirubin is part of the micellar complex in the bile and thus passes into the intestine (**Fig. 5.2.14**).

Bacterial activity in the terminal ileum and colon releases unconjugated bilirubin, which is then reduced to urobilinogen. Small quantities of urobilinogen absorbed by the intestine enter the enterohepatic circulation and are re-excreted by the liver and the kidney; 0.5–5.0 μmol per day enter the systemic circulation to be excreted as urinary urobilinogen, and may be detected using Ehrlich's aldehyde reagent. Increased amounts occur in various conditions, for example haemolytic jaundice. Urobilinogen is colourless but oxidizes on exposure to air to an orange–red urobilin. It may be detected visually if urine is allowed to stand.

Some 150–500 μmol of urobilinogen is excreted in the faeces. Here it is known as stercobilinogen. It is also oxidized on exposure to air, giving rise to stercobilin and the characteristic faecal coloration.

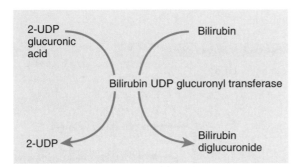

**Figure 5.2.13** Conjugation of lipid-soluble bilirubin to form water-soluble bilirubin diglucoronide

## DEVELOPMENTAL ISSUES

In the neonate, bilirubin is found only in the faeces, as the bacterial reduction mechanism for its conversion to urobilinogen does not develop fully for some months. This explains the yellow colour of babies' stools. In the adult, oral antibiotics can inhibit the bacterial reactions.

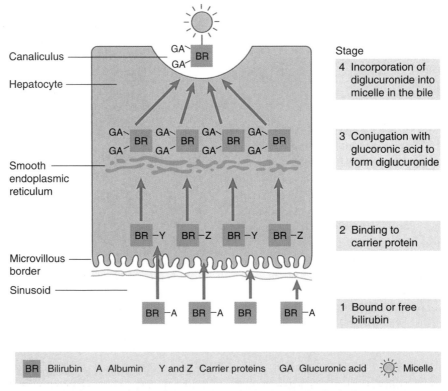

**Figure 5.2.14** Diagrammatic representation of the passage of bilirubin through the hepatocyte

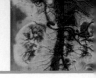

Serum bilirubin levels are measured using the Van den Bergh test. The normal ranges are as follows.

- total bilirubin: 5.0–17.0 μmol/L
- conjugated ('direct'): <3.0 μmol/L
- unconjugated ('indirect'): 2.0–15.0 μmol/L.

## CLINICAL APPLICATIONS

### JAUNDICE

Jaundice occurs when the normal metabolism of bilirubin is altered resulting in an increased serum bilirubin level. Clinically, it can be identified by a yellow coloration of the skin, sclera and other elastic tissues, which is visible in daylight at serum levels greater than 34 μmol/L. The urine may be dark due to the presence of excess bilirubin and the faeces pale due to its absence. Traditionally, jaundice has been classified as haemolytic, hepatocellular or obstructive (cholestatic). This, however, is an oversimplification and the following classification is more helpful:

**In jaundice due to increased bilirubin load** an increased production and/or breakdown of red cells may occur. As these are the precursors of haem and thus bilirubin, an increased amount of the latter is formed. The liver is unable to conjugate all the pigment so that a rise in the level of unconjugated pigment in the serum takes place. This situation occurs in various haemolytic conditions both congenital, such as hereditary spherocytosis and the haemoglobinopathies, sickle-cell anaemia and thalassaemia major; and acquired, such as severe bacterial infection or malaria or, rarely, following the administration of certain chemical preparations such as quinine or sulphonamides.

Serum levels of bilirubin are usually less than 85 μmol/L and the jaundice is mild and lemon yellow. The faeces are dark due to increased quantities of stercobilinogen but the urine rarely darkens, although the urinary urobilinogen is raised. Anaemia also accompanies the condition because of the increased breakdown of red cells.

**In jaundice due to deficiency of the transferase enzyme**, deficiency of the conjugation enzyme bilirubin uridine diphosphate glucuronyl transferase also leads to raised levels of unconjugated bilirubin. This occurs in various hereditary conditions, the most common being **Gilbert's disease**. A mild, benign, fluctuating jaundice occurs with no change in colour of the urine or faeces.

The liver of a neonate may be immature, giving rise to a temporary deficiency of transferase. The decreased conjugation rate leads to a retention of unconjugated bilirubin and the development of an orange–yellow jaundice after the first 24 hours in a full-term infant and after approximately 48 hours in a preterm infant. This 'physiological' jaundice, which is common in otherwise normal babies, usually subsides within 2 weeks.

Unconjugated bilirubin, being lipid soluble, has an affinity for nervous tissue, particularly in the newborn and, at high levels, passes into the basal ganglia and other areas of the brain and spinal cord causing disturbance of cellular metabolism and resulting in **kernicterus**. The mortality from this is high and surviving infants are usually mentally handicapped.

Treatment of rising bilirubin levels (estimated from heel-prick blood samples by a bilirubinometer) by phototherapy, which converts bilirubin to a colourless compound with no known long-term deleterious effects on the infant, is used for more severe 'physiological' jaundice. Serum bilirubin levels exceeding 340 μmol/L in full-term infants or 270 μmol/L in preterm infants are considered dangerous and exchange transfusion may be considered. Kernicterus may also develop when haemolytic disease of the newborn due to Rhesus incompatibility between the mother and infant occurs (see Chapter 4.1).

'Breast milk jaundice', with an unconjugated bilirubin level raised above 205 μmol/L, can occur in some breast-fed infants. This may last from 2 weeks until 2 months after delivery. The cause of this jaundice is not known and brain damage is unlikely. Breast feeding can usually be continued.

Jaundice in a baby persisting beyond 2 weeks of age should always be investigated further so that a treatable liver disease is not overlooked.

**In jaundice due to liver cell damage**, general damage to the liver by toxic or infective agents causes disruption of the cells with a regurgitation of bilirubin, both conjugated and unconjugated, into the blood. Infective agents include, most commonly, the viruses responsible for all types of hepatitis (A, B, C, D and E) and also yellow and glandular fevers. Toxic agents include drugs such as halothane (anaesthetic) and the monoamine oxidase inhibitors (antidepressants), to which some individuals develop sensitivity reactions. Serum bilirubin levels are variable, often greater than 340 μmol/L, and show a rise during the icteric (jaundiced) period followed by a fall during convalescence. The urine is dark due to the presence of conjugated water-soluble bilirubin, whereas the faeces are paler than normal as little bilirubin reaches the intestine due to the microscopic obstruction of the bile canaliculi.

**In jaundice due to intrahepatic obstruction**, microscopic intrahepatic obstruction leads to a regurgitation of conjugated bilirubin to the blood. In the condition of biliary cirrhosis, fibrous

**Table 5.2.1** The characteristics of different types of jaundice

| | Haemolytic | Hepatocellular | | Obstructive | |
|---|---|---|---|---|---|
| Abnormality | Increased bilirubin load | Deficiency of transferase | Cellular damage | Intrahepatic fibrous obstruction | Extrahepatic obstruction |
| Example | Hereditary spherocytosis | Gilbert's disease | Infective hepatitis | Biliary cirrhosis | Carcinoma of head of pancreas |
| **Urine** | | | | | |
| Colour | Normal | Normal | Dark | Dark | Dark |
| Urobilinogen | Increased | Variable | Variable | Absent | Absent |
| Bilirubin | Absent | Absent | Increased | Increased | Increased |
| **Faeces** | | | | | |
| Colour | Dark | Normal | Paler than normal | Pale | Pale |
| Stercobilinogen | Increased | Normal | Low | Absent | Absent |
| **Plasma** | | | | | |
| Unconjugated bilirubin | Increased | Increased | Decreased | Increased | Increased |
| Conjugated bilirubin | Normal | Decreased | Increased | Increased | Increased |

obstructions to the secretion of bile at the canaliculi occur. The onset of jaundice is gradual but high levels of serum bilirubin (greater than 510 µmol/L) may be reached after prolonged illness. The urine is dark and the faeces pale. In prolonged jaundice the skin may appear greenish in colour due to the presence of biliverdin.

Some drugs may cause intrahepatic obstruction by forming plugs within the canaliculi, thus leading to jaundice. Chlorpromazine (Largactil) is an example of this; 1–2% of patients receiving it developing jaundice.

**Jaundice due to extrahepatic obstruction** to bile flow may be caused within the biliary tree by gallstones or by external obstructions causing occlusion of the ducts, such as carcinoma of the head of the pancreas. Gallstones often give rise to an intermittent jaundice. The urine is dark and the faeces pale.

The characteristics of the different types of jaundice are shown in **Table 5.2.1**.

## NURSING MANAGEMENT OF A PATIENT WITH JAUNDICE

To a large extent, the management of jaundice is directed at eliminating the underlying cause if at all possible, for example the withdrawal of an offending agent, such as alcohol or a certain medication. However, in hepatocellular jaundice the extent of the liver damage may militate against resolution. Equally, in obstructive jaundice eliminating the cause may not always be possible. Nursing intervention focuses on both the management of the symptoms and the patient's understanding of the specific disorder involved, be it benign or otherwise. For many patients, it may be hard to come to terms with the fact that for some the jaundice has a simple resolvable cause and for others it reflects mortal disease. Time spent giving information and support to patients (and their families) who are experiencing the latter is paramount in ensuring that they can come to terms with their diagnosis.

Whatever the cause, the nursing management and care for a patient with jaundice aims to achieve comfort and rest, avoid injury, cope with the change in body image and to promote and maintain optimal appetite and nutrition.

### To achieve comfort and rest

The key priority here is to relieve itching, which effectively includes the following measures:

- Avoid extremes of heat, such as hot baths and showers, and keep the environment cool as sweating will irritate the skin further.
- Avoid using perfumed or deodorized soaps that may dry or irritate the skin; use emollients such an oilatum and aqueous cream.
- Although it may lack an evidence-base, 50 g of bicarbonate of soda added to the bath

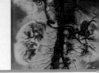

water appears to soothe the itching in many patients.

- Keep bed clothing cool and light.
- Provide distraction and diversional activity, such as reading or interaction with other patients.
- The administration of prescribed medications, which may include:
  - cholestyramine to prevent the accumulation of bile acids by binding them in the bowel and preventing their being reabsorbed
  - antihistamines, particularly at night when their action not only reduces the itching but also may help the patient sleep
  - ursodeoxycholic acid, which may be effective in some patients as it appears to protect the body from the bile salts
  - the antibiotic rifampicin, which appears to reduce itching by its action on liver enzymes. This must be used with caution, under specialist guidance, as it may be toxic to the liver.

### To avoid injury to the skin

- Understand the desire but explain the damaging effect of scratching.
- Keep nails short and smooth. If necessary provide cotton gloves at night.
- Administer medications as indicated above.

### To promote acceptance of changes in body image

- Convey an accepting attitude for the expressed feeling and concerns.
- Be a supportive listener to both patient and family.
- Provide individualized and ongoing information and explanations.

### To promote and maintain optimal appetite and nutrition

- Carry out a careful assessment of nutritional well-being.
- Provide a diet that is high in kilocalories and glucose (the latter being thought to aid liver cell recovery), limited in fat and with fat-soluble vitamin supplements as appropriate.
- Omit all poorly tolerated food.
- Monitor clinical appearance and weight as appropriate.

## Lipids

The major lipids in bile are cholesterol and lecithin (a phospholipid).

### Cholesterol

Cholesterol is a chemically unreactive hydrocarbon, insoluble in water. It occurs in cell membranes and circulates in the plasma. Cholesterol is synthesized in the liver and is also absorbed from the intestine. The latter, i.e. that absorbed, derives from endogenous cholesterol secreted in the bile, cholesterol from shed epithelial cells and from exogenous sterols in food, which are hydrolysed in the intestine. The size of the body pool is variable, normal total cholesterol for the whole body being $3.5–7.0\,\mu mol/L$. Under normal conditions, the rate of synthesis shows a diurnal rhythm. A high cholesterol intake decreases the rate of synthesis in the liver, whereas loss of cholesterol through a biliary fistula increases it. The biliary content is $1.6–4.4\,mmol/L$. Cholesterol absorbed from the intestine is esterified, (i.e. its alcohol (—OH) group is linked to an organic acid (usually a fatty acid), eliminating water) within the intestinal cells and carried as a lipoprotein or chylomicron in the lymph to the thoracic duct. From there it travels in the systemic circulation to the liver where it is rapidly assimilated. The free unesterified form is excreted from the liver cells into the bile micelles. Cholesterol is also metabolized to bile acids within the liver.

### CLINICAL APPLICATIONS

When an imbalance of the main constituents of bile occurs, namely a reduction in bile salts and phospholipids and an increase in cholesterol, cholesterol can be precipitated, leading to the formation of gallstones. When prolonged raised serum cholesterol levels occur, as in biliary cirrhosis, flat or slightly raised soft yellow areas called **xanthomas** appear on the face, neck, chest or back. These disappear as the cholesterol level falls.

### Phospholipids

Lecithin accounts for 90% of the phospholipids in bile; others are lysolecithin (3%) and phosphatidyl ethanolamine (1%). Lecithin (or phosphatidyl choline, which is an alternative name) is important in fatty acid metabolism.

Fatty acids are delivered to the liver in a free form or esterified with glycerol or cholesterol. Others are synthesized within the liver from carbohydrate or amino acid precursors. In turn, these fatty acids are metabolized to the forms in which they leave the liver, either as lipoproteins or as phospholipids containing choline, for example lecithin.

Within the bile, lecithin and its partially hydrolysed derivative lysolecithin, which has a detergent action, are incorporated into the micelles. They aid the emulsification of dietary lipids and undergo further hydrolysis within the intestine, to be excreted in the faeces. They do not enter the enterohepatic circulation.

## Other constituents of bile

### Electrolytes

The following ions are secreted into the bile: sodium, potassium, chloride, hydrogen carbonate, calcium and magnesium. These pass into the bile at the hepatocytes as a result of the osmotic effect of the actively transported bile salts. The hormones secretin and cholecystokinin (CCK), both released by the duodenal mucosa, and insulin and glucagon, both from the pancreas, also stimulate the secretion of chloride and bicarbonate. Within the gall bladder, reabsorption of water and the electrolytes occurs so that their respective concentrations are diminished disproportionately. Whereas sodium is the dominant electrolyte in hepatic bile, chloride predominates in gall bladder bile. The alkalinity of the bile aids the neutralization of the acidic food (chyme) within the intestine.

### Alkaline phosphatase

This enzyme is synthesized in the liver; another related form (i.e. an isoenzyme) is synthesized in bone. The two forms can be separated by electrophoresis. The normal serum level is 21–100 iu/L. The biological role of hepatic alkaline phosphatase is not known, although involvement in the transport of compounds into the bile has been postulated.

### Minor constituents

The following substances are found in small quantities in the bile: vitamin B12, nucleoproteins, mucin, triglycerides, free fatty acids, plasma proteins such as albumin, and free amino acids.

Vitamin B12 is stored in the liver. It has a lipotrophic effect and is necessary for protein metabolism and for formation of the erythrocytic stroma (see Chapter 4.1). It is reabsorbed into the enterohepatic circulation.

## Secretion of bile from the liver cells to the duodenum (see also Chapter 5.1)

The secretion of bile from the hepatocytes into the canaliculi takes place in different ways. First, there is a **bile-acid-dependent secretion**, which, as its name suggests, is determined by the secretion of bile acids. This involves their active transport into the canaliculi where they exert an osmotic effect that draws water, electrolytes and bile pigments across the cell membrane. The volume of bile produced is determined by the rate at which bile salts are returned to the hepatocytes by the enterohepatic circulation.

There is also a **bile-acid-independent secretion**, which involves an active sodium pump mechanism carrying water, small solutes and electrolytes into the bile.

Third, there is a **ductular secretion**, which modifies the canalicular flow of bile. This is stimulated by the hormone secretin, released from the duodenal mucosa when the acid food chyme enters the duodenum. The enzyme acts on the biliary ductules giving rise to a 'watery' bile due to increased secretion of water, sodium bicarbonate and sodium chloride. As this secretion takes place mainly during a meal, it does not result in storage of the bile in the gall bladder where water may be reabsorbed. Of the approximately 600 mL of bile secreted in 24 hours, 225 mL are bile-acid-dependent, 225 mL are bile-acid-independent and 150 mL are ductular.

The hepatic bile, produced continuously, is stored in the gall bladder between meals. Here, reabsorption of some constituents occurs, particularly of water and electrolytes, which leads to an increased concentration of five to ten times that of other constituents,

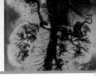

particularly bilirubin, bile salts, cholesterol, fatty acids and lecithin. Muscular contraction of the gall bladder, stimulated by the vagal nerve and the hormone cholecystokinin, produced by the intestinal wall, releases bile into the duodenum via the cystic duct and the relaxed sphincter of Oddi. Two or three cycles of bile secretion occur at each meal, resulting in approximately 500–1000 mL total secretion in 24 hours. Evacuation of the gall bladder takes place only once during a meal. The bile flow subsequent to that is directly from the liver into the intestine.

## CLINICAL APPLICATIONS

### CHOLESTASIS

Interference of the bile flow from the liver to the duodenum results in a syndrome called cholestasis – an accumulation of bile in the liver cells with a resultant retention in the blood of substances normally excreted in the bile. The effects vary with the type and duration of the obstruction. **Extrahepatic obstruction** is mechanical; examples are gallstones in the biliary ducts or carcinoma of the pancreas occluding the duct. **Intrahepatic obstructions** are due to damage of the liver itself by agents including viruses (hepatitis), alcohol and drugs. Jaundice (described earlier) will be evident, as will steatorrhoea. **Malabsorption** of other nutrients apart from fats occurs, particularly of the fat-soluble vitamins A, D, E and K and calcium, which is absorbed with fats in the form of a soap. On a long-term basis this can lead to a state of malnutrition, with vitamin and calcium deficiencies. The diet supplied to the patient should therefore be strictly controlled. Restricting the intake of fat to about 30–40 g per day makes life more tolerable as the patient passes fewer bulky stools. Medium-chain triglycerides (smaller parts of fat molecules) can be given orally to increase the energy intake because they are water soluble and absorbed directly into the blood without the need for the presence of bile salts. Intramuscular preparations of fat-soluble vitamins and calcium supplements prevent deficiency conditions.

**Pruritus** (itching of the skin) is associated with cholestasis and for many years this was thought to be due to the presence of bile salts irritating cutaneous sensory nerves. However, pruritus may well be due to an as yet unidentified serum factor, because there is a low correlation between serum bile acid levels and the presence of pruritus. Treatment involves the use of antihistamines or cholestyramine, an exchange resin said to bind bile salts in the intestine causing their faecal excretion and consequent lowering of the serum bile acid level. There is often a reluctance by the patient to take this preparation because it can produce nausea. Scrupulous skin hygiene is necessary for affected patients by the use of soft sheets, lotions such as calamine, bathing in tepid water and keeping the nails short so that scratching does not damage the skin.

**Clotting abnormalities** also occur in cholestasis. In particular, the prothrombin time is prolonged because vitamin K is not absorbed; spontaneous bruising may occur. Collection of blood by venepuncture should be as infrequent as possible. Dental care should be gentle because a hard toothbrush can cause bleeding of the gums; mouthwashes and the use of swabs may be more appropriate.

### GALLSTONES

Gallstones occur in both men and women, with a higher incidence among the latter. There is a general increase in prevalence with age so that by the seventh decade of life 22.4% of females and 11.5% of males have had gallstones.

The predominant constituent of gallstones found in Westerners is cholesterol. At present, understanding of gallstone formation remains incomplete but a major factor involves an alteration in the 'cholesterol-carrying capacity' of the bile. Normally, the bile is saturated with cholesterol and has sufficient capacity within the micelles to carry the amount present. In certain circumstances it may become lithogenic (potentially gallstone forming). This occurs when there is a reduced secretion of bile acids by the liver and thus an insufficient cholesterol-carrying capacity, so that the bile is supersaturated with cholesterol. This crystallizes out and aggregates to form a stone if an appropriate (but unknown) nucleating agent is present. Gallstones are formed in the gall bladder because the bile accumulates here between meals. Factors associated with gallstone formation are increasing age, child bearing, obesity, the use of the drug clofibrate (to treat certain hyperlipidaemias) and the long-term use of oestrogen in oral contraceptives and hormone replacement therapy. Oestrogen reduces hepatic bile acid secretion so that the bile produced is more lithogenic. A reduced bile salt pool (and thus cholesterol-carrying capacity) occurs with prolonged cholestyramine therapy for pruritus and following ileal resection when the enterohepatic circulation of bile acids is broken. There is an increased incidence of gallstones in these conditions.

Other constituents of gallstones include calcium salts of bilirubin and trace quantities of fatty acids, phospholipids, bile acids and glycoproteins. When large amounts of calcium are present the stones are radio-opaque. Only about 10% of gallstones can be seen on X-ray, thus ultrasonography and/or oral cholecystography are important diagnostic tools. Other investigative techniques include computerized axial tomography (CT scan) and endoscopic retrograde cholangiopancreatography (ERCP). Pigment stones, without cholesterol, are associated with haemolytic conditions when excessive quantities of bilirubin, particularly the less soluble unconjugated form, are present in the bile.

**Cholecystitis** is an inflammation of the gall bladder, usually in association with obstruction of the cystic duct or the neck of the gall bladder by gallstones. It may be acute or chronic, the former being the third most common cause of acute pain requiring hospital admission in the United Kingdom. Biliary colic, the pain of acute or chronic cholecystitis, is severe. It arises in the epigastrium and moves to the right side and back or shoulder. The pain lasts several hours and may be accompanied by nausea and vomiting. Jaundice may be slight or latent, that is, revealed only by bilirubin estimations. The attack may be precipitated by the ingestion of fatty foods. The pain is due to the gall bladder contracting in an attempt to overcome the blocked cystic duct. The walls are also stretched to accommodate the accumulating inflammatory exudate. Thus the splanchnic and phrenic nerve endings in the wall of the gall bladder are stimulated. Irritation of the overlying peritoneum, which is innervated by spinal nerves, gives rise to superficial pain. The diaphragm lies close to the gall bladder and stimulation of the sensory nerves supplying it, that is, the phrenic and some intercostal nerves, gives rise to the referred pain. Treatment includes bedrest, suitable analgesia (such as pethidine), antispasmodics, antibiotics if infection is present, and the maintenance of fluid and electrolyte balance by intravenous therapy. Medical treatment of gallstones involves the oral administration of the naturally occuring bile acids chenodeoxycholic and/or ursodeoxycholic acids, which dissolve the stone and reduce cholesterol saturation in the blood. This treatment, cholelitholysis, is long term and there is a tendency for stones to reoccur when treatment is stopped.

If **cholecystectomy** (surgical removal of the gall bladder) is to take place, immediately prior to surgery the stomach is emptied by nasogastric suction. During cholecystectomy, exploration of the common bile duct is undertaken to detect the presence of further stones. A T-tube is inserted to maintain the patency of the bile duct during healing and to enable observation of the biliary flow **(Fig. 5.2.15)**. Observable drainage occurs via the stem portion of the T-tube, which is brought out through the abdominal wall via either the incision or a stab wound and attached to a drainage bag. During the first 24 hours, frequent observation for haemorrhage is necessary. Small amounts of blood mixed with bile are lost during the first few hours and thereafter normally bile alone in variable quantities. The tube is clamped, so that all the bile flows through the bile duct, and is gradually shortened prior to removal. Observation of the remaining dressing is necessary to detect bile seepage. Large quantities may damage the skin and leakage into the abdominal cavity may cause peritonitis. Further advances in the treatment of gallstones include lithotripsy (fragmentation of the stones) by an extra-corporeal shock-wave technique, endoscopy to facilitate sphincterotomy and removal of common bile duct stones and the recent introduction of laparoscopic cholecystectomy (so called key-hole surgery). Chronic cholecystitis might not be caused by the presence of gallstones. Bouts of biliary colic occur at intervals accompanied usually by general digestive complaints such as nausea, flatulence and dyspepsia.

## Synthetic processes of the liver

In addition to the production of bile, which is the excretory route for some substances, the liver is also the site of many synthetic processes, some of which are unique to it.

## Plasma proteins

All plasma proteins except the immune gammaglobulins are manufactured within the liver.

### Albumin

This is the smallest plasma protein, with a molecular weight of about 69 000. About 175 mg albumin per kg body weight per day are made, or 12 g per day in an adult. About one-sixth of dietary nitrogen is utilized in this way. The synthesis is dependent on prevailing amino acid levels so the nutritional status of the individual is important. Protein-deficient diets such as those which lead to malnutrition states also lead to a lowered serum albumin. The total body pool of albumin is about 300 g, of which approximately one-third is in the blood at a level of 35–50 g/L.

Albumin is the protein mainly responsible for the maintenance of the colloidal osmotic effect of the plasma, which influences the exchange of water between the tissues and blood. The osmotic effect is due to its lower molecular weight and the quantity

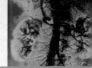

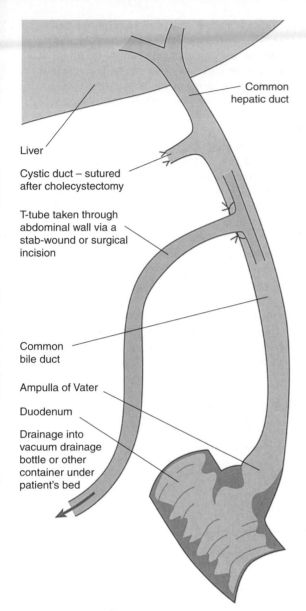

Figure 5.2.15  T-tube in position

Common hepatic duct

Liver

Cystic duct – sutured after cholecystectomy

T-tube taken through abdominal wall via a stab-wound or surgical incision

Common bile duct

Ampulla of Vater

Duodenum

Drainage into vacuum drainage bottle or other container under patient's bed

of molecules present compared with other plasma proteins.

### DEVELOPMENTAL ISSUES

#### α-FETOPROTEIN

α-Fetoprotein, with a normal concentration of less than 30 ng/mL, is similar in molecular size to albumin. It is produced by the fetal liver with a maximum level occurring at 12–16 weeks of gestation. Maternal blood levels can be measured to indicate the presence of fetal abnormalities, particularly neural tube defects. The protein passes from the fetal nervous system into the amniotic fluid and is absorbed by the mother. In

adult life the protein is produced in acute and chronic hepatitis, and more particularly by primary hepatic tumours.

### Globulins

The total serum globulin level is 18–32 g/L, of which 7–15 g/L are $\gamma$-globulins. The $\alpha_2$, $\beta$ and some $\alpha_1$-globulins are synthesized in the liver. The $\gamma$ (immune) globulins are made in the mononuclear phagocytic (reticuloendothelial) system outside the liver. The globulin molecules are much bigger than albumin, their molecular weights ranging from 90 000 to over a million. They are involved in the transport of various substances such as cortisol, oestrogen, copper (ceruloplasmin) and iron (transferrin). As with albumin, their synthesis depends on the amino acid level.

### CLINICAL APPLICATIONS

Changes in plasma protein levels occur in liver disease, usually with a decrease in serum albumin and an increase in serum globulins. These changes are detected using flocculation tests or electrophoresis. Flocculation (or turbidity) tests determine quantitative changes in the amounts of plasma albumin and globulins and measure the immunoglobulin response to liver cell damage rather than the damage itself. More accurate estimations of the proportions of plasma protein can be made by electrophoresis, a technique based on the fact that different proteins move at different rates in an electric field. This separates the albumin, $\alpha_1$-, $\alpha_2$-, $\beta$- and $\gamma$-globulins. Different patterns are obtained in different conditions. The altered albumin : globulin ratio of the plasma caused by defective hepatocellular function leads to **ascites**. This is a condition of abdominal distension due to the accumulation of fluid in the peritoneal cavity; it can be acute or chronic in onset. It generally occurs when both hepatocellular failure and portal hypertension are present. The exact mechanism is not understood and the following is a possible explanation. When the liver cells are damaged, the synthesis of albumin is decreased, leading to lowered plasma levels. As this protein is so important in the maintenance of the osmotic pressure of the plasma, a decrease leads to a lowered pressure with a consequent movement of fluid and electrolytes, particularly sodium, into the peritoneal cavity from the circulation. Portal hypertension also contributes to this movement, with a resultant depletion of effective intravascular fluid and electrolytes. This situation

529

stimulates sodium and water retention in the kidney via the renin–aldosterone system (see Chapter 5.4) as a homeostatic mechanism to restore the blood volume.

The treatment of ascites requires bedrest to decrease the metabolic activity of the liver. Restriction of fluids (to approximately 1.5 L per day) and a low-sodium diet are given and strict attention is paid to fluid balance. Daily weighing to detect the amount of water gained or lost is particularly important and it is the nurse's responsibility to ensure that this is carried out at the same time each day, preferably after the patient has emptied the bladder. Diuretic therapy may be required if weight loss is insufficient. The prevention of pressure ulcers is a priority in the patient's care plan because the skin is stretched and more liable to breakdown. Abdominal paracentesis (removal of fluid from the peritoneal cavity via a trochar and cannular) may be used as a diagnostic procedure to detect protein and electrolyte levels and the type of any cells or microorganisms present in the ascitic fluid. Generally, large quantities of fluid are not removed because of the danger of complications such as hypokalaemia, hyponatraemia, encephalopathy or renal failure due to a reduction in body fluids.

Acute ascites may occur as a result of a precipitating factor such as shock, infection or a large intake of alcohol when hepatocellular function is depressed.

### SERUM TRANSAMINASES

Two enzymes of medical significance – aspartate aminotransferase (AST, previously known as glutamic oxaloacetate transaminase, or GOT) and alanine aminotransferase (ALT, previously known as glutamic pyruvate transaminase, or GPT) – are synthesized in the liver as well as in other tissues. The reaction catalysed by these enzymes is a transamination in which the deamination of an amino acid is coupled with the simultaneous amination of a keto acid (Fig. 5.2.16).

Glutamic acid and α-ketoglutaric acid are almost always involved in any transamination reaction. The enzymes named catalyse the following reactions with the formation of two non-essential amino acids from products of carbohydrate and fat metabolism:

**Aspartate aminotransferase:**

Glutamic + oxaloacetic $\rightleftharpoons$ α-ketoglutaric + aspartic
acid         acid                  acid            acid

**Alanine aminotransferase:**

Glutamic + pyruvic $\rightleftharpoons$ α-ketoglutaric + alanine
acid         acid                  acid

There are other transaminase enzymes that catalyse reactions involving other amino acids. Reactions may be coupled so that non-essential amino acids (i.e. those that can be made in the body) can be formed from essential ones (i.e. those not made in the body and therefore necessary in the diet).

Aspartate aminotransferase is a mitochondrial enzyme. Raised serum levels may be indicative of myocardial infarction (although they may also result from damage to other organs) because the cells of the heart synthesize the enzyme and so myocardial cell damage leads to release of the enzyme into the circulation. Normal serum levels are <18 iu/L. Alanine aminotransferase is a cytoplasmic enzyme present in the heart, skeletal system and liver. In the liver the amount is less than aspartate aminotransferase but proportionately greater than that in the heart or skeletal system, thus an increase in serum level is specific for liver damage. The normal serum level is <20 iu/L. The degree of increase is indicative of the cause and thus aids diagnosis.

## Blood clotting factors

Many of the protein clotting factors involved in the blood coagulation mechanism (see Chapter 4.1) are made in the liver.

### Fibrinogen (Factor I)

This is the soluble precursor of insoluble fibrin, which forms fine strands as the basis of a blood clot.

### Prothrombin (Factor II)

This is another plasma protein and the precursor of thrombin, which is required for the conversion of fibrinogen into fibrin. The synthesis of prothrombin depends on the amount of vitamin K reaching the liver cells, as well as on their functional state. In cholestasis there is a decreased absorption of the fat-soluble vitamin K, with a resultant decrease in prothrombin production leading to delayed clotting, estimated by the measurement of the prothrombin time. Administration of intramuscular vitamin K improves the clotting mechanism.

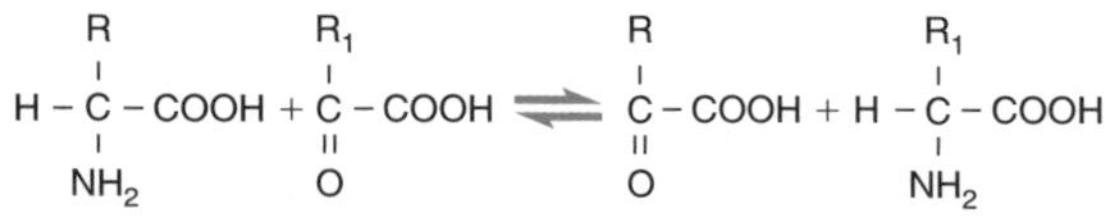

$$\underset{\text{Glutamic acid}}{H-\underset{\underset{NH_2}{|}}{\overset{\overset{R}{|}}{C}}-COOH} + \underset{}{\underset{\underset{O}{\|}}{\overset{\overset{R_1}{|}}{C}}-COOH} \rightleftharpoons \underset{\text{α-ketoglutaric acid}}{\underset{\underset{O}{\|}}{\overset{\overset{R}{|}}{C}}-COOH + H-\underset{\underset{NH_2}{|}}{\overset{\overset{R_1}{|}}{C}}-COOH}$$

**Figure 5.2.16** A transamination reaction

## DEVELOPMENTAL ISSUES

Neonates have a low prothrombin level. In the adult vitamin K is synthesized in the intestine by bacteria but this does not occur until the intestinal flora are established during the first months of life (see Chapter 5.1). Thus, in certain circumstances in which babies are prone to bleed, such as prematurity or following an operative or traumatic delivery, a synthetic analogue of vitamin K (Konakion) is given to reduce the risk of prolonged bleeding.

## Other clotting factors

The following clotting factors are synthesized in the liver: V, XI, XII and XIII. Factors VII, IX and X are also synthesized in the liver but require the presence of vitamin K (see Chapter 4.1 for full names).

## Heparin

This mucopolysaccharide is made in the liver and involved in the balance of fibrinolysis, preventing coagulation of plasma.

The liver also clears the active clotting factors from the blood, thus preventing excess clotting.

## CLINICAL APPLICATIONS

In conditions of hepatocellular damage, the synthesis of clotting factors may be impaired, resulting in a prolonged prothrombin time and spontaneous bleeding, bruising and purpura; this should be borne in mind particularly if **liver biopsy** is considered. The liver, being a vascular organ, is liable to bleed profusely, especially if the clotting mechanism is not functioning properly. It is thus vital to know the prothrombin time. If it is prolonged, treatment with intramuscular vitamin K for several days prior to the biopsy is necessary. As a precaution in case of haemorrhage, the patient's blood group should be noted and cross-matched blood made available.

Following a biopsy it is necessary for the patient to remain in bed for 24 hours, for the first 4 hours lying on the right side, thus putting pressure on the biopsy site to reduce the likelihood of bleeding. Observations of pulse and blood pressure are made, usually every 15 minutes initially, to detect possible haemorrhage. Observation of vital signs is maintained regularly for 24 hours.

## Glycogen formation and the maintenance of blood glucose levels

The liver has a short-term store of glycogen, a complex carbohydrate compound.

Glucose, absorbed from the intestine, readily diffuses from the portal circulation into the liver cells. Within the hepatocytes it is phosphorylated (i.e. a phosphate group is added) under the influence of the enzyme glucokinase to form glucose-6-phosphate. An enzyme converts this into glucose-1-phosphate, which can then be added on to the glycogen molecule by glycogen synthetase.

Liver glycogen is broken down by phosphorylase to release glucose into the blood to maintain the blood glucose level, which is vital to life (see Chapter 2.5). Alternatively, glycogen may be broken down to glucose-6-phosphate. A phosphatase enzyme, found only in the liver, catalyses the hydrolysis of glucose-6-phosphate to release glucose to the blood. The reactions involved are summarized in **Fig. 5.2.17**.

Other sources from which liver glycogen may be derived via the formation of glucose-6-phosphate

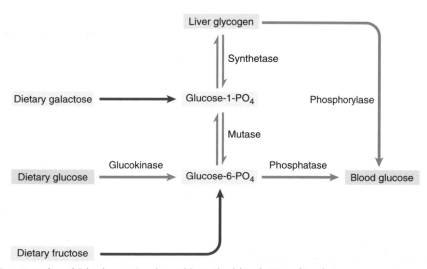

**Figure 5.2.17** Processes by which glucose is released into the blood. $PO_4$, phosphate

include fructose and galactose, pyruvic and lactic acids (products of carbohydrate metabolism), deaminated amino acids and the hydrolysis of neutral fats. Gluconeogenesis (new glucose formation from protein or fat precursors) occurs only in the liver. It is important because fasting exhausts the liver glycogen store of approximately 100 g in 24 hours.

Blood glucose is required by the cells of the body as an energy source. When glucose is withdrawn from the blood by tissues, the decreased level stimulates the release of glucose from liver glycogen to maintain the blood level. This is stimulated by the diabetogenic group of hormones that includes adrenaline (epinephrine), thyroxine, the diabetogenic factor of the anterior pituitary gland and glucagon. These hormones stimulate the activity of liver phosphorylase, thus promoting hepatic glycogenolysis (breakdown of glycogen). This action is opposed by insulin. (Chapter 2.6 contains a full discussion of the endocrine control of blood glucose levels.) Changes in blood glucose level as a result of hepatic malfunction occur in acute liver failure rather than in chronic conditions. Resultant hypoglycaemia (low blood glucose level) may lead to coma and death.

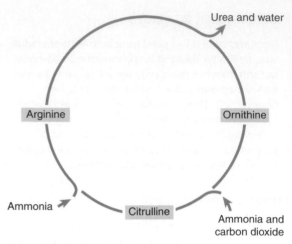

**Figure 5.2.18**    The Krebs' urea cycle

ketone bodies. Some ammonia is incorporated into newly formed amino acids.

The liver is the only tissue that converts the surplus toxic ammonia into **urea**, which is water soluble, non-toxic and can be excreted via the kidney. The formation of urea is a cyclical reaction in which two molecules of ammonia unite with one of carbon dioxide with the elimination of water. The amino acid ornithine is involved in the Krebs' urea cycle (**Fig. 5.2.18**).

Another source of ammonia is from the breakdown of protein material by the intestinal flora. The ammonia is absorbed into the portal circulation and taken up by the liver, where it is detoxified by urea formation.

## DEVELOPMENTAL ISSUES

### RED CELL PRODUCTION AND DESTRUCTION (see Chapter 4.1)

The liver is an important site of red cell formation after the third month of fetal life. However, as the bone marrow begins to act as a blood-forming organ from about 20 weeks of fetal life, the erythropoietic activity of the liver declines. In later life the liver resumes erythropoietic activity if severe marrow damage occurs.

In the adult, the Kupffer cells of the liver break down the mature erythrocytes. The haemoglobin is released and broken down as described in the section on bile pigments.

## Degradation reactions and excretory products

Like the synthetic liver reactions, metabolism occurring in the liver involves the breakdown of various substances.

## Deamination of proteins

When amino acids are broken down, usually in the liver, they are deaminated so that ammonia is released; the remaining non-nitrogenous part is further metabolized to other amino acids, glucose, fat or

## CLINICAL APPLICATIONS

It has been suggested that ammonia toxicity may be responsible for the varied changes of **hepatic encephalopathy**. The exact cause of this condition is not known but ammonia toxicity is the most widely investigated possibility. When severe liver damage occurs, the portal blood may bypass the remaining healthy liver cells by means of a collateral circulation or by passing directly through damaged hepatocytes, as in acute liver failure. This means that ammonia enters the systemic circulation without undergoing metabolism in the liver. Ammonia exerts toxic effects on tissues, particularly nervous tissue. Blood levels of up to 5000 µg/L ammonia (the upper limit of normal is 800–1000 µg/L) have been found in encephalopathy. The symptoms involve mental and neurological dysfunction, such as disturbed consciousness, personality changes, intellectual deterioration, slurred speech and a characteristic 'flapping' tremor of the hands. Encephalopathy develops more frequently in

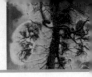

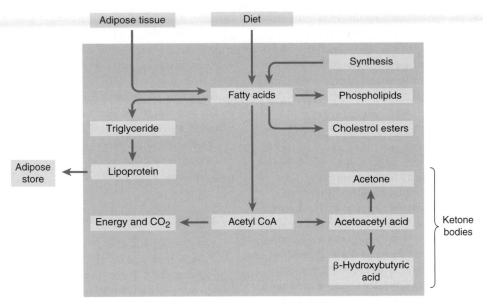

**Figure 5.2.19** An outline of fatty acid metabolism in the liver

chronic liver conditions and is reversible in its early stages.

Treatment of encephalopathy involves removal of the precipitating factor, a low-protein diet and intestinal antibiotics (to prevent ammonia being formed from protein in the gut by the intestinal flora). When treatment is commenced, a gradual increase in the amount of dietary protein given is made with the aim of establishing the upper level of protein tolerance. It is important that the nurse ensures that the correct diet is received and consumed by the patient. The nature and quantity of leftovers and the consumption of any other foods need to be recorded, so that an accurate assessment of dietary intake can be made. Neomycin is the antibiotic of choice in acute encephalopathy as it is very poorly absorbed from the gut. The synthetic dissaccharide lactulose may also be given in chronic encephalopathy. This is hydrolysed in the colon to form lactic, acetic and formic acids and carbon dioxide. The acidic medium thus produced traps ammonia, and possibly other toxic compounds.

## Breakdown of fats

The liver stores some fat in the form of neutral fat or triglycerides and also the fat-soluble vitamins A, D, E and K. The fat is derived from three sources: (i) triglycerides absorbed from the intestine and transported in chylomicrons via the lymphatics and systemic circulation; (ii) free fatty acids from the adipose tissue stores; and (iii) fat synthesized in the liver.

Within the liver, newly arrived fats are converted into fatty acids which may be metabolized in several different ways (**Fig. 5.2.19**). Triglycerides are reformed by the esterification of glycerol. These form lipoprotein by the addition of protein and pass into the systemic circulation to be deposited in the adipose tissue stores.

Other fatty acids are involved in phospholipid formation and in the esterification of cholesterol. Fatty acids are broken down by oxidation to provide energy in the form of adenosine triphosphate (ATP), an energy-rich compound, with the release of carbon dioxide. An intermediary product in this breakdown is acetyl co-enzyme A (acetyl CoA). An alternative metabolic path for acetyl co-enzyme A occurs when two molecules join to form acetoacetyl co-enzyme A, which is metabolized irreversibly in the liver to the **ketone bodies** acetoacetic acid, β-hydroxybutyric acid and acetone. Very low levels of these are found in the blood of normal individuals. They can be metabolized to produce energy in tissues other than the liver.

### CLINICAL APPLICATIONS

In abnormal conditions such as fasting or diabetes, when carbohydrate is not available as an energy source, the oxidation of fatty acids is increased to meet the energy demands. As more acetyl co-enzyme A is formed than can be metabolized to carbon dioxide with the production of energy, an accumulation of the ketone bodies occurs, leading to increased blood levels and the condition of **ketosis**. The ketones are excreted in the urine and there is often a sickly sweet odour of acetone in the expired breath, sometimes described as being akin to the smell of new-mown hay.

Fatty acids are synthesized in the liver cells from non-lipid substances, a process known as **lipogenesis**. Carbohydrates, some amino acids and fatty acids may be broken down to acetyl co-enzyme A, which is then involved in a complex series of reactions resulting in a step-by-step increase of the chain length of the fatty acids.

## Elimination of copper

The liver is the main site of copper metabolism in the body. Dietary copper is cleared rapidly from the plasma by the liver and incorporated into proteins such as cytochrome oxidase (a respiratory electron-transfer enzyme) and ceruloplasmin (a blue-coloured glycoprotein transporting copper in the blood). Copper is excreted in the bile bound to a carrier, usually a bile acid or pigment, which prevents its reabsorption by the intestine. Excess copper is toxic. In Wilson's disease, a congenital condition involving the accumulation of copper, it produces structural and functional changes to the cells of the liver, nervous system, eyes and kidneys.

## Detoxification of endogenous and exogenous compounds

The metabolism of steroid and thyroid hormones and drugs, particularly those administered orally, in the liver and their consequent excretion in the bile clear these substances from the blood and tissues. The biological effects of the compounds are curtailed and the body is protected against the intoxicating results of their accumulation.

A two-phase reaction occurs to render the substances more polar so that they can be excreted in the bile. The first phase, which takes place in the endoplasmic reticulum of liver cells, is an oxidative reaction that provides an available hydroxyl ($-OH$), carboxyl ($-COOH$) or amine ($-NH_2$) group for the second phase of conjugation, which is combination with another molecule. Substances that can be utilized in conjugation reactions include the sulphate group, the amino acid glycine, glutathione (a tripeptide of three amino acids – glutamic acid, cysteine and glycine), and acetyl and methyl derivatives. The most metabolically important conjugate is the carbohydrate derivative glucuronic acid. This can attach to a variety of chemical groups giving them a versatile ability to conjugate many different molecules. Drugs conjugated by glucuronic acid include imipramine, morphine, chloramphenicol, salicylic acid and indomethacin.

### ALCOHOL CONSUMPTION

Consumption of alcohol has long been associated with the incidence of cirrhosis of the liver. Alcohol is not stored in the body but undergoes obligatory oxidation, predominantly in the liver. A healthy individual cannot metabolize more than 160–180 g per day, but as alcohol induces (i.e. increases the activity of) the enzymes involved in

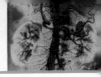

its catabolism, alcoholics may be able to metabolize more than this.

The Health Education Authority currently recommends that women drink no more than 14 units of alcohol per week, and men no more than 21 units per week. One unit of alcohol is equivalent to ½ pint (0.3 L) of beer, one measure of spirits or one glass of wine.

Ethanol is metabolized by alcohol dehydrogenase within the liver cells to acetaldehyde, which is toxic and causes membrane damage and cell necrosis. Acetaldehyde can be further broken down to acetyl co-enzyme A, which may be metabolized in the same way as it is when produced from fats or carbohydrates, to give energy, carbon dioxide and water. Hydrogen is produced when ethanol is converted into acetaldehyde. This hydrogen replaces fatty acids as a fuel so that the fatty acids accumulate, giving rise to ketosis, an increase in triglycerides, hyperlipidaemia and the formation of a fatty liver.

Alcohol can also be metabolized by a system of enzymes in the microsomes of the cell; these enzymes metabolize other drugs as well. Alcohol induces this system, which may explain the increased tolerance of the alcoholic to alcohol and also to sedative drugs. Alcohol also stimulates the formation of collagen, which disrupts the cellular structure; the resulting fibrosis impedes the passage of substances between the blood and liver cells. The damage is reversible at first if the causative agent, alcohol, is removed, but progresses to an irreversible state.

Alcohol is prohibited for patients who are convalescent or recovered from hepatitis or other infections of the liver for a period of 6–12 months. This allows the liver to regenerate as fully as possible, whereas taking alcohol during this period might lead to permanent damage.

Not only do drugs and chemical agents cause disorders of liver function, as demonstrated above, but altered liver function, as in conditions of hepatocellular failure, may affect the metabolism of drugs. Detoxification reactions may be reduced so that the pharmacological action of the drug is prolonged. Drugs that might be metabolized abnormally in liver disease include tolbutamide (an antidiabetic agent), phenytoin (an anticonvulsant), theophylline (for bronchospasm) and diazepam (a tranquillizer and sedative).

## Parenchymal dysfunction

### CLINICAL APPLICATIONS

A wide variety of reactions takes place within the liver cell. When the cells are damaged there is an alteration in the metabolism of many substances, affecting different functions and with various effects. Almost every system of the body is affected in some way.

**Cirrhosis**, a process of fibrosis and nodule formation following hepatocellular necrosis, demonstrates the wide variety of effects of liver cell failure. There are many different causes of cirrhosis, including viral hepatitis, certain metabolic conditions such as Wilson's disease, and prolonged cholestasis; consumption of alcohol is more commonly associated in Western countries, whereas protein malnutrition may be responsible in developing countries. The liver cell structure is destroyed by the causative agent. Following this, fibrous tissue is laid down, distorting the lobular structure of the liver. The healthy tissue attempts regeneration but the new growth is irregularly shaped, which distorts and thus disrupts the blood supply to the lobules. As a result of this, pressure in the portal vessels increases, leading to impaired perfusion and a decrease in the nutrient supply to the liver tissue. The effects of this type of damage to the liver are many and varied.

### Portal hypertension and collateral circulation

Nodules formed as part of the cirrhotic process exert pressure on the hepatic vessels, thus tending to decrease the rate of blood flow within the liver. The pressure of the portal system, normally 5–10 mmHg (0.7–1.3 kPa), increases with the additional resistance to the flow of blood in the vessels of the liver. When the pressure is increased above 14 mmHg (1.9 kPa), a collateral circulation occurs via tributaries of the portal vessels to the systemic circulation, with consequent bypassing of the liver by the portal blood. The main sites of joining with the systemic circulation occur in the submucosa of the stomach and lower oesophagus, the rectum and anterior abdominal wall.

### Varices

The presence of a collateral circulation in the oesophagus gives rise to varices, dilated vessels that may rupture causing bleeding that presents as haematemesis or malaena. The precise factors responsible for the rupture are unknown but an elevated portal pressure appears relevant. Bleeding in this way may precipitate liver cell failure, coma, jaundice and ascites, and may be fatal.

Initial treatment for bleeding involves the replacement of blood volume by blood transfusion. Oral neomycin is given to prevent bacterial breakdown of protein in the intestine, which would otherwise increase the load at the liver and so increase the likelihood of the development of coma. The blood from the rupture itself constitutes an increased amount of

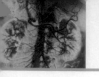

protein in the intestine. Vasopressin (Pitressin) may be given intravenously. This reduces the portal pressure and contracts the oesophageal muscle. It also stimulates intestinal contractions, which help to remove the blood from the bowel. Compression of the varices by means of a Sengstaken–Blakemore oesophageal compression tube is used infreqently as there are various difficulties associated with its use, for example obstruction of the pharynx and resultant asphyxia. Surgical intervention, creating a shunt from the portal to the systemic circulation and thus reducing portal pressure, may be performed. This procedure has varying survival rates depending on the type of shunt formed.

## Ascites

This condition was discussed on p. 530.

## Circulatory changes

The general circulation becomes hyperdynamic. An increased blood flow through the skin is observed, with consequent flushing of the extremities (palmar erythema) and bounding pulses. The cardiac output is also increased, as evidenced by tachycardia. Blood flow to the spleen is increased whereas that to the kidney is reduced, which may result in abnormal renal function. The blood pressure is low. The cause of these changes is uncertain but they may be due to the presence of a vasodilator substance in the circulation.

## Pulmonary changes

Some patients with cirrhosis may be cyanosed and it is found that their arterial blood has a reduced oxygen saturation compared with normal. Within the lungs there are microscopic arteriovenous fistulae through which the blood may be shunted, thus bypassing the alveoli (i.e. the functional units). There is also an increase in the diffusion barrier which may be related to the dilation of the blood vessels and the thickening of their walls by a layer of collagen.

## Jaundice

Jaundice is recognized as a yellow discoloration of the skin and sclera. However, jaundice (also known as icterus) is complex phenomenon that can arise when, for many different reasons, there is an excess amount of the bile pigment bilirubin in the body. Jaundice is not a disease but rather a symptom or clinical sign of an underlying disorder. Normally, bilirubin is formed by the breakdown of haemoglobin during the natural destruction of worn out red blood cells (erythrocytes). As highlighted earlier, several conditions may result in jaundice but they can be considered in certain categories:

- Haemolytic jaundice where there is an excessive disintegration of erthyrocytes.
- Hepatocelluar jaundice when, due to damage to the liver parenchyma or the absence of necessary enzymes, bilirubin is not removed from the blood and transported into the bile.
- Obstructive jaundice when there is some form of obstruction in or around the liver that blocks the passage of bile from the liver to the intestines.

Hepatocellular and obstructive causes are also known respectively as intrahepatic and extrahepatic cholestatic jaundice.

## Tissue loss

There is a loss of flesh and muscle-wasting in patients with prolonged liver cell failure, due to the inability of the liver to synthesize tissue protein. Anorexia and poor dietary habits add to the malnutrition.

## Skin changes

The appearance of vascular **spider naevi** on the face, neck, forearm and back of the hand is attributed to oestrogen excess. The arterial spider (a synonym) consists of a central arteriole from which numerous small vessels radiate, resembling spiders' legs. When sufficiently large it may be seen to pulsate.

**Palmar erythema**, a bright red coloration of the palms of the hands (often called liver palms), which are warm, also occurs in some cirrhotic patients. This may be due to oestrogen excess or to the circulatory changes.

## Endocrine changes

A fall in the circulating testosterone levels of cirrhotic males due to decreased production and increased binding by globulins has been associated with loss of body hair and testicular atrophy. **Gynaecomastia** (development of breast tissue) occurs in some males. Raised levels of oestrogens, which are normally inactivated by the liver, may be responsible for this but the mechanism is not known.

## Changes in nitrogen metabolism

Amino acids are excreted in the urine and plasma levels show a characteristic change: there is an increase in methionine, tyrosine and phenylalanine and a decrease in valine, isoleucine and leucine.

Urea production is impaired but there is a considerable reserve capacity for synthesis, which maintains the normal blood level. The failing liver cannot convert ammonia to urea.

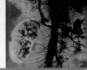

### Neurological changes

These have been discussed previously.

### Disordered blood coagulation

Failure to synthesize many of the proteins involved in blood coagulation results in prolonged bleeding. Spontaneous bruising and the appearance of purpura may occur. Care needs to be taken when operative procedures are considered, including venepuncture and liver biopsy, as well as large-scale surgery. Administration of vitamin K to decrease a prolonged prothrombin time is essential treatment.

### Fetor hepaticus

The breath of patients with severe hepatocellular disease or with an extensive collateral circulation may have a sweetish, slightly faecal odour. This is presumed to be due to the exhalation of methyl mercaptan. This compound is apparently metabolized from the amino acid methionine by the intestinal flora. As the normal demethylation reactions are reduced in a damaged liver, the methyl mercaptan passes into the systemic circulation. It is excreted in the urine as well as exhaled in the breath. The presence of fetor hepaticus may precede coma.

### Hepatitis

Hepatitis, or inflammation of the liver, can be caused by several agents such as drugs, toxic substances or one of several infective organisms. These organisms include the cytomegalovirus, the Epstein–Barr virus and the herpes simplex virus, as well as the five major hepatitis viruses: hepatitis A, B, C, D and E.

The symptoms of hepatitis A may include an influenza-like illness, nausea, vomiting, anorexia, urticarial rash, joint pains, hepatomegaly, dark urine, pale faeces and jaundice (due to liver cell damage). The length of the acute phase is variable (normally around 6–8 weeks), treatment is symptomatic and recovery is monitored by blood tests. The virus is usually transmitted via the faeco-oral route.

Hepatitis B (HBV) (originally called Australia antigen because it was first described in the blood of a native Australian) is transmitted parenterally or by sexual contact and may give rise to a subclinical infection with no symptoms. However, it generally presents as a much more virulent liver disease than hepatitis A. Individuals in whom infection has become subclinical are more likely to become chronic carriers and may infect others unknowingly.

Complications and long-term effects of hepatitis B virus infection, particularly among carriers (of whom there are an estimated 300 million in the world), include chronic hepatitis, cirrhosis and the development of primary liver cancer. Nurses and other at-risk individuals may come into contact with blood or used needles from such people so it is extremely important to be protected against this disease by vaccination and/or safe-practice techniques.

Viral hepatitis constitutes a major global health problem due to the number of individuals affected and the complications and long-term effects of infection. As the fundamental lesion in both common types of hepatitis is cellular necrosis, recovery from hepatitis depends on the balance between cell loss and cell regenerative capability, and on the loss of hepatic function.

## Investigation of the liver

### CLINICAL APPLICATIONS

A series of biochemical tests on the serum is made when investigating hepatic disease. These tests have been referred to in the relevant parts of this chapter, and are listed in **Table 5.2.2**.

### LIVER TRANSPLANTATION

Liver transplantation was first carried out in 1963. Although limited numbers of operations were performed at first, there has been a substantial increase in numbers in recent years at centres around the world. Children as young as 4 weeks old have received transplanted liver tissue. Modifications of technique have resulted in an improved survival rate of up to 80% after 1 year and 60% after 5 years. Factors include improved patient selection and timing of the operation, the introduction of immunosuppressive medication (including cyclosporin A), refinements to operative techniques (particularly the use of a venovenous bypass) and the introduction of a new preservative solution for the donor organ, which enables it to be stored for up to 24 hours rather than 6–8 hours.

Conditions for which transplants are performed include acute liver failure following viral B or drug-induced hepatitis, cirrhosis, primary hepatic malignant tumours and biliary atresia, particularly in children. When liver transplantation takes place, the donor liver must function immediately, otherwise the patient will die. There is no artifical process analogous to the haemodyalysis utilized in renal failure and transplantation. Owing to the

**Table 5.2.2** The major biochemical liver function tests

| Biochemical test | Normal range | Importance |
|---|---|---|
| Alkaline phosphatase | 21–100 iu/L | Diagnosis of jaundice<br>Presence of tumours |
| Bilirubin<br>  Total<br>  Conjugated | <br>5–17 μmol/L<br><3 μmol/L | Diagnosis of jaundice<br>Degree of liver cell damage |
| Plasma proteins<br>  Albumin<br>  Globulin | <br>35–50 g/L<br>7–15 g/L | Diagnosis of jaundice<br>Degree of liver cell damage<br>Course of chronic hepatitis and cirrhosis |
| Serum transaminases<br>  Aspartate aminotransferase (AST)<br>  Alanine aminotransferase (ALT) | <br>5–30 iu/L<br>5–30 iu/L | Early diagnosis of liver disease<br>Degree of liver cell damage |
| Prothrombin time | 10–15 s | Degree of liver cell damage |

complexity of liver function, there are many possible immediate postoperative problems, including hypoglycaemia, failure of the blood clotting mechanism and electrolyte imbalance. The nursing care of liver transplant patients is intensive and requires an understanding of the complex physiology of the liver to detect possible complications. Long-term problems include cholestasis, fistulae formation, infection and rejection of the transplanted organ.

## DEVELOPMENTAL ISSUES

The weight of the liver decreases by about 35% between young adulthood and late old age. Blood flow through the liver is also reduced. Although routine liver function tests may show little alteration, the rate of metabolism and clearance of drugs declines with age. This appears to be a consequence of the changes in liver size and blood flow. However, variation between individuals and between different drugs is also influenced by other factors, including disease state, coadministration of other drugs, and environmental factors such as smoking and nutritional status. As drugs may remain in the body longer, their therapeutic effect can be increased, which may require reduced dosages. Monitoring of the older patient in receipt of medication is particularly important when repeat prescriptions are required.

Other functional effects of ageing on the liver include changes in protein synthesis (and thus enzyme activity) and an increase in the cellular lipid content. Enhanced hepatic secretion of cholesterol and a decline in bile acid synthesis result in bile with and increased cholesterol concentration and a consequent tendency for gallstone formation. In general, the older liver is less able to respond or adapt to stressing conditions than the liver of a young person.

## Conclusion

The physiology of the liver involves all aspects of metabolism and their interrelationships. The functions of the liver are numerous and have diverse effects throughout the body, effects that are particularly noticeable when the liver is not functioning in its normal manner. The importance of the liver to the well-being of the individual cannot be over-emphasized.

## Clinical review

In addition to the Learning Objectives at the beginning of this chapter the reader should also be able to:

• Explain the causes and effects of cholestasis

• List the factors associated with the formation of gallstones

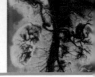

- Explain the formation of ascites and list the principles of treatment
- Understand the rationale for the nursing management of jaundice
- Teach a junior nurse the importance of preparation and care for the patient undergoing liver biopsy
- Discuss the detoxification of substances within the liver
- List the effects of cellular damage of the liver

## Review questions

1  Which two blood vessels supply the liver?
2  Which vessels are contained in the portal canals?
3  In which direction does bile flow in the cystic duct?
4  From which substance are the primary bile acids synthesized?
5  What are the characteristics of molecules that form micelles?
6  What is the fate of most of the bile salts secreted into the intestine?
7  What is the origin of the majority of bilirubin?
8  How is the gall bladder stimulated to contract?
9  What are the respective functions of the plasma proteins albumin and globulin?
10  What is the function of glycogen?
11  What is gluconeogenesis?
12  What is the purpose of conjugation of drugs and hormones in the liver?

## Suggestions for further reading

Hunter, J. (2002) *Davidson's Principles and Practice of Medicine,* 19th edn. London: Churchill Livingstone. *Medical textbook with helpful chapters on the liver and biliary system.*

Kumar, P. & Clark, M. (2002) *Kumar and Clark Clinical Medicine,* 5th edn. London: W.B. Saunders. *Medical textbook with helpful chapters on the liver and biliary system.*

Sherlock, S. & Dooley, J. (2001) *Anatomy and Function in Diseases of the Liver and Biliary System,* 11th edn. Oxford: Blackwell Scientific.

*A comprehensive and detailed account of all aspects of liver physiology, investigation and pathology.*

Smith, G.D. & Watson, R. (2004) *Gastrointestinal Nursing.* Oxford: Blackwell Scientific. *A nursing textbook with specific emphasis on gastroenterology and issues related to gastrointestinal nursing.*

Walsh, M. (2002) *Watson's Clinical Nursing and Related Sciences,* 6th edn. London: Baillière Tindall. *A good nursing reference text.*

## Reference

Moore, K.L. & Persaud, T.V.N. (1993) The digestive system. In: *The Developing Human, Clinically Orientated Embryology,* 5th edn. Philadelphia: W.B. Saunders.

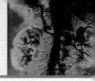

# Chapter 5.3

# Respiration

*Carol Law    Roger Watson*

---

## LEARNING OBJECTIVES

### After studying this chapter the reader should be able to:

- Discuss the ways in which the respiratory, cardiovascular and neuromuscular systems are interrelated to ensure a continuous exchange of oxygen and carbon dioxide between the atmosphere and the tissues

- Describe the role of the diaphragm and other respiratory muscles in breathing

- Describe the processes involved in inspiration and expiration

- Relate the structure of the respiratory system (lungs, thorax and airways) to the function of gas exchange

- Describe how the alveolar capillary membrane is well adapted to gas diffusion

- State why the composition of alveolar air differs from that of atmospheric or expired air

- List the factors that can increase the work of breathing

- Describe the developmental anatomy of the lung

- Discuss the effects of changes in dead space and breathing patterns on the magnitude of alveolar ventilation

- Describe the ways in which oxygen and carbon dioxide are transported around the body

- Discuss the physiological significance of the sigmoid shape of the oxygen–haemoglobin dissociation curve

- Describe how the basic rhythm of respiration is generated

- Describe how alveolar ventilation is regulated according to body needs

---

## INTRODUCTION

The processes by which the cells of the body use oxygen, produce carbon dioxide and exchange these gases with the atmosphere are collectively termed **respiration**. Efficient respiration depends on the interdependence and integration of many functions within the respiratory, cardiovascular and central nervous systems. Failure of any of these systems will result in disruption of homeostasis and rapid cell death due to oxygen starvation and build-up of toxic waste products.

In an adult, the body cells consume about 250 mL of oxygen per minute under resting conditions. This demand increases up to 30-fold during strenuous exercise. The endproduct of the energy-producing (metabolic) processes is carbon dioxide, of which approximately 200 mL per minute is produced at rest. Although we can survive without food or water

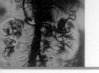

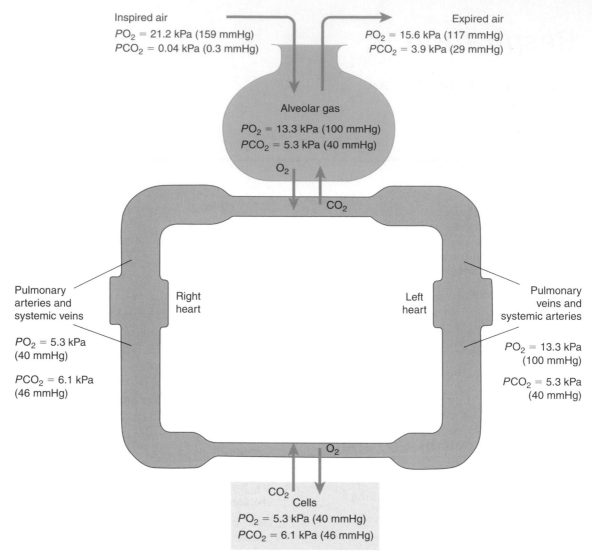

Inspired air
$PO_2 = 21.2$ kPa (159 mmHg)
$PCO_2 = 0.04$ kPa (0.3 mmHg)

Expired air
$PO_2 = 15.6$ kPa (117 mmHg)
$PCO_2 = 3.9$ kPa (29 mmHg)

Alveolar gas
$PO_2 = 13.3$ kPa (100 mmHg)
$PCO_2 = 5.3$ kPa (40 mmHg)

$O_2$

$CO_2$

Pulmonary arteries and systemic veins
$PO_2 = 5.3$ kPa (40 mmHg)
$PCO_2 = 6.1$ kPa (46 mmHg)

Right heart

Left heart

Pulmonary veins and systemic arteries
$PO_2 = 13.3$ kPa (100 mmHg)
$PCO_2 = 5.3$ kPa (40 mmHg)

$O_2$

$CO_2$ Cells
$PO_2 = 5.3$ kPa (40 mmHg)
$PCO_2 = 6.1$ kPa (46 mmHg)

**Figure 5.3.1** Schematic representation of the process of respiration showing the partial pressures of the gases involved in internal and external respiration

for days, we can live without oxygen for only a matter of minutes – primarily because the brain cells are incapable of functioning without it. Furthermore, any significant accumulation of carbon dioxide in the body would be highly toxic.

The primary function of the respiratory system is to provide an adequate supply of oxygen to the tissues and to remove the metabolically produced carbon dioxide. To maintain virtually constant levels of oxygen and carbon dioxide in arterial blood under a wide range of physiological circumstances, several complex and interrelated processes must occur. Not only must the lungs be supplied with air (**ventilation**) and blood (**perfusion**) but the two must also be evenly matched to ensure that efficient gas exchange by **diffusion** can occur.

Complex mechanisms are involved in the **transport** of oxygen and carbon dioxide around the body in blood, due to the relative insolubility of oxygen

and the toxic effects that large quantities of dissolved carbon dioxide would have on the acid–base balance in the body.

Finally, the rate and depth of breathing must be carefully **regulated** according to body requirements. In this chapter, each of these processes (summarized in **Fig. 5.3.1**) will be considered in detail. However, it is first necessary to appreciate the relationship between the structure and function of the various components of the respiratory system.

## The relationship between the structure and functions of the respiratory system

The respiratory system consists of the nose, pharynx, larynx, trachea, bronchi and lungs and the chest structures responsible for moving air in and out of

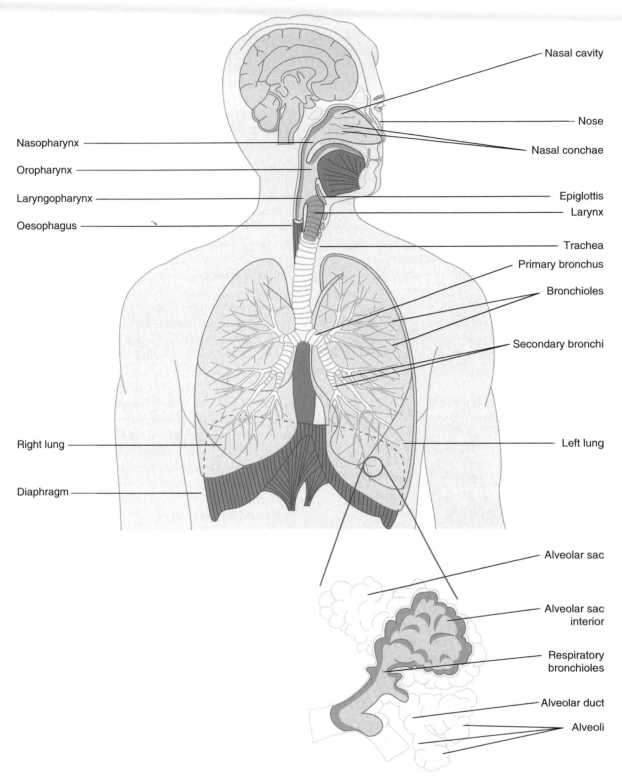

Nasal cavity

Nose

Nasal conchae

Nasopharynx

Oropharynx

Laryngopharynx

Oesophagus

Epiglottis

Larynx

Trachea

Primary bronchus

Bronchioles

Secondary bronchi

Right lung

Left lung

Diaphragm

Alveolar sac

Alveolar sac interior

Respiratory bronchioles

Alveolar duct

Alveoli

**Figure 5.3.2** Anatomy of the human respiratory system

the lungs (**Fig. 5.3.2**). The two cone-shaped lungs lie in the thoracic cage (chest), which consists of the ribs, sternum, thoracic vertebrae, diaphragm and inter-costal muscles; these structures form a protective air-tight cage around the lungs.

The basic rhythm of respiration is generated by cyclical nerve impulses passing from the respiratory centre in the medulla of the brain, down the phrenic and intercostal nerves to the diaphragm and inter-costal muscles, respectively. Cyclical excitation of these respiratory muscles results in alternate expansion and relaxation of the thoracic cage, which in turn causes air to be drawn into (**inspiration**) and expelled from (**expiration**) the lung.

## Organization of the airways

For air to reach the lungs it must pass through a series of branching airways, which become progressively more numerous and smaller in diameter (**Fig. 5.3.3**). The respiratory tract is arbitrarily divided at the level of the cricoid cartilage into upper and lower parts. The lower respiratory tract (i.e. larynx, trachea, bronchi and lungs) is primarily concerned with conduction of air to and from the alveoli of the lungs. As will be discussed later, the upper respiratory tract (nose, throat and associated structures) has several physiological functions in addition to that of air conditioning. These include swallowing, speech, appreciation of smell and conditioning of air prior to its passage through the trachea. Air may enter the respiratory passages via the nose or mouth, although very young infants, as a result of anatomical differences, are preferential nose breathers and rarely breathe through their mouths until about 3–6 months of age. It is therefore essential that their nasal passages are kept as clear as possible.

The **nasal cavity** consists of a large, irregular cavity divided by a septum. It is lined with ciliated epithelium, the surface area of which is greatly increased by the presence of bony projections, called turbinates or conchae, which project into the cavity. The ciliated epithelium ensures that air is warmed, filtered and moistened as it passes through the nose. When inspired air bypasses the nose, for example after endotracheal intubation or tracheostomy, the lower respiratory mucosa becomes dry and cessation of ciliary activity follows rapidly, predisposing to infection. It is vital to ensure that inspired air and/or oxygen is adequately warmed and moistened by using a humidifier when an artificial airway is in situ. Regrettably, in the past the inefficiency of many commercially available humidifiers resulted in severe airway damage in intubated patients. To a lesser degree, such problems can also occur in mouth breathers. The mucous membrane covering the turbinates is vascular and swells rapidly when inflamed or irritated, to the extent that the entire nasal cavity, including the paranasal sinuses, can become blocked during head colds or allergic reactions.

Having passed through the nose or mouth, air enters the **pharynx** (throat), which is also a common passageway for food and water. The pharynx is a funnel-shaped tube that starts at the internal nares (nasal passages) and extends to the level of the cricoid cartilage (the laryngeal cartilage lying immediately above the trachea). Its wall is composed of skeletal muscles and lined with mucous membrane. The uppermost portion of the pharynx (nasopharynx) has two openings from the internal nares and two from the auditory (Eustachian) tubes. The posterior wall also contains the pharyngeal tonsil or adenoid. The central portion of the pharynx (oropharynx) has an opening from the mouth called the fauces and contains two pairs of tonsils. This portion of the pharynx provides a common passageway for drink, food and air. The lowest portion of the pharynx (laryngopharynx) divides into the oesophagus (along which food is directed on its way to the stomach) and the larynx, through which air passes on its way to the trachea, bronchi, bronchioles and alveoli.

The **larynx**, or voice box, is composed of pieces of cartilage, connected by ligaments and moved by various muscles. It produces the bump in the neck called the Adam's apple which, after puberty, is larger in men than in women. It is lined with mucous membrane that is continuous with that of the pharynx and trachea. As well as being part of the airway, the larynx contains the elastic vocal cords which function in sound production. The space between the vocal cords, through which the air passes, is called the **glottis**.

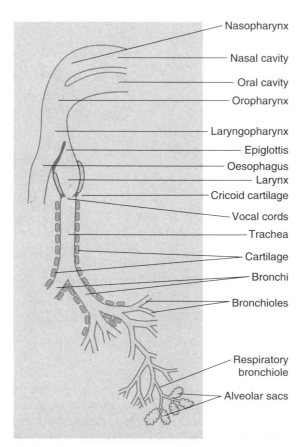

- Nasopharynx
- Nasal cavity
- Oral cavity
- Oropharynx
- Laryngopharynx
- Epiglottis
- Oesophagus
- Larynx
- Cricoid cartilage
- Vocal cords
- Trachea
- Cartilage
- Bronchi
- Bronchioles
- Respiratory bronchiole
- Alveolar sacs

**Figure 5.3.3**   Organization of the airways

## CLINICAL APPLICATIONS

Inflammation of the mucous membrane lining of the larynx produces hoarseness and loss of voice (**laryngitis**). This may be relieved by removing irritants, avoiding smoking, resting the voice, steam inhalations and cough medication. Persistent hoarseness is commonly the first symptom of laryngeal cancer. The small larynx of a child under 5 is particularly susceptible to spasm when inflamed and may become partially or totally obstructed. This produces a barking cough and inspiratory stridor (an abnormal, high-pitched sound heard on inspiration) and can cause severe respiratory distress (**croup**). A quiet environment and parental support are reassuring to the child. The value of humidifying therapy has not been established. Adrenaline (epinephrine) has been shown to decrease the need for intubation and tracheostomy (Chandler, 2002).

The **epiglottis** is a large leaf-shaped piece of cartilage lying on top of the larynx. The stem of the epiglottis is attached to the thyroid cartilage (Adam's apple) but the rest is unattached and free to move up and down like a trapdoor. During swallowing, the epiglottis forms a lid over the glottis, preventing aspiration of food or liquid into the larynx. If anything but air enters the larynx, the cough reflex attempts to expel it (see cough and sneeze reflexes p. 548).

**Valsalva's manoeuvre** involves forced expiratory effort against a closed glottis, such as occurs when straining to move a heavy object, to change position in bed or to defaecate, especially when constipated. Such straining increases intrathoracic pressure, thereby reducing venous return to the heart. On subsequent relaxation of the muscles there is a rapid increase in venous return. Whereas the performance of Valsalva's manoeuvre creates no problems for healthy people, those with cardiovascular disease are usually advised to avoid straining in this way by exhaling instead of holding their breath. This decreases the risk of the heart suddenly becoming overloaded.

The **trachea** (windpipe) is a cylindrical tube, 10–12 cm long, which is composed of 16–20 incomplete (C-shaped) rings of cartilage joined together by fibrous and muscular tissue. The cartilage, which forms the anterior and lateral walls of the trachea, provides rigidity to the trachea and prevents it collapsing and blocking air flow during inspiration when airway pressure becomes negative. The muscular portion of the trachea lies over the oesophagus, providing a flattened surface that can be stretched slightly. This facilitates movement of food boluses down the oesophagus. The trachea is lined with ciliated epithelium, which assists in filtering and warming inspired air.

## CLINICAL APPLICATIONS

### TRACHEOSTOMY

A tracheostomy is an artificial opening into the trachea, at the level of the second or third cartilaginous ring, which is kept patent by the insertion of a metal or plastic tube. A tracheostomy decreases the work of breathing by eliminating the resistance of the upper airway and reduces the dead space by about 50%, thereby increasing the efficiency of breathing. It may be performed:

- if there is severe upper airway obstruction
- if there is paralysis of the vocal cords
- to improve the efficiency of ventilation and facilitate the removal of secretions from the airways, particularly in patients who require prolonged mechanical ventilation.

Narrow-diameter tracheostomy tubes, known as mini-tracheostomies, are increasingly being used to enable the suction of secretions in patients who might be in danger of sputum retention; these avoid the need for mechanical ventilation. They can also be used to provide oxygen therapy.

Although a tracheostomy is frequently a life-saving measure, it does have certain disadvantages, in that:

- air passes directly to lower airways without being filtered, warmed and humidified in the nasal passages
- it interferes with speech production and coughing
- there is an increased danger of water entering the airways, so that care is required, especially when taking a shower.

The trachea extends from the larynx to the level of the fifth thoracic vertebra, where it divides (bifurcates) into the two **primary bronchi**. There is an internal cartilagenous ridge at the point of bifurcation, called the **carina**. This is lined with mucous membrane and is an extremely sensitive area, closely associated with the cough reflex. The right bronchus is a shorter, wider tube than the left and lies in a more vertical position. Consequently, any foreign bodies that enter the trachea are more likely to be inhaled into the right main bronchus where they may become lodged, requiring removal through a bronchoscope.

The primary bronchi enter the right and left lungs at the **hilum**. The right main bronchus divides into the right upper, middle and lower bronchi to supply the three lobes of the right lung, whereas the left main bronchus divides into left upper and left lower lobe bronchi. Each lobar bronchus then subdivides into segmental divisions. The lower airways are known as bronchi down to the smallest divisions containing cartilage – thereafter they are called **bronchioles**, which are usually less than 1 mm in diameter. The bronchi are purely conducting airways (i.e. no gas exchange occurs). There are approximately 8–13 divisions from the trachea to the smallest bronchi, with a further 3–4 divisions of the bronchioles before reaching the **terminal bronchiole**.

There may be up to 50 **respiratory bronchioles** (so-called because they are lined with thin respiratory epithelium across which gas exchange can occur) per terminal bronchiole, with an estimated 200 **alveoli** being supplied per respiratory bronchiole. The term 'small airway' usually refers to bronchi of less than 2 mm in diameter, of which there are approximately 30 000 in an adult. The continuous branching from the bifurcation in the trachea resembles a tree trunk and hence is often referred to as the **bronchial tree**.

The bronchi are composed of tissues similar to those of the trachea but, as they become progressively smaller by subdivisions inside the lungs, the cartilage becomes less well defined and irregular in shape.

The walls of the bronchioles, like those of the larger airways, are composed of rings of smooth muscle. Changes in smooth muscle tone are particularly effective in altering the calibre of the bronchioles because, unlike the trachea and bronchi, they have no cartilage in their walls to maintain rigidity. The tone of the smooth muscle is under autonomic control. It contains β-receptors, which cause relaxation of the muscle in response to sympathetic stimulation (e.g. during exercise) and to drugs such as adrenaline (epinephrine), noradrenaline (norepinephrine) and salbutamol, resulting in generalized **bronchodilation** (widening of the air passages). As this facilitates air entry to the lungs, these drugs are frequently administered to patients with bronchoconstriction. Bronchodilation also occurs in response to certain hormones and to local increases in the level of carbon dioxide.

**Bronchoconstriction** is caused by parasympathetic activity, acetylcholine, histamine and stimulation of receptors in the trachea and large bronchi by irritants such as cigarette smoke. Airway hyperresponsiveness (hyperactivity) which, together with airway inflammation, is a characteristic of asthma, is an exaggerated bronchoconstrictor response to many physical, chemical and pharmacological agents. These triggers can vary substantially in their impact from person to person and some people may have triggers in more than one category. The level of hyperresponsiveness can be determined in the laboratory by a standard inhalation challenge using methacholine or histamine. This involves measuring airway function (see p. 563) before and after the subject inhales increasing doses of a provocative agent such as histamine. Marked reductions in airflow will occur at much lower doses

in asthmatic subjects than in normal individuals. This principle is also used in reversibility testing where peak flow or spirometry is performed before and after the administration of a short-acting bronchodilator and is used in diagnosis of asthma [British Thoracic Society (BTS)/Scottish Intercollegiate Guidelines Network (SIGN) (2003)]. Additional factors influencing airway calibre are discussed later (see Resistance, p. 559).

## CLINICAL APPLICATIONS

### BRONCHOSCOPY

The bronchial tree can be examined by **fibre optic** bronchoscopy, in which a flexible, lighted catheter, through which local anaesthetic can be delivered directly to the airways, is introduced into the trachea. This technique can be used in sedated patients to examine the airways, remove airway secretions and mucous plugs, take cultures or smears, perform bronchoalveolar lavage or stop bleeding. Removal of foreign bodies and abnormal tissue is normally carried out with a rigid bronchoscope. Major nursing responsibilities include explanation of the technique to the patient and ensuring that, following administration of local anaesthetic to the upper airways, all fluid and food are withheld for several hours (see Swallowing reflex, p. 549). The nurse should also remember the importance of psychological support as bronchoscopy is often performed to establish a diagnosis such as carcinoma of the lung. The use of special chest X-rays (**bronchograms**) that involved injecting an opaque contrast medium (such as iodine) through a catheter passed into the trachea via the nose or mouth to examine the bronchial tree has largely been replaced by computerized tomography (CT) and magnetic resonance imaging (MRI).

## Functions of the airways

The volume of the nasal cavity, pharynx, larynx, trachea and bronchi (which are collectively known as the conducting airways) is approximately 150 mL in the adult. As no gas exchange can occur across these thick-walled tubes, the space within them is called the **anatomic dead space**.

Inasmuch as they constitute a dead space and offer a resistance to airflow, which increases in the presence of any form of obstruction, it might be thought that the airways are nothing but a hindrance to efficient respiration. However, they perform the vital function of protecting the delicate respiratory tissues in the alveoli by filtering, warming and humidifying the air during its passage to the lungs.

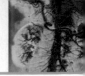

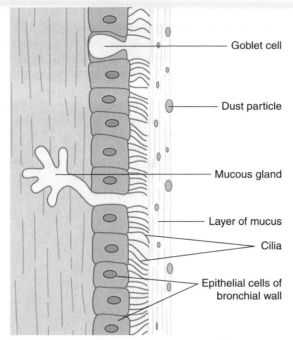

**Figure 5.3.4**  Epithelial lining of the respiratory tract. Mucus is secreted by mucous glands and goblet cells and traps inhaled particles. The cilia propel the mucus towards the pharynx (the mucociliary escalator) where it can be swallowed

Labels on figure:
- Goblet cell
- Dust particle
- Mucous gland
- Layer of mucus
- Cilia
- Epithelial cells of bronchial wall

The structure of the epithelial lining is well suited to its function as an air filter (**Fig. 5.3.4**). The epithelial glands secrete a thick, sticky substance called mucus, which lines all parts of the respiratory tract above the bronchioles. This layer of mucus waterproofs the epithelial surface (thereby diminishing water loss from the body), acts as a protective barrier against irritants and traps foreign particles. Hypertrophy of the mucous glands and excessive mucus production, as in chronic bronchitis, will occur in response to prolonged irritation of the mucosa by cigarette smoke and other pollutants.

The epithelial lining of all large airways also contains hair-like projections called cilia. These beat between 600 and 1000 times each minute, sweeping the mucus, and any trapped particles in it, towards the pharynx where it can be swallowed, broken down by digestive juices and eliminated in the faeces. This mechanism also contributes to defence against infection as many bacteria enter the body on dust particles and can be 'swept out' again in this manner. The large numbers of phagocytic cells in the epithelial lining also contribute to defence by engulfing debris, dust and bacteria. The cilia may be unable to clear the mucous blanket adequately if:

- the secretions become too thick and tenacious, as in dehydration or cystic fibrosis
- the cilia are damaged or paralysed by inadequate humidification of inspired air (this occurs especially during artificial ventilation) or exposure to irritant gases such as those in cigarette smoke
- there is excessive production of mucus, as in upper respiratory tract infections.

In any of these situations, there will be retention of secretions that are likely to contain bacteria and may therefore lead to respiratory infections. In addition, excess mucus may drain into the lower airways causing partial or complete airways obstruction and serious interference with gas exchange. Sputum retention can be a potentially life-threatening situation and requires early recognition or preferably proactive intervention to stop it happening. Diagnosis of the condition is based on evidence of respiratory distress with rapid, shallow and bubbly respirations, and it should be suspected in patients with any of the following signs:

- crackles heard through the stethoscope
- suspiciously quiet breath sounds
- the subjective report that 'there is something in my chest'.

Sputum retention is particularly likely if there is a history of lung disease or recent surgery, or if the patient is dehydrated (Hough, 1992).

## CLINICAL APPLICATIONS

### PNEUMONIA

**Pneumonia** is an acute inflammatory process of the alveoli caused by bacteria or viruses. It usually begins in the large bronchi and then spreads towards the periphery of the lung. The inflammatory process causes vasodilation of the pulmonary arterioles and capillaries with consequent leakage of plasma, fibrin and blood cells. This exudate frequently collects in the alveoli where its presence prevents adequate gas exchange – the affected part of the lung is said to be **consolidated**. The pneumococcal bacteria that are the most common cause of pneumonia are normally present in the upper respiratory tract in about 50% of the 'healthy population'. The excellent defence mechanisms afforded by the respiratory tract in health prevent these bacteria entering the lower respiratory tract and initiating the inflammatory process. It is only when the body's resistance to disease is lowered that the risk of contracting pneumonia is increased. Consequently, those most susceptible to pneumonia include older people, infants, those who smoke cigarettes, people with chronic obstructive lung disease and individuals who are immunocompromised (e.g. people with AIDS, malignancy or those taking immunosuppressive drugs, for example following an organ transplant). Intoxication with alcohol or drug abuse also increases the risk by reducing the phagocytic ability of the macrophages, interfering with normal ciliary action and depressing the cough reflex that would normally facilitate removal of bacteria and mucus from the lungs. Thus susceptible individuals could develop pneumonia when in hospital (hospital-acquired pneumonia) and at home (community-acquired pneumonia).

## Cough and sneeze reflexes

Coughing is the body's reflex mechanism for attempting to remove excess mucus or other irritants from the air passages. This reflex originates in receptors in the lining of the respiratory tract, which, when activated, cause stimulation of the respiratory centre in the medulla of the brain. The medulla regulates the special breathing pattern used during coughing. After an initial deep inspiration, a forced expiration is made. The glottis is closed during initial expiration so that no air can leave the lungs. Consequently, the pressure beneath the glottis builds up rapidly so that when it is suddenly re-opened, air rushes out at a speed that may approach 500 miles per hour (mph). This collects up liquid matter and clears the airways. Sneezing is a similar protective reflex stimulated by irritation of the nasal mucosa. It involves a series of short inspirations followed by an explosive expiration, usually with the mouth closed. The rapid spread of respiratory infections is largely due to the distance that infected droplets of water can travel during coughing and sneezing.

### CLINICAL APPLICATIONS

#### COUGHING

**Coughing** that results in expulsion of mucus (sputum) should be encouraged because it will help prevent accumulation of secretions within the lungs. **Sputum** is an abnormal excess of secretions from the airways. Laboratory analysis of sputum can be used to assist in the diagnosis of both respiratory and cardiac disorders. Specimens of sputum should be collected into a sterile container soon after waking (the overnight accumulation of secretions facilitates production of sputum rather than saliva). The amount of sputum produced, its colour, consistency and degree of effort required to produce it should be observed. Taste can also be assessed as patients often report a metallic taste in their mouth prior to an infection whilst sputum from patients with cystic fibrosis can taste salty (Law, 2000). As sputum production is potentially embarrassing for

the patient, it is essential that the nurse ensures the patient's privacy and shows no personal distaste. Precautions should also be taken to avoid cross-infection from potentially infected sputum; the nurse should ensure a sputum pot, tissues, mouth washes and hand-washing facilities are readily accessible to the patient.

Following intrathoracic surgery, the intercostal nerves are sometimes injected with a local anaesthetic to reduce pain. If this is not done, a patient may adopt a pattern of shallow breathing and inhibit the cough reflex in an attempt to minimize pain. This may delay re-expansion of the lungs or lead to obstruction of the smaller airways with subsequent alveolar collapse (**atelectasis**). Morphine and narcotic drugs should be used sparingly because they tend to depress respiration and the cough reflex. A nurse may provide support by placing her hands on the anterior and posterior chest walls in the painful areas while encouraging deep breathing and coughing.

### AIRWAY SECRETIONS

Other methods of preventing accumulation of retained secretions include:

- early mobilization and/or frequent changes of position
- maintenance of adequate fluid balance, without which secretions become thick and tenacious (see Chapter 5.4); warm drinks are especially helpful
- administration of inhalations, expectorants or mucolytic enzymes
- physiotherapy (e.g. active cycle of breathing techniques) and postural drainage
- administration of antibiotics if infective organisms are present in sputum
- use of flutter valve – a hand-held pipe-like device with a ball-bearing in the central core that oscillates during exhalation causing the airways to vibrate and so loosen secretions.

However, the role of postural drainage in the management of conditions associated with chronic sputum production has been challenged recently, especially in relation to the flutter valve (Bellone et al., 2000; Fink, 2002).

If the cough reflex is lost (during anaesthesia or unconsciousness), or if a tracheostomy or endotracheal tube is present, patients will be unable to raise their own secretions. Under these circumstances it may be necessary to use a small sterile catheter attached to a suction pump to remove secretions. During suction, care should be taken to avoid traumatizing the delicate respiratory epithelium, introducing any infection or creating too great a negative pressure in the airways, which could lead to lung collapse.

Particular care is required when applying suction to the trachea of premature neonates on the intensive care unit because they may become hypoxic very rapidly during this procedure.

## HUMIDIFICATION AND WARMING

As air passes along the upper respiratory tract it is exposed to a large surface area of highly vascular epithelium and undergoes a rapid exchange of heat and water. Lack of humidification can cause severe damage to the cilia and thereby initiate or aggravate respiratory disease. Consequently, compressed oxygen (which is completely dry) should always be warmed and humidified before being administered to patients, particularly if they are unable to breathe through their nose. Inadequate humidification of inspired gases was a major cause of lung damage in mechanically ventilated patients before the significance of humidification was appreciated. To decide whether a patient receiving oxygen via a face mask requires the oxygen to be humidified, the nurse must consider whether there is existing lung pathology, the length of administration and percentage/flow rate of oxygen being administered.

Under normal circumstances, approximately 150–200 mL of water are lost from the body in expired gas each day. If ventilation increases due to exercise, fever or lung disease, or if an individual mouth breathes, this loss will be greater and must be compensated for by increased fluid intake.

If very cold air is breathed, parasympathetic stimulation of the bronchiolar smooth muscles causes bronchoconstriction, which slows the passage of air into the alveoli and allows more time for it to be warmed up. This reflex is evident from the 'tight' feeling in the chest that is sometimes experienced when walking in cold weather. In patients with hypersensitive airways, this cold air challenge may be sufficient to provoke an attack of asthma.

## Swallowing reflex

The presence of food or water in the pharynx normally stimulates the swallowing reflex, which involves a temporary cessation of breathing and the closure of the larynx (glottis) by the lowering of the leaf-shaped piece of tissue called the **epiglottis**. If this reflex is absent (e.g. in an unconscious patient or during and after anaesthesia), food or water may be inhaled into the lungs, resulting in choking and possible airway obstruction, lung collapse or pneumonia. To minimize this risk, atropine is given preoperatively to reduce secretions, and oral food and fluid are withheld from patients postoperatively until the swallowing reflex is regained. Similarly precautions are necessary following local anaesthesia of the upper airways, e.g. for bronchoscopy.

## Speech

The airways play a vital role in the production of sound and speech. Sound is produced by the vibration of air as it passes through the vocal cords, which are two strong bands of elastic tissue stretched across the lumen of the larynx, covered by membranous folds. The glottis can be varied in shape and size to produce different levels of pitch in sound production. Normally, sound is produced during expiration, and inspiration occurs silently. Inflammation, infection or the presence of a tumour in the larynx may lead to hoarseness and loss of voice. The nasal cavities and sinuses act as resonating chambers, which alter the quality of sound.

## Smell

The olfactory receptors, which are concerned with the sense of smell, are found in the posterior portion of the nasal cavities. Their efficiency is greatly diminished by any obstruction (e.g. oedema) of the nasal passages and sinuses. It is for this reason that the common cold affects ability to smell and, as the sense of smell enhances the sense of taste, results in food seeming tasteless and less appetizing.

## Relationship of lungs to thoracic cage

The lungs are paired, cone-shaped organs lying in the thoracic cavity. They are separated from each other and the heart by the mediastinum. The lungs are attached to the thoracic cage by serous membranes called the **pleurae**. The visceral pleura covers the outer surface of each lung and is continuous with the parietal pleura, which is closely attached to the inner surface of the thoracic cage. These two membranes normally lie in intimate contact with one another, being separated only by a thin layer of pleural fluid. In effect, each lung is enclosed within its own double-walled, fluid-filled sac, by which it is attached to the thoracic cage. There is no communication between the intrapleural fluid surrounding the right and left lung because the mediastinum effectively divides the thoracic cavity into two halves (**Fig. 5.3.5**).

## Pleural fluid

The two pleural layers are effectively sealed together by a film of **pleural fluid**, which exerts a strong surface tension force that prevents separation of the

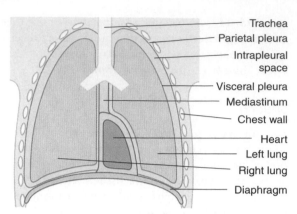

Trachea
Parietal pleura
Intrapleural space
Visceral pleura
Mediastinum
Chest wall
Heart
Left lung
Right lung
Diaphragm

**Figure 5.3.5** Relationship between the lungs, thoracic cage and pleurae. The volume of pleural fluid is exaggerated for clarity. The visceral and parietal pleurae normally lie in intimate contact with only a very thin layer of fluid between them. Note that there is no communication between the left and right intrapleural space

membranes. This seal is essential because it enables the lungs (which themselves contain no skeletal muscle) to be expanded and relaxed by movements of the chest wall.

Pleural fluid is secreted by the membranes and is basically a capillary filtrate.

### CLINICAL APPLICATIONS

#### PLEURAL EFFUSION

Anything that disturbs the normal balance of forces occurring at the capillaries, such as:

- increased capillary permeability (as in inflammatory conditions)
- increased pulmonary capillary pressure (as in left ventricular failure)
- reduced flow through pulmonary lymphatics (as in tumours and infections)

can result in excess pleural fluid formation, known as **pleural effusion**. This condition may develop gradually and not be recognized until the accumulation of fluid is great enough to compress the lung, causing difficulty in breathing (**dyspnoea**). This unpleasant symptom can be relieved by draining the pleural effusion by **chest aspiration (thoracentesis)**. This aseptic procedure is performed by a doctor using local anaesthetic. It involves passing a biopsy needle through the chest wall, between the ribs, at the affected site. Pleural effusions can be either transudates or exudates. It is therefore important that a sample of the fluid is sent for analysis to establish the cause of the effusion and

so that medical management is directed appropriately.

Nursing responsibilities include: ensuring that patients know what to expect and how best to cooperate, helping to support the patient in a stable sitting position during the procedure and observing for signs of respiratory distress and bleeding both during the aspiration and after. It is important to control the amount of fluid removed at any one time as unilateral pulmonary oedema has been described following removal of over 2 L. This can be prevented by slow aspiration with a maximum of 1200–1500 mL being removed at a time (BTS, 2003c).

## Intrapleural pressure

The relaxed volume of the lung is considerably smaller than that of the thoracic cage (**Fig. 5.3.6**). Attachment of the lung to the inside of the thorax by the pleura results in the thoracic cage being pulled inwards while the lung is expanded (**Fig. 5.3.6c**). Both the thorax and lung are elastic structures, that is, they will spring back (or recoil) to their original size as soon as any distending pressure (or force) is removed. Although the pleural fluid seal prevents the lung actually separating from the thorax, the tendency of the thorax to spring out and the tendency of the lung to collapse, produces forces pulling in opposite directions. This produces a negative pressure (relative to atmosphere) inside the intrapleural space. The resting volume adopted by the lung at the end of a normal expiration is known as the **functional residual capacity (FRC)**. This volume is usually about 3 L in an adult male and represents the lung volume that is achieved when the outward pull of the thorax is exactly balanced by the inward recoil of the lung. At the end of expiration, intrapleural pressure is about $-0.5\,\mathrm{kPa}$ ($-5\,\mathrm{cmH_2O}$). The more the lungs are expanded, the greater their tendency to spring back to their relaxed volume. Consequently, intrapleural pressure becomes increasingly negative during inspiration (**Fig. 5.3.7**).

Intrapleural pressure is sometimes referred to as **intrathoracic pressure** because it is transmitted to all structures in the thorax including the heart. The negative intrathoracic pressure assists venous return by exerting a slight 'sucking' force, sometimes called the 'respiratory pump'. This force is increased during exercise when deeper breathing is accompanied by greater negative intrathoracic pressure. Conversely, venous return may be impeded in some patients during mechanical ventilation as a result of the applied positive pressure, which is transmitted not only down the airways but also around all the thoracic blood vessels.

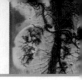

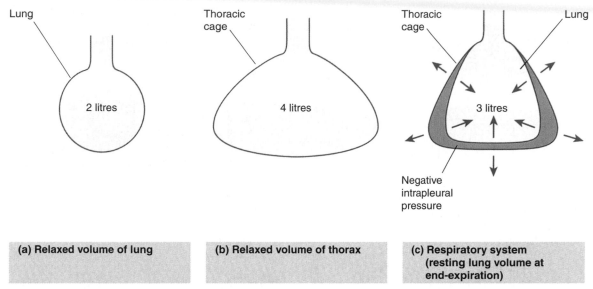

Negative
intrapleural
pressure

**(a) Relaxed volume of lung**

**(b) Relaxed volume of thorax**

**(c) Respiratory system
(resting lung volume at
end-expiration)**

**Figure 5.3.6**  Representation of the relative sizes of the isolated lungs and thoracic cage, and of the total respiratory system at rest. When the lungs are attached to the thorax by the pleura, the thorax is pulled inwards and the lung expanded; creating a negative intrapleural pressure

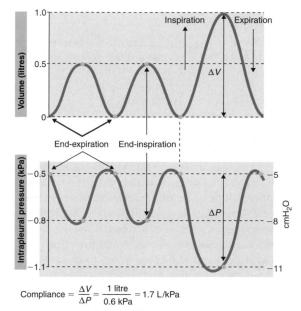

$$\text{Compliance} = \frac{\Delta V}{\Delta P} = \frac{1 \text{ litre}}{0.6 \text{ kPa}} = 1.7 \text{ L/kPa}$$

**Figure 5.3.7**  Changes of intrapleural pressure during the respiratory cycle

## CLINICAL APPLICATIONS

### PNEUMOTHORAX

If the pleural fluid seal is broken (e.g. by a spontaneous intrapulmonary air leak, during chest surgery or by a stab wound), air will be drawn into the intrapleural 'space', creating a real air-containing space between the lungs and thorax and abolishing the negative intrapleural pressure. This is called a **pneumothorax**. When a

pneumothorax occurs, the lung in the affected area collapses, the chest wall bows out and, because movement of the chest wall is no longer effective in expanding the lung, gas exchange is seriously impaired. Fortunately, because there is no continuity between the pleural fluid seal around the right and left lung, only one side will collapse, unless both sides are damaged simultaneously.

Rapid diagnosis and treatment of a pneumothorax are essential. Decreased movement of one side of the chest on inspiration (except following pneumonectomy, when this is to be expected), difficulty in breathing, sudden deterioration in condition, cyanosis and chest pain all suggest the presence of a pneumothorax and should be reported immediately.

Diagnosis is usually confirmed by a portable chest X-ray.

Treatment is aimed at restoring the lung to its original size as rapidly as possible. This is usually achieved by the insertion of a tube to draw air from the pleural space into an under water seal drainage system.

Various methods may be used to achieve drainage of a pneumothorax or pleural effusion; all are based on the same principle of encouraging air and excess fluid to escape from the pleural cavity while preventing any reflux. The basic apparatus is illustrated in **Fig. 5.3.8**. The drainage tube from the patient is connected to a long catheter, the end of which is submerged below a few centimetres of sterile water in a calibrated drainage bottle. The decrease in pressure inside the pleural cavity during

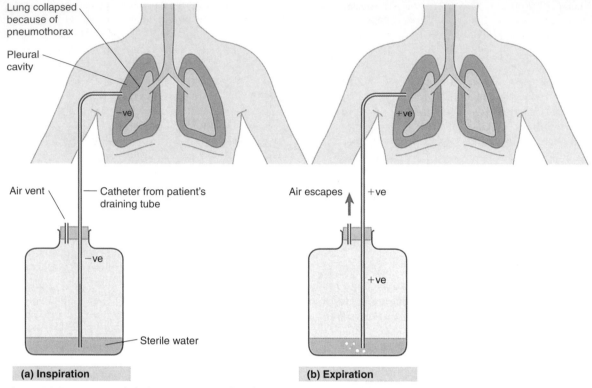

Lung collapsed because of pneumothorax

Pleural cavity

−ve

+ve

Air vent — Catheter from patient's draining tube

Air escapes +ve

−ve

+ve

Sterile water

**(a) Inspiration**

**(b) Expiration**

**Figure 5.3.8**  Water seal drainage using one bottle. During inspiration (a) the negative pressure in the pleural cavity sucks up the tube. During expiration (b) pressure in the pleural cavity and tubing becomes positive, forcing air out of the cavity

inspiration causes air to be sucked up the tube, usually to a height of about 10–20 cm. Consequently, drainage bottles must always be kept well below the level of the patient's chest, preferably on the floor, to prevent water being sucked into the chest. During expiration the rise in pressure forces air out of the pleural cavity. The water level in the tube will fall and some air will bubble out through the water and escape from the bottle via the air vent. Re-entry of air during the following inspiration is prevented by the water seal.

The magnitude of pressure swings in the pleural cavity (as reflected by the swings of water level in the tube) will depend on the amount of air present and depth of breathing. Coughing and deep breathing promote drainage. Drainage may be assisted by low-pressure suction, in which case there will be no swings in water level as the applied negative pressure will be held at a constant level.

## CHEST DRAINAGE

A patient undergoing **chest drainage** requires regular observation. Chest pain, difficulty in breathing or a rising pulse rate require immediate investigation. During drainage, the amount of air

and type and volume of fluid drained are observed and recorded.

Patency of the drainage system should be checked regularly. Blockage may be caused by the drainage tube becoming kinked, by the patient lying on it or by a clot or other debris inside the tube. There will be no oscillation ('swinging') when the lung has re-expanded. However, suction also causes oscillation to stop and the nurse therefore needs to be clear when to be concerned about 'lack of swing' and when it is expected. Furthermore, constant bubbling of the fluid in the underwater seal drainage bottle can indicate that there is either an air leak in the system or that the patient still has a pneumothorax.

If the bottle needs to be replaced, the drainage tube must first be sealed with two clamps placed close to the chest wall. Sealing in this way ensures that neither fluid nor air can accidentally enter the chest. It is imperative that clamps are removed after the bottle has been changed; failure to do so could result in a tension pneumothorax (a potentially life-threatening situation). The tube does not need to be clamped when the patient is moved but must remain below the level of the chest; a clamped drain on an unresolved pneumothorax can also lead to a tension pneumothorax. However, there may be specific medical orders to clamp a drain at set intervals to delay drainage, e.g. following installation of drugs or following pneumonectomy. A spare set of clamps should always be available in case of emergency, i.e. accidental disconnection. As a chest drain can be uncomfortable, care should be taken to support the tubes to ensure that they do not pull on the chest wall or become dislodged.

When no air remains in the pleural space, the bubbling and oscillation of water levels will cease. Re-expansion of the lung is confirmed by chest X-ray before removal of the tubes. Analgesia is usually administered prior to withdrawal of the tubes.

The wound is immediately sealed (i.e. with a purse-string suture) to facilitate wound healing and to prevent recurrence of the pneumothorax, and the patient is observed closely for several hours for any signs of leakage of air into the chest. The British Thoracic Society has published guidelines on the management of pneumothorax, chest drains and pleural disease (BTS, 2003a, b, c).

## Structure and functions of the alveoli

The epithelial lining of the airways becomes progressively less ciliated as it approaches the **alveolar ducts**. These are thin tubes of squamous epithelium branching off the terminal bronchioles and opening into the alveoli, which are tiny, cup-shaped hollow sacs. Three types of cell are found in the alveolar epithelium:

- Thin **squamous epithelial** cells, which cover most of the alveolar surface.
- Larger **cuboidal epithelial** cells (type II), which are metabolically active and responsible for both epithelial cell renewal and synthesizing **surfactant**, a phospholipid that reduces surface tension forces in the lung (see below).
- **Alveolar macrophages**. These are active phagocytic cells thought to be derived from bone marrow. They provide the chief defence mechanism against any debris or bacteria that reaches the alveoli. They migrate through the epithelium, engulf any foreign matter and are eliminated mainly in the sputum.

There are no ciliated or mucus-producing cells in the alveolar epithelium.

### DEVELOPMENTAL ISSUES

#### SURFACTANT AND THE RESPIRATORY DISTRESS SYNDROME OF THE NEWBORN

To establish efficient gaseous exchange at birth, there must be rapid clearance of liquid from the lungs and airways, expansion of the alveoli and establishment of an adequate resting lung volume. The success of this transition depends largely on the presence of adequate amounts of the phospholipid **surfactant**, which is secreted from the alveolar cells. Although surfactant is present in fetal lungs from approximately 23 weeks gestational age, it rarely occurs in sufficient quantities to prevent persistent alveolar collapse before 28–32 weeks gestational age. The surface tension of alveolar fluid is 7–14 times greater than normal in infants born with surfactant deficiency. Consequently, the lungs are very stiff (low compliance) and the alveoli may collapse almost to their original uninflated state at the end of each expiration. This condition, known as the **respiratory distress syndrome (RDS)** of the newborn, develops within a few hours after birth and remains a major cause of neonatal mortality.

The introduction of increasingly sophisticated methods of ventilatory support for newborn babies, together with the detection of surfactant deficiency before birth (by amniocentesis) and administration of maternal steroid therapy (which accelerates fetal lung development), have reduced the morbidity and mortality from respiratory distress syndrome. However, the greatest breakthrough has been the recent development of surfactant replacement therapy. Surfactant, which is derived from animal tissues or produced synthetically, is administered directly to the lungs and airways of high-risk premature infants by introducing small quantities of surfactant solution into the endotracheal tube. The dose is frequently repeated within 12–48 hours. Following several large multicentre trials, this is now standard practice for infants with surfactant deficiency at birth (Greenough, 1997).

The lungs are divided into approximately 300 million alveoli. Similarly, the pulmonary artery, which brings venous blood to the lungs for gas exchange, branches and subdivides into millions of thin-walled capillaries forming a dense network of blood vessels wrapped around each alveolus (**Fig. 5.3.9**).

### The alveolar–capillary membrane

For gas exchange to occur in the lungs or tissues, gases have to cross cellular membranes. Surfaces of the lung that are thin enough to permit rapid diffusion of gases include the alveoli, the alveolar ducts and the respiratory bronchioles, and are collectively known as the pulmonary (or alveolar–capillary) membrane (**Fig. 5.3.10b**). This membrane consists of the alveolar epithelium, the interstitium and the capillary endothelium. It is exceedingly thin, being

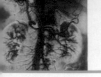

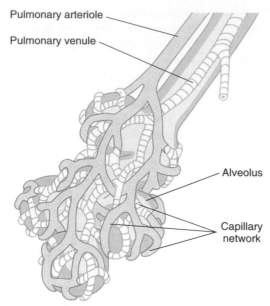

**Figure 5.3.9** Relationship between alveoli and blood vessels. Gas exchange can occur across the vast surface provided by the dense network of capillaries

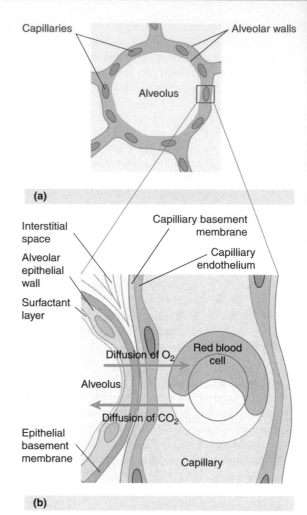

**Figure 5.3.10** Cross-section through an alveolus (a) and higher magnification (b) showing histology of part of the alveolar–capillary membrane. The dense network of capillaries forms an almost continuous sheet of blood in the alveolar walls, providing a very efficient arrangement for gas exchange

less than 0.4 μm thick in most parts, which is less than the diameter of a red blood cell. The blood travelling through the capillaries is thus brought into intimate proximity with the alveolar air, thereby facilitating diffusion (**Fig. 5.3.10a**). The function of the lung as an organ of gas exchange is also favoured by its subdivision into millions of alveoli. This arrangement vastly increases the surface area available for diffusion to about $70 \, m^2$ (some 40 times larger than the entire external body surface area).

Having considered how the structure of the lung is suited to its primary role as an organ of gas exchange, the various physiological processes that are involved in providing the tissues with oxygen and eliminating excess carbon dioxide will be considered.

## Ventilation of the lungs

Pulmonary ventilation, or breathing, is the process by which gases are exchanged between the atmosphere and lung alveoli. As discussed below, this gas exchange is dependent on the creation of pressure gradients between the lungs and atmosphere. To understand how this process occurs it is necessary to remember how gases behave.

### Behaviour of gases

Whenever a substance exists as a gas, its molecules are free to move about independently in space. This perpetual motion of gas molecules results in numerous collisions, which exert a certain pressure. Any factor that increases the number of collisions occurring (such as a rise in temperature, which increases the speed at which molecules travel) will cause a rise in gas pressure, and vice versa.

If temperature remains constant, the pressure of a gas varies inversely with the volume in which it is contained, because any decrease in volume leads to increased concentration of gas molecules and hence more collisions. Thus, if the same volume of air is drawn into three syringes (**Fig. 5.3.11**), the pressure within them can be altered, relative to atmospheric pressure, by closing the ends of the syringes and then moving the plungers to decrease (**Fig. 5.3.11b**) or increase (**Fig. 5.3.11c**) the internal volume of the syringe.

Although gas molecules are always in perpetual motion, there will be a net flow of gas from one area to another only if a pressure gradient exists. Movement

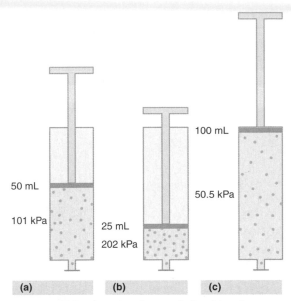

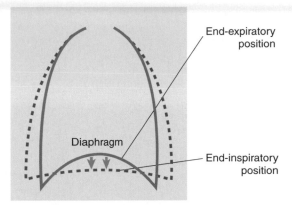

**Figure 5.3.12** Diaphragmatic movements during respiration. The dome-shaped diaphragm contracts during inspiration, pressing down on the abdominal contents and lifting the rib cage, resulting in an increase in the volume of the thorax

**Figure 5.3.11** Pressure–volume relationship of gases. Atmospheric pressure has been taken to be 101 kPa (760 mmHg). By moving the plunger down as in (b), the gas in the syringe is compressed to 25 mL (volume is halved), with corresponding rise in gas pressure. By contrast, if the plunger is withdrawn, the gas molecules will move apart to fill the 100 mL space, but pressure will be halved (c)

of gases along a pressure gradient is said to occur by **bulk flow**, movement always being from an area of high to low pressure until an equilibrium is achieved. Thus, if the syringes in **Fig. 5.3.11** are opened to the atmosphere, there would be no net exchange of gas from syringe (a), air would flow out of syringe (b), and air would flow into syringe (c), until the pressure within all returned to atmospheric (which at sea level is equal to 101 kPa or 760 mmHg).

During a breathing cycle, air flows in and out of the lungs by bulk flow. During inspiration, the thoracic cage expands due to contraction of the respiratory muscles, increasing lung volume as it does so. This causes a temporary drop in pressure inside the lungs so that atmospheric air flows into them until pressures are equivalent again. This process is reversed during expiration, when reduction in the volume of the thoracic cage due to relaxation of the respiratory muscles decreases lung volume and temporarily causes pressures within the lung to exceed that of the atmosphere.

## Inspiration

The most important muscle of inspiration is the **diaphragm**. This is a dome-shaped sheet of muscle attached to the lower ribs. When the diaphragm contracts during inspiration, it flattens, pressing down on the abdominal contents and lifting the rib cage,

thus enlarging the thoracic cage and lung, both from top to bottom and from front to back (**Fig. 5.3.12**). Because the air in the lungs now occupies a greater volume, alveolar pressure temporarily falls below atmospheric pressure. This causes air to be drawn into the lungs by bulk flow until alveolar pressure again equals atmospheric at the end of inspiration (termed 'end-inspiration'). By contrast, intrapleural pressure becomes increasingly negative throughout inspiration, due partly to the increase in the elastic recoil of the lung and partly to the reduction in alveolar pressure (**Fig. 5.3.13**).

Although the external intercostal muscles play virtually no part in expanding the rib cage during quiet breathing, they do play a vital role in stabilizing (stiffening) the rib cage. If, for example, the intercostal muscles are paralysed, much of the effort expended during breathing will be spent on distorting the rib cage rather than on effecting gas exchange.

### DEVELOPMENTAL ISSUES

Newborn infants have very compliant (floppy) chest walls, which tend to get drawn in (recessed) easily. This phenomenon is particularly marked in the presence of lung disease, rapid eye movement sleep and following premature delivery. Indrawing of the rib cage during inspiration, as the abdomen moves out, results in asynchronous or paradoxical breathing patterns. These greatly decrease the efficiency, and increase the work, of breathing.

During exercise, when requirements for gas exchanges increase, or in the presence of an upper airway obstruction that impedes the flow of gas into the lungs, the external intercostals, together with other accessory muscles of inspiration such as the sternomastoids,

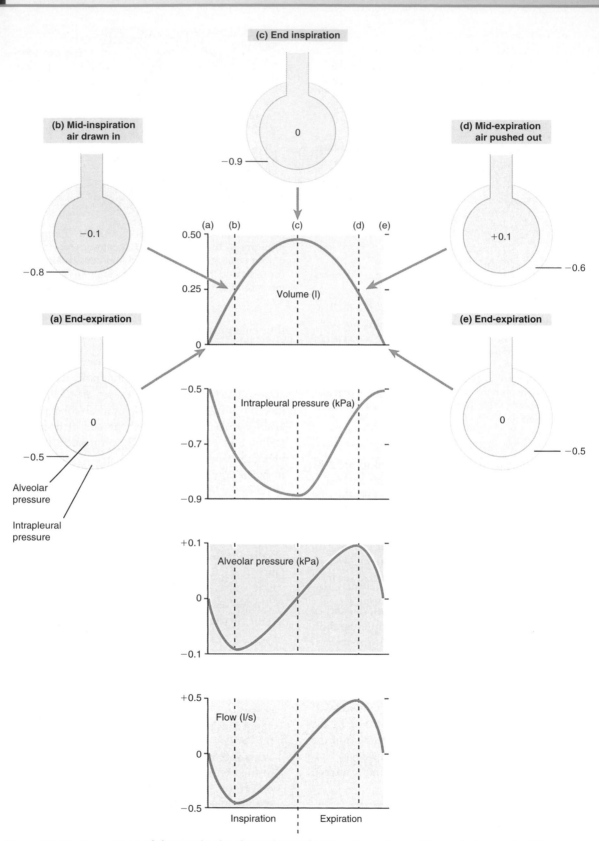

**Figure 5.3.13** Comparison of changes in alveolar and intrapleural pressure during the respiratory cycle. All pressures are given in kPa (multiply by 10 to obtain approximate values in cmH$_2$O). Note that intrapleural pressure normally remains negative throughout the respiratory cycle. By contrast, alveolar pressure is atmospheric at end-expiration (points a and e), and end-inspiration (c) (where there is no flow of gas) but becomes negative during inspiration (b) and positive during expiration (d), thereby providing the driving force to move air in and out of the lungs, as shown by the recording of airflow and volume

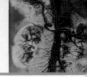

scalene and pectoralis muscles, assist in the expansion of the rib cage. Use of these accessory muscles to aid ventilation may also be observed in patients with obstructive airway disease, such as chronic bronchitis.

## Expiration

During quiet breathing, expiration is a passive process requiring no active muscle contraction. At end-inspiration, the respiratory muscles relax allowing the elastic lung and thorax to recoil to their original resting volume (**functional residual capacity**). This reduction in volume compresses the air in the lungs so that alveolar pressure temporarily exceeds atmospheric, providing the necessary driving force to push air out of the lung. Expiratory flow ceases when alveolar pressure is again equal to atmospheric pressure. During expiration, intrapleural pressure becomes progressively less negative, partly due to the progressive reduction in elastic recoil of the lung as it returns to its resting position but also because of the positive alveolar pressure during expiration (**see Fig. 5.3.13**).

Active expiratory efforts may occur if requirements for gas exchange increase (during exercise) or if the airways are narrowed. The most important accessory muscles of expiration are those of the abdominal wall. Contraction of these muscles increases abdominal pressure, which forces the diaphragm higher up into the thorax. This causes a greater compression of alveolar gas and thus facilitates expiratory flow.

## Pulmonary ventilation

The volume of air that passes in and out of the lungs during each breath is called the **tidal volume**. The total volume of air exchanged between the respiratory system and atmosphere each minute is referred to as the **minute volume** or **pulmonary ventilation**. This is determined by the tidal volume and respiratory rate, both of which vary enormously in health and disease, and according to the age of the subject.

However, in a resting adult with an 'average' tidal volume of about 500 mL and respiratory rate of 12 breaths/min, pulmonary ventilation will be approximately 6000 mL/min. However, not all the air that is inspired actually reaches the alveoli for gas exchange to occur. Approximately 150 mL of each tidal breath is 'trapped' within the **dead space** and is breathed out again during the subsequent expiration with its composition unchanged.

## Alveolar ventilation

The volume of fresh air entering the alveoli each minute is called the **alveolar ventilation**, and is calculated as follows:

$$\text{respiratory rate} \times (\text{tidal volume} - \text{dead space})$$
$$= \text{alveolar ventilation}$$
$$(\text{e.g. } 12 \text{ breaths/min} \times (500 - 150 \text{ mL})$$
$$= 4200 \text{ mL/min})$$

Thus, although pulmonary ventilation may be 6000 mL/min, only 4200 mL/min would actually be available for gas exchange. The minimal alveolar ventilation compatible with life would be about 1200 mL/min in an adult. By contrast, during maximal breathing efforts, it can temporarily be increased to as much as 10 000 L/min. Shallow rapid breathing is generally very inefficient because, the smaller the tidal volume, the greater the proportion that will be wasted in the dead space (**Table 5.3.1**). Similarly, the efficiency of ventilation will be impaired if the dead space increases, either due to attachment to some external apparatus (such as a snorkel or mechanical ventilator) or lung disease. In either situation, pulmonary ventilation will have to be increased if an adequate level of alveolar ventilation is to be maintained. When patients are being weaned from mechanical ventilation, they are usually left connected to the machine while it is switched off for gradually increasing periods of time. During these periods it is particularly important that they are observed carefully for

**Table 5.3.1** Effects of changing patterns of breathing on alveolar ventilation

| Pattern | Tidal volume (mL) | Respiratory rate/min | Total ventilation (mL/min) | Dead space ventilation (mL/min) | Alveolar ventilation (mL/min) |
|---|---|---|---|---|---|
| Rapid, shallow breathing | 200 | 30 | 6000 | 4500 | 1500 |
| 'Normal' | 500 | 12 | 6000 | 1800 | 4200 |
| Deep, slow breathing | 1000 | 6 | 6000 | 900 | 5100 |

Calculations based on a constant dead space of 150 mL. Note that total ventilation remains constant throughout, but that alveolar ventilation shows marked changes.

signs of respiratory distress. Intensive-care nurses are increasingly playing an important role in the initiation and management of extubation and criteria to support this process are being developed.

## Composition of atmospheric, expired and alveolar air

Atmospheric air consists primarily of 21% oxygen and 79% nitrogen, with negligible quantities of carbon dioxide and water vapour. The composition of alveolar air differs from that of atmospheric air for several reasons:

- As air passes along the airways it is humidified with water vapour, which causes a slight reduction in the partial pressure of the other gases present.
- Alveolar air is continually losing oxygen because it diffuses into the blood; this oxygen is replaced by carbon dioxide, which diffuses out of the blood.
- Only a fraction of alveolar gas is renewed with each breath.

Thus alveolar air contains considerably less oxygen and more carbon dioxide and water vapour than atmospheric air. As expired alveolar air is 'diluted' with atmospheric air from the dead space, the composition of mixed expired gas falls between that of alveolar and of atmospheric air (**Table 5.3.2**).

## Exchange of alveolar air with atmospheric air

The **functional residual capacity** (FRC) can be regarded as a reservoir of air in the lungs, which is diluted by successive inspirations of tidal air. Only about 12% of alveolar gas can be exchanged with fresh gas during a single breath and it usually takes about 23 seconds to renew half the gas in the lungs.

The mechanism of partial dilution means that the composition of alveolar gas remains very stable. Thus, the functional residual capacity acts as a buffer, preventing the marked fluctuations in alveolar (and hence arterial blood) gases that would otherwise occur during the respiratory cycle.

## Changes in barometric pressure

There is a progressive decrease in atmospheric pressure as the distance above sea level increases. Thus, although atmospheric air maintains a relatively constant composition, there is a fall in partial pressure of each of its constituent gases. At an altitude of 3000 metres (10 000 feet), atmospheric pressure is reduced to 70 kPa (523 mmHg). Consequently, atmospheric $PO_2$ is reduced to 21% of 70 kPa (i.e. 15 kPa or 110 mmHg) and alveolar $PO_2$ decreases to around 9 kPa (68 mmHg), i.e. 13% of 70 kPa (**see Table 5.3.2**). The subsequent reduction in the normal pressure gradient for oxygen across the alveolar–capillary membrane reduces the rate at which oxygen can diffuse into the blood. This results in a general deficiency of oxygen in the body (hypoxia) unless augmented oxygen is breathed. Rapid ascent to altitude generally results in some degree of mountain sickness due to hypoxia. However, the body can gradually acclimatize to chronic exposure to low inspired $PO_2$ (by changes in ventilation, cardiac output and composition of the blood), as demonstrated by the remarkably normal lives led by the inhabitants of the

**Table 5.3.2** Composition of atmospheric, expired and alveolar airs, expressed as partial pressures at sea level (kPa and mmHg) and as percentage concentrations

| Gas | Atmospheric air | | | Expired air | | | Alveolar air | | |
|---|---|---|---|---|---|---|---|---|---|
| | Partial pressure | | | Partial pressure | | | Partial pressure | | |
| | kPa | mmHg | % | kPa | mmHg | % | kPa | mmHg | % |
| Oxygen | 21.2 | 159.0 | 20.8 | 15.6 | 117 | 15.4 | 13.3 | 100 | 13.2 |
| Carbon dioxide | 0.04 | 0.3 | 0.04 | 3.8 | 29 | 3.8 | 5.3 | 40 | 5.3 |
| Nitrogen | 79.6 | 597.0 | 78.6 | 75.6 | 567 | 74.6 | 76.4 | 573 | 75.3 |
| Water | 0.5 | 3.9 | 0.5 | 6.3 | 47 | 6.2 | 6.3 | 47 | 6.2 |
| Total | 101.3 | 760.0 | 100.0 | 101.3 | 760 | 100.0 | 101.3 | 760 | 100.0 |

1 kPa = 7.5 mmHg
Note that since atmospheric pressure at sea level is 101.3 kPa, partial pressures of each gas expressed in kilopascals are virtually identical to their percentage concentrations within each gas mixture.
The water content of atmospheric air varies daily according to prevailing conditions.

Andes and Himalayas, who permanently live at an altitude of about 5500 m.

Atmospheric pressure increases below sea level to the extent that 10 m below the surface it is twice as great as normal (202 kPa or 1520 mmHg). This can cause increased diffusion of oxygen and nitrogen into body fluids, with subsequent interruption of normal cellular activity. More dangerously, on return to sea level, excess nitrogen that has been forced into the body fluids under pressure, re-expands, forming bubbles in body tissues. These cause severe pain, gastrointestinal distension and possible paralysis or death due to embolism. Deep-sea divers breathe reduced-concentration oxygen to prevent excess uptake of oxygen on descent, and use decompression chambers to allow the excess dissolved nitrogen to escape gradually on return to the surface.

## The work of breathing

The amount of energy expended on breathing depends on:

- the rate and depth of ventilation
- the ease with which the lungs and thorax can be expanded
- the resistance to airflow offered by the airways.

Normally, less than 1% of the resting metabolic rate is spent on breathing, but this may rise to 3% during heavy exercise and up to 50% in severe respiratory disease, resulting in exhaustion of the patient and possible respiratory failure.

## Compliance

The term 'compliance' is used to describe the distensibility of the lungs and thorax. Under normal conditions, the lungs and thoracic wall expand easily, i.e. are highly compliant.

The lungs usually require an inflating pressure (i.e. intrapleural pressure change) of only about 0.3 kPa (3 cmH$_2$O) to produce a tidal volume of 500 mL (**see Fig. 5.3.7**), whereas 100 times more pressure may be required to inflate a child's balloon to the same volume.

### CLINICAL APPLICATIONS

#### FACTORS INFLUENCING COMPLIANCE

The lungs will become stiffer (decreased compliance) if there is:

- a reduction in lung size (**atelectasis**, i.e. collapsed lung or portion of lung, or pneumonectomy)
- increased pulmonary fluid or blood (e.g. pulmonary congestion in heart failure)

- a deficiency of surfactant; this phospholipid, which is secreted by the alveolar epithelial cells, normally decreases surface tension forces, facilitating lung expansion (see p. 573).

In contrast, compliance will increase (the lungs will be more distensible) if there is a loss of elastic tissue, such as occurs with ageing and in **emphysema** due to overstretching and destruction of alveolar walls. This is not as beneficial as it might at first appear because the loss of elastic recoil results both in overinflation of the lungs (which can no longer 'spring back' as efficiently as normal during expiration) and a narrowing of the airways (which no longer have the normal degree of traction exerted on their outer walls). Consequently, active expiratory efforts, accompanied by a marked rise in the work of breathing, may be required to force air out of the lungs during expiration.

### EMPHYSEMA

**Emphysema** is generally caused by long-term irritation by environmental pollutants. However, it may also be due to imbalance between $\alpha_1$-antitrypsin and the level of circulating enzymes that break down tissue protein, such as **elastase**.

$\alpha_1$-Antitrypsin is a plasma protein secreted from the alveoli. It inhibits **elastase** and hence protects the connective tissues in the walls of the alveolar sacs from destruction, and so prevents emphysema.

Cigarette smoking not only deactivates $\alpha_1$-antitrypsin but inhibits repair of damaged lung tissue (see also 'pink puffers', p. 573).

## Resistance of the airways

**Airways resistance** can be defined as the pressure required to produce a flow of gas of one litre/second (1 L/s) through the airways. In a healthy adult, resistance is approximately 0.2 kPa/L/s (2 cmH$_2$O/L/s) during mouth breathing (note that in lung function testing, pressures are usually measured in kPa or cmH$_2$O and not in mmHg: 1 kPa = 7.5 mmHg = 10.20 cmH$_2$O). The magnitude of airways resistance is influenced by several factors, the most important of which is the calibre of the airways. The narrower the airways, the higher their resistance and the greater the pressure change (and hence the work of breathing) required to drive the airflow.

The calibre of the airways can be affected by physical, chemical or neural factors, including:

- **Changes in lung volume**. Resistance falls during inspiration and rises during expiration due to the variable intrathoracic pressure surrounding the airways (**see Fig. 5.3.13**). Destruction of elastic

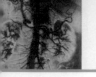

tissue and loss of recoil pressure in emphysematous lungs results in reduced traction applied to the outside of the airway walls. Consequently, airway diameter is reduced and airways resistance is significantly elevated, especially during expiration, when airway closure may occur.

- **Smooth muscle tone**. Sympathetic stimulation causes bronchodilation and a fall in resistance; parasympathetic stimulation has the reverse effect.

  Airway smooth muscle contraction is the primary abnormality in bronchial **asthma**, exacerbations of which are characterized by shortness of breath, cough and wheezing, and which reverse either spontaneously or with treatment. As a result of elevated expiratory resistance, the patient has difficulty breathing out and the lungs may become severely hyperinflated. Increased resistance is caused not only by the airway spasm but by inflammation of the epithelial lining and the production of excessive secretions.

  There has been a significant increase in the prevalence, morbidity and mortality of asthma during the past 30 years, the reasons for which remain unclear, although increasing levels of both internal and external pollutants, such as house-dust mites and car exhaust fumes, have been implicated. Of particular concern is the marked increase in the number of young women who smoke throughout pregnancy. There is now substantial evidence to suggest that babies born to such mothers have suboptimal lung growth in utero, with narrowed airways at birth and an increased tendency to wheeze during subsequent respiratory tract infections (Martinez et al., 1991; Tager et al., 1993). Effective health education to discourage all smoking during pregnancy and in the presence of young children is essential if the lung health of future generations is to be protected (Royal College of Physicians, 1992).

- **Airway obstruction**. Resistance increases if the airways become partially blocked by secretions, scar tissue (e.g. from previous inflammation or surgery) or external compression (e.g. in chronic bronchitis, cystic fibrosis, neoplasm or enlarged thyroid).

## CLINICAL APPLICATIONS

### DYSPNOEA

One of the most important symptoms of lung disease is dyspnoea. **Dyspnoea** is a subjective feeling of 'air hunger', or shortness of breath, which occurs when the demand for ventilation is out of proportion to the patient's ability to

respond to that demand and, as a result, breathing becomes difficult, laboured and uncomfortable, and is recognized as inappropriate.

Abnormalities of the lung and chest wall may both increase the demand for ventilation (e.g. if there is mismatching of the air and blood supply in the lung) and decrease the ability to respond to this demand.

As there are no objective signs of dyspnoea, which is something that only the patient can feel, it is very difficult to assess how severe it is. However, standard questionnaires may be used to grade breathlessness according to how far a person can walk on the level or upstairs without pausing for breath. These can be of particular value when following a patient's progress: the 6-minute walk is routinely used and the Borg Scale is used to measure the patient's subjective state of dyspnoea, particularly within pulmonary rehabilitation programmes.

To experience difficulty in breathing is frightening. In severe cases, as in asthma or acute pulmonary oedema, the patient is likely to be very distressed and may panic. If possible, such individuals will almost certainly want to sit upright, perhaps leaning slightly forward and supporting themselves against a piece of furniture.

Breathing tends to be most efficient when a person is sitting or standing. Functional residual capacity is approximately 0.5 L greater when in an upright position than when lying down because the doming movement of the diaphragm into the chest is less when upright and pulmonary blood volume decreases on moving from lying down to an upright position.

Severely dyspnoeic patients expend a great deal of energy in their fight to breathe effectively and soon become very weak and tired. They need to use their accessory muscles of respiration to aid ventilation and will probably breathe through their mouths because resistance to airflow is less through the mouth than through the nose. Continual mouth breathing dries the oral mucous membranes and such patients require frequent mouth care in a form they are able to tolerate.

The acute stress of dyspnoea is produced by sympathetic nervous stimulation (see Chapter 2.5), and the signs and symptoms associated with this, plus the physical exertion of breathing, produce a clinical picture of a frightened, tired patient, fighting to breathe. The patient may be pale or flushed, cold and clammy, or hot and sweating. Respiratory rate and heart rate will be raised and pupils may be noticeably dilated.

### Care of the dyspnoeic patient

It is essential that nurses caring for dyspnoeic patients take effective steps to relieve their physical problems and to prevent or alleviate unnecessary mental distress. Patients can be helped by being supported in a comfortable, upright sitting position and by being encouraged to breathe less rapidly and more deeply, since this will tend to maximize alveolar ventilation. Relaxation is extremely difficult for these patients but they should be encouraged to try and take control of their breathing. Typically, patients with chronic obstructive pulmonary disease (COPD) are tachypnoeic, anxious, using the accessory muscles of respiration, feeling short of breath and tired. These patients need to breathe like this; they should *not* be told to relax their shoulders and take deep breaths. Positioning them so that they can secure their shoulders and use accessory muscles without wasting energy by holding their shoulders up high will help. In patients who are positioned well, breathing should slow down; if not, the key is to focus on the out breath and to make each expiration slightly longer than the previous one. Nurses and physiotherapists can work together to address this challenging situation with a positive supportive approach to the management of dyspnoea. Patients should also be given appropriate explanations of what is being done medically to help. Indeed, in every situation it is immensely important that, by their words and actions, those caring for such patients instil a confidence in their ability to help in the management of that person's dyspnoea. Gift (1993) provides a framework for an holistic approach to the management of dyspnoea.

Actual medical treatment will depend on the cause of the dyspnoea and may include oxygen therapy, short- or long-acting bronchodilators, anti-inflammatory drugs, non-invasive positive-pressure ventilation or chest aspiration when pleural effusion is present.

## RESPIRATORY FAILURE

Like all skeletal muscles, the respiratory muscles can fatigue if their workload is too high. During severe respiratory disease, when the work of breathing is greatly increased, the respiratory muscles might not be able to sustain the necessary effort required to maintain adequate gas exchange and respiratory failure may ensue, requiring artificial ventilation until recovery occurs. Respiratory failure is defined as either type 1 or type 2 respiratory failure. This distinction is important because it will influence the medical management:

- type 1 failure: hypoxaemia with normal or low $CO_2$ levels
- type 2 failure: hypoxaemia with hypercapnia ($CO_2$ retention).

**Mechanical ventilation** of the lungs will also have to be employed if the respiratory muscles are paralysed by drugs (e.g. tubocurarine), disease (poliomyelitis) or trauma to the respiratory centre.

Artificial ventilation is most commonly performed using a machine that intermittently applies a positive pressure to the lungs (intermittent positive pressure ventilation; IPPV) during inspiration. Expiration is usually achieved by passive recoil of the lungs.

This type of ventilation may also be referred to as **conventional mechanical ventilation** (CMV). The patient is usually attached to the ventilator by an endotracheal tube or tracheostomy, intermittent suctioning of which is necessary to remove excess secretions from the airway (see Airway secretions, p. 548). Whereas the introduction of conventional mechanical ventilation in both neonatal and adult intensive care units (ICUs) has significantly reduced mortality in critically ill patients, its use is far from trouble free. Persistent problems associated with conventional mechanical ventilation include irreversible hypoxaemia, pneumothorax, interstitial emphysema and chronic lung damage. The latter remains a significant cause of mortality and morbidity following prolonged assisted ventilation of neonates (Ehrenkranz & Mercurio, 1992).

A growing appreciation of the need to match ventilator settings to the underlying pathophysiology of the patient has resulted in increasing use of automated methods of monitoring blood gases and respiratory mechanics on the intensive care unit (Marini, 1991). Existing rationales for conventional mechanical ventilation settings include the following:

- avoid high airway pressures (which may cause pulmonary oedema and lung damage)
- avoid high oxygen tensions (see Oxygen toxicity, p. 575)
- use appropriate distending pressure during expiration (**positive end-expiratory pressure** or PEEP) to maintain an adequate lung volume and reverse hypoxaemia.

The time taken to expire to passive resting lung volume is prolonged in patients with severe obstructive airway disease by the increased resistance to airflow, which delays lung emptying. Under these circumstances, careful adjustment of distending pressures and ventilator rates are essential to prevent progressive overinflation of the lung (sometimes referred to as intrinsic positive end-expiratory pressure) and subsequent deterioration of patient condition.

In recent years, there has been an increasing use of alternative techniques for administering assisted ventilation. These include negative extrathoracic pressure support (using adaptations of the original 'iron lung' that used to be used during polio epidemics) and high-frequency ventilation (HFV). This delivers very small tidal volumes (less than anatomic dead space) at extremely rapid rates (Clark, 1996). The use of non-invasive positive pressure ventilation (NIPPV) may avoid the need for intubation and/or admission to an intensive care unit. Biphasic positive airway pressure (BiPAP) is particularly useful in an acute exacerbation of chronic obstructive pulmonary disease, when patients typically have hypercapnia, hypoxia and acidosis and one wishes to avoid mechanical ventilation (BTS, 1997).

If respiration suddenly ceases (**respiratory arrest**), immediate action is required to re-establish the oxygen supply to the brain. It must first be ascertained whether the heart is still beating, as without this no oxygen can be transported to the brain. The **resuscitation techniques** of mouth-to-mouth respiration and external cardiac massage are described in Chapter 4.2.

## ASSESSMENT OF LUNG FUNCTION

Lung function tests are being increasingly performed in patients of all ages with respiratory disease. Some tests, such as peak expiratory flow rate (PEFR), are simple enough to perform anywhere, whereas others require complex apparatus and highly skilled staff, and are therefore restricted to pulmonary function laboratories. The assessment of respiratory rate and pattern is discussed under Control of ventilation (p. 578).

These investigations require the patient's full participation and often need to be repeated to obtain accurate results. Patients who are anxious are less likely to be able to cooperate fully. It is therefore important that they are prepared in advance, so that they understand what to expect and how they can help.

Lung function tests are rarely diagnostic in their own right because the same functional abnormalities can occur in several different diseases. However, they can provide valuable information on the type and severity of the abnormality and enable a subject's progress, response to therapy or fitness for surgery to be assessed objectively. The measurement of arterial blood gases gives the most pertinent information on lung function and is described in a later section. A brief description of some of the commoner methods of assessing lung and airway function is given below. More details can be found in reviews of the subject, for example Hancox (2001).

## LUNG VOLUMES AND CAPACITIES

A **spirometer** is used to measure the volume of air that the patient is able to expel from lungs after maximal inspiration – it plots volume against time or airflow against volume. In the past, this usually consisted of a weighted drum containing air or oxygen inverted over a tank of water. With the nose clipped, the patient breathed through a tube, which passed up inside the apparatus (**see Fig. 5.3.15**). During inspiration, air was removed from the drum, causing it to sink; during expiration the drum rose as air was added to it. The drum was usually counterbalanced so that inspiration caused an upward deflection of the pen, whereas expiration caused a downward deflection. All respiratory movements were recorded by the pen on a variable speed kymograph, enabling volume changes to be measured directly from the chart. Portable hand-held spirometers now facilitate rapid data acquisition and analysis in both primary and secondary care settings.

As a result of the negative intrapleural pressure surrounding them, the lungs still contain a considerable volume of air at the end of a normal expiration, commonly known as the functional residual capacity (FRC). This cannot be assessed by spirometry, which measures only *changes* in volume, not absolute values, but it can be measured using a gas dilution technique (West, 1985) or by whole body plethysmography (Murray, 1986). Once the functional residual capacity is known, all standard lung volumes can be computed by adding or subtracting the appropriate inspired or expired volumes measured, using a spirometer. A spirogram showing differing depths of inspiration and expiration is shown in **Fig. 5.3.14**. As described earlier (Pulmonary ventilation, p. 557), the volume of air inspired (or expired) during each breath is called the **tidal volume**.

If, at the end of normal expiration, the subject breathes in as deeply as possible, the lungs will inflate to the **total lung capacity** (TLC). The volume of air that is drawn into the lungs beyond that already present at end-expiration is called the **inspiratory capacity** (IC), and usually amounts to about 3000 mL. The **TLC** (= **FRC** + **IC**) of a healthy young adult male is approximately 6000 mL. Measurement of total lung capacity gives the best indication of lung size and is particularly useful in diseases that cause a reduction in lung volume, such as pulmonary fibrosis. An increase in total lung capacity is most frequently associated with obstructive airway disease, in which gas becomes trapped in the lungs behind narrowed airways.

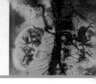

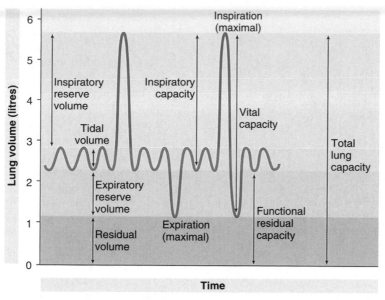

**Figure 5.3.14**  Lung volumes as measured using a spirometer. Note that only *changes* in lung volume can be measured using a spirometer. Other methods are required for measuring functional residual capacity

If, at the end of normal expiration, the subject breathes out as far as possible, a further 1000–1500 mL of air may be expelled from the lungs by active contraction of the abdominal and other expiratory muscles. This is known as the **expiratory reserve volume (ERV)**. However, no matter how much effort is exerted, some air will always remain in the lungs at the end of a maximal expiratory effort. This is known as the **residual volume (RV): (RV = FRC − ERV)** and normally amounts to approximately 1500 mL. The residual volume tends to be decreased in pulmonary fibrosis, when the lung is stiff and tends to recoil to a smaller volume, but increased in the presence of airway obstruction (due to gas trapping), or as the result of respiratory muscle weakness.

The total volume of air that an individual can forcibly expel from the lungs following a maximal inspiratory effort is called the **vital capacity (VC)** **(VC = IC + ERV)**. In a normal adult, the vital capacity is about 4500 mL. The vital capacity is a measure of an individual's ability to inspire and expire air (i.e. of the maximum **stroke volume** of the lungs) and is determined primarily by the strength of the respiratory muscles and the amount of effort that is required to expand the lungs and thoracic cage.

## ASSESSMENT OF AIRWAY FUNCTION

Although the resistance of the airways can be measured directly by plethysmography, the technique is complicated and the equipment costly. Consequently, airway function is most commonly assessed by using forced expiratory

manoeuvres. Generally, the higher the resistance the slower the rate at which air can be forced out of the lungs. Airway resistance (in obstructive airway disease) is measured indirectly from forced expiratory manoeuvres and compliance (in restrictive lung disease) measured indirectly from lung volume measurements.

The simplest forced expiratory measurement is **peak expiratory flow rate (PEFR)**, in which an individual simply takes a full inspiration and blows out as forcibly as possible into an instrument that registers the maximal flow during exhalation in litres per minute. Peak expiratory flow rate readings are usually taken at intervals to monitor a patient's progress, and the best of three attempts is recorded.

Nurses are often responsible for supervising the patient when taking this measurement. It is essential that the patient understands that it is not the *volume* of air expired that is crucial, but the greatest *rate* at which it can be expired. Individuals requiring close supervision of airway function, such as those with severe asthma or following heart or lung transplants, may be asked to record peak expiratory flow rate at home. In asthma, this is done morning and evening to identify diurnal variation, as a diurnal variation of greater than 20% on 3 or more days in one week for two weeks is diagnostic of asthma.

Alternatively, by using a spirometer and asking the subject to inhale as deeply as possible and then exhale as far and as forcibly as possible, a **forced vital capacity** (FVC) can be recorded (**Fig. 5.3.15**). The volume exhaled in the first second is called the forced expiratory volume (FEV$_1$). Normally, about 80% of the forced vital capacity

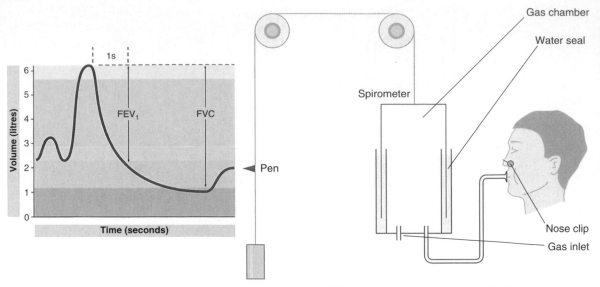

**Figure 5.3.15**  Measurement of timed forced expiratory volume (FEV$_1$) and forced vital capacity (FVC)

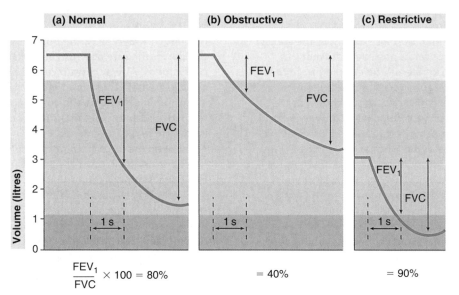

**Figure 5.3.16**  Normal and abnormal patterns of forced expiration

can be forcibly expired in 1 second, i.e. **FEV$_1$/FVC = 0.8**. Variations in this ratio are often helpful in distinguishing obstructive from restrictive types of lung disease (**Fig. 5.3.16**). In **restrictive lung diseases**, e.g. as a result of severe curvature of the spine (kyphoscoliosis) or pulmonary fibrosis, inspiration is limited by weakness of the respiratory muscles or reduced compliance (increased stiffness) of the lung or chest wall, thereby reducing the vital capacity. Such lungs also tend to recoil to lower volumes, resulting in reduction of functional residual capacity and residual volume, and hence an overall fall in total lung capacity. However, the increased traction applied to the outer airway walls holds them more widely open, thereby

facilitating expiratory airflow and resulting in a forced expiratory volume (FEV$_1$) which, while reduced compared to normal values (due to the diminished total volume of gas in the lungs), is normal or even elevated when related to the subject's actual functional residual capacity (**Fig. 5.3.16c**). A similar pattern is seen in patients who have lost some of their lung tissue following pneumonectomy.

In **obstructive lung disease** (e.g. bronchitis, asthma, chronic obstructive pulmonary disease), the forced vital capacity is also reduced, primarily because airway narrowing or closure during expiration limits the amount of gas able to leave the lungs. Hence total lung capacity is typically abnormally large due to the gas trapping.

However, the increased airways resistance (or decreased elastic recoil as in emphysema) causes a much greater reduction in forced expiratory volume than forced vital capacity, giving a low $FEV_1$/FVC ratio (**Fig. 5.3.16b**). Spirometry is being used increasingly in primary care, along with the 6-minute walk, to monitor the impact of chronic obstructive pulmonary disease over a period of time and as an objective measure within pulmonary rehabilitation programmes.

During the last 20 years, many techniques have been developed or adapted to allow lung function to be assessed in infants both when breathing spontaneously and during assisted ventilation (American Thoracic Society, 1993; Landau, 1990; Stocks, 1995). Such measurements may be useful in evaluating therapy, optimizing ventilator settings and clarifying the relationship between chronic obstructive lung disease in adults and insults to the developing respiratory system (such as passive smoking, and infection) both before and after birth.

## Exchange of respiratory gases (diffusion)

Gas exchange between the pulmonary capillary blood and the air within the alveoli occurs by diffusion. To understand this process it is again necessary to remember how gases behave and to appreciate the fine structure of the alveolar–capillary (or pulmonary) membrane (see p. 553).

## Behaviour of gases

When different kinds of molecules are present in a gas mixture (as in air, the main components of which are oxygen and nitrogen), each gas exerts its own pressure (depending on the number of molecules present) as if it were completely filling any available volume. The total pressure of a gas mixture is merely the sum of all the individual (or partial) pressures (Dalton's law of partial pressures). As air consists of approximately 21% oxygen, and atmospheric air has a total pressure of 101 kPa (760 mmHg) at sea level, the partial pressure of oxygen ($PO_2$) in atmospheric air at sea level is:

$$21/100 \times 101 = 21.2 \, kPa \, (160 \, mmHg)$$

Similarly, the partial pressure of nitrogen ($PN_2$) of this air is 79 kPa (590 mmHg).

As discussed on p. 555, movement of gases in and out of the lungs by bulk flow can only occur if there is a difference in total pressure between two areas.

However, even if no gradient of total pressure exists, net movement of any individual gas in a gas mixture can occur by the process of **diffusion**, as long as a partial pressure gradient for that particular gas exists. Providing no specific barrier to diffusion exists, a gas will move from an area of high to lower partial pressure until an equilibrium is achieved. The constant consumption of oxygen and production of carbon dioxide by the cells and the continual renewal of gas in the alveoli during ventilation maintain a perpetual pressure gradient for oxygen and carbon dioxide both within the lungs and at tissue level, thereby enabling gas exchange to occur by passive diffusion. The rate at which a gas can diffuse, and hence the amount of gas exchange that can occur in the lungs or tissues, is proportional to:

- the magnitude of the partial pressure gradient
- the solubility of the gas
- the thinness of the membrane across which the gases must move
- the surface area available for diffusion.

Mixed venous blood (i.e. blood that has supplied the tissues with oxygen and removed their excess carbon dioxide) is continually brought to the lungs via the pulmonary artery (right ventricular output). As this blood has a lower $PO_2$ and higher $PCO_2$ than the air in the lungs, gas exchange can occur by the simple process of diffusion, with oxygen diffusing into the blood for transportation to the tissues and carbon dioxide diffusing out of the blood into the air for expulsion during expiration.

As described earlier (p. 553) the structure of the alveolar–capillary membrane is ideally suited for its function as an organ of gas exchange. Under normal conditions, gas exchange in the lungs is so efficient that venous blood entering the capillaries can equilibrate with alveolar air in about 0.2 seconds. As it usually takes the red blood cell approximately 0.7 seconds to pass through the pulmonary capillaries at rest, much of the diffusing capacity of the lung is normally held in reserve. The surface area of the pulmonary membrane can be increased during exercise by the opening up, or 'recruitment', of additional capillary units. The most common cause of a reduction in surface area is poor matching of the distribution of air and blood in the lungs, but it might also be caused by alveolar collapse or surgical removal of part of the lung. Thickening of the pulmonary membrane may result from pulmonary oedema or deposition of fibrous tissues in the alveolar wall. This, like a reduction in surface area, rarely causes any problems at rest but may seriously limit gas exchange during exercise when, due to the increased blood flow through the lungs, the time available for gas exchange may be reduced to 0.3 seconds.

## Perfusion of the lungs

The pulmonary circulation begins at the main pulmonary artery, which receives venous blood pumped by the right ventricle. The pulmonary artery, which is the only artery that carries deoxygenated blood, then branches and divides, like the bronchial tree, into a series of pulmonary arterioles and finally into the dense capillary network that surrounds the alveoli (**see Fig. 5.3.9**). Following gas exchange across the pulmonary membrane, the blood is collected from the capillary bed into small pulmonary veins which eventually unite to form the four large pulmonary veins which drain into the left atrium.

## Pressures within the pulmonary circulation

The primary function of the pulmonary circulation is to bring the entire cardiac output into intimate contact with alveolar air so that gas exchange can occur. This is facilitated not only by the structural arrangements of alveoli and pulmonary capillaries but by the very low resistance of the pulmonary circulation. This means that considerably less pressure has to be exerted to pump blood around the pulmonary circulation than the systemic circulation. The systolic/diastolic blood pressure in the pulmonary artery is only about 25/8 mmHg (3.3/1 kPa), compared with 120/80 mmHg (16/10.6 kPa) in the aorta. Mean pulmonary capillary pressure is normally about 15 mmHg (2 kPa). As the osmotic pressure of plasma proteins is 25 mmHg (3.3 kPa), there is a net force of about 10 mmHg (1.3 kPa) keeping fluid within the capillaries and preventing the formation of tissue fluid within the alveoli.

### CLINICAL APPLICATIONS

#### PULMONARY OEDEMA

If pulmonary capillary pressure rises about 25 mmHg (3.3 kPa), the net flow of fluid out of the capillaries into the interstitial space will cause thickening of the alveolar–capillary membrane. Fluid may also enter the alveoli causing dyspnoea and hypoxia. This condition is known as pulmonary oedema or cardiac asthma (see also Chapter 4.2). The patient's distress is increased when lying down (**orthopnoea**) because vital capacity is reduced and the increased pulmonary blood volume causes pulmonary congestion. Such patients need to be nursed in a relatively upright position, even during sleep, to avoid paroxysmal nocturnal dyspnoea.

A rise in left atrial pressure (such as may occur in mitral stenosis or during the development of left heart failure) will precede the development of pulmonary oedema, and may be detected by measuring the **pulmonary capillary wedge pressure** (PCWP). This closely reflects left atrial pressure due to the low resistance of the pulmonary circuit and is measured by passing a fine catheter from the vena cava through the right side of the heart and into the pulmonary circulation until it becomes 'wedged' due to the diminishing calibre of the vessels (see also Chapter 4.2).

Severe acute onset of pulmonary oedema may lead to death from respiratory failure within a few hours if left untreated. Management is usually aimed at treating the primary cause and may include:

- administration of digitalis to increase contractibility of the heart
- increased concentrations of inspired oxygen
- fluid restriction and diuretic therapy
- nursing the patient in the upright position.

## Ventilation–perfusion relationships

For adequate gas exchange in the lung, not only must sufficient air and blood be delivered to the alveoli each minute, but they must be delivered in the right proportions. In a healthy adult at rest, alveolar ventilation is about 4 L/min, while pulmonary capillary blood flow is about 5 L/min. Consequently, the ventilation–perfusion ratio at rest is:

$$\frac{\text{alveolar ventilation}}{\text{pulmonary capillary blood flow}} = \frac{4 \,\text{l/min}}{5 \,\text{l/min}}$$
$$= 0.8$$

During severe exercise, when there is a greater increase in ventilation (up to 15-fold) than cardiac output (up to 6-fold), this ratio may rise to about 2.0, but it is generally kept fairly constant under widely varying conditions.

However, it is not enough to have an acceptable overall ratio of ventilation to perfusion. If 5 L of blood flowed through a completely unventilated lung each minute, and 4 L of air were delivered to the other unperfused lung, the overall ratio would still be 0.8 and yet no gas exchange could occur (**Fig. 5.3.17**).

Even in the healthiest lungs, some regional differences in ventilation–perfusion ratios occur due to the effect of gravity. Certain compensatory measures are available to facilitate matching of ventilation and perfusion. These depend on the sensitivity of the smooth muscle in the bronchioles and pulmonary arterioles to local changes in gas tensions. In relatively poorly ventilated areas of the lung, the gas will

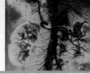

$$\text{Total:} \quad \frac{\text{Ventilation}}{\text{Perfusion}} = \frac{4}{5} = 0.8$$

**Right lung:** $\dfrac{\text{Ventilation}}{\text{Perfusion}} = \dfrac{4}{0} = \infty$   **Left lung:** $\dfrac{\text{Ventilation}}{\text{Perfusion}} = \dfrac{0}{5} = 0$

Alveolar air has composition of atmospheric air — $PO_2 = 20$ kPa (150 mmHg) $PCO_2 = 0$

$PO_2 = 5$ kPa (40 mmHg) $PCO_2 = 6$ kPa (45 mmHg) — Alveolar air has same composition as venous blood

Venous blood
$PO_2 = 5$ kPa (40 mmHg)
$PCO_2 = 6$ kPa (45 mmHg)

Arterial blood
$PO_2 = 5$ kPa (40 mmHg)
$PCO_2 = 6$ kPa (45 mmHg)

**Figure 5.3.17**  Extreme imbalance between ventilation and perfusion. Note that despite an adequate overall ventilation–perfusion ratio of 0.8, all the ventilation goes to one lung through which there is no perfusion, whereas all the blood goes to the other lung where there is no ventilation. Consequently no gas exchange occurs. Such a situation would obviously be incompatible with life (values are given in SI units, with mmHg in parentheses)

tend to have both an elevated $PCO_2$, which stimulates bronchodilation and enhances ventilation to the area, and also a decrease in $PO_2$, which stimulates pulmonary vasoconstriction, thereby diverting some of the blood flow away from the area.

In health, adequate gas exchange occurs despite regional differences and blood leaving the lungs is virtually in equilibrium with alveolar gas. However, in the presence of lung disease, the distribution of ventilation and perfusion often becomes far more uneven, which diminishes the efficiency of gas exchange and increases the work of breathing.

Inequalities of the ventilation–perfusion ratio may occur for several reasons, some of which are summarized below.

### AREAS OF HIGH VENTILATION–PERFUSION RATIO

If intrathoracic pressure should exceed pulmonary artery pressure, either due to a rise in intrathoracic pressure (e.g. during intermittent positive pressure ventilation) or a fall in pulmonary artery pressure (shock, haemorrhage), the pulmonary capillaries will be flattened, with subsequent reduction of blood flow to an area. Gas exchange will be severely impaired in such ventilated but relatively unperfused areas, which are referred to as the **alveolar dead space**.

### AREAS OF LOW VENTILATION–PERFUSION RATIO

Certain areas of the lung may take longer to fill and empty than others, for example if they are supplied by obstructed or narrowed airways. They therefore receive a disproportionately small share of the ventilation so that only limited gas exchange can occur. Such regions act as a physiological right-to-left shunt, enabling some venous blood to pass through the lungs and return to the heart virtually unchanged, resulting in a fall in arterial $PO_2$.

Mismatching of ventilation and perfusion is the most common cause of hypoxia in lung disease (p. 572). It may or may not be accompanied by hypercapnia (increased arterial $PCO_2$), depending on the individual's ability to increase ventilation, but it always increases the work of breathing.

## Transport of gases around the body

In an earlier section, it was seen how the structure of the lung is well suited to its functions in that it provides a vast surface area for gas exchange together with a very thin pulmonary (alveolar–capillary) membrane across which gases can diffuse easily. Similar structural arrangements are available in the tissues, where the thin-walled capillaries branch and divide to bring the arterial blood into intimate proximity with the cells. The cells are separated from the intracellular fluid by only the capillary membrane, the interstitial fluid and the cell membrane, none of which normally presents any barrier to diffusion. Gas exchange cannot occur across the thicker-walled blood vessels. Consequently, the composition of systemic arterial or venous blood remains unchanged as it travels to or from the tissues.

It has already been mentioned that the rate of diffusion of a gas is proportional not only to the surface area and thinness of the membrane but also to the

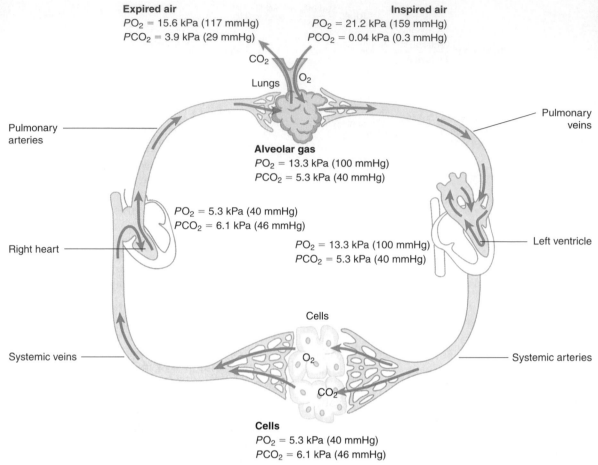

**Expired air**
$PO_2$ = 15.6 kPa (117 mmHg)
$PCO_2$ = 3.9 kPa (29 mmHg)

**Inspired air**
$PO_2$ = 21.2 kPa (159 mmHg)
$PCO_2$ = 0.04 kPa (0.3 mmHg)

$CO_2$

Lungs   $O_2$

Pulmonary arteries

Pulmonary veins

**Alveolar gas**
$PO_2$ = 13.3 kPa (100 mmHg)
$PCO_2$ = 5.3 kPa (40 mmHg)

$PO_2$ = 5.3 kPa (40 mmHg)
$PCO_2$ = 6.1 kPa (46 mmHg)

$PO_2$ = 13.3 kPa (100 mmHg)
$PCO_2$ = 5.3 kPa (40 mmHg)

Right heart

Left ventricle

Cells

$O_2$

Systemic veins

Systemic arteries

$CO_2$

**Cells**
$PO_2$ = 5.3 kPa (40 mmHg)
$PCO_2$ = 6.1 kPa (46 mmHg)

**Figure 5.3.18** Summary of oxygen and carbon dioxide pressures in inspired and expired air, and throughout the body (partial pressures are given in SI units with conversion to mmHg in parentheses). Venous blood arriving at the lungs is 'arteriolized' as it passes through the pulmonary capillary network – picking-up oxygen and losing carbon dioxide. It is then pumped back to the tissues for further gas exchange

partial pressure gradient and solubility of that gas. The constant consumption of oxygen and production of carbon dioxide in the tissues, combined with ventilation of the lungs with fresh air, provides the necessary pressure gradients to ensure adequate diffusion in the lungs and tissues (**Fig. 5.3.18**). However, gas exchange would be seriously limited if oxygen had to be transported around the body in simple solution, as only 0.23 mL oxygen can dissolve in each litre of blood for each kPa change in $PO_2$ (or 0.03 mL $O_2$/L blood per mmHg $PO_2$). Consequently, arterial blood with a $PO_2$ of 13 kPa (100 mmHg) can only carry 3 mL $O_2$/L blood in simple solution. Even if the tissues were capable of extracting all this oxygen, with a cardiac output of 5 L/min, only 15 mL oxygen would be supplied each minute, whereas even at rest the body requires 250 mL $O_2$/min.

Because carbon dioxide is about 20 times more soluble than oxygen, transport of carbon dioxide is less limited by solubility. Hence, despite the smaller pressure gradients for $PCO_2$ than $PO_2$ at lung and tissue level (**see Fig. 5.3.18**) – approximately 0.8 kPa

(6 mmHg) for $PCO_2$ compared with 8 kPa (60 mmHg) for $PO_2$ – similar quantities of both carbon dioxide and oxygen can diffuse. However, as carbon dioxide dissolves in water to form carbonic acid, the carriage of large quantities of carbon dioxide in simple solution would cause a dangerous increase in the acidity of the blood and body fluids. Consequently, both oxygen and carbon dioxide require fairly complex mechanisms to facilitate their transport around the body. These will now be considered.

## Transport of oxygen

Under normal conditions, about 99% of oxygen in the blood is bound to haemoglobin, the remainder being carried in simple solution. Despite the small contribution of dissolved oxygen to the total oxygen content of the blood, it plays a vital role in that it is this dissolved oxygen that determines the $PO_2$ of the blood and maintains the necessary pressure gradients for diffusion to occur, and not that bound to haemoglobin, which is no longer 'free' to exert a pressure.

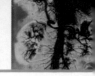

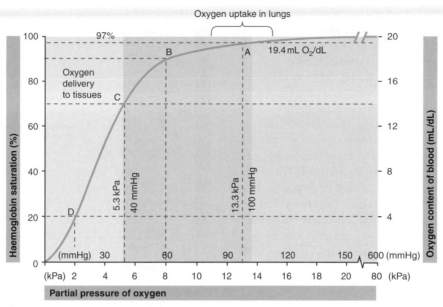

**Figure 5.3.19** The oxygen–haemoglobin dissociation curve. This oxygen dissociation curve applies when pH is 7.4 $PCO_2$ is 5.3 kPa (40 mmHg) and blood is at 37°C. The total blood oxygen content is shown, assuming a haemoglobin concentration of 15 g/dL blood (i.e. oxygen capacity of 20 mL/dL)

## Haemoglobin (Hb)

Haemoglobin is a unique conjugated protein found in red blood cells (see also Chapter 4.1). Each molecule of haemoglobin consists of four haem groups (the iron-containing pigment that gives blood its characteristic red colour) attached to four polypeptide chains (which make up the protein, globin). Each haem group is capable of combining with one molecule of oxygen by a process known as oxygenation, to give the bright red compound, oxyhaemoglobin, which gives arterial blood its characteristic colour; by contrast, reduced haemoglobin is a purple compound (hence the colour of venous blood). The normal haemoglobin complement ranges from 12 to 15 g/dL blood in women, and from 13 to 18 g/dL blood in men. (Haemoglobin concentration is expressed per decilitre of blood, rather than per litre, by clinical convention.) Each gram of haemoglobin is capable of combining with up to 1.34 mL of oxygen. Consequently, with a haemoglobin complement of 15 g/dL blood, the total amount of oxygen that could be carried (known as the **oxygen capacity** of the blood) would be around 20.1 mL/dL blood (15 × 1.34 mL). In SI units, normal haemoglobin content is 2.2 mmol/L blood and, as each molecule of haemoglobin can combine with four molecules of oxygen, the oxygen capacity would be 8.8 mmol/L (1 mmol $O_2$ = 22.4 mL). By contrast, the oxygen capacity of an anaemic individual with only 7.5 g Hb/dL will be reduced to 10 mL oxygen in the blood.

However, the actual quantity of oxygen in the blood (oxygen content) is determined not only by the haemoglobin complement but also by the $PO_2$ of

the blood. On exposure to increasing levels of $PO_2$, the oxygen content of the blood will gradually rise as more and more oxygen combines with haemoglobin. At a certain $PO_2$, when oxygen content equals oxygen capacity, the haemoglobin will be unable to take up any more oxygen and is said to be fully (100%) **saturated**, i.e.

$$\text{haemoglobin saturation} = \frac{\text{oxygen content}}{\text{oxygen capacity}} \times 100$$

## The oxygen dissociation curve

The degree to which oxygen combines with haemoglobin under varying conditions can be measured in the laboratory by exposing blood to gas mixtures with varying concentrations of oxygen. After equilibration, the haemoglobin saturation is calculated by dividing the oxygen content of each sample by the oxygen capacity of the blood. The latter is taken as the maximum oxygen content obtained in any of the samples despite any further increases in $PO_2$. For each blood sample, haemoglobin saturation is plotted against the $PO_2$, as shown in **Fig. 5.3.19**.

It can be seen that the relationship between haemoglobin saturation and $PO_2$ is not linear but **sigmoid** (S-shaped). The reason for this is that although each of the four haem groups in a haemoglobin molecule can combine with one molecule of oxygen, they do so with varying affinities. The first haem group combines with relative difficulty (but conversely 'holds on to its oxygen' more strongly when a fall in $PO_2$ occurs); the second and third haem groups have a far greater affinity for oxygen, as seen from the steep part of the curve where haemoglobin saturation increases rapidly from 25% to 75% for a relatively small change in $PO_2$; the fourth haem group combines with the greatest difficulty.

The shape of the dissociation curve is physiologically advantageous for several reasons. The blood arriving in the lungs has a $PO_2$ of 5.3 kPa (40 mmHg) or lower, and is exposed to the alveolar $PO_2$ of 13.3 kPa (100 mmHg). Consequently, oxygen diffuses across the alveolar–capillary membrane and into the plasma. This causes a rise in plasma $PO_2$ and creates a pressure gradient, enabling oxygen to diffuse into the red blood cell. However, the $PO_2$ within the red blood cell rises more slowly because the haemoglobin rapidly loads oxygen, thereby removing it from free solution. This maintains the pressure gradient and facilitates continuing rapid diffusion of oxygen until the haemoglobin is fully saturated. As $PO_2$ within the red blood cell increases from 5.3 kPa (40 mmHg) to 8 kPa (60 mmHg), there is rapid loading of oxygen with haemoglobin saturation increasing from 70% to 90% (this is on the steep portion of the dissociation curve). Thereafter relatively less oxygen is taken up per unit change in $PO_2$, with 97% haemoglobin saturation not being achieved until $PO_2$ reaches about 13.3 kPa (100 mmHg). This flat upper portion of the curve provides an excellent safety factor in the supply of oxygen to the tissues because, even if alveolar $PO_2$ should fall to 8 kPa (60 mmHg), as might occur in lung disease or when breathing at altitude, 90% of the haemoglobin leaving the lungs will still be saturated with oxygen.

As the blood enters the tissues, still with a $PO_2$ of 13.3 kPa (100 mmHg) in a healthy individual, it is exposed to a $PO_2$ of 5.3 kPa (40 mmHg). As can be seen from **Fig. 5.3.19**, the $PO_2$ of tissues (point C) lies on the steep portion of the dissociation curve, so that oxygen is readily released from the blood. Oxygen therefore diffuses from the plasma across the capillary membrane, the interstitial fluid and the cell membrane. The resultant drop in plasma $PO_2$ creates a pressure gradient between it and the red blood cell so that the oxyhaemoglobin begins to dissociate. The release of previously bound oxygen into solution enables the $PO_2$ of capillary blood to remain relatively high, thereby facilitating diffusion of oxygen into the tissues until the $PO_2$ of the tissues equals that of blood. The level of tissue $PO_2$ (5.3 kPa) falls on the steep portion of the oxygen dissociation curve (point C, **Fig. 5.3.19**), so oxygen is readily released to the tissues. If the level of tissue activity increases, its $PO_2$ may fall as low as 2 kPa (15 mmHg) (point D, **Fig. 5.3.19**). This will enable the haemoglobin to release 80% of its oxygen to the tissues, demonstrating a considerable reserve capacity above resting levels. Oxygen is loosely bound to haemoglobin (steep

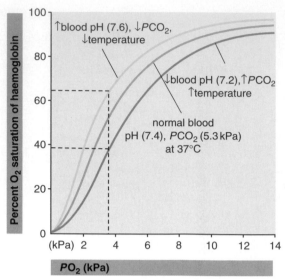

**Figure 5.3.20** Factors influencing the position of the oxygen dissociation curve. A shift of the curve to the right facilitates unloading of oxygen. Thus, at any given $PO_2$ more oxygen is released to the tissues if there is an increase in temperature or $PCO_2$ or a fall in pH (such as may occur in muscle during exercise). Conditions in the lung (fall in temperature and $PCO_2$, and rise in pH) shift the curve to the left, thereby facilitating loading of haemoglobin with oxygen at any given $PO_2$

curve) down to about 1.3 kPa (10 mmHg); below this the affinity of haemoglobin for oxygen increases (flatter curve). However, $PO_2$ seldom falls this low except in working muscles, where a special oxygen carrying protein, called myoglobin, is capable of extracting all the oxygen that the blood delivers.

The venous blood then returns to the lung, where the oxygen released in the tissues can be replaced by exposure of the pulmonary blood to alveolar air. The lower the $PO_2$ of the blood returning to the lung, the greater the pressure gradient will be for oxygen diffusion and the faster the loading of the haemoglobin will be.

## Factors influencing the oxygen–haemoglobin dissociation curve

The affinity of haemoglobin for oxygen at any given $PO_2$ is influenced by several factors that facilitate oxygen uptake in the lungs and release in the tissues, thereby maintaining a constant intracellular $PO_2$ under varying conditions. Increases in the amount of carbon dioxide and hydrogen ions ($H^+$) reduce the ability of haemoglobin to bind oxygen. Thus, for any given $PO_2$, blood entering the tissues with a $PCO_2$ of 6.1 kPa (46 mmHg) will release more of its oxygen than blood with a $PCO_2$ of 5.3 kPa (40 mmHg) (**Fig. 5.3.20**). This is sometimes expressed by saying that the curve has 'shifted to the right' with respect to the

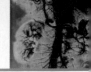

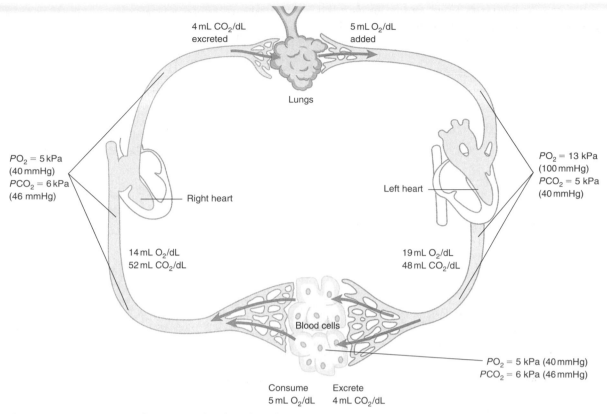

**Figure 5.3.21** Transport of oxygen and carbon dioxide

standard dissociation curve (**see Fig. 5.3.19**), which is itself based on arterial blood with a $PCO_2$ of 5.3 kPa and pH of 7.4.

In the tissue capillaries, carbon dioxide and $H^+$ bind with haemoglobin, facilitating the release of oxygen, whereas in the lungs release of carbon dioxide and $H^+$ from haemoglobin facilitates oxygen uptake. A rise in temperature also reduces the oxygen-binding ability of haemoglobin, which again facilitates oxygen delivery to active tissues.

A substance called **2,3-diphosphoglycerate** (2,3-DPG), which is a product of red blood cell metabolism, combines reversibly with haemoglobin, causing it to release more of its oxygen at any given $PO_2$. An increase in 2,3-diphosphoglycerate concentration occurs in response to chronic hypoxia (e.g. in anaemia or at altitude) and also during pregnancy, which facilitates release of oxygen across the placenta to the fetus. Maternal–fetal oxygen transfer is also facilitated by the fact that the fetus has a slightly different type of haemoglobin (fetal haemoglobin; HbF), which has an increased affinity for oxygen. This is gradually replaced by adult haemoglobin (HbA) during the first year of life.

The gas carbon monoxide (CO) is a poison because it binds very tightly with haemoglobin to form **carboxyhaemoglobin**. As carbon monoxide binds to exactly the same sites on the haemoglobin molecule as oxygen, but with a far greater affinity, it prevents oxygen transport and can cause death.

## Changes in oxygen content

So far, we have only considered the changes in haemoglobin saturation as the blood is exposed to changes in $PO_2$ around the body. However, if the haemoglobin complement of the blood is known, the **oxygen capacity** can be calculated (Hb g/dL × 1.34 mL $O_2$). As oxygen capacity is equivalent to 100% haemoglobin saturation, an axis representing oxygen content of the blood can be added to the dissociation curve (**see Fig. 5.3.19**, right-hand axis). Thus, with a haemoglobin complement of 15 g/dL, oxygen capacity (i.e. 100% saturation) = 20 mL $O_2$/dL, whereas 50% saturation represents an oxygen content of 10 mL/dL blood, and so on. Changes in oxygen content (assuming a haemoglobin complement of 15 g/dL) as blood travels around the body are summarized in **Fig. 5.3.21**. It can be seen that, under resting conditions, blood returning to the lung contains about 14 mL $O_2$/dL blood at a $PO_2$ of 5.3 kPa (40 mmHg). During passage through the lung, an additional 5 mL $O_2$/dL are loaded, due to the rise in $PO_2$, which are then released at tissue level. During exercise the haemoglobin may release up to 15 mL $O_2$/dL (if tissue $PO_2$ falls to 1.3 kPa), and therefore

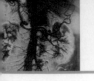

returns to the lung with only 4 mL/dL. To meet this increased oxygen consumption by the tissues, there must be a marked increase in both ventilation and cardiac output.

A muscle requires up to 50 times more oxygen during exercise than when at rest (see Exercise, p. 576). This is achieved by:

- an increase in cardiac output (and pulmonary blood flow) from 5 L/min to 30 L/min (a 6-fold increase)
- redistribution of blood, with three times as much of the cardiac output going to the active muscle than when at rest
  (together, these mechanisms increase muscle blood flow 18-fold)
- three times as much oxygen being extracted by the muscle, with haemoglobin releasing 15 mL $O_2$/dL blood during exercise, instead of the 5 mL/dL blood at rest.

This gives up to a 54-fold increase in blood flow to the muscle, which is accompanied by up to a 30-fold increase in ventilation to supply the necessary additional oxygen.

## CLINICAL APPLICATIONS

### HYPOXIA

Whenever tissues do not get sufficient oxygen to meet their needs, or are unable to utilize it, the condition is known as **hypoxia**. Note that the term **hypoxaemia** describes low arterial blood oxygen levels, whereas hypoxia refers to low oxygen levels in the tissues themselves. Hypoxia may occur for any of the following reasons:

- **Reduction in arterial PO$_2$.** Breathing at altitude and alveolar hypoventilation will reduce arterial $PO_2$ (**hypoxaemia**) and hence reduce oxygen delivery to the tissues (i.e. cause hypoxia).

  Alveolar hypoventilation is most commonly caused by diseases outside the lung (**Fig. 5.3.22**), indeed the lungs may be completely normal. However, in the presence of very severe respiratory disease, the work of breathing may be increased to such an extent that the respiratory muscles fatigue and are no longer capable of sustaining an adequate level of alveolar ventilation.

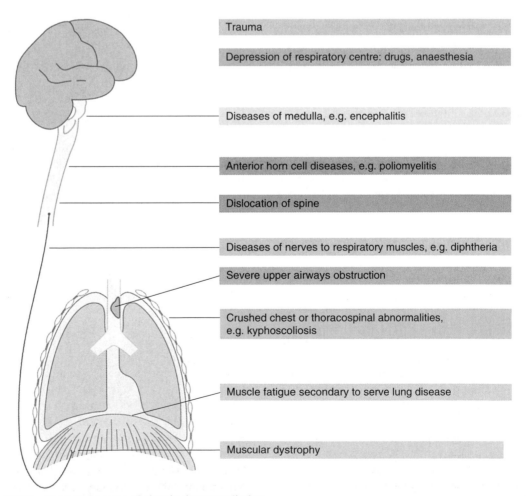

Trauma

Depression of respiratory centre: drugs, anaesthesia

Diseases of medulla, e.g. encephalitis

Anterior horn cell diseases, e.g. poliomyelitis

Dislocation of spine

Diseases of nerves to respiratory muscles, e.g. diphtheria

Severe upper airways obstruction

Crushed chest or thoracospinal abnormalities, e.g. kyphoscoliosis

Muscle fatigue secondary to serve lung disease

Muscular dystrophy

**Figure 5.3.22**　Potential causes of alveolar hypoventilation

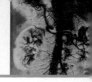

As discussed previously, one of the most common causes of hypoxaemia is ventilation–perfusion mismatch, such as occurs in chronic obstructive lung disease (COPD). In addition, despite the existence of a large reserve 'diffusing capacity' within the lungs, severe pulmonary oedema or any condition causing marked thickening of the alveolar capillary membrane may result in hypoxaemia – especially during any form of exertion.

- **Anaemic hypoxia.** Oxygen delivery to the tissues may be impeded if there is a reduction in available haemoglobin (the various causes of which are summarized in Chapter 4.1). Severe hypoxia at rest may result from a sudden loss of available haemoglobin (haemorrhage, carbon monoxide poisoning). In addition, individuals suffering from anaemia tend to have limited exercise tolerance and suffer from excessive tiredness.
- **Reduced blood supply to the tissues.** This may result from a fall in cardiac ouput (e.g. during heart failure or shock), and is known as ischaemic or stagnant hypoxia.
- **Interstitial oedema.** This increases the distance across which gases must diffuse and may result in local areas of hypoxia, necrosis and possibly gangrene.
- **An increased demand for gas exchange by the tissues.** This may occur as a result of neoplasms or during severe exercise. If the increased demand cannot be met by the normal adjustments of the respiratory and cardiovascular systems, hypoxia will occur.
- **Histotoxic hypoxia.** Even if the supply and composition of arterial blood are adequate, hypoxia may occur if there is inactivation of the enzyme cytochrome oxidase by cyanide poisoning. This prevents uptake of oxygen by the cells and rapidly leads to death.
- **Chronic hypoxia.** Various compensatory changes occur in the presence of chronic hypoxia, including: an increase in 2,3-diphosphoglycerate and an increase in the number of red cells (polycythaemia) and haemoglobin complement (unless the hypoxia is due to anaemia).

## SIGNS AND SYMPTOMS

Signs and symptoms of hypoxia may include:

- rapid pulse rate
- cyanosis (see below)
- increased respiratory rate if arterial $PO_2$ is low
- excessive tiredness and limited exercise tolerance
- systemic oedema due to pulmonary vasoconstriction, giving the patient a bloated appearance

- various effects on the brain resulting in headache, nausea, restlessness, disturbances of visual acuity, reduced mental efficiency and, if severe, possible stupor or coma.

If the brain is totally deprived of oxygen, death occurs in about 2–3 min.

### Cyanosis

If arterial blood contains more than 5 g reduced haemoglobin (Hb) per dL, it will take on a bluish hue known as **cyanosis**, which is most clearly visible in the mucous membranes. Although central cyanosis is a common clinical sign of respiratory insufficiency, it is not a reliable guide to the degree of hypoxia because it is influenced by an individual's haemoglobin complement. Thus an anaemic patient with only 7.5 g Hb/dL blood would have to have a $PO_2$ of 3 kPa (23 mmHg), i.e. a haemoglobin saturation of 33%, before 5 g Hb/dL were reduced (**see Fig. 5.3.19**). By contrast, a polycythaemic patient will show frank cyanosis with only mild hypoxia.

Peripheral cyanosis is more likely to occur when blood flow through the skin is slow, as for example in cold weather or when viscosity of the blood is increased. Generally, it is easier to observe cyanosis in fair-skinned individuals and in good lighting (see also Chapter 6.1).

### Blue bloaters and pink puffers

Generalized pulmonary vasoconstriction in response to hypoxia is in part responsible for the marked differences seen between patients with chronic obstructive airways disease, who tend to fall into two distinct categories: either 'blue bloaters' or 'pink puffers'. The blue bloaters tend to be those whose predominant problem is one of chronic bronchitis. They do not usually complain of dyspnoea but, due to wide-spread yet variable airways obstruction, have very poor matching of the blood and air supply in their lungs, which results in impaired gas exchange, hypoxia and cyanosis. In addition, generalized hypoxic vasoconstriction results in a large rise in pulmonary artery pressure (pulmonary hypertension) and right heart failure. The subsequent development of systemic oedema is responsible for their bloated appearance.

By contrast, the pink puffers, whose problem is primarily one of emphysema, are excessively dyspnoeic (puffing) on exercise but, by increasing their level of pulmonary ventilation, generally manage to maintain their blood gases within reasonable limits. Consequently, they stay 'pink' and do not usually suffer from **cor pulmonale** (right heart failure secondary to long-standing pulmonary disease, as described above).

## OXYGEN THERAPY

Although the administration of increased concentrations of inspired oxygen may be of great benefit in certain types of hypoxia, it can be of limited value or even potentially dangerous in others. It is therefore essential that the cause of hypoxia is diagnosed before oxygen is prescribed. The oxygen may be administered via face masks, nasal catheters, oxygen tents or endotracheal or tracheostomy tubes. The method of choice usually depends on the severity of illness, concentrations required, duration of treatment, need for humidification and the age and comfort of the patient (e.g. some patients feel claustrophobic behind face masks and may prefer nasal catheters). It is important to remember that oxygen is a drug, and should be treated as such with regard to its prescription, supply and administration.

Patients receiving oxygen therapy require frequent nose and mouth care because humidification may be inadequate and breathing dry gas dries and irritates mucous membranes. Oxygen masks fit closely over the nose and around the chin and should be moved frequently to relieve pressure on the underlying tissues and to prevent the formation of pressure ulcers. During administration, the patient's clinical state should be monitored, including respiratory rate, pulse rate, confusion, agitation, reduced conscious level and cyanosis. Pulse oximetry, capillary blood gas samples and arterial blood gases can be used to assess oxygenation.

**Extracorporeal membrane oxygenation (ECMO)** is an extreme life support procedure, which provides cardiopulmonary support in profound respiratory or cardiac failure using a modified heart–lung machine to support gas exchange (Cowell & Hopkins, 1991). It is generally used in patients with an 80% or greater mortality risk, who have failed to respond to conventional ventilatory therapy. Several methods of perfusion are available, the most common being the venoarterial approach in which, following cannulation, venous blood is drained from the right atrium through the right internal jugular vein and oxygenated blood returned through the right common carotid artery to the aortic arch.

In addition to total nursing care, nursing responsibilities include detection of any technical complications, such as tubing rupture, air in the circuit, accidental decannulation and so forth. Assisted ventilation is continued during the extracorporeal membrane oxygenation course but is reduced to minimal settings to prevent further pulmonary damage. Chest physiotherapy is provided to improve lung drainage.

## Benefits of oxygen therapy

Oxygen therapy may be of benefit to a patient in three different ways:

- **To correct a decreased alveolar $PO_2$**. Alveolar $PO_2$ can be increased, enabling adequate oxygen uptake by the blood despite alveolar hypoventilation or decreased barometric pressure.
- **To elevate alveolar $PO_2$**. Patients suffering from a reduction is diffusing capacity across the pulmonary membrane will benefit if augmented oxygen in breathed since the increased alveolar–arterial pressure gradient will facilitate oxygen diffusion and partially compensate for the increase in membrane thickness or reduction in surface area available for gas exchange.
- **To increase dissolved oxygen**. In the presence of an anaemic crisis or carbon monoxide poisoning, haemoglobin is no longer available to transport oxygen. Under these circumstances, the amount of oxygen physically dissolved in the blood will be critical. By breathing 100% oxygen $PO_2$ will increase to 80 kPa (600 mmHg) and at this pressure 2 mL oxygen will be dissolved per decilitre of blood. This effect can be augmented by administering oxygen at increased pressures (hyperbaric oxygen therapy) but this therapy is potentially dangerous and is generally limited to treating emergencies over brief periods of time. Hyperbaric oxygen therapy is therefore rarely used to treat respiratory failure or any chronic form of hypoxia, but is valuable in treating carbon monoxide poisoning and decompression sickness. It may also be used in the treatment of infections with anaerobic bacteria, such as gas gangrene, and as an adjunct to radiotherapy where the higher tissue $PO_2$ increases the radiosensitivity of tissues with a relatively poor blood supply. The range of disorders for which hyperbaric oxygen is being proposed is growing and now includes patients with neurological and muscular defects, e.g. autism, cerebral palsy, strokes, near drowning, sports injuries, chronic fatigue syndrome and autoimmune deficiencies.

## Limitations of oxygen therapy

Oxygen therapy is of very limited value if:

- blood is bypassing the lungs (right–left intracardiac shunt, such as may occur in 'blue babies' with congenital heart defects)
- there is generalized reduction in circulation
- there is any interference with oxygen uptake by the tissues (cyanide poisoning)
- there is chronic anaemia.

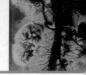

## Dangers of oxygen therapy

Despite the numerous benefits of oxygen therapy, it is not without its dangers. These are summarized below:

- Oxygen is a colourless, odourless gas, which supports combustion and therefore presents a fire risk.
- Compressed oxygen is very dry and must be humidified before reaching the patient (see above).
- By abolishing the hypoxia, oxygen therapy may completely suppress respiration in patients with chronic carbon dioxide retention (hypercapnia). (There is need for controlled adminstration of oxygen in these instances, see Control of ventilation, p. 578.)
- High concentrations of oxygen over prolonged periods may cause severe lung damage (oxygen toxicity). Inspired oxygen concentrations are therefore always kept as low as possible while maintaining reasonable blood gases. Oxygen toxicity is difficult to recognize as the signs and symptoms are similar to those of hypoxia itself. It can develop after 48 hours of exposure to inspired oxygen concentrations of 50% or higher, with most cases occurring in mechanically ventilated patients where there is little chance for dilution of oxygen by room air.
- Newborn infants, especially those born prematurely, may develop fibrosis behind the lens of the eye leading to blindness if treated with oxygen (**retrolental fibroplasia**). This condition can be prevented by constant monitoring of arterial blood gases and by keeping the arterial $PO_2$ below 8 kPa (140 mmHg).

### Long-term oxygen therapy (LTOT)

This is administered in their homes to people who have chronic hypoxia and cor pulmonale, with a $PaO_2 < 7.8$ kPa breathing air and who have had at least one episode of right sided heart failure. It should be delivered via an oxygen compressor and provides symptomatic relief, increases life expectancy and quality of life and reduces the need for hospitalization (Weg & Haas, 1998).

## Transport of carbon dioxide

Carbon dioxide is transported in the blood in three different ways:

- About 5% is carried in simple solution (0.6 mL $CO_2$ will dissolve in each decilitre of blood for every kPa of $PCO_2$, or 0.075 mL/dL/mmHg $PCO_2$).
- About 5% is carried in combination with haemoglobin.
- Approximately 90% is transported in the form of hydrogen carbonate (biocarbonate) ions.

The constant production of carbon dioxide in the cells means that the $PCO_2$ of intracellular fluid always exceeds that of the blood flowing into the tissue capillaries (**see Fig. 5.3.21**). This creates the necessary pressure gradient to enable carbon dioxide to diffuse out of the cells into the interstitial fluid, across the capillary membrane and into the plasma, where a small quantity will dissolve in simple solution, according to the equation:

$$CO_2 + H_2O \rightleftharpoons H_2CO_3$$

carbon dioxide + water $\rightleftharpoons$ carbonic acid

However, this reaction is very slow unless catalysed by the enzyme **carbonic anhydrase**, of which very little is present in the plasma although abundant supplies exist inside the red blood cell. Most of the carbon dioxide that diffuses out from the tissues diffuses into the red blood cell, where the constant and rapid production of carbonic acid 'soaks up' the carbon dioxide, thereby keeping the $PCO_2$ of the red blood cell relatively low and maintaining a pressure gradient along which carbon dioxide can move.

The total amount of carbonic acid in the red blood cell itself remains relatively low because it rapidly ionizes (dissociates) into hydrogen ($H^+$) and hydrogen carbonate (bicarbonate, $HCO_3^+$) ions. Thus:

$$H_2O + CO_2 \xrightleftharpoons[\text{anhydrase}]{\text{carbonic}} H_2CO_3 \rightleftharpoons H^+ + HCO_3^-$$

water + carbon dioxide $\rightleftharpoons$ carbonic acid $\rightleftharpoons$ hydrogen ion + hydrogen carbonate ion

The reaction shown above is a reversible one (i.e. it can proceed in either direction) and obeys the law of mass action, in that any increases in the concentration of reacting substances on the left-hand side (i.e. carbon dioxide) will drive the reaction towards the right, and vice versa. Consequently, at tissue level, when there is a continuous addition of carbon dioxide into the blood the reaction will be driven to the right, resulting in the continuous production of hydrogen ions and hydrogen carbonate ions. (By contrast, when carbon dioxide leaves the blood as it passes through the lungs, the reaction will be driven to the left.)

Hydrogen carbonate ions can pass freely across the red cell membrane. Consequently, as their concentration rises there is a net diffusion of hydrogen carbonate ions out of the cell and into the plasma along the concentration gradient. Here, they react with sodium chloride (NaCl) to form sodium hydrogen carbonate ($NaHCO_3$) and chloride ions ($Cl^-$). The hydrogen carbonate that remains in the red blood cell is transported as potassium hydrogen carbonate (bicarbonate). This net movement of negative hydrogen carbonate ions into the plasma leaves the inside of the red blood cell relatively positive. Electrical neutrality is maintained by diffusion of negatively charged chloride ions from the plasma into the red blood cells. This is sometimes known as the **chloride shift**. In addition, haemoglobin is a very effective buffer, which combines with and neutralizes many of the hydrogen ions released on ionization of carbonic acid:

$$HbO_2 + H^+ \rightleftharpoons HHb + O_2$$

oxyhaemoglobin                    reduced haemoglobin

+ hydrogen ions                          + oxygen

Not only does this prevent any marked rise in acidity in the red blood cell but it also facilitates the unloading of oxygen and the combination of carbon dioxide with haemoglobin. The haemoglobin can carry both oxygen and carbon dioxide simultaneously because carbon dioxide is attached to the amine groups in the globin part of the molecule and oxygen is carried on the haem group. However, reduced haemoglobin can carry more carbon dioxide than oxyhaemoglobin so that the unloading of oxygen in the peripheral capillaries facilitates loading of carbon dioxide. Approximately 5% of the total carbon dioxide content in blood is carried in combination with haemoglobin forming a compound known as **carbaminohaemoglobin**. The chemical reactions involved in carbon dioxide transport at tissue level are shown in **Fig. 5.3.23**.

When venous blood reaches the lung capillaries, it is exposed to the lower $PCO_2$ of alveolar air so that dissolved carbon dioxide diffuses out of the red blood cells and plasma and across the pulmonary membrane to be excreted during ventilation. The resultant fall in blood $PCO_2$ causes a reversal of all the processes that occur at tissue level (**Fig. 5.3.24**). The constant production of carbon dioxide in the red blood cell keeps the $PCO_2$ of the red cells relatively high, thus maintaining a pressure gradient between blood and alveolar air along which carbon dioxide can diffuse. In this way all the carbon dioxide released by the tissues (about 4 mL/dL blood/min at rest, or 200 mL/min when cardiac output is 5 L/min) can be delivered into the alveoli and expired. The changes in $PCO_2$ and carbon dioxide content of the blood around the body are summarized in **Fig. 5.3.21**. During exercise, much larger quantities of carbon dioxide are produced by the tissues. However, the automatic increase in alveolar ventilation and cardiac output that occurs during exercise, together with the increased rate of diffusion of carbon dioxide both at tissue level and in the lungs, normally ensure that arterial $PCO_2$ remains relatively constant, between 4.9 kPa and 5.7 kPa (37 and 43 mmHg) in an adult.

## CLINICAL APPLICATIONS

### HYPOCAPNIA

A decrease in arterial $PCO_2$ below normal levels is known as **hypocapnia**. This will occur if alveolar

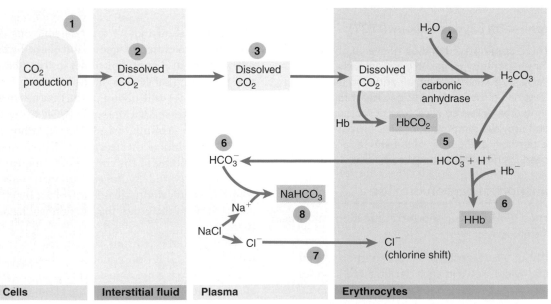

**Figure 5.3.23** Summary of the chemical reactions involved in carbon dioxide transport at tissue level. Although there is a continuous production of carbon dioxide, the numbers refer to the approximate sequence of events; 90% of carbon dioxide is carried in nue blood in the form of hydrogen carbonate ($HCO_3^-$) ions, 5% in simple solution, and 5% attached to haemoglobin as $HbCO_2$ (for key to symbols see text)

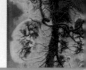

ventilation is increased above metabolic needs (**hyperventilation**), which results in a lowering of alveolar $PCO_2$, a rise in the alveolar–capillary $PCO_2$ gradient and an increase in the rate at which carbon dioxide can diffuse out of the blood. Hyperventilation can cause a marked decrease in arterial $PCO_2$ but has a far less marked effect on $PO_2$ due to the shape of the oxygen dissociation curve (**Fig. 5.3.19**). Hyperventilation may result from:

- central nervous system stimuli (pain, temperature, anxiety, salicylate poisoning)
- hypoxia (high altitude)
- excess acid in the body (metabolic disorders).

Any lowering of arterial $PCO_2$ generally decreases the stimulus to breathe and may be followed by deep, slow breathing or even apnoea, resulting in marked hypoxia of the individual and disturbances of cerebral function. For this reason, voluntary attempts to hyperventilate should never be attempted unless properly supervised. In addition, the fall in arterial $PCO_2$ will result in respiratory alkalosis. The effects of hypocapnia may be eliminated by getting the individual to rebreathe from a paper bag.

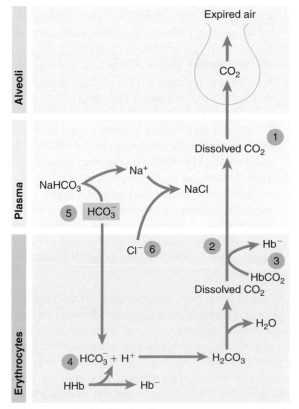

**Figure 5.3.24** Summary of chemical reactions involved in carbon dioxide transport as blood passes through the pulmonary capillaries

## HYPERCAPNIA

Any increase in arterial $PCO_2$ above normal levels is called **hypercapnia**. The two main causes of carbon dioxide retention are alveolar hypoventilation and severe ventilation–perfusion imbalance. Hypercapnia may also occur if there is either a general or local impairment of circulation, allowing carbon dioxide to accumulate in the tissues. It is important to remember that whereas hypercapnia is *always* accompanied by hypoxia (unless oxygen therapy is being given), the reverse is not true.

Any increase in arterial $PCO_2$ acts as a powerful stimulus to breathing. The rate and depth of breathing are increased and patients may experience severe dyspnoea in their attempt to eliminate carbon dioxide excess. If $PCO_2$ rises above about 10 kPa (75 mmHg), the central nervous system becomes depressed as a result of dilation of cerebral blood vessels, which causes cerebral oedema and raised intracranial pressure. Patients will suffer from headaches, lethargy and may progress to a stuporous or comatose state. Total anaesthesia and death will occur if arterial $PCO_2$ rises to 13–20 kPa (100–150 mmHg).

The only way of treating hypercapnia is to increase ventilation. If airways obstruction is a primary problem, this should be relieved by using bronchodilators, by removal of any foreign bodies or excess secretions or by performing a tracheostomy. Mechanical ventilation may be required.

## MEASUREMENT OF ARTERIAL BLOOD GASES

Of all the laboratory tests that are relevant to respiratory diseases, measurement of arterial blood gases is the most important. Knowledge of the levels of oxygen and carbon dioxide and hydrogen ion concentration (pH) in the arterial blood can help to determine the nature and severity of the disease and the response to various forms of treatment. The alveolar–arterial oxygen difference ($A–aDO_2$), which in health should be very small, may be measured to assess the efficiency of gas exchange across the pulmonary membrane.

By using suitable electrodes, the $PO_2$, $PCO_2$ and pH of blood can be determined electronically using very small samples. Blood samples may be taken from the radial, femoral or brachial arteries and should be taken immediately to the laboratory in a heparinized, iced receptacle, ensuring that no contamination with room air occurs.

Normal ranges for arterial blood gases are:

- $PO_2$: 10.6–13.3 kPa (80–100 mmHg)
- $PCO_2$: 4.6–6.9 kPa (35–45 mmHg)

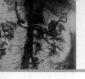

- pH: 7.35–7.45
- oxygen saturation 94–100% (96% breathing room air)
- Base excess 0 ± 2 mmol/L.

In the past 40 years there have been rapid technological advances in the development of non-invasive devices to support the monitoring of hypoxia and hypercapnia. These instruments can measure **transcutaneous** oxygen and carbon dioxide tensions, and oxygen saturation by **pulsed oximetry,** simply by attaching small disposable electrodes or light-sensitive monitors to the finger or earlobe. **Capillary blood gas analysis** can now be performed – the accuracy appears to be good and the procedure is less painful and has fewer potential complications than arterial stabs, although it is still invasive. Similarly, end-expiratory carbon dioxide levels can be measured by placing a small catheter in one nostril to allow analysis of gas. Such methods are being increasingly used by clinicians to evaluate and monitor patients with cardiopulmonary disorders. Many of the problems of monitoring the rapidly changing oxygenation and ventilation of acute and chronically ill patients by intermittent arterial blood gas analysis have been overcome by the facility to perform continuous non-invasive measurements. However, nurses still need to assess patients as a whole and not just rely on the technology available. A patient's problem may be solved simply by being sat upright so the lungs can fully expand, or the patient might have normal saturation levels but raised carbon dioxide levels and be on verge of respiratory arrest.

### RESPIRATORY FAILURE

Respiratory failure is said to occur when the lung fails to oxygenate the arterial blood adequately and/or prevent undue retention of carbon dioxide. Although there are no absolute values of the levels of arterial blood gases that indicate respiratory failure, an arterial $PO_2$ of less than 8 kPa (60 mmHg) is usually indicative of this condition:

Signs and symptoms of respiratory failure include:

- disorientation
- headache
- weakness
- malaise
- tachycardia
- cyanosis
- hypertension
- stupor.

Treatment consists of providing adequate oxygenation and reversing acidosis using augmented inspired oxygen and/or assisted ventilation (see Mechanical ventilation, p. 561) with additional medical management being directed by whether the patient has type 1 $PCO_2$ < 6.7 kPa (50 mmHg) or type 2 $PCO_2$ > 6.7 kPa (50 mmHg) respiratory failure.

## Control of ventilation

Respiration is largely an involuntary act resulting from the automatic generation of rhythmic breathing by the respiratory centre in the brainstem. The respiratory muscles are innervated by the phrenic nerve to the diaphragm (which originates from the IIIrd, IVth and Vth cervical nerves) and the intercostal nerves, to the intercostal muscles (which originate from the thoracic portion of the spinal cord, T1–12). Spinal transection above C3 results in total respiratory paralysis, whereas if the damage occurs in the thoracic portion of the spinal cord diaphragmatic breathing can continue, although the intercostal muscles will be paralysed resulting in a loss of stability of the chest wall.

Respiratory rhythm generated in the brain is conveyed to the spinal cord through three anatomically separate pathways:

1. The **voluntary pathway**, which runs in the dorsolateral region of the spinal cord. The voluntary control of breathing is accomplished by descending pathways from the cerebral cortex to the medullary respiratory centre.
2. The **involuntary pathway**, which runs in the ventrolateral part of the cord. Interaction between voluntary and involuntary breathing occurs at spinal level. Certain lesions of the brainstem or spinal cord may destroy voluntary control of breathing but leave automatic control unaffected, or vice versa, depending on the exact location.
3. **Tonic influences** on the respiratory motor neurones arise from a nucleus in the upper medulla and help to determine the degree to which various respiratory muscles are relaxed or contracted. The axons from this nucleus run in close proximity to the ventrolateral rhythmical pathways.

Even during passive expiration, nerve impulses pass to the respiratory muscles, which maintain their tone thereby helping to maintain the stability of the chest wall and posture. However, as inspiration starts, there is a rapid increase in the number of impulses arriving at the respiratory muscles, so that the force of inspiration gradually increases and thoracic expansion occurs. Then, at the end of inspiration, a sudden reduction in the number of impulses results in relaxation of the inspiratory muscles, and expiration usually

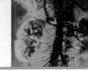

follows passively by elastic recoil of the lungs and thoracic cage. After a given period of time (2–3 seconds in the resting adult), the barrage of impulses returns and the cycle is repeated.

The level of ventilation must be continously adapted according to changes in body requirements (e.g. exercise) or atmospheric conditions (e.g. high altitude) if adequate oxygenation is to be maintained. It is likely that several mechanisms are involved and that at any given moment in time, respiration is being controlled not by any single factor but by several interrelated events.

## Central rhythm-generating mechanisms

The respiratory nerves receive their impulses via synaptic connections in the spinal cord from neurones whose cell bodies lie in the medulla and pons in a portion of the lower brainstem known as the **respiratory centre**. These neurones control the automatic system responsible for the periodic nature of inspiration and expiration, and so transection of the brainstem above this level leaves the mechanism for generating rhythmic breathing essentially intact.

It has been found that certain neurones in the medulla record in perfect synchrony with inspiration, and stimulation of such neurones results in sustained inspiratory effort. These have been called the **inspiratory neurones**. Similarly, other groups of neurones (the **expiratory neurones**) discharge synchronously with expiration. Interaction between these two groups of neurones is apparently responsible for the inherent rhythmicity of impulses in the medulla that continues, albeit somewhat irregularly, even when all known afferent stimuli have been abolished. It therefore appears that these cells do have the capacity for self-excitation, although they are dependent on various inputs if a smooth and regular respiratory rhythm is to be maintained.

It is believed that the inspiratory neurones may be arranged in a loop in such a way that, when one of these neurones becomes excited, it sends a signal around the circuit stimulating all other neurones and finally becoming restimulated itself (**Fig. 5.3.25**). Fibres from this circuit carry impulses down the spinal cord where they synapse with the nerves supplying the inspiratory muscles to cause contraction. The faster the inspiratory neurones transmit their impulses around the circuit, the more frequent will be the impulses arriving at the respiratory motor units, thereby increasing the force of muscle contraction and hence the depth of inspiration. Not only do excitatory nerve impulses pass out of the circuit to the respiratory muscles, but inhibitory impulses are transmitted to the expiratory neurones. This reduces or stops any expiratory activity during inspiration.

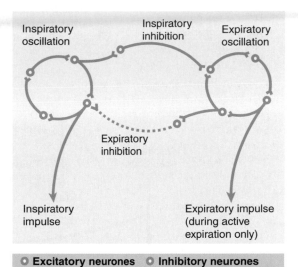

**Figure 5.3.25** Diagrammatic representation of possible interactions between inspiratory and expiratory neurones

The expiratory neurones are probably organized in a similar manner, although impulses are usually only transmitted down the spinal cord to the expiratory muscles during active expiration, since no muscle contraction is necessary to effect passive expiration. Oscillation of the impulse around the expiratory circuit causes self-excitation of all the expiratory neurones and transmission of inhibitory impulses to the inspiratory neurones.

Thus, these two groups of neurones mutually inhibit one another so that when one is oscillating the other stops, and vice versa.

At the transition between inspiration and expiration, large numbers of respiratory neurones suddenly either stop or start discharging and this is accompanied by equally rapid changes in muscle activity. The current explanation for this rapid transition between inspiration and expiration is based on some inhibitory threshold mechanism which, once activated or inactivated, rapidly 'turns off' either the inspiratory or expiratory neurones and hence the activity of the appropriate muscles. It is thought that, once this inhibitory threshold is reached, inspiration is suddenly switched off, enabling expiration to occur. During expiration, the inhibition on the inspiratory cells will gradually decrease until a new lower threshold is reached, enabling the 'on switch' for inspiration to be reactivated. The level at which the thresholds are set may be altered according to various inputs from the brain and rest of the body, thereby allowing deeper respiration to occur before inspiration is switched off.

A schematic representation of the way in which the basic rhythm of respiration may be controlled is shown in **Fig. 5.3.26**.

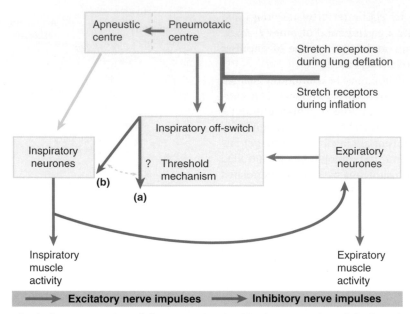

**Figure 5.3.26** Hypothetical representation of the system involved in the generation of rhythmic breathing. Inspiration will only occur if the 'inspiratory off-switch' is *not* activated, i.e. when it is at position (a). Once the combined inspiratory inhibitory effects reach a certain threshold level, inspiration is switched off (moves to position (b)). Once inspiration has ceased, expiratory neurones are no longer inhibited and active expiratory effort can occur if necessary

## Influence of the pontine respiratory centres

The medullary neurones receive an input from two separate areas in the pons: the **apneustic centre**, which stimulates the inspiratory centre (but which appears to play a relatively small role in the intact animal) and the **pneumotaxic centre** (or nucleus parabrachialis), which has an inhibitory effect on the inspiratory neurones, either directly or by its inhibitory influence on the apneustic centre. If the pneumotaxic centre is destroyed, the unopposed action of the apneustic centre will cause prolonged inspiration with only occasional brief expiratory efforts. However, if the entire pons is destroyed an essentially normal balance between inspiration and expiration occurs, providing vagal input is intact.

### CLINICAL APPLICATIONS

#### FAILURE OF THE RESPIRATORY CENTRE

Despite the duplication of neurogenic mechanisms that help to ensure that respiration will continue even if one part of the respiratory centre is damaged, occasionally all these mechanisms fail simultaneously. Potential causes include barbiturate overdose, cerebral contusion, severe hypoxia or paralysis of the respiratory muscles by:

- damage to anterior horn cells, which relay nerve impulses to the respiratory muscles (poliomyelitis)

- drugs that block the transmission of nerve impulses at the motor endplates (e.g. tubocurarine, which is used during general anaesthesia as a muscle relaxant).

Management of respiratory centre failure is extremely difficult and, in general, the only effective treatment is to use artificial ventilation until recovery occurs (see Mechanical ventilation, p. 561). However, in some cases the damage may be irreversible and recovery, therefore, impossible.

## Regulation of respiratory centre activity

Although the basic rhythm of respiration is set and coordinated by the respiratory centre in the medulla, the rhythm can be modified by numerous different inputs according to changing body requirements.

### Voluntary control of breathing

Voluntary control over breathing patterns can be demonstrated during breath holding or hyperventilation, although the duration of such efforts is usually limited by the intensity of the involuntary chemical stimuli that they induce. Nevertheless, in the absence of proper supervision, or as a result of anxiety states, hyperventilation may be carried to extremes, resulting in a marked reduction of arterial $PCO_2$, a slowing or cessation of respiration, and respiratory alkalosis.

Complex control of the respiratory system is necessary during speech and singing. Whenever nerve

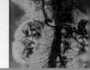

impulses are transmitted from the brain to the vocal cords, simultaneous impulses are transmitted to the respiratory centre to control the flow of air between the vocal cords. Marked changes in respiration are also seen in emotional states (e.g. laughing and crying). Finally, cortical factors may play an important role in preparing the body for additional activity and may contribute to the rise in ventilation that occurs during exercise.

Mental alertness and wakefulness have a stimulating effect on breathing, whereas sleep, sedatives, some anaesthetics and alcohol usually reduce both the rate and depth of ventilation.

## Chemoreception

As the main function of breathing is to maintain homeostasis by providing the body with oxygen and eliminating carbon dioxide, it is hardly surprising that the respiratory system is highly responsive to small changes in arterial $PO_2$ and $PCO_2$.

### Peripheral chemoreceptors

The carotid bodies and similar vascular structures around the aortic arch contain **chemoreceptors**. A chemoreceptor is a receptor that responds to a change in the chemical composition of the blood or fluid surrounding it. These receptors sense the levels of $PO_2$ and $PCO_2$ and hydrogen ion concentration ($[H^+]$) in the blood and relay the information (via the glossopharyngeal and vagal nerves) to the respiratory areas in the brain (**Fig. 5.3.27**). Denervation of these structures abolishes the response to hypoxia and decreases the response to hydrogen ion concentration and hypercapnia. Whereas homeostasis of arterial oxygen depends on peripheral arterial chemoreceptors, the response to hypercapnia is primarily dependent on other receptors found in the brainstem and known as **central chemoreceptors**.

### Central chemoreceptors

For many years, it was believed that the central response to hypercapnia was due to the direct effect of carbon dioxide on the rhythm-generating mechanisms in the brainstem. However, there is increasing evidence that specific receptor sites, known as central chemoreceptors, are situated just under the ventral surface of the medulla (Duffin, 1990). The actual mechanism by which they exert their control has been the subject of much controversy. However, it now appears that when arterial $PCO_2$ rises, carbon dioxide diffuses from the cerebral blood vessels across the blood–brain barrier and into the cerebrospinal fluid (CSF), which bathes the entire brain,

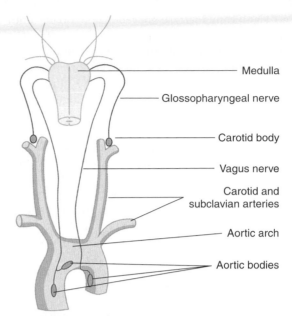

**Figure 5.3.27** Peripheral chemoreceptor systems involved in the control of breathing

including the central chemoreceptors. The blood–brain barrier is relatively impermeable to hydrogen ions or hydrogen carbonate (bicarbonate) ions, but dissolved carbon dioxide crosses easily. However, once in the cerebrospinal fluid, the carbon dioxide liberates hydrogen ions according to the reaction:

$$CO_2 + H_2O \rightleftharpoons H_2CO_3 \rightleftharpoons H^+ + HCO_3^-$$

It is the rise in hydrogen ion concentration that causes the stimulation of the chemoreceptors, which in turn send excitatory impulses to the inspiratory neurones to increase their rate of discharge. The resultant hyperventilation reduces arterial $PCO_2$ in the blood and hence $PCO_2$ of the cerebrospinal fluid, so that homeostasis can be maintained. Conversely, any fall in arterial $PCO_2$, and hence fall in hydrogen ion concentration within the cerebrospinal fluid, inhibits the rate of discharge of the respiratory neurones, leading to a reduction in ventilation. Thus, it can be seen that the $PCO_2$ in the blood regulates ventilation by its effect on the hydrogen ion concentration of the cerebrospinal fluid.

## Chemoreceptor reflexes

### Hypoxia

Under normal circumstances, the ventilatory response to hypoxia is weak. Increased levels of inspired oxygen will only reduce ventilation by about 20%, whereas when the $PCO_2$ is within normal limits, no significant increase in ventilation occurs until arterial oxygen drops below 8 kPa (60 mmHg). The hypoxic drive can only increase ventilation to 50% above resting values. The central chemoreceptors are not sensitive to changes in arterial $PO_2$. Indeed, in the absence of the peripheral chemoreceptors, hypoxia depresses ventilation – presumably by direct action on the respiratory centre.

The relatively weak hypoxic drive under normal conditions is not surprising. Increasing ventilation does little to increase oxygen delivery to the tissues due to the shape of the oxygen dissociation curve (see Fig. 5.3.19), and increasing ventilation in response to hypoxia, in the presence of a normal $PCO_2$, would eliminate excess carbon dioxide from the body and hence depress breathing.

The only two circumstances in which the hypoxic reflex assumes particular importance are:

- At altitude when, after a few days acclimatization, there is a decrease in the buffering capacity of the blood and cerebrospinal fluid (see p. 581). This enables the hypoxic drive to act unopposed by the accompanying fall in $PCO_2$, which would normally have a depressant effect.
- In chronic lung disease, when the hypercapnic drive has been depressed.

### Hypercapnia/changes in hydrogen ion concentration

The most powerful factor regulating alveolar ventilation is arterial $PCO_2$. Whenever arterial $PCO_2$ rises, respiration is stimulated, whereas a fall in arterial $PCO_2$ below the normal level of 5.3 kPa (40 mmHg) results in a reduction in alveolar ventilation. In healthy subjects, a 3- to 4-fold increase in ventilation occurs if a mixture of air containing 5% carbon dioxide and normal levels of oxygen is breathed. Ventilation may be increased up to 15-fold if the inspired concentration of carbon dioxide is raised to 15%. However, no further increases occur above this level, as very high levels of arterial $PCO_2$ depress the entire central nervous system, including the respiratory centre, and can prove lethal. The sensitivity of this feedback mechanism is such that, despite marked variations in tissue activity throughout the day, arterial $PCO_2$ rarely changes by more than 0.4 kPa (3 mmHg), except during sleep when it may rise a little more. The increase in ventilation that occurs in response to a rise in $PCO_2$ results in increased excretion of carbon dioxide, thereby enabling arterial $PCO_2$ to return towards normal levels, and vice versa.

Any rise in the hydrogen ion concentration in arterial blood (fall in pH) acts as a powerful stimulus to breathing. However, the maximum increase that will occur purely in response to a fall in pH is about 5-fold (i.e. only about one-third of that which can be induced in response to carbon dioxide). Although it is difficult to separate the ventilatory response to hydrogen ion concentration from that caused by any accompanying change in $PCO_2$, the response to hydrogen ion concentration can be seen in patients with metabolic disorders, such as diabetes mellitus. Such patients frequently hyperventilate in response to their low blood pH (caused by excess acids in the blood) despite the fact that this 'blows off' excess carbon dioxide, resulting in a low arterial $PCO_2$ ($PaCO_2$), which would depress respiration under normal circumstances.

Undoubtedly, the predominant effect of changing arterial $PCO_2$ is on the central chemoreceptors, whereas hypoxia stimulates the peripheral receptors. Quantitative assessment of their relative importance and interactions is difficult because $PCO_2$ and hydrogen ion concentration stimulate both peripheral and central mechanisms, whereas hypoxia stimulates the peripheral but depresses the central mechanisms. However, it is clear that the peripheral chemoreceptors are responsible for about one-third of the ventilatory response to hypercapnia and are also the chief site at which interaction between the effects of $PCO_2$, $PO_2$ and hydrogen ion concentration occurs.

### Vagal influences

Numerous stretch receptors in the lung are sensitive to the degree of lung expansion. Impulses from these receptors pass via the vagus to the respiratory centres in the medulla, where they have an inhibitory effect on inspiration during lung inflation and an inhibitory effect on expiration during lung deflation. These reflexes therefore help to maintain the rhythmicity of breathing and to prevent excessive changes in lung volume.

Vagal input is thought to play a much larger part in controlling breathing and maintaining lung volume in young babies, in whom the brainstem (and hence pontine control) is more poorly organized. The **Hering–Breuer reflex** is vagally mediated and results in temporary apnoea if the lung is overinflated. This reflex is easily elicited in babies and young children, and during general anaesthesia, but appears to have no physiological significance in older, awake subjects during tidal (normal resting) breathing.

If the vagi are cut, a highly characteristic pattern of deep, slow breathing occurs. This is because, if the inhibitory effects of the vagus on inspiration are removed, it will take longer to reach the necessary threshold before inspiration can be 'switched off'. The activity of the pons (which normally acts as a central relay station for vagal input) becomes more

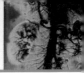

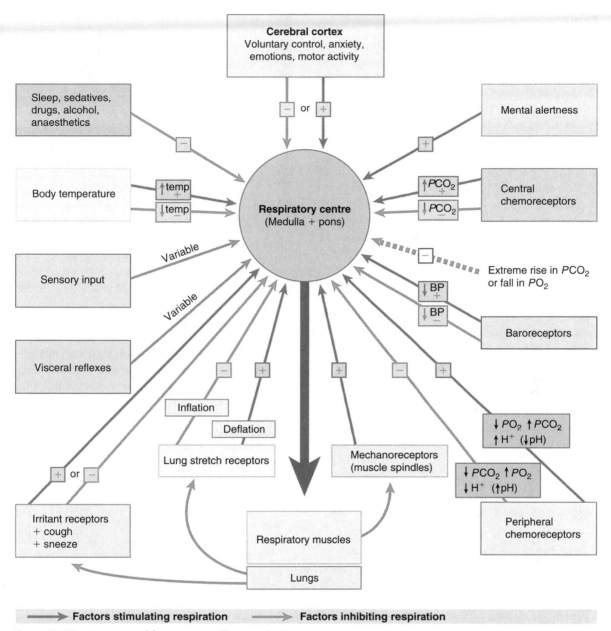

**Figure 5.3.28** Summary of factors controlling respiration

important if there is any decrease in vagal input. Other reflexes, including those arising from baroreceptors and diaphragmatic muscle spindles, and from temperature, pain and visceral (swallowing, coughing, sneezing) receptors, may also contribute to the regulation of breathing rate and pattern.

Although chemoreceptors seem to be primarily involved in changing the *level* of ventilation, receptors in the lungs and airways may be more important in regulating the *pattern* of breathing. Stretch receptors in the airways may be important in producing a combination of tidal volume and respiratory rate that achieves adequate alveolar ventilation while minimizing the work of breathing. Very rapid, shallow breathing is inefficient both because of the wasted energy spent on ventilating the dead space and because the energy required to overcome airways resistance increases with increasing flows. Similarly, very deep breaths result in a disproportionate increase in the energy required to stretch the lungs and chest wall. These reflexes can be overcome by cortical control, for example during speech, and by other reflexes, such as the protective cough and sneeze reflexes.

The regulation of respiration by the interaction of multiple factors is summarized in **Fig. 5.3.28**. Under normal circumstances, this system ensures that homeostasis of the blood gases and hydrogen ion concentration can be maintained at all times, despite widely varying circumstances.

## Exercise

During exercise, ventilation increases in almost direct proportion to the amount of work being performed by the body. There are two distinct components in the ventilatory response to exercise: an immediate increase when exercise first starts, and a slower rise to plateau level as exercise is maintained. Pulmonary ventilation may rise up to 120 L/min in a fit individual (i.e. a 20-fold increase over resting levels) (**Fig. 5.3.29**). The physiological mechanisms involved in this are still poorly understood. The initial increase in ventilation is thought to be too rapid to involve the chemoreceptor system, especially as no significant changes in blood gases occur during exercise due to the increased ventilation and cardiac output. The speed of this initial reaction strongly suggests a neurological mechanism, which could be due either to a direct drive from the cerebral cortex or to stimulation of the respiratory centre by stimulation of proprioceptors in the exercising muscles and joints.

The cause of the subsequent slow rise in ventilation and the factors sustaining ventilation when the plateau has been reached remain unexplained. There is some evidence that peripheral oxygen chemosensitivity is increased with exercise. Alternatively, the deeper, more rapid breathing that occurs during exercise could cause more marked oscillations in blood gases during the breathing cycle than normal, which may stimulate the peripheral chemoreceptors even though the mean arterial levels of $PCO_2$, $PO_2$ and hydrogen ion concentration remain constant.

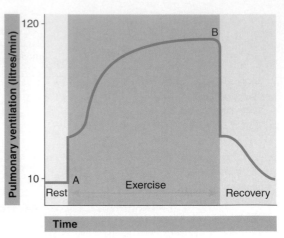

**Figure 5.3.29** Changes in ventilation during exercise. There is a sudden increase in ventilation at the very onset of exercise (A) and an equally rapid, although larger, decrease in ventilation immediately the exercise ceases (B)

## CLINICAL APPLICATIONS

### CHRONIC LUNG DISEASE

Some patients with chronic lung disease have a poor response to hypercapnia. This is partly due to mechanical obstruction to breathing in that they are incapable of increasing their work of breathing any further. However, in some patients (the 'blue bloaters'), there is a true reduction in response to $PCO_2$. At one time this was thought to be due to changes in the buffering capacity of the blood and cerebrospinal fluid in response to chronic carbon dioxide retention, but this is no longer considered to be an adequate explanation. It is known that there is a wide variation in normal response to carbon dioxide and it may be that the peripheral chemoreceptors in 'blue bloaters' develop a reduced responsiveness to carbon dioxide, similar to the fall in peripheral chemosensitivity seen in people living at altitude. These patients no longer respond to rising $PCO_2$ and become dependent on the hypoxic drive to breathe.

Administration of augmented oxygen in this situation can eliminate this drive and cause a total cessation of breathing (apnoea). It is therefore important to establish the ventilatory status of a patient with chronic lung disease when administering oxygen and for appropriate monitoring of the ventilatory status to take place as oxygen is being administered. In patients with chronic obstructive pulmonary disease without type 1 failure, the risk of hypercapnia is often overstated and undertreatment of serious hypoxaemia can result in death (Bateman & Leach, 1998).

This risk is reduced by administering oxygen in minimal concentrations compatible with adequate oxygenation of arterial blood. The Venturi-type mask is usually used for patients for whom it is important to know the exact percentage of oxygen being administered because it enables the flow of oxygen to be mixed continuously with air to ensure the percentage of oxygen prescribed is delivered, i.e. there is a fixed flow rate. Thus, Venturi-type masks are designed to provide a specified fractional concentration of oxygen ($FiO_2$), which cannot be exceeded by the patient or the attendants. When using nasal cannulae, the concentration of oxygen delivered cannot be guaranteed because it depends on factors such as patient's breathing pattern, whether the patient breathes through the nose or the mouth, and nasal resistance – 2 L by nasal cannulae could actually deliver up to 40% oxygen in some patients, i.e. there is variable performance. In patients with chronic lung disease, a low percentage should be administered to supplement oxygen levels

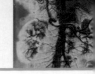

without increasing carbon dioxide levels. A rising $CO_2$ or falling pH indicates the need to lower the oxygen concentration or support ventilation.

Oxygen should not be withheld from acutely ill patients with chronic obstructive lung disease as it might need to be prescribed for other reasons, e.g. cardiac failure, and not to treat their lung condition. The National Institute for Clinical Excellence (NICE) guidelines on the management of chronic obstructive pulmonary disease (COPD) for adults in primary and secondary care recommend that oxygen should be given to keep the $SaO_2$ above 90% and that arterial blood gases should be measured and the inspired oxygen concentration noted in all patients with an exacerbation of COPD. It is imperative that the percentage of oxygen to be delivered is prescribed, as oxygen is a drug and should be treated as such. Therefore nurses adjusting the percentage of oxygen should do so within a patient group direction (PGD) or protocol.

The response of patients to oxygen therapy should be noted at frequent intervals by observing their state of consciousness, the frequency and depth of breathing and by measuring the $PCO_2$ and pH of their arterial blood. Saturation levels provide a non-invasive measure but should not be relied on solely.

Other patients with chronic lung disease, the 'pink puffers', retain their carbon dioxide sensitivity, remaining relatively well oxygenated at the expense of considerable, often distressing, effort.

Severely hypoxic patients, especially those in whom respiration is being driven primarily by a lack of oxygen, frequently exhibit a striking pattern of periodic breathing known as **Cheyne–Stokes respiration**. This is characterized by periods of apnoea lasting approximately 15–20 seconds, alternating with periods of hyperventilation of about the same duration. It seems to result from relative insensitivity of the respiratory control mechanisms to small changes in $PO_2$. Such insensitivity may be due to prolongation of circulation time from lung to brain, as may occur in cardiac failure. The period of hyperventilation raises arterial $PO_2$ so that peripheral chemoreceptors are no longer stimulated, and breathing then stops until the $PO_2$ has fallen sufficiently to reactivate the receptors, when the cycle begins again. Cheyne–Stokes breathing is frequently seen at high altitude (especially during sleep), in anaesthetized individuals who are allowed to breathe spontaneously and in some patients with severe cardiorespiratory disease or brain damage.

## ASSESSMENT OF RESPIRATORY RATE AND RHYTHM

The rate of respiration varies according to the size of the individual, the metabolic demands of the body and the mechanical properties of the lung and chest wall. As described above, the respiratory control centre in the medulla receives a constant barrage of information from receptors all over the body and normally adjusts the rate and depth of breathing to achieve the necessary level of alveolar ventilation with the least investment of energy.

Respiratory rates generally tend to decrease with increasing body size. Thus, newborn infants have a 'normal' rate of about 40 breaths per minute, whereas in adults it is generally between 10 and 15 breaths per minute. However, it should be stressed that there is considerable individual variation and changes in respiratory rate can only provide vital warning signs of respiratory (or cardiac) problems if an accurate record has previously been kept for that particular patient. The depth of respiration (tidal volume) normally increases with increasing body size.

Although respiration is generally an involuntary act, it is easily influenced by subjective factors, particularly if a patient is aware that his or her pattern of breathing is being observed. Consequently, it is usually more satisfactory if respirations are assessed when the patient thinks the pulse rate is still being counted. While counting respiratory rate it is also vital to observe:

- the depth and regularity of breathing
- the presence of any breath sounds (wheezing, stridor)
- the presence of any chest recession or uneven chest movements
- the amount of effort required by the patient to breathe, including whether or not the patient is mouth breathing and/or using accessory muscles to aid ventilation (see Dyspnoea, p. 560).

Adequate assessment of the above usually requires a full minute's observation.

A normal respiratory rate is termed **eupnoea**; **tachypnoea** refers to an increased respiratory rate, and a cessation of respiration is called **apnoea**.

## ABNORMALITIES OF RESPIRATORY CONTROL DURING SLEEP

Sleep fluctuates cyclically through four stages of quiet, or non-rapid eye movement (non-REM) sleep and the stage of rapid eye movement (REM). The cycle periodicity is 90 to 120 minutes in adults but much shorter in newborn infants, who may spend up to 50% of sleeping time in REM sleep. This is associated with dreaming and is typically

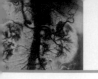

characterized by irregular and rapid breathing with frequent periods of apnoea lasting up to 20 seconds in healthy adults and children and 10 seconds in infants. The decrease in intercostal muscle tone and reduction in laryngeal activity during REM sleep may result in paradoxical (asynchronous) breathing movements and a reduction in resting lung volume in newborn infants (Gaultier, 1995). Disorders of breathing during sleep may underlie a wide variety of problems, including sleep apnoea, the sudden infant death syndrome, certain types of insomnia and excessive day-time sleepiness. In recent years there has been an increasing use of automated polygraphic cardiorespiratory monitors to perform 'sleep studies' on patients suspected of suffering from sleep apnoea and related disorders.

## SLEEP APNOEA

An apnoeic episode is defined as cessation of airflow at the nose and mouth lasting at least 10 seconds. **Sleep apnoea syndrome** is diagnosed in adults if there are at least 30 apnoeic episodes during a 7-hour period of nocturnal sleep. By simultaneously measuring airflow and the movements of the chest wall and abdomen, three distinct types of apnoea have been defined:

- **Central apnoea** is defined as a cessation of airflow accompanied by cessation of all respiratory movements. Several defects in metabolic control systems have been described in patients with central sleep apnoea. Damage to the respiratory neurones has been implicated in sleep apnoea or hypoventilation, which may complicate infectious, vascular or neoplastic disorders of the brainstem. Defects in peripheral or central chemoreceptors have been demonstrated in patients with primary (idiopathic) central hypoventilation.
- **Upper airway (obstructive) apnoea:** airflow is absent, despite continuing respiratory efforts. This may occur in patients with enlarged tonsils or adenoids, laryngeal stenosis or micrognathia (abnormally small jaw).
- **Mixed apnoea:** has characteristics of both central and obstructive apnoea.

Guidelines on the management of obstructive sleep apnoea/hypopnoea syndrome (OSAHS) were recently published by the Scottish Intercollegiate Guidelines Network (SIGN, 2003). These indicate that continuous positive airway pressure (CPAP) is the first-choice therapy for someone with moderate or severe obstructive sleep apnoea/hypopnoea syndrome who has sufficient symptoms to require intervention. It acts as a pneumatic splint to maintain upper airway patency during all phases of sleep breathing. Most patients require lifelong treatment.

## SUDDEN INFANT DEATH SYNDROME

Sudden infant death syndrome (SIDS) is the sudden, unexpected death of an apparently healthy baby in whom post-mortem history reveals no adequate cause of death. Sudden infant death syndrome was responsible for 1400 deaths in the United Kingdom in 1990 (i.e. 1.7 per 1000 live births) but fell to 0.7/1000 in 1994, the lowest incidence since records began, following the introduction of the 'back to sleep' campaign and, by 2000, death rates from sudden infant death syndrome in England and Wales were 0.47 per 1000 for boys and 0.33 for girls. Sudden infant death syndrome remains the most common cause of death in infants between 1 week and 2 years, with peak incidence occurring at 1–4 months. The cause of sudden infant death syndrome remains unclear, researchers think that there are likely to be a number of different causes or that a combination of factors affects a baby at a vulnerable stage of development (Platt & Pharoah, 2003). However, several valuable observations have emerged as a result of investigations over the past 15 years and it has been suggested (Department of Health, 1993, 2000; Dwyer et al., 1991; Fleming et al., 1990) that risk of cot death will be reduced if:

- babies are put down to sleep on their backs
- parents do not smoke (during pregnancy and postnatally) in the same room as the baby
- babies are not allowed to become overheated (i.e. avoid excessive clothing/bedding or high room temperatures)
- babies are placed in the feet-to-foot position to prevent them wriggling down under the covers
- the GP is contacted early if a baby appears unwell.

It has also been shown that although apnoea may provide the final common pathway, an increased incidence of apnoea during early life is not associated with subsequent SIDS. Furthermore, although giving apnoeic monitors to parents who have experienced a previous sudden infant death or whose baby is thought to be at increased risk due to abnormal breathing patterns may provide much needed reassurance, there is no scientific evidence that the use of such monitors in any way diminishes the risk of sudden infant death syndrome. One of the major problems of most apnoeic monitors is that they only monitor respiration from chest and/or abdominal movements, whereas it has been shown that infants suffering from apparent life-threatening episodes often have obstructive

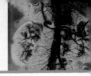

apnoea, in which there may be increased respiratory movements, despite lack of any airflow into or out of the lungs. Ideally, non-invasive monitoring of blood gases, pulse rate and airflow should be performed in addition to surface recordings of respiratory movements. However, such intensive monitoring may be very intrusive to normal home life and should be reserved for those infants deemed to be at high risk of a life-threatening event and whose parents have been fully instructed in infant resuscitation techniques. The health visitor will play a vital role in supporting and reassuring the family during this sort of intervention.

## Respiration and the regulation of hydrogen ions

Respiration and carbon dioxide transport have profound effects on the acid–base status (or pH) of the body. Hydrogen ions ($H^+$) are far more reactive than any other positively charged ions in the body and it is the concentration of hydrogen ions that determines the acidity of blood and body fluids.

Even small changes away from the normal hydrogen ion concentration will affect the structures of proteins. Enzymes are particularly susceptible to changes in the pH of the surrounding medium and, whereas small changes may drastically reduce their efficiency, larger alterations will result in a life-threatening disruption of metabolism. Consequently, the intake and production of hydrogen ions in the body, which may vary considerably according to diet, level of exercise, drugs or disease, must be matched by an efficient system of buffering these ions in the body fluids and their controlled excretion by the lungs and kidneys, to ensure that homeostasis is maintained.

Before considering the regulation of hydrogen ion concentration it is important to understand the notation of pH. If you have not already studied the section on pH in Chapter 1.2, it would probably be a good idea to turn to it now before continuing with the remainder of this chapter.

The normal pH of blood is 7.4 (i.e. it has 0.000 000 04 mol $H^+$/L) and it is therefore a slightly alkaline fluid. The range of pH compatible with life is only 7.0–7.8 and, in a healthy adult, arterial blood pH is almost always maintained between 7.35 and 7.45. The clinical use of the pH scale may be replaced in future by expressing hydrogen ion concentration directly in nanomoles per litre (nmol/L), where 1 nanomole = $10^{-9}$ moles. Arterial blood normally has a hydrogen ion concentration of 40 nmol/L (range 36–45 nmol/L). The range compatible with life lies between 16 and 100 nmol $H^+$/L.

## Buffer systems

The pH of blood is normally kept within fairly narrow limits by two buffer systems. These are:

- the haemoglobin in red blood cells
- the carbonic-acid–hydrogen-carbonate system in plasma.

Buffers are systems that minimize any change in overall pH by accepting hydrogen ions when hydrogen ion concentration rises (i.e. pH falls) and by donating hydrogen ions when hydrogen ion concentration falls (i.e. pH rises).

### Haemoglobin

Plasma proteins and haemoglobin play a vital role in maintaining a constant blood pH despite the continous addition of carbon dioxide into the blood at tissue level and its removal as blood passes through the lungs.

At tissue level, the following reaction occurs as carbon dioxide enters the red blood cell:

$$CO_2 + H_2O \rightleftharpoons H_2CO_3$$

If the carbonic acid were allowed to dissociate into free hydrogen ions and hydrogen carbonate ions, there would be a marked rise of hydrogen ions in the red blood cell and consequent disruption of its function. However, haemoglobin reacts with carbonic acid forming potassium hydrogen carbonate and reduced haemoglobin:

$$\underset{\substack{\text{carbonic}\\\text{acid}}}{H_2CO_3} + \underset{\substack{\text{potassium}\\\text{haemoglobin}}}{KHb} \rightleftharpoons \underset{\substack{\text{reduced}\\\text{haemoglobin}}}{HHb} + \underset{\substack{\text{potassium}\\\text{hydrogen}\\\text{carbonate}}}{KHCO_3}$$

Reduced haemoglobin acts as a much weaker acid than carbonic acid and therefore binds its hydrogen more tightly, preventing a rise in hydrogen ion concentration.

As the blood passes through the lungs, carbon dioxide is released into alveolar air. Potentially, this could result in a marked decrease of hydrogen ion concentration in the blood, because the reaction:

$$H^+ + HCO_3^- \rightleftharpoons H_2CO_3 \rightleftharpoons H_2O + CO_2$$

is driven to the right by the continuous excretion of carbon dioxide. However, under these circumstances some of the reduced haemoglobin dissociates to release hydrogen ions, thereby maintaining a constant level of carbonic acid (and hence hydrogen ions) in the blood:

$$HHb + KHCO_3 \rightleftharpoons KHb + H_2CO_3$$

In addition, this 'releases' the potassium haemoglobin to buffer more hydrogen ions when the blood passes through the tissues again. The efficiency of this buffer system depends on alveolar ventilation being regulated according to body needs, so that only the correct amount of carbon dioxide is excreted at any given time.

## The carbonic-acid–hydrogen-carbonate system

Although carbonic acid is a stronger acid than reduced haemoglobin, it is still considerably weaker than many of the acids ingested or produced by the body during metabolism. Consequently, together with its salts, potassium and sodium hydrogen carbonate (bicarbonate), it can buffer acid produced during metabolism, ingested in the diet or released in diabetes. In addition, the hydrogen carbonate ion has the advantage that, because it can be converted to carbonic acid and then excreted as carbon dioxide and water, any excess acid can be removed from the body, providing ventilation can be adjusted adequately.

If excess hydrogen ions are added to the body, e.g. lactic acid formed during exercise, the hydrogen carbonate ions will 'mop up' excess hydrogen ions to form carbonic acid and a neutral salt. The carbonic acid can then be prevented from releasing any of *its* hydrogen ions by the action of the haemoglobin buffering system, i.e:

$$H_2CO_3 + KHb \rightleftharpoons HHb + KHCO_3$$

Once the blood reaches the lung, these reactions are reversed, so that the hydrogen carbonate ions are converted into carbonic acid, resulting in excretion of carbon dioxide and production of water. However, to do this, ventilation must be increased above normal levels and the additional excretion of carbon dioxide (which came not from the tissues but from the 'pool' of hydrogen carbonate ions in the blood) will result in a reduction in blood hydrogen carbonate ions (base deficit) and a temporary reduction in its buffering power. Although the level of blood hydrogen carbonate ions is initially affected by dietary intake, secondary changes may occur as a result of its role as a buffer. The numbers of hydrogen carbonate ions will decrease if additional hydrogen ions are added to the blood or if hyperventilation occurs resulting in excessive loss of carbon dioxide and water from the body. The hydrogen carbonate ion concentration will rise if there is retention of carbon dioxide or any loss of hydrogen ions.

The level of hydrogen carbonate ions (which is ultimately regulated by the kidney) plays a vital role in maintaining blood pH at its normal level. The ratio of hydrogen carbonate ions to carbonic acid must be maintained at 20 : 1 if the pH of the blood is to remain at 7.4. The $PCO_2$ of blood determines the amount of carbonic acid (i.e. dissolved carbon dioxide).

The way in which blood pH is determined by the ratio of bicarbonate to dissolved carbon dioxide (i.e. base to acid) can be demonstrated by the **Henderson–Hasselbach** equation, which states:

$$blood\ pH = 6.1 + \log\left(\frac{[hydrogen\ carbonate]}{[CO_2\ in\ solution]}\right)$$

The numeral '6.1' merely represents a logarithmic constant describing the degree to which carbonic acid dissociates into hydrogen carbonate ions and hydrogen ions (i.e. how 'strong' an acid it is). Logarithms are used on the right-hand side of the equation to allow for the fact that the concentration of hydrogen ions on the left is expressed logarithmically (i.e. as pH). At a normal arterial $PCO_2$ of 5.3 kPa (40 mmHg), there are usually 26 mmol/L of hydrogen carbonate ions and 1.3 mmol/L of dissolved carbon dioxide, resulting in a hydrogen carbonate : carbonic acid ratio of 20 : 1:

$$pH = 6.1 + \log\frac{26}{1.3}$$
$$= 6.1 + \log 20$$
$$= 6.1 + 1.3$$
$$= 7.4$$

Any increase in hydrogen carbonate ions or fall in carbonic acid (i.e. $PCO_2$) will cause an increase in the ratio and a rise in pH (i.e. increased alkalinity of the blood, or alkalosis). Conversely, any reduction in the ratio, whether by a fall in hydrogen carbonate ions or a rise in $PCO_2$, will decrease pH (increased acidity of the blood, known as acidosis).

The buffer systems in the blood provide a highly efficient mechanism for responding to immediate changes in hydrogen ion concentration and help prevent any marked fluctuations in pH despite the variations in intake or production of acids in the body. However, they are a temporary expedient, and can only continue to function if there is some means by which excess acid or base can be excreted from the body. The two organs most active in this capacity are the lungs as described below, and the kidneys, which function in more long-term control (see Chapter 5.4).

## The role of the respiratory system

The respiratory system plays a vital role in maintaining blood pH in that alveolar ventilation is normally adjusted very precisely to the level of $PCO_2$ and hydrogen ion concentration in arterial blood (see Control of ventilation, p. 578).

Any increase in $PCO_2$ or hydrogen ion concentration, and hence fall in pH, is sensed by central and peripheral chemoreceptors and results in a rapid increase in alveolar ventilation, thus speeding the reaction:

$$H^+ + HCO_3^- \rightarrow H_2CO_3 \rightarrow CO_2 + H_2O$$

which causes an increased excretion of carbon dioxide and hydrogen ions from the blood. By contrast, any fall in the level of $PCO_2$ or hydrogen ion concentration depresses the respiratory drive. In this way, the respiratory system, acting with the blood buffers, normally provides a highly efficient mechanism for maintaining blood pH within a narrow range in response to short-term changes.

However, the overall increase or decrease in hydrogen carbonate ion concentration resulting from such changes in the level of alveolar ventilation has to be compensated for by the kidney. The role of renal control also assumes great importance in the presence of respiratory disease when alveolar ventilation cannot be increased sufficiently to excrete excess carbon dioxide. Renal control of acid–base balance and acid–base disturbances is described in Chapter 5.4.

## DEVELOPMENTAL ISSUES

The airways of the lung begin their development at about 3–4 weeks postfertilization as an outgrowth from the foregut lined by epithelium of endodermal origin. This outgrowth (called the laryngotracheal bud) appears just behind the pharynx, and differentiates over the next 4 weeks into the future larynx, glottis and trachea. The distal portion divides into two lung buds. These become invested with mesenchyme and subsequently differentiate to form the airways, cartilage, muscle, blood vessels, lymphatics and other connective tissue elements of the lungs and bronchial tree.

As the lung buds develop, they divide first to form two branches on the left and three on the right, i.e. the five-lobed pattern typical of the human lung. As hollow bronchial tubes branch and branch again, the numerous blind-ended tubules give the lung the pseudoglandular appearance that characterizes the first embryonic phase. Following the embryonic phase in humans, three phases of lung development can be recognized:

- **Pseudoglandular,** during which the preacinar branching pattern of the airways is established.
- **Canalicular,** when vascularization of the mesenchyme rapidly increases and the

respiratory portion of the lung begins to develop.
- **Terminal sac or alveolar,** when additional respiratory bronchioles develop and there is differentiation of the future respiratory units into a single terminal bronchiole, with its respiratory bronchioles, alveolar ducts and alveoli.

The adult pattern of airway branching is complete by weeks 16–18 of gestational age and the fetal airway mucosa is functional by 24 weeks gestation. However, primitive alveolar development does not commence until about 20 weeks gestation and there is rarely sufficient surfactant production to establish a stable lung volume before 28–32 weeks gestation. There is continuing rapid growth and multiplication of the alveoli throughout the first few years of life.

## CONGENITAL ANOMALIES

The most common congenital anomalies of the respiratory system include:

- **tracheo-oesophageal fistula:** communication between trachea and oesophagus, often associated with oesophageal atresia
- **tracheomalacia:** congenital absence or weakness of the tracheal cartilagenous rings resulting in functional tracheal stenosis (narrowing) or obstruction
- **bronchomalacia:** weakness/absence of bronchial cartilagenous rings resulting in narrowing of the bronchi, often associated with abnormal lobar distension due to gas trapping, i.e. **congenital lobar emphysema**
- **congenital diaphragmatic hernia:** represents 8% of all major congenital anomolies and is left-sided in approximately 90% of cases. There is usually reduced lung growth on the affected side resulting from severe compression of the developing lung by the abdominal contents
- **congenital pulmonary hypoplasia:** characterized by a reduced number of peripheral airways with relatively few, poorly differentiated alveoli, and may not be compatible with life. Pulmonary hypoplasia is frequently associated with a reduction in amniotic fluid due to accompanying anomalies of the fetal renal system or prolonged rupture of membranes.

## THE INFLUENCE OF AGE ON THE RESPIRATORY SYSTEM

The respiratory system of the newborn infant is not simply a miniaturized version of that found later in life. Changes in the relationship between the lungs and thoracic cage throughout life may

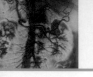

at least partially explain the increased vulnerability of the very young (and the very old) to respiratory infections (Stocks, 1995).

As explained previously, resting lung volume is normally determined by the balance between the tendency of the lung to recoil inwards and that of the chest to recoil outwards, a negative pleural (distending) pressure developing in the pleural space between the two. In infants, the chest wall is much more compliant (floppy) than in older subjects and hence exerts far less traction on the lung (i.e. transpulmonary pressure at end-expiration is less negative than in an adult). This allows the lung to deflate to a lower lung volume, where peripheral airway function and gas exchange may be impaired.

These low distending pressures and the subsequent tendency for the small airways to close, combined with the absolute small diameter of the airways, render the infant and small child very vulnerable to airway obstruction. Indeed, certain viruses that cause little more than inconvenience to the older child and adult can produce life-threatening events in the young infant (e.g. bronchiolitis). The low recoil of the rib cage also influences its stability and allows it to distort more readily (i.e. chest wall recession) in the presence of any airway obstruction or lung stiffening. This in turn greatly decreases efficiency and increases the work of breathing (Papastamelos, 1995).

Growth of the lung occurs as a result of both increase in size and number of alveoli during the first few years of life. However, the adult complement of approximately 300 million alveoli is normally achieved by 2–4 years of age, subsequent lung growth being achieved purely by increase in alveolar size. Lung growth ceases at about 16 years of age in girls whereas in boys it may continue until about 20–25 years. Although there are well described sex differences for respiratory function, these only become markedly apparent after puberty, with males having relatively greater static lung volumes, respiratory muscle strength and spirometric values thereafter. The significant functional advantages that boys gain during this rapid period of growth and development may in part explain clinical observations that boys with chronic lung disease (e.g. cystic fibrosis, asthma) tend to fare better than girls during and after puberty.

The relatively low transpulmonary pressures distending the resting lung volume in infants are also found in older people. However, in the latter, this is not due to a floppy chest wall, which becomes increasingly rigid with age, but a gradual increase in lung compliance as the airways and alveoli become less elastic due to gradual destruction of the tissues. As a result there is an increase in residual volume and functional residual capacity but a decrease in vital capacity. The latter may be reduced by as much as 35% in a 70-year-old compared with a healthy 30-year-old. This process is accelerated by increased exposure to environmental pollutants, such as tobacco smoke. Although some decrease in respiratory performance can be expected in old age, cigarette smoking accelerates this; the decline in expiratory airflow slows when smoking ceases to the rate of a non-smoker, although the lost function is never recovered.

Accompanying the changes in lung elasticity (see Emphysema, p. 559), there is a gradual decrease in blood levels of oxygen, diminished ciliary action of the respiratory epithelial lining and decreased activity of the alveolar macrophages. The combination of these age-related factors, together with a gradual reduction in mobility and exercise, all contribute to the increased susceptibility of older people to bronchitis, emphysema, pneumonia and other respiratory disorders.

## Conclusion

In conclusion, the complexity of the human respiratory system arises from the fact that, although energy production is accomplished by every cell of the body, oxygen cannot diffuse efficiently across skin, tissue and bone to reach all the cells of an individual in the quantities required. Consequently, oxygen must be transported to the cells in the blood, which also carries away the waste products of metabolism – carbon dioxide and water. Hence the lungs are several steps away from the process of cellular respiration. Nevertheless, the unique relationship between the structure and function of the respiratory system, together with the way in which the various processes such as ventilation, perfusion and cardiac output are regulated, ensure that the cardiopulmonary system can respond almost instantaneously to enormous increases in the demand for oxygen above basal metabolic rates. These processes not only provide adequate exchange of oxygen and carbon dioxide to meet the ever-changing needs of the human body, but help regulate the acidity of body fluids and hence maintain homeostasis.

In health, the efficiency of the respiratory system is such that breathing remains a largely subconscious activity. Nevertheless, the lungs are the only internal organ in direct communication with the external environment and as such, are easily damaged. Currently, over one million people in the United Kingdom live with some form of lung disease and respiratory disease remains a major cause of morbidity and mortality, especially in the first year of life and in the elderly.

Despite its complexities, the study of respiratory physiology is fundamental, not only to understanding how our own bodies work but also to improving the care, treatment and ultimately the prevention of the numerous respiratory diseases that currently cause so much suffering and reduced quality of life.

## Clinical review

In addition to the Learning Objectives at the beginning of this chapter the reader should be able to:

- Assess an individual's respiratory status and recognize the significance of these observations
- Describe how a pneumothorax might occur and the principles of treatment for this condition
- Discuss the importance of even distribution of gas and blood flow through the lungs and describe the causes and effects of ventilation–perfusion imbalance
- Describe methods commonly used to assess lung function
- List causes of inspiratory failure
- Enumerate the causes of hypoxia and hypocapnia
- Explain why infants and elderly people are particularly vulnerable to respiratory infections

## Review questions

1. What are the two phases of respiration?
2. Describe the position and structure of the trachea
3. What are the defence mechanisms of the respiratory tract?
4. What happens to intrapleural pressure during inspiration?
5. Outline the events leading to inspiration
6. What happens to the diaphragm during inspiration?
7. When are the accessory muscles of respiration used?
8. What is the dead space?
9. How do gases move between the alveoli and the blood?
10. How do the blood pressures in the pulmonary circulation differ from those in the systemic circulation?
11. What are the consequences of the shape of the oxygen–haemoglobin dissociation curve?
12. What are the consequences of shifting the oxygen–haemoglobin dissociation curve to the right?
13. Which enzyme catalyses the synthesis of carbonic acid?
14. What does the chloride shift achieve?
15. Why is cortical control of breathing necessary?
16. Why is it necessary to regulate the concentration of hydrogen ions?

## Suggestions for further reading

Bourke, S.J. (2003) *Lecture Notes on Respiratory Medicine*, 6th edn. Oxford: Blackwell Publishing.
*Provides a good introduction to the essentials of respiratory medicine.*

Casey, G. (2001) Oxygen transport and the use of pulse oximetry. *Nursing Standard*, **15**(47); 46–53.
*An up-to-date and readable article on pulse oximetry.*

Chernick, V. & Kendig, E.I. (eds) (1999) *Kendig's Disorders of the Respiratory Tract in Children*, 2nd edn. Philadephia: W.B. Saunders.
*A large, expensive but comprehensive textbook covering all aspects of infectious and non-infectious respiratory diseases in infants and children.*

Esmound, G. (2001) *Respiratory Nursing*. Edinburgh: Bailière Tindall.
*Provides a good insight into key issues relating to the care and management of people with respiratory disease.*

Fox, V.J (1996) Thoracic surgery. In: Rothrock, J.C. (ed) *Perioperative Nursing Care Planning*, 2nd edn. St. Louis: C.V. Mosby.
*A chapter (ch. 15) on thoracic surgery within a manual designed for use by nurses involved in perioperative care, which provides guidelines on patient assessments, common perioperative problems, nursing diagnoses and interventions, and methods of evaluating nursing care.*

Jevon, P. (2000) Measuring peak expiratory flow. *Nursing Times*, **96**(38); 49–50.
*An up-to-date and readable article on peak flow.*

Jevon, P. & Ewens, B. (2001) Assessment of the breathless patient. *Nursing Standard*, **15**(16); 48–53.
*An up-to-date and readable article on assessment of respiratory function.*

McAllister, J. (2002) Chronic obstructive pulmonary disease: Foundation. *Nursing Times*, **98**(35); 41–44.

McAllister, J. (2002) Chronic obstructive pulmonary disease: diagnosis and assessment. *Nursing Times*, **98**(36); 27–30.

McAllister, J. (2002) Chronic obstructive pulmonary disease: Nursing care and implications for nursing. *Nursing Times*, **98**(37); 43–46.
*A series of three very readable articles on chronic obstructive pulmonary disease (COPD).*

Murray, J.F. (1986) *The Normal Lung*. Philadelphia: W.B. Saunders.
*A medium-sized, readable textbook on respiratory physiology.*

Shuldham, C. (ed) (1998) *Cardiorespiratory Nursing*. London: Stanley Thomas.
*A comprehensive text addressing key aspects of respiratory care from a nursing perspective.*

West, J.B. (2003) *Respiratory Physiology – The Essentials*, 7th edn. Baltimore: Lippincott, Williams and Wilkins.
*A popular paperback textbook covering all aspects of respiratory physiology.*

West, J.B. (2003) *Pulmonary Pathophysiology – The Essentials*, 6th edn. Baltimore: Williams and Wilkins.
*The accompanying volume to West's Respiratory Physiology dealing with the pathophysiology of a wide range of respiratory diseases.*

## Useful websites

The British Thoracic Society: www.brit-thoracic.org
*Has details of guidelines for the management of a range of respiratory conditions as well as those already cited in this chapter.*

Lung and asthma information agency: www.sghms.ac.uk/depts/laia.htm
British Lung Foundation: www.lunguk.org/index.htm
Asthma UK: www.asthma.org.uk/

## References

American Thoracic Society/European Respiratory Society (1993) Respiratory mechanics in infants: Physiologic evaluation in health and disease. *American Review of Respiratory Diseases*, **147**; 474–496.

Bateman, N.T. & Leach, A.M. (1998) Acute oxygen therapy. *British Medical Journal*, **317**; 798–801.

Bellone, A., Lasoli, R., Rashi, S., Guzzi, L. & Adone, R. (2000) Chest physical therapy in patients with acute exacerbation of chronic bronchitis: Effectiveness of three methods. *Archives of Physical Medicine and Rehabilitation*, **81**; 558–560.

British Thoracic Society/Scottish Intercollegiate Guidelines Network (2003) British & guidelines on the management of asthma. *Thorax*, **58**; Supplement V, 1–79.

Byard, R.W. (1991) Possible mechanisms responsible for the sudden infant death syndrome. *Journal of Paediatrics and Child Health*, **27**; 147–157.

Chandler, T. (2002) Croup. *Paediatric Nursing*, **14**; 41–48.

Clark, J.S., Votteri, B., Ariagno, R.L. et al. (1992) Noninvasive assessment of blood gases. *American Review of Respiratory Diseases*, **145**; 220–232.

Clark, R.H. (1996) High-frequency ventilation. *Journal of Pediatrics*, **124**; 661–670.

Cowell, R. & Hopkins, S. (1991) Neonatal EMCO. *Nursing Times*, **87**; 36–37.

Department of Health (1993) *Report of the Chief Medical Officer's Expert Group on The Sleeping Position of Infants and Cot Death*. London: HMSO, pp. 1–113.

Department of Health (2000) *Reduce Risk of Cot Death*. London: HMSO.

Duffin, J. (1990) The chemoreflex control of breathing and its measurement. *Canadian Journal of Anaesthesia*, **36**; 933–942.

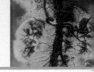

Dwyer, T., Ponsonby, A.L.B., Newman, N.M. & Gibbons, L.E. (1991) Prospective cohort study of prone sleeping position and sudden infant death syndrome. *Lancet*, **337**; 1244–1247.

Ehrenkranz, R.A. & Mercurio, M.R. (1992) Bronchopulmonary dysplasia. In: Sinclair, J.C. & Bracken, M.B. (eds) *Effective Care of the Newborn Infant*. Oxford: Oxford University Press, pp. 399–424.

Fink, J.B. (2002) Positioning versus postural drainage. *Respiratory Care*, **47**; 769–777.

Fleming, P.J., Gilbert, R., Azaz, Y. et al. (1990) Interaction between bedding and sleeping position in the sudden infant death syndrome: A population base case-control study. *British Medical Journal*, **301**; 85–89.

Gaultier, C. (1995) Cardiorespiratory adaptation during sleep in infants and children. *Pediatric Pulmonology* **19**(2); 105–117.

Gift, A.G. (1993) Therapies for dyspnoea relief. *Holistic Nursing Practice*, **7**; 57–63.

Greenough, A. (1997) Replacement surfactant therapy. *Professional Care Mother and Child*, **7**; 99–100.

Hancox, B. (2001) *Pocket Guide to Lung Function Tests*. Sydney: McGraw-Hill.

Hough, A. (1992) Making sense of sputum retention. *Nursing Times*, **88**(36); 33–35.

Landau, L.I. (1990) New diagnostic approaches to lung disease. *Current Opinions in Pediatrics*, **2**; 487–494.

Law, C. (2000) A guide to assessing sputum. *Nursing Times NTPlus Supplement*, **96**; 7–10.

Lebowitz, M.D. (1991) The use of peak expiratory flow rate measurements in respiratory disease. *Pediatric Pulmonology*, **11**; 166–174.

Marini, J.J. (1991) Assessment of the breathing workload during mechanical ventilation. In: Benito, S. & Net, A. (eds) *Pulmonary Function in Mechanically Ventilated Patients* (*Update in intensive care and emergency medicine 13*). Berlin: Springer-Verlag, pp. 62–80.

Martinez, F.D., Morgan, W.J., Wright, A.L. et al. (1991) Initial airway function is a risk factor for recurrent wheezing respiratory illnesses during the first three years of life. *American Review of Respiratory Diseases*, **143**; 312–316.

Murray, J.F. (1986) *The Normal Lung*, 2nd edn. Philadelphia: W.B. Saunders.

Papastamelos, C., Panitch, H.B., England, S.E. & Allen, J.L. (1995) Developmental changes in chest wall compliance in infancy and early childhood. *Journal of Applied Physiology*, **78**; 179–184.

Platt, M. & Pharoah, P. (2003) The epidemiology of sudden infant death syndrome. *Archive of Diseases in Children*, **88**(1); 27–29.

Royal College of Physicians (1992) *Smoking and the Young. A Report of a Working Party of the Royal College of Physicians*. London: Royal College of Physicians.

Scottish Intercollegiate Guidelines Network (SIGN) (2003a) British Guidelines on Management of Asthma. *Thorax*, **58**; Supplement V.

Scottish Intercollegiate Guidelines Network (SIGN) (2003b) *Management of Obstuctive Sleep Apnoea/Hyperapnoea Syndrome in Adults. A national clinical guideline*. Edinburgh: Scottish Intercollegiate Guidelines Network.

Stocks, J. (1993) Assessment of lung function in infants. *Perfusion*, **8**; 71–80.

Stocks, J. (1995) Developmental physiology and methodology. In: Silverman and Taussing: 'Early Childhood Asthma'. *American Journal of Respiratory and Critical Care Medicine*, **151**; S15–S17.

Tager, I.B., Hanrahan, J.P., Tosteson, T.D. et al. (1993) Lung function, pre- and post-natal smoke exposure, and wheezing in the first year of life. *American Review of Respiratory Diseases*, **147**; 811–817.

Weg, J.G. & Haas, C.F. (1998) Long-term oxygen therapy for COPD. *Postgraduate Medicine*, **103**.

West, J.B. (1985) *Respiratory Physiology – The Essentials*. Baltimore: Williams & Wilkins.

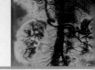

# Renal function

*Susan M. McLaren*

## LEARNING OBJECTIVES

After studying this chapter the reader should be able to:

- Describe the anatomical features of the kidney and lower urinary tract
- List the functions of the kidneys in humans
- Review the regional structures and mechanisms that subserve filtration, reabsorption and secretion in the nephron
- Discuss the mechanisms involved in the formation of concentrated and dilute urine

- Describe the major influences in the regulation of body water, sodium and potassium balance
- Discuss the role of the kidney in the regulation of acid–base balance
- Describe the process of micturition
- Describe the volume and composition of the body fluid compartments and explain how major imbalances can arise

## INTRODUCTION

The kidney is an organ that fulfils a vital role in maintaining the volume and composition of the body fluids and is thus a major regulator of the internal environment; indeed, it is frequently referred to as 'the ultimate regulator of homeostasis'.

In this chapter, the physiological mechanisms which subserve normal renal function, and thus homeostasis, are examined. Consideration is also given to the problems that arise when normal renal mechanisms are altered by disease.

## Gross anatomy of the kidney

In humans, the kidneys are paired, compact organs that lie one on either side of the vertebral column at the level of the 12th thoracic to the 3rd lumbar vertebrae. Situated behind the peritoneum, they are attached by adipose tissue to the posterior abdominal wall.

Supporting connective tissue covers the anterior surfaces of each kidney, renal blood vessels, aorta and the adrenal glands. **Figure 5.4.1** represents a coronal section of the kidney and upper ureter. Each kidney is covered by an external capsule of fibrous connective tissue. Renal arteries, veins, lymphatics and nerves enter and leave at a medial indentation known as the **hilum**. Also entering at the hilum is the funnel-shaped upper end of the ureter, which expands to form an internal cavity known as the **renal pelvis**. Beneath the capsule lie two distinct areas of tissue, the outer **cortex** and inner **medulla**. The medulla consists of 8–18 wedge-shaped tracts of tissue known as the **medullary pyramids**. At the tips of these medullary pyramids, papillary tissue projects into minor **calyces**, which are hollow projections of the renal pelvis. Urine draining from tiny ducts in the papillary tissue passes from the minor into the major calyces, finally reaching the renal pelvis where the lining of transitional

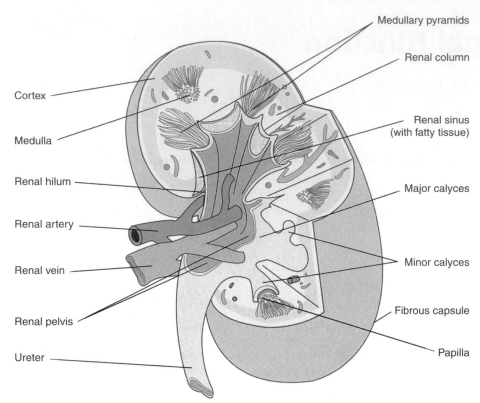

Cortex

Medulla

Renal hilum

Renal artery

Renal vein

Renal pelvis

Ureter

Medullary pyramids

Renal column

Renal sinus
(with fatty tissue)

Major calyces

Minor calyces

Fibrous capsule

Papilla

**Figure 5.4.1**  Anatomy of the kidney

epithelium distends to accommodate it. Contractions of the smooth muscle in the walls of the calyces and pelvis propel urine downwards into the ureter.

## The nephron

Each kidney contains approximately 1–1.5 million nephrons. Each nephron consists of a tuft of blood vessel, the **glomerulus**, within the invagination of a tubule 6 cm long, lined throughout by a columnar epithelium (**Fig. 5.4.2**). Five anatomically distinct regions can be distinguished in the tubule of each nephron: Bowman's capsule, the proximal convoluted tubule, the loop of Henlé, the distal convoluted tubule and the collecting ducts.

### The glomerulus and Bowman's capsule

Bowman's capsule forms the spherical, dilated upper end of the tubule that surrounds the glomerulus; the entire structure is only 150 nm in diameter. All glomeruli lie in the cortex and originate from an afferent arteriole. They give rise to an efferent arteriole that branches (on leaving Bowman's capsule) into a dense capillary network surrounding the renal tubule.

Total glomerular capillary surface area is vast, at 5000–15 000 cm²/100 g tissue. Research suggests that the glomerular capillaries are one hundred times more permeable to water and solutes than extrarenal capillaries and that they contain 'pores' of 75–100 nm diameter. The capillary endothelium rests on a basement membrane, on the other side of which rests the epithelium lining Bowman's capsule. A wealth of electron microscopy evidence has confirmed that this epithelium has a unique, podocytic architecture (Greek *podus* = foot), that is to say, the cells are elongated and divide towards the base to form pedicels (foot processes) which rest on the basement membrane (Pavenstädt et al., 2002). A well-developed cytoskeleton supports the cell body and foot processes, with an actin-based contractile system present in the latter. Foot processes of adjacent podocytes interdigitate and are separated by filtration slits 30–40 nm wide. Fine diaphragms containing rectangular pores 4 × 14 nm, which permit fluid flow, appear to bridge the filtration slits. The protein nephrin is a vital structural component of the slit diaphragm and must be intact for normal glomerular filtration to take place. Congenital or acquired abnormality or absence of nephrin can contribute to extensive proteinuria (Tryggvason & Wartiovaara, 2001). The entire structure, comprising the capillary endothelium, basement membrane and podocytic epithelium, constitutes the selective filtration barrier, as shown in **Fig. 5.4.3**.

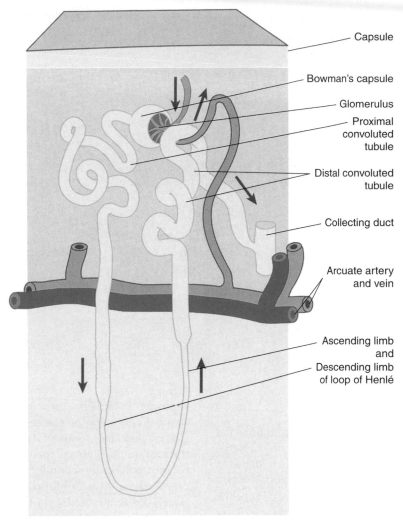

**Figure 5.4.2** Microanatomy of nephron

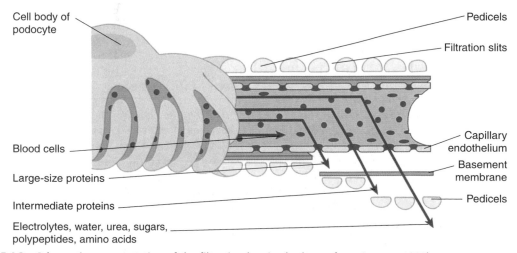

**Figure 5.4.3** Schematic representation of the filtration barrier (redrawn from Creager, 1983)

## The proximal convoluted tubule

Following Bowman's capsule, the proximal convoluted tubule extends for a length of 12–24 mm through the cortex. This region is 50–65 nm in diameter and lined by large columnar epithelial cells, which are modified on the internal surface to form a brush border of microvilli, which increases the surface area inside the proximal tubule where most of the solute reabsorption takes place.

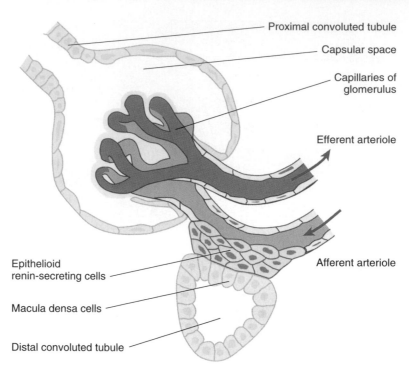

**Figure 5.4.4** Anatomy of a renal corpuscle

## The loop of Henlé

Extending from the proximal convoluted tubule, the thin-walled descending limb of the loop of Henlé moves down into the medulla and then makes a U-turn, moving back into the cortex via a thicker-walled ascending limb. In both limbs of Henlé's loop, the columnar cells are flatter and they contain fewer microvilli on the internal (luminal) surfaces.

## The distal nephron

The ascending limb of the loop of Henlé leads into the distal convoluted tubule, the first part of which folds back in proximity to the afferent arteriole, where it forms a region known as the **macula densa** (**Fig. 5.4.4**). Specialized epithelial cells of the macula densa monitor the sodium chloride concentration of fluid flowing through this area and comprise part of the juxtaglomerular apparatus.

The distal convoluted tubule is comparatively short (4–8 mm) and leads into the collecting ducts, which join together as they move through the medulla, finally opening at the tips of medullary papillae into the calyces of the renal pelvis.

## Cortical and juxtamedullary nephrons

Two types of nephron are present: superficial cortical nephrons and juxtamedullary nephrons. Comprising seven-eighths of the total, cortical nephrons lie in the superficial areas of the cortex. The juxtamedullary

nephrons, comprising only one-eighth of the total, lie in deeper areas of the cortex. They have larger glomeruli, longer loops of Henlé with a thin and thick ascending limb and their efferent arterioles give rise not only to the peritubular network previously described but also to looped capillaries, which lie closely alongside the loop of Henlé, known as the **vasa recta**. Current evidence suggests that the renal medullary circulation encompassing the vasa recta and associated capillary network, is important in the control of sodium excretion and blood pressure (Mattson, 2003) (see p. 617).

## Renal blood supply

Twenty-five per cent of the cardiac output is delivered to the kidneys each minute. In terms of blood flow rate, this is 400 mL/min/100 g at rest, higher than that of any other tissue.

The two renal arteries arise from either side of the abdominal aorta, enter at the hilum and divide in the renal tissue to form interlobar arteries between the pyramids (**Fig. 5.4.5**). Arcuate arteries arising from these give rise to cortical interlobar arteries, which branch and ultimately give rise to afferent arterioles supplying each glomerulus.

Efferent arterioles emerging from the glomerulus form a dense peritubular capillary network. Venous plexi drain this capillary bed around the tubule, delivering venous blood via the inter lobular, arcuate and interlobar veins to the renal vein. A renal vein

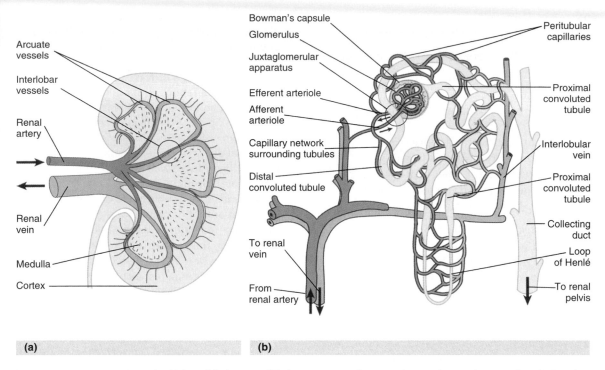

**Figure 5.4.5** Cross-section of a kidney (a) showing (b) the anatomy of a juxtaglomerular nephron with associated blood vessels

leaving the hilum returns venous blood to the inferior vena cava.

## Renal nerve supply

The kidneys are richly innervated by sympathetic nerve fibres (see Chapter 2.4). A few parasympathetic fibres are also present. Sympathetic nerve fibres supply the smooth muscle of the arterioles and the juxtaglomerular apparatus. Stimulation of these nerves brings about vasoconstriction, reduced renal blood flow, a reduced glomerular filtration rate and the release of renin from the juxtaglomerular apparatus.

In addition, the kidney is supplied with afferent nerve fibres that mediate the sensation of pain. Stimulation of these fibres occurs when the renal capsule is distended, such as may be caused by bleeding, inflammation associated with glomerulonephritis or pyelonephritis, and obstruction by calculi. Ischaemia caused by renal artery occlusion may also stimulate the pain fibres.

## Juxtaglomerular apparatus

Two major cell types are found here (see Fig. 5.4.4):

- **Renin-secreting cells**, which are located in the wall of the afferent arteriole and are derived from smooth muscle cells.

- **Macula densa cells**, which are found in the epithelium lining the first part of the distal convoluted tubule. These cells monitor the sodium chloride concentration of fluid as it flows through this area of the nephron.

### DEVELOPMENTAL ISSUES

The embryological development of the kidney is closely related to that of the reproductive system (see Chapter 6.3). On approximately the twenty-third day of embryonic life, a cluster of mesoderm cells at the level of the ninth somite divide to form a solid nephrogenic cord. Subsequently, this develops a lumen, giving rise to the nephric duct, which opens into the cloaca of the embryo. At 5 weeks, a ureteric bud grows from the mesonephric duct, giving rise to the ureter, pelvis, calyces and collecting tubules of the kidney. The remainder of the kidney develops from the metanephrogenic cap, an area of mesoderm surrounding the bud. Vesicles form, extending to form nephrogenic tubules, one end of which fuses with the collecting tubules and the other forms the glomerulus. Initially, the developing kidney lies in the pelvis but gradually ascends and rotates to the loin as the ureteric bud lengthens. The renal artery forms at 3 months' gestation. The bladder is formed from the primitive urogenital sinus which lies above the mesonephric duct.

## Renal function

Four main functions are performed by the kidney:

1. Removal of the nitrogenous waste products of metabolism.
2. Regulation of acid–base and other electrolyte balances.
3. Maintenance of water balance.
4. Production of erythrogenin (renal erythropoietic factor; see Chapter 4.1) and the biologically active form of vitamin D (1,25-dihydroxycholecalciferol; see Chapter 2.5).

The first three of these functions are achieved by processes of ultrafiltration, reabsorption and secretion in the nephron. An ultrafiltrate of plasma is produced at the glomerulus. As this flows through regionally specialized areas of the nephron, water and vital solutes, including glucose, electrolytes, amino acids and vitamins, are conserved by reabsorption. Waste products of metabolism, including urea, creatinine, uric acid, sulphates and nitrates, remain in the filtrate. These, together with secreted metabolites, and water and electrolytes that are surplus to requirements, reach the terminal collecting ducts and renal pelvis as the excretory products, urine. This is finally conveyed via the ureter into the lower urinary tract for elimination.

In the adult, approximately 180 L of plasma are filtered each day by the kidneys; 99% of the water, glucose, sodium ions ($Na^+$), hydrogen carbonate ions ($HCO_3^-$), chloride ions ($Cl^-$) and amino acids filtered is subsequently reabsorbed in the nephrons. The final volume of urine produced each day by an adult in health is in the range 1–1.5 L, although its volume and composition vary depending on fluid intake, diet and extrarenal losses of water and electrolytes, for example in sweat and expired air. Over a 24-hour period, total fluid intake balances fluid output, as can be seen in **Table 5.4.1**.

Some of the properties and the composition of urine in a healthy adult are summarized in **Table 5.4.2**. The levels of protein and glucose listed are not detectable by routine methods of ward investigation. Normal urine is clear, with a pale yellow tinge caused by the presence of urochrome pigments.

### CLINICAL APPLICATIONS

A number of disorders are characterized by the presence of abnormal urinary constituents (Fletcher & Ayub, 2002). **Glomerulonephritis** and its sequel, the **nephrotic syndrome**, feature pathological changes in the glomeruli. Alterations in the permeability properties of the filtration barrier then result in **proteinuria**, which may be

so severe that hypoproteinaemic oedema is precipitated. **Glycosuria** is a characteristic feature of diabetes mellitus and bile pigments may appear in the urine in hepatic disorders when jaundice is present, imparting a brown coloration to the urine. Other variations in colour due to the presence of abnormal constituents include white (chyle, pus), pink or red (myoglobin, haemoglobin) and brown or black (levadopa, methyl dopa). Abnormal odours caused by metabolic changes or infection include sweet/fruity (ketones) and ammoniacal (bacterial infection).

'**Polyuria**' is the term used to describe a persistent output of urine that is greater than 2 L per day. In healthy individuals it can occur when a high fluid intake is in excess of body requirements. It may also be a feature of disorders such as diabetes mellitus, diabetes insipidus and early chronic renal failure. In all of these, the ability to form a concentrated urine in the nephron is impaired.

'**Oliguria**' is the term used to describe a urine output in the range 100–400 mL/24 hours; **anuria** is a range of 0–100 mL/24 hours. Both of these symptoms are caused by the reduced glomerular filtration rate that characterizes hypovolaemia and different stages of acute and chronic renal failure.

**Table 5.4.1** Water balance in an adult over a 24-hour period (from Valtin, 1979)

| Intake (mL/day) | | Output (mL/day) | |
| --- | --- | --- | --- |
| In oral fluids | 1500 | In urine | 1500 |
| In food | 1000 | In faeces | 200 |
| Water of metabolic oxidation | 500 | Insensible: skin lungs | 900 400 |
| Total | 3000 | | 3000 |
| *Recycling of gastrointestinal fluid* | | | |
| **Secreted** | | **Reabsorbed** | |
| Saliva | 1500 | | |
| Gastric juice | 2500 | | |
| Bile | 500 | | |
| Pancreatic juice | 700 | | |
| Intestinal juice | 3000 | | |
| Total | 8200 | | 8000 |
| Therefore, 200 mL lost in faeces | | | |

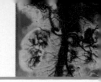

**Table 5.4.2** The composition of urine in an adult (from Valtin, 1979)

| | |
|---|---|
| pH | 5.0–6.0 |
| Osmolality | 500–800 mosmol |
| Specific gravity | 1.003–1.030 |
| Urea | 200–500 mmol/L |
| Creatinine | 9–17 mmol/L |
| Sodium ions | 50–130 mmol/L |
| Potassium ions | 20–70 mmol/L |
| Organic acids | 10–25 mmol/L |
| Protein | 0–50 mg/24 h |
| Urochrome | Traces |
| Glucose | 0–11 mmol/L |
| Cellular components (epithelial cells, leucocytes) | <20 000/L |

nephrotic syndromes, has identified structural areas of damage to the filtration barrier that could contribute to proteinuria. For example, in congenital nephrotic syndrome a defect in the protein nephrin, a component of the filtration slits occurs. This rare autosomal recessive disease is marked by nephrosis immediately after birth. In contrast, acquired minimal change nephrotic syndrome is marked by effacement of the foot processes of podocytes and partial loss of nephrin from the filtration slits (Tryggvason & Wartiovaara, 2001).

Haemoglobinuria may occur in nephrotic syndrome when red blood cells traverse the damaged filtration barrier, haemolysing in urine and releasing detectable amounts of haemoglobin. Alternatively, haemoglobin may be released from red blood cells if haemolysis occurs in the bloodstream as a result of haemolytic diseases or blood transfusion reactions. As haemoglobin has a relative molecular mass of 68 000, which is near the limits of pore size, it can cross the healthy filtration barrier in small quantities and appear in the urine.

## Glomerular filtration

Glomerular filtration is the first stage in urine production. Ultrafiltration of plasma takes place across the barrier of the glomerular endothelium, basement membrane and podocytic epithelium of Bowman's capsule into the intracapsular space. Blood cells are retained by the fenestrated glomerular endothelium and the basement membrane prevents the passage of larger plasma proteins. Finally, the diaphragms bridging filtration slits act as a fine filter impeding proteins the size of albumin or greater from entering the intracapsular space (Tryggvason & Wartiovaara, 2001). Overall, the selective permeability of the barrier prevents the filtration of blood cells and protein macromolecules with relative molecular mass greater than 70 000. In other respects, the filtrate has approximately the same solute concentrations, pH and osmolality as plasma. Very small amounts of albumin of relative molecular mass 69 000 are filtered each day.

**CLINICAL APPLICATIONS**

If the filtration barrier is damaged by diseases such as the nephrotic syndrome, or by trauma, then the effective 'pore' size may be increased and large molecules above relative molecular mass 70 000 may then appear in the urine, e.g. proteins (proteinuria, albuminuria) and red or white blood cells. Recent research on selected inherited and acquired forms of glomerulopathies leading to

**Fluid filters out of the glomeruli into Bowman's capsule because a pressure gradient exists between the two areas.** If a hydrostatic pressure difference exists across any porous membrane, water will flow across from the side of higher pressure to that of lower pressure, dragging with it molecules that are smaller than any pores in the membrane.

In effect, the forces involved in glomerular filtration are the forces that govern fluid exchanges between other systemic capillaries and tissues (see Chapter 4.2). Hydrostatic pressure in the glomerular capillary is the major force moving fluid out of the capillary. In lower mammals this has a value of approximately 45 mmHg, but it may be higher in humans. Two forces oppose movement of fluid from the capillary: the colloid osmotic pressure exerted by plasma proteins (25 mmHg) and the hydrostatic pressure in Bowman's space (10 mmHg). The net ultrafiltration pressure is therefore low:

$$45 - (25 + 10\,\text{mmHg}) = 10\,\text{mmHg}$$

In addition to their unique permeability characteristics, other important differences exist between glomerular and systemic capillaries.

Due to the movement of fluid exclusively *out* of glomerular capillaries, the oncotic pressure rises along the length of the capillary until it equals the hydrostatic pressure. At this point no further filtration can take place, i.e. filtration equilibrium is reached. This factor limits the fraction of plasma filtered to one-fifth (120 mL) of the total 600 mL entering the glomerular capillaries per minute.

Hydrostatic pressure decreases only very slightly along the glomerular capillary length. It falls markedly in systemic capillaries.

As a consequence of these differences, note that in systemic capillaries the balance of forces favours a movement of fluid out at the arteriolar end and back at the venous end. In glomerular capillaries, fluid moves exclusively out and across the filtration barrier. **The glomerular filtration rate (GFR) is defined as the volume of plasma filtered through the glomeruli in 1 minute.** In health, the balance of forces in the glomerular capillaries limits the volume of plasma filtered to about 120 mL/min. However, as the glomerular filtration rate is decreased by acute or chronic renal and cardiovascular disorders, its measurement is used to assist in diagnosis, and to monitor the progression of such illnesses.

## Measurement of the glomerular filtration rate

To measure the glomerular filtration rate, it is necessary to estimate the renal clearance of a harmless chemical marker that is freely filtered by the glomerulus and is neither secreted nor reabsorbed in the nephron, i.e. the amount of marker that finally appears in the urine depends only on the rate at which it is filtered at the glomerulus. Furthermore, while the glomerular filtration rate is being measured, plasma concentrations of the marker must remain constant.

**Renal clearance** is defined as the volume of plasma from which the kidneys remove the marker in 1 minute. For such a marker, which is freely filtered and unmodified during its transit through the nephron, clearance is equal to the glomerular filtration rate.

The glomerular filtration rate is most conveniently and routinely estimated in humans by measuring the clearance of creatinine, an endproduct of muscle metabolism. Creatinine has the advantages of continuous internal production, and its plasma levels are virtually constant over a 24-hour period. Set against these are the disadvantages that 10–15% of urinary creatinine is secreted into the proximal convoluted tubule, which results in a tendency of this technique to overestimate glomerular filtration rate and the need for 24-hour collections of urine, which are often difficult to collect. The method for estimating creatinine clearance is as follows: urine is collected from the patient over a 24-hour period, during which time a blood sample is taken. Creatinine concentrations are then measured in both samples by routine biochemistry and the glomerular filtration rate is calculated from the urine volume excreted per minute ($V$), concentration of creatinine in mg/mL urine ($U$) and the plasma concentration of creatinine in mg/mL ($P$).

### Calculation of the glomerular filtration rate

For solutes such as creatinine, which are freely filtered at the glomerulus and neither secreted nor reabsorbed in the nephron, the amount filtered from the plasma must equal the amount that is excreted in the urine.

**Filtered creatinine**. The amount of creatinine filtered at the glomerulus depends on the glomerular filtration rate in mL/min and the plasma concentration of creatinine ($P$) in mg/mL, i.e.:

$$\text{creatinine filtered} = \text{GFR} \times P$$

**Excreted creatinine**. The amount of creatinine excreted depends on the urine flow rate ($V$) in mL/min and the urine concentration of creatinine ($U$) in mg/mL, i.e.:

$$\text{creatinine excreted} = U \times V$$

The amount of creatinine filtered from the plasma equals the amount excreted in the urine. Therefore:

$$\text{GFR} \times P = U \times V$$

and:

$$\text{GFR (mL/min)} = U \times V/P$$

As it varies with body size, the normal range of glomerular filtration rate in humans is expressed per 1.73 m$^2$ surface area. In view of the disadvantages associated with the estimation of glomerular filtration rate via creatinine clearance, a number of other approaches have been developed utilizing the plasma creatinine in combination with other important variables, e.g. age, gender, ethnicity, body weight (Manjunath et al., 2001).

## Regulation of renal blood flow and glomerular filtration rate

As described earlier, the hydrostatic blood pressure in the glomerulus is the main force that brings about the ultrafiltration of plasma, moving fluid out of the glomerular capillary across the filtration barrier and into Bowman's space. It would be logical to expect the hydrostatic pressure, and therefore the glomerular filtration rate, to vary directly according to changes in the arterial blood pressure. However, both remain fairly constant over a range of arterial systolic blood pressures, extending from 80 mmHg to 180 mmHg. How then is the glomerular hydrostatic pressure controlled and why does it, and the glomerular filtration rate, show such small changes when the arterial blood pressure varies over such a wide range?

Consider first the structure of the afferent and efferent arterioles supplying each glomerulus. A thin layer of smooth muscle, richly supplied with sympathetic nerve fibres, is present in the walls of these blood vessels. Acting like a sphincter, the degree of muscle contraction controls the diameter of the arterioles and

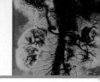

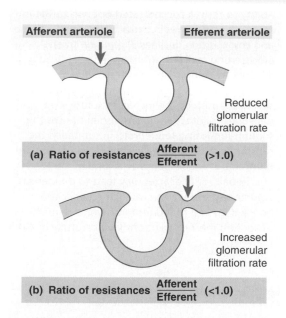

**Afferent arteriole**  **Efferent arteriole**

Reduced glomerular filtration rate

**(a) Ratio of resistances** $\dfrac{\text{Afferent}}{\text{Efferent}}$ **(>1.0)**

Increased glomerular filtration rate

**(b) Ratio of resistances** $\dfrac{\text{Afferent}}{\text{Efferent}}$ **(<1.0)**

**Figure 5.4.6** Changes in glomerular filtration brought about by altered resistance in arterioles

thereby the resistance to blood flow. If the afferent arteriole is constricted, glomerular hydrostatic pressure and glomerular filtration rate will decrease; whereas constriction of the efferent arteriole raises the glomerular hydrostatic pressure and glomerular filtration rate (**Fig. 5.4.6**).

A number of factors, including the following, are known to influence changes in the diameter of the afferent and efferent arterioles.

## Sympathetic nervous stimulation

**Sympathetic nerve fibres** supply the renal arterioles. Stimulation of these nerves in situations of emotional stress, pain, shock, haemorrhage and vigorous exercise causes constriction of the afferent arterioles, reducing the renal blood flow and glomerular filtration rate. In life-threatening situations, reduction in blood flow to the kidney makes additional blood available to perfuse such vital structures as the brain and heart.

In a healthy individual, resting in a supine position, the sympathetic nerves transmit few impulses to the renal blood vessels. Changes in posture, such as standing up, cause a transient pooling of blood in the veins and, as a result, the venous return and cardiac output decrease. To maintain the systemic blood pressure, this triggers a compensatory reflex response by the sympathetic nervous system, producing constriction of blood vessels supplying the skin and visceral organs including the kidney. Due to autoregulation, no changes in glomerular filtration rate accompany this alteration in renal blood flow. Autoregulatory mechanisms adjust the degree of constriction in the afferent/efferent arterioles such that

glomerular hydrostatic pressure and glomerular filtration rate remain stable.

**Angiotensin II** is a powerful vasoconstrictor produced following the release of the hormone renin from the juxtaglomerular apparatus in the kidney (see Chapter 2.5). Renal blood vessels are highly sensitive to the effect of angiotensin II, which causes constriction of the afferent arteriole and a decrease in the glomerular filtration rate. (In juxtamedullary nephrons, constriction of efferent arterioles results from angiotensin II.)

**Atrial natriuretic hormone (ANH)** opposes the effects of angiotensin II on vascular smooth muscle, producing vasodilation in systemic blood vessels. Atrial natriuretic hormone dilates the afferent arteriole, increasing glomerular filtration rate.

**Nitric oxide (NO)** is synthesized from L-arginine by at least three forms of the enzyme nitric oxide synthase; the different forms are present in different regions of the kidney. Nitric oxide synthesis is involved in the control of renal blood flow, glomerular filtration rate, tubular reabsorption and possibly in renin release. Nitric oxide causes vasodilation; reduction in its synthesis by enzyme inhibition reduces blood flow in the renal cortex and medulla (see p. 617 for a discussion of the impact of angiotensin II, atrial natriuretic hormone, nitric oxide and other factors on the regulation of medullary blood flow and sodium balance).

## Autoregulation

The kidney is able to regulate its own blood flow over a wide range of arterial blood pressures from 80 mmHg to 180 mmHg. This phenomenon is termed **autoregulation** and it has been shown to persist in isolated, perfused, denervated kidneys. It suggests that the kidney possesses internal mechanisms that maintain the glomerular filtration rate by altering the diameter of the afferent and efferent arterioles whenever the systemic blood pressure changes. One factor that appears to play an important role in autoregulation is prostaglandin $E_2$ ($PGE_2$). This is synthesized by interstitial cells in the renal medulla and has been shown to cause renal vasodilation, increasing renal blood flow and glomerular filtration rate. These effects oppose those of sympathetic nerve stimulation described earlier. It seems likely that prostaglandins and angiotensin II are only two of a number of factors probably involved in the phenomenon of autoregulation.

Autoregulation has its limitations and it does not sustain the renal blood flow and glomerular filtration rate when the sympathetic nerves are stimulated. Neither will it maintain the glomerular filtration rate during shock when the systolic blood pressure is less than 80 mmHg, which is outside the autoregulatory range.

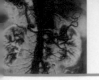

## DEVELOPMENTAL ISSUES

### AGE AND RENAL FUNCTION

At birth, the glomerular filtration rate is only 30 mL/min per m$^2$, and the volume of urine passed each day is only 20–50 mL. Although the glomerular filtration rate rises steadily afterwards as the infant matures, up to the age of 3 months the low glomerular filtration rate restricts the rate at which water can be excreted. This is one reason why babies are so vulnerable to circulatory overload and oedema when undergoing fluid replacement therapy.

At the other end of the spectrum, degenerative vascular changes associated with ageing lead to alterations in renal function. Histological evidence reveals marked subintimal thickening of renal arterioles and elastic reduplication of the tunica media, which narrows the vascular lumen. In addition, patchy areas of cortical atrophy are evident, marked by tubular degeneration, shrinkage of glomeruli and deposition of collagen inside Bowman's capsule. These changes may be exacerbated by the presence of vascular disease affecting the kidney.

Inevitably, structural degeneration results in altered renal perfusion, filtration and the ability to concentrate or dilute urine. In an 80-year-old person, the renal plasma flow has declined from 600 mL/min (the value in a young adult) to 300 mL/min, and the glomerular filtration rate has fallen by 50% to 60–70 (mL/min)/1.73 m$^2$. As a result of the decline in glomerular filtration rate, creatinine clearance also falls by 50% but the plasma creatinine concentration remains unchanged due to a diminution in muscle mass associated with ageing. Regional perfusion also alters in the ageing kidney; a relative fall in cortical blood flow is found while medullary flow is preserved. Reduction of glomerular filtration rate in older people must be taken into consideration when drugs that are excreted unchanged by the kidney are prescribed, e.g. digoxin and sulphonamides. Reduced excretion of a drug can lead to an elevation of its concentration in the plasma, increasing the likelihood of toxic effects. The same problem applies in the oliguric/anuric stages of renal failure. Therefore, for older patients, it may be necessary to reduce the dosage of these drugs to minimize the risk of toxicity. However, at both ends of the age spectrum, the changes in glomerular filtration rate usually only cause problems during illnesses that demand that the kidney responds rapidly in the excretion of water, electrolyte and acid or base loads.

Other dimensions of renal function are also impaired in old age. There is a fall in renal responsiveness to antidiuretic hormone and the ability to form a concentrated or dilute urine in response to changes in extracellular fluid volume and composition declines. Plasma renin and aldosterone concentrations are also reduced by 30–50% in older people, with a diminution in the ability to conserve sodium ions. A mild osmotic diuresis caused by the increased solute load delivered to intact nephrons also enhances the sodium-ion-losing tendencies. In summary, the responses of the kidney to sodium ion deficit are blunted but the response to a sodium ion load is also impaired. The latter may lead to dangerous volume expansion with vascular complications, hence the need to monitor intravenous infusions of sodium-ion-rich solutions very carefully in older patients.

## CLINICAL APPLICATIONS

### GLOMERULAR FILTRATION IN RENAL FAILURE

For most excretory products to be eliminated by the kidney, they must first be filtered. If the filtering mechanism is impaired by renal, ureteric or cardiovascular disorders, the ability of the kidney to excrete nitrogenous waste products and regulate water, electrolyte and acid–base balance will also be impaired. As a consequence of severely impaired filtration, the concentrations of excretory products in plasma (such as urea and creatinine) increase, precipitating uraemia, and the urine output falls. If during this time the individual is maintained on a normal dietary intake then the failure to excrete urea and fluid and electrolytes that are surplus to requirements produces serious problems. The severity of these problems depends on a number of factors:

- the extent to which the glomerular filtration rate is reduced
- the total number of functioning nephrons that remain
- whether it is possible to control the uraemia, fluid and electrolyte problems by limiting protein, fluid and electrolyte intake
- the temporary or permanent nature of the renal damage.

Unfortunately, overt symptoms of renal failure may not appear until the glomerular filtration rate has fallen below 30 mL/min, by which time the blood urea levels have quadrupled (normal 3.0–7.0 mmol/L) and the individual is uraemic and oliguric. One major consideration, then, is whether the uraemia can be controlled by limiting the protein intake or if alternative routes for the excretion of nitrogenous wastes must be provided by dialysis.

## ACUTE RENAL FAILURE

In acute renal failure there is an abrupt cessation of normal renal function, which in most cases is apparent as a drastic fall in the glomerular filtration rate. As a result, oliguria or anuria is present in the early stages, together with uraemia. Fortunately, the loss of renal function is frequently reversible. The reduction in glomerular filtration rate and resulting oliguria are brought about by various causes:

### Prerenal causes

- Reduced renal perfusion due to low cardiac output in shock, heart failure, severe dehydration and haemorrhage.
- Constriction of the afferent arteriole, which occurs in these emergency situations as an autonomic reflex response to divert blood to other vital organs.

Both the above factors reduce the glomerular hydrostatic pressure and thus the major force for glomerular filtration.

### Renal causes

- Tubular obstruction, which may be brought about by sloughing necrosis (acute tubular necrosis; ATN) of the epithelium lining the nephron due to ischaemic or toxic damage. This causes the hydrostatic pressure in Bowman's capsule to rise, reducing the glomerular filtration rate.
- Back leakage of filtered fluid through the damaged tubular epithelium may occur, causing oliguria.
- Constriction of the afferent arteriole by sympathetic nerve stimulation (see Prerenal causes).

If the cause is postrenal, the reduced glomerular filtration rate and oliguria are caused by an obstruction in the lower urinary tract. Prostatic hypertrophy, bilateral ureteric strictures, stones in the renal pelvis or ureter, and compression of the ureter and bladder by external neoplasms are the precipitating causes. Obstruction to the flow or urine generates a back pressure that eventually raises the hydrostatic pressure in the Bowman's capsule, reducing the glomerular filtration rate.

## CHRONIC RENAL FAILURE

In the chronic form of renal failure, the number of functioning nephrons is irreversibly reduced due to the progression of diseases such as pyelonephritis, glomerulonephritis, hypertensive disease and diabetic nephropathy. Glomerular damage, with distortion of the cortex and medulla due to fibrosis and scarring, are common features of these disorders. The progression from health to illness, in contrast to acute renal failure, is slow, taking place over months to years. The glomerular filtration rate falls slowly. In the early stages of chronic failure, loss of the ability to concentrate urine causes polyuria but in the terminal stages of the glomerular filtration rate is reduced to such a level that oliguria and severe uraemia occur.

## PROBLEMS IN OLIGURIC/ANURIC RENAL FAILURE

It is beyond the scope of this text to give a detailed consideration of the problems arising in the oliguric/anuric stages of acute or chronic renal failure, when the glomerular filtration rate is severely reduced. Three major problems will be briefly discussed here.

### Failure to excrete a fluid load

Oliguric patients who fail to excrete a fluid load rapidly expand their body fluid compartments, precipitating dyspnoea and peripheral oedema due to heart failure, unless their water intake is restricted. Fluids should be given to replace extrarenal losses and the urinary losses over a 24-hour period. Assuming an insensible loss of 1 L per day, and a gain of 600 mL water from oxidative metabolism, the fluid intake in a totally anuric patient should not exceed $1000 - 600$ mL $= 400$ mL.

Expansion of the extracellular fluid compartment is exacerbated in the presence of a positive sodium balance, therefore in anuria or very severe oliguria, restricting the sodium intake may be necessary. As a general rule, positive sodium balances are avoided by restricting the dietary intake where necessary.

### Failure to maintain electrolyte balance

In the severely oliguric or anuric patient who fails to maintain electrolyte balance, failure to excrete a potassium load may result in fatal hyperkalaemia, and failure to excrete the hydrogen ions of 'fixed' acids may result in metabolic acidosis. Restricting the dietary potassium intake, administration of sodium/potassium ion exchange resins, and the provision of a high-energy carbohydrate diet that minimizes potassium ions produced from tissue breakdown, may be adequate measures to control the patient's serum potassium ion level. A high-energy carbohydrate diet with restricted protein content may also reduce the production of 'fixed' acids from protein and lipid metabolism.

## Uraemia

A complex array of problems is associated with **uraemia**, including anorexia, nausea, vomiting due to gastrointestinal irritation, and bleeding from the gut wall. Uraemic irritation of the skin may cause pruritus, and muscle cramps and stomatitis may be present. The effects of uraemia on the central nervous system include irritability, confusion, drowsiness and coma, and may lead to death.

Uraemia can be controlled conservatively by:

- Decreasing the protein intake to curtail the production of urea and other nitrogenous wastes.
- Preventing the catabolism of protein stores in muscle by supplying a high-energy carbohydrate diet.

Guidelines for dietary protein and energy intakes in different types and levels of severity of acute and chronic renal failure are available (Bihl, 2001; Toigi et al., 2000).

Any sources of infection should be eliminated to prevent catabolism. In the presence of severe uraemic symptoms, uncontrollable fluid overload, hyperkalaemia and metabolic acidosis, the only options available are to institute continuous or intermittent renal replacement therapy via haemofiltration, haemodialysis or peritoneal dialysis according to clinical indication (Kellum et al., 2002). In those patients with chronic renal failure, when the return of normal renal function cannot occur a renal transplant offers the only hope of escape from lifelong intermittent dialysis. Ideally, dialysis should be instituted before severe uraemia sets in; it is mandatory once the glomerular filtration rate falls below 3 mL/min.

## Tubular reabsorption and secretion: the modification of the glomerular filtrate

In the first stage of urine production, during the process of **glomerular filtration**, an ultrafiltrate is formed of approximately the same solute concentrations, osmolality and pH as plasma. Blood cells and protein macromolecules of a relative molecular mass greater than 70 000 are not filtered.

During the second stages in the production of urine – **tubular reabsorption and secretion** – the filtrate is greatly modified as it moves along the nephron. Vital solutes that must be conserved, such as glucose, amino acids and electrolytes, are reabsorbed, together with water. They pass from the lumen of the nephron across the epithelial layer, to be transported away by peritubular blood capillaries. A few substances are actually secreted into the filtrate in the reverse direction, including hydrogen ions, ammonia and drug metabolites.

By the time the final excretory product – urine – drains from the collecting duct into the renal pelvis, it is greatly reduced in volume and contains nitrogenous waste products together with electrolytes that are surplus to body requirements.

The vast extent of solute reabsorption accomplished by nephrons can be illustrated by considering the volumes and quantities involved. During the course of one day, 180 L of plasma are filtered through the kidneys. These 180 L contain about 500 g sodium bicarbonate, 100 g amino acids, more than 1 kg sodium chloride and 270 g glucose. Only negligible amounts of these solutes appear in the 1–1.5 L of urine eliminated each day.

Some variation exists in the volume of fluid and type of solutes reabsorbed in different regions of the nephron. By far the greatest degree of reabsorption occurs in the proximal convoluted tubule, where two-thirds of the filtrate is removed. Glucose and amino acids are reabsorbed almost exclusively here, whereas water and electrolytes are also reabsorbed in more distal areas. A summary of the degree of regional specialization in reabsorption in the nephron is given in **Fig. 5.4.7**.

In this section, some of the transport mechanisms by which reabsorption and secretion take place are described, together with some of the major disorders that impair them. Reabsorption of hydrogen carbonate ions and excretion of hydrogen ions are considered separately in the section on acid–base balance (see p. 604). Similarly, factors that regulate sodium and potassium balance are also described later.

## Transport mechanisms in the nephron

For any substance to be reabsorbed from the nephron, it must be transferred across the plasma membranes and cytoplasm of the epithelial cell into interstitial fluid, and from there into the peritubular blood capillaries. In the case of secretion, the reverse applies. The tubular transport mechanisms that permit reabsorption and secretion are either passive or active.

### Passive transfer
**Passive transfer** is defined as the movement of non-electrolytes and ions across cell membranes according to the chemical and electrical gradients that prevail. In effect, these solutes move 'downhill', from an area of high to an area of low chemical concentration or electrical potential. In addition to passive movement down a concentration gradient, charged solutes such as ions must also negotiate electrical gradients and move across a 'polarized' membrane to the side that is

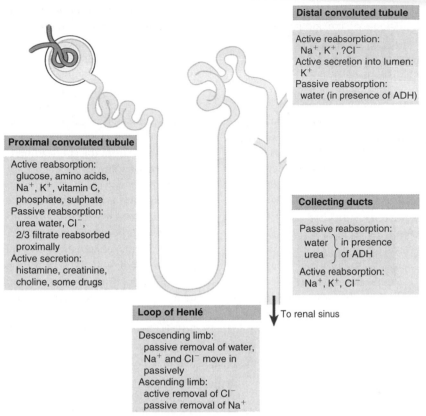

**Distal convoluted tubule**

Active reabsorption:
  Na$^+$, K$^+$, ?Cl$^-$
Active secretion into lumen:
  K$^+$
Passive reabsorption:
  water (in presence of ADH)

**Proximal convoluted tubule**

Active reabsorption:
  glucose, amino acids,
  Na$^+$, K$^+$, vitamin C,
  phosphate, sulphate
Passive reabsorption:
  urea water, Cl$^-$,
  2/3 filtrate reabsorbed
  proximally
Active secretion:
  histamine, creatinine,
  choline, some drugs

**Collecting ducts**

Passive reabsorption:
  water ⎱ in presence
  urea ⎰ of ADH
Active reabsorption:
  Na$^+$, K$^+$, Cl$^-$

**Loop of Henlé**

To renal sinus

Descending limb:
  passive removal of water,
  Na$^+$ and Cl$^-$ move in
  passively
Ascending limb:
  active removal of Cl$^-$
  passive removal of Na$^+$

**Figure 5.4.7** Regional specialization in reabsorption and secretion in the nephron. Note the occurrence, throughout the nephron, of: the exchange of sodium ions (Na$^+$) for hydrogen ions (H$^+$), reabsorption of hydrogen carbonate ions (HCO$_3^-$) and ammonia (NH$_3$) secretion (see Acid–base balance, p. 604). ADH, antidiuretic hormone

oppositely charged. In a polarized membrane there is a distribution of electrical charge such that one side of the membrane is positively charged and the other side negative; this is called a **potential difference**. Ions with a negative charge will move passively across the membrane to the side that is positively charged, and vice versa. No energy is used in the process of passive transfer, although setting up the gradients in the first place requires energy. All living cells have an intracellular ionic composition that is different from their environment, and a negative electrical potential operates across the plasma membrane (this is discussed further in Chapter 2.1).

## Active transfer

In contrast to passive movements, **active transfer** is defined as the 'uphill' movement of solutes against an unfavourable chemical or electrical gradient. In this case, solutes are moved from an area of low to an area of high concentration, and ions are transported against an unfavourable electrical potential. A direct use of energy in the form of adenosine triphosphate (ATP) is consumed in powering the active transport of solutes against unfavourable gradients. However, *net* movement of an ion may take place down a

favourable concentration gradient but still require energy if a greater unfavourable electrical gradient is also present, and vice versa.

Both active and passive mechanisms may be involved in the reabsorption of solutes across the epithelium of the nephron, but the overall process is called 'active' as long as one of the steps involves active transport.

A number of models have been put forward to explain active transport across cell membranes, but such are the limitations of experimental techniques at present that they are difficult to prove. Nevertheless, an active 'pump' mechanism must have some sort of 'carrier' mechanism for binding a specific solute on one side of the cell membrane and discharging it on the other, with energy supplied in the form of adenosine triphosphate to move the solute plus carrier. In fact, the enzyme sodium/potassium ATPase mediates the transport of sodium ions and potassium ions across the plasma membrane in all cells, not just the kidney epithelium. This is a protein (as are all enzymes) with specific binding sites for sodium ions and potassium ions. It extrudes sodium ions from the cell and moves potassium ions inside. Complex, interacting hormonal mechanisms exert varying effects on sodium/potassium ATPase-dependent sodium transport in different regions of the kidney (Feraille & Doucet, 2001).

Little is known about the nature of other membrane carriers but it seems likely that they too are proteins and are part of the plasma membrane. Carriers mediate not only active transport but some passive transfer systems too, when the favourable concentration gradient is the driving force that moves the carrier across the membrane. An interesting feature of carrier-mediated active transfer systems is that they may be interdependent, and that more than one solute can use each carrier. This is certainly the case where glucose is reabsorbed in the nephron in conjunction with other sugars; and glucose transport is linked to the active transport of sodium ions.

## Glucose

**Glucose** is reabsorbed in the proximal convoluted tubule against a concentration gradient by active transport. The carrier system for glucose also transports other sugars such as galactose, mannose, xylose and fructose. An interesting feature is that glucose transfer is linked to the active transport of sodium ions, a phenomenon known as **cotransfer**. Glucose is preferentially bound by a sugar carrier mechanism, so that in the presence of an increased glucose concentration, reabsorption of the other sugars is decreased.

Active transport systems such as that involved in glucose reabsorption can only operate up to a certain limit, known as the **transport maximum ($T_m$) value**. In healthy individuals with plasma glucose concentrations in the range 4.2–6.7 mmol/L, virtually all the filtered glucose is reabsorbed. However, the maximum rate at which the carrier systems can reabsorb glucose is 375 mg/min. At any plasma glucose level that exceeds the critical renal threshold of 10 mmol/L, so much glucose is filtered that the carrier system is saturated and unable to reabsorb the load. As a result, glucose appears in the urine. In health, the plasma glucose concentration is maintained in the normal range, mainly by the hormone insulin, so that glycosuria does not normally occur. Glycosuria is therefore a feature of diabetes mellitus in which plasma glucose levels are elevated due to insulin deficiency.

## Phosphate

**Phosphate** is also actively reabsorbed in the nephron, mainly in the proximal tubule, by a system with a transport maximum. Plasma phosphate levels are low, at 1.0 mmol/L, so a large part of the phosphate that is absorbed from the gut each day is excreted in the urine to maintain balance. In effect, this means that alterations in renal phosphate reabsorption play a vital role in controlling the total body phosphate pool. Phosphate reabsorption is linked in some way to glucose transport because, if the carrier system for glucose is saturated, an increased amount of phosphate appears in the urine.

A number of hormones are known to exert a regulatory role on phosphate reabsorption in the nephron. Parathyroid hormone, vitamin D and calcitonin all promote the excretion of phosphate in urine. In hyperparathyroidism, the excessive secretion of parathyroid hormone promotes calcium loss from bone and reabsorption from the gut, leading to hypercalcaemia. Increased quantities of calcium are then filtered by the kidney and eventually calcium deposits appear in the epithelium lining the nephron and also inside the tubules. Together with the reduction in renal phosphate reabsorption, this predisposes to the formation of calcium phosphate calculi. In contrast, severe hypoparathyroidism is marked by increases in the plasma phosphate concentration (phosphataemia) due to the increase in phosphate reabsorption in the nephron.

## Sulphate and vitamin C

**Sulphate** and **vitamin C** are both actively reabsorbed in the proximal convoluted tubule by systems that are also linked in some way to glucose transfer. Saturation of the carrier system for glucose decreases both sulphate and vitamin C reabsorption.

## Proteins

Proteins with a molecular mass <70 000 that cross the filtration barrier are reabsorbed in the proximal convoluted tubule by endocytosis, a process that involves binding at the apical pole of the tubular epithelial cell, vesicular internalization and degradation by lysosomes. The proteins megalin and cubilin, present in the luminal membrane of the tubular cells, play a vital role in binding these filtered proteins (Verroust & Kozyraki, 2001).

## Amino acids

Amino acids are actively reabsorbed, almost entirely in the proximal convoluted tubules, by systems that show a transport maximum for each amino acid that is transferred. Several carrier mechanisms have been identified.

Amino acid transport is independent of glucose transfer but, as yet, the exact mechanisms involved are not fully understood.

A number of rare inherited disorders, for example, cystinuria and Fanconi's syndrome, are caused by defective amino acid reabsorption and feature aminoaciduria – the presence of amino acids in the urine.

## Active mechanisms for reabsorption

Sodium and potassium ions are actively reabsorbed throughout the nephron, as shown in **Fig. 5.4.8**.

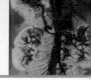

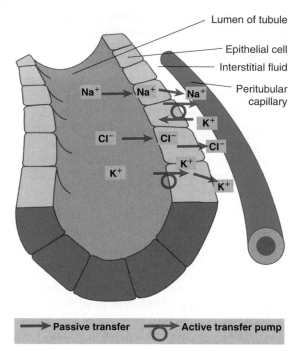

Figure 5.4.8 Ion transport in the proximal convoluted tubule

following the combination of antidiuretic hormone with receptors in the basolateral membrane of the collecting duct cell. An intracellular signal is generated via cyclic adenosine monophosphate (AMP), which results in the transfer of AQ2 water channels from a store in cytoplasmic vesicles to the apical cell plasma membrane, where they facilitate water reabsorption. As antidiuretic hormone declines, AQ2 are retrieved by endocytosis and returned to storage vesicles, returning the apical cell membrane to its water-impermeable resting state (Marples et al., 1999). At the basolateral membrane, where AQ3 and AQ4 are permanently sited, an exit channel is formed allowing water to pass out into the interstitial space, from where it is absorbed into the capillary network surrounding the nephron.

Abnormalities in aquaporin formation or regulation appear to be associated with the syndrome of inappropriate antidiuretic hormone secretion, congestive cardiac failure and cirrhosis, which are marked by water retention and/or oedema. Polyuric conditions, such as polydipsia and diabetes insipidus, may also be associated with aquaporin disturbances (Knepper et al., 1997) (see p. 613).

Chloride ions are passively reabsorbed in the proximal convoluted tubule but must be actively transported elsewhere. Potassium ions are normally secreted in the distal convoluted tubule. Mechanisms concerned with the reabsorption of hydrogen carbonate ions are described in the section on acid–base balance (see p. 618).

### Passive transport

**Urea**. The transfer of urea across the tubular epithelium is unusual in that it is passively reabsorbed in the proximal and distal tubules and collecting ducts but secreted into the loop of Henlé. In effect, there is some recycling of urea between the nephron and medullary tissue, a process that is discussed later in the sections on the formation of concentrated and dilute urine (see p. 610).

**Water**. Water is passively reabsorbed throughout the nephron along the osmotic gradients created by the transport of other solutes, notably sodium ions. In the distal regions of the nephron, water reabsorption is controlled by antidiuretic hormone (ADH) under conditions described on p. 607. Comparatively recently, the aquaporins were recognized as proteins constituting a family of water channels that mediate the flow of water across cell membranes. At least seven types of aquaporin (AQ) have been identified on the basis of their amino acid structure. In the nephron, AQ1 is localized to the epithelium of the proximal convoluted tubule and loop of Henlé; AQ2, AQ3 and AQ4 to the epithelium of the collecting ducts. Mechanisms of aquaporin action are best illustrated by events

### Tubular secretion

Tubular secretion is the reverse of reabsorption, entailing the movement of solutes from the peritubular capillary, across the epithelial cell, into the lumen of the nephron. Both active and passive transport mechanisms facilitate this process. Actively secreted solutes include drugs such as penicillins, sulphonamides and chlorothiazides. In addition, active secretion of thiamine, choline, creatinine and histamine also takes place. However, active secretion is not the main route of removal for any of these substances, for all are primarily eliminated by glomerular filtration.

The circumstances under which potassium ions are passively secreted into the distal convoluted tubule are described in the section on potassium balance (see p. 614).

### Countercurrent multiplication and exchange: the formation of concentrated and dilute urine

In the proximal convoluted tubule, water is passively reabsorbed along the osmotic gradient largely set up by the active transport of sodium ions. In contrast to this, water reabsorption in the distal convoluted tubule and collecting ducts is controlled by antidiuretic hormone (ADH). When the osmolality of plasma rises, signalling a physiological requirement for water, antidiuretic hormone is secreted into the circulation from the posterior pituitary and renders the epithelium lining the distal tubule and collecting duct permeable to water. As a result, water moves passively out of these areas, drawn by the osmotic effects of trapped solutes in the medullary interstitial fluid (interstitium) outside. It is subsequently transported away by peritubular blood capillaries, into the circulation. Under these circumstances, enough water is reabsorbed to return the osmolality of plasma to normal (285 mosmol/kg $H_2O$) and a concentrated urine is formed.

In the absence of antidiuretic hormone, the distal tubule and collecting duct are almost impermeable to water, so that virtually no reabsorption takes place and a dilute urine is eliminated.

Before considering the release mechanisms and actions of antidiuretic hormone in greater detail, we must first consider how solutes such as urea, sodium and chloride ions are trapped in the medullary interstitium around the nephron, creating a gradient of increasing osmolality, 300–1200 mosmol/kg $H_2O$, through the renal medulla (**Fig. 5.4.9**).

The trapping of solutes in the medullary interstitial fluid forms the basis of the **countercurrent theory**, advanced to explain how concentrated

urine is formed by the passive reabsorption of water. According to this theory, the U-shaped countercurrent arrangement of the loop of Henlé and vasa recta operates to cycle or trap solutes in such a way that the osmolality of the medullary interstitium is increased. Furthermore, due to countercurrent multiplication in the loop of Henlé, the fluid reaching the distal convoluted tubule is dilute. This is subsequently concentrated by passive reabsorption of water when tubular fluid is exposed to the medullary osmotic gradient exclusively under the influence of antidiuretic hormone.

## The loop of Henlé: countercurrent exchange and the formation of concentrated urine

Fluid leaving the proximal convoluted tubule is approximately isosmolal with plasma, at 300 mosmol/kg $H_2O$. In the descending limb of the loop of Henlé, the epithelium is relatively permeable to water, which moves out passively under the influence

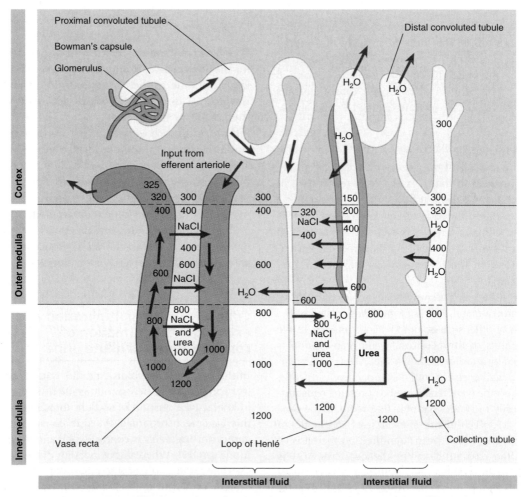

**Figure 5.4.9**   Countercurrent mechanism and urine concentration. Concentrations are in milliosmoles

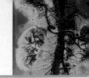

of the hyperosmotic medullary interstitium and is removed by peritubular capillaries. It is not known exactly how much water is lost from the descending limb but the contents become increasingly concentrated towards the tip of the loop and attain the same osmolality as the interstitium by the time the U-bend is reached.

In the thick ascending limb of the loop of Henlé, the epithelium is impermeable to water. However, chloride ions are actively transported out of this area into interstitial fluid accompanied passively by sodium ions. As ions are removed from the tubular fluid and water is not, the fluid delivered to the distal convoluted tubule is dilute and has an osmolality of approximately 100 mosmol/kg $H_2O$.

The chloride and sodium ions move through the interstitium and diffuse passively back into the descending limb. Urea also diffuses passively into the descending limb; both these mechanisms contribute to the increased concentration of tubular fluid at the bend of the loop.

This cyclic movement of ions from the ascending limb across to the descending limb without the simultaneous transport of water multiplies the concentration of solutes in the descending limb, hence the term countercurrent multiplication. The longer the loop of Henlé, the greater will be the concentration at the tip of the loop. In essence, the countercurrent operation of the loop of Henlé continuously moves ions into the interstitial fluid of the medulla and raises its osmolality, such that the gradient shown in **Fig. 5.4.9** exists. Countercurrent multiplication also ensures that a dilute fluid reaches the distal convoluted tubule.

In the presence of antidiuretic hormone, the epithelium lining the distal convoluted tubule and collecting duct becomes water permeable. Water then moves out passively by osmosis into the medullary interstitium until the osmolality of the interstitium equilibrates with that of the tubular fluid. Water is eventually reabsorbed into the peritubular capillaries and transported away into the circulation. Urine that is concentrated in this way flows out of the collecting duct into the renal pelvis and from there down the ureter to the bladder.

## Formation of dilute urine

The stages are the same as those described above until the dilute fluid reaches the distal convoluted tubule. In these circumstances, antidiuretic hormone is absent and the epithelium lining the distal tubule and collecting duct is virtually impermeable to water, so that very little water is reabsorbed despite the huge osmotic gradient operating between the tubule and interstitium outside. As a result, a dilute fluid reaches the collecting ducts and a dilute urine is excreted.

## The vasa recta

Juxtamedullary nephrons possess a U-shaped capillary network closely surrounding the loop of Henlé. By acting as countercurrent exchangers, these blood vessels also help to trap solutes in the medullary interstitium which, combined with the actions of the loop of Henlé, raises the osmolality of interstitial fluid.

Blood moving down the descending limb of the vasa recta (**see Fig. 5.4.9**) gains solutes that move passively into the limb from their higher concentration in the medulla outside. At the same time, the descending limb loses water passively, due to the osmotic gradient existing between the interstitium and capillary blood.

In the ascending limb of the vasa recta, the reverse process takes place. As blood flows through this region towards the cortex, the external gradient diminishes. As blood has gained solutes in the descending limb, such that its osmolality approaches 1200 mosmol/kg $H_2O$, these solutes now pass out from their high concentration in blood into the region of lower concentration in the medulla outside. At the same time, water moves back into the ascending limb by osmosis.

The *net* result is that the vasa recta remove water from the inner regions of the kidney, but solutes are recycled in the medulla, helping to raise the osmolality of the interstitial fluid. Blood leaving the vasa recta has an osmolality of 325 mosmol/kg $H_2O$, having gained a small amount of solutes.

## The role of urea

In addition to increasing the water permeability of the distal tubules and collecting ducts, antidiuretic hormone also increases the permeability of the terminal collecting ducts to urea. By the time fluid reaches this area of the nephron, water has been reabsorbed in the distal tubule; it therefore contains a high concentration of urea. Urea moves out of the collecting duct, down its concentration gradient into the medullary and papillary interstitium until the concentrations are the same. The effect of this movement of urea into the interstitium under the influence of antidiuretic hormone is that it too raises the osmolality of this area, aiding the urine-concentrating mechanism. Eventually, a large part of the urea is secreted back into the loop of Henlé as part of a recycling process, and some is removed by the vasa recta. Knepper et al. (2003) suggested that, in addition to urea recycling and ion movement, the presence of hyaluronan (a gel-like glycosaminoglycan) in the

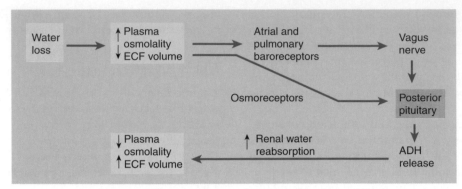

**Figure 5.4.10**   Stimuli to antidiuretic hormone secretion

medullary interstitium might contribute to the generation of the osmotic gradient that facilitates urine concentration.

## Water balance: control of the secretion of antidiuretic hormone

The actions of antidiuretic hormone on the distal convoluted and collecting ducts controls water balance. In the presence of antidiuretic hormone, a concentrated urine is formed and water is conserved to meet body requirements. In the absence of antidiuretic hormone, a dilute urine is formed to unload water that is in excess of body needs.

Antidiuretic hormone is synthesized by cells of the supraoptic nucleus in the hypothalamus and is then transported along axons for storage in the posterior pituitary (see Chapter 2.5). A number of mechanisms are responsible for triggering the secretion of antidiuretic hormone into the circulation (**Fig. 5.4.10**):

- Primary factors:
  - osmoreceptors
  - pressure receptors (baroreceptors).
- Secondary factors:
  - pain
  - emotional stress
  - hypoxia
  - severe exercise
  - surgery, anaesthetics such as cyclopropane and nitrous oxide
  - angiotensin II.

Osmoreceptors trigger the secretion of antidiuretic hormone in response to:

- Dehydration produced by water loss that increases the osmolality of plasma.
- 'Relative' dehydration: no net loss of water but a gain of sodium ions that raises plasma osmolality.

In an individual deprived of water, the plasma osmolality rises and antidiuretic hormone is secreted from the posterior pituitary, resulting in water reabsorption

in the distal nephron. A reduced volume of concentrated urine is produced and the plasma osmolality is returned to normal (285 mosmol/kg $H_2O$). In contrast, in an individual who consumes a large volume of water, the dilution of plasma decreases its osmolality and secretion of antidiuretic hormone is inhibited. As the distal nephron remains impermeable to water in this situation, a large volume of dilute urine is eliminated.

Precisely where the osmoreceptors are located remains unclear but the available evidence suggests that they are near the supraoptic nucleus or adjacent areas of the hypothalamus and third ventricle.

**Pressure receptors (baroreceptors)** are also involved. Secretion of antidiuretic hormone is also stimulated by changes in the circulating volume; a reduction of 8–10% in blood volume due to haemorrhage evokes secretion. Conversely, there is some evidence to suggest that expansion of the plasma volume inhibits the secretion of antidiuretic hormone. The pressure receptors are located in the walls of the atria and large pulmonary blood vessels, and the nerve impulses that trigger the release of antidiuretic hormone are relayed by the vagus nerve (see also atrial natriuretic hormone, p. 615).

### Thirst

Alterations in fluid balance that trigger the sensation of **thirst** also increase the secretion of antidiuretic hormone. Thus, thirst is experienced when the plasma osmolality rises and when the extra- and intracellular fluid volumes are decreased. It is not known whether the osmoreceptors involved are the same as those that stimulate the secretion of antidiuretic hormone.

Angiotensin II is a hormone produced in response to a decrease in blood volume and this appears to bring about the sensation of thirst by combining with receptors in an area of the third ventricle known as the lamina terminalis (Fitzsimmons, 1998). The role of the renin–angiotensin–aldosterone system, which complements the actions of antidiuretic hormone in controlling the extracellular fluid volume, is discussed later.

## CLINICAL APPLICATIONS

### IMPAIRED CONCENTRATION

Damage to the medullary countercurrent system, inadequate secretion of antidiuretic hormone and osmotic diuresis all result in a reduced ability to **concentrate** urine. Polyuria is the consequence of this, as long as the glomerular filtration rate is not critically reduced at the same time.

**Damage to the medullary countercurrent system**. Progression of chronic renal disorders, such as pyelonephritis, results in **distortion** of the medullary tissue and **damage** to the loop of Henlé and its associated blood capillaries. As a result, hyperosmolality of the medulla cannot be maintained and so urine cannot be concentrated.

**Inadequate secretion of antidiuretic hormone**. This may be caused by deficient secretion of antidiuretic hormone, as is found in the disorder known as **diabetes insipidus**. Individuals afflicted with this disorder may eliminate 5–20 L of urine each day.

A psychological condition known as **polydipsia** (excessive water drinking) results in a dilution of the plasma, lowering its osmolality, and causing inhibition of antidiuretic hormone secretion.

**Solute (osmotic) diuresis**. In the *early* stages of chronic renal failure there is a reduction in the number of functioning nephrons. As a result, an increased amount of solute is delivered to those nephrons that are still functioning normally. The osmotic pressure exerted by this increase in solute concentration in remaining nephrons prevents the reabsorption of water and, as a result, large volumes of urine are eliminated.

In the *late*, 'diuretic', phase of acute renal failure, which follows recovery from oliguria, the ability to reabsorb solutes, particularly sodium and potassium ions, is impaired. Again, this results in the elimination of large amounts of urine.

In diabetes mellitus the elevated blood glucose concentration brings about a glucose load in the nephron that exceeds the reabsorptive capacity, causing an osmotic diuresis.

In the majority of these conditions, continued water and electrolyte losses due to polyuria must be balanced by adequate replacement therapy, or dehydration, hyponatraemia and even hypovolaemic shock may supervene.

### IMPAIRED DILUTING ABILITY

The ability to form a **dilute** urine is impaired in the following conditions:

- **Renal failure**. The diluting ability is impaired in early acute **renal failure** and late chronic renal failure once the glomerular filtration rate has fallen below 30 mL/min.

- **Liver failure**. A failing liver may no longer metabolize hormones such as aldosterone efficiently. The plasma concentrations of the hormone rise, resulting in an increase in the reabsorption of sodium ions and water from the nephron. This impairs normal diluting mechanisms.

- **Heart failure**. In **heart failure**, aldosterone secretion is enhanced due to the low cardiac output, which reduces renal perfusion and triggers renin release from the juxtaglomerular apparatus. The retention of sodium ions and water due to the actions of aldosterone on the nephron impairs the normal diluting mechanism.

- **Excessive secretion of antidiuretic hormone**. Rarely, excessive secretion of antidiuretic hormone by tumours of the lung, brain or pancreas may result in increased water reabsorption from the nephron.

A major problem for the patient who cannot dilute urine is that failure to excrete a fluid load results in expansion of the extracellular fluid volume and may lead to oedema. If the fluid intake is not restricted, signs of water intoxication may become apparent, including anorexia, muscle weakness and confusion. Heart failure may be worsened or precipitated by prolonged circulatory overload.

### ACTIONS OF DIURETIC DRUGS ON THE NEPHRON

As their name suggests, diuretic drugs are used to promote diuresis, augmenting the excretion of solutes and water and increasing the volume of urine eliminated by the kidneys. Conventionally, diuretics are widely used for the treatment of fluid retention and oedema in heart failure, liver disorders and renal disorders such as the nephrotic syndrome.

**Osmotic diuretics**, such as mannitol, are inert substances that are freely filtered at the glomerulus and are not reabsorbed in the tubule of the nephron. The osmotic effects exerted by filtered mannitol prevent the reabsorption of water, increasing urine flow rate and volume. Mannitol can promote a diuresis even when the glomerular filtration rate is reduced. For this reason, it is used to prevent acute renal failure occurring in patients who are hypovolaemic and potentially oliguric, for example following haemorrhage. Atrial natriuretic hormone may also prove to be a useful diuretic in the prevention of acute renal failure.

In contrast, **thiazide diuretics** such as hydrochlorothiazide inhibit the reabsorption of sodium and chloride ions in the ascending loop of Henlé and proximal and distal nephron, thereby promoting water loss.

The **loop diuretic**, furosemide (Lasix), which is related to the thiazides, acts in a similar way, enhancing the excretion of chloride ions. However, both drugs produce an increase in the excretion of potassium ions so that it is necessary to provide potassium ion supplements during the therapy. Furosemide is a very potent diuretic and the diuresis it evokes may reach 10 L/day in a grossly oedematous patient. Its action must therefore be monitored very closely by observing strict fluid balance recordings; any impending signs of dehydration should be immediately reported.

**Potassium-sparing diuretics**, such as spironolactone, act as antagonists to the hormone aldosterone, resulting in decreased reabsorption of sodium in the distal convoluted tubule and hence promoting sodium and water loss. Decreased sodium ion reabsorption is balanced by potassium ion retention at this site and potassium ion supplements are not necessary with these drugs. Potassium retention is one potentially toxic side-effect of drugs that act as aldosterone antagonists.

## The renin–angiotensin–aldosterone system

The operation of the renin–angiotensin–aldosterone system (RAAS) plays an important part in the maintenance of the extracellular fluid volume, sodium and potassium balance and the regulation of blood pressure.

Renin is a proteolytic enzyme secreted into the circulation by the juxtaglomerular apparatus of the kidney; its source appears to be the granular epithelioid cells in the wall of the afferent arteriole. Renin cleaves an $\alpha_2$-globulin in plasma – **angiotensinogen** – to form the decapeptide (i.e. composed of 10 amino acids) angiotensin I. As blood circulates through the lungs and kidneys, this is converted by an enzyme in these two sites into the octapeptide, angiotensin II (**Fig. 5.4.11**). Angiotensin II brings about the following physiological effects:

- increased peripheral resistance in arterioles and small arteries, increasing systemic blood pressure
- aldosterone release from the adrenal cortex, which increases the reabsorption of sodium ions and water in the nephron
- thirst.

The operation of the entire system is summarized in **Fig. 5.4.11**. Angiotensin II exerts a negative feedback effect on renin release.

### Renin release

Renin is released from the juxtaglomerular apparatus in response to:

- A fall in perfusion pressure in the afferent arteriole. This stimulus is probably mediated by receptors (baroreceptors) in the wall of the afferent arteriole as the blood pressure falls.
- A decrease in the delivery of sodium and chloride ion to the distal convoluted tubule, which is detected by macula densa cells. This takes place whenever blood pressure and volume are decreased and the glomerular filtration rate is reduced. A low flow rate of fluid through the nephron also allows more time for sodium and chloride ion reabsorption, reducing their concentration by the time fluid reaches the distal convoluted tubule.
- An increase in the activity of the renal sympathetic nerve supply in shock and haemorrhage, which brings about renin release via a direct action on the juxtaglomerular cells and also constriction of the afferent arteriole.

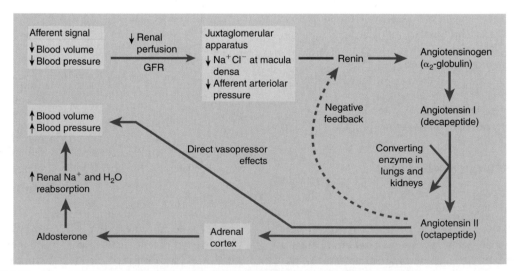

**Figure 5.4.11**    The renin–angiotensin–aldosterone system. GFR, glomerular filtration rate

- A fall in the plasma concentrations of sodium and potassium ions increases renin release, and vice versa.

A reduction in plasma sodium ion concentration brought about by excessive losses due to vomiting, sweating and severe diarrhoea may be compensated in part by increased aldosterone secretion, which promotes renal sodium reabsorption.

The role of renin in the maintenance of normal blood pressure is not fully understood, and even more difficult to assess is its role in the aetiology of hypertension. Atrial natriuretic hormone inhibits renin release.

## Atrial natriuretic hormone (ANH)

In recent years it has become clear that a number of complementary feedback loops operate to maintain the volume and composition of extracellular fluid. The synergistic actions of both antidiuretic hormone and the renin–angiotensin–aldosterone axis increase the extracellular fluid volume, maintain its sodium content and elevate systemic blood pressure in response to a homeostatic challenge. The existence of a third feedback loop involving a 'natriuretic hormone' that modulated the operation of the other two axes was postulated for a number of years, but the hormone proved elusive. In 1985, De Bold, reviewing the evidence obtained from earlier animal studies (that an extract of rat atrial muscle could induce diuresis and natriuresis) confirmed this to be a peptide hormone of 28 amino acids – atrial natriuretic hormone (ANH) – suggesting an important and hitherto unsuspected endocrine role for the heart.

### Secretion and release

Atrial natriuretic hormone is synthesized in secretory granules within atrial myocytes. Release from the secretory granules is accompanied by cleavage of the prohormone (126 amino acids), generating α-atrial natriuretic hormone (the active hormone) and one other fragment that undergoes further cleavage to form three other short peptides with vasodilatory and natriuretic properties. Atrial natriuretic hormone is secreted into interstitial fluid, reaching circulating blood via the coronary sinus (Saito et al., 1987; Seul et al., 2003). The major stimulus to release of the hormone is an increased right atrial pressure due to the distension brought about by an increased circulating volume associated with sodium loading. The atrial myocytes acting as volume (pressure) receptors, which secrete the hormone, show increased activity in the atrial epicardium where distensional forces are greatest. Release of the hormone appears to be directly proportional to mechanical load.

In healthy individuals, the normal plasma concentration of atrial natriuretic hormone ranges from 10 to 70 pg/mL, and there appears to be a continuous low, basal release of the hormone (Needleman & Greenwald, 1986). However, early studies found that increasing the dietary intake of sodium for 3–5 days doubled the plasma concentration of the hormone and rapid volume expansion resulted in an atrial-natriuretic-hormone-induced natriuresis and diuresis (Trippodo, 1987).

Plasma concentrations of atrial natriuretic hormone are increased during normal pregnancy, presumably due to the expansion in circulating volume that occurs. Increased plasma concentrations of the hormone have also been demonstrated in clinical conditions associated with fluid overload, or elevated cardiac filling pressures or both, notably valvular heart disease, congestive cardiac failure and chronic renal failure (Cantin & Genest, 1987). Recent studies by Capellin et al. (2001) have suggested that the atrial natriuretic hormone subfragments produced by cleavage of the prohormone are useful diagnostic markers for congestive cardiac failure.

Receptors for atrial natriuretic hormone have been identified in a number of tissues, including the renal cortex and medulla, with specific localization to glomeruli, loops of Henlé and collecting duct membranes, the adrenal cortex, pituitary gland, third ventricle of the brain, eye, lung, intestinal and vascular smooth muscle.

### Renal effects

The renal effects of atrial natriuretic hormone are to raise the glomerular filtration rate, leading to natriuresis and diuresis. In the early studies by Richards et al. (1988) effects in healthy volunteers were relatively more selective for natriuresis than diuresis, and an increased excretion of calcium ions and magnesium ions also occurred.

The elevation in glomerular filtration rate is caused by dilation of the afferent arteriole with concurrent efferent constriction. Other important intrarenal effects of atrial natriuretic hormone that explain its natriuretic properties are to increase renal medullary blood flow; to reduce tubular sodium ion transport, opposing the sodium-retaining effects of aldosterone; and to inhibit renin secretion by macula densa cells in the walls of the afferent arteriole.

### Extrarenal effects

Atrial natriuretic hormone has been shown to bind to cells in the zona glomerulosa of the adrenal cortex, where it directly blocks aldosterone secretion. The inhibitory effects of atrial natriuretic hormone

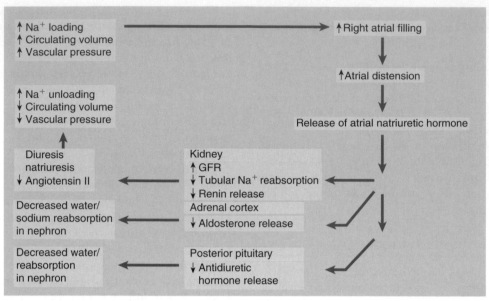

**Figure 5.4.12**   The effects of atrial natriuretic hormone

on renin secretion also remove a primary stimulus for aldosterone release, angiotensin II.

When given in pharmacological doses, atrial natriuretic hormone also inhibits the release of antidiuretic hormone by the posterior pituitary, hence formation of a dilute urine occurs. Atrial natriuretic hormone also inhibits the vasopressor effects of angiotensin II on vascular smooth muscle, lowering systemic blood pressure. Effects on vascular smooth muscle affects arteries and veins; in addition, atrial natriuretic hormone appears to have negative inotropic properties so that its combined effects are to reduce cardiac workload by reducing venous return and peripheral resistance (Saito et al., 1987). It could be considered to function in the control of cardiac filling pressures (Trippodo, 1987).

In summary, the actions of atrial natriuretic hormone (**Fig. 5.4.12**) appear to oppose those of antidiuretic hormone and the renin–angiotensin–aldosterone axis, and it may serve solely to modulate over-rapid expansion of vascular volumes, pressures and short-term sodium balance. Considerable debate still surrounds its biological effects at low plasma concentrations in individuals who have normal cardiovascular function and volume homeostasis.

Atrial natriuretic hormone may have a more complex role in central nervous system control of extracellular fluid volumes and composition, hence its function as a neurotransmitter/neuromodulator is currently under investigation. Future applications in therapeutics remain to be clarified but its role in the genesis and treatment of essential hypertension are a focus for research. Atrial natriuretic hormone has been evaluated in the management of acute renal failure caused by tubular necrosis, where its diuretic and natriuretic

properties through increased glomerular filtration rate could prevent further deterioration in tubular function. A reduced need for dialysis but no impact on mortality was reported in selected studies, benefits not replicated in others (Bihl, 2001).

## Hypertension and the kidney

Hypertension is secondary to a definable cause in only 10% of cases and, of these, renal disorders account for the majority. Renal causes of hypertension may be considered in three categories.

### Renovascular hypertension

Stenosis of the renal artery, which is most commonly brought about by arteriosclerosis, causes this form of hypertension. Plasma renin activity is elevated in 65% of the patients suffering from this disorder. The reduction in renal perfusion brought about by renal artery stenosis leads to renin release, culminating in the formation of angiotensin II, which elevates blood pressure via direct effects on arterioles and via aldosterone, increasing sodium and water retention and hence the circulating volume.

### CLINICAL APPLICATIONS

#### RENAL PARENCHYMAL HYPERTENSION

This form of hypertension is commonly found in individuals suffering from chronic renal failure. Many of these patients have normal plasma renin levels, although in a few cases slight elevations have been detected. It is possible that this form of hypertension may be associated with failure to excrete a salt load or with an increased sensitivity to angiotensin II.

### RENOPRIVAL HYPERTENSION

Renoprival hypertension occurs in those patients whose kidneys are totally non-functioning or have been removed and who are undergoing permanent haemodialysis. In this situation, renin cannot be involved in the cause of hypertension but it is possible that, following nephrectomy or chronic renal damage, a renal vasodilator, which lowers the systemic blood pressure, is lost. This vasodilator may be prostaglandin $E_2$ ($PGE_2$), which is produced in healthy individuals by interstitial cells of the renal medulla. The observed effects when prostaglandin $E_2$ is administered to normotensive and hypertensive individuals are a lowering of the blood pressure and promotion of the renal excretion of sodium and water. It may be involved in the autoregulation of renal blood flow and glomerular filtration rate.

As yet, a role for renin in the cause of essential hypertension is speculative, as plasma renin activity is elevated in very few individuals suffering from this disorder. However, the malignant phase of hypertension is associated with increased renin secretion. Strategies for reducing the hypertension associated with increased renin secretion include:

- restriction of dietary sodium intake
- administration of diuretics in the presence of oedema
- reduction of plasma renin activity by administration of drugs that block the effects of the sympathetic nervous system, e.g. propranolol, oxprenolol, acebutalol
- inhibition of the enzyme that converts angiotensin I into angiotensin II by drugs such as captopril.

The lack of atrial natriuretic hormone as a factor contributing to the development of essential hypertension in some individuals is currently under investigation.

## Sodium balance

In health, sodium balance is regulated exclusively by the kidneys, the plasma sodium concentration remaining within the narrow limits of 135–146 mmol/L. In the face of any challenge to sodium balance, rapid adjustments are made by the kidney to prevent sodium depletion or overload.

Of the filtered load of sodium (approximately 1 kg/24 hours), 67% is reabsorbed in the proximal convoluted tubule and a further 33% is reabsorbed in the remainder of the nephron, mainly in the loop of Henlé.

If the glomerular filtration rate rises, sodium excretion will be increased and, if it falls, sodium retention will result. Compensatory mechanisms must then be brought into operation to prevent excessive sodium losses or gains whenever the glomerular filtration rate alters. These include:

- autoregulation, which stabilizes the glomerular filtration rate, preventing sodium depletion or overload
- reabsorption of a constant percentage of the filtered sodium (67%) in the proximal convoluted tubule, despite changes in filtration rate.

### Challenges to sodium balance

In response to an increased intake of sodium in the diet or intravenously, the following mechanisms act to readjust the balance; the *reverse* takes place if the sodium intake is reduced or excessive sodium losses occur in sweating, prolonged vomiting or diarrhoea.

In the presence of a sodium load, the glomerular filtration rate increases to increase the amount of sodium excreted in the urine. The increase in glomerular filtration rate is probably brought about by expansion of the extracellular fluid volume, which increases the blood pressure and release of atrial natriuretic hormone.

Tubular reabsorption of sodium decreases in the nephron if the intake of sodium is increased. Two hormonal factors are responsible here: sodium loading decreases aldosterone secretion and increases atrial natriuretic hormone secretion, both of which restore sodium balance by reducing tubular sodium reabsorption and increasing the urinary sodium excretion.

Also involved in alterations in tubular sodium reabsorption are the systemic and local mechanisms that regulate blood flow to the renal medulla and within it. Although changes in the resistance of cortical vessels affect the downstream medullary blood flow, it appears that the latter can be regulated independently. Approximately 10% of renal blood flow perfuses the medulla via efferent arterioles of the juxtamedullary nephrons, which give rise to vasa recta and a capillary network.

Current research suggests that systemic and local factors that increase medullary blood flow through vasodilation can reduce tubular sodium reabsorption, leading to a natriuresis, diuresis, reduced extracellular fluid volume and a decline in arterial blood pressure. Hypothetically, increased medullary blood flow involving the vasa recta could bring this about by causing a washout of the medullary interstitial osmotic gradient, which would change driving forces for sodium and water reabsorption in juxtamedullary

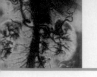
nephrons. Another possibility is that increased medullary blood flow may increase interstitial hydrostatic pressures, reducing tubular sodium absorption (Mattson, 2003).

Systemically circulating atrial natriuretic hormone and locally produced prostaglandins, kinins, nitric oxide and adenosine can all increase medullary blood flow, whereas the actions of renal sympathetic nerve stimulation, antidiuretic hormone and angiotensin II reduce it. Actions of the latter three factors in reducing medullary blood flow would promote the conservation of sodium and water, in line with their other renal and systemic effects. However, as yet the interrelationships between factors that regulate cortical and medullary blood flow under differing homeostatic conditions are incompletely understood.

## Potassium balance

Net reabsorption of potassium takes place in the nephron; only 10–20% of the filtered load of potassium is excreted in health. Most of the filtered potassium is reabsorbed in the proximal convoluted tubule and loop of Henlé. In a healthy person taking a normal diet, potassium is secreted into the distal convoluted tubule, whereas further reabsorption of potassium takes place in the collecting ducts. Alterations in distal reabsorption or secretion of potassium are seen where the dietary intake of potassium varies. In the presence of a low intake, net secretion of potassium is reversed in favour of reabsorption in the distal tubule. If the potassium intake is high, enhanced secretion into the distal tubule takes place.

Other factors that increase potassium excretion in the distal nephron include the hormones aldosterone and cortisol. Both act to promote the reabsorption of sodium, particularly in the distal nephron, at the expense of potassium, which is excreted. Thus hypokalaemia is a feature of Cushing's disease and primary aldosteronism (where hypersecretion of adrenocorticotrophic hormone (ACTH) and aldosterone, respectively, occurs) and is responsible for the severe muscle weakness, flaccid paralysis, cardiac arrhythmias and alkalosis that feature in these disorders.

Acid–base disorders also affect potassium excretion in the nephron. In acidotic states, potassium excretion is decreased, whereas in alkalosis it is enhanced.

## Acid–base balance

It is essential that the pH of blood is maintained within the narrow limits of 7.35–7.45 because the activities of enzymes that govern intracellular chemical reactions are dependent on an optimum pH range, as are the structures of other proteins. Deviation outside the normal pH range may produce fatal changes

in metabolism; the pH range compatible with life is 7.0–7.8.

Each day, the pH of blood is maintained in the face of a massive acid onslaught. Over a 24-hour period, 10 000–20 000 mmol carbon dioxide are produced by oxidative metabolism and converted to the weak acid, carbonic acid in a reaction catalysed by the enzyme carbonic anhydrase:

$$H_2O + CO_2 \rightleftharpoons H_2CO_3 \rightleftharpoons H^+ + HCO_3^-$$

In addition to this daily source of hydrogen ions are the fixed acids such as sulphuric and phosphoric acid, which are derived from protein and lipid metabolism, respectively. A fixed acid production of 40–70 mmol each day is a feature of the high meat protein diet typical of Western civilizations.

How then, is the threat of acidaemia controlled? Three systems of body defence are employed:

- blood buffer systems
- the lungs
- the kidneys.

## *Buffers* (see also Chapters 1.2 and 5.3)

Buffers are chemicals that resist changes in pH on dilution or on addition of acid or alkali. They usually consist of either of the following pairs in solution:

- a weak acid with one of its salts
- a weak base with one of its salts.

For blood pH to be maintained in the range 7.35–7.45, the ratios of weak acid to salt concentration must be preserved in all the buffer pairs in body fluids. Major buffer pairs in humans include:

- Hydrogen carbonate (bicarbonate)/carbonic acid pair, predominantly located in extracellular fluid: $[HCO_3^-]/[H_2CO_3]$.
- Hydrogen phosphate/dihydrogen phosphate pair, predominantly located in intracellular fluid: $[HPO_4^{2-}]/[H_2PO_4]$.
- Protein/acid protein pair, located in plasma and intracellular sites including haemoglobin: [protein]/[acid protein].

All buffers in extra- and intracellular fluid are in equilibrium with each other, with the result that addition of hydrogen ions to any individual system is eventually reflected in changes throughout all the buffer systems. Addition of hydrogen ions to the hydrogen carbonate system, the major extracellular buffer, will ultimately result in alterations in all the other buffer pairs. It follows, therefore, that regulating the hydrogen carbonate buffer pair $[HCO_3^-]/$ $[H_2CO_3]$ ratio will ultimately control the ratio of [salt]/[acid] in all other buffer systems and maintain

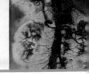

the hydrogen carbonate/carbonic acid ratio at 20 : 1 and the pH of the blood at 7.4.

The capacity of the buffering systems in humans is vast and 1000 mmol of hydrogen ions can be buffered before the pH in the body fluid compartments falls to fatal levels.

## The lungs (see Chapter 5.3)

The lungs play a vital role in controlling the threat to hydrogen ion homeostasis from carbonic acid accumulation, by eliminating 10 000–20 000 mmol carbon dioxide each day.

Carbon dioxide formed as a result of metabolism diffuses from the tissues into the erythrocytes and, in the presence of the enzyme carbonic anhydrase, is converted to carbonic acid. Hydrogen ions resulting from this are extensively buffered by haemoglobin.

The reverse process takes place in the lungs, and carbon dioxide is unloaded in expired air. Suppression of carbon dioxide unloading for as little as half an hour would produce a fatal lowering of blood pH. However, adjustments in ventilation can adjust the pH in minutes following the introduction of an acid load.

As soon as the pH declines below normal limits, the respiratory centre in the brainstem is stimulated and the ventilation rate is increased, unloading carbonic acid as water and carbon dioxide in expired air. This restores the $[HCO_3^-]/[H_2CO_3]$ ratio to 20 : 1.

## The kidneys

The kidneys provide the third line of defence in maintaining hydrogen ion homeostasis. Unlike the other two defence systems, which become effective almost immediately, the renal mechanisms involved in acid–base balance take hours to days to complete.

The renal mechanisms that operate against acidaemia include:

- Reabsorption of virtually all filtered hydrogen carbonate ions to restore the buffering capacity in extracellular fluid.
- Excretion of the hydrogen ions of fixed acids.
- Reclamation of the hydrogen carbonate ions originally consumed in buffering fixed acids.
- Excretion of the anions of fixed acids that cannot be converted into carbon dioxide and therefore cannot be removed by respiration.
- Compensation for acidosis by increasing tubular hydrogen ion secretion, and vice versa in alkalotic states.

### Reabsorption of hydrogen carbonate

Eighty to ninety per cent of the hydrogen carbonate that is filtered is **reabsorbed** in the proximal convoluted tubule; the remainder is reabsorbed throughout the other areas of the nephron. The mechanism concerned with hydrogen carbonate ion reabsorption is shown in **Fig. 5.4.13**. The process for conserving hydrogen

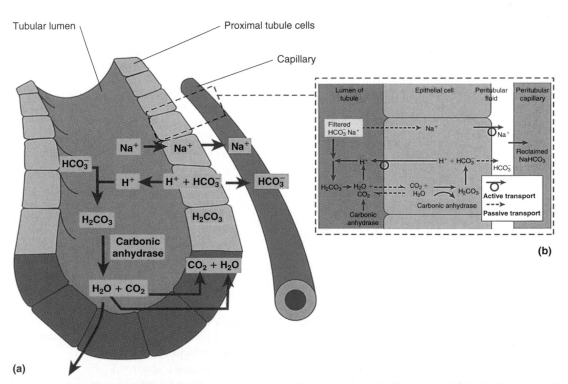

**Figure 5.4.13**  (a) $H^+$ ion secretion and bicarbonate reabsorption by the proximal convoluted tubule, (b) chemical reactions occurring at the cellular level

carbonate ions are used to generate carbon dioxide in the tubular fluid in the presence of the enzyme carbonic anhydrase. In turn, the carbon dioxide formed in the tubular fluid is used to generate hydrogen carbonate ions inside the tubular epithelial cell and it is this ion that is reabsorbed, not the hydrogen carbonate ion originally filtered. One hydrogen carbonate ion is reabsorbed together with a sodium ion in exchange for each hydrogen ion actively transported out into the tubular fluid, as shown in **Fig. 5.4.13**. Several factors affect the renal conservation of hydrogen carbonate ions.

## CLINICAL APPLICATIONS

If the **arterial** $P\text{CO}_2$ rises due to lung disorders that cause hypoventilation, the blood pH will fall and the patient will develop a respiratory acidosis. In this situation, renal hydrogen carbonate ion reabsorption is increased to return the blood pH to normal limits. Exactly the reverse takes place when an individual hyperventilates; the increased unloading of carbon dioxide precipitates a respiratory alkalosis. Here, the kidney compensates by reducing hydrogen carbonate ion reabsorption.

An increase in the **serum potassium concentration** reduces the renal reabsorption of hydrogen carbonate ions by disturbing the mechanism shown in **Fig. 5.4.13**. The reason is that fewer hydrogen ions can be secreted if, due to an increased serum potassium, more potassium ions enter the tubular cells from the blood. If hydrogen ions cannot be secreted, then $\text{HCO}_3^-$ cannot be reabsorbed. The reverse occurs if the serum potassium ion concentration falls.

## Replacement of hydrogen carbonate used in buffering fixed acids; excretion of H⁺ of fixed acids

Fixed acids, including phosphoric and sulphuric acids, are derived from the metabolism of lipids and proteins, respectively. As soon as these acids are formed, they are buffered by the hydrogen carbonate buffer system in plasma as follows:

sulphuric + sodium → disodium + water + carbon
  acid      hydrogen    sulphate           dioxide
           carbonate

phosphoric + sodium → disodium + water + carbon
  acid      hydrogen    hydrogen         dioxide
           carbonate  phosphate

The carbon dioxide formed is unloaded in expired air through the lungs and the two salts – disodium hydrogen phosphate and disodium sulphate – are filtered into the nephron. The role of the kidney is to recover the hydrogen carbonate ions originally used in buffering these fixed acids, to unload hydrogen ions and to excrete the anions of the fixed acids (sulphate and phosphate) that cannot be converted into carbon dioxide and eliminated via respiration. There are two ways of achieving by the kidney:

**1. Renal excretion of ammonium ions.** Disodium sulphate formed by the buffering of sulphuric acid is filtered into the nephron. **Figure 5.4.14** summarizes the reactions that subsequently take place in all areas of the nephron. Inside the epithelial cell, hydrogen ions and hydrogen carbonate ions are produced by the same intracellular reactions previously described. Ammonia ($\text{NH}_3$) is also produced in the epithelial cells by the metabolism of glutamine, an amino acid. Ammonia is fat soluble and easily diffuses across the cell membrane into tubular fluid, where it accepts actively secreted hydrogen ions, forming ammonium sulphate that is excreted in urine. The reabsorption of sodium and internally produced hydrogen carbonate ions into peritubular fluid and blood is dependent on the active secretion of hydrogen ions into tubular fluid. In fact, a large proportion of the ammonium ions ($\text{NH}_4^+$) excreted in urine are in the form of ammonium chloride. The *net* results of the process outlined in **Fig. 5.4.14** are as follows:

- indirect replenishment of stores of hydrogen carbonate ions originally used in buffering fixed acids by intracellular generation in the epithelial cell
- excretion of hydrogen ions
- reabsorption of sodium ions
- excretion of the sulphate anion $\text{SO}_4^{2-}$ of sulphuric acid.

In acidotic states, more ammonia is produced by the tubular cells and this enables more hydrogen ions to be excreted in the form of ammonium ions. In chronic renal failure, when renal tissue is damaged and the cells can no longer form ammonia, less hydrogen ions can be excreted and a metabolic acidosis may ensue.

**2. Formation of titratable acid.** Disodium hydrogen phosphate formed from the hydrogen carbonate buffering of phosphoric acid is filtered into the nephron. Hydrogen carbonate ions are generated by the intracellular mechanisms shown in **Fig. 5.4.15** and are reabsorbed with sodium ions in exchange for hydrogen ions, which are actively secreted. The hydrogen ions are then combined with sodium hydrogen phosphate in tubular fluid to form sodium dihydrogen phosphate – **titratable acid** – which is excreted. Again, the ultimate result of this process is that:

- hydrogen carbonate ions are reabsorbed, replenishing those originally consumed in buffering phosphoric acid
- sodium ions are reabsorbed
- hydrogen ions are excreted
- the fixed acid phosphate anion ($\text{PO}_4^{2-}$) is excreted.

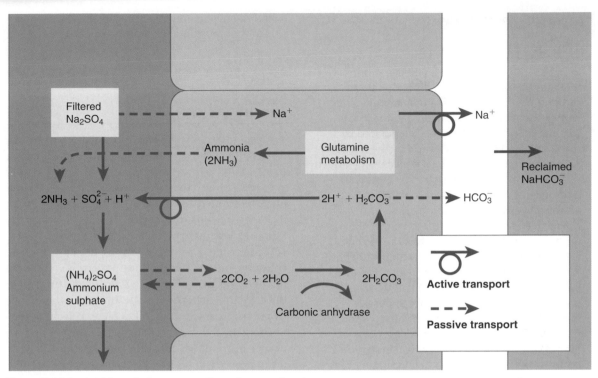

**Figure 5.4.14** Acid–base balance: excretion of ammonium ions

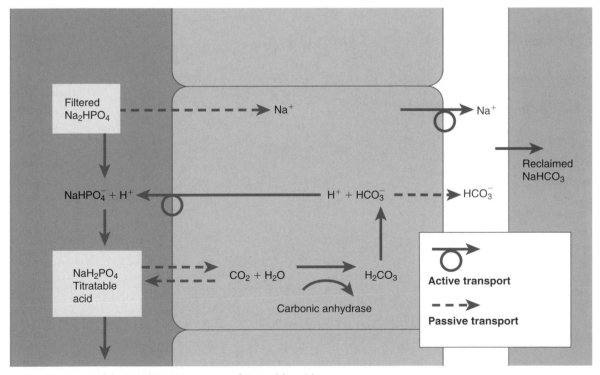

**Figure 5.4.15** Acid–base balance: excretion of titratable acid

Thus, in an indirect way, the hydrogen carbonate ions originally used in buffering fixed acids have been reclaimed and hydrogen ions excreted, restoring the acid–base balance.

More titratable acid is excreted in urine in acidotic states. As the hydrogen ion concentration in blood rises,

eventually the intracellular hydrogen ion concentration also increases, enhancing the active secretion of hydrogen ions into urine.

Approximately 75% of the daily fixed acid load is excreted as ammonium ions, the rest as titratable acid.

## CLINICAL APPLICATIONS

### ACID–BASE DISTURBANCES

In health, the lungs, kidneys and blood buffers regulate the ratio of hydrogen carbonate to carbonic acid at 20 : 1, so maintaining blood pH within normal limits. The hydrogen carbonate component of this buffer pair is regulated by the kidney and the carbonic acid by the lungs. Acid–base imbalances occur if either the hydrogen carbonate component is altered by metabolic disorder, or the carbonic acid component is affected by respiratory disturbances.

Any decrease in arterial pH to below 7.35 (i.e. an increase in hydrogen ions to above 45 nmol/L) is termed **acidosis**, whereas a rise in pH to above 7.5 (i.e. a decrease in hydrogen ions to below 32 nmol/L) is called **alkalosis**. It is not always possible to classify a disturbance as purely metabolic or respiratory because mixed disorders frequently occur. For example, an overdose of aspirin (which is acidic) will cause metabolic acidosis, but this stimulates the respiratory centre and the hyperventilation that follows frequently results in profound respiratory alkalosis.

## The lower urinary tract (Fig. 5.4.16)

### The ureters

The two ureters are hollow tubes that extend from the renal pelvis to the posterior wall of the bladder. In an adult, each ureter is approximately 30 cm long and lies behind the peritoneum. The wall of the ureter is formed by layers of smooth muscle, lined inside by mucous membrane. The renal pelvis is the funnel-shaped upper end of the ureter.

Urine formed in the nephrons drains from tiny collecting ducts into hollow projections (calyces) of the renal pelvis. Urine passes down from here through the ureters into the bladder, where it is stored before micturition takes place. Peristaltic contractions in the muscle walls of the ureters help to propel urine down into the bladder. Back-flow of urine from the bladder is prevented by the oblique

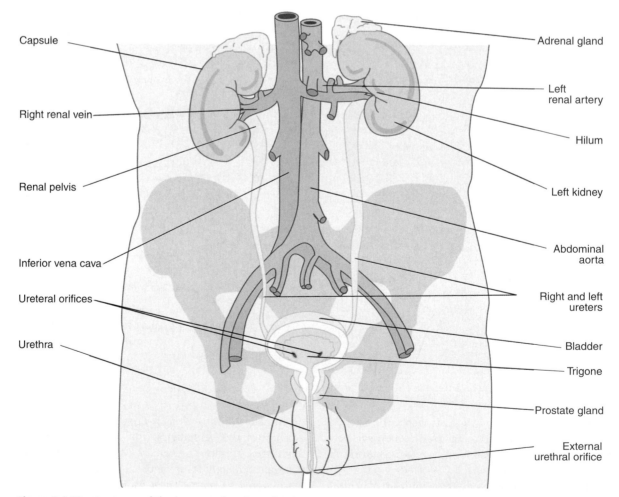

**Figure 5.4.16** Anatomy of the lower male urinary tract

angle taken by the ureters as they pass through the bladder wall.

## The bladder

The bladder is a hollow, highly muscular organ that, when empty, lies low in the pelvis and expands upwards and forwards in the abdomen as it fills. It is lined by a transitional epithelium that allows stretching as the bladder fills and is able to withstand the hypertonicity of urine. Beneath this lies a sheet of smooth muscle known as the **detrusor**.

At the base of the bladder, the smooth muscle fibres form an internal sphincter that surrounds the urethra. As the detrusor contracts, the internal sphincter also contracts, widening the neck of the urethra and allowing urine to enter. At the same time, the levator ani muscles of the pelvic floor relax, 'funnelling' the bladder base and helping urine to flow into the urethra.

The trigone is a triangular area formed by the openings of the ureters and bladder neck. Smooth muscle fibres at the apex of this area help to form the internal sphincter.

## The urethra

The urethra extends from the neck of the bladder to the external urethral opening (meatus). Due to the tone of surrounding smooth muscle and the activity of the external sphincter, no urine enters the urethra except when micturition takes place. A stratified squamous epithelium lines the internal surface of the urethra and its lower part is surrounded by the external sphincter, which is formed from striated muscle (**Fig. 5.4.17**).

In the female (**Fig. 5.4.17a**), the urethra is approximately 4 cm long, running down and along the anterior wall of the vagina; the external meatus opens in front of the vaginal orifice. In the male (**Fig. 5.4.17b**) the urethra is 20 cm long and penetrates the prostate gland (the prostatic glands and ejaculatory duct open into it) before running the length of the penis. Three distinct regions are present: the prostatic, membranous and spongy areas. The external sphincter is situated in the membranous region.

## Micturition

Micturition requires the coordinated activity of parasympathetic, sympathetic and somatic nerves. It is controlled by higher brain centres in the cerebral cortex, basal ganglia and reticular formation. A centre for the reflex control of micturition is situated in the second, third and fourth sacral segments of the spinal cord. It connects with nerve tracts that descend from, and ascend to, the higher centres, and also with parasympathetic and somatic nerves that supply the bladder and sphincters.

### Parasympathetic nerve supply

Motor (efferent) and sensory (afferent) parasympathetic nerves pass in the pelvic splanchnic nerve to and from the bladder. The sensory fibres supply the detrusor and, as the bladder distends, impulses are relayed by these nerves to the sacral segments of the spinal cord. From here they are transmitted in the ascending ventral columns of the cord to the higher centres concerned with the control of micturition. As a result of this passage of impulses, the individual becomes aware of the need to pass urine.

Parasympathetic motor nerve fibres relay to the bladder from the sacral segments of the spinal cord. These nerves supply the detrusor muscle and the internal sphincter and, when stimulated during micturition, bring about contraction of the detrusor muscle and relaxation of the internal sphincter.

Acetylcholine (ACh) is the chemical transmitter that relays the signal from the parasympathetic nerve fibres to the smooth muscle cells of the detrusor; contraction of the detrusor follows this. If the drug atropine is administered, for example as a premedication, acetylcholine is prevented from combining with receptors in the muscle cell membrane. As a result, the nerve impulses that cause contraction of the detrusor are blocked and retention of urine may occur.

### Sympathetic nerve supply

The sympathetic nerve supply consists of sensory (afferent) and motor (efferent) fibres but their role in micturition in humans appears to be minor.

Sympathetic motor fibres originate from the lower thoracic and upper regions of the spinal cord. It is thought that stimulation of these nerves inhibits contraction of the detrusor and closes the internal sphincter.

Sympathetic sensory fibres relay impulses from the bladder to the thoracic region of the spinal cord and these are transmitted upwards in the spinothalamic tracts to higher centres. The sensory nerve fibres relay impulses in response to painful stimuli; they are

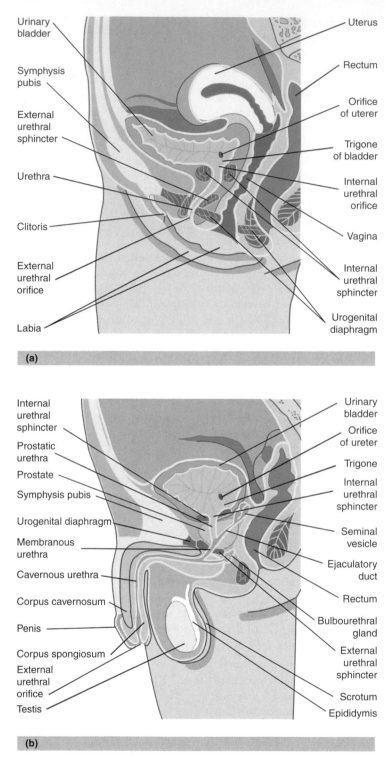

Figure 5.4.17    Anatomy of the urethra in (a) the female and (b) the male

stimulated by overdistension, spasm and inflammation caused by bladder infections, stones or carcinoma.

the sensory fibres supply the wall of the urethra and the motor nerves the external sphincter.

### Somatic nerves

Somatic sensory and motor nerve fibres supply the bladder in the pudendal nerves. More specifically,

### The mechanism of micturition

As urine accumulates, it causes the bladder to distend increasing the wall tension. This stimulates stretch receptors that generate impulses which are transmitted via the parasympathetic sensory nerves to the sacral centre. When small volumes of urine are present in the bladder, an individiual is not aware of any distension. This is because the impulses reaching the sacral centre are prevented from travelling upwards to the cortex by inhibitory impulses descending from these higher centres. However, the presence of approximately 250 mL urine in the bladder sufficiently increases the intensity of impulses to the sacral centre to overcome the descending inhibition. Nerve impulses are then relayed upwards to the sensory cortex and the individual becomes aware of the need to pass urine. Micturition is postponed until the time and place are socially acceptable. When these are satisfactory, inhibition exerted by the motor cortex on the spinal centre is lifted and micturition takes place. Contraction of the detrusor and relaxation of the internal sphincter are brought about by impulses relayed in parasympathetic motor nerves. As soon as urine enters the urethra, stretch receptors are stimulated and generate impulses in sensory afferent nerves to the sacral centre. By reflex, this produces inhibition of the somatic motor nerves that maintain the external sphincter closed while the bladder is filling. As the external sphincter relaxes, urine passes out through the meatus. The detrusor contracts until the bladder is empty, helped by a volley of excitatory impulses relayed down from the higher centres.

Expulsion of urine is also helped by contractions of the abdominal muscles and the performance of Valsalva's manoeuvre, that is, forced expiration against a closed glottis. Control of micturition is learned in infancy and is usually attained at about 2 years of age, when the infant acquires the power to inhibit spinal reflexes and contract the external sphincter at will.

## CLINICAL APPLICATIONS

### DISORDERS THAT IMPAIR MICTURITION

For normal micturition to take place, the following criteria must be met:

- An intact nerve supply to the urinary tract at all levels, including the higher centres.
- Normal muscle tone in the detrusor, sphincters, periurethral and pelvic floor muscles, together with maintenance of an acute angle between the urethra and posterior bladder wall.
- Absence of any abnormal obstruction to the outflow of urine in any part of the upper or lower urinary tract.
- Normal bladder capacity.
- Absence of any psychological or environmental factors which may impair micturition.

## ABNORMAL MICTURITION: SOME DEFINITIONS

**Frequency** is defined as the passage of urine on seven or more occasions during the day and more than twice each night. It is a characteristic feature of the uninhibited neurological bladder, cystitis, lower urinary tract obstructions and conditions in which bladder capacity is reduced due to intrinsic or extrinsic tumours, or pregnancy.

**Urgency** is most commonly described as a strong desire to micturate. This can become irrepressible and lead to uncontrolled voiding of urine – urge incontinence (see below).

**Retention** is an inability to pass urine despite experiencing the desire to do so. It may be associated with frequency, overflow or incontinence and be preceded by a reduced or interrupted flow of urine. The bladder becomes distended, tense and often painful.

**Obstruction** of the lower urinary tract, for example by prostatic hypertrophy, fibroids and strictures, or compression due to external tumours may all cause retention of urine.

**Postmicturition dribbling** after the bladder has apparently emptied is a common feature of obstructive disorders due to prostatic hypertrophy in males and the presence of bladder tumours or calculi. It may also occur as a complication following prostatectomy or, in young men, may be caused by failure of the bulbospongiosus muscle to evacuate the urethral bulb during micturition.

**Incontinence** is defined as the passage of urine at unsuitable times in unacceptable places, due to loss of the voluntary control of micturition. It is a symptom of one or more underlying disorders, which can be reversible or persistent.

**Urge incontinence** is characterized by frequency and urgency due to involuntary bladder contractions. Underlying causes include detrusor instability (common in older adults), uninhibited neurogenic bladder (defective cortical regulatory pathways) and sensory urgency attributable to infection, extrinsic compression/obstruction caused by constipation or a tumour (Royal College of Physicians, 1995).

**Stress incontinence** is the leakage of urine that follows a rise in intra-abdominal pressure due to sudden exertion, coughing, sneezing, bending or even hitting a tennis ball! Laxity and weakness in the muscles supporting the bladder neck, urethra and pelvic floor, or damage to the urethral sphincter are common causes. In males, this can occur after prostatectomy and in females after muscular stretching during childbirth or at the menopause, when mucosal turgor is diminished due to decreased oestrogen secretion. Loss of muscle tone as part of the ageing process can also lead to stress incontinence.

**Overflow incontinence** is essentially a dysfunction of voiding, characterized by symptoms such as hesitancy, frequency, postmicturition dribbling and retention of urine. Underlying causes include neurogenic bladder of the reflex, autonomous, motor and sensory types, attributable to lesions at or above sacral segments S2–S4 (Royal College of Physicians, 1995). Side-effects of medication (hypnotic and diuretic drugs), outflow obstruction due to prostatic enlargement, bladder tumours and faecal impaction are other possible causes.

## ASSESSING INCONTINENCE

Assessment of incontinence is an essential prerequisite to effective management, bearing in mind that more than one type of incontinence may be present in the same individual, presenting a complex symptomatology. Assessment can encompass medical/surgical history, neurological examination, micturition patterns and symptoms, fluid balance (frequency–volume charts), urinalysis, postvoiding residual volumes of urine, medication, body mass index, perineal and rectal examination, pelvic and vaginal examination in women. Contributory factors of social and environmental origin should be noted, together with the presence of chronic disability. Urodynamic investigation can offer more definitive, diagnostic evidence in the identification of physiological causes of incontinence (Button et al., 1998).

## MANAGING INCONTINENCE

Management of incontinence encompasses a wide range of therapeutic options, many of which are beyond the scope of this text. Shah & Leach (2001), Laycock & Haslam (2002) and the Cochrane Review by Roe et al. (1999) offer more detailed information of significant clinical relevance.

Urge incontinence can be treated using bladder training, which involves a gradual voluntary increase in the intervals between voiding until frequency is reduced to 4-hourly intervals. Anticholinergic drugs such as tolterodine, which block acetylcholine-mediated detrusor contraction, can be effective alone or their effects augmented in combination with bladder training, as shown in a recent multicentre study by Mattiasson et al. (2003). When an overactive detrusor is refractory to these treatments, sacral nerve stimulation can bring improvement (Abrams et al., 2003).

Stress incontinence can be significantly improved or cured using pelvic floor exercises to improve muscle tone and bulk. Other treatments, which offer varying success rates, include behavioural therapy (biofeedback using vaginal cones), periurethral/transurethral injection therapy and nerve stimulation. Surgical approaches using pubovaginal slings and retropubic suspension techniques have been reported to achieve 82–84% success rates (Kobashi & Leach, 1999).

Overflow incontinence requires treatment of the underlying cause, which may require surgery in obstructive disorders. Timed voiding schedules, together with pharmacotherapy, can be helpful in the management of sensory neurogenic bladder and stimulation of reflex voiding through gentle suprapubic tapping can assist in the care of reflex neurogenic bladder. Other approaches to management of incontinence resulting from neurological disorders, include intermittent self-catheterization and, in males, the use of a sheath connected to a urinary drainage bag.

## URINARY TRACT INFECTION

The term **'significant bacteriuria'** is used to denote the presence of at least $10^5$ colony-forming bacterial units per millilitre of voided urine and indicates that a urinary infection has occurred, as it is unlikely that contaminants could account for this level of colonization. However, Asscher (1980) has maintained that this definition is limiting when applied to urinary infections and suggests instead that: 'if in a symptomatic subject, pus cells are present and pure growth of an organism is obtained, then urinary tract infection is present, regardless of bacterial numbers.' In 1979, the Medical Research Council Bacteriuria Committee defined three states of urinary tract infection:

- **Cystitis**: an inflammation caused by the presence of bacteria in the bladder or urethra, associated with frequency, dysuria, loin pain and fever.
- **Covert bacteriuria**: bacteria are present in the bladder urine but no symptoms of cystitis are present.
- **Pyelonephritis**: a localized inflammation of the kidneys resulting in scarring, one cause of which is bacteria ascending from the lower urinary tract. This is accompanied by loin pain, fever, dysuria.

The organisms that commonly cause urinary infections are *Escherichia coli* and *Streptococcus faecalis*; the former has been established as the cause of 25% of all hospital-acquired infections. Both these bacteria are common in the normal gut flora and colonize the perineum. *Staphylococcus albus*, found in the skin flora, is another frequent cause of infection. Other, less frequent, organisms that cause urinary infections include *Bacillus proteus* and *Pseudomonas aeruginosa*.

## Symptoms of infection

These include frequency and urgency, as irritation of the pressure receptors in the bladder wall causes the detrusor to contract when only small volumes of urine have collected. A debilitating dysuria or abdominal pain may be present together with pyrexia, shivering, a raised erythrocyte sedimentation rate and leucocyte count. The urine looks cloudy, smells offensive and contains pus cells and leucocytes. Serious complications can arise from a urinary tract infection, including pyelonephritis, which can cause chronic renal failure, and bacteraemia, which can lead to septicaemia.

## Defence mechanisms

Normally, bladder urine is a sterile fluid but some microorganisms may enter the urethra in both sexes. As the female urethra is short (4 cm), it is relatively easy for microorganisms to enter from the perineal skin surface.

A number of protective mechanisms in the bladder and urethra are known to prevent the entry and growth of bacteria. Immunoglobulins IgA and IgG, which are synthesized locally and secreted by the mucosa, are present in human urine and increased in concentration if an infection occurs. Lactic acid secreted by the mucosal cells also helps to inhibit bacterial growth and, in males, prostatic fluid contains an antibacterial agent. Another important defence mechanism is that the bladder empties completely during micturition and so no residual urine remains to provide a reservoir for bacterial growth, although approximately 1 mL of urine may remain in the compressed folds of the mucosa. If a residual urine accumulates, for example in an autonomous or automatic bladder or obstructive disorder, the risk of infection is significantly increased, as is that of stone formation. The optimal pH for bacterial growth is 6–7; inhibition of growth occurs at pH values below 5.5 and above 7.55 (normal urine pH 5–6).

## Sources of infection

An increased risk of bladder infection exists if residual urine is present to provide a potential reservoir for bacterial growth, and in any situation in which microorganisms could be pushed through the urethral meatus and ascend to the bladder.

An infection could thus be a sequel to any of the following:

- bladder catheterization and cystoscopy
- urethral trauma during childbirth or intercourse
- a vaginal discharge
- obstruction of the lower urinary tract
- any condition requiring prolonged bedrest, when urinary stasis may occur.

In addition, any individual suffering from immune depression is at risk of developing a urinary tract infection, for example while taking a course of cytotoxic or corticosteroid drugs, or in the presence of uraemia. Other vulnerable groups include neonates who have an immature immune system, older people and diabetic patients.

## Diagnosis

The presence of urinary tract infection is confirmed by taking a midstream specimen of urine (MSU) for culture and sensitivity. An MSU is a specimen of urine that is not contaminated by organisms outside the urinary tract. Before taking the sample, the perineum and urethral meatus in females and the penis in males should be cleaned. To obtain a midstream specimen of urine, the patient first micturates into either a toilet or non-sterile container to clear contaminants from the lower urethra and its meatus and then stops urination in midstream. On recommencing micturition, 30–50 mL urine is collected in a sterile container. This is then removed and the patient completes passing urine into the non-sterile receptacle. The specimen is sent to the laboratory immediately in a sterile container, labelled correctly, for culture and sensitivity tests.

## Management

After culture and sensitivity of the infecting organism, an appropriate antibiotic is prescribed, usually for a period of 7–10 days. However, in the case of chronic infections, relatively longer-term antibacterial drugs may be given, for example cotrimoxazole (Septrin) for 3 weeks. Other important aspects of management are to increase the fluid intake to 2.5–3 L a day to aid expulsion of bacteria from the urinary tract, unless fluid restrictions are essential. Scrupulous attention to perineal hygiene is required, particularly so in patients who are suffering from faecal incontinence. Analgesia is prescribed for abdominal or loin pain and the patient should be advised to avoid intercourse until the symptoms have disappeared. As a prophylactic measure it is vital that an adequate fluid intake of at least 2 L daily is attained by immobile, bedridden patients in whom urinary stasis is likely to occur, and that remobilization is attempted as soon as the patient's condition allows. A repeat midstream specimen of urine is taken when treatment is complete, to confirm that the infection has been eradicated.

### Catheterization

In hospital, the prevalence of patients with a urinary catheter in situ is high (12.6%) and the procedure shows a strong positive correlation with the presence of bladder infection (Mulhall, 1990). Despite the inception of closed drainage systems, a survey by Meers (1981) reported that 41% of patients suffering a hospital-acquired bacteriuria were catheterized. The risk of acquiring bacteriuria has been estimated at 5–8% for each day the catheter is in situ (Mulhall, 1988) and over 90% of patients undergoing longer-term catheterization develop significant bacteriuria within 4 weeks (Slade & Gillespie, 1985).

Problems resulting from catheterization are not only confined to local or systemic infection but also include tissue damage and pain, all of which can exert a negative impact on recovery (Platt et al., 1983).

Unfortunately, closed drainage systems are not impervious to the entry of microorganisms, which can gain access either during the insertion procedure, if the closed system is subsequently contaminated or by migration between the catheter surface and urethral epithelium. A number of risk factors that may affect the progression of symptomless bacteriuria to overt urinary tract infection and septicaemia have been identified. Byrne (1989) has identified several intrinsic factors, unique to the patient, which may be involved, notably the production and composition of protective bladder/uroepithelial mucus and the patient's immune status.

Some catheter materials may, by virtue of their chemical composition and physical properties, produce more local inflammation, encrustation and bacterial colonization than others. Encrustation occurs only on the surfaces of catheters and balloons exposed to urine, not on those in contact with the bladder or urethral mucosa (Getliffe & Mulhall, 1991).

Infection by urease-producing microorganisms produces the alkaline urine that induces precipitation of ammonium magnesium phosphate and calcium phosphate encrustation. The coarse surfaces of these deposits can cause pain and unpleasant trauma to the urethra when the catheter is removed, in addition to producing catheter blockage. The latter can lead to urinary retention and incontinence leakage around the catheter. Encrustation can also provide a focus for bacterial colonization and becomes an effective barrier protecting microorganisms from

therapeutic agents; electron microscopy studies of encrusted catheters have shown microorganisms lying beneath mineral deposits (Cox, 1989). A similar phenomenon has been observed in relation to the formation of biofilms on catheters and other invasive devices made of inert materials. Here, the composition of the catheter and its surface properties can favour the growth of microorganisms as a functional consortia within a polysaccharide glycocalyx. The latter may protect microorganisms from antibacterial drugs and host defence mechanisms (Brown, 1988; Prosser, 1987).

Other factors exerting a direct influence on catheter-associated infection relate to asepsis during insertion procedures and strategies used to minimize exogenous contamination thereafter. Some surveys have identified problems in these areas of nursing management, notably incorrect positioning of drainage bags, breakage of the closed drainage system and poor attention to handwashing practices before and after meatal cleansing and bag emptying (Crow et al., 1988).

It is vital that bladder catheterization is undertaken only when absolutely necessary (**Table 5.4.3**) and that the catheter is removed as soon as possible. General measures that could minimize the risk of sepsis are summarized below:

• Ensuring catheters are of the appropriate length, diameter, balloon size and materials for each individual, i.e. the smallest that will drain effectively, bearing in mind the anticipated duration of catheterization. A catheter that is

| **Table 5.4.3** Indications for bladder catheterization |
|---|
| To relieve retention associated with lower urinary tract obstruction or neurological disorders |
| To provide preoperative bladder decompression prior to abdominal surgery |
| To obtain an accurate estimate of urine output in critically ill and/or unconscious patients |
| To irrigate the bladder in infections and clot retention and to install antimicrobial drugs in the former |
| To alleviate incontinence of urine when other methods have failed |
| To alleviate painful urination, incontinence, severe skin problems, pressure sores in palliative care |
| To facilitate postoperative drainage following urological or gynaecological surgery |

too large may block the drainage of the paraurethral glands, leading to local abcess or stricture formation.

- Avoiding overinflation of the balloon, which could lead to local bladder irritation, painful contractions and an increased residual volume that favours infection.
- Selecting catheters made of solid silicone and hydrogel, which appear to cause less encrustation, inflammation, urethral trauma and stricture formation. This is particularly important if longer-term use is not anticipated.
- Avoiding any breach of the closed drainage system.
- Employing rigorous asepsis during insertion and bag emptying; handwashing is vital.
- Positioning drainage bags to avoid reflux and to facilitate the effects of gravity. Drainage bags should be positioned well clear of floors or other sources of contamination.

- Avoiding long-term use of prophylactic antibiotics or locally applied antibacterial creams/lotions because these permit the emergence of resistant bacterial strains and bladder irrigations involve a breach of the drainage system. Antibiotics are effective in treating a single episode of infection, however.
- Maintaining a high fluid intake to encourage diuresis if the clinical condition of the patient permits this.
- Removing encrusted deposits. This can be achieved by irrigation using acidic solutions. Benefits here must be weighed against the potential for adverse effects, which include the removal of bladder surface mucus, epithelial exfoliation, chemical cystitis and breach of the closed drainage system.

These issues are discussed in depth by Getliffe & Mulhall (1991).

---

## Clinical review

In addition to the Learning Objectives at the beginning of this chapter, the reader should be able to:

- List the causes of acute and chronic renal failure, and relate these to the pathophysiological changes that occur

- Identify the major problems that arise during renal failure and review their management

- Explain the mode of action of diuretic drugs

- Identify problems that result from micturition disorders and review their nursing management

- Identify the symptoms of fluid and electrolyte imbalance and describe how they may be alleviated

- Explain the effects of ageing on renal function

---

## Review questions

1   Which structures enter and leave the kidney at the hilum?
2   Which tubular structure lies between the glomerulus and the collecting duct?
3   How does the renal arterial supply subdivide to supply the nephrons?
4   What happens when the sympathetic nervous supply to the kidney is stimulated?
5   How does the renal filtrate differ from the blood in the glomerulus?
6   Which forces oppose movement of fluid into the Bowman's capsule?
7   Which factors regulate glomerular filtration rate?
8   What does reabsorption achieve?
9   How are substances transported across membranes against concentration gradients?
10   How is water reabsorbed in the nephron?
11   What does the action of antidiuretic hormone achieve?
12   What is angiotensinogen?

13 What stimulates the release of renin?

14 Which aspects of renal function maintain sodium balance?

15 How does the buffering response of the kidney differ from the responses of the blood and lungs?

16 How does urine move from the kidney to the bladder?

17 How do the external and internal sphincters of the bladder differ?

18 When do we know that our bladder is filling?

## Suggestions for further reading

Bacallao, R.L. & Carone, F.A. (1997) Recent advances in the understanding of polycystic kidney disease. *Current Opinion in Nephrology and Hypertension*, **6**; 377–383.

Bonegio, R. & Lieberthal, W. (2002) Role of apoptosis in the pathogenesis of acute renal failure. *Current Opinion in Nephrology and Hypertension*, **11**; 301–308.

Bridoux, F., Hugue, V., Coldefy, O. et al. (2002) Fibrillary glomerulonephritis and immunotactoid (microtubular) glomerulopathy are associated with distinct immunologic features. *Kidney International*, **62**; 1764–1775.

Burton, M.D. & Rose, D. (1999) *Clinical Physiology of Acid–Base and Electrolyte Disorders*. London: McGraw-Hill.
*An overview of the mechanisms subserving acid–base balance, integrating renal and respiratory function. Good review of common clinical acid–base disorders and aspects of treatment. Highly recommended for readers working in critical care settings.*

Carr, S. (2002) Evaluating renal function. *British Journal of Renal Medicine*, **Spring**; 10–12.

Christensen, E.I. & Birn, H. (1997) Hormone, growth factor, and vitamin handling by proximal tubule cells. *Current Opinion in Nephrology and Hypertension*, **6**; 20–27.

Closs, E.I. (2002) Expression, regulation and function of carrier proteins for catonic amino acids. *Current Opinion in Nephrology and Hypertension*, **11**; 99–107.

Donald, W., Seldin, M.D. & Giebisch, G. (2000) *The Kidney: Physiology and Pathophysiology*, 3rd edn. New York: Lippincott, Williams and Wilkins.
*An in-depth review of mechanisms underpinning normal and abnormal renal function.*

Eladari, D., Chambrey, R., Pezy, F. et al. (2002) pH dependence of $Na^+$/myo-inositol cotransporters in rat thick limb cells. *Kidney International*, **62**; 2144–2151.

Giebisch, G.H. (2002) A trail of research on potassium. *International Society of Nephrology*, 1498–1509.

Glynne, P. (2003) *Acute Renal Failure in Practice*. London: Imperial College Press.
*An excellent contemporary review of the management of acute renal failure. Of interest to those working in renal units and related primary care settings.*

Hilpert, J., Wogensen, L., Thykjaer, T. et al. (2002) Expression profiling confirms the role of endocytic receptor megalin in renal vitamin D3 metabolism. *Kidney International*, **62**; 1672–1681.

Holcslaw Mitchell, P., Hodges, L.C., Muwaswes, M. & Walleck, C. (1988) *AANN'S Neuroscience Nursing*. Norwalk, CT: Appleton-Lange.

Johnson, D.W. (2000) Growth factors in progressive renal disease. *Nephrology*, **5**; 251–261.

Khan, S.R., Glenton, P.A., Backov, R. & Talham, D.R. (2002) Presence of lipids in urine, crystals and stones: Implications for the formation of kidney stones. *Kidney International*, **62**; 2062–2072.

Laycock, J. & Haslam, J. (2002) *Therapeutic Management of Incontinence and Pelvic Pain*. London: Springer.
*Emphasis on therapeutics, with a very helpful discussion on pain and its management.*

Muramatsu, Y., Tsujie, M., Kohda, Y. et al. (2002) Early detection of cysteine rich protein 61 (CYR61, CCN1) in urine following renal ischemic reperfusion injury. *Kidney International*, **62**; 1601–1610.

Oliveira-Souza, M., Malnic, G. & Mello-Aires, M. (2002) Atrial natriuretic peptide impairs the stimulatory effect of angiotensin II on $H^+$–ATPase. *Kidney International*, **62**; 1693–1699.

Palacín, M., Estévez, R., Bertran, J. and Zorzano, A. (1998) Molecular biology of mammalian plasma membrane amino acid transporters. *The American Physiological Society*, **78**(4); 969–1034.

Peters, H., Noble, N.A. & Border, W.A. (1997) Transforming growth factor-B in human glomerular injury. *Current Opinion in Nephrology and Hypertension*, **6**; 389–393.

Reilly, R.F. & Ellison, D.H. (2000) Mammalian distal tubule: Physiology, pathophysiology, and molecular anatomy. *Physiological Reviews*, **80**(1); 277–298.

Roe, B., Wilson, K. & Palmer, M. (1999) *Bladder Training for Urinary Incontinence* (Cochrane Review). The Cochrane Library, Issue 2. Oxford: Update Software.

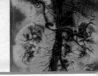

Shah, J. & Leach, G. (2001) *Urinary Incontinence*, 2nd edn. Oxford: Health Press.
*Concise and informative update encompassing aetiology, assessment and management of incontinence.*

Sutton, T.A., Fisher, C.J. & Molitoris, B.A. (2002) Microvascular endothelial injury and dysfunction during ischemic acute renal failure. *Kidney International*, **62**; 1539–1549.

Taal, M.W. & Brenner, B.M. (2001) Evolving strategies for renoprotection: Non-diabetic chronic renal disease. *Current Opinion in Nephrology and Hypertension*, **10**; 523–531.

Thorup, C. & Persson, A.E.G. (1998) Nitric oxide and renal blood pressure regulation. *Current Opinion in Nephrology and Hypertension*, **7**; 197–202.

Valtin, H. & Schafer, J. (1995) *Renal function*. New York: Lippincott, Williams and Wilkins.
*Update of the classic renal physiology text, concise, clear, accessible and affordable; highly recommended.*

Vize, P.D., Woolf, A.S. & Bard, J.B.L. (2003) *The Kidney: From Normal Development to Congenital Disease*. San Diego: Elsevier Science.
*A comprehensive review of the development of the kidney and mechanisms involved in the aetiology of congenital disease.*

Warnock, D.G. (1997) Sodium transporters in health and disease. *Current Opinion in Nephrology and Hypertension*, **7**; 372–376.

# References

Abrams, P., Blaivas, J.G., Fowler, C.J. et al. (2003) Lower urinary tract. *British Journal of Urology International*, **91**; 355–359.

Asscher, A.W. (1980) *The Challenge of Urinary Tract Infections*. London: Academic Press.

Bihl, G. (2001) Non-dialytic management of acute renal failure in the ICU. *British Journal of Renal Medicine*, **Summer**; 6–8.

Brown, M.R.W. (1988) Resistance of bacterial biofilms to antibodies: A growth related effect. *Journal of Antimicrobial Chemotherapy*, **22**; 777–783.

Button, D., Roe, B., Webb, C. et al. (1998) *Continence: Promotion and Management by the Primary Health Care Team. Consensus Guidelines*. London: Whurr.

Byrne, D. (1989) Interaction of urinary tract protein with enteric bacteria. *Journal of Urology*, **141**; 250A.

Cantin, M. & Genest, J. (1987) The heart as an endocrine gland. *Hypertension*, **10**; 1118.

Cappellin, E., Gatti, R., Spinella, P. et al. (2001) Plasma atrial natriuretic peptide (ANP) fragments proANP (1–30) and proANP (31–67) measurements in chronic heart failure: A useful index for heart transplantation? *Clinica Chimica Acta*, **310**; 49–52.

Cox, A.J. (1989) Infection of catheterised patients: Bacterial colonisation of encrusted Foley catheters shown by scanning electron microscopy. *Urology Research*, **17**; 349–352.

Creager, J.G. (1983) *Human Anatomy and Physiology*. Belmont, CA: Wadsworth.

Crow, R.A., Mulhall, A.B. & Chapman, R. (1988) Indwelling catheterisation and related nursing practice. *Journal of Advanced Nursing*, **13**; 489–495.

De Bold, A.J. (1985) Atrial natriuretic factor: A hormone produced by the heart. *Science*, **230**; 767.

Féraille, E. & Doucet, A. (2001) Sodium-potassium-adenosine-triphosphatase-dependent sodium transport in the kidney: Hormonal control. *Physiological Reviews*, **81**(1); 345–418.

Fitzsimons, J.T. (1998) Angiotensin, thirst, and sodium appetite. *Physiological Reviews*, **78**(3); 583–585.

Fletcher, S. & Ayub, W. (2002) Urinalysis – a valuable tool. *British Journal of Renal Medicine*, **Summer**; 10–12.

Getliffe, K. & Mulhall, A.B. (1991) The encrustation of indwelling catheters. *British Journal of Urology*, **67**; 337–341.

Kellum, J.A., Mehta, R.L., Angus, D.C. et al. (2002) The first international consensus conference on continuous renal replacement therapy. *Kidney International*, **62**; 1855–1863.

Knepper, M.A., Saidel, G.M., Hascall, V.C. & Dwyer, T. (2003) Concentration of solutes in the renal inner medulla: interstitial hyaluronan as a mechano-osmotic transducer. *American Journal of Physiology Renal Physiology*, **284**; F433–F446.

Knepper, M.A., Verbalis, J.G. & Nielsen, S. (1997) Role of aquaporins in water balance disorders. *Current Opinion in Nephrology and Hypertension*, **6**; 367–371.

Kobashi, K.C. & Leach, G.E. (1999) Stress urinary incontinence. *Current Opinion in Urology*, 9; 285–290.

Laycock, J. & Haslam, J. (2002) *Therapeutic Management of Incontinence and Pelvic Pain*. London: Springer.

Manjunath, G., Sarnak, M.J. & Levey, A.S. (2001) Prediction equations to estimate glomerular filtration rate: An update. *Current Opinion in Nephrology and Hypertension*, **10**; 785–792.

Marples, D., Frokiaer, J. & Nielsen, S. (1999) Long-term regulation of aquaporins in the kidney. *The American Physiological Society*, **276**(45); F331–F339.

Mattiasson, A., Blaakaer, J., Hoye, K., Wein, A.J. & the Tolterodine Scandinavian Study Group. (2003) Simplified bladder training augments the effectiveness of tolterodine in patients with an overactive bladder. *British Journal of Urology International*, **91**; 54–60.

Mattson, D.L. (2003) Importance of the renal medullary circulation in the control of sodium excretion and blood pressure. *The American Physiological Society*, **284**; R13–R27.

Meers, P.D. (1981) National Survey of Infection in Hospitals. Part 2: Results. Part 3: Urinary Tract Infection. *Journal of Hospital Infection,* **2**(Suppl.); 23–28.

Mulhall, A.B. (1990) Catheterisation. *British Medical Journal,* **301**; 1216.

Mulhall, A.B. (1988) Bacteriuria during indwelling urethral catheterisation. *Journal of Hospital Infection,* **11**; 253–262.

Needleman, P. & Greenwald, J.E. (1986) Atriopeptin: a cardiac hormone intimately involved in fluid, electrolyte and blood pressure homeostasis. *New England Journal of Medicine,* **314**; 828.

Pallone, T.L. & Mattson, D.L. (2002) Role of nitric oxide in regulation of the renal medulla in normal and hypertensive kidneys. *Current Opinion in Nephrology and Hypertension,* **11**; 93–98.

Pavenstädt, H., Kriz, W. & Kretzler, M. (2003) Cell biology of the glomerular podocyte. *The American Physiological Society,* **83**; 253–307.

Platt, R., Polk, B.F., Murdoch, B. & Rossner, B. (1983) Reduction of mortality associated with nosocomial urinary tract infection. *Lancet,* **1**; 893–897.

Prosser, B. (1987) Method of evaluating effects of antibiotics upon bacterial biofilm. *Antimicrobial Agents and Chemotherapy,* **31**; 1502–1506.

Richards, A.M., McDonald, D. & Fitzpatrick, M.A. (1988) Atrial natriuretic hormone has biological effects in man at physiological plasma concentrations. *Journal of Clinical Endocrinology and Metabolism,* **67**(6); 1134–1138.

Richards, A.M., Nicholls, M.G. & Ikram, H. (1986) Renal haemodynamic and hormonal effects of human atrial natriuretic peptide in healthy volunteers. *Lancet,* **1**; 545.

Roe, B., Wilson, K. & Palmer, M. (1999) *Bladder Training for Urinary Incontinence* (Cochrane Review).

The Cochrane Library, issue 2. Oxford: Update Software.

Royal College of Physicians (1995). *Incontinence: Causes, Management and Provision of Services.* London: Royal College of Physicians.

Saito, Y., Nakao, K. & Nishimura, I.K. (1987) Clinical application of atrial natriuretic peptide in patients with congestive heart failure. *Circulation,* **76**; 115.

Seul, K.H., Han, J.H., Kang, K.Y. et al. (2003) Regulation of ANP secretion by cardiac $Na^+/Ca^{2+}$ exchanger using a new controlled atrial model. *The American Physiological Society,* **284**; R31–R40.

Shah, J. & Leach, G. (2001) *Urinary Incontinence,* 2nd edn. Oxford: Health Press.

Slade, N. & Gillespie, W.A. (1985) *The Urinary Tract and the Catheter: Infection and Other Problems.* Chichester: Wiley.

Toigi, G., Aparicio, M., Attman, P-O. et al. (2000a) Expert Working Group report on nutrition in adult patients with renal insufficiency (Part 1). *Clinical Nutrition,* **19**(3); 197–207.

Toigi, G., Aparicio, M., Attman, P-O. et al. (2000b) Expert Working Group report on nutrition in adult patients with renal insufficiency (Part 2). *Clinical Nutrition,* **19**(4); 281–291.

Trippodo, N.C. (1987) An update on the physiology of atrial natriuretic factor. *Hypertension,* **10**; 1–22.

Tryggvason, K. & Wartiovaara, J. (2001) Molecular basis of glomerular permselectivity. *Current Opinion in Nephrology and Hypertension,* **10**; 543–549.

Valtin, H. (1979) *Renal Dysfunction: Mechanisms Involved in Fluid and Solute Imbalance.* Boston: Little Brown.

Verroust, P.J. & Kozyraki, R. (2001) The roles of cubilin and megalin, two multiligand receptors, in proximal tubule function: Possible implication in the progression of renal disease. *Current Opinion in Nephrology and Hypertension,* **10**; 33–38.

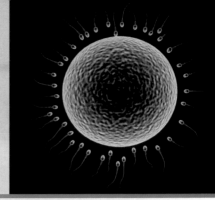

# Section 6

# Protection and survival

# Innate defences

*Sharon L. Edwards*

## LEARNING OBJECTIVES

After studying this chapter the reader should be able to:

- Describe the structure of the epidermis and dermis

- Outline the appendages of the skin

- Relate the structure of the skin to its protective functions

- Briefly describe skin changes during fetal development

- Detail areas of practice relating to the skin such as assessment, prevention of breakdown, wound healing and imbalances of the skin

- Discuss temperature homeostasis, thermoregulation and heat regulation mechanisms

- Detail the imbalances of temperature control: (hyper)pyrexia, hyperthermia, hypothermia

- Describe how to assess body temperature, the sites, equipment and diurnal variations

- Describe the body's innate defences against bacteria

- Detail how microorganisms gain entry to the body, the surface membrane barriers, the cells and molecules of innate immunity, and how an increase in body temperature prevents the spread of infection

- Discuss the role of inflammation as an innate defence mechanism

- Outline how innate immunity stimulates the specific immune response

## INTRODUCTION

Humans are constantly faced with a hostile army of microorganisms swarming their skin. Considering the persistent invasion of bacteria and viruses, it is surprising that humans stay healthy most of the time. This chapter is concerned with body defences that are present at birth and do not vary. Whether the body is protecting itself from mechanical, chemical, physical or microbiological trauma the response remains the same.

The human body, if it is to survive, must be protected against environmental influences that could do it harm. The protective defences include an intact skin, the ability to control body temperature, which can be

increased in an attempt to destroy bacteria, and the innate defences themselves – a group of defence mechanisms are contained within the outer and some inner coverings of the body. These processes function to maintain homeostasis and are the first line of defence against bacteria.

## The anatomy of the skin

Human skin is surprisingly versatile. It is waterproof, stretchable, washable and crease resistant. It also invisibly repairs small cuts, grazes, burns and lasts a lifetime. It is the largest organ of the body, and together

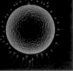

with its appendages (sweat and oil glands, hairs and nails), makes up a complex set of organs that fulfils several functions, the major one of these being protection. Together, these organs form the integumentary system.

The skin forms the largest sensory organ and covers the entire body. Its total surface area (which can be calculated from nomograms) is 1.5 m² to 2.0 m², depending on the height and weight of the individual. It weighs about 4 to 5 kg (9–11 pounds) and accounts for 7% of total body weight.

The skin varies in thickness from 1.5 to 4.0 mm or more in different parts of the body. It also varies in its degree of pigmentation. Throughout the body, exposed areas are generally darker than areas that are normally kept covered. The skin also varies in its degree of hairiness (hirsutism) over different areas of the body and between individuals.

The skin is made up of three distinct regions: the **epidermis**, **dermis** and **hypodermis**. The epidermis is composed of **epithelial cells** and forms the outermost protective cover of the body. It contains no blood vessels or nerve endings. Nutrients reach the epidermis by diffusion through the tissue fluid from blood vessels in the dermis.

The underlying dermis is composed of **connective tissue**. It is tough, makes up the bulk of the skin and contains the blood vessels and nerve endings (Fig. 6.1.1).

The hypodermis is the deep tissue, consisting mainly of adipose tissue or fat store, and anchors the skin to the underlying muscles. This layer thickens when a person gains weight.

## Epidermis

### The cells of the epidermis

The epidermis includes specialized cells: keratinocytes, melanocytes, Langerhans' cells and Merkel cells:

- **Keratinocytes** are produced from keratin, a small, insoluble, fibrous protein molecule made up of 18 amino acids. It is keratin that gives the epidermis its toughness and its protective properties. Keratinocytes arise in the deepest part of the epidermis, from the layer of basal cells (the stratum basale) that undergo continuous mitosis. The keratinocytes are pushed towards the surface by the production of new cells beneath them. By the time the keratinocytes reach the free surface of

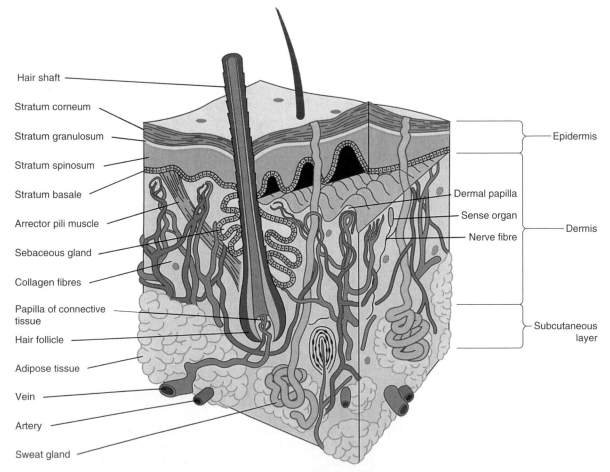

**Figure 6.1.1** Microscopic structure of the skin. The epidermis is raised at one end to show the dermal papillae

the skin they are dead. Millions of these dead cells rub off the skin surface every day, giving a new epidermis every 25–45 days.

- **Melanocytes** synthesize the pigment **melanin** and are found in the deepest layer of the epidermis. They form a pigment shield that protects the keratinocyte nucleus from the damaging effects of ultraviolet (UV) radiation in sunlight. The differences in skin colouring are due to the variation in melanocyte activity and the speed of melanin breakdown.
- **Langerhans' cells** arise from bone marrow and migrate to the epidermis. They help to activate the immune system.
- **Merkel cells** are relatively small in number and act as sensory receptors for touch.

## The layers of the epidermis

Structurally, the epidermis and dermis form two distinct layers, yet they function as a single layer. The epidermis is formed of **squamous epithelial tissue** and this is usually made up of five layers of cell types **(Fig. 6.1.2)**. It is therefore a stratified epithelium, with cells being produced in the basal layer and moving through the other layers over a period of approximately 35 days.

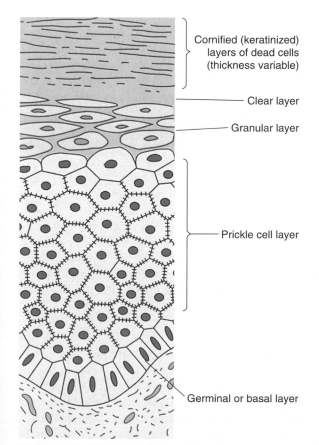

Cornified (keratinized) layers of dead cells (thickness variable)

Clear layer

Granular layer

Prickle cell layer

Germinal or basal layer

**Figure 6.1.2**  Cell layers of the epidermis

1. The **basal layer** (stratum basale) is the single-cell layer nearest to the dermis. Cell division occurs in this basal layer, which, as a result, is sometimes called the **germinal layer** (stratum germinativum). The cells in the basal layer dip down into the dermis to surround sweat glands and hair follicles. After injury, for example burning, as long as that part of the dermis that contains the hair roots or sweat glands is retained then some epidermal regeneration can occur from the remaining basal cells.

   **Keratinocytes** in the basal layer begin the process of **keratinization**, which progresses throughout the layers of the epidermis until cells in the horny layer are keratinized, i.e. filled with the protein keratin. Keratinization is most evident in those areas subjected to the greatest friction, for example, the palms and soles. It is absent from areas that are not exposed to external stresses, for example, inside the lips. Callosities are formed when keratinization occurs in excess.

2. The **prickle layer** (stratum spinosum), which lies above the basal layer, is several cells thick. The cells in this layer are attached to desmosomes, which prevent cell separation (something that might otherwise occur as a result of surface stresses). To facilitate the protein synthesis that occurs in keratinization, the cells are rich in ribonucleic acid (RNA). In addition, this layer contains Langerhans' cells, which arise from bone marrow precursors.

3. The **granular layer** (stratum granulosum) consists of cells containing cytoplasmic granules. These contain a precursor of keratin called keratohyaline, which contributes to keratin aggregation. The cells contain a waterproofing glycolipid that is secreted into the extracellular space and slows water loss across the epidermis.

4. The **clear layer** (stratum lucidum) is present only in thick skin, such as that on the palms of the hands and soles of the feet. The cells here are starting to undergo nuclear degeneration and contain eleidin, a gel-like substance, that is the precursor of keratin.

5. The **cornified (horny) layer** (stratum corneum) forms the surface layer of cells. All the cells in this layer are dead and are constantly being shed from the body's surface. **Up to one million of these cell flakes, formed of keratin, are shed every 40 minutes, amounting to approximately 1 g lost per day.** This layer of dead cells provides a durable layer for the body, protecting deeper cells from a hostile environment and from water

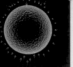
loss rendering the body relatively insensitive to biological, chemical and physical assaults. The process by which cells are shed is called **desquamation**, or **exfoliation**.

## The normal flora of the skin epidermis

There may be up to three million microorganisms on each square centimetre of skin most; of these are **commensals**. A harmless association exists between humans and their commensal microorganisms, to the sole benefit of the latter. The bacteria commonly present as commensals on the skin are *Corynebacterium* species and *Staphylococcus epidermis* (Gould, 1991).

### CLINICAL APPLICATIONS

The skin does not provide a very hospitable environment for bacteria unless they have become adapted through evolution to live there and commensals have, in general, become adapted to live off human skin scales and the slightly acid secretions produced by the skin. The microorganisms tend to live in the deeper layers of the stratum corneum, near to their food source. Hence, they are not normally shed during desquamation. The application of strong deodorants and the use of strong soaps, which alter the skin pH from acid to alkaline, upset the fine balance that exists between pathogens (disease producing microorganisms) and our skin, killing or inhibiting the normal flora and leaving the area open to potential colonization by pathogens.

Babies are born with little or no resident microbial flora. During a normal delivery, a baby picks-up organisms during the passage down the vagina. A resident population of commensals makes it harder for pathogens to survive and so a neonate is particularly prone to skin infections until the skin becomes colonized. If skin is poorly cared for, the normal microbial commensals may be overcome and pathogens may colonize the area. Microorganisms thrive in moist conditions, and so the axillae and groins provide favourable areas for their growth.

Individuals live in harmony with commensals as long as the skin remains an intact barrier. However, if these microorganisms are given the opportunity to invade the dermis, or the normally sterile body cavities, for example the bladder, these normally harmless bacteria may then act as opportunistic pathogens.

## Dermis

The dermis is formed of loose **areolar connective tissue (Fig. 6.1.3)** of mesenchymal origin. It is a fibrous elastic bed, supporting and providing nourishment for

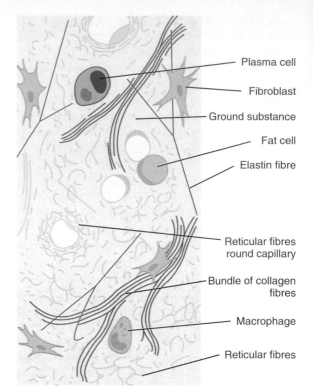

**Figure 6.1.3** Loose (areolar) connective tissue

the epidermis and its appendages (the hairs, sweat glands, blood vessels, lymphatic vessels and nerve endings) **(see Fig. 6.1.1)**. The dermis ranges in thickness from about 0.5 mm in the eyelid, penis and scrotum to over 4 mm thick on the soles of the feet and the palms of the hands. It gives mechanical strength to the skin.

The dermis is formed of two distinct layers, the **papillary layer** and the **reticular layer**. The papillary layer lies next to the basal layer of the epidermis and forms a series of undulations called dermal papillae (or rete pegs), which alternate with the epidermis. In fact, the two layers slot into one another rather like two pieces of corrugated paper **(see Fig. 6.1.1)**. A polysaccharide gel further serves to bind the two layers together. This cellular arrangement prevents the epidermis shearing off the dermis when shearing forces are applied to the skin. The deeper reticular layer contains fewer blood vessels and is less reactive.

Like all true connective tissues, the dermis is formed of a **ground substance** or matrix, **fibres** and **cells**.

## Ground substance

The ground substance supports fibres and cells and fills the spaces between them. Substances in solution travelling between blood vessels and cells must cross through this matrix. The gel is made up of hyaluronic acid, mucopolysaccharides and chondroitin sulphate, and is synthesized by the cells suspended in it. Certain microorganisms, for example *Streptococcus pyogenes* and *Clostridium perfringens*, produce an enzyme called hyaluronidase, which can lyse (dissolve) the hyaluronic acid in the ground substance and thus open-up tracks in the dermis for dissemination of infections.

## The fibres

There are three main fibres, all produced by mesodermal fibroblasts:

1. **Collagen fibres.** Collagen is a fibrous protein with the tensile strength of steel wire of the same diameter. The fibres lie parallel to one another in the dermis in bundles. Apart from its strength and protective function, the major characteristic of collagen is that it binds water avidly, so much so that the dermis contains 18–40% of the total body water. The mucopolysaccharides in the ground substance aid in this function. This water can be mobilized in dehydration or haemorrhage.

   Ascorbic acid is necessary for collagen formation and hence an adequate intake is essential for efficient wound healing.

### DEVELOPMENTAL ISSUES

The water-binding properties of collagen decrease with age and it is thought that the wrinkled appearance of the skin in elderly people is due not so much to degeneration of elastin fibres (as was previously thought) as to decreased water-holding power of the collagen and mucopolysaccharides.

### CLINICAL APPLICATIONS

Although the bundles of collagen fibres run in diverse directions, in certain areas they tend to lie in the same direction. Wherever possible, surgeons make their incisions in the direction in which the fibres lie (the line of cleavage).

2. **Reticular fibres** form a loose framework in the dermis and envelop the collagen bundles. They help to disperse mechanical forces applied to the dermis.
3. **Elastin fibres** are branching yellow fibres. They are elastic but may rupture when stretched by pregnancy, obesity or prolonged ascites. When this occurs, silvery linear scars appear, called striae or **stretch marks**.

## The cells

These are either resident (synthesizing ground substance or fibres) or blood-borne and transient:

- **Fibroblasts** lie between the bundles of collagen and synthesize collagen and elastin. Their numbers increase considerably during wound healing.
- **Tissue macrophages or histiocytes** are wandering phagocytic cells (derived from the monocytes in blood). They engulf particles and matter and are protective in function.
- **Tissue mast cells** produce histamine, prostaglandin and other inflammatory mediators, and are found in connective tissues. They occur only transiently in blood following their release from their site of synthesis in bone marrow and are non-functional in blood.
- **Transient cells** include neutrophils, lymphocytes and monocytes. They move constantly between the blood vessels of the dermis, moving out of the blood in large numbers as part of the inflammatory reaction which occurs in response to trauma and infection. Normally, the dermis is free from bacteria.

### Skin colour

The three pigments that contribute to skin colour are melanin, carotene and haemoglobin. These pigment-producing cells are present in the dermoepidermal junction over the entire skin.

Melanin, which colours hair, originates from melanocytes near the hair papillae, and there is a biochemical difference in the melanin produced by blondes, brunettes and redheads, which results in different tones of hair pigment colour. The melanin in the iris of the eye, too, differs structurally between individuals. Melanin production is influenced by sunlight. After exposure of skin to sunlight, new melanin is not formed immediately. Erythema (reddening of the skin) due to inflammation occurs initially and this lasts approximately 2 days. Then melanin production is evident as the skin colour changes from pink to brown. Melanin production is under genetic control, and is regulated by melanocyte-stimulating hormone (MSH), secreted from the anterior lobe of the pituitary gland.

Haemoglobin gives the pinkish hue of fair skin, which is due to the crimson colour of oxygenated haemoglobin in the red blood cells circulating through the dermal capillaries.

## Blood vessels

The cutaneous blood vessels **(Fig. 6.1.4)** lie entirely within the dermis and have an essential role in transporting nutrients to, and waste substances from, the dermal tissues. They are also of major importance in the regulation of body temperature. (This latter topic will be discussed in greater detail later in the chapter). The skin is capable of accommodating varying amounts of blood. The number of vessels carrying blood at any one time varies with the environmental

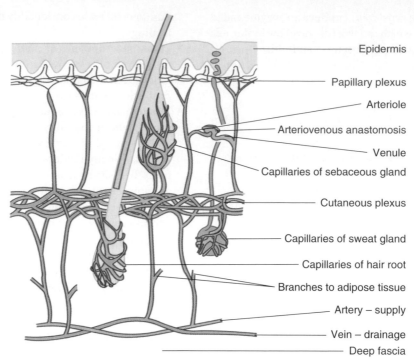

**Figure 6.1.4** Cutaneous blood flow

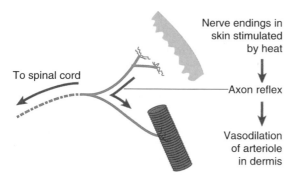

**Figure 6.1.5** Axon reflex

temperature. When body temperature rises, the sympathetic vasoconstrictor tone is reduced leading to vasodilation, allowing blood to circulate to the deeper capillary beds. A larger volume of warm blood enters the superficial vessels, promoting heat loss. When the environmental temperature drops, the sympathetic nerves are stimulated and so vasoconstriction occurs; vasodilation results from sympathetic inhibition in warm conditions **(Fig. 6.1.5)**.

Under normal conditions, there is always a certain amount of background vasoconstrictor tone. Circulating adrenaline (epinephrine) and noradrenaline (norepinephrine) enhance the vasoconstrictor effect of the sympathetic nerves.

## Lymphatic vessels

Lymphatic vessels are found throughout the dermis and have a major role in draining excess tissue fluid

and any plasma proteins that may have leaked into the tissues. Up to 15% of all tissue fluid can be drained via this route, fluid which, due to the nature of capillary dynamics, cannot be reabsorbed back into the venous circulation in the capillary bed. The lymphatic vessels are important in maintaining circulating volume by reducing the accumulation of interstitial fluid and returning the drained fluid to the cardiovascular system via the great veins.

## Nerve supply

The skin is the largest sensory organ in the body. Its dermis contains sensory nerves whose cell bodies lie in the dorsal root ganglia. These afferent nerves may then either link with a reflex arc and/or travel up the spinal cord in specific spinal pathways for each sensory modality to the sensory cortex, where the information they carry is interpreted.

Sensory receptors, in general, are specialized so that they each respond to a different form of energy – chemical, mechanical or thermal – thus the modalities of touch/pressure, cold, warmth and pain can be consciously appreciated.

The receptors act as **transducers**, and convert the energy into action potentials. The skin contains three main types of sensory nerve ending **(Fig. 6.1.6)**: **naked nerve endings**, **encapsulated endings** (Pacinian corpuscles, Meissner's corpuscles and Krause's end-bulbs) and **expanded endings** (Ruffini's organs). These are in addition to petrichial sensory endings that supply hair follicles (see Chapter 2.2).

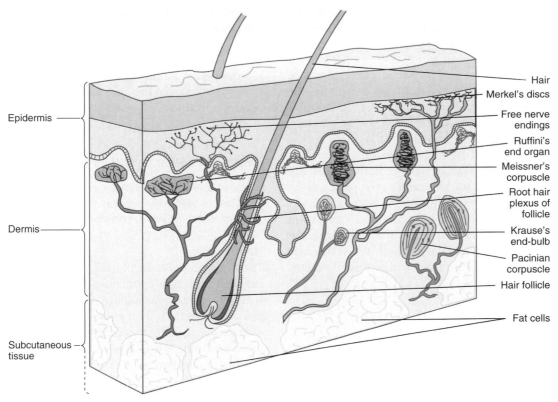

**Figure 6.1.6** Sensory receptors in the skin

## Appendages of the skin

Along with the skin, the integumentary system includes extensions or appendages including the hair follicles, and hair, nails, sweat glands and sebaceous (oil) glands. Each plays an important role in maintaining homeostasis.

### Hair

Hair is formed of fibrous protein (largely keratin) and is exclusive to mammals. It functions to protect the skin from ultraviolet light, extremes of temperature and from trauma. Owing to the presence of nerve endings around hair follicles, hair also acts as a tactile organ. To a certain extent, in human society, it serves sexual display purposes. Hair is very durable and can resist decay for thousands of years: Egyptian mummies show traces of head hair. Hair follicles develop during weeks 12–18 of fetal life, and the total number of hairs decreases with age.

### Hair follicles

The **hair follicle** lies in the dermis, surrounded by its blood and nerve supply. The basal layer of the epidermis dips down to surround it **(Fig. 6.1.7)**. The shaft of the hair projects beyond the surface of the skin. In the centre of the shaft is the medulla, containing loosely packed keratinized cells and air spaces. Surrounding the shaft is the **cortex**, formed of keratinized cells that are cemented together and contain

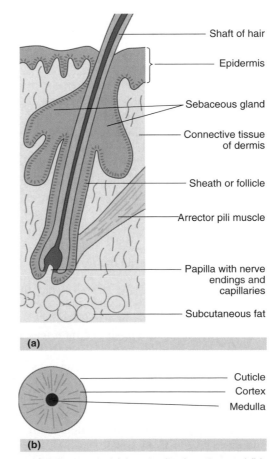

**Figure 6.1.7** Hair in (a) longitudinal section and (b) cross-section

granules of melanin. The melanin is secreted by melanocytes, which are concentrated around the germinal base of the hair. If air spaces occur in the cortex, the hair will appear grey or silver.

The **cuticle** surrounds the cortex and is formed of overlapping pigment-free cells which, under the microscope, look rather like fish-scales. These scales can be prised off the cortex and hence the hair may be damaged by the technique of 'back-combing' it.

The lower end of the shaft in the dermis is distended to form the **bulb**. If a hair is pulled sharply out of the scalp, the bulb at the end can be seen quite clearly. Cell division occurs in the bulb and hence this area is affected by cytotoxic drugs. A small bundle of muscle fibres is attached to the portion of the shaft near the bulb called the **arrector pili muscle**. When this contracts, the hair is pulled more vertically in the dermis.

### Types of hair

Human hair is of three types:

- **Lanugo** is fine, long, silky non-pigmented hair present in the first 7–8 months of fetal life, after which time it is shed in utero. Premature babies may be born still covered in lanugo. This can be a cause of distress to parents, who may need to be reassured that the presence of lanugo at this stage is normal and that it will soon disappear. In malignant disease, it occasionally happens that lanugo may replace terminal hair (see below) following chemotherapy.
- **Vellus** is short hair similar to lanugo. It is colourless, forms the child's body hair and remains on the adult female's face.
- **Terminal hair** is found on the adult head and pubis. When, as a result of disease such as Cushing's syndrome, a person becomes hirsute, it is terminal hair not vellus that appears on the face. This is much more noticeable and can cause distress.

### Hair production

Hair production is influenced by several factors:

- **Racial factors**. In Caucasians, straight hair tends to be round, and curly hair oval in cross-section. In people of African descent, hair is flat in cross-section. These ribbon-shaped hairs tend to spiral, producing crinkly hair.
- **Hormonal factors**. The level of androgens is a critical factor in hair growth. Testosterone stimulates beard growth but not that of head hair. It is testosterone, in conjunction with an inherited predisposition, which produces male-pattern baldness.
- **Genetic factors**. Hair colour and texture are inherited characteristics. The tendency to

premature balding or greying is familial. Hair tends to grow in cycles of activity, and at any one time about 85% of scalp hairs are in an actively growing stage, which lasts for about 2 years. This active period is followed by a period of rest, then regression. Out of the total of about 100 000 hair growing scalp follicles, about 70–100 scalp hairs are lost daily.

### CLINICAL APPLICATIONS

The rate of hair loss may be increased by such factors as severe illness, very low calorie diets, exposure to radiation and childbirth.

### Nails

These are protective keratinized plates resting on the stratified squamous epithelium that form the highly sensitive and vascular nailbed. The nails protect the tips of the fingers and toes from injury. The nail root extends deeply into the dermis towards the interphalangeal joint. Nails can give an indication of certain diseases to the observer. This will be discussed later.

### Sweat glands

Sweat glands produce **sweat** when the skin surface temperature rises above 35°C. They have a minor role in ridding the body of some waste substances and a much more important role in helping to bring about heat loss.

Sweat is composed of 99% water, with a small amount of sodium chloride, urea, lactic acid and potassium in solution. It is hypotonic with reference to plasma, containing fewer electrolytes and very little glucose. It is usually acid in reaction. The specific gravity of sweat is normally about 1.004, but this varies with the rate of secretion, the level of the hormone aldosterone in the blood and acclimatization to extreme heat.

Sweat forms a minor excretory route for some drugs, allergens and substances such as garlic. Sweat glands have a cholinergic sympathetic innervation. There is always some slight activity, with a resultant insensible loss of some 400–500 mL per day. This loss is not all via the sweat glands.

In a temperate climate, approximately 500 mL of sweat each day is produced in addition to the insensible loss. This amount varies with the degree of activity and the environmental temperature. Sweat production can rise to 12 L/day in very hot climates. Sweat production also increases in stressful and emotional states. The evaporation of sweat from the skin surface requires latent heat from the surface of the skin and is thus a method of heat loss. The areas most active in this thermoregulatory sweating are the face, trunk, axillae, palms and soles. The evaporation of

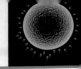

1 L of sweat from the skin requires 2400 kJ (580 kcal) of heat, and it is the evaporation of sweat that causes heat to be lost (not simply the production of sweat). Sweat will not evaporate if the environment is already laden with water vapour.

There are two distinct types of sweat gland (sometimes known as sudoriferous glands) in the skin, each of which has a separate function:

- **Eccrine glands**: these glands are well developed only in humans. In the adult, there are between 3 and 4 million sweat glands, not all of which are active at the same time. The distribution of glands throughout the body is uneven; there are over $400/cm^2$ on the hands and feet and only $70/cm^2$ on the back. They are formed as coiled tubular downgrowths from the epidermis, each having its own blood supply and innervation from cholinergic sympathetic fibres (**see Fig. 6.1.1**).
- **Apocrine glands**: these glands are responsible for the individual's distinctive odour. They are related to the hair follicles, being situated near the sebaceous glands. Apocrine glands are mainly present in the areas of the pubis, genitalia, areola, axillae, umbilicus and external auditory canals. The apocrine glands are ten times larger than the eccrine glands and the openings of their coiled ducts are just visible to the naked eye.

  The secretion from these glands is scanty and sticky. It is odourless when first secreted but is quickly acted upon by bacteria and then gives rise to a distinctive, rather unpleasant, smell. In childhood, the apocrine glands are non-functional but at puberty they begin actively to secrete, stimulated by the sex hormones. Their secretion does not seem to be under the control of the nervous system, although secretion increases in stress and so there may be some sympathetic nervous influence.

  Apocrine secretions may contain pheromones – sexually attractant substances. Human females are thought to produce fatty acid pheromones in their vaginal secretions in the middle of the menstrual cycle and it is possible that the apocrine glands secrete a similar substance. The individual secreting the pheromone is unable to detect its presence.

### Sebaceous glands

These are formed as outgrowths of the developing hair follicles (**see Fig. 6.1.7**). They start to produce their secretions at about 15 weeks of fetal life. Their activity, which is low in childhood, increases during puberty. These glands are particularly plentiful over the scalp and face where there may be up to $900/cm^2$, and also over the middle of the back, the auditory canal and

genitalia. There are very few sebaceous glands on the hands and feet. Over the forehead of a person with particularly active sebaceous glands, more than 2 g of slightly acid sebum may be produced each week.

**Sebum** is a mixture of triglycerides, waxes, paraffins and cholesterol. The sebaceous glands are holocrine glands, their secretion being formed by the disintegration of the glandular cells. New lobes of the gland are therefore continually reforming. Most, but not all, of the glands open onto a hair shaft.

---

**CLINICAL APPLICATIONS**

The function of sebum is to waterproof the skin; in addition, it is thought possible that it protects from fungal and bacterial infections: athlete's foot, for instance, occurs in an area between the toes where there are no or very few sebaceous glands and a damp environment. The skin forms a dry barrier and pathogenic bacteria on its surface often die simply through desiccation. Sebum production is stimulated by a rise in temperature and by androgens; it is inhibited by oestrogen.

---

A child has very small sebaceous glands, which are few in number, and hence babies and children are prone to chapping of the skin on exposure to damp conditions. This predisposes to nappy rash. In old age, the number of sebaceous glands diminishes, with resulting potential skin-care problems.

## Hypodermis

This layer is sometimes called the superficial fascia and not always considered as part of the skin, but it shares the skins protective functions. It contains most (up to 60%) of the body's stores of fat.

### Subcutaneous fat

**Adipose tissue**, or fat, forms a valuable store of triglycerides for the body, and this is a potential source of energy; 60% of the total body fat stores are subcutaneous, and this fat insulates the body and prevents heat loss from the core. Fat also protects from trauma, in that it acts as a shock absorber. Blows to the body surface cause lateral displacement to the skin due to the presence of subcutaneous fat, and hence the full force of the blow is not transmitted to the deeper structures.

Fat distribution, under the skin, differs between the sexes. This difference becomes evident at puberty: females have greater deposits on the upper limbs, breasts and buttocks than do males. Generally, the adult female has greater fat stores than the male – some 15 kg as opposed to the male's 7.5 kg. Diet, genetic factors and sex hormones determine fat stores.

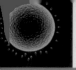

Adipose tissue has very little ground substance, the tissue being divided into lobes by septa, which carry the blood vessels and the nerves. The cells that make up adipose tissue are large and consist of a flat nucleus surrounded by a large single fat globule. When fat is broken down (catabolized), considerable metabolic water is produced – a factor of importance to humans in starvation.

### Brown fat

Some fat appears to be dark in colour. Microscopically, each brown fat cell contains many droplets of fat (instead of a single globule), many mitochondria and some pigment. Brown fat tissue is also more vascular than adipose tissue. The fact that the cells contain many small droplets of fat means that brown fat forms a more readily and rapidly available energy supply. The presence of many mitochondria suggests that the tissue is capable of an increased rate of metabolism.

---

#### CLINICAL APPLICATIONS

Brown fat has an important role in the neonate as it provides an easily mobilized energy source. The neonate has a large body surface area relative to its weight and it is also unable to shiver. The newborn baby therefore has the potential problem of inability to conserve body heat and a propensity to lose too much heat. Thus, the neonate uses the brown fat stored around the back of its neck and kidneys, free fatty acids being liberated from this in response to cold, noradrenaline (norepinephrine) and the hormone glucagon.

Brown fat breakdown increases oxygen consumption and brings about localized energy release. It loses its importance in thermal regulation as the child develops muscular control and hence uses muscular activity and shivering as a method of heat production. It is possible that some individuals may retain their stores of brown fat into adulthood, within the para-aortic, renal and peritoneal fat depots, and that such individuals may be less prone to obesity. They may also be able to lose weight more easily.

---

## The functions of the skin

### Protection

The skin as the outer covering protects the body from trauma, entry of bacteria, the loss or gain of water and from harmful radiation in sunlight. It protects from all the minor mechanical blows that the environment deals, for example pressure and friction. When intact,

the skin is virtually impermeable to microorganisms. It gives rise to protection in four different ways:

- **Physical barrier**: The continuity and keratinization of the skin work together with its acid mantle to deter bacterial invasion. The waterproofing glycolipids of the epidermis block the diffusion of water and water-soluble substances between cells, preventing both their loss from and entry into the body through the skin.

  The skin protects us from all minor mechanical blows dealt by the environment, for example pressure and friction. In addition, it protects us from chemicals (weak acids, alkalis) and most gases (although some gases developed for use in chemical warfare can be absorbed through the skin). The skin also protects against some forms of radiation, such as alpha-rays (which cannot penetrate skin at all) and, to a lesser extent, beta-rays (which can penetrate a few millimetres of skin but are unable to reach the underlying organs).

- **Chemical barrier**: The skin secretions and melanin provide these. The low pH of skin secretions (acid mantle) retards the multiplication of bacteria. Many bacteria are killed outright by bactericidal substances in sebum. In addition, the skin cells secrete a natural antibiotic called human defensin that punches holes in bacteria. The melanin produced within the skin gives protection from ultraviolet radiation.

- **Biological barrier**: These include the Langerhans' cells of the epidermis, which are active elements of the immune system. The Langerhans' cells present foreign substances or antigens to the lymphocytes to activate the immune response. The macrophages in the dermis dispose of viruses and bacteria that have managed to penetrate the epidermis.

- **Absorption**: Certain fat-based molecules can be absorbed through the skin, for example oestrogens, fat-soluble vitamins (A, D, E and K), steroids, methyl salicylate, glyceryl trinitrate (GTN). Such substances can be administered as either ointments or gels, or transdermally via slow-release skin patches. The patches should be applied to clean, non-hairy skin to facilitate absorption, which will depend on the site and its blood flow.

### Cutaneous sensation

The skin forms the largest sensory organ of the body and is richly supplied with cutaneous sensory receptors (part of the nervous system). Nerve endings are found in the dermis and are more concentrated in certain areas (e.g. the fingertips and lips).

They are sometimes classified as exteroceptors because they respond to stimuli arising outside the body. These include:

- **Meissner's corpuscles** (in the dermal papillae) allow awareness of a caress or the feel of our clothing against our skin.
- **Pacinian receptors** (in the deeper dermis or hypodermis) alert awareness to bumps or contacts involving deep pressure.
- **Root hair plexuses** report on wind blowing through our hair and a playful tug at an arm or leg.
- **Painful stimuli** (irritating chemicals, extreme heat or cold, touch) are sensed by bare nerve endings that occur throughout the skin.

In addition, skin hairs are supplied by nerve endings sensitive to touch. Through awareness of these sensations appropriate behavioural action can be taken.

## Temperature regulation

Contributing to the maintenance of a constant core temperature is a major function of the skin and overall control is by the hypothalamus of the brain. In temperate and hotter climates the problem is mainly one of losing the heat produced by metabolism. Homeostasis is achieved via conduction, convection and radiation of heat from the skin surface. Dilation or constriction of the blood vessels, which supply the skin, so increasing or decreasing its blood flow can vary this heat loss. Heat is also lost by the evaporation of sweat.

The skin protects the body from excessive heat loss in cold weather by decreasing both the blood supply to the skin surface and the production of sweat. The organs lying deeper in the body are further insulated from the environment by subcutaneous connective tissue and fat.

Temperature regulation is described in more detail later in this chapter.

## Excretion

There is a very small amount of gas exchange through the skin, a negligible amount of carbon dioxide being lost in this way – about 0.5% of that lost through the lungs. The skin also serves as a minor excretory route for urea, ammonia and uric acid in body sweat, although most of these substances (wastes) are excreted in urine. Profuse sweating is an important avenue for water and salt (sodium chloride) loss.

## Vitamin D synthesis

The term 'vitamin D' actually refers to a group of sterols. The vitamin obtained from fish-liver oils and dairy produce should more correctly be called vitamin $D_3$, or cholecalciferol. It is synthesized when ultraviolet light falls on uncovered skin and acts on the 7-dehydrocholecalciferol present in the dermis, converting it to pre-vitamin $D_3$. This is then slowly converted into vitamin $D_3$.

The synthesis of vitamin D from 7-dehydrocholecalciferol indirectly promotes calcium absorption from the gut. In the United Kingdom, dietary intake usually provides an adequate supply of vitamin D and in this situation the production of vitamin D by the skin is not essential for health. A full discussion of calcium metabolism can be found in Chapter 2.6. This is a further example of a mechanism that maintains a stable internal environment. In this case, vitamin D helps to maintain an adequate amount of calcium in body fluids.

## Energy and water reserve

The skin forms a reserve of energy and water for use in emergencies. To restore a fall in blood volume (e.g. in haemorrhage), fluid can be reabsorbed from the dermis via capillary dynamics. Subcutaneous fat forms an energy reserve, which can be called upon in starvation.

### DEVELOPMENTAL ISSUES

The epidermal layers of the skin are derived from ectoderm, whereas the dermis is formed from mesenchyme, the precursor of connective tissue. The ectodermal cells proliferate to form the protective periderm and it is from these cells that the vernix (the cheesy covering of the skin before birth) is formed. Vernix protects the fetal skin from the effects of being continually surrounded by amniotic fluid.

Melanoblasts, the precursors of melanocytes, are formed during early fetal life from cells of the neural crest (Moore, 1983). Ultraviolet radiation is necessary for the formation of melanin so this process cannot start until after birth.

By 11 weeks of fetal life, the mesenchymal cells in what is to be the dermis have started to produce both collagen and elastin fibres. The dermal papillae are forming and capillary loops and sensory nerve endings are developing.

Hair growth starts at 12 weeks, with the formation of a hair bud by the basal epidermal cells. This extends into the dermis to form a hair bulb by 14 weeks. Two weeks later the hair shaft is beginning to grow from mesenchymal cells and the hair papilla is present. By 18 weeks the hair shaft has grown sufficiently to pierce the epidermis and arrector pili muscles are present. Sebaceous glands begin their development at about 16 weeks on the lateral margins of the developing hair follicles. They contribute to the formation of the vernix mentioned earlier.

As the hairs are developing so too are the sweat glands, which similarly derive from a bud. The gland is initially formed of a solid, cylindrical down growth which, by 18 weeks, develops a lumen and starts to coil.

Fingernail development starts at about 10 weeks, toenails forming a little later. The epidermis on the dorsal surface of each finger or toe becomes thickened into an area called a nail fold. Nail folds develop laterally and proximally on each digit. Eventually cells grow up from the proximal nail folds and become keratinized to form the actual nail or the nail plate.

## CLINICAL APPLICATIONS

### ASSESSMENT OF THE SKIN

The skin is of great importance in the defence of the body and, as such, knowledge of the anatomy of the skin has application in nursing practice. It reflects physiological and pathological changes in other areas of the body and skin changes can be used to aid both nursing and medical diagnosis.

Loss of homeostasis in body cells and organs shows itself on the skin in many ways. The skin is an organ from which a huge amount of information about a patient's nutritional status, fluid balance, circulation, emotional state and age can be obtained. The skin can provide clues leading to the diagnosis of a patient's health problems and to an evaluation of the effectiveness of a patient's health care.

### Age

From the simple observation of the skin it is possible to gain a fairly accurate impression of a person's age. Skin tends to become drier or more wrinkled with age. The care given to the skin may determine the general state of grooming. The latter may give a clue to a patient's physical or mental state. For example, in elderly people, toenails may be neglected because of arthritis, a condition that makes it difficult for the patient to reach them.

### Observation of the skin

The skin can give a clear indication as to the patient's physical state. It may indicate signs of shock, anaemia, high temperatures, reduced oxygen or the presence of a particular disease or condition.

### Skin colour

The colour of the skin is of great importance in assessment. The following changes can occur:

**Pallor** of the skin is dependent on blood flow through the surface vessels. When blood flow to the skin surface is reduced, pallor will occur due to the vasoconstriction of peripheral blood vessels commonly observed when the body is maintaining homeostasis. In response to a stimulus the body redirects blood away from the periphery to the central major organs, as occurs in compensated shock (Edwards, 2002). Pallor occurs in other conditions, such as myocardial infarction and exposure to a cold environment. During stress, adrenaline (epinephrine) causes selective vasoconstriction and noradrenaline (norepinephrine) causes the blood vessels of the systemic circulation to constrict. Hence, anxiety and pain may lead to the appearance of pallor.

In **anaemia**, surface vessel blood flow is adequate but the haemoglobin concentration of the blood is low. The oxygen saturation monitor is not a good estimate of an anaemic state because all the haemoglobin present in the blood will be fully saturated, producing a normal reading. The most accurate method of assessment in this instance is by looking at the mucous membranes, for example, inside the lips or lower eyelid. Here the blood vessels lie nearer the surface and colour can therefore be more clearly observed.

**Flushing** is when there is an increased blood flow of normal haemoglobin content to the surface of the skin leading to the red appearance of the skin. In hot weather, cutaneous vessels dilate to facilitate heat loss from the skin surface. In inflammation (which will be discussed later), vasodilation occurs over the affected area, and redness is a characteristic feature of the process.

**Cyanosis** occurs when more than 5 g/dL (0.74 mmol/L) of haemoglobin is in the reduced state. Cyanosis, a blue coloration, occurs relatively frequently in patients with polycythaemia but is rarely seen in those who are anaemic. Cyanosis occurs in individuals suffering from diseases that result in a reduced amount of oxygen being carried by the blood (hypoxaemia; see Chapter 5.3).

Cyanosis may be central, occurring over the face or lips, or peripheral, when the extremities are affected. The latter usually indicates inadequate or sluggish blood flow in the peripheral tissues. Cyanosis is difficult to assess in patients whose skin pigments may obscure the condition. The inside of the lips, palms of the hands and soles of the feet may give some indication of the problem.

**Jaundice** is an abnormal yellow skin tone, which is usually a sign of a liver disorder. It is caused by the accumulation of abnormal levels of bilirubin in the blood. Bilirubin is the waste product of red blood cell breakdown by the spleen. The majority (99%) is excreted as bilirubin in bile; the other 1% is excreted in the urine as urobilinogen. If the bilirubin cannot be excreted in the bile due to an obstruction, some of the excess is excreted in the urine or deposited in body tissues.

The earliest signs of jaundice can therefore be detected in the urine. Subsequently, a yellow discoloration of the skin is most easily recognized in the conjunctiva, before leading to changes in skin colour. Jaundice is evident when plasma bilirubin levels rise above 34 mmol/L (the normal level is less than 19 mmol/L). A slightly yellow appearance may be apparent in the skin in the later stages of malignant disease when cachexia exists.

## Scars

The presence of scars, striae and bruising on the skin can be significant. Injection marks may give a clue to drug abuse or to conditions requiring prophylactic medication by injection, such as diabetes or haemophilia. Small bruises like dark purple purpura, which are evident in septicaemia, should be considered in relation to the patient's condition.

## Palpation of the skin

How the skin feels to the touch can give information about the patient's fluid balance, state of nutrition and health.

### Moderate and severe dehydration

This can be assessed by gently but firmly pinching up a fold of skin on the back of the hand or on the inner forearm. In a well-hydrated person, it will return immediately to its normal position. In the patient who is in an advanced state of dehydration, the fold of skin may stay pinched for up to 30 seconds. This phenomenon happens to a lesser extent with advancing years.

### Oedema

Oedema is an abnormal collection of fluid in the tissues that can either collect in the interstitial or intracellular spaces. The causes of oedema are varied, and are summarized in **Table 6.1.1**. Oedema is a problem of fluid distribution and does not necessarily indicate fluid excess (McCance & Huether, 1998). It is usually associated with weight gain, swelling and puffiness, tight-fitting clothes and shoes, limited movement of an affected area, and symptoms associated with an underlying pathological condition.

Oedema is recognized by pressing firmly over a bony prominence, such as the medial malleolus of the ankle, for about 5 seconds. Waterlogged tissue retains the imprint of the finger (so-called **pitting oedema**).

### Obesity

This can be assessed by palpation. Skinfold calipers can be used to measure superfluous subcutaneous fat. Obese skin feels flabby and may wobble when pushed. A previously obese patient who has experienced rapid weight loss may have folds of skin on the abdomen and buttocks.

### Temperature

A reasonable estimate of relative temperature can be obtained by feeling the skin, which will feel warm over an inflamed area – a characteristic sign of inflammation – or over an area of increased blood flow. When circulation to a specific area of the skin is increased in the presence of swelling over the area and pain in the calf of the leg, a deep vein thrombosis may be provisionally diagnosed.

It is usual to employ the back of the hand for testing skin temperature. This area has a more constant blood flow than the pads of the fingers, which may be warm from activity or from touching something warm. Additionally, the nerve endings here are more sensitive to changes in temperature.

## Observation of the appendages of the skin

### Nails

In iron-deficiency anaemia the nails become concave and spoon-shaped; this is called **koilonychia**. **Paronychia** is the name given to infection of the margin of the nail. The nail may show numerous small vertical haemorrhages (splinter haemorrhages) with subacute bacterial endocarditis (SABE) or injury to the nail. **Clubbing** describes a condition in which the fingertip and nail appear expanded, rather like a drumstick where the nail curves over the tip of the finger. Clubbing is due to an increase in vascularity of the chronically hypoxic peripheral tissue. Clubbing is associated with congenital heart disease and chronic respiratory conditions.

### Hair

**Alopecia** is hair loss. It occurs in some treatments, such as radiotherapy or chemotherapy, that affect rapidly dividing cells, such as those in the hair follicle. Alopecia also occurs in conditions such as ringworm. Abnormal patterns of hair distribution may be observed, which may be due to hormonal conditions or to drug therapy, for example long-term steroid or androgen administration. Further information

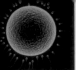

**Table 6.1.1** The causes of oedema (modified from Edwards 2003a,b)

| Interstitial oedema | Intracellular oedema |
|---|---|
| **Caused by:**<br>Changes in capillary dynamics and oedema forms by:<br>• increases in hydrostatic pressure<br>• reduction in oncotic pressure<br>• blocked lymphatic system<br>• the stimulation of the inflammatory immune response | **Caused by:**<br>A lack of oxygen to cells due to:<br>• pressure ulcers<br>• myocardial infarction (internal and invisible)<br>• any of those caused by interstitial oedema |
| **Observed in:**<br>• trauma<br>• head injury (cerebral oedema)<br>• surgery/anaesthetic<br>• renal/liver disease<br>• pancreatitis<br>• burns<br>• Gastrointestinal disorders: ulcers, hernia, irritable bowel syndrome, inflammatory bowel disease, ulcerative colitis<br>• infection/sepsis<br>• pulmonary oedema<br>• drugs<br>• hypertension<br>• heart failure<br>• malnutrition<br>• anaphylaxis | **Observed in:**<br>• hypovolaemia/hypotension<br>• myocardial infarction/cardiac arrest<br>• shock<br>• deep vein thrombosis<br>• pulmonary embolism<br>• acute tubular necrosis<br>• pressure ulcers<br>• cerebral thrombosis (clot) |

These two processes are not mutually exclusive. Interstitial oedema can result in swelling that cuts off blood supply, leading to intracellular oedema. Intracellular oedema can lead to cellular damage, which will stimulate the release of mediators and the inflammatory response.

can be obtained by observing whether the hair looks cared for and clean.

### Use of the sense of smell

Normal skin is odourless. People who do not pay sufficient attention to their personal hygiene may develop a characteristic odour that results from bacterial decomposition of the eccrine, and in particular the apocrine, secretions. Skin infections may lead to quite characteristic smells, for example, the mousy smell that occurs with gangrene infections.

### Use of hearing

Hearing is vital in assessing one particular condition – surgical emphysema. When air enters the tissue spaces in the skin (this may, for example, occur around the entry point of an intercostal drainage tube if there is a small leak) a distinctive crackling can be heard (and felt) when pressure is applied to the area.

### Breaking of the innate skin barrier

There are times when the innate skin barrier to the entry of infection is broken to administer necessary treatments. Breaking of skin is a common procedure in clinical practice and often required when the patient's condition demands the administration of intravenous (IV) fluids via a cannula, invasive haemodynamic monitoring, or both. The skin may also be broken for administration of feeding lines directly into the gastrointestinal tract, or for peritoneal dialysis and during surgery **(Table 6.1.2)**.

Intact, the skin is a formidable barrier against the entry of microorganisms but, when it is broken, its ability to prevent pathogens entering the body is severely reduced. As invasive procedures are a common occurrence in clinical practice, nurses need to be aware that meticulous observation and assessment must be given to the insertion site. Its condition needs to be documented and any changes reported to the relevant healthcare professional.

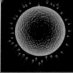

**Table 6.1.2** Breaking the innate skin barrier

| Insertion | Used for | Practical issues |
|---|---|---|
| Intravenous cannula insertion into a vein generally the radial | Administration of IV fluids or drugs, e.g. antibiotics | Ensure sterile procedure as do not want to transfer commonsals from the skin into the vein<br>Observe regularly for signs of inflammation at the site of insertion |
| Central venous pressure monitoring – a catheter placed into the jugular or superior vena cava into the right atrium of the heart | Administration of IV fluids, drugs, parenteral nutrition or to measure right-sided heart pressures | The most common complications include: pneumothorax, hydrothorax, and ventricular arrhythmias; infection and air embolism, all of which should observe for during and after insertion |
| Pulmonary artery dilution catheter – a dilution catheter is placed in the same way as a CVP, but the line is longer and goes through the heart and sits in the pulmonary artery | In addition to the use of the CVP, PAP, PAWP, CO and SVR are measured in critical care areas | Meticulous observation of the insertion site is paramount<br>The implications of entry of bacteria through the skin in this instance may have serious consequences, e.g. sepsis |
| PEG or jejunostomy tube – a gastrostomy/jejunostomy tube is used and held in place with an inflated balloon | Where long-term feeding is anticipated due to upper gastrointestinal obstruction, chronic illness such as AIDS, or when the use of nasal gastric tube is restricted | Placed through the skin into the stomach or jejunum while the patient is sedated<br>Care of insertion site is imperative to prevent the entry of bacteria from the skin or other areas |
| Peritoneal dialysis – the insertion of a catheter into the peritoneum using it as the dialysing membrane for osmosis and passage of solutes | When there is inadequate renal function and the body is unable to rid itself of waste products | A sterile procedure, which involves a small incision into the abdomen, and the peritoneum, is punctured<br>Care of the insertion site is of great importance as it is a life saving procedure for the patient, any infection will require treatment |
| All surgical and some invasive diagnostic procedures | Treatment of certain conditions/illnesses or as a diagnostic tool | All areas need to be checked and document any change or sign of inflammation |

Co, cardiac output; CVP, central venous pressure; IV, intravenous; PAP, pulmony artery pressure; PAWP, pulmonary artery wedge pressure; PEG, percutaneous endoscopically placed gastrostomy; SVR, systemic vascular resistance.

### Breakdown of the skin

The skin can break down due to interference to its blood supply. The blood flow to an area of superficial tissue ceases, due to pressure occluding or collapsing the capillaries and small blood vessels, or by sliding and shearing against a resistant surface. As a result there is insufficient delivery of oxygen and nutrients to the cells, and the resultant ischaemia leads to cell death and tissue necrosis and pressure ulceration **(Fig. 6.1.8)**.

During hypoxic injury, oxygen levels in the blood flow fall below the critical level required to maintain cell viability (Edwards, 2002). The interrupted supply of oxygenated blood to cells leads to anaerobic metabolism and to loss of

adenosine triphosphate (ATP) and cellular membrane disruption.

*Anaerobic metabolism*

Nutrients such as glucose and fatty acids, as well as oxygen, enter the cell across the cell membrane. Hypoxic injury results in an inadequate flow of nutrients and oxygen to the cell. If tissue perfusion continues to be insufficient, the reduced oxygen in the cell resorts to anaerobic metabolic pathways for energy production. This produces several changes in cell function:

* mitochondrial activity is diminished due to a lack of oxygen for glycolysis leading to the formation of excessive free radicals

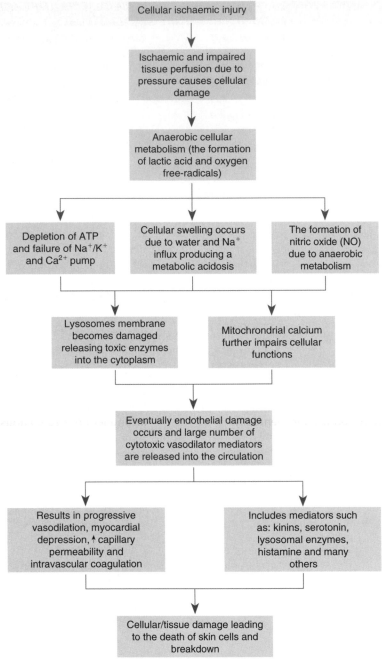

**Figure 6.1.8** Cellular changes following hypoxic/ischaemic injury (redrawn from Edwards, 2002). ATP, adenosine triphosphate

- cellular adenosine triphosphate stores are used up rapidly.

The endproducts are lactic acid and nitric oxide which can build up rapidly to high concentrations in the cell and blood, lowering their pH. There is also a reduction in energy available for cell work.

*The loss of adenosine triphosphate*
As oxygen levels fall in the cell, there is ultimately a reduction in adenosine triphosphate for cellular work (Edwards, 2002). Without intervention

oxygen deprivation will be accompanied by cellular membrane disruption leading to electrolyte disturbance. Without sufficient supplies of adenosine triphosphate the plasma membrane of the cell can no longer maintain normal ionic gradients across the cell membranes and the sodium/potassium and calcium pumps can no longer function.

Thus, one of the most rapid effects of hypoxia and a shortage of adenosine triphosphate is destruction of the normal ionic gradients across the cell membrane, with a rapid efflux of potassium from the cell and movement of sodium and calcium into the cell. The increased sodium in the interior of cells also result in water entering the cell, driven by osmotic forces and causing cellular swelling and distortion that can interfere with organelle function (Buckman, 1992). The cytoplasmic membrane of cells becomes increasingly permeable to larger-molecular-weight proteins, not simply due to direct cellular injury but also due to the systemic intracellular energy debt.

If preventive interventions are not initiated, e.g. pressure-relieving devices, intracellular acidaemia becomes extreme and cellular dysfunction becomes intemperate. This leads to intracellular lysosome membrane disruption and intracellular calcium ion release and if permitted to continue may lead to skin cell damage and death.

When a pressure ulcer forms, a hyperaemic inflammatory area surrounds it. In severe cases, the subcutaneous fat also necroses.

A severely debilitated patient can develop cellular death in the skin after just half-an-hour of unrelieved pressure. When this occurs, the dermal–epidermal junction is sheared and deeper blood vessels are damaged. As a result, necrosis can occur in the deeper tissues while the surface skin initially appears normal, but eventually results in a deep pressure ulcer.

## Patients at risk of skin death and pressure ulcer formation

A pressure ulcer usually occurs over bony prominence, such as the bottom, hip or heel, because here body weight is concentrated on a smaller area of skin and so the degree of tissue compression is greater. Pressure ulcers are a potentially avoidable complication of bedrest and decreased mobility. Patients who are at more risk of developing pressure ulcers include:

- **Immobilized patients**: Some patients are not able to move because they may be paralysed, unconscious, in pain, too weak, too obese, too heavily sedated or have musculoskeletal mobility problems. In addition, patients may have restricted movement due to constraints such as intravenous lines, traction or other equipment. It is these patients who are more likely to experience tissue damage as a result of sustained pressure unless they are helped to move and so redistribute their weight.

  Although thin patients are obviously at risk, obese people are also prone to pressure ulcer formation. They may be unable to easily shift their body weight and fat cells readily break down when subjected to pressure. Elderly people, because of the multipathological basis of their degenerative illnesses and the loss of elasticity of their skin, tend to be particularly vulnerable.

- **Poorly nourished or dehydrated patients**: These patients are often thin and in negative nitrogen balance, with skin that is already in a poor condition. Cell death may be due to vitamin deficiency (especially of vitamin C), leading to poor healing properties. A reduced protein intake will reduce the ability of cells to divide and reduce the skin's white blood cell population residing in the deep tissues of the skin. This will further reduce wound healing, enhance the breakdown of the skin and increase the likelihood of infection.

- **Patients subjected to mechanical injury**: Mechanical injury may result from, for example, a too-tight plaster cast, crumbs in the bed, wrinkles in the sheet, hard lavatory paper, damage from the nurse's sharp fingernails, watch or rings and poor lifting techniques. Shearing forces may also occur when strapping or dressing tape is removed roughly. Hard support surfaces, such as operating tables, commodes, and trolleys may also inflict mechanical damage.

- **Incontinent or oedematous patients**: Skin that is habitually moist at the surface or water-logged in the dermis is prone to pressure ulcers because it becomes soft and fragile. Similarly, problems may occur when two moist body surfaces are juxtaposed and so subjected to friction, e.g. under heavy breasts and between obese thighs. Clothing that is slippery and non-absorbent, and which causes the patient to sweat (e.g. nylon), may increase the risk of ulcer formation, either from excess skin moisture or from shearing forces produced during slipping down the bed.

- **Patients with infection or who are very ill**: Skin infections or generalized sepsis increase the risk of tissue damage as a result of pressure. Febrile conditions increase the body's metabolic rate and therefore oxygen demand in an area that is already potentially hypoxic. Patients, who already have circulatory problems, for example anaemia, atherosclerosis or hypoxaemic conditions, and those with malignant disease, are similarly susceptible to skin death and pressure area problems. Shock, with its associated peripheral circulatory failure, can predispose to rapid cellular death (Edwards, 2001b).

## Wound healing

After injury to the body has occurred, healing of the wound takes place to restore the intact

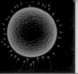

barrier provided by the skin. The healing process and the inflammatory process, although described separately here, overlap to a considerable degree.

When the edges of a wound are closed, for example after a surgical incision, healing is likely to be rapid, and is sometimes said to occur by **primary or first intention**. If this is not possible, for example when there is a deep and wide ulcer or a gaping wound, the healing process takes longer and occurs by the formation of granulation tissue from the bottom of the wound; this is sometimes referred to as healing by **secondary intention**.

### Healing of a surgical wound (Fig. 6.1.9)

By 8 hours after surgery, a blood clot with its fibrin framework has filled the incision track. Necrosis occurs on either side of the incision and extends for 100–200 μm. This is due to the disturbance in the blood supply to the surrounding tissues brought about by the incision. By 16 hours after surgery, epidermal cells have started to invade the boundary between the living and the necrotic tissue. Eventually, after about 40–80 hours, the two ends of epithelial cells unite in the dermis below the level of the incision. This severs the connection between the necrotic area and the living area. The necrotic area forms the scab and, when the underlying epithelium becomes keratinized, the scab will be shed.

Fibroblasts in the area are stimulated to produce collagen fibres and capillaries grow into the area from surrounding vessels; as a result a soft, pink, delicate tissue called **granulation tissue** fills the wound area. As the fibroblasts mature and form more collagen, both the cells and the fibres start to shrink, causing some contraction of the area and eventual obliteration of some of the capillaries. The end result is a firm fibrous epithelial scar.

For the first 3–5 days postoperatively, the tensile strength of the wound is low. It can be measured experimentally by estimating the force required distracting the edges of a wound. The rate of increase in strength is maximal between days 5 and 12 postoperatively, when collagen formation is occurring rapidly. The remaining gain in strength occurs gradually over subsequent weeks, as collagen continues to be deposited for up to 80 days postoperatively.

By this time up to 70–80% of the original strength is regained and the scar has retracted, appearing smaller and whiter. The role of sutures in securing wound adherence is thus complete by 12–14 days after surgery, as by this time sufficient collagen has been formed to ensure skin healing.

### Criteria for wound healing

To promote healing, certain criteria should be met. When considering wound healing it is essential that the wound be exposed to as natural a physiological environment as possible. Such an environment involves:

- A moist environment, which is necessary for epidermal growth.
- Removal of excess exudate. This avoids maceration of the wound surface and promotes the removal of debris, toxins and microorganisms.
- Exclusion of bacteria.
- Insulation of the wound to provide a constant temperature of 37°C. Wound temperature drops at every dressing change, with a consequent slowing in the rate of cell division.
- Occlusive dressings: vascularization is promoted in granulation tissue under anaerobic conditions. Occlusive dressings also provide better pain relief.
- Exclusion of foreign bodies, which prolong inflammation. Dressings must not, therefore, shed particles.
- Dressings that do not stick to the wound in any way. Nor should new granulation tissue grow into the dressing material, only to be torn away at the next dressing change.

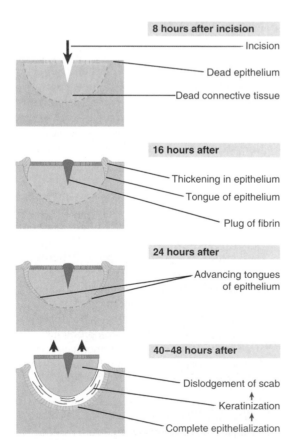

**Figure 6.1.9**    The stages of wound healing

Many factors play a part in the success or failure of wound healing and it can be difficult to ascertain the cause of failure in any one patient. A major nursing responsibility is to ensure that optimal conditions for healing are promoted in all patients.

## Homeostatic imbalance of the skin

### Psoriasis

Psoriasis is a skin condition characterized by rapid and excessive production of keratinized cells, which form silvery flakes on the skin surface and which result in excessive desquamation.

### Acne

Acne may be caused by streptococci, staphylococci or *Corynebacterium acnes* within the hair follicle. These bacteria act on sebum and liberate free fatty acids from it, which cause the wall of the hair follicle to burst thus allowing the bacteria to come into contact with epidermal tissue. This results in inflammation in the epidermis: leucocytes come to the defence of the tissue, pus formed of living and dead leucocytes and bacteria is produced, and pustules develop. The condition can be treated with:

- tetracycline
- ultraviolet light, which has a bactericidal effect
- the administration of oestrogen in females
- the use of the keratolytic agents (which exert a peeling effect on the skin) such as resorcinol, sulphur, salicylic acid or tretinoin (Retin-A; Porth, 1990).

### Changes in pigmentation

Pigmentation is affected by oestrogen production, which causes the marked darkening of the nipple, the surrounding areola and linea nigra in pregnancy. It occasionally causes patchy brown pigmentation of the face in pregnancy, which can be upsetting for those affected; this phenomenon is sometimes referred to as the 'mask of pregnancy'.

Albinism is an autosomal recessive hereditary condition characterized by a lack of ability to produce melanin in the skin, hair and eyes due to lack of the ability to synthesize the precursor enzyme tyrosinase. Albino skin is pink, the hair pale or white. Consequently, sufferers have no protection from ultraviolet light and, unless precautions are taken, such as constant wearing of dark glasses, retinal problems may develop.

### Vitamin D deficiency

Problems of vitamin $D_3$ deficiency (rickets in children and osteomalacia in adults) can occur when dietary intake is insufficient (i.e. below 2.5 g per day for adults and 10 g per day for children and pregnant women). Dietary intake in the United Kingdom is usually adequate but, with the increasing emphasis on the need to cut intake of saturated fats found in dairy produce, it is possible that deficiencies could occur.

Deficiencies can also occur when the body is deprived of sunlight, for example if sunlight is prevented from reaching the body by atmospheric pollution or excessive clothing. Dark-skinned immigrants to temperate countries are particularly at risk if their dietary intake of vitamin $D_3$ is inadequate because they are no longer able to supplement it by ultraviolet-stimulated synthesis of vitamin $D_3$, as would have been possible in their sunnier countries of origin.

### Organic solvents and heavy metals

Organic solvents such as acetone, dry-cleaning fluid, paint thinner and heavy metals such as lead, mercury and nickel can be absorbed through the skin. They should therefore never be handled with bare hands. If it occurs, the effects of absorption can be devastating and sometimes lethal. Absorption of organic solvents through the skin into the blood can cause the kidneys to shut down and can also cause brain damage. Absorption of lead results in anaemia and neurological defects.

### Burns

Burns are a devastating threat to the body, primarily because of their effects on the skin. A burn is tissue damage inflicted by intense heat, electricity, radiation or certain chemicals, all of which denature cell proteins and cause cell death in the affected areas. The immediate threat to life resulting from severe burns is a catastrophic loss of body fluids containing proteins and electrolytes. As fluid seeps from the burned surfaces, dehydration and electrolyte imbalance result. These lead to renal shut down, and circulatory shock due to inadequate blood circulation due to reduced blood volume (Edwards, 1998b).

The fluids lost must be replaced immediately. In adults, this is estimated by calculating the percentage of body surface burned using the rule of nines. This method divides the body into eleven areas, each accounting for 9% of total body areas, plus an additional area surrounding the genitals accounting for 1% of body surface area **(Fig. 6.1.10)**.

In addition, burns patients require thousands of extra food calories daily to replace lost proteins and allow tissue repair. Infection becomes the main threat and is the leading cause of death in burn victims. Bacteria, fungi and other pathogens easily invade areas where the skin barrier is

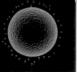

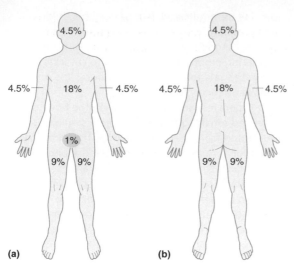

**(a)**        **(b)**

**Figure 6.1.10** Estimation of burn injury: the rule of nines (redrawn from McCance & Huether, 1998)

destroyed, and they multiply rapidly in the nutrient-rich environment of dead tissues and protein-containing fluid.

Burns are classified according to their severity (depth) as first-, second- (partial thickness burns) and third-degree burns (full thickness burns):

- First-degree only: the epidermis is damaged, localized redness, swelling and pain, heal quickly in 2–3 days without special attention. Includes sunburn.
- Second-degree burns: injure the epidermis and the upper region of the dermis. Symptoms are those of first-degree burns but blisters also appear. If complications do not occur, regeneration takes place with little or no scarring in 3–4 weeks.
- Third-degree burns: involve the entire thickness of the skin. Nerve endings are destroyed and so the burned area is not painful. These burns usually require skin grafting, as healing takes too long.

Burns are considered critical to life if any of the following conditions exist:

- over 25% of the body has second-degree burns
- over 10% of the body has third-degree burns
- there are third-degree burns of the face (possible burns to the respiratory passageways, which can swell and cause suffocation), hands or feet.

### Skin cancer

The majority of tumours that arise in the skin are benign and are unlikely to spread to other body areas. However, some skin tumours are malignant or cancerous and invade other body areas. The most common predisposing factor for skin cancer

is overexposure to ultraviolet radiation in sunlight. There are different types of skin cancer:

- Basal cell carcinoma: the least malignant and most common skin cancer. Cells of the stratum basale proliferate, invading the dermis and hypodermis. Basal cell carcinoma occurs in sun-exposed areas. It is slow growing and metastasis rare.
- Squamous cell carcinoma: arises from the keratinocytes of the stratum spinosum. It grows rapidly and metastasizes to adjacent lymph nodes if not removed.
- Malignant melanoma: cancer of the melanocytes. This is the most dangerous skin cancer. Its incidence is increasing rapidly. One-third of tumours develop from pigmented moles.

The ABCD rule for recognizing a melanoma is as follows:

A = asymmetry: the two sides of the pigmented spot or mole do not match
B = border: irregularity the borders of the lesion are not smooth but exhibit indentations
C = colour: the pigmented spot contains several colours (blacks, browns, tans and sometimes blues and reds)
D = diameter: the spot is larger than 6 mm in diameter.

## Temperature regulation

A change in body temperature is a common occurrence both in the community and in hospital. Such a change may alert nurses to the presence of infection, thermoregulatory dysfunction, deterioration in a patient's condition or hypothermia, and so its detection is vital if therapeutic intervention is to be instigated early. Accurate monitoring of temperature is important as both abnormally high and abnormally low values can have deleterious effects on the body.

If body temperature is to be regulated at an optimal level, a balance must be achieved between heat gained and heat lost by the body. Overall control is exerted via the heat-regulating centre in the hypothalamus of the brain. Humans are homeothermal, that is, they maintain a constant core temperature of about 37°C independent of the environment. They are capable of living at environmental temperatures ranging from −52°C to +49°C.

The maintenance of body temperature within the normal range is necessary for life. The temperature is controlled by the hypothalamus in the brainstem, which maintains temperature homeostasis. This includes the ability to increase heat production and conserve heat or to increase heat loss, thus ensuring that body temperature remains between 35.5 and 37.5°C. This process is known as **thermoregulation**.

The homeostatic process of thermoregulation whereby the body temperature is kept within acceptable limits, regardless of the environmental conditions, is governed by physiological mechanisms within the body. Body temperature is regulated almost entirely by nervous feedback control mechanisms and almost all of these operate through a temperature-regulating centre located in the hypothalamus.

To maintain set point temperature, receptors are continually sending information about environmental and body temperature to the hypothalamus (control centre). In extreme heat or cold, when the body temperature may be higher or lower than set point temperature, the hypothalamus maintains the appropriate level. This is achieved by interpreting the information received and passing regulatory commands to effector cells, which then activate either heat loss or heat conservation mechanisms to adjust the body temperature so that it matches the set point temperature.

## Core and peripheral temperature

The term **core temperature** refers to that inside the skull and the abdominal organs. The skin over the trunk, when the body feels comfortably warm, may be 33–34°C and the core temperature of 37°C is reached about 2 cm below the body surface. When feeling comfortably warm, the toes may be at 27°C, arms and legs at 31°C, and the forehead at about 34°C. There is thus a temperature gradient between the deep tissues and the skin or, in other words, between the core and the periphery.

The temperature of the body is not the same all over: if the environmental temperature is cooler than body temperature, the skin and peripheries are normally several degrees cooler than the core (organs, blood and deeper tissues). The temperature of the skin varies according to the temperature of the environment and thus if the air temperature is high, the peripheral temperature will also rise and may be almost equal to that of the core. This has an effect on heat-transfer mechanisms (described below). The ability of the blood vessels near the surface of the skin to constrict or dilate is crucial to thermoregulation and measurement, and monitoring of the difference between peripheral and core temperature is indicated in the management of some patients. This difference may also be used to give an indication of the effectiveness of warming procedures in cases of hypothermia.

## Heat-regulation mechanisms

The body is continuously producing heat as a by-product of metabolism and this heat must be lost to the environment at the same rate as it is produced if body temperature is to remain constant. When environmental conditions are either too warm or too cold, the body must control the gains or losses to maintain homeostasis. Temperature homeostasis is achieved through heat-transfer, heat-loss and heat-gain mechanisms.

## Heat-transfer mechanisms

Heat-transfer mechanisms function to maintain a balance between heat production and heat loss. Four processes are involved: radiation, conduction, convection and evaporation.

### Radiation

Loss of heat by radiation comprises energy loss in the form of infrared heat rays. This is heat lost from the body to any surroundings that are cooler than the body itself; this loss increases as the temperature of the surroundings decreases. Over half the heat lost from the body in temperate climates is as a result of radiation. The exact amount varies with body temperature and skin temperature. Little heat is lost through radiation if the air temperature is equal to, or higher than, skin temperature.

### CLINICAL APPLICATIONS

Heat rays leave the warm body and potentially warm objects in their path. If the objects encountered by the rays are light in colour or shiny, then the heat is reflected back. This is the principle upon which aluminium foil 'space-blankets' are based when these are used to warm neonates and those suffering from hypothermia.

### Conduction

The direct transfer of energy through physical contact, for example sitting on a cold chair, is referred to as conduction heat loss. Although heat loss through direct contact is not a very effective mechanism, loss of heat by conduction to air does represent a sizeable proportion of the heat lost under normal conditions.

Heat is conducted to any solid in direct contact with the skin, as long as the surface temperature of the object is lower than that of the skin. For example, heat is lost to cold tile floors from the soles of the feet, and from the buttocks to a lavatory seat. In general, conduction is not a major method of heat loss from the body.

## Convection

Movement of air molecules, due to heat, is known as convection. For removal of heat from the body by convective air currents to occur, the heat must first be conducted to the air and then carried away by the convection currents.

### CLINICAL APPLICATIONS

Fan therapy works by increasing heat loss through conduction and convection because the warmed air is constantly being replaced by cool air. Fans that are used to cool patients who are pyrexial work by increasing the efficiency of convection currents, but fanning is generally not recommended directly onto the skin surface because of the risks associated with chilling and drying of the skin (Edwards, 1998a).

Conversely, the use of a space blanket creates a layer of warm air around the body, thus reducing heat loss.

Air coming into contact with naked skin is warmed by it; the warm air rises and is replaced by cooler air. The efficiency of this convection as a method of heat loss depends on the skin blood flow, the temperature difference between the skin and the air, the airflow and the total area of exposed skin.

## Evaporation

When water evaporates, it changes from a liquid to a vapour and heat energy is used in the process of evaporation. Water evaporates from the skin and lungs at a rate of about 600 mL/day. This is termed **insensible loss** and at rest accounts for roughly one-fifth of the body's heat loss. The sweat glands responsible for perspiration have a very wide range of activity, ranging from virtual inactivity to secretory rates of 2–4 L/hour. When the body becomes overheated, large quantities of sweat are secreted onto the surface of the skin by the sweat glands to provide rapid evaporative cooling of the body. Heat loss through evaporation becomes increasingly important when the ambient temperature is the same as the skin temperature, because little or no heat is lost through radiation, conduction or convection.

Water is lost continually and insensibly from the surface of the body. It evaporates when the environmental temperature is higher than that of the body surface, and in so doing takes heat from the body. The evaporation of 1 L of water requires 2400 kJ (580 kcal) of heat. Sweat loss can vary between 500 mL and 12 L (1–24 pints) per day; evaporation of 12 L of sweat requires 30 000 kJ (approximately 7000 kcal) of heat. Evaporation of sweat can no longer

occur when the environmental humidity is high. Heat loss via evaporation normally accounts for about 15% of the heat loss that has to occur to achieve balance.

## Heat-loss mechanisms

When temperatures rise above the set point, the hypothalamus reduces the stimulation to the sympathetic nervous system in an attempt to increase heat loss. The thermostatic area of the hypothalamus increases the rate of heat loss from the body in the following ways:

- sweat glands are stimulated to increase their output, perspiration flows across the body surface and evaporation heat loss is accelerated
- depth and rate of respiration are increased, causing increased heat loss through evaporation from the lungs
- peripheral vasodilation takes place, causing warm blood to flow closer to the surface of the body, greatly increasing loss of heat from the skin through radiation and convection
- activities that produce heat are decreased, for example muscle contraction.

In extremely warm temperatures, clothing is removed to expose more of the body surface and thus maximize heat loss, intake of hot food and drinks is restricted and less exercise is undertaken. Furthermore, postures that encourage maximum heat loss are adopted, for example arm and legs spread wide when sunbathing.

## Heat-gain mechanisms

When the core temperature falls below the normal range, special mechanisms are set in motion to conserve the heat already in the body and to generate heat production to maintain core temperature.

### Heat-conservation mechanisms

Heat is conserved in the following ways:

- peripheral vasoconstriction decreases blood flow to the dermis of the skin, thus reducing heat loss through radiation, convection and conduction, and the skin cools
- hairs on the body stand on end (piloerection), trapping air next to the skin so that the transfer of heat via radiation is reduced
- sweating ceases, thus reducing heat loss through evaporation
- voluntary behavioural measures, such as wearing warm clothing.

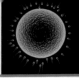

In cold weather, people tend to undertake activities that generate heat, for example, exercising and clapping their hands together. They also try to prevent heat loss, for example by increasing insulating layers in the form of extra clothing. As little of the body surface area as possible is exposed to the cold environment, and huddled postures may be adopted in order to reduce the surface area exposed.

### Heat-generation mechanisms

There are three heat-generation mechanisms:

1. **Shivering**: increases the tone of the skeletal muscles throughout the body, causing characteristic muscle contraction. Body-heat production during severe shivering can rise by a factor of four to five.
2. **Chemical heat production (thermogenesis)**: results from the release by the sympathetic nervous system of adrenaline (epinephrine) and, to a lesser extent, noradrenaline (norepinephrine), which cause an increase in cellular metabolism (thermogenesis); the effects are immediate.
3. **Hormonal heat production**: the hormone thyroxine increases the rate of cellular metabolism throughout the body but, unlike thermogenesis, this does not occur immediately.

Metabolism is the major way in which heat is gained in the body. Organs such as the liver produce a more or less constant amount of heat through their oxidative processes. The amount produced by skeletal and cardiac muscle varies with their activity; but after a prolonged bout of exercise, for example, body temperature may rise to 39°C.

If no heat were to be lost by the body, metabolic processes produce an amount sufficient to raise the body temperature by 1°C per hour, at rest. Activity might raise that figure to 2–3°C per hour. Thus, it can be seen that the problem for humans in general, is one of losing heat rather than gaining it. The resting metabolic rate varies throughout life: it is higher in babies and children, and tends to drop slightly in old age. It is usually up to 10% lower in females than in males, and is affected in both sexes by thyroxin production.

There are occasions, when changes in temperature occur, when the homeostatic mechanisms described above are unable to generate enough heat or cause enough heat to be lost to maintain normal temperature, as a result of which the body temperature either increases (pyrexia, hyperpyrexia or hyperthermia) or decreases (hypothermia). All of these conditions may require hospital treatment and can be fatal.

Heat is gained from the external environment when the ambient temperature is higher than that of the body. Thus, heat is gained from the sun, a coal fire or radiator, mainly by radiation and conduction, and a hot bath can raise body temperature.

### Diurnal variations

Generally, body temperature is lower during the night than during the day. It starts to rise from about 5 a.m. to 11 a.m. The early morning oral temperature ranges from 36.3°C to 37.1°C. After 11 a.m., body temperature tends to level out, until about 5 p.m., by which time it may have risen by 0.5–0.7°C from the early morning level. After this time, the body temperature starts to fall, until 1 a.m. A stable period then follows until the next cycle starts at 5 a.m. (Edwards, 1998a). This pattern varies slightly between individuals but it is interesting to note that it persists for a time even when night shifts are worked.

> **CLINICAL APPLICATIONS**
>
> The normal daytime pattern is retained in nurses who work on night-duty for, say, one week in every four. However, those who go on night-duty for 3 months at a time will experience a reversal of their temperature biorhythms.

It is vital that body temperature is retained at a more or less constant level if a stable internal environment is to be maintained for the optimal functioning of cellular enzymes. The respiratory and other cellular proteins are not only pH specific but also temperature specific and so fail to function efficiently once the body temperature differs from its normal level.

As already mentioned, balance must be achieved between heat gained by the body and heat lost. The various factors that may influence both sides of this equation are shown in **Table 6.1.3**.

**Table 6.1.3** Balance between heat gained and heat lost (from Marieb, 2001)

| Heat gained or produced | Heat lost |
|---|---|
| Basal metabolism | Radiation |
| Muscular activity (shivering) | Conduction/ convection |
| Thyroxine and adrenaline (epinephrine) (stimulating effects on metabolic rate) | Evaporation |
| Temperature effect on cells | |

As long as heat production and heat loss are balanced, body temperature remains constant.

## CLINICAL APPLICATIONS

### HOMEOSTATIC IMBALANCE OF TEMPERATURE CONTROL

Fever results from infection by bacteria, viruses or protozoa or from the presence of necrotic tissue (e.g. in gangrene, following myocardial infarction or with a large, deep pressure ulcer), all of which produce pyrogens that affect the temperature regulating centre. In addition, brain damage, cerebral tumour or head injury may directly affect the function of the temperature-regulating centre.

### Pyrexia (fever) and hyperpyrexia

Pyrexia (body temperature between 37.6 and 40°C) and hyperpyrexia (temperature >40°C) are conditions in which the thermoregulatory mechanisms are intact but the body temperature is high. Infection is the most common cause of pyrexia but there other causes as well. A number of drugs have been associated with the occurrence of pyrexia, for example, diuretics, antiseizure therapy, analgesics, anti-arrhythmics and antibiotics (Edwards, 1998a). Other causes of pyrexia include neoplasm, surgery, acute myocardial infarctions, heart failure, haemolysis (seen in reactions to blood transfusions) and hyperthyroidism.

In fever, the thermostat of the hypothalamus (which is normally set at 37°C) functions as if it has been reset to a new, higher level. As a result, heat production is increased and heat loss inhibited in order to raise the core temperature to the new level. With each rise in temperature of 0.5°C, tissue oxygen requirements increase by 7% and so heart rate and respiratory rate both increases. At this stage, the patient feels cold until the core temperature reaches the new, higher level; warm bed clothing is appreciated. The cutaneous blood vessels are constricted, with resultant pallor; the patient may shiver or experience rigors, and generally feels cold and unwell **(Table 6.1.4)**. These responses are independent of the ambient temperature and their net result is that the patient's core temperature is raised, and the patient becomes pyrexial.

### The stages and patterns of pyrexia

There are four stages associated with pyrexia:

1. The **chill stage** is the cold stage when the hypothalamic thermostat is reset to a higher level and before the body temperature has risen to this point. The patient feels chilly, may have goose pimples and is cool to touch and pale.
2. The **plateau** is the hot stage when the body temperature has been raised to a level equal to the hypothalamic set point. The patient feels hot, warm to touch, is flushed and has raised heart and respiratory rates.
3. The **difervescence stage** is that stage when the temperature returns to normal, heat is dissipated through heat-loss mechanisms, including active sweating. The skin remains warm to touch and flushed until eventually body temperature drops to a normal level.
4. The **crisis stage** occurs if the temperature fails to respond to treatment. If the microorganism responsible cannot be eradicated, and if thermoregulation mechanisms can no longer control heat loss; death may ensue.

These stages **(see Table 6.1.4)** account for the discomfort experienced by patients with high temperatures. They also explain why a patient developing a high temperature may initially feel cold and want to wrap up rather than be uncovered.

### Beneficial and detrimental responses to pyrexia

Pyrexia can be beneficial and is an important host defence mechanism. A body temperature of 40.9°C will kill some *Pneumococcus* and *Gonoccoccus* organisms. The high temperature causes a reduction in serum levels of iron, zinc and copper and this inhibits the replication of certain microorganisms. Pyrexia as a result of viral infection increases interferon production by the infected cells, which then enters non-infected cells to inhibit infiltration by the invading virus. The activity of phagocytes and leucocytes is increased at temperatures between 38°C and 40°C, thus improving the infection-fighting ability of the immune system (Bruce & Grove, 1992). Furthermore, high temperatures cause the breakdown of lysosomes (involved in the intracellular digestive system), which allows cells to digest and remove unwanted substances such as bacteria) in infected cells, thereby destroying cells and preventing them from initiating viral replication.

However, pyrexia can also be detrimental to the patient, whose basal metabolic rate will be increased, eventually leading to exhaustion. As a result, the glycogen stores in the liver become reduced and lead to nitrogen wastage (as protein is used for energy) and, if prolonged, may result in debility, impaired healing and delirium. If patients have compromised cardiopulmonary function, the effects of increased metabolic, heart and respiratory rates can be quite dangerous. These effects can lead to an increase in carbon dioxide production and oxygen consumption.

Dehydration may result from fluid loss during sweating and from the lungs due to increased respiratory rate, leading to hypovolaemia and electrolyte imbalance (Bruce & Grove, 1992) and this can be life threatening. In addition, the

**Table 6.1.4** The first three stages of pyrexia (from Edwards, 1998a)

| Stages | Process |
| --- | --- |
| Stage 1 – the cold stage | • Begins when the hypothalamic thermostat is reset to a higher level.<br>• All the mechanisms for heat production and conservation are activated. During this stage there is a rapid and steady rise in temperature (10–40 min)<br>• It includes a raised metabolic rate because of sympathetic stimulation and shivering, which leads to an increased heart, respiratory rate and thirst. Vasoconstriction conserves body heat, the patient feels chilly, has goose bumps, is cool to touch and is pale |
| Stage 2 – the hot stage | • The heat-producing mechanisms have raised the body temperature to a level that equals the hypothalmic set point<br>• The temperature remains constant at this new higher level<br>• The length of time at this stage depends on how long it takes to eradicate the bacteria/virus responsible<br>• Heat is maintained throughout this stage – includes a flushed skin warm to touch, the patient feels hot, heart and respiratory rates remain raised. The hot stage ends when the underlying cause of the pyrexia has been treated, leading to a decrease in the hypothalamic set point |
| Stage 3 – the defervescence stage (heat dissipating) | • Begins when the hypothalamic set point is normal<br>• Characterized by the heat-loss mechanisms vasodilation, sweating, inhibition of heat production mechanisms like shivering<br>• The skin is warm to touch and flushed<br>• The end result is a drop in body temperature to a normal level |

patient will feel uncomfortably hot and sweaty, with a loss of appetite, weakness and malaise, apathy and confusion (Bruce & Grove, 1992).

### Management of pyrexia and hyperpyrexia

Some researchers have criticized management of an abnormally high temperature using cooling methods such as tepid sponging or fanning. Bruce & Grove (1992) argue that, ultimately, these methods are of no use because sensory nerves in the skin relay messages back to the hypothalamus, which stimulates a compensatory response that can create a new temperature spike that is as high as, or higher than, the original one. Provoking heat-generating activities such as shivering may compromise unstable patients by depleting their metabolic reserve. Bruce & Grove (1992) argue that the best way to treat a high temperature is to use antipyretic drugs such as aspirin or paracetamol. These prevent the hypothalamus from synthesizing prostaglandin E and thus inhibit the set point of temperature rising further.

A rigor occurs when the hypothalamic set point temperature has risen in response to a microorganism and the body is attempting to achieve that temperature by generating heat through excessive shivering. In this instance, it is best to apply extra clothing and allow the body temperature to rise.

### Hyperthermia

**Hyperthermia** is defined as an increase in body temperature, with increased cellular metabolism, oxygen consumption and carbon dioxide production, but where the body fails to activate compensatory cooling mechanisms (Morgan, 1990). This condition is caused by problems of the central nervous system and does not respond to antipyretic therapy.

Hyperthermia causes cerebral metabolism to increase and the brain has great difficulty keeping up with the increase in carbon dioxide production. Cerebral vasodilation occurs, which may increase intracranial pressure and is thus dangerous in neurologically compromised patients. A temperature between 41°C and 43°C produces nerve damage, coagulation, convulsions and death. Unless effective cooling measures are initiated, irreversible brain damage and death will occur (Holtzclaw, 1993).

Hyperthermia also presents in five other conditions: heat cramps, heat exhaustion, heat stroke, malignant hyperthermia and neuroleptic malignant syndrome (NMS) **(see Table 6.1.5)**. Heat cramps and exhaustion, even though they can be severe, do not generally warrant admission to hospital and those at risk can be taught ways to avoid it. However, heat stroke, malignant hyperthermia and NMS must be

**Table 6.1.5** The conditions that present in hyperthermia (modified from Edwards, 2003c)

| Condition | Clinical features | Causes |
|---|---|---|
| Heat cramps | • Sweating<br>• Sodium loss when an individual has consumed large quantities of water but not taken any salt replacement | Strenuous physical exercise in high temperatures |
| Heat exhaustion | • Profound vasodilation<br>• Profuse sweating<br>• Decrease in blood volume<br>• Dehydration<br>• Hypotension | Malfunction of the thermoregulatory system |
| Heat stroke | • Skin becomes hot and dry<br>• Sweat glands are inactive<br>• Body temperature climbs to 41–45°C<br>• Destruction of brain, liver, skeletal muscle and kidney cells | • The thermoregulatory system ceases to function<br>• Excessive heat storage |
| Malignant | • High temperature above 40°C<br>• Temperature does not respond to antipyretic drugs | • Inherited muscular disorders<br>• Administration of drugs (anaesthetic agents, diuretics, analgesics, and antibiotics) |
| Neuroleptic | • High temperature above 40°C<br>• Muscular rigidity<br>• Akinesia<br>• Impaired consciousness | • Rare<br>• Psychotropic drugs used to treat psychosis (phenothiazines, butyrophenones) |

recognized quickly, as, untreated, they may be fatal.

### Management of hyperthermia

Cooling methods are valuable in hyperthermia, heat stroke and malignant hyperthermia because the body fails to activate compensatory cooling methods. Moreover, these conditions generally do not respond well to antipyretic therapy (Morgan, 1990). Aggressive cooling should be commenced early, as temperatures of above 41°C causes cell, tissue and eventually organ damage (Bruce & Grove, 1992). Cooling techniques commonly used include packs of ice water, cold water, cooling mattresses, fanning and tepid water sponging.

In malignant hyperthermia the above methods of cooling may be beneficial but the addition of dantrolene sodium will give a more marked improvement (Donnelly, 1994). In heat stroke, cooling methods are the intervention of choice because heat production in the body is higher than heat loss, creating an increase in temperature which is overwhelming the regulatory system. Neuroleptic malignant syndrome (NMS) is a life-threatening condition that requires cooling methods and may also require additional resuscitative measures.

### Hypothermia

**Hypothermia** is defined as a core temperature of less than 35°C and affects virtually all-metabolic processes in the body (Fritsch, 1995). Degrees of hypothermia are classified as follows:

• mild: body temperature 32–35°C
• moderate: 28–31.9°C
• severe: 20–27.9°C
• profound: <20°C.

In hypothermia, peripheral vasoconstriction shunts blood away from the cooler skin to the core in an effort to decrease heat loss. This peripheral vasoconstriction leads to peripheral tissue ischaemia, which causes the hypothalamus to stimulate shivering in an effort to increase heat production. Severe shivering occurs at core temperatures below 35°C and will continue until the core temperature rises or drops further to 30–32°C. At 34°C, thinking becomes sluggish and coordination is impaired.

At 31°C the individual becomes lethargic, heart and respiratory rates decline, cardiac output is diminished, and there is confusion, hyperactivity and exaggerated tendon reflexes (Holtzclaw, 1993). Cerebral blood flow is decreased. Metabolic rate declines, further

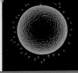

decreasing core temperature. This has an effect on drug metabolism as the drug half-life is increased (Fritsch, 1995). Sinus node depression occurs with slowing of conduction through the atrioventricular node, and premature ventricular contractions (ectopics) are common. There is also an increased risk of atrial fibrillation and other arrhythmias.

In severe hypothermia, pulse and respiration may be undetectable and the blood coagulates more easily. Dehydration is common after a lengthy exposure to the cold. Loss of consciousness and the absence of neurological reflexes follow. As the temperature falls below 20°C, hypothermic patients become unable to regulate their body heat and the thermoregulatory mechanisms fail (Holtzclaw, 1993). Ice crystals form on the inside of cells, causing them to rupture and die.

Attention must be paid to the degree and time period of exposure of the patient (Fritsch, 1995). Thus, the length of time hypothermia has taken to occur is significant in that it can influence outcomes. After 12 hours there will be significant fluid loss from the blood, due to shifts of fluid from the extracellular space to other fluid spaces and from cold-induced diuresis (Danzl & Pozos, 1994). In addition, there is a marked increase in mortality. The period over which the hypothermia has occurred is also significant when rewarming patients as the time span of hypothermia will determine the best method of achieving rewarming. There are five different types of hypothermia: accidental, therapeutic, induced, inadvertent and postanaesthetic.

**Accidental hypothermia** is defined as a core body temperature below 35°C that occurs accidentally, for example from sudden immersion in cold water or prolonged exposure to cold environments. Environmental causes are common in older adults, the very young, those who have suffered trauma, homeless people, overdose patients, in drug and alcohol misuse, which diminishes the conscious perception of cold, and in those with mental health problems. It may occur in accidents involving immersion in cold water or near drowning. Accidental hypothermia is a potential problem for four main groups of people:

- those who experience accidents in circumstances likely to produce a fall in body temperature, such as divers or mountaineers
- very young babies (older babies also may be at risk because they have a relatively large surface/volume ratio which facilitates heat loss)
- elderly people

- people who sleep without shelter: in this group, susceptibility may be further increased by misuse of alcohol and other drugs.

The survival time of those immersed in water at 5°C is 20–30 minutes; at 15°C, survival time is about 1–2 hours (Edwards, 1999a). In neonates, problems occur with a temperature-regulating centre that is not fully operational and an inability to shiver. A baby exposed to cold may kick to try to increase heat production but this may lead to kicking off the bedclothes, so accelerating heat loss. In spite of the hypothermia, the baby may appear deceptively pink and healthy. This is because dissociation of oxygen from haemoglobin does not occur so rapidly at low temperatures. The baby may also exhibit cold vasodilation, which was referred to earlier.

Older adults are particularly at risk of accidental hypothermia because they have poor responses to extremes of environmental temperature as a result of slowed blood circulation, structural and functional changes in the skin, and overall decrease in heat-producing activities. They also have a decreased shivering response (delayed onset and decreased effectiveness), slowed metabolic rate, decreased vasoconstrictor response, diminished or absent sweating and a decreased perception of heat and cold. If they also have psychological problems (e.g. a recent bereavement and/or loneliness), a sedentary lifestyle, low income, poor nutritional intake and a reduced ability to care for themselves, the risks are further increased.

The term **therapeutic hypothermia** generally refers to a deliberately induced state of hypothermia, which is used to slow a patient's metabolism and thus preserve ischaemic tissue during some types of major surgery, thereby preserving function (Edwards, 1999b). However, hypothermia that occurs inadvertently during surgery is also termed therapeutic hypothermia because it presents during a therapeutic procedure. Both types of hypothermia can sometimes extend into the postoperative period. Therapeutic hypothermia is therefore classified into the following three categories **(Table 6.1.6)**:

- **induced hypothermia**
- **inadvertent, intraoperative or unintentional hypothermia**
- **postanaesthesia or postoperative hypothermia.**

Normally, when the body temperature falls, shivering occurs. This is a protective mechanism that functions to raise core temperature. The ability to shiver, however, gradually decreases as the core temperature falls below 34°C. Muscle weakness then occurs, as the core temperature

**Table 6.1.6** Categories of therapeutic hypothermia (from Edwards, 1999b)

| Type | Causes | Nursing considerations |
|---|---|---|
| Induced | Intentional lowering of body temperature used in:<br>• neurosurgery<br>• treatment of hyperthermia<br>• cardiac surgery | To increase the body temperature gradually at 1°C per hour |
| Inadvertent | • Exposure of body cavities to a cool environment<br>• Irrigation of body cavities with room temperature solutions<br>• Inhalation of unwarmed anaesthetic agents<br>• Use of drugs that impair thermoregulatory mechanisms and prevent body movement<br>• Skin preparations that are allowed to dry on skin, increasing the loss of body heat by evaporation | Effective means of prevention have been sought, e.g. scoring checklist devised by Tudor as an assessment tool to help nurses identify those patients at risk. A score of six or more indicates the use of heat-retaining devices, e.g. blankets, towels and hats, while a score of 10 or more indicates the use of heat-generating devices, e.g. blood warmers, humidifiers and warming blankets |
| Postanaesthesia | • May be an extension of induced hypothermia<br>• Leads to reduced cardiac function and temperature regulation | Monitoring blood pressure, assessing respiratory rate and ausculating cardiac sounds in patients who are hypothermic immediately after surgery It is thin, older adults who are particularly at risk |

drops further. Activity becomes difficult as muscular movements become uncoordinated, and dulling of mental faculties become evident.

Consciousness is lost at a body temperature of 30–32°C. At 22–28°C, cardiac arrhythmias occur, and at 18–22°C the heart stops. The ability spontaneously to bring about cessation of heat loss and to initiate heat production is lost at 28°C. At this temperature, however, gradual rewarming of the patient in hospital may still permit survival. Hypothermia of 26–28°C may be induced surgically to enable the circulation to be stopped for relatively long periods. The oxygen needs of the tissues are substantially reduced at low temperatures (the Bohr effect), for example at 28–30°C, the metabolic rate is reduced by half.

*Management of hypothermia*

Accidental hypothermia is more likely to occur in the community than in hospital. It will, however, require a stay in hospital. Advanced age is a known risk factor. Older patients often experience more severe temperature drops and rewarming difficulties due to limited cardiac reserve, reduced cardiac output, a diminished muscle mass, lower basal metabolic rate and impaired ability to sweat. All contribute to alterations in heat generation, conservation and dissipation. An ageing autonomic nervous system often results in

a decreased ability to shiver, low resting peripheral blood flow, reduced vasomotor tone and decreased peripheral vascular reactivity to cold. In addition, many older patients take daily doses of antihypertensive medications, which have a vasodilating effect that can increase the loss of body heat (Dennison, 1995).

Hypothermia in older adults is usually preventable. Nurses in the community can aid prevention by, for example, giving advice on obtaining financial assistance with heating bills, involving family members and/or social services and discussing Meals on Wheels or cooking aids.

Restoring the hypothermic patient to normothermia by **rewarming** is vital to prevent the complications associated with hypothermia, which can be fatal (Edwards, 1999a). However, raising body temperature to normal can double a patient's oxygen consumption and prompt and effective assessment and evaluation of the patient's physiological response is crucial. The instigation of appropriate rewarming techniques is a critical intervention to minimize hypothermic shivering, which increases metabolic rate, oxygen consumption and myocardial workload.

The process of rewarming should proceed no faster than 1–2°C per hour. If a patient is rewarmed too rapidly, oxygen consumption,

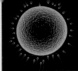

**Table 6.1.7** Methods of rewarming following hypothermia (Edwards, 1999a)

| Type | Method used | Recommended | Nursing implications |
| --- | --- | --- | --- |
| Passive external | Uses normal metabolic heat production: <br>• blanket <br>• space blanket | Mild (32–35°C) <br>Moderate (28–31.9°C) <br>Onset of less than 12 hours <br>Has limited value in profound hypothermia (<20°C) | Temperature should be taken half-hourly, then every 1–2 hours until the temperature is above 35°C <br>Other vital signs such as blood pressure, heart rate and respiration to be monitored <br>Cautious use of intravenous fluids avoidance of vigorous movement that contributes to heat loss through convection and may reduce temperature further if not closely monitored <br>If temperature fails to rise, active external rewarming should be commenced |
| Active external | Achieved by using: <br>• hot baths <br>• hot air blowers <br>• radiant heat <br>Can also be used as an adjunct to active internal rewarming | A slow hypothermia over a 12-hour period that is mild or moderate <br>Not recommended alone in the treatment of severe hypothermia | The patient's vital signs and peripheral temperature must be closely monitored or rewarming shock may occur <br>If the patient has a persistently low blood pressure or if the core temperature continues to fall, active internal rewarming should be started |
| Active internal | Warming is achieved using invasive methods such as: <br>• warm fluid for gastric/peritoneal lavage <br>• cardiopulmonary bypass | These techniques are highly invasive and only indicated in extreme cases | The use of warmed gases to the respiratory tract via an endotracheal tube if the patient is ventilated, and warmed intravenous fluids via a blood warmer are the easiest methods <br>If warmed oxygen is used, it should be humidified as well <br>The aim is to reduce the risk of cardiac arrest, by reducing the time that the patient's core temperature is below 32.2°C |

myocardial demand and vasodilation increase faster than the heart's ability to compensate and death can result. Taking account of the patient's core temperature and the duration of the hypothermia, rewarming should be started with intravenous fluid administration, monitoring of blood results and the electrocardiograph (ECG). Urine output should be measured and any drugs administered with caution as the half-life of many drugs is greatly extended. There are three methods of rewarming a hypothermic patient: passive external, active external and active internal rewarming **(Table 6.1.7)**.

All three methods of rewarming allow the deep tissues of the body to be warmed safely, as they allow the lungs and heart to be rewarmed first. The advantage of active internal rewarming, is that it avoids the peripheral vasodilation associated with surface rewarming, and allows correction of any fluid deficits. A disadvantage is

that after-drop may be observed after internal active rewarming is discontinued – a decrease in temperature of as much as 2°C may occur as blood circulates to the peripheries, cools and then returns to the core (Edwards, 1999a). Thus, when active internal rewarming methods are discontinued, passive and active external rewarming are necessary to prevent such an after-drop. Active internal rewarming is most effective when the hypothermia has developed in less than 12 hours, and is moderate or severe in nature.

Regular **observations and blood tests** are necessary to monitor the patient's condition, particularly blood glucose levels, potassium and arterial blood gases.

**Respiratory observation** during hypothermia is vital to detect hypoxia leading to inadequate cerebral perfusion. There may be changes in a person's behaviour and/or level of consciousness.

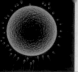

Very early signs of cerebral underperfusion include the inability to think abstractly or perform simple mental tasks, restlessness, apprehension, uncooperative behaviour and irritability. Short-term memory may also be impaired. There may be changes in blood pressure, pulse rate and the colour of mucous membranes. Oxygen saturation measurement using a probe on the patient's finger will indicate whether saturation is normal, i.e. between 98 and 100%. However, a patient may experience a significant drop in oxygen supply but with minimal effect on oxygen saturation and so careful observation is important.

Hypothermia initiates a **cold diuresis**. Peripheral vasoconstriction shunts blood to the core, creating a relatively hypervolaemic state here and this suppresses the secretion of antidiuretic hormone (ADH). As a result, urinary output is increased, leading to hypovolaemia. Renal function is dependent on adequate renal perfusion, which is determined by the blood pressure, cardiac output, vascular tone and acute tubular necrosis and renal failure may result (Fritsch, 1995). If the hourly urine output falls below 0.5 mL/kg for more than 2 hours, this may indicate that cardiac output is low and the doctor needs to be informed. The urinary output should be at least 30 mL/hour. Patients need to be catheterized to enable accurate measurement of urine output at hourly intervals.

**Blood glucose levels** should be closely monitored. As body temperature decreases and shivering stops (at around 30°C), hyperglycaemia occurs, insulin secretion decreases and the cells become more resistant to insulin that is present (Fritsch, 1995). Hyperglycaemia may be resistant to treatment until the patient's core temperature is above 30°C, as below this temperature glucose and insulin utilization is minimal; if insulin is administered, rebound hypoglycaemia may occur during rewarming and so this is generally avoided in the hypothermic patient. However, if hypoglycaemia occurs during rewarming, it should be corrected.

**Serum potassium** blood levels should be monitored, as alterations in potassium levels may occur as temperature decreases. Alterations in the sodium–potassium pump within body cells may result in an increased potassium level outside the cell (extracellular) during hypothermia. During rewarming, the sodium–potassium pump returns to normal and the potassium moves back inside the cell (intracellular) and hypokalaemia may follow. If the patient's cardiac signs are being monitored, changes to the T wave are an early warning sign of hypokalaemia.

**Acid–base balance** by arterial blood gas analysis is necessary because, as temperatures fall, acid–base changes occur. Hyperventilation occurs during early hypothermia causing respiratory alkalosis. As the temperature decreases, respiratory failure leads to a progressive respiratory and metabolic acidosis (Holtzclaw, 1993). However, measurement of arterial blood gases is invasive and requires puncturing an artery or obtaining a specimen from an arterial line.

**The electrocardiograph (ECG)** should be monitored, as a slow heart rate and unusual QRS and T complexes are common in hypothermia. In addition, the incidence of cardiac arrest increases with decreasing temperature and active internal rewarming is indicated; continuous basic life support may be necessary. Ventricular and atrial fibrillation, asystole and electromechanical dissociation have all been reported as cardiac arrest rhythms due to hypothermia. Defibrillation may not be successful at lower body temperatures but should still be attempted.

*The consequences of hypothermia*
A number of consequences of hypothermia need to be considered in the management of patients. These are summarized in **Table 6.1.8**.

## ASSESSMENT OF BODY TEMPERATURE

Assessment of temperature is necessary to identify abnormalities in temperature regulation, to ensure the correct treatment is promptly instigated. There are four types of thermometer in common use **(Table 6.1.9)**.

Resources on the ward often determine selection of thermometer. However, in terms of patient comfort, the single-use chemical thermometer is the preferred choice. Some patients find it uncomfortable to have an oral temperature taken using a glass thermometer or electronic thermometer and they can be unsafe for patients who are restless, disorientated or shivering. While tympanic membrane probes are relatively safe and comfortable, there is a slight risk of trauma to the tympanic membrane (eardrum).

It must be remembered that many standard thermometers do not record temperatures below 35°C, and low-reading mercury, electronic or light-reflecting thermometers are necessary for accurate measurement of hypothermia (Haskell et al., 1997).

### Taking the temperature

#### Time of day

Certain times of the day are better than others for temperature recording (Holtzclaw, 1993). There is a diurnal variation in body temperature in

**Table 6.1.8** The consequences of hypothermia (Edwards, 1999a)

| Consequences | In hypothermia | Rewarming | The nurse's role |
|---|---|---|---|
| Shivering occurs in an effort to increase heat production. | Peripheral vasoconstriction shunts blood away from the skin in an effort to decrease heat loss<br>• Produces peripheral tissue ischaemia<br>• Body movement increases, energy is used to produce heat, causing a raised metabolic rate, leading to increased oxygen consumption (400–500%), increased carbon dioxide production and myocardial work | It may also occur during rewarming | It is important that nurses monitor and control shivering to avert the increased metabolic demand and the discomfort this creates |
| Rewarming shock | Shock may occur if peripheral warming occurs before central warming and cold acidic blood is returned to the heat causing myocardial depression | Shock may also occur during rewarming if circulating volume is inadequate | Vigilant temperature and haemodynamic monitoring is imperative to avoid this |
| Impaired immunity | Vasoconstriction and the decrease in oxygen supply to the tissues reduce the body's ability to kill microorganisms; wound healing may also be affected | | Nurses need to be vigilant regarding infection control practices on hypothermic patients |
| Acidosis | • Acids from the waste products of metabolism accumulate in the stagnant blood in the periphery<br>• The fall in blood pH results in a metabolic acidosis, which depresses the activity of all vital organs, especially the cardiovascular system | The waste products return to the heart during rewarming | • Urine testing to determine pH balance of urine will give some indication of acid base status of the blood<br>• Vital signs such as respiratory rate increase in acidosis to remove excessive acids as carbon dioxide |
| Nutritional needs | Postoperative hypothermic patients do not advance to solid food intake quickly and this may delay healing and lengthen the stay in hospital | Due to stress, the gastrointestinal tract may not function immediately | Poor wound healing, loss of nitrogen and protein increases the patient's risk of wound infection |
| Pharmacokinetics | Temperatures of 30°C have effects on the half-life of drugs. There is increased protein binding of administered drugs, with the result that their effects are often diminished | The drugs are released from the protein binding, may lead to toxicity | The use of all drugs should be restricted and carefully monitored during the rewarming process |

**Table 6.1.9**   Equipment used to measure body temperature (Edwards, 1997)

| Type of thermometer | Positive | Negative |
|---|---|---|
| Glass mercury thermometers | • Glass mercury thermometers are cheap<br>• Disposable covers are available to minimize cross-infection | • Require disinfecting after use<br>• Takes longer to use (2 min orally, 3 min axilla)<br>• They may break, exposing people to small amounts of mercury vapour<br>• Unsuitable for oral temperature recording in patients who have seizures, as well as those who are unconscious or confused |
| Single-use chemical thermometers: small temperature-sensitive dots that change colour with increasing temperature | • Left in place for 1 min for oral recordings and 3 min for axilla and rectal recordings<br>• Is ready to read 10 seconds after removal<br>• Will record temperatures between 35.5 and 40.5°C. They are particularly suitable for people with badly fitting dentures or sore mouths<br>• Require no cleaning reducing the risk of cross-infection | • Difficult to read subtle changes in temperature<br>• Does not read low-grade temperature such as hypothermia, need a special type of thermometer to do this |
| Electronic thermometers provide a reading in digital format | • Uses a disposable cover<br>• A signal indicates when the maximum temperature has been reached, to prevent premature removal<br>• Are accurate and easy to use | They are more expensive than glass or single-use thermometers |
| Tympanic membrane uses infra-red reflectance thermometry that detects heat radiated as infra-red energy from the tympanic membrane of the ear | • Correlates well with pulmonary artery temperature<br>• Inserted into the ear a digital recording is obtained in a matter of seconds<br>• Can be undertaken quickly, with no discomfort | Otitis media or the presence of wax or hair in the ear canal may influence recordings. If the patient has been lying on one ear, causing more heat to be retained, this may also influence the recording |

humans, owing to diurnal rhythms, and body temperature is most likely to be elevated at the peak of the diurnal cycle, which is between 5.00 and 8.00 p.m. Thus, to detect pyrexia, it is preferable to record the temperature in the evenings. Temperature recording in hospitals is sometimes ritualized but it may not be necessary for it to be done so frequently. Daily recordings will be most effective if carried out between 5.00 and 8.00 p.m.

### Sites

The pulmonary artery temperature is the most accurate measure of core body temperature. However, this form of temperature measurement is extremely invasive and only available in critical care settings. Temperature sites in close proximity to the brain (e.g. tympanic membrane, mouth) best reflect the thermal environment of the brain **(Table 6.1.10)**. This is particularly relevant to the oral temperature, as the oral cavity is in close proximity to the sublingual artery, which is in direct contact with the brain and hypothalamus. None of the sites given in **Table 6.1.10** is ideal in every respect, and the notion that one site is a more accurate reflection of core temperature than another is erroneous (Edwards, 1997). The type of information required and the patient's safety, comfort and convenience also influence the choice of site.

**Table 6.1.10** Sites available for measuring body temperature (Edwards, 1997)

| Site | Advantages | Disadvantages |
|---|---|---|
| Oral | The most common and most accessible site for temperature recording | • Affected by factors, e.g. hot or cold drinks, exertion, talking, while the thermometer is in situ, and by smoking (involves the inhalation of heat)<br>• Early morning estimations will usually be up to 0.5°C lower than early evening readings due to diurnal temperature variations<br>• In females, postovulation readings will be slightly higher than preovulation ones |
| Axilla | • A convenient site and comfortable for the patient<br>• A safer area to record body temperature, it avoids trauma in patients who may accidentally bite the thermometer<br>• It is a valuable site if the thermometer is used correctly<br>• To obtain an accurate reading, it should be left for at least 10 minutes and the same axilla should be used for each measurement | • Thought to be a less accurate reflection of core body temperature (The temperature in the axilla is generally 0.5°C below oral temperature and so if this site is used, it should be noted on the chart)<br>• Recordings can be inaccurate in thin patients (poor contact between the thermometer and the skin in the axilla) and in obese people (the presence of adipose tissue prevents close contact with the blood supply)<br>• Excessive sweating or axillary air pockets may lead to inaccuracies |
| Rectal | • Core temperature is most accurately reflected in the rectum<br>• Rectal temperatures are uncomfortable and embarrassing for the patient and can cause rectal trauma | • Affected by heat generated by faecal bacteria and consequently might be inaccurate (Rectal temperature will, on average, register a temperature of up to 0.5°C higher than the oral temperature; one reason for this is thought to be the extra metabolic heat that is produced in the rectum by the bacterial colonization of the area)<br>• Rarely used in the UK, only for patients acutely ill or unconscious |
| Tympanic membrane | • This is close to the hypothalamus and gives an accurate reflection of core temperature<br>• It provides a rapid recording and is comfortable for the patient<br>• The probe should not touch the tympanic membrane and so the risk of trauma is small | • Affected by the presence of earwax, hairs. The position of the patient may also affect the accuracy<br>• Care when positioning the thermometer probe is important. It should fit snugly in the ear canal to prevent air affecting the reading |
| Peripheral temperature | The toe temperature is an inexpensive and non-invasive way of monitoring tissue perfusion and is a useful guide to determining the severity of shock | Not widely used in all clinical practice areas, requires monitoring using a temperature probe |

Normal body temperature varies between 35 and 37.5°C and varies from site to site. The difference between core temperature and oral and ear temperatures is about 0.5°C. The temperature in the axilla is approximately 1°C below core temperature. Thus, if the core temperature is 37°C, the temperature in the mouth and ear would be 36.5°C, and that in the axilla 36°C. The temperature should not be recorded immediately after bathing or physical exercise because it may be raised in response to immersion in hot water and heat production from active muscular work.

## Innate defences

Despite the myriad of microorganisms that live around and on us, we stay amazingly healthy most of the time. Microorganisms can survive either on the surface of the human body and in body cavities, where they absorb food and release enzymes but remain outside human cells, or by infecting (invading) human cells where they not only survive (intracellularly) but also replicate, utilizing the host-cell energy sources. Both intracellular and extracellular microorganisms grow, reproduce and can infect other individuals. Many different species invade humans: some are relatively harmless, some helpful; others cause disease, and this leads to a constant battle between the invading pathogen and the immune system. In some cases microorganisms can even cause the death of their host.

To survive such infections the human body relies on two systems that respond immediately to protect it from all foreign substances. These two systems act both independently and cooperatively. One of these systems is the **innate (non-specific) immune system**. 'Innate' means 'present at birth'. The innate immune response is the same for every microorganism attacking the body. It responds immediately to protect the body from all foreign substances. The innate immune system erects two barriers that prevent entry to microorganisms:

1. The external body membranes, which includes an intact skin and mucosae.
2. The generation of chemical signals when the external defences are penetrated. These trigger the production and action of phagocytes, antimicrobial proteins, natural killer cells, inflammation and an increase in temperature.

The second protective system is the **acquired specific immune response**, which mounts an attack against particular foreign substances, and is different for each microorganism. This immune response is the subject of Chapter 6.2. **Even though these two defence mechanisms are considered separately in this text, the specific and non-specific defences always work hand in hand.**

## Gaining entry into the body

Before a pathogen can invade the host and cause infection, it must first attach to and penetrate the surface epithelial layers of the body. Organisms gain entry into the body by active or passive means. This might involve burrowing through the skin, being ingested in food, inhaled into the respiratory tract or penetrating an open wound. Whatever their mode of entry, they have to pass across physical barriers, such as the dead layers of the skin or living epithelial cell layers, which line the cavities in contact with the exterior such as the respiratory, genitourinary or gastrointestinal tracts. The majority of pathogens enter via these routes.

In many instances, our innate defences alone are able to destroy pathogens and ward off infection and innate defences effectively reduce the workload of the acquired immune system by preventing entry and spread of microorganisms in the body. **Table 6.1.11** summarizes the most important innate, non-specific defence mechanisms.

## Innate surface membrane barriers/secretions

The first line of defence against the invasion of disease causing microorganisms is the skin and the mucous membranes, and the secretions these membranes produce. These are highly effective as long as the epidermis or epithelial membranes are unbroken.

### The skin

The skin is the most effective barrier preventing entry of microorganisms into the body. The skin is highly effective as long as the epidermis is unbroken. It provides a watertight barrier protecting the internal organs from infection. The acid nature of the skin secretions (pH of 3–5) inhibits bacterial growth, and the sebum the skin secretes contains chemicals that are toxic to bacteria. The skin contains keratin, a protein that presents a formidable physical barrier to most microorganisms that swarm on the skin.

### Vaginal secretions

The acid medium of the vagina (pH 4.0–4.5) is maintained by the resident bacterial flora, notably *Lactobacillus*. This organism acts upon the glycogen in the vagina to produce lactic acid, which forms a hostile environment for many fungi, bacteria and viruses. If non-prescribed douches or vaginal deodorants are used, the acid environment of the vagina is disturbed and pathogens may colonize the area. The fungus, *Candida albicans* may supervene and produce vaginal thrush. In postmenopausal females, the production of glycogen in the vagina decreases, less acid is produced and a senile vaginitis may occur. This condition can be treated with oestrogens.

**Table 6.1.11**  Summary of the innate immune defences (modified from McCance & Huether, 1998)

| Elements | Protective mechanism |
| --- | --- |
| **Surface membrane barriers** | |
| Intact skin epidermis: | As long as the epidermis is unbroken it presents a formidable physical barrier to most microorganisms that swarm the skin |
| • acid mantle | • Skin secretions (perspiration and sebum) make epidermal surface acidic, which inhibits bacterial growth; sebum also contains bactericidal chemicals |
| • keratin | • Provides resistance against acids, alkalis and bacterial enzymes |
| Intact mucous membranes: | Form mechanical barriers to all areas of the body open to the exterior e.g. digestive, respiratory, urinary, reproductive, ears and secret secretions which contain phagocytes and is a weak acid to destroy pathogens |
| • mucous | • traps microorganisms in respiratory and digestive tract |
| • nasal hairs | • filter and trap microorganisms in nasal passages |
| • cilia | • propel debris-laden mucous away from the respiratory passages |
| • gastric juice | • contains concentrated hydrochloric acid and protein-digesting enzymes that destroy pathogens in stomach |
| • acid mantle of vagina | • inhibits growth of bacteria and fungi in female reproductive tract |
| • tears, saliva | • continuously lubricate and cleanse eyes and oral cavity; contain lysozymes, an enzyme that destroys microorganisms |
| • urine | • normally acid pH inhibits bacterial growth; cleanses the lower urinary tract as it flushes from the body |
| **Non-specific cellular and chemical defences** | |
| Phagocytes | Engulf and destroy pathogens that breach surface membrane barriers; also contribute to immune response and may use additional oxidizing chemicals to ensure the death of an invading microorganism |
| Natural killer cells | Promote cells lysis by direct cell attack against virus-infected or cancerous body cells. Do not depend on a specific antigen recognition as they act against any target. They will kill viruses infected in body cells before the immune system is activated. They are not phagocytic, they attack the target cell membrane and release certain chemicals that disintegrate the nucleus rapidly |
| Inflammatory response | This is the natural tissue response to injury. Disposes of pathogens and dead tissue cells and promotes tissue repair. Chemical mediators released attract phagocytes to the area |
| Antimicrobal proteins: | |
| • interferons | • proteins released by virus-infected cells that protect uninfected tissue cells from viral take-over; mobilize immune system |
| • complement | • lyses microorganisms, enhances phagocytosis by opsonization and intensifies inflammatory and immune responses |
| Pyrexia | Systemic response initiated by pyrogens; high body temperature inhibits microbial multiplication and enhances body repair processes |

## Urine

The constant downward flow of urine through the ureters and bladder and the acid pH of urine tend to militate against ascending infections. The acid urine will kill most bacteria and the act of micturition irrigates the urethra. These are effective responses in the long male urethra, but less so in the female. The adult female urethra is only 2 or 3 cm long and hence forms a relatively short and readily available portal of entry for organisms into the bladder.

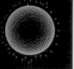
## The stomach mucosa

The hydrochloric acid (pH 3) produced by the stomach and protein-digesting enzymes will kill most organisms entering the stomach in food and drink, or in swallowed sputum, as most organisms are unable to survive in such an acid environment. Some organisms can, however, resist this strong acid, for example, tubercle bacilli, enteroviruses, helicobacteria and salmonella. Milk and proteins are both effective buffers against gastric acid and so some organisms (if ingested with these foodstuffs) may be protected from the gastric acid. This explains how, in spite of gastric defences, typhoid and dysentery can still occur.

To a certain extent, the small and large intestines rely on the stomach's bactericidal activity. The resident flora of the large intestine – *Esherichia coli*, non-haemolytic streptoccocci, anaerobic *Bacteroides* – all contribute to the normal function of the area. Their role becomes more evident when they are removed by the administration of broad-spectrum antibiotics. The area is then open to colonization by pathogens (e.g. *Staphylococcus pyogenes*). Superinfections, such as methicillin-resistant *Staphylococcus aureus* (MRSA), which may be resistant to antibiotics can be fatal in debilitated patients.

The small and large bowels are both liberally supplied with patches of lymphoid tissue throughout their length. In the specific immune response (see Chapter 6.2), plasma cells from these areas produce immunoglobulins (IgA) and these provide local defence.

## Saliva

The buccal cavity is lined with a fairly tough mucous membrane, which is irrigated by a constant backward flow of saliva (i.e. directed towards the throat). The flow of saliva also prevents organisms from entering the salivary glands, and traps organisms, which can then be swallowed.

The resident bacteria in the mouth are in general harmless; indeed, α-haemolytic *Streptococcus* is of positive benefit because it produces hydrogen peroxide, which helps to clean the mouth. The tonsils, formed of lymphoid tissue, further defend the oral cavity. However, the tonsillar epithelial covering is very thin and so is easily traumatized. Tonsillar infections are not uncommon, especially in childhood.

### The eye

The conjunctival sac is constantly irrigated with tears produced by the lachrymal glands. The lachrymal fluid washes the external eye surfaces and produces tears. Tears contain components of complement (see later) and more lysozyme than any other body fluid. The eye infections that occur when vitamin A is deficient do so as a result of the decrease in lysozyme secretion in this condition. Blinking is a defensive reflex, which helps to rid the eye of irritants and to distribute the tears. In conditions such as facial nerve paralysis or unconsciousness, this reflex is lost and it becomes necessary to prevent the conjunctiva drying or becoming ulcerated by keeping the eye closed and irrigated regularly.

### The nose and upper respiratory tract

The nose is lined with small mucous-coated hairs, which trap small-inhaled particles and the mucosa of the upper respiratory tract is ciliated. The cilia sweep dust and bacteria-laden mucus upward towards the mouth to be swallowed, thus preventing it from entering the lower respiratory passages where the warm, moist environment provides an ideal site for bacterial growth. Should any organisms reach the alveoli they are engulfed and destroyed (phagocytosis; **see Fig. 4.1.9, p. 000**) by alveolar macrophages. The hilum of the lung is well supplied with lymph nodes, which act as a further filter. Sneezing is a protective reflex that expels irritants. Coughing is a defensive reflex which removes particulate matter or excess mucus in the lower tract.

### Cells of the innate immune system

Even though the surface barriers are quite effective, they are breached occasionally by small cuts and nicks resulting from brushing teeth, or shaving. When this happens, and microorganisms manage to invade deeper tissues, the internal innate defences come into play.

## Cellular and chemical defence mechanisms

The body uses an enormous number of innate defensive cellular devices to protect itself. These include the destructive power of phagocytes and natural killer cells and the involvement of antimicrobial proteins, mast cells, basophils and dendritic cells.

## Phagocytes

**Phagocytes** engulf bacteria (**see Fig. 4.1.9**, p. 356). They confront pathogens that get through the skin and mucosa into the underlying connective tissues. The two main types of phagocytes are **neutrophils** and **macrophages**.

### Neutrophils

These are often called **polymorphonuclear leucocytes** (PMLs). They are mobile phagocytes that comprise the majority (approximately 60%) of blood leucocytes (white cells). The chemotaxic agents for neutrophils include protein fragments released when complement is activated (e.g. C3a and C5a) (Roitt et al., 2001). Their granules contain peroxidase, alkaline and acid phosphatases and defensins (antimicrobial peptides), which are important for the killing of microorganisms. They are produced in the bone marrow and their main function is to patrol the body via the bloodstream in search of invading microbes. Polymorphonuclear leucocytes are an essential part of the innate immune system, wiping out many infections before they have a chance to multiply.

The polymorphonuclear leucocytes are very short lived, surviving for no more than a few days. They move towards sites of infection attracted by various chemicals, which includes some bacterial products and substances that escape from cells when they are damaged (mediators). Therefore, these cells are pivotal cells in stimulating the inflammatory response (Lydyard et al., 2000).

### Macrophages

Macrophages develop as monocytes in the bone marrow. Once released from marrow, monocytes circulate for 1 or 2 days in the blood, making up 6% of the white blood cells (leucocytes). They then squeeze between the cells of the blood-vessel wall (a process called **diapedesis**) and migrate into the tissues. There they develop into macrophages. Macrophages are part of a widely distributed, tissue-bound phagocytic system called the **mononuclear phagocyte system** (previously called the reticuloendothelial system). Their function is to dispose of microorganisms and dead body cells through the process of phagocytosis. Macrophages can either be:

- **Free macrophages**: these migrate from the blood to the tissues in search of foreign invaders or cellular debris. These cells are known as **monocytes** for the short period that they are in the blood and have limited function while they are contained in the cardiovascular system.

- **Fixed macrophages**: such as the Kupffer cells in the liver or alveolar macrophages of the lungs, which are permanent residents of particular organs.

Activated macrophages release interleukin-1 (IL-1), a costimulator that enhances the activation of T cells (cells of specific cell-mediated immunity) and costimulates T cells to liberate interleukin-2 (IL-2) and to synthesize more interleukin-2 receptors. Interleukin-2 is a key growth factor for T cells, acting as a local hormone. It sets up a positive feedback cycle that encourages activated T cells to divide even more rapidly. This process is a clear example of how the innate and specific immune responses function in unison (see later).

### The phagocytic process

A phagocyte moves towards a microorganism and attaches to its surface. **Endocytosis** of the pathogen then occurs leading to it becoming enclosed in a vacuole (**phagosome**). This phagosome then becomes fused with a lysosome to become a phagolysosome, where the foreign material is degraded. The residual material is then removed by **exocytosis** (**see Fig. 4.1.9, p. 000**).

A phagocyte's attempt to destroy a bacterium is not always successful because the phagocyte has to first adhere or cling to the particle. This is made possible because the phagocyte recognizes the particle's external carbohydrate signature, although this can be particularly difficult with microorganisms such as the pneumococcus, which has an external capsule made from complex sugars. These pathogens can sometimes elude capture because the phagocyte cannot bind to their capsules. Adherence to the capsule in such instances can be facilitated by **complement**. Complement proteins and **antibodies** coat foreign particles, a process called **opsonization** ('to make tasty') by providing sites to which phagocyte receptors can bind (Lydyard et al., 2000).

### Natural killer cells

Natural killer cells (NKCs) are found throughout the tissues of the body but mainly in the blood and lymph. They kill viruses before the immune system is activated and will act spontaneously against any target. These cells are not phagocytic. Instead, their mode of killing involves attacking the target cell's membrane and releasing cytolytic chemicals to disintegrate the microorganism's membrane and nucleus very rapidly. Natural killer cells also secrete potent chemicals that enhance the inflammatory response.

### Mast cells and basophils

**Basophils** are granulocyte white blood cells and are present in very low number in the circulation. They

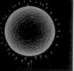

transform into **mast cells** once they migrate into the tissues.

Mast cells are found in connective tissues throughout the body, close to blood vessels and particularly in the areas of the respiratory, urogenital and gastrointestinal tracts. When activated, mast cells do not release substances that attack the invaders directly, but instead release mediators, such as histamine and later prostaglandins (the latter are not preformed and so are not released immediately). This release of chemicals simulates an organized attack by the immune system at the site of infection. The mediators attract other white blood cells and are essential in the development of an **acute inflammatory response**. The effect of the mediators is instantaneous and causes local blood vessels to dilate, the vascular permeability of the capillaries to increase and the attraction of leucocytes to the site of degranulation (see later).

### Dendritic cells

Dendritic cells (DCs) are so called because their surface membrane is similar in appearance to the dendrites of the nervous system. Their function is to present antigens to lymphocytes and, as such, these dendritic cells are at the interface of the innate and acquired immune systems. They recognize microbial antigens through innate receptors and are able to present peptide antigens to the T and B lymphocytes. It is thought that this interaction in the B-cell follicles of lymphoid tissue is important in B-cell survival (Lydyard et al., 2000).

## Innate molecular defence against organisms

A variety of molecules mediate protection against pathogens during the period before specific immunity develops. These include **complement**, **interferon**, **acute-phase proteins** and **cytokines**, all of which are present in blood and tissue fluid. Most of these molecules, which play a role in the innate immune system also, have functions associated with the specific immune system. Antibodies can activate the complement system and cytokines, released by macrophages, are involved in activation of antigen-presenting cells critical to triggering T-lymphocyte responses. Cytokines also play a role in acute inflammation. Thus the immune response to microorganisms is continuous with both systems being intimately involved and synergistic.

### *The complement system*

Although part of innate defences, the complement system has very close links with the acquired immune system, particularly with antibodies. In fact, the name 'complement' derives from the early understanding that the system 'complemented' antibodies in the destruction of bacteria (Walport, 2001).

Complement is a system that consists of more than 30 proteins. These proteins are found in plasma and on cell surfaces. They work in a cascading sequence with the end function bacterial destruction. However, along the way to this goal, they initiate other processes that are very important in the functioning of the immune response to antigens. Three pathways can be followed to lead to the ultimate end result of bacterial cell lysis (death). These are the classical pathway, the alternative pathway and the mannan-binding lectin (mb-lectin) pathway. However, the latter pathway links up to the classical pathway quite early in the sequence.

The **classical pathway** was the first complement pathway discovered, and it consists of nine stages (**see Fig. 6.1.11**). The proteins in the pathway were numbered according to the order in which they were identified, which explains their rather strange ordering: the fourth complement factor discovered was actually found to be the second factor in the sequence. Of all the complement factors, C3 is the most pivotal because all the other pathways converge at this point. However, each of the three pathways is initiated by different activators.

### The classical pathway

The classical pathway is activated by combinations of antigen and antibody – the **antigen–antibody immune complexes**. C1 consists of three factors: C1q, C1r, and C1s. This combination is known as the **recognition unit** of the complement system because

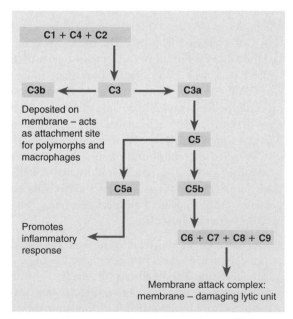

**Figure 6.1.11** Simplified complement pathway

they recognize an antigen in combination with immunoglobulin and this initiates the classical pathway of the complement system. C1, as the first protein in the sequence, recognizes the Fc region of immunoglobulin when there are enough of them in close proximity to each other (hence the need for the antigen–antibody complex, which ensures that this condition is met). Immunoglobulin G (IgG) is a very good initiator of the complement system because it readily forms such complexes, but immunoglobulin M (IgM) is even better at binding to C1 because, being a pentamer, it has ten potential Fc binding sites, all in close proximity to each other – and that is before they bind to antigen.

Once C1 has bound to sufficient immunoglobulin Fc sites, one of its three components, C1s, cleaves (i.e. splits) the next complement in the sequence, which is C4, into C4a and C4b. C4b first binds to the bacterial surface and then binds to C2, which is then in turn cleaved by C1s into C2a and C2b. C4b and C2b bind together, forming the C4b–2b complex, which is an active enzyme capable of cleaving C3 into C3a and C3b. C3b is a very important molecule because it coats the surface of the bacteria.

To give an example of the cascade effect of the complement system, one molecule of C4b–2b can cleave up to 1000 molecules of C3 to form a huge number of C3b molecules, which coat the bacterial surface. The other product of C3 cleaving, C3a, is an inflammatory mediator. C3 is the most abundant complement protein in plasma, so, at this stage, the main effect of complement activation is to cover the bacterial cell surface with large quantities of C3b. Here it forms a tightly bonded coating all over the surface and this prepares the bacterium for its eventual destruction by acting as an opsonin. The three complement factors C4, C2 and C3 are collectively known as the **activation unit of the complement system**.

The next factor in the complement system, C5, is then enabled to bind to C3b. Once this has occurred, C5 is then cleaved by C2b to give C5a and C5b. C5b in turn initiates the terminal stages of the complement system, leading to **lysis** of the bacterium. One molecule of C5b binds to a single molecule of C6. This C5b–6 complex is then able to bind to a molecule of C7. The resulting C5b–6–7 complex then binds to C8 and C9. This whole unit (C5b–6–7–8–9) is then turned into a membrane attack unit, which is **hydrophobic** and able to make a hole through the membrane of Gram-negative bacteria. C8 initiates the process by which this hole is kept open. It induces a change in C9, causing it to make a ring of 10–16 molecules and thereby making a pore-like structure. This pore facilitates the passage of water and solutes out of the cell. In effect, the cell has been punctured and the bacterium has been killed. This is quite a dramatic scenario, but at the moment, the applause for this aspect of the complement system has to be somewhat muted. Although the membrane attack complex appears potentially to be of significant importance, unfortunately, to date, the only bacteria against which it has been found to be effective are the Gram-negative *Neisseria* species. This is the bacterium, which, in one or other of its two forms, can either cause a vicious form of bacterial meningitis, or the sexually transmitted disease, gonorrhoea. So, although the complement system's lysing capabilities are by no means negligible, they appear to be effective only against a few pathogenic organisms (*Neisseria* and a few viruses). The other effects of the complement system, particularly the opsonizing and inflammatory roles, appear to be of far more importance to the well-being of the host.

Other indirect effects of the complement system occur prior to the membrane attack complex being activated, for example, increased vascular permeability enabling components of the immune system to enter the blood and allowing them to move to other areas of the body where they are needed. C3a and C5a are **anaphylotoxins** and mediate anaphylotoxin-type biological effects by stimulating degranulation of mast cells and the release of vasoactive amines from the same cells. This includes the release of histamine and leukotrienes, leading to a subsequent increase in vascular permeability. In addition, mast cells are a source of a particular important cytokine – tumour necrosis factor-$\alpha$ (TNF-$\alpha$), which causes local inflammation (Seymour et al., 1995). C3a and C5a are also chemotactic agents. They mediate the recruitment of inflammatory cells and their movement towards sites of inflammation and infection. C3 and C4 bind to complement receptors and so help in the opsonization of pathogenic organisms, as well as the removal of immune complexes. C3b and C4b augment antibody responses and are also capable of enhancing immunological memory (Walport, 2001). Thus, the importance of the complement system as part of the immune defences cannot be overstated.

As well as the sequential progression of the classical complement pathway, amplification takes place at each stage, so that even though the initial activation may occur because of only a few bacterial antigen–antibody immune complexes, the subsequent amplification at each step ensures a very dramatic response, albeit only at a local level (Nairn & Helbert, 2002).

## The alternative pathway

This pathway is activated by a wide variety of antigens, such as Gram-negative bacteria, viruses and fungi, tumour cells, apoptotic cells (cells that have undergone cell death) and C-reactive protein, which is bound to ligand (Walport, 2001).

The alternative pathway functions because C3 is an unstable molecule and is continually being activated at a low level – usually in plasma. Although normal cells of the body possess complement inhibitors on their surfaces, which prevent C3 activation on host cells, the surfaces of pathogens lack such complement inhibitors and are therefore at risk of activating the complement system (Nairn & Helbert, 2002). The alternative pathway requires two specific factors, called **factor B** and **factor D**. Factor D splits factor B into Ba and Bb, which proceed to activate and cleave C3 into C3a and C3b, and then to form an enzyme called C3bBb. This enzyme is quite unstable and can easily dissociate (break apart). However, another molecule called **properdin** (factor P) binds to the C3bBb enzyme and prevents this dissociation. Once the stable C3bBb complex binds to further C3b, it is able to cleave C5 and then progress towards cell lysis as part of the classical pathway (Seymour et al., 1995).

### Mannan-binding lectin pathway

This pathway is initiated due to the ability of mannan-binding lectin to bind to carbohydrates that are present on the surface of bacteria. Once the lectin portions have bound to the bacterium, the complex formed indirectly activates the complement components C4 and C2, which proceed to activate C3.

It can now be seen how C3 is the pivotal complement factor in this system, as all three pathways lead to C3 activation.

Before leaving the complement system, it is of interest to note that it can also interact with other enzyme cascades, namely the coagulation, kinin and fibrinolytic systems (see Chapter 4.1).

In summary, the complement system provides a major mechanism for destroying foreign substances in the body. Complement is a group of at least 30 plasma proteins that normally circulate in the blood and body fluids in an inactive state. It can be activated either directly by certain molecules associated with microorganisms, or by antibodies bound to a pathogen or any other antigen. When complement is activated:

- chemical mediators that amplify virtually all aspects of the (acute) inflammatory process are unleashed
- neutrophils are attracted to the site of microbial attack (chemotaxis)
- attachment of the microorganisms to the phagocyte (opsonization) is enhanced
- the membrane attack complex is activated, killing the microorganism through lysis.

This powerful system of inflammation and destruction can cause extensive damage to host cells if uncontrolled. Through the long process of evolution, our own cells have become equipped with proteins that inactivate complement, limiting its membrane-damaging ability to the immediate vicinity of the activation site. The complement system is also tightly regulated by inhibitory/regulatory proteins. Although complement itself is part of innate immunity, it enhances both innate and specific immune defences.

## Acute-phase proteins

These are a group of plasma proteins important in innate defence, mainly against bacteria and in limiting tissue damage caused by infection, trauma, malignancy and other diseases, e.g. rheumatoid arthritis. In addition, they maximize activation of the complement system and opsonization of invading pathogens. They include:

- C-reactive protein (CRP)
- serum amyloid protein A (SAA)
- mannose-binding protein (MBP).

## Interferon

Interferons (IFNs) are proteins involved in protection against viral infections. Viruses are essentially nucleic acids surrounded by a protein coat and lack the cellular machinery to generate adenosine triphosphate or synthesize proteins. Viruses do their damage in the body by invading tissue cells and taking over the cellular metabolic machinery they need to reproduce themselves.

The virus-infected cells can do little to save themselves, but they can help protect other cells that have not yet been infected by secreting interferon. There are two different types of interferon, type I and II. Type I inhibits protein synthesis in virally infected cells preventing mRNA translation and DNA replication; type II enhances natural killer cell function and the phagocytic function of macrophages. Interferon's protection is not virus specific, thus interferon produced against particular viruses protects us against a variety of other viruses.

## The inflammatory response

The inflammatory response incorporates the action of macrophages, mast cells and all types of white blood cells, as well as dozens of chemical substances that kill pathogens and help repair tissue. These protective mechanisms recognize surface carbohydrates unique to infectious organisms (bacteria, fungus and viruses).

Activation of the inflammatory response (IR) represents a major physiological event in the body

(Huddleston, 1992). It is triggered whenever body tissues are injured, for example physical trauma, intense heat and irritating chemicals, as well as to infection by viruses, fungi and bacteria. Acute inflammation is caused by the release of inflammatory mediators from microbes, damaged tissue, mast cells and other leucocytes. The inflammatory response:

- protects the body from invading microorganisms and prevents the spread of damaging agents to nearby tissues
- limits the extent of blood loss and injury
- removes and disposes of dead cells, other debris and pathogens
- promotes rapid healing of involved tissues (as such, inflammation is closely associated with wound healing).

Chemicals called **leucocytosis-inducing factors**, which are released by injured cells, promote rapid release of neutrophils from red bone marrow and, within a few hours, the number of neutrophils in the bloodstream may multiply by up to five times. This leucocytosis is a characteristic sign of inflammation. Neutrophils usually migrate randomly but inflammatory chemicals act as homing devices or, more precisely, chemotactic agents, that attract them and other white blood cells to the site of injury. The mediators cause four characteristic features of inflammation: these are redness over the area (**rubor**), oedema (**tumor**), heat (**calor**) and pain (**dolor**). If the swollen area is a joint following injury movement may be hampered temporarily, forcing the injured part to rest, so aiding healing.

The main cells involved in an acute inflammatory response are mast cells and neutrophils. Others include eosinophils, basophils, lymphocytes and microbes, which may release endotoxins and/or exotoxins, both of which are **inflammatory mediators**. When damaged, the cells release mediators such as histamine, prostaglandins, cytokines leading to capillary dilation and increased vascular permeability (**Table 6.1.12**).

Following an insult or injury, there is a systemic response that produces extensive inflammation by attracting nutrients, fluids, clotting factors and large numbers of neutrophils and macrophages to the damaged site. The ultimate goal of an inflammatory response is to clear the injured area of pathogens and dead tissue cells so that tissue can be repaired. Once this is accomplished, healing usually occurs quickly. Damaged or injured tissue releases inflammatory chemicals into the extracellular fluid. Injured tissue cells, phagocytes, lymphocytes, mast cells and blood proteins are all sources of these inflammatory mediators. The most important inflammatory mediators are: histamine, kinins, prostaglandins, complement and cytokines, especially interleukin-1.

## Vasodilation

The mediators all have individual inflammatory roles (**see Table 6.1.12**). They all promote smooth muscle contraction and dilation of the small blood vessels in the area increasing blood flow to the area. This leads to localized hyperaemia, accounting for the redness and heat of an inflamed area.

## Cell migration

The pattern of cell migration to the site of injury is complex but is determined by interactions between circulating leucocytes, phagocytes and the endothelium of blood vessels (**Fig. 6.1.12**). The process is controlled by signalling molecules (selectins, chemokines, integrins), which are expressed on the surface of the endothelium, e.g. cell adhesion molecules (ICAMs) and occur principally at the venules (Roitt et al., 2001). The initial interactions are represented by a three-step model:

1. **Tethering**: the leucocyte is slowed in the circulation by interactions between E-selectin and carbohydrate groups (CDIS), which cause it to roll along the endothelial surface (a process known as margination or pavementing). While tethered in this way, the leucocytes can receive signals from the endothelium to activate cell migration.
2. **Triggering**: the leucocyte can now receive signals from chemokines bound to the endothelial surface, or by direct signalling from endothelial surface molecules. The longer a cell rolls along the endothelium, the more time it has to receive sufficient signals to trigger cell migration. Activation of leucocytes via chemokine receptors initiates the next stage.
3. **Adhesion**: the leucocytes develop a firm adhesion to the endothelium using their surface integrins. The triggering upregulates integrins (CR3 or LFA-1) so that they can bind to cell adhesion molecules (ICAMs), induced on the endothelium by inflammatory cytokines.

## Increased vascular permeability

The liberated chemicals increase the permeability of local capillaries. The enlarged pores in the capillary allow the cells and other contents of the blood to escape in the fluid exudate. The small protein molecules in the exudate exert an osmotic effect in the tissues. Consequently, fluid-containing proteins such as clotting factors and phagocytes, leucocytes and antibodies transfer from the blood into the interstitial tissue spaces.

**Table 6.1.12**  Inflammatory mediators (Roitt et al., 2001)

| Mediator | Origin | Action |
| --- | --- | --- |
| Histamine | Mast cells and basophils | Increased vascular permeability, smooth muscle contraction, chemokinesis |
| 5-hydroxytryptamine (5HT; serotinin) | Platelets, mast cells | Increased vascular permeability, smooth muscle contraction |
| Platelet-activating factor (PAF) | Basophils, neutrophils, macrophages | Mediator release from platelets, increased vascular permeability, smooth muscle contraction, neutrophil activation |
| Neutrophil chemotactic factor (NCF) | Mast cells | Neutrophil chemotaxis |
| Interleukin-8 | Monocytes and lymphocytes | Polymorph and monocyte localization |
| C3a | Complement C3 | Mast cell degranulation, smooth muscle contraction |
| C5a | Complement C5 | Mast cell degranulation, neutrophil and macrophage chemotaxis, neutrophil activation, smooth muscle contraction, increased capillary permeability |
| Bradykinin | Kinin system (kininogen) | Vasodilation, smooth muscle contraction, increased capillary permeability, pain |
| Fibrinopeptides and fibrin breakdown products | Clotting system | Increased vascular permeability, neutrophil and macrophage chemotaxis |
| Prostaglandin $E_2$ ($PGE_2$) | Cyclo-oxygenase pathway, mast cells | Vasodilation, potentiates increased vascular permeability produced by histamine and bradykinin |
| Leukotriene $B_4$ ($LTB_4$) | Lipoxygenase pathway mast cells | Neutrophil chemotaxis, synergizes with $PGE_2$ in increasing vascular permeability |
| Leukotriene $D_4$ ($LTD_4$) | Lipoxygenase pathway | Smooth muscle contraction, increasing vascular permeability |

The table lists the major inflammatory mediators that control blood supply and vascular permeability or modulate cell movement.

## Migration of cells from the blood into damaged/infected tissues

Different sets of adhesion molecules and chemotaxic agents are used for each type of cell movement from the blood to the tissues. There is a clear distinction between the flow of leucocyte traffic, which occurs at the site of inflammation. The first to arrive are the **neutrophils** and these are the major cell type present for several days (Roitt et al., 2001). Within an hour of the inflammatory response beginning, neutrophils have collected at the injury site and are actively devouring bacteria, toxins and dead tissue cells.

**Monocytes** follow neutrophils into the area. Initially, these are fairly poor phagocytes, but within 8–12 hours of leaving the bloodstream and entering the tissues they swell and become activated **macrophages** with insatiable appetites. Macrophages are central to the final disposal of cell debris as an acute inflammation subsides. T lymphocytes usually arrive later, having been produced as part of the specific immune response.

## Movement of fluid

The net result of the local movement of fluid out of the circulation is that blood flow slows in the dilated vessels and any toxins in the tissue spaces are diluted. The movement of fluid or exudate causes the local oedema, or swelling. This swelling can lead to a loss of circulating volume and a relative rather than a true hypovolaemia (Edwards, 1998b). In addition, the

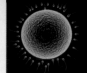

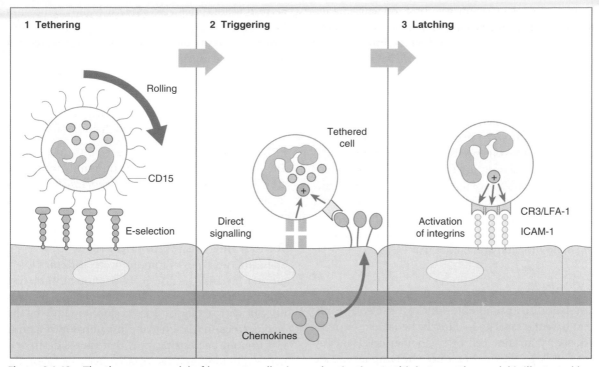

**Figure 6.1.12** The three-step model of leucocyte adhesion and activation. In this instance the model is illustrated by a neutrophil, although different adhesion molecules would be used by other leucocytes in different situations. See the text for a detailed explanation of the three stages (redrawn from Roitt et al., 2001)

swelling may in turn press on adjacent nerve endings contributing to pain.

## Pain

As described above, pain experienced as part of the inflammatory process can result from swelling due to the movement of extracellular fluid into the interstitial space and pressure on the local nerve endings as well as the effects of the release of prostaglandin and kinins. Some non-steroidal anti-inflammatory drugs, for example, aspirin, paracetamol and ibuprofen, produce their analgesic (pain-relieving) effects by inhibiting prostaglandin synthesis (Galbraith et al., 1999).

Prostaglandin has many functions, one of which is to sensitize nerve endings at the peripheral level. This action provokes primary afferent fibres involved in pain (nociceptors) and triggers an action potential in these fibres characterized by depolarization (exchange of sodium and potassium ions across the neuronal membrane), which ascends along the neuronal path to the cerebral cortex. The perception of pain is experienced when the action potential reaches the area of the brain that allows recognition of the pain sensation.

In addition, if there is an inflammatory response at the injured site, C fibres sense chemicals released by damaged tissues (e.g. bradykinins, histamine, prostaglandins). C fibres then produce peptides (substance P and neurokinins A and B; the **axon effect**), which stimulates a nociceptive signal to the brain.

Sympathetic nerves release noradrenaline (norepinephrine), acetylcholine and adenosine, adding to the effect.

## The progression of the inflammatory response

The progression of the acute inflammatory reaction depends on whether the antigen or the infectious agent is cleared. If it is not, a chronic inflammatory reaction develops. In this instance, few neutrophils are seen but there are large numbers of T cells and macrophages, which dominate at sites of prolonged or chronic inflammation. Pus may accumulate in the wound. Pus is a mixture of dead or dying neutrophils, broken-down tissue cells and living and dead pathogens.

## Termination of the inflammatory response

Once the offending insult has been removed or controlled, inhibitors dampen inflammation and tissue repair mechanisms become activated. Inhibitors of the pro-inflammatory cytokines include soluble receptors, anti-inflammatory cytokines, components of the haemostatic system (see Chapter 4.1) and glucocorticoid hormones. Glucocorticoid hormones are potent anti-inflammatory agents, inhibiting production of nearly all pro-inflammatory mediators. As the inflammatory phase is neutralized by these anti-inflammatory molecules, repair of the damage begins and involves various cells including fibroblasts and macrophages, both of which make the collagen required to mend tissues.

However, a lack of regulation of the inflammatory response can lead to an uncontrolled intravascular inflammation that ultimately harms the body. This process predisposes the victim to excessive stimulation of inflammatory pathways leading to a severe and prolonged increase in vascular permeability (Edwards, 2002). The mediators become overstimulated and toxic to other cells, damaging tissues, vessels, organs far away from the initial injury (Huddleston, 1992). As overfilling of the 'third space' becomes critical, oxygen diffusion from capillary to cell is impaired producing hypoxic damage to organs. If the pathophysiological changes cannot be reversed or slowed, organ dysfunction and failure may ensue.

## Cytokines

Cytokines are small soluble proteins, secreted by a cell, that have the capacity to alter the behaviour or properties of that same cell or of another cell (Janeway et al., 2001). Cytokines produced by lymphocytes are often called **lymphokines**. Most cytokines produced by T-cell lymphocytes are called interleukins (IL). However, the main cytokine released by CD4 T cells is interferon-γ (IFN-γ), which can block viral replication and can even help to eliminate viruses from infected cells without killing the cell. Although most cytokines have varying biological effects, they have more specific physiological roles. Some important examples of cytokines are shown in **Table 6.1.13**.

Cytokines are part of an extracellular signalling network that controls every function of the innate and specific immune response including:

- inflammation
- defence against virus infections
- proliferation of specific T- and B-cell clones and regulation of their differentiated function.

The production of these regulatory molecules is transient and tightly regulated. There are groups of cytokines with a variety of names: interleukin (ILs), interferons (INFs), colony stimulating factors, tumour

necrosis factors (TNF), growth factors and chemokines (see Table 6.1.13). Sometimes confusion with these molecules occurs due to the fact that cytokines can have multiple functions:

- Cytokines share similar functions
- They are rarely produced alone, and rarely act alone
- A complex network where production of one cytokine will influence the production of, or response to, several others.

The following relate to innate immunity, but there are clear links between the cytokines of innate immunity and the relationship to cell activation of specific immunity.

### Tumour necrosis factor (TNF)

There are two types of tumour necrosis factor (TNF): tumour necrosis factor α is a protein molecule synthesized mainly by activated macrophages, whereas tumour necrosis factor β is produced mainly by the T-helper cells. In relation to the inflammatory response, it is tumour necrosis factor α that causes death and necrosis in tumour cells. Tumour necrosis factor α is produced by activation of macrophages, lymphocytes, mast cells and basophils. In addition to its direct killing effects it also induces macrophages to produce interleukin-1β and interleukin-6. These endogenous pyrogens can induce endothelial cells in the hypothalamus to secrete prostaglandin E, which increases smooth muscle contraction (shivering) and blood vessel constriction which induces pyrexia (Roitt et al., 2001).

### Interleukin-1

There are two forms of interleukin-1: α and β. The major secreted form of interleukin-1β is produced by tissue macrophages and several other cells such as hepatocytes, endothelial cells and keratinocytes. Interleukin-1β has the same effect as tumour necrosis factor α. It induces pyrexia and shivering through actions on the hypothalamus and on smooth muscle and also induces hepatocytes to produce complement components and acute phase proteins which exacerbate the inflammatory response. Interleukin-1α

**Table 6.1.13** The cytokine groups (Roitt et al., 2001)

| Name | Abbreviation | Examples |
| --- | --- | --- |
| Interleukin (currently numbered 1–22) | IL | IL-1, IL-2, etc. |
| Interferons | IFN | IFNα, IFNβ, INFγ |
| Tumour necrosis factor | TNF | TNFα, TNFβ |
| Growth factors | GF | NGF, EGF |
| Colony stimulating factors | CSF | M-CSF, G-CSF, GM-CSF |
| Chemokines | – | RANTES, MCP-1, MIP-1α |

increases B-cell proliferation and is a cosignal for T-cell activation during the immune response. Activation of the macrophages is the major source of interleukin-1 in inflammation.

## Interleukin-6

This cytokine is produced during the inflammatory response and tends to arise later in the inflammatory response than tumour necrosis factor α or interleukin-1β, both of which are produced by macrophages. Interleukin-6 is the major cytokine responsible for terminal differentiation of B lymphocyte cells into plasma cells that secrete immunoglobulin at high rates. During inflammation, interleukin-6 is also produced by hepatocytes and Kupffer cells, and thus is especially important for the induction of acute-phase proteins and complement components in the liver.

All of these pyrogens create the inflammatory response by increasing the set point of the hypothalamic thermoregulatory centre.

## High temperature or fever

Inflammation represents a localized response to invading microorganisms. A high temperature or fever is a systemic response to invading microorganisms. As previously discussed, body temperature is regulated by a cluster of neurones in the hypothalamus, commonly referred to as the body's thermostat. However, in the event of invading pathogens, the thermostat is reset upward in response to chemicals called **pyrogens**, which, as described above, are secreted by leucocytes and macrophages after exposure to bacteria and other foreign substances in the body.

It is the cytokines interleukin-1, tumour necrosis factor α and interleukin-6 that directly effect the hypothalamus to regulate body temperature (Roitt et al., 2001). Interleukin-1 and interleukin-6 act as circulating mediators of the acute-phase pyrexial response. Distant effects of macrophage-derived cytokine include effects on thermoregulatory centres in the central nervous system, on muscle and fat stores, and on the neuroendocrine system.

## The relationship between innate and specific immunity

It is believed that specific immunity is not possible without the assistance of the mechanisms of innate immunity. This is proposed to occur in a number of ways.

Macrophages and dendritic cells are phagocytes and are also responsible for 'presenting' antigens to T cells to initiate both cell-mediated and antibody-mediated adaptive immune responses. In addition, the cytokines released by activated macrophages are part of a signalling network that controls every function of the innate and specific immune response including: inflammation, defence against viral infection, proliferation of specific T- and B-cell clones and regulation of their differentiated function. Although some links between innate and acquired immune responses are now well established, there are others that are still only understood in part and these are the subject of ongoing research (Roitt et al., 2001).

### CLINICAL APPLICATIONS

### SUPPRESSION OF THE INNATE IMMUNE RESPONSE

The innate immune response can be suppressed, and certain factors are known to reduce the innate immune response. Reduction in immune response might be due to an individuals' general condition and/or his or her inability to take nutrition for some reason, for example, fasting practices in hospital. It might also be due to prescribed treatments or drug therapies. It is therefore important to be vigilant in relation to infection control practices as patients' immune systems can be severely reduced, putting them at risk of obtaining a hospital-acquired infection.

Some practices that occur in the community and in hospital can serve to reduce the innate immune defences and put patients at risk of developing hospital-acquired infection **(Table 6.1.14)**.

**Table 6.1.14** Hospital practices that may reduce the innate immune response

| Hospital practices | Effect on the immune system |
|---|---|
| Steroid therapy | Reduces the immune response |
| Antacids (e.g. gaviscon) and H$_2$-receptor drugs (ranitidine) | These can reduce the acid environment within the stomach that normally kills bacteria and viruses that attempt to enter the body by this route |
| Insertion of intravenous lines | An intact epidermis is a first line of defence against microorganisms and, as such, prevents entry of bacteria through this route |
| Prescription of some broad-spectrum antibiotics | These can reduce the normal flora in the vagina, saliva (candida or thrush) and in the gut (diarrhoea) |

## Non-steroidal anti-inflammatory drugs (NSAIDs)

Non-steroidal anti-inflammatory drugs (NSAIDs) are prescribed to relieve pain and to reduce inflammation. Examples include aspirin, paracetamol and ibuprofen. They work by reducing the release of prostaglandin during the inflammatory response. Prostaglandins have a number of roles in the body. They:

- stimulate the inflammatory response, which leads to swelling and pressure on localized nerve endings resulting in pain
- stimulate the clotting cascade, so any interference with its release might induce bleeding from the nose vagina and from wounds
- control renal blood flow; if prostaglandin is reduced then glomerular filtration rate (GFR) will be reduced, leading to sodium and water retention
- send messages to the brain so that pain is felt.

This provides the basis for the information required by patients about the side-effects, restrictions and considerations associated with taking NSAIDs. NSAIDS are acid; they increase the acidity of the stomach and can lead to the formation of ulcers. Thus strict adherence to administering these drugs after meal times is essential (Galbraith et al., 1999). In addition, it is essential that patients taking NSAIDS should not take more than one type at a time, as for example, protein-bound anticoagulants such as aspirin displace other drugs from protein sites, causing more free anticoagulants. It should also be noted that these drugs reduce the inflammatory response and so healing mechanism may also be delayed.

## Broad-spectrum antibiotics

These antibiotics not only destroy the invading bacteria but also devastate the normal flora present in the mucous membranes. Broad-spectrum antibiotics destroy resident flora living in the mouth and vagina, allowing organisms (commonly the fungus *Candida albicans*, which causes thrush and is usually held in check by lactobacilli in normal flora) to colonize, leading to fungal infections.

## Antacids

Antacids neutralize the acidity of the gastric juice and can give rise to an increase in production of bacteria living in the stomach, small and large intestine, which can lead to diarrhoea.

## The administration of chemotherapy and radiotherapy

Both chemotherapy and radiotherapy can destroy the actively dividing cells in bone marrow that produce neutrophils, monocytes and lymphocytes. The administration of chemotherapy and radiotherapy can lead to patients becoming neutropenic, which leads to an increased risk of septicaemia (Green & Youll, 2001). Holmes (1997) showed that in patients receiving chemotherapy who were neutropenic, the patients' own natural flora of microorganisms caused 85% of infections. Lymphocytes are particularly susceptible to irradiation, with resultant suppression of the immune response.

## Steroids

Steroid hormones are synthesized by the adrenal cortex and hydrocortisone (cortisol) is the naturally occuring hormone. Corticosteroids are anti-inflammatory and suppress the immune response. The suppression of the immune processes can result in an increased susceptibility to infection and impaired wound healing (Galbraith et al., 1999).

## Reduced nutritional intake

Nutritional (e.g. glucose, fats, protein, vitamins and minerals) intake is required to produce the cells and molecules of innate immunity. During and following exposure to a bacterium, the cells and molecules of innate immunity may become depleted and, if nutrients are not available, new molecules and cells cannot be produced, reducing the body's innate defences protection against infection. In addition, with fasting practices often observed on the wards, the inflammatory process cannot be switched off due to reduction in anti-inflammatory molecules. Such events may lead to serious complications.

The nutritional requirements for wound healing include an adequate protein intake. Proteins supply the amino acids necessary for repair and regeneration of tissues, and produce many of the proteins involved in the innate immune response. Fibrous tissue is protein based and hence scar tissue will have poorer tensile strength in those who are protein depleted. Vitamin A is necessary for re-epithelialization and vitamin C is required for collagen synthesis and capillary integrity. Zinc deficiency is thought to be associated with delayed wound healing. Zinc supplements have been shown to promote venous ulcer healing in those who were zinc depleted.

Nutrition affects the body's ability to fight infection and a patient admitted to hospital may have suppressed nutrition before admission, or

### Table 6.1.15 Nutritional factors that affect the innate immune response

| Nutritional element | Effect on the immune system |
|---|---|
| Undernourishment | Causes changes in phagocytes and in the levels of circulating complement |
| Vitamin E | Assists to stimulate immunoglobulin production enhancing humoral and cell-mediated immunity |
| Copper | Is important in maintaining lymphocyte functioning |
| Zinc | Is implicated in the prevention of wound infections, as it plays a role in the immune response as it is required in DNA/RNA synthesis |

obtain poor nutritional support while in hospital (Edwards, 2000). In addition, certain hospital practices can exacerbate bad nutrition and hence the patient's immune response:

- preoperative patients only need to be fasted between 4 and 6 hours
- postoperative feeding should be initiated immediately; leaving fasting until the return of bowel sounds is traditional, ritualistic and unnecessary
- the prescription of 5% dextrose solution to maintain nutrition promotes malnutrition: 1 L of 5% dextrose solution contains only 170 kcal.

The innate immune system requires nutrients to construct its major proteins. Patients who are not taking sufficient nutrients may be at risk of reducing their immune response and acquiring an infection (Table 6.1.15).

## DEVELOPMENTAL ISSUES

### CHANGES ASSOCIATED WITH AGEING

Many body processes deteriorate with increasing age. The innate immune response is no exception to this and so elderly people are at greater risk from developing complications as a result of this deterioration.

### SKIN CHANGES

Hair greys as air enters the cortex of the shaft. The sebaceous glands produce less sebum so both the hair and skin become drier. With the loss of sebum goes the loss of the protection from infection which its acidity confers. Pigmentation of the skin alters and blotchy pigmented (liver) spots may appear on the backs of the hands, due to an alteration in the size of the melanocytes.

### INCREASED RISK OF INFECTION

Fibroblast activity decreases with age, with consequent poor collagen formation and slowing of healing. The elderly are especially vulnerable to infection as they have a reduced innate immune response. Elderly people in the community or in hospital may not have eaten well due to frailty and ill-health. If admitted to hospital, these patients are at particular risk of infection and well-planned care is essential in such circumstances if hospital-acquired infection is to be prevented. A number of assessment tools are available.

### REDUCED HEALING PROCESSES

Collagen fibres in the skin decrease in number become cross-linked and stiff and, as one of their functions is to bind water, the skin becomes progressively wrinkled, loses its elasticity and acquires a 'plumped out' appearance. Alongside this, elastin fibres rupture and lose their elasticity and there is a loss of subcutaneous fat. The skin becomes thinner in areas not exposed to sunlight and less resistant to trauma. Bruising may result from quite minor injuries. Mitosis occurring in the basal layer of the epidermis is slowed in old age and hence delayed wound healing results.

### REDUCED ABILITY TO MAINTAIN BODY TEMPERATURE

Temperature regulation is affected due to an impaired ability to sense changes in the ambient temperature and impaired hypothalamic mechanisms. Decreased metabolic processes, together with problems with mobility and exercise compound the problem. Sweat gland production decreases because the number of glands diminishes.

### Stress

One of the earliest responses to injury is neuroendocrine activation, which is intimately linked to the stress response. The neuroendocrine response is to protect the body from the effects of injury. It occurs in response to cytokine release and is involved in cellular immunity. These cytokines are released at the

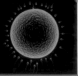

site of injury and enhance the activity of the body's own immune and non-specific responses. One of the cytokines – interleukin-1 (IL-1) – is released from activated macrophages and damaged endothelium, and may play a role in linking the immune response to the neuroendocrine system (Huddleston, 1992). Interleukin-1 stimulates the sympathetic nervous system, hypothalamus, pituitary and adrenal glands. The increased sympathetic activity affects almost all elements of the cardiovascular system and stimulates a series of events that leads to stimulation of the peripheral sympathetic nervous system and adrenal medulla resulting in the release of numerous hormonal substances into the circulation such as the catecholamines and glucocorticoid and mineralcorticoid hormones (see Chapter 2.7).

The stress response leads to a reduction in protein and other nutrients available for the production of innate immune system molecules and cells. In the longer term, it can lead to a reduction in phagocytes, interferon, complement and an overall reduction of the body's innate defence mechanisms.

### CLINICAL APPLICATIONS

#### INFECTION CONTROL

As mentioned above, people who are ill may have a reduced innate immune response. It is important to ensure that all patients are protected from infection and, to achieve this, it is crucial that health workers understand the nature of microorganisms and the principles and practice of infection control. Discussion of these topics is beyond the scope of this text and readers are strongly recommended to refer to texts such as Wilson (2001).

### Conclusion

This chapter has discussed innate body defences that, in health, are possessed by everybody and function to protect us from mechanical, chemical, physical or microbiological trauma.

Innate defence mechanisms prevent pathogenic microorganisms from entering the body. They include the maintenance of an intact skin barrier, surface membrane barriers and secretions, phagocytic and other immune cells, molecular defences and the inflammatory immune response. All these, and the raised body temperature that occurs in infection, are first lines of defence against infection and function to maintain homeostasis.

The chapter has also outlined how these innate defences can be reduced by healthcare practices that break the skin defence barrier, the effects of continued pressure on the skin and wounds caused by surgical procedures, trauma and disease, inadequate nutrition and certain prescribed treatments and drug therapies. Conditions relating to the body's inability to maintain body temperature have also been described.

Perhaps the most important message of this chapter is that nurses and other healthcare professionals need to understand that the function of the innate defence mechanisms is often reduced in clinical practice. Clear understanding of the reasons for the particular vulnerability of ill people underlines the need for proactive measures, based on sound rationale, to prevent and control the spread of infection.

### Clinical review

In addition to the Learning Objectives at the begining of this chapter, the reader should be able to:

• Discuss areas of practice relating to innate defences

• Detail how some treatments and stress can reduce the effect of innate immunity

• Outline how nurses in practice can use this knowledge to prevent the spread of infection using infection control practices

### Review questions

1   List the main innate defences of the body:
   • Surface membrane barriers/secretions
   • Cellular and chemical defence mechanisms
   • Innate molecular defence against organisms

2　What is the significance of the inflammatory immune response to innate immunity in relation to, inflammatory mediators, healing, pain, NSAID therapy, and swelling?

3　Outline the interventions often observed in practice that potentially suppresses innate immune defences.

4　Explain how age effects innate immune defences.

5　In light of this chapter, discuss the importance of infection control practices.

## References

Bruce, J. & Grove, S. (1992) Fever: Pathology and treatment. *Critical Care Nurse*, **12**(1); 40–49.

Buckman, R.F. (1992) Pathophysiology of haemorrhagic hypovolaemia and shock. *Trauma Quarterly*, **8**(4); 12–27.

Danzl, D.F. & Pozos, D.S. (1994) Accidental hypothermia. *The New England Journal of Medicine*, **331**(26); 1756–1760.

Dennison, D. (1995) Thermal regulation of patients during the perioperative period. *AORN Journal*, **61**(5); 827–832.

Donnelly, A.J. (1994) Malignant hyperthermia: Epidemiology, pathophysiology, treatment. *AORN Journal*, **59**(2); 393, 395, 398–405.

Edwards, S.L. (1997) Measuring temperature. *Professional Nurse*, **13**(2); S5–S7.

Edwards, S.L. (1998a) High temperature. *Professional Nurse*, **13**(8); 523–526.

Edwards, S.L. (1998b) Hypovolaemia: Pathophysiology and management options. *Nursing in Critical Care*, **3**(2); 73–82.

Edwards, S.L. (1999a) Hypothermia. *Professional Nurse*, **14**(4); 253–258.

Edwards, S.L. (1999b) Uses of therapeutic hypothermia. *Professional Nurse*, **14**(6); 405–409.

Edwards, S.L. (2000) Maintaining optimum nutrition. In: Manley, K. & Bellman, L. (eds) *Surgical Nursing: Advancing Practice*. Edinburgh: Churchill Livingstone.

Edwards, S.L. (2001a) Regulation of water, sodium and potassium: Implications for practice. *Nursing Standard*, **15**(22); 36–42.

Edwards, S.L. (2001b) Shock: Types, classifications and exploration of their physiological effects. *Emergency Nurse*, **9**(2); 29–38.

Edwards, S.L. (2002) Physiological insult/injury: Pathophysiology and consequences. *British Journal of Nursing*, **11**(4); 263–274.

Edwards, S.L. (2003a) The formation of oedema. Part 1: Pathophysiology, causes and types. *Professional Nurse*, **19**(1); 29–31.

Edwards, S.L. (2003b) The formation of oedema. Part 2: Cellular response to tissue damage. *Professional Nurse*, **19**(3); 155–158.

Fritsch, D.E. (1995) Hypothermia in the trauma patient. *AACN Clinical Issues*, **6**(2); 196–211.

Gailbraith, A., Bullock, S., Manias, E., Hunt, B. & Richards, A. (1999) *Fundamentals of pharmacology: A Text for Nurses and Health Professionals*. Edinburgh: Addison Wesley.

Gould, D. (1991) Skin bacteria: What is normal? *Nursing Standard*, **5**(52); 216–228.

Green, P. & Youll, J. (2001) Promoting comfort through surgery, chemotherapy and radiotherapy. In: Kinghorn, S. & Gamlin, R. (eds) *Palliative Nursing: Bringing Comfort and Hope*. Edinburgh: Ballière Tindall.

Haskell, R.M., Boruta, B., Rotondo, M.F. & Frankel, H.L. (1997) Hypothermia. *Advanced Practice in Acute Critical Care – Clinical Issues*, **8**(3); 368–382.

Holmes, S. (1997) *Cancer Chemotherapy – A Guide for Practice*, 2nd edn. Surrey, UK: Asset Books.

Holtzclaw, B.J. (1993) Monitoring body temperature. *Clinical Issues in Advanced Practice Acute and Critical Care*, **4**(1); 44–55.

Huddleston, V. (ed) (1992) *Multisystem Organ Failure: Pathophysiology and Clinical Implications*. St Louis: Mosby Year Books.

Janeway, C.A., Travers, P., Walport, M. et al. (2001) *Immunobiology*, 5th edn. New York: Garland Publishing.

Lydyard, P.M., Whelen, A. & Fanger, M.W. (2000) *Instant Notes on Immunology*. Oxford: BIOS Scientific.

McCance, K.L. & Huether, S.E. (1998) *Pathophysiology: The Biologic Basis for Disease in Adults and Children*, 2nd edn. St Louis: Mosby.

Marieb, E.N. (2001) *Human Anatomy and Physiology*, 5th edn. San Fransisco: Benjamin/Cummings Publishing Co.

Moore, K. (1983) *Before We Are Born: Basic Embryology and Birth Defects*, 2nd edn. Philadelphia: W.B. Saunders.

Morgan, S. (1990) A comparison of three methods of managing fever in the neurologic patient. *Journal of Neuroscience Nursing*, **22**(1); 19–24.

Nairn, R. & Helbert, M. (2002) *Immunology for Medical Students*. St Louis: Mosby.

Porth, C.M. (1990) *Patho-physiology: Concepts of Altered Health States*, 3rd edn. Philadelphia: J.B. Lippincott.

Roitt, I.M., Brostoff, J. & Male, D. (2001) *Immunology*, 6th edn. Edinburgh: Mosby.

Seymour, G.J., Savage, N.W. & Walsh, L.J. (1995) *Immunology: An Introduction for the Health Sciences*. Roseville, Australia: McGraw-Hill.

Walport, M.J. (2001) Complement: part 1. *New England Journal of Medicine*, **344** (14); 1058–1066.

Wilson, J. (2001) *Infection Control in Clinical Practice*, 2nd edn. London: Ballière Tindall.

# Acquired defences

*Peter S. Vickers*

## LEARNING OBJECTIVES

After studying this chapter the reader should be able to:

- Describe the nature and characteristics of the acquired (specific) defence mechanism

- Define the term 'antigen'

- Explain how an immune complex forms

- Outline the role of the major histocompatability complex (MHC) and human leucocyte antigens (HLA) within the context of the immune system

- Describe the anatomical features of the lymphatic system

- Discuss the importance of the lymphatic system in the formation, and reabsorption, of interstitial fluid

- Describe the functions of the lymph glands in relation to the immune system

- Outline the development of lymphocytes

- Compare and contrast the development and methods of function of the cell-mediated and humoral immune systems

- Describe the characteristics of a typical antibody

- Name the classes of immunoglobulins and state where each is to be found and their functions

- Explain the ways in which interaction between antigen and antibodies conveys immunological protection to the body

- Outline the ways in which interaction between cell antigens and immunologically competent T lymphocytes conveys immunological protection

- Explain how the primary and secondary responses to infection underpin the effectiveness of the immune system and the process of immunization

- Compare and contrast the features of artificially induced active and passive immunity (immunization)

- Relate the different types of hypersensitivity to their effects upon the body

- Define tumour surveillance and discuss aspects of cancer immunotherapy

- Demonstrate knowledge of primary immunodeficiencies

- Outline the nature of secondary immunodeficiencies and their increasing importance in world health

## INTRODUCTION

The human body is constantly under attack from organisms out to destroy it. This may sound dramatic but it is true. Infectious microorganisms, toxins and pollutants are some of the harmful substances from which the body has to defend itself. Fortunately, we have evolved and developed many defences to repel and destroy these harmful substances. Some of these defences, such as the skin, have already been discussed (see Chapter 6.1); the defence mechanisms associated with phagocytic blood cells, such as macrophages and monocytes, have also been discussed (see Chapters 4.1 and 6.1).

This chapter is concerned with a particular part of the defence mechanism – the **acquired immune system**. It is called the 'acquired immune system' because it does just that – through the function of the cells of this system we acquire immunity to harmful substances, rather than relying upon generic immunity present from birth (or from before birth). To acquire this immunity, the immune system first of all has to come into contact with a particular (or specific) infectious organism. Another name for the acquired immune system is the **specific immune system** because it confers specific immunity to a specific organism or harmful substance. Similarly, another name for it is the **adaptive immune system**, because it is capable of adapting to particular, or specific, threats.

This acquisition of specific immunity can be seen to good effect following immunization against an infectious disease such as polio or whooping cough. **Immunization** is not a modern procedure, the first recorded practice of it was by Edward Jenner in 1796. At that time, much of the world was plagued by smallpox, which is caused by a virus (vaccinia) with often fatal consequences. Even those who survived were often seriously disfigured by the pox scars. Jenner noticed that milkmaids were often prone to get a similar disease called cowpox (caused by a similar vaccinia virus to the one that causes smallpox) but without the serious consequences that smallpox causes to humans. These milkmaids were infected by cowpox as a result of handling the cows in their charge, particularly during milking. At the same time, Jenner observed that these same milkmaids who had been infected by cowpox did not become affected with smallpox. After much thought and deliberation he came to the conclusion that infection by cowpox somehow conferred immunity to smallpox. The next stage for Jenner, as for all good scientists and researchers, was to try and prove – or disprove – his theory. This he did by vaccinating a child with the fluid from the cowpox blisters of a milkmaid and then later infecting him with fluid from the blisters of someone with smallpox. Jenner found that this child did not go on to develop smallpox and concluded that his theory was correct, and that it was possible to confer immunity upon someone by stimulating their defences with a similar, but less serious, microorganism. So began the history of immunization, a topic that will be discussed in more detail later in this chapter. Another name for immunization is **vaccination**, which comes from the Latin word for cow – *vacca* – and was so called because the first immunization/vaccination antigens were from cowpox. The name of the virus – vaccinia – also comes from the same Latin word. (It is interesting to note that today Jenner's experimental procedure would not have received ethical approval because it is now considered totally unacceptable to put someone at risk for the sake of research.)

This first successful attempt at immunization to a disease is an excellent example of acquired immunity. Initially, the child had no defence against the smallpox virus but, after coming into contact with the less virulent cowpox virus (a near-relative of smallpox), he developed, or acquired, immunity to smallpox.

Immunology – the study of the immune system – is still a relatively new branch of bioscience and medicine. Although some of the mechanisms and components of immunity, such as antibodies and blood cells, have been known for some time, it is only recently that so much research has been undertaken into the immune system. Without a doubt, the onset of HIV and AIDS in the 1980s was the trigger for much of this research and it is now accepted that the immune system is a complicated and wonderful system that underpins much of our current understanding of disease and disease processes generally, not just those diseases caused by infectious microorganisms.

This chapter will describe the body's acquired immune defences and explain how they all work together with the innate immune defences (Chapters 4.1 and 6.1) to give the body a good chance of surviving the continuous and continuing assaults to which it is subjected by microorganisms, toxins and other pollutants.

## The nature of acquired immunity

Higher vertebrates have evolved immune systems that are able to find ways of attacking and destroying specific harmful organisms, toxins and other substances. This distinguishes them from the lower orders of animal and insect life that possess only innate immunity. In addition, the immune systems of higher vertebrates possess another property that distinguishes acquired immunity from innate immunity, namely **immunological memory**, through which the immune system remembers how to fight specific harmful substances and which, upon subsequent infections by the same organism, can direct the appropriate components of the immune system to destroy them rapidly.

What are the components of the immune defences and how do they work? Many of these components and their modes of action, for example skin, leucocytes, phagocytes, certain chemicals such as lysozyme in tears and hydrochloric acid in the stomach, as well as the inflammatory process, are discussed in Chapter 6.1. The current chapter will concentrate on those components and processes that form the acquired immune system, and the way in which both the acquired and innate immune systems combine to provide such a high level of immunity for the body.

The major components of the acquired system are another type of white blood cell – the **lymphocytes**. In adults, the lymphocytes originate in the bone marrow and, as well as destroying invading organisms, they also control the very complicated network and processes of an immune response. Some of the lymphocytes, the **B-cell lymphocytes** are responsible for the production of **immunoglobulins** – also known as **antibodies**. These immunoglobulins have the ability to bind onto **antigens**, a name derived from the term '**antibody-generator**'. These antigens can be invading microorganisms such as bacteria, viruses, protozoa and fungi, as well as other non-self matter (i.e. matter that does not originate from within a particular host body), such as molecules of toxins and pollutants. All these antigens contain within them, or on their surfaces, small, specific and unique clusters of molecules (usually polypeptides, glycoproteins or glycolipids) that occur in particular molecular conformations or shapes. These specific and unique molecular conformations, also known as antigenic determinants or **epitopes**, do not normally occur on the cells and macromolecules of the host's own body. This is a very important point when considering the ability of the host to mount an immune response. Each antigen may have several different or identical epitopes, but together they possess a shape/conformation that is unique to that antigen. For example, the intestinal bacterium *Escherichia coli* will possess epitopes that are unique to that type of bacterium; they will be different to the epitopes present on, for example, another intestinal bacterium called *Salmonella typhi,* although some contain similar, or shared epitopes.

**Immunoglobulins** (or antibodies) also possess specific receptors that can bind onto the corresponding antigenic epitope, very much like two pieces of a jigsaw coming together. Immunoglobulins possess the ability to 'mix and match' their receptors so that there are specific antibodies that can bind to specific antigens (Roitt, 2001). However, immunoglobulins on their own are unable to destroy antigens. For that, the body needs other components of the immune system, such as the phagocyte. Immunoglobulins, however, do have an important role to play because they are able to hold the antigen in place to prevent it escaping so that the phagocytes are able to destroy it. Just like antigens, all the cells of the body possess unique molecular receptors on their surface. This is important because, as well as the immunoglobulins having receptors on one end that can bind to the antigenic receptors, on the other end they have receptors that can bind to specific cells of the host – in this instance to the phagocyte. By binding to the phagocyte and to the antigen at the same time, the immunoglobulin is able to capture the antigen and attach it to the phagocyte until it is phagocytosed. This is not the only role for immunoglobulins (the other roles will be discussed later in this chapter). Immunoglobulins are composed of protein and are found in the gammaglobulin fraction of blood plasma protein. Some immunoglobulins circulate within the blood and are known as humoral antibodies – forming part of the **humoral immune system** – whereas some of them are found on the cells of the immune system and form part of the **cell-mediated immune system.**

## Antigen–antibody complexes (immune complexes) (Fig. 6.2.1)

When antigens and antibodies interact, they form an **immune complex**; also known as an **antigen–antibody complex**. Immune complexes occur with the binding of antibody to soluble antigen. As antibodies possess two or more binding sites for antigen, they can link to two or more antigens. If several antibodies bind to several antigens, there may be cross-linking, in which two or more antibodies bind to the same antigen as well as binding to other antigens. When this occurs, these immune complexes are normally easily cleared by the **mononuclear phagocytic system** (previously known as the reticuloendothelial system) but if they remain in the circulation, they can cause type III hypersensitivity. Large immune complexes are found wherever there is sufficient antibody to cross-link the antigen. These large complexes are able to trigger the complement system (see Chapter 6.1) and it is easier for them to be recognized by other components of the immune system. When the opposite occurs and antigen is in excess of antibodies then small, soluble immune complexes form. These are capable of being deposited in small blood vessels and damaging them.

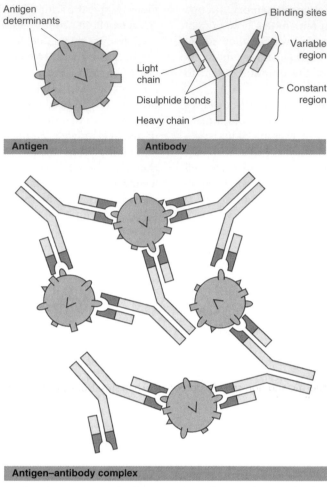

**Figure 6.2.1** The formation of an immune complex between an antigen and an antibody

Antigens that cause an immune response are known as **immunogens (immune-response generators)** but not all antigens are immunogens. Some of them are small (i.e. of low molecular weight) and non-immunogenic. These are called **haptens**. To stimulate an immune response in the host, they must combine with larger immunogenic molecules, usually proteins, known as carriers to form a complex. The complex is recognized by the immune system as 'non-self' and an immune response is mounted. These complexes are more easily phagocytosed than are single antigens. In addition, these immune complexes can trigger the complement cascade, which is part of the innate immune system. There is a downside to immune complexes, unfortunately. They can trigger autoimmune disorders such as systemic lupus erythromatosis (SLE), as well as causing hypersensitivity reactions (Janeway et al., 2001). Normally, the immune complexes are cleared by phagocytes and they cause little damage to the host's tissues. However, sometimes this clearance can fail, leading to hypersensitivity and systemic lupus erythematosus, amongst other disorders. The effects are also seen

in chronic infections, such as bacterial endocarditis. In this case, for some reason the immune response is incapable of fully clearing the infection. There is thus a persistent release of bacterial antigen as well as a high antibacterial antibody response. This leads to widespread immune complex injury to the small blood vessels in various organs, including the kidneys (Janeway et al., 2001).

The work of immunoglobulins and other immune components will be discussed in more detail later in the chapter, but for now it is important to accept that the innate and acquired immune systems need to work in a synchronized and highly organized way to provide adequate levels of protection against all invading non-self matter such as microorganisms (Fig. 6.2.2).

## Major histocompatability complex

To understand the functions of the acquired immune system, it is necessary, first of all, to make a slight detour and look at the role of the major histocompatability complex (MHC).

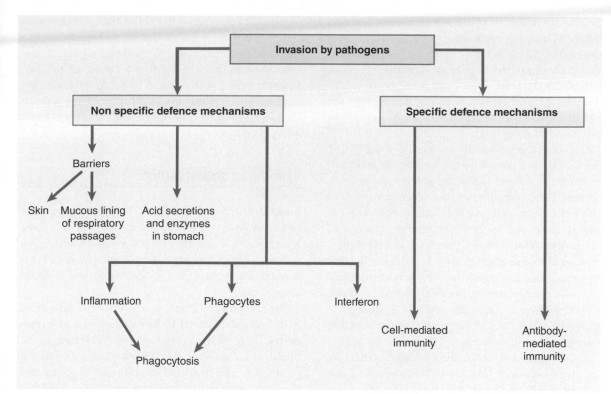

**Figure 6.2.2** Summary of specific and non-specific defence mechanisms. Non-specific mechanisms prevent entry of many pathogens and act rapidly to destroy those that manage to cross the barriers. Specific defence mechanisms take longer to mobilize but are highly effective in destroying invading microorganisms

The major histocompatibility complex is a cluster of genes on the short arm of chromosome 6. These genes code for the molecules that form antigenic receptors on the surface of the white blood cells in the body (Klein & Sato, 2000). The major histocompatibility complex is found in all higher vertebrates and in humans the genes in this region are designated as those coding for human leucocyte antigens (HLA). So it is also known as the human leucocyte antigen region.

Within this region, there are three classes of major histocompatibility complex molecules, known as MHC I, MHC II, and MHC III. All have important roles to play in the functioning of the immune system. MHC class I molecules consist of three types, known as HLA-A, HLA-B and HLA-C. MHC class I molecules present antigen derived from proteins in virus-infected cells. Once a cell is infected with a virus, the virus breaks up into its component parts of protein capsule and DNA strand. During viral replication, viral proteins are synthesized within the infected cell. Many viruses replicate, using the cell's protein-synthesizing machinery in the cytoplasm; others, the retroviruses, enter the cell's nucleus forcing it to code for hundreds of copies of viral capsule proteins and viral DNA. Peptide fragments of these viral proteins that have been made by the cell's DNA, bind to MHC class I molecules, which then find their way to the surface of the cell. In this way, the cell's own recognition surface receptors become altered because of their proximity to these combined viral peptides and MHC class I molecules, which are also now on the cell surface. Because of the altered state of the surface receptors on the cell, the immune system recognizes the infected cells as non-self and so they are destroyed, along with the viruses inside them (Janeway et al., 2001). A type of white cell, designated cytotoxic T (TC), destroys infected and malignant cells. They recognize and destroy these abnormal cells in one of two ways. The first depends upon the fact that all nucleated cells in the body normally express MHC class I molecules on their surface but that sometimes they lose their ability to express these molecules correctly. This may be as a result of damage by an infecting organism, such as the herpes virus, as in the above description, or it may be as a result of malignancy. If there are no pure MHC class I molecules on the cell surface, there is no signal given out to prevent the cell from being destroyed by the cytoxic T cells. This destruction of a cell is effected by the natural killer (NK) cell inserting a perforin molecule into the abnormal cell membrane and then injecting it with cytotoxic enzymes. The second way developed by the immune system to destroy abnormal cells, such as virally infected cells, is by the direct binding of the cytotoxic T cell to the target cell. This triggers a cascade of intracellular biochemical changes in the target

689

cell, which eventually activates a proteolytic enzyme known as caspase. Following several further biochemical reactions, the target cell is induced to commit suicide, a process known as apoptosis (Nairn & Helbert, 2002). MHC class I genes are expressed by all nucleated somatic (i.e. body) cells, although the level of expression of these genes varies depending upon the actual tissue type.

MHC class II genes are more specialized than MHC class I genes and are only expressed by some cells of the immune system, including B-cell lymphocytes, activated T-cell lymphocytes, macrophages and dendritic cells. Other cells are also able to express MHC class II molecules if they are in the presence of gamma-interferon (IFN-γ). Interferon is a **cytokine** – a chemical messenger, released by white cells, that can activate macrophages. The function of both these classes of major histocompatibility complex molecules is to present pathogen-derived peptides to T-cell lymphocytes. This in turn initiates the adaptive, or acquired immune response (Klein & Sato, 2000).

As is the case with MHC class I molecules, there are three major types of MHC class II molecules. These are known as HLA-DP, HLA-DQ and HLA-DR. These molecules present antigenic molecules, i.e. peptides, to the T-cell receptor on the surface of helper T-cell lymphocytes. The MHC class II molecules bind to these antigenic peptides within the cell and transport them to the cell surface where they can trigger the initiation of the immune response. However, they operate on different infecting organisms to those presented by the MHC class I molecules. There are several types of pathogenic organisms, such as Leishmania and the mycobacteria (which cause tuberculosis) that replicate inside intracellular vesicles in macrophages. Within the vesicles, these pathogens are broken down into peptide fragments by acidic enzymes. The peptide fragments in turn bind with MHC class II molecules and are transported to the cell surface (Janeway et al., 2001). Again, the cell is destroyed because the cytotoxic cells do not recognize the affected cell as 'self'. In the meantime, the full might of the immune system has been initiated.

Thus it can be seen that these first two classes of major histocompatibility complex molecules both present the peptide fragments of infecting organisms to initiate the immune response and/or to destroy infected or damaged cells.

The third type of major histocompatibility complex molecules, class III, consist of genes that encode for some complement factors, and also for cytokines (chemical messengers secreted by blood cells) such as tumour necrosis factor-α (TNF-α), all of which have important functions in immunity (Janeway et al., 2001). The role of cytokines and complement are explored more fully in Chapter 6.1.

An understanding of the major histocompatibility complex system is important in understanding the immune system because the acquired immune system relies so heavily upon the ability of its constituents being able to bind to either receptors on antigens such as microorganisms, or being able to bind to affected receptor molecules on the surface of infected cells.

## The lymphatic system

It has already been stated that the acquired immune system is based mainly upon one class of cell – the lymphocytes – and that only the higher vertebrates possess an acquired immune system. The reason for this is that only the higher vertebrates possess a lymphatic system.

The lymphatic system is a specialized system of lymph vessels (similar to blood vessels) and lymph nodes. It can be thought of as a parallel system to the blood circulatory system but it does not have a pump, like the heart, which pumps blood around the body. Instead the lymph is agitated around the body by a combination of the smooth muscular walls of the lymph vessels and the flexing and relaxing of the diaphragm during breathing and other striated muscles as the individual moves around (**Fig. 6.2.3**).

The peripheral lymphatic system is made up of lymphatic vessels and lymphatic capillaries, as well as encapsulated organs (i.e. organs situated within their own 'capsule'). These include the secondary lymphoid tissues of the spleen, tonsils and lymph nodes. In addition, the lymphatic system also includes unencapsulated, diffuse lymphoid tissue in the gastrointestinal tract, the urogenital tract and the lungs.

The lymph vessels and capillaries form a network throughout the body that is at least as extensive as the vascular system and that connects the tissues of the body to the lymphoid organs, such as the spleen, and the lymph nodes. The lymphatic vessels contain a fluid known as lymph, which drains into the lymphoid organs from nearby body organs. To be more specific, the lymph originates from plasma leaking from the blood capillaries. The lymphatic capillaries, which lie within the interstitial spaces, start as blind-ended vessels. Lymphatic capillaries have some anatomical similarities with blood capillaries in that their walls consist of a layer of endothelial cells. However, lymphatic capillary walls do not have a basement membrane. This lack of a basement membrane allows substances of relatively large molecular weight, such as plasma proteins, to enter the lymphatic capillaries between the endothelial cells of the capillary walls. Fluid and solutes enter the lymph system along the whole length of the capillaries.

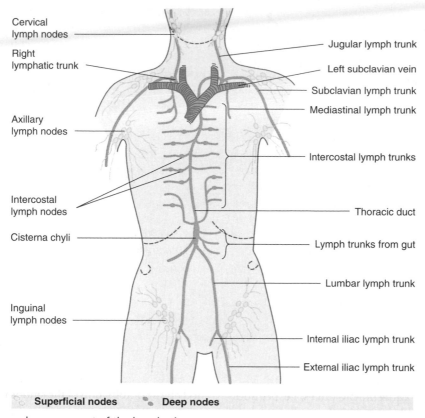

Cervical lymph nodes

Right lymphatic trunk

Axillary lymph nodes

Intercostal lymph nodes

Cisterna chyli

Inguinal lymph nodes

Jugular lymph trunk

Left subclavian vein

Subclavian lymph trunk

Mediastinal lymph trunk

Intercostal lymph trunks

Thoracic duct

Lymph trunks from gut

Lumbar lymph trunk

Internal iliac lymph trunk

External iliac lymph trunk

Superficial nodes      Deep nodes

**Figure 6.2.3**   General arrangement of the lymphatic system

Mayerson (1963) discussed how some hormones of large molecular weight travel to the blood by way of the lymphatic system, and suggests that this system of fluid seepage actually evolved to relieve the high intravascular pressure that is necessary in the body to allow the whole vascular system to be adequately perfused with blood. Hydrostatic pressure at the arterial end of capillaries forces water and solutes with a molecular weight of less than 68 000 moles into the interstitial spaces. In this process, the water and solutes are transported across the membranes of the lymphatic vessels and capillaries and then returned to the blood circulatory system. Most of this plasma is returned to the blood capillaries at the venous end, where there is less hydrostatic pressure (see Chapter 4.2), but some plasma remains in the lymphatic system to be carried around the body. Within a 24-hour period, about half of all plasma proteins enter the interstitial fluid and if these plasma proteins were not constantly being routed via the lymphatic system, the interstitial fluid would increase. This, in turn, could result in oedema – the accumulation of fluid in tissues. This effect can sometimes be seen in patients with breast cancer in which there is involvement of the axillary lymph nodes. The patient may develop gross oedema of the arm in which the lymph nodes are situated, as a result of the failure of the lymphatic drainage process, due to blockage by the enlarged lymph nodes.

The rate of lymph formation and its flow depends upon the rate at which interstitial fluid is accumulated. This is normally 2–4 litres over 2 hours and ensures a constant turnover of the interstitial fluid. This turnover is important in the effective migration of immune cells and the filtering of harmful toxins and infecting organisms from the blood.

The lymphatic capillaries in this network join together (like tributaries of a river) to form larger lymphatic vessels – just as in the blood circulatory system. These larger lymphatic vessels contain smooth muscle in their walls and also have one-way valves to prevent backflow of the lymph. Lymph flows through the vessels by means of skeletal muscle contraction in the limbs, pulsation of adjacent arteries and negative intrathoracic pressure. In addition, lymphatic vessels themselves contract rhythmically, with their rate of contraction being proportional to the volume of lymph in the vessels.

Throughout the lymphatic system are situated lymph glands, like railway stations on a railway network. Afferent lymphatic vessels (i.e. those entering the gland) feed the lymph into the lymph glands and efferent lymphatic vessels (i.e. those leaving the gland) drain the lymph from the lymph glands.

All the lymph eventually arrives at two large lymph ducts. One of them is called the **thoracic duct** and this receives lymph from the lower limbs, the digestive

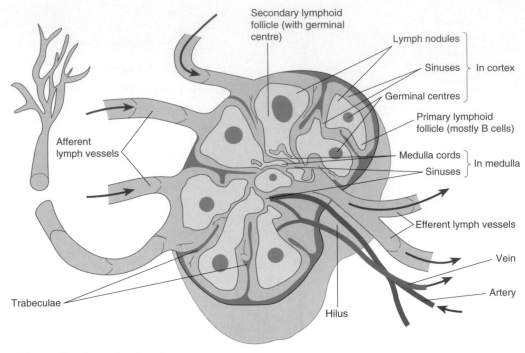

**Figure 6.2.4**   Section through a lymph node

tract, the left arm and the left side of the thorax, head and neck. The other large lymph vessel, called the **right lymphatic duct**, receives lymph from the right arm and the right side of the head, neck and thorax. The two lymph ducts then empty into the great veins in the neck, thus restoring the fluid and proteins to the venous circulation.

## Lymphoid tissue

As well as lymphatic vessels, the lymphatic system contains lymphoid tissue. This consists of lymph glands, called lymph nodes, which are approximately the size and shape of a broad bean, and lymphoid tissue, found in specific organs, particularly the spleen, bone marrow, lung and liver.

Lymph enters the lymph glands via the afferent lymphatic vessels, from where it makes its way via the marginal sinuses to the trabeculae, which extend into the central part of the gland. The gland itself is made up of a meshwork of reticular cells. The lymph, which at this stage contains antigens from infected cells and tissues as well as antigen-bearing dendritic cells, passes through this meshwork and the antigenic substances are trapped. Note that antigens entering the body at any point are swept rapidly towards a lymphoid organ or lymph node. Within the lymph node, B-cell lymphocytes are located in the primary lymphoid follicles as well as the secondary lymphoid follicles containing the germinal centres. Within the germinal centres, the B cells are proliferating after encountering their specific antigen and cooperating

T cell. The B cells at the centre of the secondary follicles are actively dividing, whilst those at the periphery are antibody forming (**Fig. 6.2.4**).

T-cell lymphocytes are to be found in the paracortical area of the gland. In addition, large numbers of phagocytic macrophages are found, along with antibody-secreting plasma cells, in the medulla of the gland. Macrophages and other antigen-presenting cells spend most of their lives migrating through the tissues until they encounter antigens. These are then phagocytosed and transported to the nearest lymph node. Macrophages in the gland also encounter trapped foreign antigen-bearing cells within the meshwork of reticular cells and, having ingested these, they partially break them down (phagocytosis), thus expressing antigen sites to the T-cell lymphocytes. This carrying of partially ingested antigens to the lymph glands, as well as the partial ingestion within the lymph nodes, ensures presentation of antigen receptor to the lymphocytes for recognition and initiation of the immune process.

The 'cleansed' lymph then leaves the lymph gland via the efferent lymphatic vessel, which is situated at the hilum of the gland. Lymphocytes migrate from the blood circulatory system within the gland. They migrate through the walls of the smallest venous capillaries in the lymph node. Lymphocytes spend only a few minutes in the blood during each circuit, compared to several hours spent in the lymphoid system. Once they are antigen-primed in the lymph nodes, lymphocytes are also found migrating through the body tissues. They circulate through the body until they encounter the antigen for which they are expressing the appropriate receptor, following which they are able to initiate the immune process.

## Other lymphoid organs

The spleen is an organ that is situated just behind the stomach and is about the size of a fist. It collects antigen from the blood for presentation to phagocytes and lymphocytes, and also collects, and disposes of, dead red cells. Approximately 70% of lymph passes through the spleen.

The gut-associated lymphoid tissues (GALT) include the tonsils, adenoids, appendix and Peyer's patches in the small intestine. These collect antigen from the epithelial surfaces of the gastrointestinal tract. Peyer's patches are the most highly organized of these tissues, in which the antigen is collected by specialized epithelial cells – the multifenestrated, or M, cells. In Peyer's patches, the lymphocytes form a follicle with a large central dome of B-lymphocytes, which is surrounded by smaller numbers of T-lymphocytes. This same formation of lymphocytes is found in the bronchial-associated lymphoid tissue (BALT) and other mucosa (mucosal-associated lymphoid tissue; MALT) where they protect the respiratory epithelium (Janeway et al., 2001). According to Janeway et al. (2001), the mucosal immune system is estimated to contain as many lymphocytes as the rest of the body.

The lymph nodes, spleen and mucosal-associated lymphoid tissue share the same basic architecture, and operate on the same principle, namely trapping antigen from sites of infection and presenting it to lymphocytes to stimulate the acquired immune system and, consequently, the innate immune system (Janeway et al., 2001).

Each of the lymphoid organs filters fluid from particular parts of the body. The spleen filters the bloodstream, the lymph nodes filter the lymph draining from the intercellular system and the diffuse lymphoid tissues filter lymph from the gut, lungs and urogenital organs.

The anatomy of the lymphoid system thus enables lymphocytes to protect the tissues and vessels of the body. It holds lymphocytes in antigen 'traps' in the lymph nodes and other lymphoid organs, and it brings them into close proximity with other immune cells. This is essential for the cell-to-cell communication that recruits, directs and regulates a coordinated immune response.

Lymph glands are the major centres for lymphocyte proliferation and antibody production as well as for filtering the lymph. Carbon particles introduced artificially have been shown to accumulate in the lymph glands distal to the point of introduction. Although this is a very efficient mechanism for filtering out

unwanted and dangerous antigens within the body, there is a major drawback. Malignant cells, if they invade lymphatic vessels, can be carried away in the lymph until their progress is impeded by the filtering effect of the lymph glands, where they become deposited and can give rise to a secondary tumour.

Normally, lymphatic vessels cannot be seen with the naked eye and lymph glands cannot be palpated. However, when bacteria are carried away from a focus of infection by the lymphatic vessels, this can give rise to inflammation in the lymphatic vessels themselves and subsequently in the lymph glands into which they drain. For example, when the focus of infection is superficial, such as in the hand, the inflamed lymphatic vessels may be seen as red streaks extending up the arm, and the lymph glands in the axilla may be tender, hard and enlarged.

## Lymphocytes

All blood cells are derived from precursor cells known as pluripotent haemopoietic stem cells (HSCs), which later develop into all the different types of blood cells (see Chapter 4.1 for more information on the development of blood cells). Lymphocytes are white blood cells and therefore develop from haemopoietic stem cells. Lymphocytes are actually developed from a common lymphoid progenitor.

There are two major classes of lymphocyte, T-cell lymphocytes and B-cell lymphocytes, and both classes are crucial to the development of acquired immunity. Each class is responsible for certain discrete and complimentary processes within acquired immunity, working together, along with other parts of the immune system, to ensure a very high level of protection. T-cell lymphocytes are concerned with cell-mediated immunity and B-cell lymphocytes are concerned with humoral immunity.

### Cell-mediated immunity (T-cell lymphocytes) (Fig. 6.2.5)

T-cell lymphocytes originate in the bone marrow but they do not remain there; at a certain stage they leave the bone marrow as immature lymphocytes. These immature lymphocytes find their way to the thymus. The thymus is situated in the chest in babies and is a large organ (relative to size), although it atrophies (shrinks) with age. It is architecturally highly organized, consisting of numerous lobules, an outer cortex and an inner medulla. The complete development of the thymus is attained by the twelfth week of gestation.

The cortex of the thymus contains densely packed small lymphocytes, whereas the medulla contains more dispersed lymphocytes (Stiehm et al., 2004).

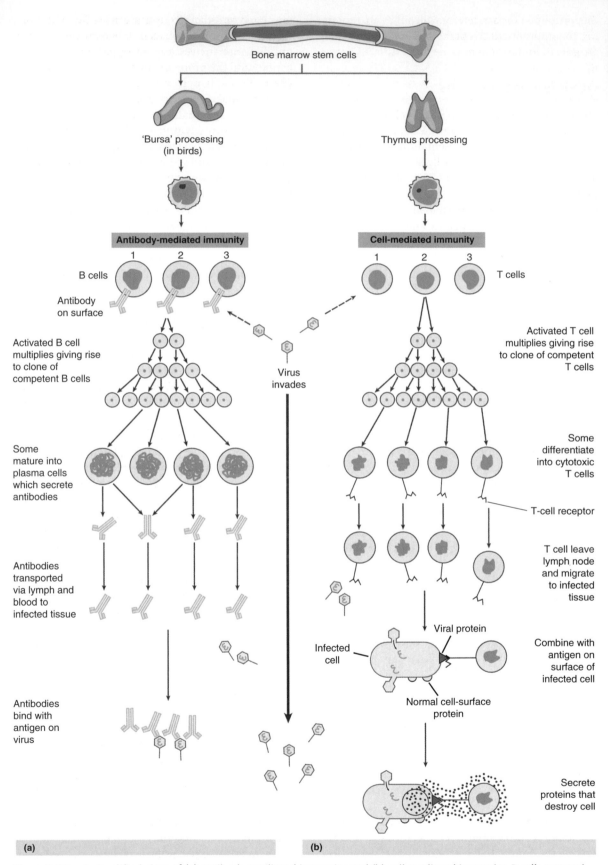

**Figure 6.2.5** A simplified view of (a) antibody-mediated immunity and (b) cell-mediated immunity. B cells respond to specific antigens on the virus and give rise to plasma cells, which produce specific antibodies. T cells respond to antigens on the surface of infected cells; they leave the lymph nodes and destroy the infected cells

The lymphocytes that develop within the thymus are the ones that we call T-lymphocytes, because they are thymus-dependent lymphocytes. Within the thymus, the stem cells mature and differentiate into their various subclasses, such as T-helper cells. In addition, they also become able to recognize and differentiate 'self' cells from 'non-self' cells. 'Self' cells are cells that originate and belong to an individual, whereas 'non-self' cells are cells that come from outside the individual. The T-cell receptor on the surface of the lymphocyte allows the T cells to distinguish 'self' from 'non-self' cells. To do this, the T-cell receptor binds with the peptide and peptide-binding part of the human leucocyte antigen molecule (Klein & Sato, 2000). Lymphocytes within the thymus are known as **thymocytes**.

It might be helpful to think of the thymus as a school for T-cell lymphocytes in which the cells take part in learning experiences as they mature, and in which they also are guided to different careers after they leave the 'school'. Even though the thymus starts to degenerate at puberty, T cells continue to develop in the thymus throughout life (Delves & Roitt, 2000).

The development of the lymphocytes within the thymus is complex and fascinating. For a start, most of them will die in there. This is because the immature lymphocytes that enter the thymus are programmed to die unless they instantly receive signals for them to start to differentiate (Klein & Sato, 2000). Most T-cell development occurs in the cortex of the thymus, as the lymphocytes go through the several stages of development, as well as differentiation to perform one of several tasks once they are mature. During these stages of development, the lymphocytes start to express different CD markers (cluster of differentiation). To make these different receptors, the cells have to assemble a functional gene within their DNA for each T-cell receptor, and also ensure that each T cell expresses receptors of one specific type (Janeway et al., 2001).

Thymic epithelium produces several hormones (e.g. thymosin, thymopoeitin and thymostimulin), which act on the immature lymphocytes in the thymus and stimulate them to proliferate and develop the ability to recognize the huge numbers of antigens that the host will encounter throughout life (McCance & Huether, 2002).

During maturation, the T cells produce new proteins that are inserted into the plasma membrane of the cell. These proteins are classified as CD antigens. There are at least 150 different CD antigens (McCance & Huether, 2002). For example, CD3 antigens are on T cells that interact with T-cell receptors, CD4 antigens are on T-helper cells and are adhesion molecules for class II human leucocyte antigen binding, whereas CD8 antigens are found on T-cytotoxic and T-suppressor cells and are adhesion molecules for class I HLA binding. As they enter the thymic cortex, the thymocytes have an opportunity to match these new CD receptors with HLA–peptide complexes. Most of the thymocytes do not make this connection and so do not receive a signal to justify their further existence, and therefore they die (apoptosis). Only a minority avoid apoptosis and proceed further into the thymus. In the medulla, the surviving thymocytes come into contact with lots of macrophages and dendritic cells (antigen-presenting cells) that display large numbers of HLA–peptide ligands. Consequently, these thymocytes have a second opportunity to find a match for their receptors (Klein & Sato, 2000). Only if the thymocytes make a second match are they allowed to proceed to become mature lymphocytes and leave the thymus as naïve T-cell lymphocytes (i.e. cells that have not yet come into contact with a pathogenic organism or other antigenic stimulator). Only 1% of the lymphocytes that enter the thymus actually reach this stage. Although this system may seem wasteful, it does ensure that most of the thymocytes that are self-reactive (i.e. could potentially destroy 'self' cells), and therefore might cause an autoimmune response, are destroyed before they can do any harm.

These naïve, but mature, lymphocytes, which are antigenically committed (primed) but non-self-reactive, leave the thymus through the blood and lymphatic vessels and are now ready to react with any antigen they encounter in the body with which they can bind (McCance & Huether, 2002). Once bound with an antigen, the T-cell lymphocytes are stimulated to proliferate. When this antigen binding had taken place, the T-cell lymphocyte is no longer a naïve cell but is considered fully mature.

T-cell lymphocytes have different functions to perform within the acquired immune system, and the functions that they perform are dependent upon the differentiation they underwent within the thymus. The type of CD receptor a T cell carries determines its function. The major functions performed by the T-cell lymphocytes are:

- **Cytotoxicity (cell-destruction):** this function is performed by the T-cytotoxic lymphocytes that possess many CD8 receptors. These cells mediate the direct cellular killing of target cells (McCance & Huether, 2002). These target cells may be virally infected 'self' cells, tumours or 'non-self' grafts, such as kidney transplants. The T-cytotoxic lymphocytes bind to the target cell and release toxic substances into the target cell, which are capable of destroying it. If the target cell is a virally infected 'self' cell, that cell is destroyed, as are the viruses that have

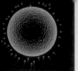

infected it. In this way the viruses are unable to go on to invade other 'self' cells.

- **Control of the immune system:** this is a task undertaken by the T-helper and T-suppressor lymphocytes. T-helper cells are coated with many CD4 receptors, and these cells stimulate the immune system, both the acquired immune system and many parts of the innate immune system, to proliferate in response to antigenic appearance in the host's body. There are two types of T-helper cell. Type 1 T-helper cells secrete two chemical messengers – interleukin-2 (IL-2) and γ interferon (IFN-γ), whereas type 2 T-helper cells secrete interleukins-4, 5, 6 and 10 (IL-4, IL-5, IL-6 and IL-10). These chemicals are known as **cytokines**, although those secreted by lymphocytes are also known as **lymphokines**. Cytokines are small soluble proteins secreted by a cell (often, but not always, a T lymphocyte) that have the capacity to alter the properties of that or another cell (Janeway et al., 2001). As their functions are relatively non-specific, they are described in Chapter 6.1. All cytokines have a pivotal role to play in influencing particular types of response by the immune system. For example, the production of γ-interferon activates the macrophages, which are able to kill intercellular organisms such as bacteria. Although these cytokines are many, and their functioning is complex, for the purposes of this part of the chapter, it is possible to simplify matters and say that the production of cytokines by T-helper 1 cells induces cell-mediated immunity, which includes macrophage and T-cell cytotoxic activity, whereas T-helper 2 cell cytokine production and T-helper 3 regulatory cells facilitate humoral (B cell) immunity and allergic reactions (Delves & Roitt, 2000; Goldsbie et al., 2003).

  The body is usually very efficient at stimulating immune activity in response to antigens but there is a need for balances and checks to prevent the overstimulation of immunological activity. This function is performed by the T-suppressor cells. Many studies have identified CD8 T-suppressor cells, but there appears to be no unique receptor marker for T-suppressor cells, and so immune suppression may actually be a task performed by a combination of T-helper and T-cytotoxic cells by means of a negative feedback mechanism (Male, 1991).

- **Memory:** a special quality of the acquired immune system is its ability to remember immunogenic receptors that have been previously detected by the immune system. By means of cloning it is then able to produce a group of lymphocytes that can stimulate the parts of the immune system that are able to

counter these antigens immediately when that antigen is detected in the future. T-memory lymphocytes are responsible for a rapid response to a second, and subsequent, antigenic challenge (McCance & Huether, 2002). This process is known as the secondary immune response. One cytokine – IL-2 – is a major T-cell growth factor and another – IL-15 – has been implicated in maintaining CD8 T-memory lymphocyte cells (Janeway et al., 2001). Memory cells are long-lived and there is always a constant number of T-memory cells for a given antigen in circulation (Janeway et al., 2001).

- **Delayed hypersensitivity:** once thought to be a discrete T-lymphocyte subset, this reaction is now thought to be due to an imbalance between T-helper type 1 and T-helper type 2 lymphocytes (in which T-helper 1 cells outnumber T-helper 2 cells) (Kay, 2001). Delayed hypersensitivity is responsible for such disorders as contact dermatitis.

There is a further type of lymphocyte, which appears to express only the earliest markers of T-cell differentiation. These are known as **null cells or natural killer (NK) cells.** The natural killer cells do not bind antigen, nor are they induced to proliferate by contact with an antigen. They bind to chemical changes on the surfaces of virally infected cells or malignant cells, rather than antigen receptors (McCance & Huether, 2001). Although they are lymphocytes, natural killer cells are usually classified within the innate immunity system and have also been described in Chapter 6.1 (**Fig. 6.2.6**).

## Humoral immunity (B-cell lymphocytes)

Like T-cell lymphocytes, B-cell lymphocytes originate in the bone marrow in the adult but, unlike the T cells, they mature also within the bone marrow. For a long time, it was not known where this class of lymphocytes matured in humans, but it was known that in birds they matured in a lymphoid organ known as the Bursa of Fabricius. It was therefore decided that humans must have an equivalent organ to the Bursa of Fabricius, and so these lymphocytes were known as bursa-dependent lymphocytes, or B-cell lymphocytes. After many years spent in a fruitless search for the human bursa-equivalent organ, it was found that the B-lymphocytes, as well as originating from within the bone marrow, also mature there. As bone marrow begins with a 'B', fortunately there was no need to change the name, so they remained as B-cell lymphocytes.

As with the T-cell lymphocytes, the B cells need to undergo a maturation process in which they have to

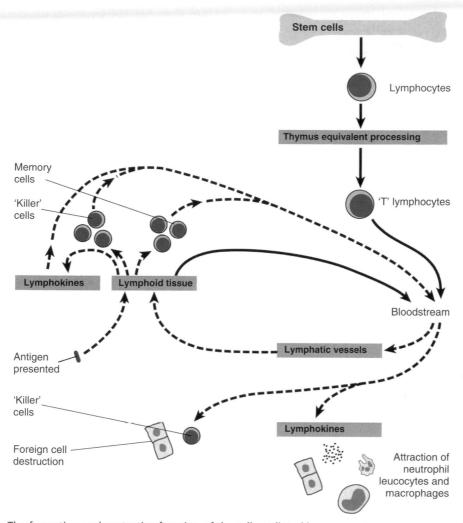

**Figure 6.2.6**   The formation and protective function of the cell-mediated immune system

survive a negative selection process. Again like the T cells, this is an attempt to ensure that the antigen receptors on their surface membrane do not display self-reactivity (Nairn & Helbert, 2002). During this process, those lymphocytes that are autoreactive to the host cells and tissues are destroyed, leaving only non-autoreactive naïve lymphocytes behind to go on to the next stage of maturation and selection. This is a very important process because any self-reactivity of the B cells, as with any T-cell self-reactivity, may result in **autoimmunity**. The actual mechanism of the B-cell negative-selection process within the bone marrow is similar to that process that is undergone by the T cells during their maturation and differentiation within the thymus. In addition, the B cells undergo a positive selection process in which those lymphocytes that are able to respond to non-self antigens are preserved, and those that are not are left to die. The B cells that have survived this negative selection find their way to the peripheral lymphoid organs where they may encounter actual non-self

antigens for which they have specificity. Again, this is important because with the great diversity of possible receptors that can be generated on the surface of the B cells, those that can recognize and respond to non-self antigens have to be cherished, especially as an individual can express only a small fraction of the total possible receptor types in a lifetime (Janeway et al., 2001). It is thought that more than 100 million different antigens may be recognized by the B-cell lymphocytes. The goal is for all those B cells that survive these two processes to be useful and fully functioning members of the immune system. B cells are able to become activated if the need should arise, for example, following infection by a microorganism that carries the specific antigenic receptor that is a match, and they then differentiate into antibody-producing plasma cells. Those B cells that do not encounter their specific antigen will die within a few weeks (Nairn & Helbert, 2002). The vast majority of B cells (95%) die within the bone marrow during these selection processes (Seymour et al., 1995).

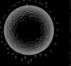
## Clonal selection theory

Once activated by an antigen, the lymphocytes give rise to clones of antigen-specific cells. These cells then mediate acquired immunity. The theory of **clonal selection** was first proposed by Macfarlane Burnet as long ago as 1950 to explain why antibodies are only produced in great numbers for those antigens to which an individual is exposed, even though the lymphocytes are capable of producing antibodies to almost any antigen (remember, it has been calculated that lymphocytes can produce antibodies to about 100 million different antigens). To cover all possibilities and permutations, although an individual carries lymphocytes with antigen receptors of only one specificity (i.e. capable of bonding to only one specific antigen), the specificity of each lymphocyte is different. In effect the many millions of lymphocytes an individual possesses at any one time can theoretically collectively carry an equivalent number of receptors of different antigen specificity (known as the lymphocyte receptor repertoire) (Janeway et al., 2002). During their lifetime, only the lymphocytes that actually come into contact with an antigen to which they can bind (i.e. those that possess the appropriate specific antigen receptor) are able to divide and proliferate – to clone themselves – many times over to produce a large number of lymphocytes with the same antigen-specific receptors, all prepared to play a part in the destruction of that particular antigen. Because these cells have divided asexually, each daughter cell will be a mirror image of the mother cell, their own daughter cells, and so on. This avoids swamping the body with lots of lymphocytes carrying antigen receptors that are not needed. The process is known as clonal expansion. Maturation and differentiation also take place at this time, and some of these lymphocytes become memory cells, able to carry the 'blueprint' of their specific antigenic receptors throughout their lifetime and as they divide the population is maintained for the future. In this way they are always ready to spring into action the next time their particular antigen makes an appearance.

## Differentiation of B cells

Mature B cells are of two types, either B-memory cells (with a similar role to play as the T-memory cells) or antibody-secreting plasma cells. The antibodies secreted by the plasma cells are also known as **immunoglobulins**, and their role is to assist other components of the immune system in the destruction of non-self antigens. The plasma cells, which carry the immunoglobulins, are much larger than naïve B cells and remain in lymphoid tissue for the duration of their short life. The immunoglobulins are soluble molecules and there are five different classes of them. They are serum glycoproteins and are produced by the plasma cells in response to the immune system coming into contact with an immunogen. Immunoglobulins can occur as soluble proteins in the circulation or they can be found on the surface of mature B cells, where they act as surface receptors (Nairn & Helbert, 2002). Each mature B cell (plasma cell) has about 100 000 surface immunoglobulin molecules in its surface membranes. Remember that an immunogen is an antigen that always produces an immune response, whereas antibodies are immunoglobulins that react specifically with the immunogen that stimulated their production (Nairn & Helbert, 2002).

## Immunoglobulin structure

All immunoglobulins (Igs) have the same basic structure, being made up of light (L) and heavy (H) molecular chains (Nairn & Helbert, 2002). The categories of light and heavy refer to molecular weight, with heavy chains having a molecular weight of between 50 000 and 70 000 daltons, and light chains having a molecular weight of approximately 25 000 daltons. A basic immunoglobulin consists of two heavy chains and two light chains, which are linked by non-covalent and disulfide bonds **(Fig. 6.2.7)**. As mentioned previously, there are five different classes of immunoglobulin, each of which has a slightly different structure. The heavy chains differentiate these five different immunoglobulin classes, and each of the classes is named after their respective heavy chain, to which are assigned lower case Greek letters (Nairn & Helbert, 2002). These are: gamma ($\gamma$), alpha ($\alpha$), mu ($\mu$), delta ($\delta$) and epsilon ($\varepsilon$), and their equivalent immunoglobulin names are IgG, IgA, IgM, IgD and IgE. There are only two classes of light chain and these are also given lower case Greek letters: kappa ($\kappa$) and lambda ($\lambda$). Both these

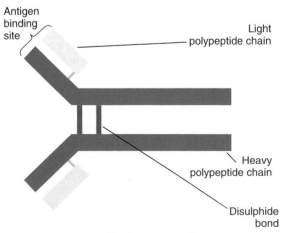

**Figure 6.2.7**  Generalized structure of an immunoglobulin molecule

classes of light chain are found in all five immunoglobulin classes but any one immunoglobulin contains only one type of light chain. In addition, both IgG and IgA can be divided into subclasses, respectively $IgG_1$, $IgG_2$, $IgG_3$, $IgG_4$, $IgA_1$ and $IgA_2$.

In **Fig. 6.2.7**, it can be seen that there are two distinct ends to an immunoglobulin, which is roughly in the shape of the letter 'Y'. The end that only contains the two heavy chains is known as the Fc region (standing for **f**ragment **c**rystallizable). This region is capable of binding to surface receptors on phagocytic cells, such as macrophages, and various other cells, as well as fixing complement, thereby initiating the complement sequential cascade (the complement system is discussed in Chapter 6.1). The other end of the immunoglobulin, containing both light and heavy chains, is known as the Fab (**f**ragment **a**ntigen-**b**inding) region. This region, as its name implies, is capable of binding to antigen. Thus it can be seen that the immunoglobulin can bind phagocytic cells to receptors on antigens, and this allows for the antigen to be held fast and prevented from escaping when it is being phagocytosed. The Fab region is also known as the variable region, because it can change its receptors so easily between different B cells. The Fc region is known as the constant region, because there are only a few different classes.

The Fab region of an immunoglobulin is fascinating because it has the ability to change its shape between different B cells so that it can potentially bind to any of the $10^8$ possible antigens previously mentioned. It achieves this through variation of the genes within the B-cell DNA. This variation occurs during embryological development, giving rise to the potential for a diverse population of B cells. The whole ordering of diversification/variability within immunoglobulins is very complicated, but for now it is enough to be aware that the genes that code for the receptors at the Fab end of the immunoglobulin are produced through random re-arrangements to produce a receptor to fit any of the potential $10^8$ different antigens. Once this re-arrangement is successful, the B cell is committed to that single specificity for the rest of its life.

## Functions of immunoglobulins

The primary function of an antibody is to bind antigen (Roitt, 2002). Within this primary function, the main functions of antibodies are to protect the host by neutralizing bacterial toxins, neutralizing viruses, opsonizing bacteria and activating components of the inflammatory response (McCance & Huether, 2002). Antibodies rarely act in isolation but rather join with other components of the immune system to effect antigen destruction. This is particularly apparent with the opsonization of bacteria. Sir Almoth Wright, in

1903, was the first to call immunoglobulins 'opsonins' (from the Greek '*opson*' meaning a dressing or a relish) because he claimed that they prepared the bacteria as 'food' for the phagocytes (Roitt, 1994). In effect, the immunoglobulins make the bacteria susceptible to phagocytosis. Opsonization is necessary because many bacteria possess an outer capsule, making them resistant to phagocytosis unless antibody is produced against them (McCance & Huether, 2002). As well as being opsonins themselves, immunoglobulins initiate the complement system, which also has a role in opsonization.

A second role of the immunoglobulin is the neutralization of bacterial toxins. These toxins are produced by the bacteria and make them more pathogenic, thus causing more harm to the host. When this happens, the immunoglobulins function as antitoxins and are able to form **toxin–antitoxin complexes** (the same as antigen–antibody complexes). This occurs by the antitoxic immunoglobulins cross-linking with the bacterial toxins. This means that the immunoglobulins occupy the binding sites of the toxins, which are then unable to bind to the cells of the host – thus they are neutralized. Once formed, these complexes are either phagocytosed or washed out of solution in body fluids (McCance & Huether, 2002).

The immunoglobulins similarly neutralize viruses by binding on to the viral surface receptors, so preventing them from in turn binding onto the host's cells. Again, the neutralized viruses may be phagocytosed or washed out. Thus the immunoglobulins can prevent the viruses from infecting cells of the body. If a virus escapes the immunoglobulins and enters a cell then the immunoglobulins have very little effect on it but, fortunately, as discussed earlier, another part of the immune system – the T cells – can take over and destroy any virus-infected cells.

The fourth role of immunoglobulins is that of activating components of the inflammatory response. The immunoglobulin acts as a 'bridge', with the Fab end binding specifically to antigen and the Fc end informing the non-specific components of the inflammatory response of the identification of an antigenic substance within the body. They do this by binding to these non-specific immune system components. Mononuclear phagocytes, neutrophils, natural killer cells, eosinophils and mast cells express receptors for the Fc end of immunoglobulins. These cells are capable of interacting with the immunoglobulins and so commence such activities as phagocytosis, tumour cell lysis and mast cell degranulation (Roitt, 2001).

## Classification of immunoglobulins

The five classes of immunoglobulin have slightly different structures and undertake different functions.

## Immunoglobulin G

This is the most important immunoglobulin involved in the secondary immune response. It is the most abundant of the immunoglobulins in serum – constituting about 75% of total serum immunoglobulin (Seymour et al., 1995). It has the smallest molecular weight (approximately 150 000 daltons) and it divides into four subclasses: namely $IgG_1$, $IgG_2$, $IgG_3$ and $IgG_4$. $IgG_1$ makes up 65% of the total IgG in the body, with $IgG_2$ comprising 23%, $IgG_3$ making up 8% and $IgG_4$ only 4%. IgG has the longest half-life of all immunoglobulins (i.e. it survives in serum for the longest time). This half-life is about 20–21 days, although $IgG_3$ only has a half-life of 7 days.

Because of its low molecular weight, IgG is found equally within the intravascular and extravascular areas of the body, thus its effects are far reaching. It plays a major role against blood-borne infective organisms as well as those invading the tissues. This low molecular weight also means that IgG can cross the placental barrier to give a high degree of temporary passive immunity to the newborn child. Maternal IgG disappears by the age of 9 months, by which time the infant is producing its own IgG. However, some infants are unable to make their own IgG and have a condition known as **hypogammaglobulinaemia**, which requires life-long, regular infusions of IgG and rapid antibiotic therapy to maintain their health, and even life. There is also a condition known as transient hypogammaglobulinaemia of infancy, in which the child does not make sufficient IgG until they are over 18 months of age. Again, these children will need supportive therapy in the form of IgG infusions and rapid antibiotic therapy, but only until they have their own functioning IgG antibodies. By the age of 12 months, most children are usually producing about 80% of the adult level of IgG.

IgG mediates the immune system in several ways. It is important for activating the complement system. $IgG_1$ and $IgG_3$ also bind to macrophages via the Fc receptor, and so enhance phagocytosis. $IgG_2$ and $IgG_4$ bind to killer cells and mediate antibody-dependent cell-mediated cytotoxicity (ADCC) against cells already coated with antibody. IgG also binds to platelets, which aids the inflammatory response by leading to platelet aggregation. $IgG_2$ is important in the immune responses against encapsulated bacteria (Nairn & Helbert, 2002; Roitt, 2001; Seymour et al., 1995).

## Immunoglobulin M

IgM is the predominant antibody involved in the primary immune response, as well as being involved in the early stages of the secondary immune response. IgM is the largest immunoglobulin in terms of molecular weight and is, in actual fact, a pentamer. This means that each IgM is composed of five immunoglobulin units of two heavy chains and two light chains. These five units are held together by a J (joining) chain. IgM weighs approximately 970 000 daltons. Because it is a pentamer, it has ten potential antigen-binding sites, as opposed to the two sites that most of the other immunoglobulins possess and, as a result of this feature, it is the most efficient antibody at agglutinating (combining) bacteria and also activating the classical pathway of the complement system – which occurs once it has bound to its target antigen.

Due to its size, IgM is restricted almost entirely to the intravascular spaces and it is often involved with the immune response to complex, blood-borne infectious organisms. IgM is also found on B-cell surfaces, and it is the major antigen-binding molecule by which B cells identify antigen (Nairn & Helbert, 2002; Roitt, 2001; Seymour et al., 1995). IgM has a half-life of only 7 days, approximately one-third of that of IgG. By the age of 12 months, an infant has 75% of its IgM levels.

## Immunoglobulin A

There are two types of IgA, serum and secretory. IgA constitutes about 15% of total serum immunoglobulins, but as Roitt (2001) points out, 'it is generally accepted that the secretory form of the protein is, in the functional sense, the most important' (p. 75). In fact, secretory IgA is the major immunoglobulin found in external body secretions, such as saliva, breast milk, colostrum, tears, nasal secretions and sweat, as well as the secretions of the respiratory, gastrointestinal and genitourinary tracts. Secretory IgA is usually found as a dimer, i.e. two immunoglobulin molecules held together by a J-chain. In addition to the two IgA molecules and J-chain, secretory IgA has a molecule of a secretory component. This secretory component allows for the easy transfer of secretory IgA across the epithelial cells into the secretions, as well as protecting the IgA from the proteolytic attack mounted by enzymes secreted by bacteria. Secretory IgA has a molecular weight of approximately 380 000 daltons, whereas serum IgA has a molecular weight of 160 000 daltons. The half-life of IgA is, like that of IgM, only 7 days.

The main function of secretory IgA (sIgA) is to prevent antigens crossing the epithelium. Because sIgA is a dimer, it has four binding sites for antigen and so can aggregate antigen, which can then be readily destroyed by other components of the immune system. In addition, aggregated sIgA can activate the complement system but, unlike IgA and IgM, it does not activate the classical pathway of the complement system. Rather, it activates the alternative pathway. Secretory IgA plays an important role in the protection of the host's body against respiratory, urinary and bowel infections. In addition, because it is present in such large quantities in colostrum and breast milk, it performs a vital role in the prevention of neonatal gut infections – hence the importance of the promotion of breastfeeding.

There are two subclasses of IgA: namely $IgA_1$ and $IgA_2$. $IgA_1$ is the major subclass of IgA in serum, comprising some 80–90% of total IgA within the serum. It is also present in certain secretions (tears, saliva, nasal secretions and breast milk). In these secretions it constitutes 70–95% of the total IgA. However, in spite of this figure, overall, secretory IgA is predominantly made up of $IgA_2$ (for example, $IgA_2$ makes up some 60% of total IgA in the colon), whereas serum IgA is predominantly made up of $IgA_1$. The reason for the difference is that $IgA_1$ can be cleaved by proteases released by bacteria found in many secretions, whereas $IgA_2$ is protected by the addition of the secretory component (Nairn & Helbert, 2002; Roitt, 2001; Seymour et al., 1995).

## Immunoglobulin E

IgE makes up less than 0.01% of the total serum immunoglobulins but is found on the surface of mast cells and basophils. Immunoglobulin E has a half-life of only 2 days and a molecular weight of 190 000 daltons. It has a very high avidity (binding potential) to tissue mast cells and circulatory basophils, and the binding of IgE to Fc receptors on these cells in the presence of antigen can trigger an allergic reaction. This reaction consists of the activation of the mast cell, degranulation of the cell and the release of mediators such as histamine. This degranulation of the mast cell and release of preformed vasoactive amines helps to cause an acute inflammatory response. This in turn leads to the classical signs of allergic reactions, such as those seen in hay fever and asthma, namely the migration of polymorphonuclear neutrophils and eosinophils, leading directly to redness and oedema. Immunoglobulin E is also responsible for sensitizing cells on mucosal surfaces, such as the conjunctival, nasal and bronchial mucosa. This gives rise to other symptoms of an allergy, including rhinitis and conjunctivitis.

It is believed that this immunoglobulin originally evolved as a means of protection against parasitic infection, for example tapeworms and other intestinal worms, and in many parts of the world, this is still a very important role. In more developed countries, however, its presence is now observed mainly in allergic conditions (Nairn & Helbert, 2002; Roitt, 2001; Seymour et al., 1995).

## Immunoglobulin D

Little is known about the functions of IgD. It is chiefly found on B-cell surface membranes and it acts as a receptor molecule. It is also known that it has a molecular weight of 184 000 daltons, a half-life of only 2 days and that it constitutes less than 1% of total serum immunoglobulins. It is thought to be involved in antigen-triggered lymphocyte differentiation but work is ongoing in trying to decipher and understand this particular immunoglobulin (Fig 6.2.8).

## Primary and secondary responses to infection

Without the ability of the acquired immune system to 'remember' previous encounters with an antigen, each time an individual came into contact with a particular antigen there would be a risk of a serious, if not fatal, illness. This **immune memory** is crucial to the safe functioning and defence of the body, because it allows it to mount an immediate immune response against the antigen, without waiting for the immune system to work out a way of destroying that antigen each time it is encountered.

How does the immune system gain this memory of a specific antigen? The first time the immune system encounters an antigen it mounts a primary (or first) immune response. With the primary immune response, there is always a long time period before a response can be made. This is known as the 'lag' phase because the response lags some way behind the encounter with the antigen. During this time there are no detectable antibodies produced by the mature B-cell lymphocytes because they must first differentiate into plasma cells following contact with an antigen. This period can be likened to an industrial process that is being started up from scratch. Planning has to occur, machinery has to be put in place, materials ordered and delivered, and a workforce trained. There is always a delay before production can come on line. In the case of the primary immune response, this lag phase can take anything from 5–10 days before there has been sufficient production of antibodies to make a difference. During this period, the host can become very sick indeed, and may even die.

Another aspect of the primary immune response is that the major immunoglobulin class produced at this stage is IgM. IgM has a low affinity for an antigen, i.e. it does not bind to it very well. Eventually, smallish amounts of IgG are produced and, hopefully, the antigen is destroyed. What is important, however, is that at the same time the memory cells are retaining a memory of this specific antigen and,

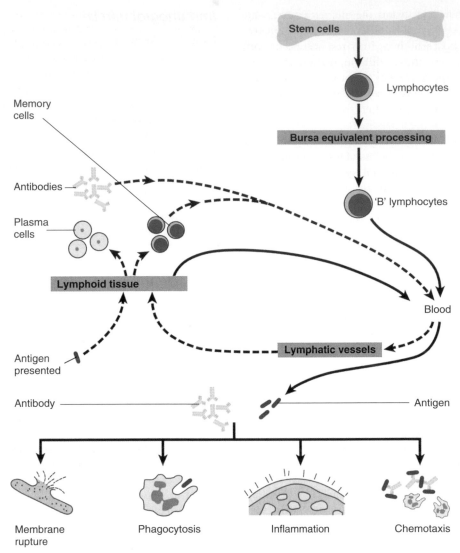

**Figure 6.2.8** The formation and protective function of the humoral immune system

because of a long half-life and subsequent cloning, this memory will stay with the host for a long time. In fact, each time the host is infected by that same antigen, the memory cells are reinforced.

Now, if that same antigen does subsequently make an appearance, then, assuming that the memory cells are working effectively, the body is capable of mounting a secondary immune response. In this scenario, the response is much quicker **(Fig. 6.2.9)**. To continue with the analogy with an industrial process, it is as if once the firm has started production it takes a break, perhaps shuts down for a holiday. After the holiday, the industrial process needs to be restarted. Production, however, can come on line very quickly because the machinery is already set up, the raw materials are already in store and the workforce is already trained. It is the same with the secondary immune response. Because there are many more memory cells carrying the memory of this antigen than the first B-cell population, the production of

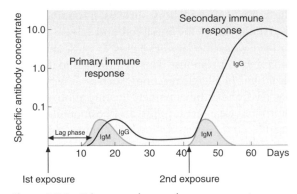

**Figure 6.2.9** Primary and secondary responses to infection

antibodies can take place very quickly, so that there is a very short lag phase. There are usually only from 1–3 days before sufficient antibodies are produced to affect the outcome of the disease. In addition, the major antibody class produced during the secondary immune response is IgG, although occasionally IgA or IgE may be produced, depending on the nature of the antigen and its route of entry (Nairn & Helbert, 2002). IgG is produced in huge quantities very quickly and has a high affinity for an antigen. As a result, the response is very rapid and effective, and the antigen is often destroyed even before there are any symptoms perceived by the host.

Often a host encounters the same antigen frequently and this serves to reinforce the immune response. This is known as a 'booster' response. Sometimes there can be a very long gap between the first encounter with an antigen and a subsequent one. To deal with this the immune system has long-term immunological memory, which is thought to result from clonally expanded, antigen-specific B- and T-cell lymphocytes that are capable of persisting in a resting state for many years, and sometimes for the lifetime of a host (Nairn & Helbert, 2002).

This immunological memory and the primary and secondary immune responses are the basis for the success of immunization or vaccination.

## CLINICAL APPLICATIONS

### IMMUNIZATION

More than 70 bacteria, viruses, fungi and parasites have been identified as pathogenic infectious organisms capable of causing serious diseases in humans (Ada & Ramsey, 1997). Vaccines are available against some of these and work is in progress to find vaccines for almost all the bacteria and viruses, and about half of the parasites (Ada, 2001).

Immunization or vaccination is either the process of transferring antibodies to an individual who is lacking them (passive immunization), or the process of inducing an immune reaction in an individual (active immunization). The second process is possible because of the primary and secondary responses to infection outlined above. Immunizations induce the primary response by exposing the immune system to an infectious organism. This infectious organism is either inactivated (killed) or attenuated (weakened) so that it is no longer infectious, but it still possesses the antigenic receptors that stimulate the immune system.

There are several requirements for an effective vaccine. The first, and most important, is that it is safe; it must not cause significant illness or death. In addition, it must do its job – it must be effective in protecting the body against the particular pathogenic organism. Finally, it must give sustained protection, if at all possible, ideally for life, but at least for several years (Janeway et al., 2001). For this to happen, both T- and B-cell

lymphocytes must be stimulated to provide an immune response, creating a memory population. If a vaccine is effective, it provides herd **immunity** to a population. This term means that by reducing the number of people in a population who are susceptible to a particular disease-causing organism, there is a fall in the natural reservoir of infected people in that population. This then reduces the risk of transmission of the infectious organism so that even individuals in that population who have not been vaccinated are also protected against that organism (Janeway et al., 2001).

### Passive immunization

In passive immunization, the individual is actually injected with the antibodies. There are two types of passive immunization that are natural and very common. The mother transfers IgG antibodies across the placenta to the fetus. Whatever organisms the mother is immune to, the newborn baby will also be immune to them. The second form of passive immunization takes place during breast feeding, when the mother passes IgA antibodies to the baby in her colostrum and milk.

Remembering that IgG has a short half-life, and that IgA has an even shorter half-life, then it can be seen that passive immunization is also short lived, and lasts only as long as it takes for these antibodies to be cleared from the body. This type of immunization will not normally provoke an immune response in the recipient's body and therefore there will be no immunological cover for subsequent exposure to that particular antigen.

Passive immunization may also be given in the form of gamma-globulin (antibody) infusions when an individual has not developed active immunity from vaccination and is at risk from infection by, for example, tetanus. Passive immunization may also be indicated when a person has reduced or no immunity (is immunocompromised) following cytotoxic chemotherapy, radiation therapy, or bone marrow transplantation, or when the patient has a primary or secondary immunodeficiency. Again, the immunity gained by this passive route is short-lived and there is a risk of allergic reaction to the gamma-globulin infusion.

An important use of passive immunity in healthcare practice is following a susceptible individual's exposure to serum-borne hepatitis B antigens. Another common use is to give a Rh-negative mother antibodies against Rh antigens to prevent her manufacturing her own antibodies, with the aim of preventing a Rh incompatibility reaction in future pregnancies (see Chapter 4.1).

## Active immunization

Active immunization is the process of presenting antigen to the immune system to induce an immune response against it. This is the type of immunization that takes advantage of the primary and secondary responses to immunity.

The antigen presented to the immune system is made as safe as possible by either using a whole microorganism and making it weaker whilst keeping it alive (known as a live-attenuated vaccine), or killing it and possibly just using part of the microorganism (known as an inactivated vaccine). In fact, all that is required to initiate some sort of immune response are the antigen receptors.

Live, attenuated vaccines have traditionally been made by repeatedly passing the infectious agent in either tissue culture or animal hosts, and selecting the least infectious each time, until it was sufficiently weakened and non-infectious to be safe but at the same time maintained its immunogenicity, i.e. its ability to provoke an immune response. A second method has been to use chemicals such as formalin to destroy the microorganism's infectivity.

These days, other methods are also used. Only parts of the organism, usually the surface receptors, are used for the vaccine. Alternatively, some vaccines use recombinant DNA technology to produce surface antigen, thereby making the organism safe. An example of this is the vaccine against hepatitis B virus.

As mentioned, parts of the microorganism are all that are needed to initiate an immune response. These are known as subunits. The response from these subunits is predominantly an antibody response (Nairn & Helbert, 2002). Although these are safer than vaccines based on whole organisms, it has been found that a single, isolated component of a microorganism on its own does not normally produce an effective vaccine. This is because the vaccine needs to be able to activate more than one cell type to elicit an effective immune response. These types of vaccines are often used for bacteria with a polysaccharide capsule around them. Types of bacteria with an outer capsule composed of polysaccharides include *Neisseria meningitides* and *Streptococcus pneumoniae*, both of which are capable of causing severe, and possibly fatal, disease. Although polysaccharide vaccines on their own can be used, children under 2 years of age cannot be effectively immunized using only polysaccharide vaccines because they are T-cell independent antigens. Children at this age are unable to make enough T cells to make them effective against these microorganisms. To overcome this, the bacterial polysaccharides are chemically conjugated (or linked) to protein carriers that are recognized by T-helper cells. These conjugate vaccines are very effective, as can be seen by the vaccine for *Haemophilus influenzae* type B. This microorganism is a cause of meningitis and serious chest infections. To elicit an effective immune response, the polysaccharide of the bacterial capsule is combined with tetanus toxoid protein. The two components of the vaccine are then able to provoke both B- and T-cell immune responses, to provide very effective immunity against this pathogenic microorganism.

Another approach to making safe and effective vaccines is by adding adjuvants to purified antigen. On their own, purified antigens are not normally very immunogenic. Adjuvants are substances that enhance the immunogenicity of antigens (Janeway et al., 2001). Tetanus toxoids are not immunogenic but, once linked to aluminium hydroxide (alum), they become effectively immunogenic. A toxoid is a preparation of a bacterial exotoxin that no longer produces disease following treatment, for example with formalin. One of the earliest vaccines given to infants is the triple vaccine for diphtheria, tetanus and pertussis (DTP). Both tetanus and diphtheria toxoids have poor immunogenicity but pertussis toxin works on its own because it has adjuvant properties. By combining the three components, diphtheria, tetanus and pertussis, the triple vaccine gives immunity against the three diseases of diphtheria, tetanus and whooping cough (pertussis).

Inactivated (killed) vaccines are vaccines that consist of microorganisms often treated in such a way that they are unable to replicate. Although these vaccines produce an immune response, live-attenuated microorganisms are much more potent because, by replicating, they stimulate a greater and longer-lasting immune response. In fact, it is this inability to replicate and therefore not provoke a long reaction and immune response that means that inactivated vaccines have to be repeated, whereas live vaccines may only need to be administered once. Unfortunately, attenuated viruses may sometimes revert to a wild pathogenic strain because of the multiple gene mutations possible in their DNA. The type 3 Sabin polio vaccine strain only differs from a wild-type strain by 10 out of a total of 7429 nucleotides, and so there is the possibility of mutations occurring in the attenuated virus which may cause the virus to revert to a neurovirulent strain, and so cause the paralytic disease poliomyelitis, also known as infantile paralysis (Janeway et al., 2001). Attenuated viral vaccines are also a risk when administered to immunodeficient individuals, when they can behave as virulent, opportunistic infecting agents. To overcome this problem, recombinant DNA technology is being attempted by replacing the wild-type genes with mutated 'safe' genes (Janeway et al., 2001). This same approach is being attempted in the development of bacterial vaccines, for example with *Salmonella typhii*, which causes typhoid.

The route by which the vaccines are administered is also important. At the moment, most vaccines are given by intramuscular injection, which is painful and expensive. In addition, there is an immunological problem with this method, because it does not mimic the usual route of entry of many important pathogens. These infect either mucosal surfaces or enter the body through the mucosa and include respiratory and enteric pathogens. Research is ongoing to develop vaccines that can be administered to the mucosa, either by the oral route or by nasal inhalation (Janeway et al., 2001). The effectiveness of live-attenuated polio vaccine is an illustration of entry via the oral route of an established vaccine.

A new development in vaccination, called DNA vaccination, is another way forward. In this method, minute metal projectiles are coated with DNA, which encodes a viral immunogen. These are then administered by 'shooting' them into muscle using a biological ballistic gun, known as a biolistic gun. This method has been effectively used in animals, but has yet to be tested in humans (Janeway et al., 2001).

## Immunization schedule

Each country has its own vaccination schedules for children but all agree that it is important to vaccinate children early, before they come into contact with too many pathogenic infecting organisms. The current schedule for the United Kingdom is given in **Table 6.2.1**.

The vaccines given at 4 years are given as preschool boosters. This is very important because when children start school they mix with many other children, some of whom may be carriers of these infections, equally, they might come into contact with some children who have no immunity to these infections.

There are few contraindications to these vaccines. It is, however, very important that live vaccines are not given to those who are immunocompromised or are suspected of being immunocompromised. This includes people with primary or secondary immunodeficiencies. In addition, those living in families where a close family member is immunosuppressed or immunodeficient should not be given live vaccines, because of the risk to the immunocompromised family member. Exceptions are those with HIV infection, who can safely be given MMR.

For most children, the only contraindications are if the child is experiencing an acute febrile illness, in which case the immunization is deferred, or if they have previously had a severe generalized or local reaction to that same vaccine.

**Table 6.2.1** The UK immunization schedule Dept of Health August, 2004

| When to immunize | What is given | How it is given |
| --- | --- | --- |
| Two, three and four months old | Diphtheria, tetanus, acellular pertussis, inactivated polios vaccine and Hib (DTaP/IPV/Hib) | One injection |
| | Men C | One injection |
| About 13 months | MMR (measles, mumps and rubella) | One injection |
| Three years four months to five years old (pre-school) | Diphtheria, tetanus, acellular pertussis, inactivated polio vaccine (dTaP/IPV) | One injection |
| | MMR | One injection |
| 10 to 14 years old (and sometimes shortly after birth) | BCG (against tuberculosis) | Skin test, then if needed, one injection |
| 13 to 18 years old | Diphtheria, tetanus, and inactivated polio vaccine (Td/IPV) | One injection |

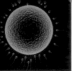
In the 1980s, there was a scare that the pertussis component of the DTP vaccine caused neurological problems. The uptake of the pertussis vaccine declined drastically and this led to pertussis epidemics. It is now accepted that the pertussis vaccine is safe and it is only contraindicated for children with an evolving neurological problem. In this case, immunization against pertussis should be deferred until the outcome of the neurological problem is clear.

A similar situation has recently arisen in the United Kingdom regarding the MMR vaccine, following some research that appeared to link it to the onset of autism and Crohn's disease. Although these results have not been replicated, much parental unease was generated, which resulted in a demand for the single measles, mumps and rubella vaccines, rather than the MMR. At the moment, this issue has yet to be resolved, as no one appears prepared to compromise. Whatever the merits of the two cases, what is not in doubt are the benefits of immunization in preventing serious disease – and measles is potentially a very serious disease, which can be fatal. The worry is that, as with pertussis in the 1980s, there may be a measles epidemic in the near future because of the decreasing uptake of the MMR vaccine by some worried parents and the refusal by the medical establishment and the government to offer single vaccines.

Some people have other concerns with the MMR vaccine, because the measles, mumps and rubella components of the vaccine are produced in egg embryos and one preservative that has been used contains a mercury-based substance. There have been concerns that there may be a risk of an anaphylactic reaction in children who are egg sensitive. This is not, however, a reason for not giving the MMR vaccine, as these reactions are very rare and may not even be due to the egg protein. If children are thought to be at risk, they should receive the MMR vaccine under strict medical conditions, with an anaphylactic kit available, and with observation for 2 hours afterwards.

There is one other point to note about the immunization schedule. It has already been mentioned that children do not start to make their immunoglobulins until shortly before they are born, and it is not until several months after birth that they have adequate numbers of their own B cells. Because of this, ideally, the immunization schedule should not commence until the infant is about 6 months of age, when there are sufficient self-immunoglobulins present to respond to the vaccines. Prior to this age, most of the immunoglobulins in an infant's body are of maternal origin. However, it was thought that the benefits of delaying the immunizations was offset by the need to give the infants protection at as early an age as possible, as anyone who has looked after infants with severe whooping cough, diphtheria, meningitis or any of the other childhood diseases will agree. In addition, the schedule has accelerated in recent years, so that more vaccines are given over a shorter period. This occurred because of the recognition that one of the most frequent reasons for poor vaccine uptake was the movement of families with young children, so that they may move out of the area before the completion of the immunization schedule.

# Hypersensitivity

The immune system has many checks and balances to maintain its effectiveness and functions. Sometimes, however, these checks and balances fail and an excessive immune response occurs. This can cause problems, some of them severe. Inappropriate immune responses can manifest in one of four ways:

1. An exaggerated response against environmental antigens – **allergy**. When antigens provoke an allergic response, they are known as allergens (allergy-generating).
2. A misdirected response against the host's own cells – **autoimmunity**.
3. An immune response that is directed against non-self antigens, such as blood transfusions and organ transplants, which are beneficial to the host – **alloimmunity**.
4. An immune response that is not of sufficient strength to protect the host – **immune deficiency**.

All four of these types of immune system abnormality have the potential to be serious, or even life threatening (McCance & Huether, 2002). Three of these conditions – allergy, autoimmunity and alloimmunity – all come under the heading of **hypersensitivity**. One definition of hypersensitivity is 'an altered immunologic reaction to an antigen that results in a pathologic immune response after re-exposure' (McCance & Huether, 2002, p. 227).

The classification of different types of hypersensitivity in use today is the Coombs and Gell classification (Gell & Coombs, 1975), in which there are four types. The first three types involve the humoral system – antibodies – and the fourth type is a function of cellular immunity.

## Type 1 hypersensitivity – immediate hypersensitivity

This type of hypersensitivity is linked to immunoglobulin E (IgE) and is mediated through the degranulation of mast cells and basophils. This degranulation produces an allergic response and the disorders that come under this classification, such as allergic rhinitis, asthma and atopic eczema, are some of the most common causes of ill-health. The term 'allergy' was first used in 1906 by Von Pirquet but, according to Kay (2001), the term has now come to be used with IgE-mediated allergic disease. Another term often used to describe IgE-mediated disease is 'atopy' (from the Greek word 'atopos', meaning 'out of place'). People with atopy have a hereditary predisposition to produce IgE antibodies against common environmental allergens and have one or more atopic diseases, such as asthma and eczema (Kay, 2001) **(Fig. 6.2.10)**.

In this class of hypersensitivity, reactions occur when an environmental antigen (e.g. house-dust mite faeces, peanuts, grass pollens or animal dander) interact with IgE, which is bound to tissue mast cells or basophils via their Fc receptors. The first time this occurs, there are no problems but the individual becomes sensitized to the antigen, so that for all subsequent exposures to that antigen, an allergic reaction is triggered. This subsequent exposure of the tissue mast cells and circulating basophils to the specific antigen causes cross-linking of the surface antigen-specific IgE molecules, which in turn triggers degranulation and the release of vasoactive compounds from these cells (Chapel & Haeney, 1993). The most potent of these compounds is histamine, which causes smooth muscle contraction, and endothelial cell contraction (Seymour et al., 1995). This in turn leads to increased vascular permeability and thence to oedema. Histamine also acts on the secretory cells, causing increased secretions (e.g. tears and mucosal secretions). Histamine acts through special histamine receptors (called $H_1$-receptors) on target cells, and it causes contraction of bronchial smooth muscle, thereby contributing to bronchial constriction, as well as vasodilation leading to increased blood flow into the area. There are also $H_2$-receptors on target cells in the host tissue, and histamine interacts with these to increase gastric secretions. Histamine may also affect the immune response by its interaction with $H_2$-receptors on most cells of the immune system. Histamine also works with another product of mast cell and basophil degranulation, namely eosinophil chemotactic factor of anaphylaxis (ECF-A), to attract eosinophils into areas of allergic inflammation. As well as ECF-A, other vasoactive compounds are released. These are lumped together under the name of slow reacting substances of anaphylaxis (SRS-A) and include prostaglandins, leukotrienes, thromboxanes and platelet-activating factors. The response from these is similar to the response seen from histamine and ECF-A, but there is a slower reaction time and the response is much longer lasting.

The target tissues of type I hypersensitivity contain large numbers of mast cells and are found in the gastrointestinal tract, skin and respiratory tract, which makes understandable the various allergic disorders, such as asthma, eczema, urticaria and gut allergies.

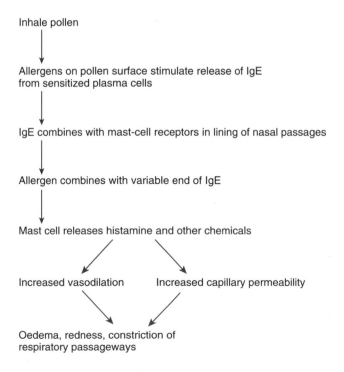

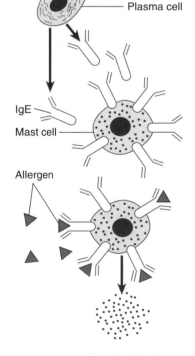

**Figure 6.2.10**   A common type of allergic response

The most serious form of atopy is acute systemic anaphylaxis, which can be fatal if not treated quickly and effectively.

## CLINICAL APPLICATIONS

### Anaphylaxis

Anaphylaxis is a reaction, which is usually IgE mediated (as are all type I reactions), and in which there is a massive release of histamine and other vasoactive substances. This reaction is triggered by a severe allergic reaction in a sensitized individual. The common causes of anaphylaxis include (Barkin & Rosen, 1999):

- insect bites and stings
- antibiotics, particularly antibiotics such as penicillin
- foods such as shellfish, peanuts, eggs, milk and beans
- drugs, including insulin, aspirin, narcotics and adrenocorticotrophic hormone (ACTH)
- inhaled allergens, such as dust, pollen and animal dander
- local anaesthetics
- biologic agents, including gamma globulin and vaccines
- latex
- diagnostic agents, such as radiological contrast media.

However, allergic reactions to diagnostic agents, local anaesthetics, aspirin and narcotics such as morphine, are not IgE mediated. These antigens are known as anaphylactoid agents. Anaphylactic-causing antigens may cause a severe anaphylactic systemic reaction by being ingested, inhaled or injected, with injected agents (including bee and wasp stings), having the highest risk of causing an anaphylactic reaction.

Once an anaphylactic reaction is set in train the course of the reaction is very rapid, with acute vasodilation and consequent fluid loss from the intravascular spaces. This is caused by increased capillary permeability and is followed by rapid onset circulatory collapse, hypotension and oedema.

Following ingestion of an allergen, angio-oedema may occur, with swelling of the subcutaneous and mucous membranes in the facial area, with or without laryngeal, pharyngeal and glossal oedema. This is either a localized reaction or it occurs as part of systemic anaphylaxis. It is important, however, to be aware that, although rare, unexplained angio-oedema can be due to a hereditary disorder that is caused by $C_1$ esterase inhibitor deficiency.

The signs and symptoms of anaphylaxis can be divided into three stages, although if not arrested, the progression through these stages is very rapid indeed.

1. **Early stage:** flush, tachycardia, feeling of fullness in the throat, cough, tight chest, nausea.
2. **Progressing stage:** pruritus, hypotension, stridor, wheeze, abdominal pain, vomiting.
3. **Late stage:** angio-oedema, diarrhoea, laryngeal obstruction, respiratory arrest, cardiac arrest.

In treating anaphylactic shock, the three main priorities initially are maintaining the airway, giving oxygen, and basic life support if a cardiac or respiratory arrest has occurred.

The main drug used to treat anaphylactic shock is adrenaline (epinephrine), which should be given intramuscularly (IM) immediately the reaction occurs and before any attempt to insert an intravenous (IV) cannula, if one is not already *in situ*. Adrenaline (epinephrine) should then be given either by the IV or intraosseous (IO) route. If stridor is present, 5 mL of nebulized adrenaline (epinephrine) 1:1000 can be given. For children, IV adrenaline (epinephrine) of 0.1 mL/kg of 1:10 000 is given or, if it is given via an endotracheal (ET) tube, then the dose is 0.1 mL/kg of 1:1000. If IM adrenaline (epinephrine) is given, the dose depends upon the age and weight of the individual. As a guide, an infant aged less than 1 year will be given 0.05 mL of 1:1000 adrenaline (epinephrine), whereas a child of 6–12 years will be given 0.5 mL of adrenaline (epinephrine) 1:1000 and an adult will receive 0.5–1 mL of adrenaline (epinephrine) 1:1000 IM. These doses of adrenaline (epinephrine) can be repeated several times at 10-minute intervals. In addition, hydrocortisone and chlorpheniramine can be given to ease the symptoms. In cases of intractable anaphylaxis, intravenous aminophylline is administered. For volume expansion to counteract hypovolaemia, colloids are given and repeated as necessary.

Following a severe anaphylactic reaction, the patient needs to be transferred to a high-dependency or intensive care unit for very close monitoring.

## Allergies and the 'hygiene hypothesis'

One of the puzzles of recent years has been the rising prevalence of atopic diseases, particularly asthma and eczema, in the Western industrialized countries. Increases in levels of pollution were thought to be the reason for this increase in levels of atopic diseases, but work by Von Mutius et al. (1994) demonstrated that children in the former East Germany had a significantly lower prevalence of asthma and allergic reactions to allergens than children living in the former West Germany. These differences occurred in spite of the much higher levels of industrial atmospheric pollution in the former East Germany. This report led to the formation of the hypothesis that the higher standard of living in West Germany, including central heating, fitted carpets, double glazing and home insulation, could be an underlying major factor in the rising levels of asthma in the children in West Germany. This study linked with work by Strachen (1989), who demonstrated that there was an inverse association between the number of children living in a household and the prevalence of hay fever. This led Strachen to put forward the theories that declining family sizes, improved household amenities and higher standards of personal hygiene have reduced opportunities for cross-infection to occur in families with young children. Following these and similar reports, the **hygiene hypothesis** came into being, which states that exposure to bacteria, and other antigens, in early life decreases the risk of allergies. This is supported by observations that children with asthma tend to live in cleaner houses than those without asthma. In addition, it has been found that growing up on farms, with subsequent higher levels of exposure to livestock and dirt, actually decreases the risk of asthma, which is also rare in areas where tuberculosis (TB) is common (Davey & Seale, 1996). The latest reports (Sherrif et al., 2002a, b) have demonstrated that increased levels of hygiene in a family were linked to higher rates of asthma and eczema when children were 30 to 42 months old. The authors suggest that children who become dirty are exposed to more bacteria and other infectious agents and that this exposure primes the immune system and protects these children from disease. In addition Sherrif et al. (2002a) consider the possibility that parents who are obsessed with cleanliness may also be reluctant to allow their children to play outdoors where they could come into contact with infectious organisms. As this limits their contact with other children, a valuable source of cross-infection is lost. So this situation could potentially affect their immune systems as well as their socialization skills.

What is the biological explanation underpinning this hypothesis? As described earlier in this chapter, the T-helper cells occur in two populations known as T-helper 1 and T-helper 2 cells. At birth, most individuals produce T-helper cells with a bias towards T-helper 2 cytokine production. The hygiene hypothesis put forward by its proponents is based upon the theory that exposure to infectious organisms that initiate a T-helper 1 response early in life moves the immune response away from T-helper 2 immune responses. T-helper 2 cells have a vital role in the establishment of IgE-mediated responses and type I hypersensitivity. By promoting T-helper 1 responses rather than T-helper 2 responses, there is thus less risk of type I

hypersensitivity developing. It was mentioned above that asthma is rare in areas where tuberculosis is common. According to the hygiene hypothesis, this is because *Mycobacterium tuberculosis* (the cause of tuberculosis) and other bacterial infections stimulate T cells to secrete a particular cytokine called $\gamma$-interferon (IFN-$\gamma$), which is capable of inhibiting T-helper 2 responses. The hygiene hypothesis suggests that this deviation from T-helper 2 to T-helper 1 response would be expected to work when the immune responses to potential allergens are developing. Most of these responses occur in the early months of life as the individual is meeting a whole range of new (to them) infectious organisms. Thus this process can only really operate early in life (Nairn & Helbert, 2002).

## Type II hypersensitivity – antibody-mediated hypersensitivity

These hypersensitivity reactions normally manifest themselves as the destruction of a target self-cell through the antibody acting against an antigen on the cell's plasma membrane (McCance & Huether, 2002). The reactions are caused by either IgG or IgM (but not IgE) binding to the surface cells. This antibody binding frequently damages red blood cells and cells of solid tissue. There are four mechanisms by which type II hypersensitivity occurs. However, all four mechanisms begin with IgG or IgM binding to tissue-specific antigens.

The first mechanism has two ways of achieving cell destruction: by complement-mediated lysis and by opsonization. With this action, IgM or IgG reacts with antigen on the cell surface. This activates the complement system that lyses – kills – the cell. For example, people with autoimmune haemolytic anaemia have their circulating erythrocytes destroyed by this method. Similarly ABO mismatched blood transfusions lead to the destruction of the transfused red blood cells (these reactions are discussed in some detail in Chapter 4.1).

The second method of type II cell destruction is phagocytosis of the cell by mononuclear phagocytes. This mechanism depends upon the IgG or IgM coating the target cell, which then facilitates their phagocytosis. Haemolytic disease of the newborn is an example of a disorder caused by this particular mechanism of type II hypersensitivity.

The third mechanism is antibody-dependent cell-mediated cytotoxicity (ADCC). This involves the destruction of target cells by natural killer cells. Natural killer cells are non-antigen-specific cytotoxic cells. This mechanism works because antibody bound to the target cell surface antigens is recognized by the natural killer cells, which then release toxic substances that destroy the cell.

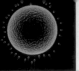

The fourth mechanism is different to the other three mechanisms of type II hypersensitivity because, with this mechanism, the cell is not destroyed but is damaged, which causes it to malfunction. IgG or IgM bind to the target cell and, in so doing, the antibodies occupy the receptors that would normally be free to bind to the various ligands (molecules), which are required to ensure normal cellular functioning. An example of this is Grave's disease, an autoimmune disease that causes hyperthyroidism because the autoantibodies produced stimulate the thyroid to overproduce hormone.

## Type III hypersensitivity – immune complex disease

Immune complexes (antigen–antibody complexes) have already been discussed. For the most part, they disappear quickly from the circulation although in some individuals they can be present for a long time in the blood, where they cause serious clinical conditions. This situation can occur when the immune-complex-clearing processes are saturated because of continuous and excessive production of these immune complexes. In addition, if there is a deficiency in the complement system, then these clearance processes cannot function.

The damage caused by immune complexes that have not been cleared is due to the activation of the innate immune system, namely the process of inflammation. Soluble small immune complexes that contain more antigens than antibodies (IgG) enter the blood circulation system and form circulating immune complexes. These complexes cause damage to the blood vessels, particularly when they lodge on the basement membrane of the blood vessel. Once lodged there, they activate the complement system. One of the functions of the complement system is chemotaxis, which causes the migration of neutrophils to the area. Once the neutrophils have reached the place where the immune complex is lodged, they release their granules containing lysosomal enzymes that damage the blood vessels. This blood vessel inflammation is known as vasculitis, and immune complexes are one of the causes of vasculitis. If the antigen that helps to form the immune complexes that are not cleared from the system is only localized, then only localized damage will occur, causing such reactions as Arthus reaction or farmer's lung. However, if these immune complexes circulate in the blood, they cause damage in any specific areas where they may lodge. These occur particularly in the kidneys, the skin and the joints.

### Kidney damage

When type III hypersensitivity involves the kidneys, renal failure can ensue. Kidney involvement is common because the blood pressure in the glomeruli is much higher than in the general circulation – about four times higher. A higher blood pressure increases the number of immune complexes that are left behind in an area. This deposition of large numbers of immune complexes may be due to a complement receptor – CR1 – which is also expressed by synovial cells. This may explain the involvement of joints in type III hypersensitivity. Once the immune complexes have been deposited in the glomeruli, they produce inflammation, which leads to two possible syndromes – nephrotic syndrome and nephritis.

When the immune complexes lodge in the glomerular basement membrane, they initiate the complement system and this damages the basement membrane, allowing proteins to leak into the urine. Proteinuria is one of the classic signs of renal damage.

### Arthus reaction

This is a localized reaction in the skin caused by type III hypersensitivity. It is often associated with an injection, for example of tetanus toxoid, which triggers the reaction. It manifests as a localized, hard, hot, painful and red swelling. These are, in fact, the classical symptoms of inflammation. The reaction usually peaks in 3 to 8 hours and causes no long-lasting damage, but it can be very painful.

Treatment of type III hypersensitivity usually consists of corticosteroids to reduce the inflammation. Another possible treatment in severe disease, particularly where B-cell proliferation is present, is the use of the very toxic drug, cyclophosphomide. This drug impairs DNA synthesis, which prevents rapid proliferation of cells. It is sometimes used in severe cases of systemic lupus erythromatosus, an autoimmune disease that produces a high level of antibodies against the individual's own DNA. Systemic lupus erythromatosus is a type III hypersensitivity and, as well as renal, skin and joint involvement, it can also affect the central nervous system and the placenta.

## Type IV hypersensitivity – delayed hypersensitivity

Unlike the other three classes of hypersensitivity, which are concerned with antibodies, type IV hypersensitivity is concerned with cell-mediated immune response. It was once thought that there was a specific type of T cell, the T-delayed hypersensitivity lymphocyte that mediated this type of hypersensitivity. It is now known that type IV hypersensitivity is characterized by T helper-1 cells. These cells initiate, and drive, an inflammatory response, which is also mediated by macrophages (Nairn & Helbert, 2002).

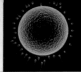

Delayed hypersensitivity reactions usually take place from 2 to 10 days after exposure to an antigen, and it can be a reaction to a variety of antigens that are not easily destroyed, such as hepatitis B virus and *Mycobacterium tuberculosis*. It is also a reaction to environmental antigens, such as nickel and plant extracts (causing contact dermatitis), and autoantigens, for example pancreatic islet cell antigens in insulin-dependent diabetes mellitus (IDDM).

Type IV reactions involve memory T cells from a prior exposure and are initiated by tissue macrophages recognizing an antigen and causing an inflammatory response. Dendritic cells then present this antigen to memory T cells from a prior exposure. The T-cells proliferate and migrate to the site of the inflammation. Both the T cells and the macrophages secrete tumour necrosis factor (TNF) and it is this that stimulates much of the damage in delayed hypersensitivity.

Several autoimmune diseases are caused by type IV hypersensitivity. These include rheumatoid arthritis, type 1 diabetes mellitus (IDDM), coeliac disease and multiple sclerosis. The type IV reactions affect different sites in the body in each of these autoimmune disorders.

## Graft rejection

Graft rejection is another reaction caused by delayed hypersensitivity and antibody-mediated mechanisms. Graft rejection refers to the rejection of a transplanted organ or bone marrow as a result of an immune reaction. Because all cells carry antigens that identify them as belonging to self, the immune system will attempt to destroy any cells coming from outside the body. This is to the advantage of the body, as most non-self cells and antigens cause problems. However, there are times when it is necessary to transplant non-self cells in to the body. Examples of these include kidney transplants, heart and lung transplants and bone marrow transplants. Rejection takes place by T-cytotoxic cells that recognize the non-self antigens on the surfaces of cells that have been transplanted. The region of the DNA that codes for the genes involved in graft rejection is the major histocompatibility complex/ human leucocyte antigen (MHC/HLA) region, which has already been discussed. To prevent rejection of the graft, it is important to get as close a human leucocyte antigen match as possible. The human leucocyte antigen region is generally unique to an individual but it is sometimes possible to obtain quite good matches. The best match comes from an identical sibling, whose major and minor histocompatability antigens will completely match those of the recipient. Transplants between identical siblings are known as syngeneic transplants and usually no problems with graft rejection ensue.

Sometimes autologous (i.e. self) transplants are undertaken, particularly with bone marrow transplantation. In these types of transplants, bone marrow is removed from a leukaemia patient. These cells are then purged of leukaemic cells and the patient undergoes chemotherapy and radiotherapy to destroy the remaining bone marrow. Following this procedure, the purged bone marrow is returned to the patient. As the cells are still that patient's cells, there are no problems with graft rejection.

The third type of transplantation is known as an allogeneic transplant, in which the transplant procedure takes place between non-identical siblings or even unrelated people who are found to have a close match of human leucocyte antigens. With non-identical siblings, there is a one in four chance of each sibling being a match for major histocompatability antigens with the recipient. There may, however, be some differences between the minor histocompatability antigens. Non-related donors may also be used, either as live or cadaver donors. Again care is made to achieve as close a match as possible. The donations of bone marrow from non-related people are known as matched unrelated donor (MUD) transplants. However, with allogeneic transplants, there is always a risk of rejection.

The fourth type of transplant is being considered due to shortage of human donors. It takes place between different species and is known as xenogeneic transplants. These carry the highest risks of rejection. At the moment there is a lot of interest in the use of specially bred pigs for use as donors for solid organ transplantation. Work is ongoing in this field and attempts are being made to breed pigs containing human genes in an attempt to overcome some of the most difficult aspects of graft rejection. However, there is still concern about the risk of transplanting porcine viruses into humans alongside the transplanted organ.

There are two types of rejection following transplantation – acute and chronic. Acute rejection can occur a matter of days, or maybe a few weeks, after the transplant. Acute rejection takes place when there is human leucocyte antigen incompatibility, and the survival of the graft is often related to the degree of human leucocyte antigen mismatching, particularly at the HLA-DR loci (Nairn & Helbert, 2002). Acute rejection can also occur when there are mismatched minor histocompatability antigens. It takes several days for a response to occur with an allogeneic match, and for the T-cytotoxic cells to proliferate and migrate into the donated graft.

However, if chronic rejection occurs, this initially takes place several months, or even years, after the transplant. Sometimes, chronic rejection is caused by a reoccurrence of the existing autoimmune disease that necessitated the transplant in the first place.

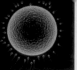
In some cases, there is actually no evidence of any damage caused by the acquired immune system.

Because of the risk of rejection in a non-syngeneic solid organ transplant, the recipient will need to be on life-long immunosuppressive therapy. This is to reduce the damaging effects of the immune system on the donated graft. At the same time, it is important not to totally suppress the immune system, otherwise there would be a very high risk of infections and a risk of tumours. Azathioprine, which is an antiproliferative drug, is often used for life-long suppression (Nairn & Helbert, 2002).

### Stem cell transplants

Another type of transplant, namely stem cell transplant, has been used to treat several haematological and immunological disorders, for example haematological malignancies such as leukaemia, reduced myeloid cell production such as aplastic anaemia, and immunodeficiency disorders such as severe combined immunodeficiency.

Stem cells are obtained from bone marrow, peripheral stem cells or cord blood. There has been a lot of success with these types of transplants in immunological disorders but they have been less successful in haematological disorders, where severe conditioning by cytotoxic drugs and/or radiotherapy is essential. If there is not a good match between recipient and donor, there is a risk of graft rejection taking place.

However, there is another rejection risk with these types of transplant, and that is graft-versus-host disease (GvHD). This occurs due to the lack of a fully functioning immune system in the recipient, so that the T cells in the donated stem cells are immunologically stronger than the T cells in the donor. Thus the donated T cells can attack and destroy the recipient's tissues because they recognize the recipient's cells as non-self. This is life threatening but removing most of the T cells from the donated stem cells before transplantation greatly reduces the risk of GvHD. In addition, if GvHD does occur, it is possible to use immunosuppressive drugs, although these will have the effect of delaying graft take by the body.

Acute GvHD can occur from 11 days to 4 weeks after the transplant and involves the skin, gastrointestinal tract, lungs and liver. Severe acute GvHD carries a mortality risk of 70%, although better immunosuppression, human leucocyte antigen matching and conditioning treatment have reduced the risks considerably since the pioneering days of bone marrow transplants. GvHD can also develop into a chronic disorder. This is not as severe as acute GvHD and mainly affects the skin and liver, with some gut involvement.

## Autoimmune disease

Autoimmune diseases are the result of an acquired immune response being mounted against the body's own cells (self-antigens). They are caused by autoreactive T cells – cells that react against the host's own antigens – thereby damaging the tissues of the body, a result of hypersensitivity reaction. These hypersensitivity reactions can be of type II, type III or type IV.

The autoimmune response involves T cells and antibodies. These particular antibodies, which react against self-tissues, are called **autoantibodies**. Actually, most individuals produce some autoantibodies, even when perfectly healthy. These are usually at a very low level and have a poor affinity for binding to autoantigens. Although it is possible that the autoantibodies found in healthy people could cause autoimmune diseases, the evidence appears to demonstrate that it is actually the T cells that initiate autoimmune disease (Nairn & Helbert, 2002).

Autoantigens, being part of the body itself, are very difficult to clear from the body, unlike non-self antigens such as bacteria and viruses, which can be cleared reasonably easily. Thus, once an autoimmune disease has been initiated it tends to be present for a long time. This sustained response leads to a chronic disease. In the process of the response, the immune system causes chronic inflammatory injury to the tissues of the body. Autoimmune diseases are actually very common and can affect any organ of the body. In addition, they can occur at any age.

The mechanism by which potential autoreactive T cells were eliminated during their time in the thymus has already been described. So the question needs to be posed as to how some T cells can become autoreactive and provoke autoimmune disease. One possible explanation is that process and virulence of the destruction of potential autoreactive T cells varies, so that it is possible for some to escape destruction (Klein et al., 2000). Another explanation, however, for the appearance of autoreactive T cells in the body beyond the thymus stage is the activation of potentially autoreactive T cells by infectious agents (Kamradt & Mitchison, 2001). Kurtzke (1993) has drawn together the evidence to implicate infectious organisms as a cause of autoimmune diseases such as multiple sclerosis and type 1 diabetes mellitus (IDDM). Many mechanisms have been postulated to explain how infection could lead to autoimmune disease. These include the relevance of sequestered autoantigens because of tissue damage and a structural similarity between some microbial antigens and autoantigens. This latter theory is known as **molecular mimicry** and it is felt that this similarity of shape between the antigens could play a leading role in the activation of autoreactive T cells (Kamradt & Mitchison, 2001). Some T cells are certainly capable of recognizing both a microbial peptide and a self-peptide if they possess a similar amino acid sequence; remember that antigens are peptides. However, it may be too simplistic to assume that autoimmunity is a result of cross-reactivity between a microbial peptide and a self-peptide because, as yet, there is no in vivo evidence that this molecular mimicry can actually initiate autoimmune disease. In fact, it is known that infections may be capable of activating a population of protective cells as well as initiating autoimmunity (Kamradt & Mitchison, 2001). Gibbon et al. (1997) have reported that multiple infections during an individual's first year of life are actually associated with a significant reduction in the risks of having one particular autoimmune disease, namely type 1 diabetes (see the hygiene hypothesis, p. 709).

Some individuals may carry a genetic susceptibility to autoimmunity. The human genome project has thrown up many possible linkages to diseases, and autoimmune diseases are no exception. Several possible loci have been identified for susceptibility to multiple sclerosis, type 1 diabetes, systemic lupus erythromatosus and Crohn's disease (Kamradt & Mitchison, 2001). The regions of the chromosomes that have been identified as linking to this susceptibility to autoimmune diseases have included some that span the areas where genes for cytokines, cytokine receptors and other immunoregulatory molecules have been found (Concannon et al., 1998; Mein et al., 1998). However, there remain difficulties in both determining and deciphering these genetic links.

One of the important theories surrounding auto-antibody production, and hence autoimmune disease, is that unregulated autoantibody production results from poor or inadequate T-suppressor cell function (Isenberg & Morrow, 1995). In fact, either a decrease in active numbers of T-suppressor cells or a decrease in activity of T-suppressor cells have been reported in patients with almost all types of autoimmune disorders. The immunoregulatory role of T-helper and T-suppressor cells has already been discussed in this chapter, and autoimmune disease is a result of an imbalance between these two types of T cell.

There are other factors, which influence the course of autoimmune diseases, and a summary of all the factors would include (Isenberg & Morrow, 1995):

- advanced age
- female hormones
- susceptible genetic background
- infections
- environmental factors (e.g. chemicals, toxins, sunlight)
- tissue damage

| Table 6.2.2 Autoimmune disorders and the organs they attack | |
| --- | --- |
| **Organ/tissue** | **Autoimmune disease** |
| Adrenal gland | Addison's disease |
| Pancreas | Insulin-dependent (type 1) diabetes mellitus |
| Joints | Rheumatoid arthritis |
| Red blood cells | Autoimmune haemolytic anaemia<br>Pernicious anaemia |
| Central nervous system | Multiple sclerosis |
| Jejunum | Coeliac disease |
| Thyroid | Graves' disease<br>Hashimoto's disease |
| Heart and joints | Rheumatic fever |
| Vertebrae | Ankylosing spondylitis |
| Neuromuscular function | Myasthenia gravis |
| Non-organ specific | Systemic lupus erythematosus |

- poor diet
- stress.

The pervasiveness of autoimmune diseases is apparent from **Table 6.2.2**.

As well as the chronic autoimmune diseases, there are also acute autoimmune disorders that have a limited span of destruction and may not lead to a chronic condition. One such disorder is Kawasaki's disease in children, which is considered to be an immune 'over-response' to a viral infection, leading to fever, macular rash, desquamation of skin, and oedema. This condition usually settles down after several days but it may, in a very few cases, lead to other acute or long-term complications.

## Insulin-dependent diabetes mellitus (type 1 diabetes)

This condition results from autoimmune damage to the β cells in the pancreatic islets of Langerhans. The role of the β cells is to secrete insulin, which aids in the take-up of glucose from the blood into the tissues. Children presenting with this disease have been found to have islet antibodies. The pancreatic islets are invaded by T cells and the islets are destroyed. This is an example of type IV hypersensitivity and it

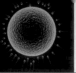

is one of the few autoimmune diseases where the gender ratio is roughly 1:1 male:female.

## Systemic lupus erythematosus (SLE)

This is a result of type III hypersensitivity in which there is production of antibodies against cellular DNA and other cell nuclear compounds. Systemic lupus erythematosus is an extreme example of the gender differences as displayed in autoimmune diseases, as the male:female ratio is 1:20. This is one autoimmune disease that has a very strong link to sex hormones, in this case oestrogen, which has the effect of increasing antibody production, which in turn increases the risk of raised autoantibody production. Systemic lupus erythematosus is non-organ-specific and joint, skin, kidney and central nervous system involvement is seen. One of the defining symptoms of the disorder is a butterfly-shaped rash on the face.

## Rheumatoid arthritis

Rheumatoid arthritis is the result of a type IV hypersensitivity reaction in which the synovial membrane, which lines the joints and tendon sheaths, is very badly inflamed – sometimes up to 100 times its normal size (Nairn & Helbert, 2002). Chronic inflammatory cells, such as T cells and macrophages, invade the synovium of the joints. Most of the symptoms – swelling and pain – are caused by the cytokines tumour necrosis factor (TNF) and interleukin-2 (IL-2), which are secreted by T cells and macrophages. The T-cell cytokines stimulate B cells in the synovium to produce **rheumatoid factor.** This is an autoantibody that is also a natural antibody found in the body. This rheumatoid factor is often produced during any chronic infection, whether rheumatoid arthritis is present or not. In rheumatoid arthritis, the rheumatoid factor may increase inflammation in the joint by producing immune complexes.

## Tumour surveillance and cancer immunotherapy

Although tumour cells are actually self-cells, some small differences in their antigenic receptors distinguish them from 'normal' self-cells. This makes them recognizable to the components of the immune system and hence they become susceptible to attack and destruction by the immune system. These tumour antigens are, like other cell antigens, expressed on the surface membranes. There are several types of tumour antigen, and examples include developmental proteins, lineage-specific proteins, viral proteins and genetic-abnormality proteins (Nairn & Helbert, 2002).

It has already been mentioned that viral proteins, when they have infected a cell, combine with major histocompatibility complex antigen receptors on the cell surface to alter the configuration of the identification receptors on these infected cells. It is now known that several cancers, for example leukaemia and cervical cancer, are caused by viral infections. Epstein–Barr virus (EBV) causes lymphoma and the human papilloma virus is implicated in cervical cancer.

The immune system has, as part of its defence against tumours, a tumour surveillance role, in which it was thought that T cells roam the body searching for tumour cells and killing them. It has been identified that people who are immunosuppressed for any reason are more likely than immunocompetent people to develop malignancies. One example is cervical cancer, which is 100 times more common in immunosuppressed women than in immunocompetent women (Nairn & Helbert, 2002). This ability of the immune system to detect precancerous and malignant cells and kill them, however, appears to have its limitations (Janeway et al., 2001). Not all tumours are recognized by the immune system. The major tumour types recognized by the immune system appear to be the virus-associated tumours, such as Epstein–Barr virus lymphoma and cervical cancer caused by the human papilloma virus. The new antigens in spontaneous cancers that are derived from multiple genetic alterations/translocations are not normally recognized by the immune system. This is because they probably lack the distinctive antigen receptors that are needed to elicit a primary T-cell immune response (Janeway et al., 2001).

Although not as successful as was once assumed, the immune system does attempt to destroy other types of cancers, apart from virus-associated cancers, by recognizing the antigens on the cell surfaces. This is mainly a T-cell response as antibody responses are not particularly effective at killing most solid tumours. However, T cells that infiltrate tumours are capable of killing them. These T cells are known as tumour-infiltrating lymphocytes (TILs) and are specific for tumour antigen (Nairn & Helbert, 2002).

The great majority of tumour cells are able to successfully evade the immune system. Because tumour cells are proliferative (i.e. dividing rapidly to produce more malignant cells), these cells are able to mutate rapidly and so acquire one or more of the immune-system-evasion processes. This then gives these cloned tumour cells an advantage over normal, non-malignant cells (Nairn & Helbert, 2002).

Some of the immune responses to tumours have already been discussed, such as T cells and natural killer cells. There is another way in which malignant cells can be effectively damaged and killed. This is based on the fact that, because tumour cells are rapidly

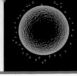

dividing and growing, they need a very good supply of oxygen, which means that they are very vascular. It is possible for the immune system to damage the blood supply to the tumours, thereby starving them of oxygen. It is believed that one of the cytokines – tumour necrosis factor – is capable of doing this, and experiments with mice appear to show that this is feasible. At the moment, however, its importance in humans has yet to be determined (Nairn & Helbert, 2002).

## Cancer immunotherapy

The previous section highlighted the fact that the majority of tumours possess low immunogenicity. In other words, they are poor at eliciting a response from the immune system. It is now believed by many in the field that enhancing the immunogenicity of tumours is one way ahead for the treatment of cancers. There have been many attempts at immunotherapy for cancer treatment but most have failed. However, attempts that have had some success can be classified into two groups – passive and active cancer immunotherapy. For further detail of these therapies see Nairn & Helbert (2002).

Gene therapy is gaining in importance in the treatment of many different diseases, such as severe combined immunodeficiency. In tumour immunotherapy, cytokine gene therapy is being explored in an attempt to localize the cytokines to where they are needed, i.e. the site of the tumour. The idea is to reduce their systemic effects.

Another way of preventing the tumour cells from escaping the attention of the immune system is by inserting tumour antigen into the presenting cells, or by extracting lymphocytes from the tumour and stimulating them with tumour antigen. The treated cells are then re-infused.

In these ways the immune system can be manipulated to increase its effectiveness against tumour cells. It must be stressed that, at the moment, a lot of this work is experimental and has been achieved mainly in studies with mice (Janeway et al., 2001; Nairn & Helbert, 2002). It is thought by many that the future of cancer treatment lies here, along with improvement of the other three modalities of cancer therapy, namely chemotherapy, surgery and radiation therapy.

## Immunodeficiencies

The immune system is very complex and capable of responding rapidly to any threat to the individual. Any deficiency in the immune system, even a minor one, can often have devastating effects on the ability of the body to deal with infections and other threats to its well-being. There are two classifications of immune deficiencies:

1. primary immunodeficiency
2. secondary immunodeficiency.

Both classes are characterized by similar signs and symptoms, particularly multiple infections, and sometimes tumours.

## Primary immunodeficiencies

Study of the immune system is still relatively new and, because of this, more and more is still being found out about it, how it works and what happens when it does not work. Ten years ago, about 70 different primary immunodeficiency disorders had been identified; now the figure is more than 95 (IUIS, 1999; Ochs et al., 1999). A primary immunodeficiency disorder is one in which the cause of the immunodeficiency is not external, such as an infection, a toxin or a chemical. Most of these disorders are inherited disorders and the defect may affect one or more components of the immune system (Buckley, 2000). Since 1993, when the human genome project began, the genetic abnormalities in several primary immunodeficiencies have been identified. The genes that code for immune functioning are spread throughout the genome. However, because of the single nature of the XY chromosomes in males, as opposed to the XX chromosomes in females, and the fact that there are a considerable number of genes of the immune system on the X chromosomes, there is a clear dominance of X-linked immunodeficiency in males. In addition, spontaneous new mutations in these X-linked genes are relatively frequent (Buckley, 2000).

The first recorded immunodeficiency disorder was by Glanzmann and Riniker in 1950, who presented the cases of two infants in Switzerland who had died from what they called 'essentielle lymphocytophthise' (idiopathic lymphocytophtisis). It is now accepted that what they described was the first recorded account of children with severe combined immunodeficiency (SCID). There are three major genetic causes of primary immunodeficiency. These are genetic mutations, polymorphisms and polygenic disorders (for more detail of these, see Nairn & Helbert, 2002).

Primary immunodeficiencies are classified according to the component of the immune system that is affected. There are two major groupings: deficiencies of innate immunity and deficiencies of acquired immunity, although because of the way the components interact, deficiency in one part of the immune system can affect other parts.

B-cell (humoral) immunodeficiencies are deficiencies that affect the production of immunoglobulins, or antibodies. One of note is, Bruton's disease, or

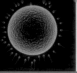

X-linked agammaglobulinaemia. As its name suggests, this is inherited as an X-linked recessive disorder. In this disorder, there are no circulating B cells, plasma cells or germinal centres in the lymph nodes. The treatment for Bruton's X-linked agammaglobulinaemia is regular immunoglobulin infusions and prompt administration of antibiotics, as well as antibiotic prophylaxis.

The most common inherited form of immunoglobulin efficiency is selective IgA deficiency. It is estimated that about 1 in 600 to 1 in 800 people have this deficiency (Janeway et al., 2001; Seymour et al., 1995). The genetic basis of IgA deficiency is unknown. Because of the importance of secretory IgA in mucosal secretions, a deficiency of this immunoglobulin tends to lead to bacterial gastrointestinal tract infections, as well as respiratory infections such as chronic lung disease. However, some people have such mild symptoms, if any, that they do not suspect that they have any disorder of the immune system. Treatment is concerned with killing the infectious organisms; therefore the short-term and prophylactic administration of antibiotics is the treatment of choice, along with nutrition and skin care. It is important to note, however, that patients with IgA deficiency should *not* be given γ-globulin infusions because there is a high risk of developing anti-IgA antibodies.

### Immunoglobulin therapy

This is a type of passive immunotherapy and consists of immunoglobulin that has been pooled from several thousand donors. Unfortunately, due to the appearance of new variant Creutzfeld–Jacob disease (vCJD), the United Kingdom no longer manufactures immunoglobulins or sends any plasma for the manufacture of γ-globulin infusions elsewhere. The plasma donors for γ-globulin preparations are rigorously screened for any diseases, particularly including HIV and hepatitis antibodies. During the manufacturing process, the γ-globulin is purified to destroy any pathogenic organisms. These purification steps include pasteurization and the adding of detergents. However, nothing done to the γ-globulin is guaranteed to remove the prions responsible for vCJD.

Once manufactured and considered safe, the γ-globulin can be given either by intravenous infusion or by a subcutaneous infusion.

### T-cell (cellular) and combined immunodeficiencies

Because of the regulatory role of T cells, most defects of T cells result in some degree of failure of the production of antibodies by the B cells. Thus, most T-cell disorders are combined disorders, being a combination of T- and B-cell immunodeficiencies. Because both arms of the cellular immune system are affected, children with a T-cell or combined immunodeficiency will suffer from infections with all types of infectious organisms, i.e. bacterial, viral, fungal and protozoal. In addition, many of the infectious organisms that cause infections in T-cell deficient children are opportunistic. Opportunistic infections are caused by microorganisms that do not normally cause problems in an immunocompetent person but, once they enter an immunodeficient host, they take the opportunity to cause major, sometime fatal, problems. *Cytomegalovirus* (CMV) and *Pneumocystis carinii* are examples of opportunistic infecting organisms, as is the fungus *Aspergillus*. The conditions are usually so severe that, without effective treatment and cure of the defect, children rarely attain adulthood.

Some of the most serious immune disorders are those that come under the heading of severe combined immunodeficiency (SCID). Without successful treatment, children with severe combined immunodeficiency will normally die before they reach their first birthday. The most severe type of severe combined immunodeficiency is reticular dysgenesis. This is a defect of T cells, B cells and granulocytes – most of the white blood cells in fact. It is a condition that leads to the death of the infant shortly after birth; death being due to overwhelming infections.

An interesting immune deficiency disorder, which does not have a hereditary origin, is DiGeorge syndrome, which is also known as thymic aplasia. This is due to the lack of a thymus, which obviously prevents the maturation and differentiation of T cells from taking place. In 90% of the cases of DiGeorge syndrome, there is a microdeletion at chromosome 22q11.2 and affected children have many problems as well as their immunodeficiency, including abnormal facies, congenital heart disease and hypoparathyroidism (Gennery et al., 2002; Segni & Zimmerman, 2002).

The signs and symptoms of severe immunodeficiency disorders can be classified into those features that are highly suspicious of an immune deficiency and those that are moderately suspicious.

Those signs and symptoms that are frequently present and highly suspicious include:

- chronic infections
- recurrent infections
- opportunistic infecting organisms
- incomplete clearing of infections
- incomplete response to infections.

Those signs and symptoms that are frequently present and moderately suspicious include:

- skin rash/eczema/candida
- failure to thrive/anorexia

- diarrhoea
- hepatomegaly
- recurrent abscesses
- evidence of autoimmunity.

Any child, or adult, seen with a combination of these signs and symptoms should be considered as possibly having an immune deficiency of some sort, and should be tested accordingly.

## CLINICAL APPLICATIONS

Children with severe combined immunodeficiency, or any of the other severe immune deficiency disorders, must be isolated immediately and placed in a reverse barrier nursing environment to protect them from any infectious organisms. They need to receive antibiotic, antiviral and antifungal drugs, usually via an intravenous route. Because of the failure to thrive, adequate nutrition is of critical importance and this may be by total parenteral nutrition (TPN). These treatments, however, are only palliative. Without curing the immune deficiency, the children will not survive long.

Since 1968, the treatment of choice has been bone marrow transplantation from a sibling donor with matching antigens of the major histocompatibility complex region. Because these disorders are genetic in origin, unfortunately there are very few siblings available to act as bone marrow donors. Consequently, the great majority of children diagnosed with severe combined immunodeficiency died as infants. However, since 1982, the use of mismatched haploidentical bone marrow transplants has transformed the chances of survival of children with severe combined immunodeficiency. A mismatched haploidentical transplant is usually obtained from a parent. Because of the way in which genes are inherited, this means that there is only half a match of the major histocompatibility complex antigens. These transplants are very difficult to perform successfully and the fact that so many children have survived is a testament to the skill of all concerned. Even so, in the early days many of the children died during the transplant procedure. However, with the advent of better immunosuppressive drugs, better techniques in the purging of T cells from the donor bone marrow, and better medical and nursing care, the survival rate now in Europe is about 70% for children having mismatched transplants. In recent years, the advent of worldwide donor lists has allowed unrelated donors who are matches to provide bone marrow for these children and for people with other disorders such as leukaemia. The matched unrelated donor transplants (or

MUDs) have further increased the survival chances of these children. In addition, the relatively recent use of peripheral stem cell transplants and the transplanting of stem cells from umbilical cord blood have also seen more children survive. Consequently, the outlook for children with these severe immunodeficiency disorders is much brighter than it was, even a few years ago. Of course, this all depends upon the child being identified as having a severe immune deficiency disorder at a very young age, and being referred to one of the specialist centres that is able to treat them (Vickers, 1999).

The treatment of adenosine deaminase (ADA) severe combined immunodeficiency with bone marrow transplants has always posed problems, and particularly in the United States, treatment of children with adenosine deaminase deficiency has also included, as an alternative to bone marrow transplantation, enzyme replacement therapy. Unfortunately this treatment has to be continually repeated at regular intervals, and so cannot be considered a cure. Because adenosine deaminase deficiency is the result of a single gene fault, it became a candidate for one of the first attempts at gene replacement therapy. Some success was obtained by inserting the gene into white cells obtained from the patient and returning them. In 2000, it was reported that gene therapy had been successfully performed on a child with another single-gene defect severe combined immunodeficiency, in France (Hacein-Bey-Abina et al., 2002; Rosen, 2002). In this case, the gene was inserted successfully into the stem cells. In 2002, successful gene therapy was performed in the United Kingdom on a child with X-linked SCID. From the beginning of this century onwards there have been international reports of success with the use of gene therapy using stem cells in children with single gene SCID (Rosen 2002, Hacien-Bey-Abinea et al., 2002, Aiuti et al., 2002 and Aiuti et al., 2003). Despite some initial setbacks (Chinon and Puck, 2004), the results so far are promising and there is now some optimism that gene replacement therapy will help children and possibly adults with immunodeficiency disorders. However, it must be remembered that these early successes with gene replacement therapy have been with single gene disorders. Many of the immunodeficiencies have a multi-gene defect, and these will be much harder to treat.

## Secondary immunodeficiencies

Secondary immune deficiencies are so called because they are secondary to an external factor. Most people are aware of one particular secondary immunodeficiency, namely acquired immunodeficiency syndrome (AIDS) caused by the human immunodeficiency virus (HIV) but there are many other causes of secondary immunodeficiencies. One of the major causes of immunodeficiency globally is protein deficiency due to malnutrition or such disorders as Kwashiorkor disease. In developed countries, apart from HIV, the major causes of secondary immunodeficiencies are iatrogenic, i.e. caused by medical personnel/treatment. These particularly include immunodeficiencies that occur following steroid or cytotoxic drug therapy for various diseases (Seymour et al., 1995). Secondary immunodeficiencies are much more common than primary immunodeficiencies but their signs and symptoms are very similar, including susceptibility to opportunistic infections, anorexia, diarrhoea, and increased risk of tumours.

Secondary immunodeficiencies are associated with a multitude of factors, including:

- infections, including HIV, hepatitis, measles, mumps, tuberculosis, congenital rubella, cytomegalovirus (CMV) and infectious mononucleosis (glandular fever)
- medications, including corticosteroids, cytotoxic drugs, immunosuppressive drugs such as cyclosporin and azathioprine, and even antibiotics
- stress, including psychological and physical stress
- malnutrition
- so-called recreational drugs, such as cocaine and heroin
- alcohol
- neoplasms (cancers), e.g. Hodgkin's lymphoma, leukaemia
- disorders of the endocrine system, e.g. diabetes
- autoimmune diseases
- ageing
- environmental chemicals such as polychlorinated biphenyls (PBCs) and dioxin
- burns and other traumas
- pregnancy
- anaesthesia and surgery
- kidney disease
- irradiation.

Treatment of secondary immunodeficiencies consists of removing or treating the cause (if at all possible) and supportive therapy until the immune system rights itself. If other diseases are causing the immunodeficiency, then these have to be tackled. Unfortunately, there are some secondary immunodeficiencies for which this does not apply. The best known of these is AIDS, although if a cure were ever found for it, then it in turn would become a transient immunodeficiency.

## HIV and AIDS

AIDS has become the fourth largest cause of death throughout the world. It has been estimated that, by the end of 2001, more than 60 000 000 people will have been infected, of whom about 20 000 000 had already died (UNAIDS, 2001). That leaves 40 000 000 people still living with AIDS or HIV. It was also estimated that in 2001 there were 5 000 000 new HIV infections (averaging at 16 000 a day), and there were 3 000 000 deaths. Of these 3 000 000 deaths, 580 000 were children aged less than 15 years. However, there is great regional variation with sub-Saharan Africa having an estimated 28 100 000 people living with HIV or AIDS (Davey & Seale, 2002).

AIDS is caused by a particular type of virus, called a retrovirus. In a retrovirus, instead of the lipoprotein envelope surrounding viral DNA, it surrounds viral RNA. Before production in the cell DNA can be taken over, the viral RNA has to become viral DNA. The lipoprotein shell surrounding the viral RNA expresses certain viral glycoprotein receptors. These receptors are mainly composed of glycoprotein gp160, which, in turn, consists of two components, namely gp 41 and gp120, which resemble major histocompatibility complex class II. The gp120 molecule is the receptor that is able to bind to CD4 receptors on the surface membrane of the host cell. This simple fact is the reason why HIV is such a dangerous virus and causes major problems to the immune system of the host. CD4 receptors are present in large numbers on the surface membranes of T-helper cells, and T-helper cells are the cells that help to regulate the immune system and stimulate it to proliferate in response to an infection. As HIV infects T-helper cells and kills them, the immune system cannot respond properly to other infectious organisms. The more the CD4 T-helper cells are destroyed, the more effective the HIV infection becomes and the sicker the host becomes. Eventu-ally, there will be too few T-helper cells in the body to be able to fight an infection, such as tuberculosis, *Pneumocystis carinii* pneumonia (PCP) and other opportunistic infections, as well as more common infections. Other cells carry CD4 receptors and so may be infected. These include macrophages, monocytes and neurones, but the major problems come from the infection and destruction of the T-helper cells.

HIV is passed in body fluids from one person to another, with the major sources of this transference of body fluids being sexual activity (particularly unprotected sex), intravenous needle sharing when taking drugs, and perinatal infection from placental transfer, blood exchange during vaginal delivery or through breast milk.

The signs and symptoms of HIV infection might not become apparent for several years after the actual infection. Initially, the infected person may get flu-like symptoms. For several years after infection, the virus may be dormant. During this time, the infected person may not show any symptoms but the virus may be reproducing and the infected host will themselves be infectious to others within 2 weeks of being infected. The period from initial infection to sero-conversion is known as the 'window period' and lasts for about 2 to 4 weeks. Seroconversion is the time when antibodies to HIV occur. These then remain detectable for life. During the time when the infected person is showing no signs or symptoms of infection, the HIV integrates into the host cells but does not replicate. However, the viruses provide a 'reservoir of infection' because while they are not replicating they cannot be recognized by the immune system and destroyed. When the immune system responds to infection by another organism, HIV replication then takes place due to signals from the T-cell receptors or from cytokines. Eventually, full-scale replication will take place and the infected host will start to experience the signs and symptoms of AIDS itself.

The signs and symptoms of AIDS are the same as for any immune deficiency; chronic and recurring infections – often by opportunistic organisms, for example, *Candida*, rashes, loss of weight, recurrent abscesses, evidence of autoimmunity and neoplasms.

There are two major types of HIV – HIV-1 and HIV-2. These are distinguished by their genetic differences, global distribution and clinical signs and symptoms. HIV-1 is the cause of the global AIDS epidemic, whereas HIV-2, found in West Africa, has a slower development and a milder course. In addition, the transfer of HIV-2 from mother to baby is rare. As well as HIV-1 and HIV-2, there are at least ten subtypes of the virus. This obviously has implications when looking for successful drug therapies and vaccines. What will work in one part of the world may not work elsewhere. Add to this the ability of HIV to mutate rapidly and it is obvious that trying to treat HIV and AIDS brings many problems. This ability to mutate rapidly and often, enables the virus to evade the immune system. This evasion occurs because the initial immune response to any novel infectious organism is slow and weak, but is much stronger with subsequent exposures. However, the mutation means that the immune system is continually coming up against what it perceives as new infectious agents, and consequently it generates the primary immune response time and time again, rather than commencing the much more effective secondary response. Any non-mutated strains of HIV are gradually eliminated by the immune system but the continuous waves of newer mutations replace these, thereby preventing the immune system from completely clearing the virus from the body (Davey & Seale, 2002).

The treatment of HIV infection and AIDS is a four-pronged attack on the disease. These four prongs are:

1. drug therapy
2. vaccine
3. immunomodulation
4. palliation.

Over the past few years, there have been many advances in drug therapy for the treatment of HIV infection and AIDS. Antiretroviral drugs are now used in combinations of three or four different drugs. These combinations have the collective title of HAART – highly active antiretroviral therapy – and have been able to arrest the progress of HIV infection, and even reverse the immune incompetence (Candy et al., 2001).

Vaccines are, in many ways, considered to be the holy grail by AIDS researchers and therapists. A huge amount of research is ongoing, but so far the difficulties have surmounted the hopes and aspirations. At the moment, no single vaccine has been produced that can cope with all the variations and mutations of HIV. Because of the rapid and frequent mutations, and the different subtypes, finding the definitive vaccine has so far proved elusive, as the vaccine needs to be effective against a range of mutations that may be present in one host at any one time, in addition to new mutations.

Immunomodulation is an attempt to boost the immune system. It has been found that a combination of interleukin-2 (IL-2), and antiretroviral drugs can reduce the number of latently infected T cells and also reduce the levels of HIV RNA in the body (Nairn & Helbert, 2002). This combination is under development at the moment, but needs to undergo many drug trials to show that the clinical improvements it brings outweigh its side-effects.

Palliative care includes the use of antibiotic, anti-viral and antifungal drugs to deal with infections and to try to prevent them becoming fatal. Other palliative measures include addressing nutritional needs, social and psychological care, stress reduction, immunizations, maintaining CD4 counts and education.

## Prognosis

Even 15 years ago, a diagnosis of HIV infection was equivalent to giving a death sentence. Now, with the greatly increased knowledge about the disease and the development of antiretroviral drug therapy, HIV has, for many in the Western world, become a disease one lives with, in much the same way as one lives with a chronic disease. The prognosis is continually improving. In the less-developed world, however, where the drugs are difficult to get hold of and are comparatively very expensive, where there are not the same medical and social support systems in place and where good nutrition and lack of stress are not available, then AIDS remains a malignant and ever-present killer.

## Conclusion

This chapter has attempted to explain the ways that the acquired immune system functions, and to demonstrate its importance to the well-being of individuals and of populations.

Immunology is a dynamic subject. New knowledge of the immune system and of therapies to cope with disorders associated with the immune system is continually being published. For example, the section in this chapter on gene therapy for immune deficiencies had been completed when the very next day came news of more successes. Consequently, that section had to be amended to keep it up to date. Since the completion of the chapter, other news stories have included the declaration that 51 European nations have now been declared officially free of polio after 3 years without an indigenous case. This eradication is the result of immunization. There has also been the prediction that it may be possible to vaccinate against asthma and arthritis, and also the discovery of a defective gene (ADAM 33) linked to asthma that could lead to earlier, and better, methods of diagnosis and treatment of asthma. Furthermore, there is the hope that a vaccine against many HIV strains has now been found and is to undergo human trials, as well as a gene (CEM 15) having now been found that appears to provide a natural defence against HIV and may within 10 years be used in HIV therapy. All these may, or may not, be of value in future therapies. Even if they are found to be of value, it will be several years before they become accepted therapies. There is now so much progress being made that it is impossible to predict the future in this discipline; but then even 10 years ago few would have predicted the state of knowledge and the therapies that are now being used. This is what makes immunology such an exciting specialty in medicine.

## Clinical review

In addition to the Learning Objectives at the beginning of this chapter, the reader should be able to:

- Describe the role of the major histocompatibility complex in the functioning of the immune system and its importance to the success of organ, blood and marrow transplants

- Compare and contrast the development and method of function of the cell-mediated and humoral immune systems

- Outline the mechanisms by which autoimmunity occurs and give examples of diseases of established autoimmune aetiology

- Describe the functions of lymph glands and outline the clinical implications of the functions

- Describe the clinical manifestations of anaphylactic shock, outlining the underlying care of each

- Outline some possible ways in which autoimmunity may occur, and give examples of disorders of known autoimmune aetiology

- Explain the role of the cell-mediated immune system in the rejection of transplanted tissue

- Outline the causes of both primary and secondary immunodeficiencies

- Explain the rationale for the signs and symptoms of immunodeficient disorders

## Review questions

1   What is formed by the binding together of an antibody and an antigen?
2   How do leucocytes deal with immune complexes?
3   How does humoral immunity differ from cell-mediated immunity?

4   How would you describe autoimmunity?

5   How do T-helper cells and T-suppressor cells differ?

6   What do T-killer cells do?

7   Where are major histocompatibility complex proteins found?

8   Which cells are responsible for humoral immunity?

9   What are memory cells responsible for?

10  Describe an immunoglobulin molecule?

11  Which common condition is caused by the interaction of antigens with IgE antibodies?

12  What is the essential difference between passive and active immunization?

13  Why do autografts cause less problems than allografts?

14  Which cells are particularly affected by HIV?

## Suggestions for further reading

All of the books referenced in the text are well worth referring to for further information but the ones included in this section are of especial note.

Abbas, A.K. & Lichtman, A.H. (2001) *Basic Immunology: The functions of the Immune System*. Philadelphia: W.B. Saunders.
*A shorter textbook that emphasizes the basic concepts and principles of human immunology.*

Arshad, S.H. (2002) *Allergy: An Illustrated Colour Text*. Edinburgh: Churchill Livingstone.
*A very clear and colourful introduction to all aspects of allergies.*

Davey, B., Halliday, T. & Horst, M. (2001) *Human Biology and Health: An Evolutionary Approach*, 3rd edn. Buckingham: Open University Press.
*This very readable book includes an excellent chapter on the immune system related to infectious diseases.*

Davey, B. & Seale, C. (2002) *Expressing and Explaining Disease*, 3rd edn. Buckingham: Open University Press.
*This book contains several chapters which are directly related to the immune system, including allergies, autoimmune disease and AIDS. Very readable, and presents a holistic approach.*

IPOPI (1995) *The Story of Primary Immunodeficiencies*. London: International Patient Organisation for Primary Immunodeficiencies.
*This book tells the story of primary immunodeficiencies from the patients' and parents' perspectives. It is a moving testament to the courage of all concerned. For information on this book contact the Primary Immunodeficiency Association (PIA).*

Isenberg, D. & Morrow, J. (1995) *Friendly Fire: Explaining Autoimmune Disease*. Oxford: Oxford University Press.
*Lives up to its name by giving very clear explanations of autoimmune diseases.*

Janeway, C.A., Travers, P., Walport, M. et al. (2005) *Immunology*, 6th edn. New York: Garland Publishing.

*Complements the Nairn and Helbert book 'Immunology for Medical students', but is much more technical and scientific. Includes a CD Rom. A 'must have' for the specialist immunology nurse.*

Kirkwood, E. & Lewis, C. (1989) *Understanding Medical Immunology*, 2nd edn. Chichester: John Wiley.
*Although an 'old' textbook, this is still one of the best, simple introductions to the immune system for nurses, and is a good springboard for progression to further, more modern texts.*

Martin, P. (1978) *The Sickening Mind: Brain, Behaviour, Immunity and Disease*. London: HarperCollins.
*This very readable book looks at the effect of the brain on immunity and the immune system on the brain. It has a very good section on stress and immunity.*

Nairn, R. & Helbert, M. (2002) *Immunology for Medical Students*. St Louis: Mosby.
*This is an excellent book, which is well presented and includes clinical material and diagnostic techniques.*

Roitt, I. (2001) *Roitt's Essential Immunology*, 10th edn. Oxford: Blackwell Science.
*A highly readable text with a supporting website at www.roitt.com*

Roitt, I., Brostoff, J. & Male, D. (2001) *Immunology*, 6th edn. St Louis: Mosby.
*Another excellent text by Roitt, this time in partnership with Brostoff and Male – all renowned in the field of immunology. Also contains a free CD with three animations.*

Stiehm, E.R., Ochs, H.D. & Winklestein, J.A. (2004) *Immunologic Disorders in Infants and Children*, 6th edn. Philadelphia: W.B. Saunders.

The following papers complement the ones referred to in the text. Of particular mention are the series of papers on advances in the immune system published in the *New England Journal of Medicine* during 2000 and 2001.

Busse, W.W. & Lemanske, R.F. (2001) Asthma. *New England Journal of Medicine*, **344**(15); 1140–1144.

Crystal, R.G. (1995) Transfer of genes to humans: Early lessons and obstacles to success. *Science*, **270**; 404–410.

Davidson, A. & Diamond, B. (2001) Autoimmune diseases. *New England Journal of Medicine*, **345**(5); 340–350.

Deeg, H.J. & Storb, R. (1984) Graft-versus-Host Disease: Pathophysiological and clinical aspects. *Annual Review of Medicine*, **35**; 11–24.

Delves, P.J. & Roitt, M. (2000) The Immune System: Part 2. *New England Journal of Medicine*, **343**(2); 108–117.

Hirschhorn, R. (1977) Defects of purine metabolism in immunodeficiency diseases. *Progress in Clinics in Immunology*, **3**; 67–83.

Hirschhorn, R. (1993) Overview of biochemical abnormalities and molecular genetics of adenosine deaminase deficiency. *Pediatric Research*, **33**(1); S35–S41.

Hoare, S., El-Shazali, O. & Clark, J.E. et al. (2002) Investigations for complement deficiency following meningococcal disease. *Archives of Diseases of Childhood*, **86**; 215–217.

Kay, A.B. (2001) Allergy and allergic diseases: Part 2. *New England Journal of Medicine*, **344**(2); 109–113.

Klein, J. & Sato, A. (2000) The HLA System: Part 2. *New England Journal of Medicine*, **343**; 782–786.

Lekstrom-Hines, J.A. & Gallin, J.I. (2000) Immunodeficiency diseases caused by defects in phagocytes. *New England Journal of Medicine*, **343**(28); 1703–1714.

Macdougall, C.F., Cant, A.J. & Colver, A.F. (2002) How dangerous is food allergy in childhood? The incidence of severe and fatal allergic reactions across the UK and Ireland. *Archives of Diseases of Childhood*, **86**; 236–239.

Noonan, N.A. & Senner, A.M. (1994) Gene therapy techniques in the treatment of adenosine deaminase deficiency severe combined immunodeficiency syndrome. *Journal of Perinatal and Neonatal Nursing*, **7**(4); 65–78.

Pappas, B.E.K. (1999) Primary immunodeficiency disorders in infancy. *Neonatal Network*, **18**(1); 13–22.

Smith, F.O. & Thomson, B.G. (2000) Umbilical cord blood collection, banking and transplantation: Current status and issues relevant to perinatal caregivers. *Birth*, **27**(2); 127–135.

Strachen, D.P. (2000) Family size, infection and atopy; the first decade of the 'hygiene hypothesis'. *Thorax*, **55**(suppl 1); S2–S10.

Vickers, P.S. (1990a) A bleak inheritance. *Nursing*, **4**(22); 18–21.

Vickers, P.S. (1990b) Severe combined immunodeficiency syndrome. *Nursing*, **4**(23); 32–35.

Vickers, P.S. (1990c) Mismatched bone marrow transplants. *Nursing*, **4**(24); 33–36.

Von Andrian, U.H. & Mackay, C.R. (2000) T-cell function and migration. *New England Journal of Medicine*, **343**(14); 1020–1033.

Walport, M.J. (2001) Complement: Part 2. *New England Journal of Medicine*, **344**(15); 1140–1144.

Zinkernagel, R.M. (2001) Maternal antibodies, childhood infections and autoimmune diseases. *New England Journal of Medicine*, **345**(18); 1331–1344.

## Useful websites

www.ImmuneDisease.com
*Offers in-depth information for consumers and health-care professionals on immunology and primary immuno-deficiency diseases.*

www.vcfs.net/
*For information on the 22q11 Group (velo-cardio-facial Syndrome – DiGeorge syndrome).*

www.hebw.uwcm.ac.uk
*Microbiology lectures – lecture 25 is on the principle and practice of immunization.*

www.ebandolier.com
*Information on intravenous immunoglobulin therapy.*

www.doh.gov.uk
*A whole series of documents, some of which are concerned with immunization.*

www.generalpractice.co.uk
*For information on immunizations.*

www.molbiol.ox.ac.uk/www/pathology/
*Lots of information on the immune system.*

www.rheumatology.org.research/guidelines/
*Information on arthritis and rheumatism.*

www.ebmt.org
*The website of the European Blood and Marrow Transplant group, including the nurse's group.*

www.ingid.org
*The website for the International Nursing Group for Immunodeficiencies.*

www.edcenter.med.cornell.edu/CUMC_PathNotes/Immunopathology/
*Introduction to the normal immune system and problems that can occur.*

www.nhsdirect.nhs.u.../immunisationschedule.as
*As its name suggest, gives an update on immunization schedules.*

## Useful address

PIA (Primary Immunodeficiency Association)
Alliance House, 12, Caxton Street, London,
SW1H 0QS
*The patient's association for immunodeficiency in the UK*

## References

Ada, G.L. (2001) Vaccines and vaccination. *New England Journal of Medicine*, **345**(14); 1042–1053.

Ada, G.L. & Ramsey, A.J. (1997) Vaccines, vaccination and the immune response. Philadelphia: Lippincott-Raven.

Aidoo, M., Terlouw, D.J., Kokzak, et al. (2002) Protective effects of the sickle cell gene against malaria morbidity and mortality. *European Journal of Pediatrics*, **161**; 233–234.

Aiuti, A., Ficaro, F., Cattaneo, F. et al. (2003) Gene therapy for adenosine deaminase deficiency. *Current Opinion in Allergy and Clinical Immunology*, **3**(6); 461–466

Aiuti, A., Slavin, S., Aker, M. et al. (2002) Correction of ADA-SCID by stem cell gene therapy combined with nonmyeloablative conditioning. *Science*, **296**; 2410–2413.

Barkin, R.M. & Rosen, P. (1999) *Emergency Pediatrics: A Guide to Ambulatory Care*, 5th edn. St Louis: Mosby.

Bruton, O.C. (1952) Agammaglobulinaemia. *Pediatrics*, **9**; 722–728.

Buckley, R.H. (2000) Primary immunodeficiency diseases due to defects in lymphocytes. *New England Journal of Medicine*, **343**(18); 1313–1324.

Candy, D., Davies, G. & Ross, P. (2001) Clinical paediatrics and child health. Edinburgh: W.B. Saunders.

Chapel, H. & Haeney, M. (1993) *Essentials of Clinical Immunology*, 3rd edn. Oxford: Blackwell Scientific Publications.

Chinen, J. & Puck, J.M. (2004) Successes and risks of gene therapy in primary immunodeficiencies. *Journal of Allergy and Clinical Immunology*, **113**(4); 595–603.

Concannon, P., Gogolin-Ewens, K.J., Hinds, D.A. et al. (1998) A second-generation screen of the human genome for susceptibility to insulin-dependent diabetes mellitus. *Nature Genetics*, **19**; 292–296.

Crystal, R.G. (1995) Transfer of genes to humans: Early lessons and obstacles to success. *Science*, **270**; 404–410.

Davey, B. & Seale, C. (2002) *Experiencing and Explaining Disease*, 3rd edn. Buckingham: Open University Press.

Delves, P.J. & Roitt, I.M. (2000) The immune system: Part 1. *New England Journal of Medicine*, **343**(1); 37–49.

Gell, P.G.H. & Coombs, R.R.A. (1968) *Clinical Aspects of Immunology*, 2nd edn. Philadelphia: FA Davis.

Gennery, A.R., Barge, D., O'Sullivan, J.J. et al. (2002) Antibody deficiency and autoimmunity in 22q11.2 deletion syndrome. *Archives of Diseases in Childhood*, **87**; 26–29.

Gibbon, C., Smith, T., Egger, P. et al. (1997) Early infection and subsequent insulin dependent diabetes. *Archives of Diseases in Childhood*, **77**; 384–385.

Glanzmann, E. & Riniker, P. (1950) Essentielle Lymphocytophthise: Ein neues Krankheitsbild aus der Säuglingspathologie. *Annals of Paediatrics*, **175**; 1–32.

Hacein-Bey-Abina, S., Le Diest, F., Carlier, F. et al. (2002) Sustained correction of X-linked severe combined immunodeficiency by ex vivo gene therapy. *New England Journal of Medicine*, **346**(16); 1185–1193.

Isenberg, D. & Morrow, J. (1995) *Friendly Fire: Explaining Autoimmune Disease*. Oxford: Oxford University Press.

IUIS Scientific Committee (1999) Primary immunodeficiency diseases: report of an IUIS Scientific Committee. *Clinical and Experimental Immunology*, **118**(suppl 1); 1–28.

Janeway, C.A., Travers, P., Walport, M. et al. (2005) *Immunobiology*, 6th edn. New York: Garland Publishing.

Kamradt, T. & Mitchison, N.A. (2001) Tolerance and autoimmunity. *New England Journal of Medicine*, **344**(9); 655–664.

Kassianos, G. (2001) *Immunization – Childhood and Travel Health*, 4th edn. London: Blackwell Sciences.

Kay, A.B. (2001) Allergy and allergic diseases: Part 1. *New England Journal of Medicine*, **344**(1); 30–37.

Klein, L., Klugmann, M., Nave, K.A. et al. (2000) Shaping of the autoreactive T-cell repertoire by a splice variant of self-protein expressed in thymic epithelial cells. *Nature Medicine*, **6**; 56–61.

Klein, J. & Sato, A. (2000) The HLA system: Part 1. *New England Journal of Medicine*, **343**(10); 702–709.

Kurtzke, J.E. (1993) Epidemiologic evidence for multiple sclerosis as an infection. *Clinical and Microbiological Review*, **6**; 382–427.

Male, D. (1991) *Immunology: An Illustrated Outline*, 2nd edn. London: Gower Medical Publishing.

Mayerson, H.S. (1963) The lymphatic system. In: *1976 Readings from the Scientific American. Immunology*. San Francisco: W.H. Freeman.

McCance, K.L. & Huether, S.E. (2002) *Pathophysiology: The Biologic Basis for Disease in Adults and Children*, 4th edn. St Louis: Mosby.

Mein, C.A., Eposito, L., Dunn, M.G. et al. (1998) A search for type 1 diabetes susceptibility genes in families from the United Kingdom. *Nature Genetics*, **19**; 297–300.

Nairn, R. & Helbert, M. (2002) *Immunology for Medical Students*. St Louis: Mosby.

Noonan, N.A. & Senner, S.A.M. (1994) Gene therapy techniques in the treatment of adenosine deaminase deficiency severe combined immunodeficiency syndrome. *Journal of Perinatal and Neonatal Nursing*, **7**(4); 65–78.

Ochs, H.D., Smith, C.I.E. & Puck, J.M. (1999) *Primary Immunodeficiency Diseases: A Molecular and Genetic Approach*. Oxford: Oxford University Press.

Roitt, I.M. (1994) *Essential Immunology*, 8th edn. Oxford: Blackwell Scientific Publications.

Roitt, I.M. (2001) *Roitt's Essential Immunology*, 10th edn. Oxford: Blackwell Scientific Publications.

Rosen, F. (2002) Successful gene therapy for severe combined immunodeficiency. *New England Journal of Medicine*, **346**(16); 1241–1242.

Salisbury, D.M. (1996) *Immunisation Against Infectious Disease*. London: The Stationery Office.

Segni, M. & Zimmerman, D. (2002) Autoimmune hyperthyroidism in two adolescents with DiGeorge/velocardiofacial syndrome (22q11 deletion). *European Journal of Pediatrics*, **161**; 233–234.

Seymour, G.J., Savage, N.W. & Walsh, L.J. (1995) *Immunology: As Introduction for the Health Sciences*. Roseville, Australia: McGraw-Hill.

Sherrif, A., Golding, J., ALSPAC Study Team (2002a) Factors associated with different hygiene practices in the homes of 15 month old infants. *Archives of Diseases in Childhood*, **86**; 30–35.

Sherrif, A., Golding, J., ALSPAC Study Team (2002b) Hygiene levels in a contemporary population cohort are associated with wheezing and atopic eczema in preschool infants. *Archives of Diseases in Childhood*, **87**; 26–29.

Stiehm, E.R., Ochs, H.D. & Winklestein, J.A. (2004) *Immunologic Disorders in Infants and Children*, 5th edn. Philadelphia: W.B. Saunders.

Strachen, D.P. (1989) Hay fever, hygiene and household size. *British Medical Journal*, **299**;1258–1259.

UNAIDS (2001) *AIDS epidemic update*. Geneva: United Nations.

Vickers, P.S. (1999) *Severe Combined Immunodeficiency: A Chronic Disease and a Paediatric Emergency?* PhD thesis.

Von Mutius, E., Martinez, F.D., Fritzsch, C. et al. (1994) Prevalence of asthma and atopy in two areas of West and East Germany. *American Journal of Respiratory and Critical Care Medicine*, **149**; 358–364.

Walport, M.J. (2001) Complement: Part 1. *New England Journal of Medicine*, **344**(14); 1058–1066.

# Chapter 6.3

# Reproduction

*Rosamund A. Herbert*   *Ruth Walker*

## LEARNING OBJECTIVES

After studying this chapter the reader should be able to:

- Describe the mechanisms involved in the determination of the sex of an individual

- Describe the normal physiology of the male and female reproductive systems

- Demonstrate how disruption of normal function can lead to abnormal states or disease.

- Discuss the complex anatomical and physiological integration necessary for the optimum functioning of the male and female reproductive systems to ensure continuation of the species

## INTRODUCTION

Reproductive biology is the science of the transmission of life. It is essential that animals reproduce to ensure the survival of their species. The efficient and complex reproductive system in humans has enabled us to evolve and survive for several million years. The mechanisms involved in reproduction will be discussed in this chapter.

The function of the reproductive system is to produce gametes (germ cells) and to provide the optimum conditions for the fusion of two gametes, one from the male and one from the female. The human female also has to provide a life-support system for the first 9 months of a new individual's life; thus her body must adapt and provide a suitable environment during that time.

Research into many aspects of human reproductive physiology is ongoing. For ethical reasons, most of this research has been conducted on animals, and great care must be taken in extrapolating conclusions from animal experiments to humans. Humans are very much 'animals with culture' and, in many instances, social and cultural influences greatly modify our basic instincts and behaviour. This is especially true in some aspects of reproductive biology.

Nevertheless, pure research into reproductive physiology is progressing, particularly in areas applicable to medicine and many advances have been made over the last 30 years. For example, research by Steptoe and Edwards in the 1970s enabled an infertile woman to have a baby by the development of a method to extract a mature ovum, fertilize it in vitro (in a laboratory)

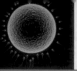
and return it to the mother. In vitro fertilization and embryo transfer are common procedures now.

Before discussing the male and female reproductive systems in detail, it is appropriate to consider how the sex of an individual is determined.

## The determination of the sex of an individual

In each human somatic cell there are 46 chromosomes, that is, 23 pairs. These are divided into 22 pairs of autosomes and one pair of sex chromosomes; the latter are given the names X and Y due to the shape of the chromosomes. The human female has the complement XX in all her cells and the male XY in all his cells (see Fig. 6.4.1, p. 778). The genetic sex of an individual is determined when the two gametes (the ovum and sperm) fuse at the time of fertilization.

The formation of gametes (germ cells) is known as **gametogenesis** and the type of cell division that results in the formation of gametes is **meiosis**. Meiotic cell division is unique to reproductive cells and gamete production (meiosis is considered in detail in Chapter 6.4).

Meiosis begins in immature reproductive cells and involves two successive nuclear divisions. The end-result is four haploid daughter cells, each containing 23 chromosomes. One of the most important aspects of meiosis is the halving of the chromosome number: each gamete must contain the haploid number of chromosomes so that when the male and female gametes fuse the resulting zygote will have the full complement of 46 chromosomes – the same number as each parent.

During the first division of meiosis, when the homologous pairs split, each resulting gamete receives one sex chromosome. The gametes from the female will all contain one X chromosome, whereas those from the male will contain *either* an X chromosome or a Y chromosome. The chromosomal sex of an individual is determined by the nature of the two gametes that unite at the time of fertilization, that is, by the sex chromosomes carried in the gametes from the parents (**Fig. 6.3.1**). So the chromosomal or genetic sex of the offspring is determined by the spermatozoon (the male gamete).

There is general agreement now that, in females, one of the two X chromosomes is inactivated in all body cells soon after fertilization (see Chapter 6.4). This is thought to be a device to compensate for the extra genetic information carried by the female on the second X chromosome. The small Y chromosome in the male was originally thought to carry very little genetic information. Recent work has shown that relatively short regions at either end of the Y chromosome are still identical to corresponding regions on the X chromosome, but the majority (95%) of the Y chromosome is a 'male specific region' of DNA and is responsible for differentiating the sexes: it includes testis specific genes that may have a role in male fertility (Willard, 2003).

For each mating there is, in theory, a 50% chance (two out of four) that a female will result and a 50% chance that a male will result. However, the observed sex ratio at birth shows that usually more males are born than females. The exact ratio varies from place to place and from time to time but, at present, in England and Wales the ratio at birth is approximately 106 males to every 100 females. It is not known what factor or factors favour conception by Y spermatozoa.

However, more than the sex chromosome complement is involved in the determination of the gender of an individual. For example, for an individual to be truly male he needs an XY chromosome complement, normal male gonads (testes) and genitalia and the presence of normal quantities of male hormones. True females need an XX chromosome complement, normal female gonads (ovaries) and genitalia and the presence of normal quantities of female hormones.

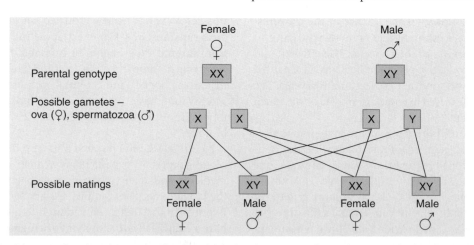

**Figure 6.3.1** Diagram showing the mechanism by which the chromosomal sex of an individual is determined

## DEVELOPMENTAL ISSUES

In embryological life, the male and female gonads are derived from the same site in the body and the primitive gonads are initially identical in both sexes. During the seventh week of embryonic life in genetic males, testes begin to develop. Testicular differentiation is the central event in the sex determination of humans. A gene on the Y chromosome has been identified that is able to induce testis differentiation. This isolated gene has been termed SRY (sex-determining region on the Y chromosome) and activates the male developmental pathway. Once testes have been formed all other differences between the sexes are secondary effects due to hormones or factors produced by the gonads. The absence of this testis determining factor (TDF) results in the undifferentiated gonad becoming an ovary, but this does not occur until about the thirteenth week of embryonic development. The steps leading to development of normal ovarian function are likely to be more complex and other genes are also involved in the process.

The primitive genital tracts, composed of the Müllerian (paramesonephric) ducts and the Wolffian (mesonephric) ducts, are also identical initially in XX and XY embryos **(Fig. 6.3.2)**. After 7–8 weeks the normal male tract begins to develop

from the Wolffian ducts in a male XY embryo, and the Müllerian ducts regress. Hormones produced by the fetal testes are responsible for these changes. The fetal testes are capable of secreting two distinct classes of hormones, which act directly on adjacent structures before being secreted into the systemic circulation to produce more generalized effects. One of these secretions, from the Leydig cells, is an androgen (male hormone, dihydrotestosterone) and it causes development of the Wolffian duct into the vas deferens, seminal vesicles and other male sexual organs. However, it does not inhibit the Müllerian duct; the other testicular hormone, produced by the Sertoli cells, does this. This is a peptide hormone (*not* an androgen) known as the Müllerian-inhibitory factor or hormone.

The female genital tract develops later from the Müllerian ducts, and the presence or absence of ovaries seems to have little or no obvious effect on its development. However, it is possible that the presence of high levels of oestrogens within the fetal ovaries may have some, as yet undefined, role to play in the development of the female reproductive system.

The development of the external genitalia in the male depends upon androgenic stimulation before the twelfth week. In the absence of androgen the external genitalia are those of a female, irrespective both of the chromosomal sex

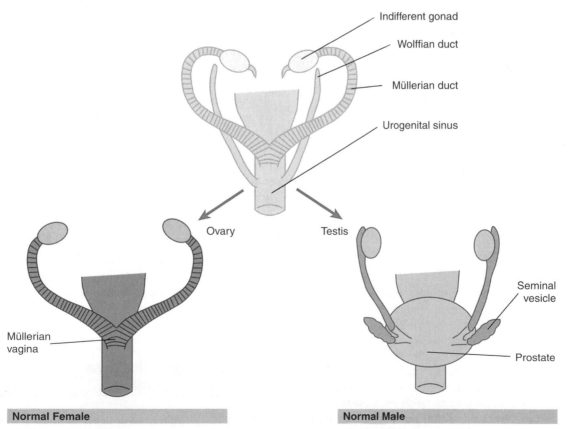

**Figure 6.3.2**   Differentiation of Müllerian and Wolffian ducts in male and female embryos

and even of gonadal sex. Thus the sexual differentiation of the gonads appears to be primarily dependent on chromosomal make-up, but the later differentiation of the genital tract and external genitalia largely depends upon the presence or absence of fetal testicular hormones. Gradually, during intrauterine life, the ovaries or testes descend from their original position high in the abdomen. In the female the ovaries and their associated tubes come to lie within the pelvis; in the male the testes normally descend into the scrotum before birth, by the eighth fetal month. The production of male gametes (**spermatogenesis**) occurs optimally just below body temperature, and the temperature within the descended testes is approximately 35°C.

Testicular descent is controlled by at least two hormones, and the evidence supports the view that Müllerian-inhibiting factor initiates transabdominal migration, whereas testosterone mediates inguinoscrotal descent. Occasionally, the testes may be retained within the abdomen (**cryptorchidism**) or their descent may be arrested at the abdominal end of the inguinal canal. If the condition is bilateral and the testes are not lowered during childhood (this can be done by hormone therapy using human chorionic gonadotrophin or surgery), the male will be sterile. An undescended testis left in the abdomen may undergo malignant changes, when it is thought that the higher body temperature causes degeneration of the tubular epithelium in the testes. Undescended testicles are a known risk factor for testicular cancer.

The sex hormones secreted even during embryonic life have effects on other aspects of the embryo's development and play a vital role in the development of sexual dimorphisms (i.e. exists in two forms in the two sexes) in the brain. In experimental animals there is clear evidence that the early embryonic brain is similar in both sexes and that conversion to the male type occurs ostensibly under the influence of testosterone at an early stage of development.

Extensive sexual differentiation of the brain has profound physiological and behavioural consequences. It seems that hormones can permanently alter the 'wiring diagram' if present at the appropriate stage of brain development, leading to differences between male and female brains in later life. Certainly work done with rats has shown that if testosterone is present in the blood during an early critical period, the animal will be permanently masculinized and also defeminized. The timing of the steroid action is crucial. Studies have shown that there are sexually

dimorphic nuclei (SDN) in the anterior part of the hypothalamus: this has been studied extensively in rodents, but similar changes are thought to exist in the interstitial nuclei of the anterior hypothalamus (INAH) in humans. These brain dimorphisms result from effects of circulating hormones during development. So sex steroids act early in development to organize neural pathways responsible for reproductive behaviour. A large range of animal behaviours are sexually dimorphic (i.e. males and females behave quite differently) but in humans these behaviours are more complex and often not very distinct. The differences between human male and female brains are small, but they do exist, and there will be a continuum of developmental differences *and* behavioural differences, with varying degrees of masculinization or feminization. The complex process of sexual differentiation, as just described, helps to explain the many variations in male and female differentiation that are observed clinically and also explains manifestations of intersex states. Aberrations of sexual development can arise either from changes in sex chromosomes or sex chromosome complement (see Chapter 6.4) or from abnormalities in sex differentiation due to hormonal or environmental causes. Congenital adrenal hyperplasia (CAH), or adrenogenital syndrome (AGS) as it is also called, is an example of this; a metabolic error can lead to overproduction of androgen in the adrenal glands and this change results in partial masculinization of the external genitalia. The changes that occur at puberty to differentiate males from females are also hormone dependent and will be discussed later in this chapter.

Thus, when considering the determination of sex of an individual, this can be considered in several ways – the genotypic sex (i.e. the genetic make-up) and the phenotypic sex (how the individual looks with his/her individual primary and secondary sexual characteristics). In addition, there is the gender identification, the subjective perception of one's sex, and this will result from a combination of the effects of the gonadal hormones (both in utero and throughout life) and the societal and cultural influences. Prenatal exposure to androgens could influence development of gender role behaviours. Gonadal hormones control our behaviour throughout life. During development they determine whether we will show male- or female-typical behavioural patterns. In adults they affect sexual behaviour.

## The functioning of the male reproductive system

A discussion of male reproductive physiology can be divided into three sections: the production of spermatozoa (the male gametes), the endocrine function of the testis, and the endocrine control of these processes. A brief description of the male reproductive system will be given first.

The male genital system consists of two testes and their ducts, several accessory glands and the penis **(Fig. 6.3.3)**. The **testes** are situated in the scrotum. The tubules and ducts from each testis unite to form the **epididymis (Fig. 6.3.4)** and from here the **vas deferens** (ductus deferens) travels up into the pelvis, passes anterior to the public symphysis and then loops around the ureter. At this point, the vas deferens enlarges to become the ampulla. A **seminal vesicle**, one of the accessory sex glands, joins each vas at the lower end of the ampulla. The duct is then known as the **ejaculatory duct**. The two ejaculatory ducts (one from each ampulla and testis) fuse with the urethra in the middle of the prostate gland. The resultant duct, known as the **prostatic urethra**, is a common duct for both urination and the carriage of semen. The ducts from two additional accessory glands, the **bulbourethral glands** (Cowper's glands), join the urethra which enters the penis.

The **penis** is an elongated organ composed of mainly vascular spaces making up the erectile tissue and consists of three cylindrical bodies: two dorsal corpora cavernosa and ventrally one corpus spongiosum **(Fig. 6.3.5)**. The penile urethra, which is lined with mucus-secreting glands, traverses the corpus spongiosum to the external urethral meatus. The head, or **glans penis**, is usually covered by the **prepuce**, or foreskin.

## Spermatogenesis

The production of spermatozoa, or spermatogenesis occurs in the seminiferous tubules of the testis **(see Figs 6.3.4 and 6.3.6)**. Each testis is divided into many compartments, each containing one or more minute **seminiferous tubules**. Within each testicular compartment, connective tissue containing the **Leydig cells** (or **interstitial cells**) surrounds the seminiferous tubules. The Leydig cells are concerned with the synthesis and release of androgenic (male) hormones.

There are two types of cell in the seminiferous tubule of an active testis: the germ cells and the Sertoli cells **(see Fig. 6.3.6)**. At any one time, the germ cells are at various stages of development but they all originate from **spermatogonia**. The spermatogonia undergo continuous mitotic divisions to ensure a constant

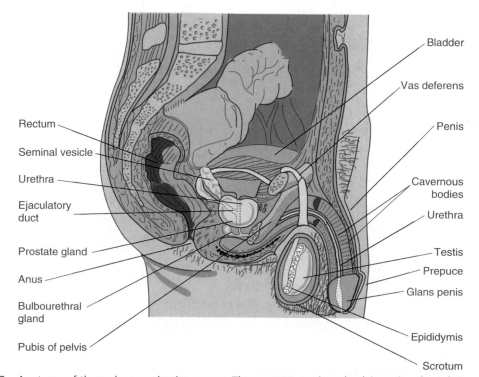

**Figure 6.3.3**  Anatomy of the male reproductive system. The scrotum, penis and pelvic regions have been cut sagittally to show their internal structures

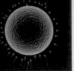

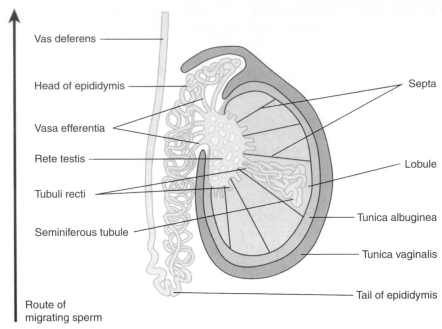

Vas deferens

Head of epididymis

Vasa efferentia

Rete testis

Tubuli recti

Seminiferous tubule

Route of
migrating sperm

Septa

Lobule

Tunica albuginea

Tunica vaginalis

Tail of epididymis

**Figure 6.3.4**   Structure of one testes

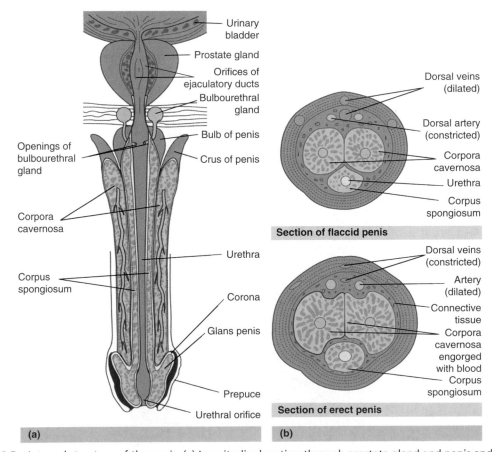

Urinary
bladder

Prostate gland

Orifices of
ejaculatory ducts

Bulbourethral
gland

Bulb of penis

Crus of penis

Openings of
bulbourethral
gland

Corpora
cavernosa

Corpus
spongiosum

Urethra

Corona

Glans penis

Prepuce

Urethral orifice

(a)

Dorsal veins
(dilated)

Dorsal artery
(constricted)

Corpora
cavernosa

Urethra

Corpus
spongiosum

**Section of flaccid penis**

Dorsal veins
(constricted)

Artery
(dilated)

Connective
tissue

Corpora
cavernosa
engorged
with blood

Corpus
spongiosum

**Section of erect penis**

(b)

**Figure 6.3.5**   Internal structure of the penis. (a) Longitudinal section through prostate gland and penis and
(b) cross-section through flaccid and erect penis. Note that the erectile tissues of the corpora cavernosa and corpus
spongiosum are engorged with blood in the erect penis

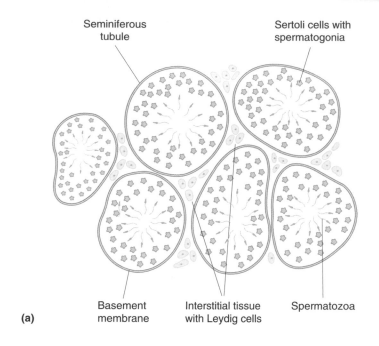

Seminiferous tubule

Sertoli cells with spermatogonia

Basement membrane

Interstitial tissue with Leydig cells

Spermatozoa

**(a)**

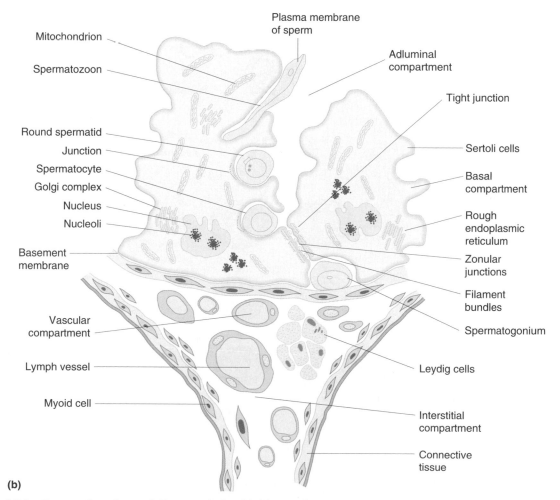

Mitochondrion

Spermatozoon

Plasma membrane of sperm

Adluminal compartment

Tight junction

Round spermatid

Junction

Spermatocyte

Golgi complex

Nucleus

Nucleoli

Basement membrane

Sertoli cells

Basal compartment

Rough endoplasmic reticulum

Zonular junctions

Filament bundles

Spermatogonium

Vascular compartment

Lymph vessel

Myoid cell

Leydig cells

Interstitial compartment

Connective tissue

**(b)**

**Figure 6.3.6**   Cross-section of a seminiferous tubule with (a) a small section enlarged and (b) showing the microscopic structure of the testis. (Adapted from Pond C (ed) 1992, Reproductive Physiology Animal Physiology, Book 1. Oxford: Ou Press.)

**supply of germ cells.** Some of these cells mature and increase in size to become primary **spermatocytes**. These primary spermatocytes undergo the first meiotic division to become secondary spermatocytes, which then contain only the haploid number of chromosomes. The secondary spermatocytes undergo the second division of meiosis to become **spermatids (Fig. 6.3.7)**.

The spermatids are in close association with the Sertoli cells. The **Sertoli cells** are polymorphic cells (occurring in many shapes) that are attached to the basement membrane but extend into the lumen of the seminiferous tubule **(see Fig. 6.3.6)**. The Sertoli cells surround the developing sperm cells and synchronize the events of spermatogenesis. The Sertoli cells also secrete critical proteins (e.g. growth factors,

androgen-binding protein and inhibin) that are important for testis function and spermatogenesis. They also have a phagocytic function, enabling any cellular constituents to be recycled.

Special tight junctions between the Sertoli cells help to form the important blood–testis barrier, which helps prevent any of the man's white blood cells from coming into contact with the haploid sperm. An immune response could be triggered by contact with his 'foreign' haploid sperm. Such a response may lead to reduced male fertility as can occur, for example, as a result of the inflammatory response elicited by mumps.

The spermatids, still in close association with the Sertoli cells, undergo transformation from relatively

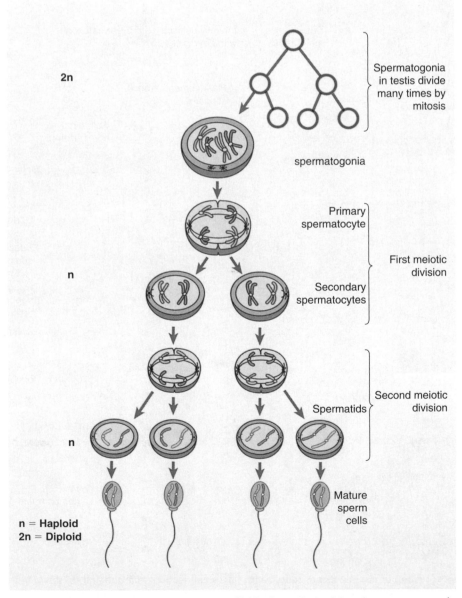

**Figure 6.3.7** Spermatogenesis. The primary spermatocyte divides by meiosis giving rise to two secondary spermatocytes and then four spermatids, which differentiate to form mature sperm cells with a haploid complement of chromosomes. For clarity only two chromosome pairs are shown

simple cells into the highly specialized **spermatozoa**. Changes occur in both the nucleus and cytoplasm of the cell. The chromatin of the nucleus condenses to become the head of the spermatozoon; the Golgi apparatus contributes towards the formation of the **acrosome** (which contains hyaluronidases and proteinases that help the spermatozoon penetrate both the mucus plug of the cervix and the ovum); one of the centrioles in the cell lengthens to form the tail, and the mitochondria aggregate in the middle section of the spermatozoon, thereby providing the structures necessary for the high-energy production needed for propulsion. Any superfluous cytoplasm is lost **(Fig. 6.3.8)**.

Once the spermatozoa have been produced, they are released from the Sertoli cells into the lumen of the seminiferous tubule. However, they are not functionally mature at this stage; completion of the maturation process occurs while the spermatozoa are stored in the epididymis. The total time taken for the production of mature spermatozoa from spermatogonia is approximately 70–100 days.

### DEVELOPMENTAL ISSUES

After puberty and throughout adult life, spermatogenesis occurs continuously. The normal human male may manufacture several hundred million spermatozoa per day. With advancing age, the seminiferous tubules undergo gradual involution and in the testes of a 70-year-old, many tubules show extensive atrophy and are depleted of germ cells but still contain Sertoli cells.

Once fully formed, the spermatozoa are pushed out of the seminiferous tubules along the tubuli recti and into the rete testis and then via the vasa efferentia into the head of the epididymis **(see Figs 6.3.4 and 6.3.9)**. The **epididymis** is a long, coiled tube (if unravelled it would be approximately 6 m long) and is divided into sections – the head, body and tail – all closely

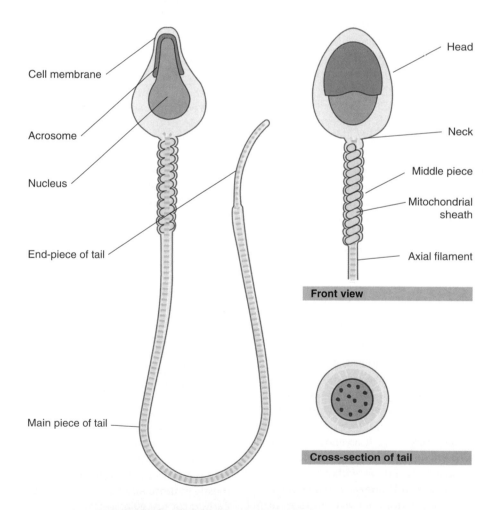

**Figure 6.3.8** Structure of the mature spermatozoon with a small cross-section of the tail enlarged to show the 9 + 2 arrangement of the axial filaments

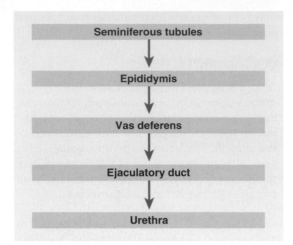

**Figure 6.3.9** Route followed by spermatozoa from synthesis to ejaculation

applied to the posterior surface of the testis. The cilia in the tubuli recti beat and the smooth muscle around the tubules contracts, moving the spermatozoa towards the epididymis.

The time spent by the spermatozoa in the epididymis is an organized delay: it allows them to mature before ejaculation. It is thought that the secretory columnar epithelium of the epididymis secretes hormones, enzymes and nutrients that may be important for sperm maturation. The growth of the epithelium of the epididymis is dependent on adequate levels of male sex hormones.

The tail of the epididymis is the main storehouse for the spermatozoa, although some may be stored in the vas. Storage is necessary because spermatogenesis is a continuous process, whereas ejaculation occurs at irregular intervals. If no ejaculation occurs, the spermatozoa in the epididymis ultimately degenerate and undergo liquefaction. It is also thought that the epithelial cells of the ducts may have phagocytic properties and may be able to remove abnormal spermatozoa. The spermatozoa mature in their abilities both to move and to fertilize ova during the passage through the excretory ducts, but the exact nature of this maturation process is not known. Spermatozoa can be stored in the genital ducts for as long as 42 days.

The vas deferens (or ductus deferens) is a muscular tube that begins in the scrotum as a continuation of the tail of the epididymis and ends in the pelvis by joining with the duct of the seminal vesicle in the formation of the ejaculatory duct. It ascends from the scrotum in the spermatic cord. The **spermatic cord** also contains blood vessels and nerves that supply the testes, and also muscular and connective tissue extensions from the anterior abdominal wall. In cases of torsion of the testis, the blood and nerve supply to the testis can be cut off and, if not corrected quickly, may necessitate an orchidectomy (removal of the testis).

The wall of the vas deferens is composed of an outer layer of loose connective tissue and three layers of smooth muscle with an abundant autonomic nerve supply. This arrangement accounts for the ability of the vas to contract quickly and efficiently during ejaculation. In addition to these peristaltic contractions, the spermatozoa are able to 'swim' by means of two-dimensional bending waves that pass from the front to the back end of their tails. The tails of the spermatozoa are composed of a central filament containing a pair of microfibrils surrounded by a circle of nine fibrils.

## CLINICAL APPLICATIONS

The vas deferens is ligated and cut during the operation of **vasectomy** for sterilization of the male. Small sections of both vas are usually removed from the epididymal end. Men having undergone a vasectomy may remain fertile for 6–8 weeks after the operation because spermatozoa may remain viable within the genital tract for this period (the duration of fertility after vasectomy also depends on the frequency of ejaculation). Therefore, additional contraceptive methods are needed for at least a couple of months after surgery. Men are usually required to go back to the clinic twice with a specimen of their ejaculate to check that there are no spermatozoa in it before sterility is assured. With the vas occluded, the man is sterile, but there should be no changes in either somatic or psychological sexual characteristics. These characteristics are androgen dependent and the secretion of these hormones from the interstitial cells of the testis into the bloodstream is not altered by the procedure. The postvasectomy changes that occur in the seminiferous tubules are variable: sometimes complete degeneration of the cells occurs, but more often some spermatogenesis continues, although the spermatozoa are destroyed by liquefaction and replaced by new cells. Antibodies to the spermatozoa may also be produced. Normal ejaculation still occurs, with the emission of fluids from the accessory sex glands, minus the spermatozoa, of course. Reversal of vasectomy is possible in some instances but may not lead to a return of fertility.

**Testicular cancer** is one of the rarer cancers, although it is still the most common cancer in young men in the United Kingdom and it occurs mostly in those aged between 19 and 44. If found early, most testicular cancers can be cured; so men's awareness of testicular cancer should be enhanced and they should be encouraged to perform a quick, simple examination regularly to

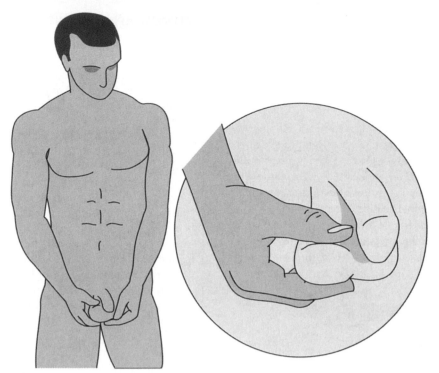

**Figure 6.3.10**  Testicular self-examination

check that there are no swellings, lumps or hardness on the testicles (Whiteford & Wordley, 2003). **Figure 6.3.10** shows how to perform testicular self-examination.

## TESTICULAR SELF-EXAMINATION

The best time is following a warm bath or shower, as the scrotal sac is relaxed and the contents can be felt more easily.

1. Hold the scrotum in the palms of the hands so that the thumb and fingers of both hands are free to feel the testicles.
2. Examine each testicle individually. Only gentle pressure is required to do this. First examine the epididymis: this should feel soft and slightly tender to the touch. Then find the spermatic cord, which goes up from the top of the epididymis: it should feel like a firm smooth tube. Finally, feel the testicle itself: it should be smooth with no lumps.
3. Consult the doctor if there are any changes. A lump may not necessarily be cancer, but the doctor should be asked.

## The role of the accessory sex glands

The accessory sex glands provide a transport medium, with the necessary nutrients, for the spermatozoa to leave the male and enter the female.

## The seminal vesicles

These two glands are so called because they were originally thought to store the spermatozoa, but that is *not* their function; they are secretory glands. They are located behind the prostate gland and lateral to each ampulla of vas. Each vesicle is a muscular convoluted tube lined by secretory epithelium with a maximum capacity of 3 mL.

The secretion of the seminal vesicles is an alkaline, viscid, yellowish fluid containing, amongst other compounds, fructose, globulin, ascorbic acid and prostaglandins. It forms the fluid vehicle for the spermatozoa. Its secretory activity is under the control of the testicular hormones and in old age the vesicles diminish in size because of decreased hormone stimulation.

## The prostate gland

The prostate gland is situated around the bladder neck and the first part of the urethra, into which its secretions pass **(Fig. 6.3.11)**. Its actual size varies considerably. At puberty, the prostate gland increases rapidly in size and in the normal adult its shape is likened to a chestnut, with an approximate 3 cm diameter in all directions; it remains fairly constant in size until middle age when it may involute or, more often, undergo benign hypertrophy, which frequently results in urological problems. The main glandular tissue is situated in the lateral and posterior portions (known as the outer zone) of the prostate, whereas the inner zone (the middle of the gland) consists mainly of mucosal glands.

The **prostatic secretion** consists of a thin, slightly acidic, milky fluid containing enzymes, for example acid hydrolase, acid phosphatase, protease and fibrinolysin; it is also rich in calcium and citrates. It is responsible for the characteristic odour of semen. Prostatic secretion is thought to stimulate the motility of the spermatozoa, coagulate the fluid from the seminal vesicles and go some way towards neutralizing the prevailing vaginal acidity. As with the secretions of the seminal vesicles, prostatic secretory activity is dependent on adequate stimulation by the testicular hormones. Any reduction of this stimulus results in involution of the gland and its secretory elements.

## DEVELOPMENTAL ISSUES

Virtually every man over the age of 40 has some degree of benign enlargement of the prostate now known as benign prostatic hypertrophy (BPH). The inner zone of the gland hypertrophies in particular and projects into the bladder, impeding the passage of urine by elongating and distorting the prostatic urethra (see Fig. 6.3.11). Benign prostatic hypertrophy is thought to be due to a disturbance of the ratio and quantity of the circulating androgens and oestrogens in the more advanced years of life.

## CLINICAL APPLICATIONS

The term **prostatism** refers to the urinary problems associated with lesions of the prostate. The common symptoms that manifest, usually between the ages of 60 and 70 years, include difficulty in initiating micturition, a poor urinary stream and urinary urgency and frequency with nocturia. Prostatism can result in incomplete voiding with stasis, infection and back pressure, resulting in renal damage. Drugs that work by relaxing the muscles of the bladder neck and prostatic urethra (e.g. α-blockers) are helpful in the treatment of benign prostatic hypertrophy. Approximately 1 in 10 men in the West require surgical treatment for prostatic enlargement (the condition has a racial distribution, being common in Western white races, rarer in Indian races and extremely rare in males of African descent). Treatment for benign hypertrophy usually involves removal or destruction (e.g. with microwave energy or laser ablation) of the enlarged lobe of the prostate. Particularly in the case of inner lobe enlargement, the removal can be performed transurethrally, i.e. via the urethra. After transurethral resection of the prostate, ejaculation may be impaired but erection should be possible.

Hormone dependency also occurs in carcinoma of the prostate, which more often involves enlargement of the outer or posterior part of the gland. The incidence of prostate cancer is increasing and it is one of the most common two male cancers (the other being lung cancer). It

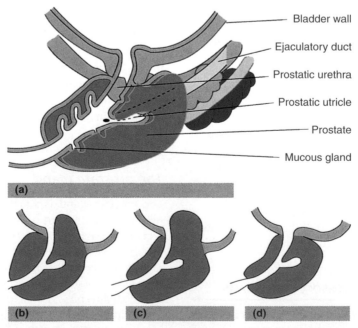

**Figure 6.3.11** The normal prostate gland (a) showing the effects of hypertrophy of (b) the lateral and middle lobes, (c) the middle lobes and (d) the lateral lobes

appears to be androgen dependent, thus treatment of this carcinoma can consist of giving large doses of anti-androgens, and sometimes oestrogens and/or orchidectomy to reduce the relative levels of circulating androgens. Radical surgery is only appropriate for a few patients because the carcinoma has often spread by the time of diagnosis; urinary symptoms do not occur until the disease is well advanced as it is associated with enlargement of the outer zones. Radiotherapy is also frequently used. Controversy still exists with regard to the value of screening for prostate cancer using prostate specific antigen (PSA) (Lewey, 2002).

## The bulbourethral glands

The bulbourethral, or Cowper's, glands are small globular glands and are roughly pea sized. They lie between the lower prostate and the penis and their ducts open into the urethra. They secrete mucus that serves as a lubricant prior to ejaculation.

## The composition of semen

Semen, or seminal fluid, consists of spermatozoa, the secretions of the genital tract, especially the epididymis, and the secretions of the associated accessory glands. The bulk of the semen (approximately 60%) originates from the seminal vesicles. The pH of the combined secretions is slightly alkaline (pH 7.2–7.4), the acid prostatic secretions being neutralized by the other components. The pH of semen is important because spermatozoa are rapidly immobilized in an acid medium. The pH of the vaginal secretions is acid (approximately pH 4.5) and the alkaline semen neutralizes the inhibitory effect of the acid vagina. The seminal fluid also contains fructose as an energy source for the spermatozoa. Semen is also rich in hyaluronidase, an enzyme that causes breakdown of mucopolysaccharides and facilitates passage through the cervical mucus and the chemicals surrounding the ovum.

The average volume of ejaculate is 3 mL (range 2–6 mL) and contains approximately 300 million spermatozoa.

### CLINICAL APPLICATIONS

The number, morphology and motility of the spermatozoa give an indication of the fertility of the male and are used clinically in the assessment of infertility. The normal is considered to be:

- volume of ejaculate: 2–6 mL
- density of spermatozoa: 60–150 million/mL
- morphology: 60–80% normal shape
- motility: 50% should be motile after incubation for 1 hour at 37°C.

A specimen of semen for investigation is obtained by masturbation. The volume and density will depend on the previous period of abstinence from sexual intercourse: frequent ejaculations lead to a progressive reduction in the spermatozoa count in the semen. Values outside these normal ranges may be an indication of infertility. Spermatozoa may be stored at −70°C for weeks or even months, and their motility and fertilizing ability reappear when unfrozen. This property is sometimes used when specimens are used for assisted reproduction or artificial insemination either by husband or donor.

Sperm from men undergoing chemotherapy for cancer may also be stored, because infertility sometimes results from the treatment.

## The endocrine function of the testis

The testes are responsible for spermatogenesis, as already discussed, but they also function as an endocrine gland. The interstitial cells of Leydig (see Fig. 6.3.6) synthesize, store and secrete androgens, principally testosterone. Very small quantities of oestrogens are also produced but their role, in the male, is obscure. Approximately 95% of the androgen is produced in the testis and the remainder in the adrenal glands.

### Testosterone

Testosterone is a steroid molecule synthesized from cholesterol (Fig. 6.3.12). Total plasma levels of testosterone in the adult male are 12–30 nmol/L (in the adult female the testosterone level is 0.5–2.0 nmol/L, of adrenal origin). Most of the testosterone is loosely bound with plasma proteins once it is released into

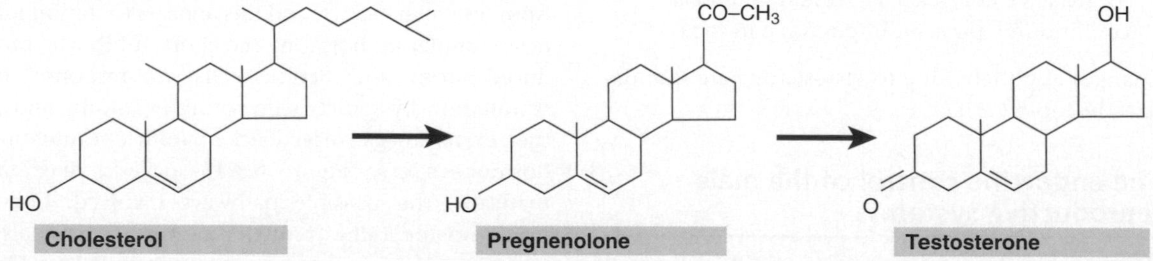

**Figure 6.3.12**  Pathways for the synthesis of testosterone

the blood; it circulates in the plasma before becoming fixed to the target tissues and then it is finally metabolized and excreted by the liver.

Testosterone has widespread effects on the body, both on the reproductive organs and on the somatic tissues. Most of the effects of testosterone (and other androgens) can be directly related to the fact that it is an important anabolic agent, synthesizing complex molecules from simpler ones. Once in the cells, testosterone stimulates an increase in the synthesis of proteins; it probably directly influences the DNA and RNA in the cell. Its major functions are:

1. Stimulating the growth of the seminiferous tubules. Testosterone is therefore an important regulator of spermatogenesis.
2. It is necessary for the development and maintenance of the accessory sex organs, including the penis and prostate gland.
3. It is responsible for the changes that occur at puberty. These include:
   (i)   the development of a typical male physique, for example muscle development
   (ii)  the stimulation of epiphyseal growth in the long bones and the subsequent fusion of the epiphyses – there is thus an initial growth spurt at puberty when testosterone levels increase, followed by cessation of growth in the late teens
   (iii) the growth of facial and body (chest, axillary and public) hair and recession of the scalp line
   (iv)  the lowering of the voice pitch due to a thickening of the vocal cords and enlargement of the larynx
   (v)   increased sebum secretion in the skin, which may predispose towards the development of acne
   (vi)  the mild retention of sodium, potassium, calcium, phosphate, sulphate and water by the kidneys
   (vii) the development and maintenance of libido (female libido is probably also androgen dependent).
4. Testosterone may also be partly responsible for the changes in male behaviour after puberty, for instance increased aggression, but social conditioning plays an important part too.

Changes at puberty due to testosterone are summarized in **Table 6.3.1.**

## The endocrine control of the male reproductive system

Three levels of hormones are involved in the control of the male reproductive system: hypothalamic

| **Table 6.3.1**   Major functions of testosterone at puberty |
| --- |
| Development of male physique |
| Stimulation of epiphyseal growth |
| Growth of facial and body hair |
| Lowering pitch of voice |
| Increased sebum secretion (skin) |
| Mild electrolyte retention (kidneys) |
| Development of libido |

hormone, anterior pituitary hormones and testicular hormones. Both spermatogenesis and androgen production are controlied by the anterior pituitary hormones, the gonadotrophins, namely **follicle-stimulating hormone (FSH)** and **luteinizing hormone (LH)**. The latter is sometimes also known as interstitial cell stimulating hormone (ICSH) in the male. Follicle stimulating hormone acts primarily on the seminiferous tubules as a stimulus for spermatogenesis. However, small quantities of luteinizing hormone are also required for the completion of spermatogenesis. Luteinizing hormone stimulates the production of androgen from the interstitial cells of Leydig, as its alternative name indicates **(Fig. 6.3.13)**.

The release of these gonadotrophins is in response to a stimulus from the hypothalamus, and the release of both follicle stimulating hormone and luteinizing hormone appears to be controlled by one hypothalamic releasing hormone, known as **gonadotrophin releasing hormone (GnRH)**. The exact nature of the feedback control system is still uncertain but it involves negative feedback acting at either or both hypothalamic and pituitary levels. If a male is castrated (i.e. has his testes removed) there is a marked increase in the levels of plasma gonadotrophins. This suggests that there is normally some negative feedback, and it is thought that testosterone levels are one of the stimuli involved; for example, relatively high levels of testosterone exert an inhibitory effect on the hypothalamus (and possibly the anterior pituitary), reducing the release of gonadotrophin releasing hormone (and follicle stimulating hormone and luteinizing hormone).

**Inhibin**, a protein hormone, has been isolated from testicular extracts and this appears to inhibit follicle stimulating hormone secretion. Inhibin is produced from the Sertoli cells in response to stimulation by follicle stimulating hormone, and it then exerts a negative feedback on follicle stimulating hormone release. **Figure 6.3.13** suggests, diagrammatically, the possible pathways involved. Other regulatory peptides (protein hormones) have also been identified, but they are not included in **Fig. 6.3.13** because their effects in vivo are not confirmed.

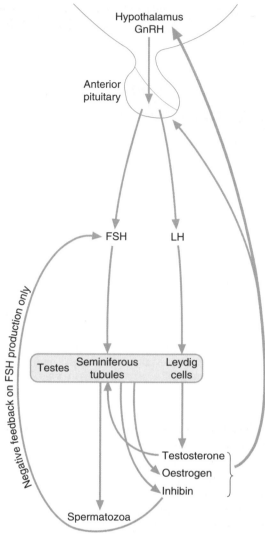

**Figure 6.3.13** Possible pathways controlling the release of male reproductive hormones. FSH, follicle stimulating hormone; GnRH, gonadotrophin releasing hormone; LH, luteinizing hormone

## The functioning of the female reproductive system

The discussion of female reproductive physiology will be divided into the following sections: the production of ova (the female gametes) and ovulation, the menstrual cycle and its relationship with ovulation and, finally, the events leading to fertilization and a brief review of pregnancy. A brief description of the anatomy of the female reproductive system will be given first.

The female genital system consists of two ovaries, two uterine tubes, the uterus, vagina and the external genitalia or vulva **(Figs 6.3.14 and 6.3.15)**. It is completely separate from the urinary system, unlike that of the male. The two ovaries, lying close

to the lateral wall of the pelvis, are suspended from the posterior layer of the broad ligament by mesentery, through which blood vessels, lymphatics and nerves pass to and from the ovaries. The broad ligament is a fold of peritoneum passing from the uterus to the side wall of the pelvis.

The **uterine tubes** (also known as oviducts or Fallopian tubes) lie in the upper margin of the broad ligament. Each uterine tube is approximately 10 cm long and has an outer smooth muscle coat and an inner mucous membrane. Both tubes have an outer funnel-shaped part, known as the **infundibulum**, the lumen of which communicates with the peritoneal cavity. The finger-like projections, or fimbriae, 'catch' the released ovum from the ovary. When fertilization occurs it usually takes place within the ampulla. Peristaltic waves occurring in the uterine tubes, together with the movements of the cilia on the epithelium, are responsible for moving the ovum into the uterus. Some non-ciliated cells in the epithelium secrete nutrients for the ovum.

The uterine tubes are slightly flattened and inverted and lead into the uterus or womb. In the adult the **uterus** is a pear-shaped structure with an upper expanded section known as the **body of the uterus** and a lower cylindrical section known as the **cervix** or neck of the uterus. In the non-pregnant state, it measures about 7.5 cm in length, 5 cm in breadth at its upper border and 2.5 cm in thickness. The part of the uterus that projects above the level of entry of the uterine tubes is known as the **fundus** (this part is used in the palpation of the uterus during pregnancy). The uterus is normally flattened dorsoventrally **(see Fig. 6.3.15)** and is supported in position by the broad, round and uterosacral ligaments.

The greater part of the wall of the uterus is composed of a mass of smooth muscle, the **myometrium**, and the cavity, which is normally collapsed, is lined by a mucous membrane, the **endometrium**.

### DEVELOPMENTAL ISSUES

From the time of puberty until the menopause the endometrium undergoes monthly cyclical changes in response to hormonal secretions from the ovary (described later).

The endometrium is a very vascular tissue, the nature of which is important in understanding menstruation **(Fig. 6.3.16)**. The surface epithelium of the endometrium contains numerous tubular uterine glands.

The cervix of the uterus does not exhibit the same cyclical activity as the body of the uterus but the nature of the mucous secretions from the glands in

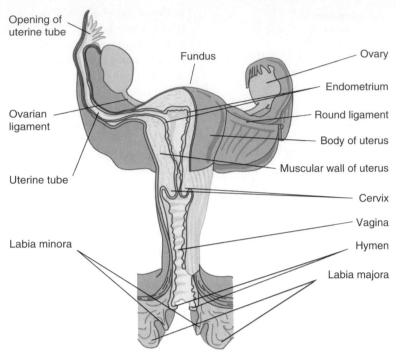

**Figure 6.3.14** Anterior view of the female reproductive system with some structures cut open to expose internal structure. *Note*: there is not normally 'space' in the vagina. The walls are usually collapsed against each other. The space is drawn in for clarity

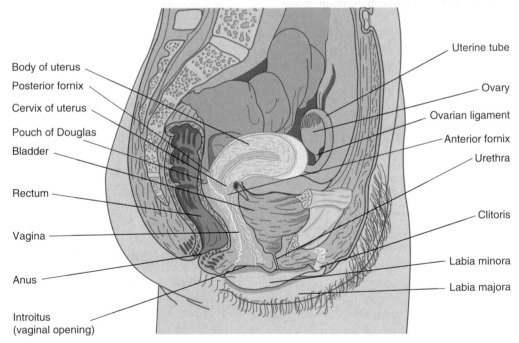

**Figure 6.3.15** Median sagittal section of the female pelvis

this region varies during the cycle. Normal columnar epithelial cells of the cervix may exhibit metaplasia (a change in form) and, under the influence of some other stimulus, as yet undefined but possibly viral in nature, the changes can become neoplastic (i.e., cancerous).

## CLINICAL APPLICATIONS

Precancerous or cancerous changes can be detected easily by examination of cervical cells taken in a smear test (the Papanicolaou (Pap) test). Other screening methods are being

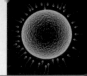

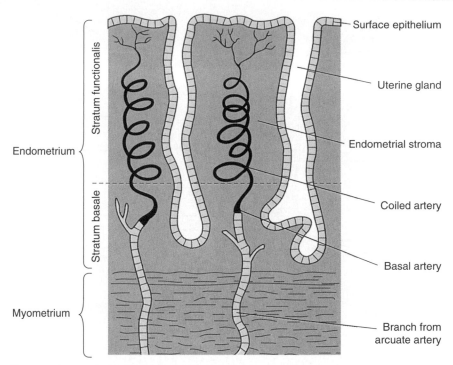

**Figure 6.3.16** The vascular supply to the endometrium

Labels in figure:
- Surface epithelium
- Uterine gland
- Endometrial stroma
- Coiled artery
- Basal artery
- Branch from arcuate artery
- Stratum functionalis
- Stratum basale
- Endometrium
- Myometrium

developed such as liquid-based cytology (LBC) and may replace the traditional Papanicolaou smear (Crouch, 2003a). The cervix can also be examined directly by means of a colposcope, which is inserted vaginally (this procedure is called a colposcopy). It is often possible to remove abnormal areas by laser treatment performed on an outpatient basis.

The cervix leads into the **vagina**, which is a tubular organ, about 8 cm long, with an outer muscle and elastic coat. It is thus capable of expanding or stretching, as occurs during sexual intercourse or childbirth. **Figure 6.3.14** shows the position of the vagina: there is not normally any 'space' or gap between the vaginal walls, they are shown like this for clarity in the diagram. During reproductive life, the vagina is colonized by Döderlein's bacilli (*Lactobacillus* species). These bacilli ferment glycogen to produce lactic acid, which renders the vaginal environment acid, with a pH in the region of 4.5; this serves to inhibit the growth of pathogenic bacteria and fungi such as *Candida albicans* (also known as thrush), which otherwise invade the genital tract. Treatment with antibiotics often has the effect of 'killing' good bacteria, such as the Döderlein's bacilli, and therefore increasing vaginal pH and allowing the *Candida* to flourish.

There are no glands in the vagina. The vagina opens into the vulva, with the vaginal orifice lying between the urethra anteriorly and the anus posteriorly (**Fig. 6.3.17**). Two small glands, **Bartholin's glands**, are situated at each side of the external orifice of the vagina; occasionally cysts occur in these glands; they may also become infected (Bartholin's abcess).

The **vulva** is composed of the mons pubis, the inner labia minora, the outer labia majora and the clitoris. The **clitoris** is a small erectile organ, the female homologue of the male penis, situated at the anterior junction of the labia minora. The **hymen** is a membranous partition partially blocking the orifice of the vagina. Its extent, even in virgins, is very variable and, if present, it is almost always ruptured with the use of internal tampons or at first coitus (sexual intercourse).

## Oogenesis and the ovarian cycle

The production of ova, or **oogenesis**, occurs in the ovaries. The **ovaries** vary in size and appearance according to the age of the female and the stage of the reproductive cycle. In the adult they are approximately 4 cm long, 2 cm wide and 1 cm thick. They have an irregular outer appearance resulting from deposition of scar tissue where follicles have previously ruptured.

The outer surface of the ovary is formed of a layer of columnar cells and is known as the germinal epithelium. This is a misnomer; it was originally thought that the ova were produced in this layer but this is not so. Next there is a poorly defined layer of fibrous connective tissue – the tunica albuginea – and then the cortex where the female germ cells (oocytes)

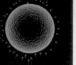

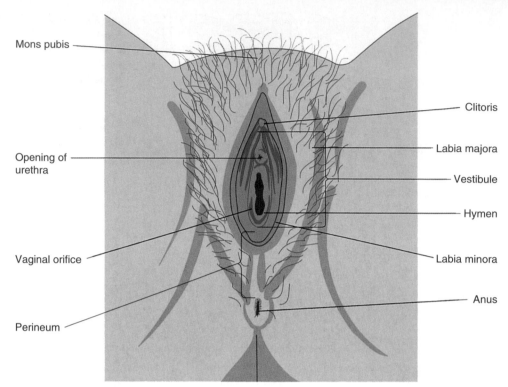

Figure 6.3.17   The vulva

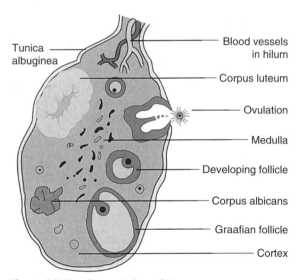

Figure 6.3.18   General plan of the ovary

are located and develop. The innermost layer is the vascular medulla (**Fig. 6.3.18**).

## DEVELOPMENTAL ISSUES

The adult ovarian cortex contains two types of structure – the follicles and the corpora lutea. The follicles contain the **oocytes**, which are all at different stages of development at any one time. During fetal life, several million germ cells develop; however, by the time of birth only 200 000 or so remain and, during a female's

reproductive life (that is, 30–40 years), only about 400 ova will be released. This is an example of programmed cell death. The number of germ cells is continually being reduced by cell degeneration or atresia.

A **follicle** consists of the developing oocyte and its surrounding follicular cells, and changes occur in both during the ovulatory cycle. The changes are easier to understand if considered separately.

The follicular cell changes will be considered first. The primoridial follicle (**Fig. 6.3.19a**) consists of flat cuboidal cells and these divide to form several layers of granulosa cells in the primary follicle (**Fig. 6.3.19b**). Amorphous material begins to accumulate between the granulosa cells and the oocyte, known as the **zona pellucida**. Outside the follicle the interstitial cells change to become the theca folliculi, which is then invaded by capillaries. The inner layer of the theca produces oestrogens. The follicle continues to increase in size and an antrum, or cleft, appears, which fills with follicular fluid. At this stage the structure is known as the **secondary follicle** (**Fig. 6.3.19c**). After a further period of maturation the granulosa cells split: one layer forms the corona radiata around the oocyte and the other outer layer, the membrana granulosa. The two layers are continuous at the cumulus oophorus. At this stage the whole structure is called a **Graafian follicle**, after the Dutch physiologist, de Graaf, who first described it in the

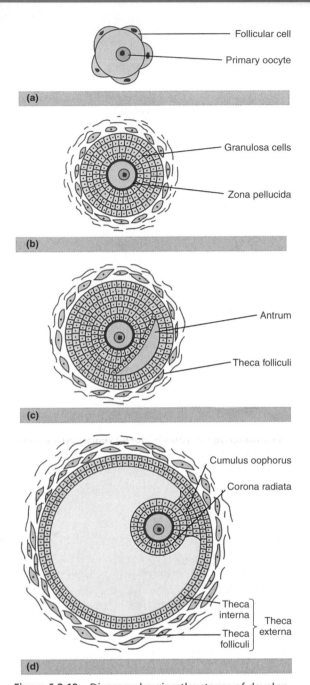

**Figure 6.3.19** Diagram showing the stages of development in the follicle. (a) Primordial follicle, (b) primary follicle, (c) secondary follicle and (d) Graafian follicle

seventeenth century (**Fig. 6.3.19d**). Gradually, the Graafian follicle moves towards the surface of the ovary.

Simultaneously, a mature **ovum** is developing within the follicle. The primordial germ cells differentiate into **oogonia** and, by the third month of the intrauterine life, they begin to undergo mitotic division to form primary **oocytes**. The primary oocytes are located in the primordial follicle. The first meiotic division occurs at this stage. Meiosis in the primary oocyte begins in utero and division up to the

diplotene stage of prophase I is completed shortly before birth. Then there is a long resting phase; in the case of the human oocyte it may be anywhere between 10 and 50 years. Thus the first meiotic division is not completed until around the time of ovulation.

In each ovarian cycle some 20 or so oocytes become selectively reactivated and proceed through meiotic division. However, usually only one continues through to the Graafian follicle stage, probably from alternate ovaries. The first meiotic division is completed before ovulation, giving a **secondary oocyte** (with only 23 chromosomes, one of each pair known as haploid) and the **first polar body** (a polar body is a minute cell containing one of the nuclei formed during meiotic cell division but virtually no cytoplasm; the secondary oocyte retains the major portion of cytoplasm). The second meiotic division begins almost immediately, but stops again at metaphase II and there is another, comparatively short, resting phase until fertilization. So the secondary oocyte (with the first polar body still in the zona pellucida) is released from the Graafian follicle at ovulation. Completion of the second meiotic division is dependent upon fertilization, that is, penetration of the ovum by a spermatozoon (**Fig. 6.3.20**).

As is apparent, the production of mature female gametes differs from the production of spermatozoa. In the male, meiosis does not begin until around puberty and then continues without interruption, whereas in the female it commences before birth and has two resting phases. Also, the secondary spermatocytes share equal amounts of chromatin and cytoplasmic material, whereas in the female there is loss of genetic material via the polar bodies.

The exact mechanism of **ovulation** – the release of the ovum from the Graafian follicle (in fact, as a secondary oocyte) – is not fully understood but it probably results from increasing quantities of follicular fluid, which raises the pressure and cause the follicle to burst. Prostaglandins may well be involved in the process of follicular rupture. Several other biologically active substances have been found in follicular fluid, for example the cytokines inhibin and activin, follistatin, interleukins and various growth factors [see Coad & Dunstall (2001) for a fuller discussion of this]. The hormone inhibin, found first in males, has been isolated in relatively high concentrations in female follicular fluid and it appears that inhibin is at least one of the factors that determine the number of follicles released at ovulation. In this way interference with the action of inhibin might contribute to the regulation of fertility.

The follicle, a fluid-filled mass, just before rupture is approximately 2 cm in diameter – large enough to be picked up by an ultrasound scan. The secondary oocyte, together with its follicular cells of the

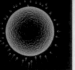

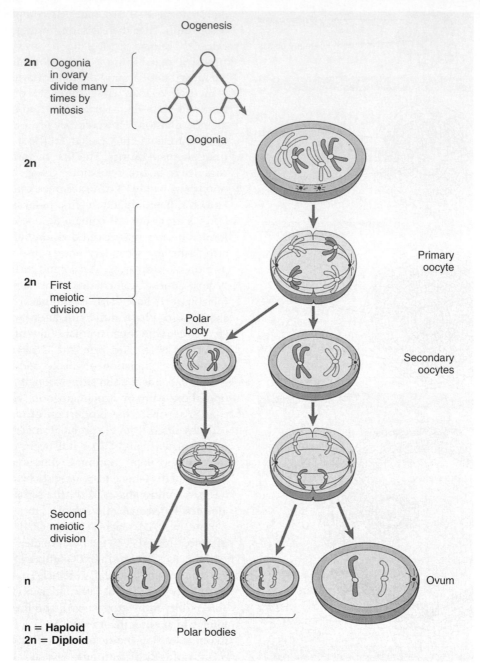

**Figure 6.3.20** Oogenesis. In the female only one functional ovum is produced, the other three cells produce polar bodies that degenerate. For clarity, only two chromosomes pairs are shown

cumulus, is released into the abdominal cavity, after which it is usually trapped by the fimbriae of the uterine tube. After ovulation the follicle collapses and the membrana granulosa becomes folded.

It is difficult to be certain on clinical grounds that ovulation has occurred: up to 10% of ovarian cycles can be anovulatory, that is, no follicle ruptures. The only absolute proof is pregnancy, but a regular cycle and dysmenorrhoea (see The menstrual cycle, p. 748) are indications that cycles are ovulatory. Some women notice lower abdominal pain for a brief period at ovulation, known as **mittelschmerz** (German for middle

pain). The pain may be bilateral or unilateral. It is usually cramp-like and lasts a day or so and is often replaced by a dull ache. The cause of the pain is uncertain: it may be due to some local irritation within the pelvis caused by the presence of follicular fluid and blood, or from the ovary itself. Most women have some microscopic bleeding into the vagina at that time and a few experience overt bleeding; this is probably due to a temporary fall in sex hormone production between the time of the follicle rupturing and before the establishment of a corpus luteum (**Fig. 6.3.21**).

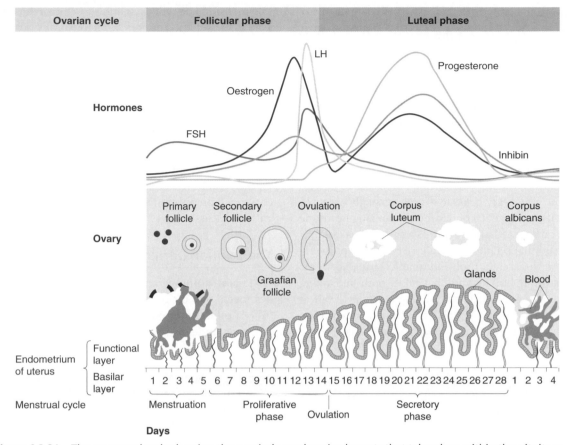

**Figure 6.3.21** The menstrual cycle showing the precisely synchronized events that take place within the pituitary, ovary and uterus. The cycle repeats about every 28 days if fertilization does not take place

The collapsed follicle becomes an endocrine gland and is termed the **corpus luteum** or yellow body (the yellowish carotenoid pigment, lutein, is formed within the cells). Both the granulosa and theca cells proliferate. The corpus luteum secretes the steroids oestrogen and, most significantly, progesterone: both play an important role in the reproductive cycle and in the maintenance of pregnancy should fertilization occur (androgens are also secreted from the stroma of the ovary). The corpus luteum, however, has a finite life, the length of which depends on whether pregnancy occurs. If no pregnancy ensues, the lutein cells degenerate after approximately 12–14 days and hormone production is reduced. Accompanying this degeneration, the corpus luteum becomes infiltrated by fibroblasts that produce scar tissue and it becomes known as the **corpus albicans** (the white body). If pregnancy occurs, the corpus luteum persists and continues to secrete oestrogen and progesterone until about the third month of gestation; this is essential to ensure the pregnancy is maintained. After this period the placenta assumes this function (see later).

The cycle of events previously described is known as the **ovarian** or **ovulatory cycle**. The cycle lasts approximately 28 days in most women, although it can vary between 21 and 35 days. It is usually divided into two phases:

- The **follicular phase**, during which the ovarian follicles grow, mature and finally rupture; during this time the theca interna cells secrete oestrogen.
- The **luteal phase**, during which the formation, development and degeneration of the corpus luteum occurs; the granulosa lutein cells secrete progesterone and the theca lutein cells secrete oestrogens (see Fig. 6.3.21).

The luteal phase of the cycle lasts approximately 14 days, although slight variations do occur amongst different individuals and from cycle to cycle in one individual; the follicular phase is more variable and accounts for the wide range in cycle length. To determine the timing of ovulation it is conventional to count *back* 14 days from the first day of the next menstruation, however researchers looking at the 'fertile window' in women found a range of 7–19 days from ovulation to the next period (Wilcox et al., 2000).

Successful release of a secondary oocyte from a mature Graafian follicle depends on the appropriate level of circulating gonadotrophins from the anterior pituitary and this is first achieved around the time of puberty (during the years from birth until puberty some follicular growth and activity occur in the ovary but follicles degenerate before completing their development).

The gonadotrophins involved are **follicle stimulating hormone** (FSH) and **luteinizing hormone** (LH). Follicle stimulating hormone stimulates the initial development of the follicles, but the process is *not* completed to the Graafian follicle stage. Subsequent release of luteinizing hormone leads to completion of follicular growth, ovulation and development of a corpus luteum. Luteinizing hormone then maintains the corpus luteum, stimulating the release of progesterone and oestrogens. It is now generally accepted that it is a surge in the level of luteinizing hormone that causes ovulation. There is a smaller peak in follicle stimulating hormone release but this is probably due to the secretion of only one releasing hormone from the hypothalamus that raises both luteinizing hormone and follicle stimulating hormone levels at the same time **(see Fig. 6.3.21)**. (A fuller description of the hormonal control is given after discussion of

the menstrual cycle.) Ovulation predictor kits are available over the counter at chemists for women to use at home; they work by measuring levels of luteinizing hormone. The test detects the sudden surge or increase of luteinizing hormone around the middle of the cycle; ovulation occurs 24–36 hours after the surge and this is the time of peak fertility. To increase chances of becoming pregnant, the couple should have intercourse during the 2 to 3 days around the time of peak fertility.

Ovulation is not an event in isolation; other parts of the female reproductive system are undergoing changes in preparation for fertilization. These changes will be discussed later.

## The ovarian hormones (see Table 6.3.2)

The main hormones produced by the ovaries are oestrogens and progesterone, as well as small quantities of other hormones such as androgens, inhibin, cytokines and growth factors. Under the influence of

### Table 6.3.2 Principal female reproductive hormones

| Endocrine gland and hormone | Principal target tissue | Principal actions |
|---|---|---|
| **Hypothalamus** | | |
| Gonadotrophin releasing hormone (GnRH) | Anterior pituitary | Stimulates release of FSH and LH |
| **Anterior pituitary** | | |
| Follicle-stimulating hormone (FSH) | Ovary | Stimulates development of follicles; with LH, stimulates secretion of oestrogens and ovulation |
| Luteinizing hormone (LH) | Ovary | Stimulates final development of follicle; stimulates ovulation; stimulates development of corpus luteum |
| Prolactin | Breasts | Stimulates milk production (after breast has been prepared by oestrogens and progesterone) |
| **Posterior pituitary** | | |
| Oxytocin | Breasts | Stimulates release of milk into ducts |
| | Uterus | Stimulates contraction |
| **Ovary** | | |
| Oestrogens | General | Growth of body and sex organs at puberty; development of secondary sex characteristics (breast development, broadening of pelvis, distribution of fat and muscle) |
| | Reproductive structures | Maturation; monthly preparation of the endometrium for pregnancy; makes cervical mucus thinner and more alkaline |
| Progesterone | Uterus | Completes preparation of and maintains endometrium for pregnancy |
| | Breasts | Stimulates development of lobules and alveoli of mammary glands |
| Inhibin | Anterior pituitary | Inhibits secretion of FSH |

follicle stimulating hormone and luteinizing hormone from the anterior pituitary, the levels of oestrogens and progesterone vary during the ovarian cycle, as seen in **Fig. 6.3.25**.

## Oestrogens

The oestrogens are hormones produced by the theca interna of the ovary during the follicular phase and from the theca lutein cells in the luteal phase (they are also produced in the placenta during pregnancy). The three main oestrogens produced are all steroid molecules, each with 19 carbon atoms, and are synthesized from cholesterol (**Fig. 6.3.22**).

**Oestradiol** is the most potent of the oestrogens, followed by **oestrone** and finally **oestriol**. Seventy per cent of the oestrogens are bound to plasma proteins, principally to sex-hormone-binding globulin (SHBG). The plasma oestrogen levels vary during the monthly ovarian cycle, as shown in **Fig. 6.3.21**. There are two peaks in plasma levels of oestrogens: the larger peak occurs just before ovulation and the smaller one during the luteal phase.

Oestrogens produce many changes in the body, which combine together to facilitate fertilization. For example, oestrogens are necessary for the development and maintenance of the uterine tubes, uterus, cervix, vagina, labia and for priming the duct tissue in the breast. Oestrogens also increase the motility of the uterine tubes and the excitability of the uterine muscle (these changes will be dealt with in greater detail in the next section). In animals, oestrogens

heighten the female's awareness, particularly to male-associated smells, and increase visual acuity and touch sensitivity. Sensitivity to pain is decreased with raised oestrogen levels, a factor that may facilitate coitus and may be significant at the end of pregnancy when oestrogen levels are high. (It has also been suggested that raised endorphin levels at the end of pregnancy may account for this decrease in sensitivity to pain.)

Females of many species, including humans, produce odoriferous substances, **pheromones**, attractive to males. Some pheromones are produced in sweat (see Chapter 6.1) and some in or around the vagina in response to oestrogenic stimulation. It has been suggested that a relatively common phenomenon in women can be explained by the existence of pheromones; namely, women living together, particularly room-mates and very close friends, show highly significant synchrony in their menstrual cycles. It is possible that some substance secreted in sweat is responsible. However, the significance of pheromones in humans is far from certain and, in general, visual cues are probably of greater significance in attracting a mate in our species. However, oestrogen is also responsible for all the obvious attributes of femininity, for example breast growth and the female pattern of body fat deposition in the buttocks giving the female curved outline. Oestrogen is involved in mood changes, too. Oestrogen alters neurochemical pathways controlling both mood and behaviour. Human females are generally sexually receptive throughout the cycle, unlike most animals that exhibit an oestrous cycle.

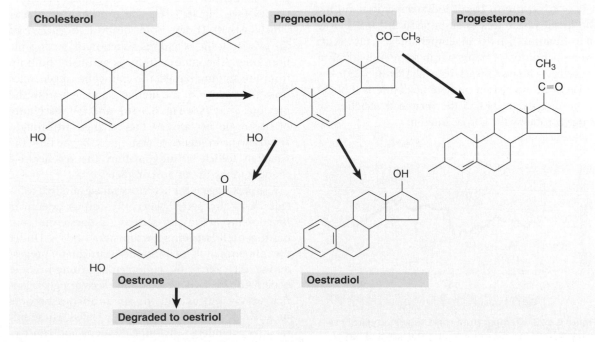

**Figure 6.3.22** Pathway for the synthesis of ovarian hormones

## CLINICAL APPLICATIONS

Oestrogen also has a protective effect on the cardiovascular system. The incidence of coronary heart disease in premenopausal women is much lower than in men. Oestrogen appears to inhibit the uptake and degradation of low density lipoproteins by the coronary vessel endothelium and so reduce atherosclerosis formation.
Oestrogen exerts other beneficial effects on the vascular system too (Coad & Dunstall, 2001).

### Progesterone

Progesterone is a hormone produced by the granulosa lutein cells of the corpus luteum during the luteal phase of the ovarian cycle (see Fig. 6.3.21). During pregnancy it is produced by the placenta. It is a steroid molecule with 21 carbon atoms and is an important intermediate in the synthesis of many steroids (see Fig. 6.3.22).

All the changes produced by progesterone can be thought of as facilitating gestation and it often acts on oestrogen-primed tissue; for example, progesterone increases the thickness of the endometrium, depresses myometrial activity, decreases cornification of the vagina and increases the secretory gland tissue in the breast (this effect is minimal during a normal cycle). Premenstrual water retention, which may be associated with clinically detectable oedema, is attributed to the increased level of progesterone in the second half of the cycle.

Progesterone is also responsible for the slight rise in body temperature during the luteal phase. There is a 0.2–0.6°C rise in basal body temperature during the luteal phase that is sustained until just before menstruation. The rise in temperature usually occurs over a period of 24 hours but in some individuals it can take 3–4 days to reach its peak (Fig. 6.3.23). The cause of the increased body temperature is thought to be directly related to the increased secretion of progesterone by the corpus luteum.

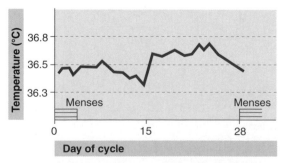

**Figure 6.3.23** Temperature chart showing typical rise in basal body temperature during the luteal phase of the menstrual cycle

If the basal body temperature is recorded daily (i.e. taken each morning on waking before any activity or refreshments are taken), it can be used as an indication of ovarian progesterone production and thus, by observing the timing of the rise, gives an *approximate* guide to the timing of ovulation. This method is used to time ovulation retrospectively by women who want to conceive and also by those who do not (as it can be incorporated with the natural methods of birth control, enabling sexual intercourse to be avoided until 3–4 days after ovulation). This 'typical' pattern of change in temperature during the menstrual cycle is not seen in all women even with ovulatory cycles.

### Androgens

Small quantities of androgens are produced from the stroma of the ovary but have little significance. Androgens of adrenal origin have a greater influence on the body.

## The menstrual cycle

The hormones released by the ovaries have functional and structural repercussions throughout the body, but particularly on the reproductive system. The changes occurring in the endometrium of the uterus constitute the menstrual cycle, which terminates in the loss of blood per vagina, i.e. menstruation. The length of the cycle is said to be approximately 28 days but its actual length may vary considerably, and 24–32 days is quite normal.

The menstrual cycle is usually divided into three phases: the proliferative, secretory and menstrual phases (see Fig. 6.3.21). The **proliferative phase**, which lasts 10–11 days, coincides with the growth of the ovarian follicles and the secretion of oestrogenic hormones. The endometrium is gradually built-up from the stratum basale, the epithelium regenerates from the stumps of the uterine glands left from the previous cycle (see Fig. 6.3.16), and the vascularity of the stroma increases. All these changes are brought about by the influence of oestrogens. By the time the Graafian follicle is fully mature, the regenerative changes in the uterus are complete.

The next stage is the **secretory phase** and this coincides with the period when the corpus luteum is functionally active and secreting progesterone and oestrogens. It lasts for approximately 14 days. Under the influence of these hormones, particularly progesterone, the cells of the endometrial stroma become oedematous, the glands dilate and secrete a glycogen-rich watery mucus and the spiral arteries become increasingly prominent and tightly coiled. These spiral arteries undergo rhythmic dilations and contractions which are under the control of the ovarian hormones. The endometrium is approximately 5 mm thick at this stage.

After approximately 12–14 days, if fertilization has not occurred, the corpus luteum begins to degenerate and the secretion of ovarian hormones wanes. Thus the hormonal support to the endometrial tissue is withdrawn; there is a loss of water and a decreased blood flow to the endometrium due to spasm of the spiral arteries (see Fig. 6.3.16), which ultimately leads to endometrial necrosis (death of the tissue). However, when the endometrial arteries dilate again, bleeding occurs into the stroma of the necrotic endometrium. Thus blood enters the lumen of the uterus and menstruation, or the menstrual phase, commences. The endometrium produces prostaglandins in increasing amounts during the secretory phase and these reach a peak at the time of menstruation. It is possible that prostaglandins are involved in the initiation of menstruation and the shedding of the endometrium.

The **menstrual loss** (or **menses**) is composed of blood and epithelial and stromal cells of the endometrium discharged per vagina (the most common cause of a positive blood urinalysis in women is contamination of urine with menstrual loss). By the end of menstruation the endometrium is only 0.5 mm in thickness. There are usually between 3 and 7 days of external bleeding, which is referred to as the **menstrual phase** of the cycle. For convenience, day one of the menstrual cycle is taken from the first day of menstrual bleeding, although this is really the end of the previous cycle. Endometrial regeneration, and hence the next cycle, can begin as early as the third day of menstrual bleeding. The endometrium regenerates from the remaining glandular, stromal and vascular elements in the stratum basale, hence the reason for the separate blood supply.

The mean **menstrual blood loss** is approximately 50 mL, although there is a wide individual variation of 10–80 mL. Sometimes, small, darkly coloured 'clots' of blood are observed in the menstrual blood, but these are usually aggregations of red blood cells in a mass of mucoid material or even glycogen. The 'clots' are not harmful and are more common when bleeding is excessive. Menstrual blood collected from within the uterine cavity does not contain any fibrinogen and therefore is incapable of clotting. The damaged endometrial cells secrete proteolytic and fibrinolytic enzymes, which stop the formation of fibrin and clot formation.

## CLINICAL APPLICATIONS

Excessive menstrual flow, **menorrhagia**, can lead to iron-deficiency anaemia due to depletion of iron stores. The iron status of women seems to be very delicately balanced. A woman taking a normal diet with a haemoglobin concentration of 12 g/dL and a roughly regular cycle, will remain in iron balance only if her blood loss does not exceed 65 mL (Wilson & Rennie, 1976). Thus, women who experience heavy menstrual bleeding may need to be advised to increase the foods they eat that contain iron (e.g. red meat, wholewheat products, egg yolks, green vegetables), folic acid (e.g. sprouts and broccoli) and vitamin C (e.g. citrus fruits). If this fails, intermittent courses of iron therapy may be necessary. Women with an intrauterine contraceptive device in situ often experience an increased menstrual loss and thus may become iron deficient.

The absence of menstruation, or **amenorrhoea**, is usually a sign of failure to ovulate and there are many possible causes. If a woman never establishes menstruation this condition is known as primary amenorrhoea. The cause may be chromosomal, for example Turner's syndrome, or due to endocrine imbalances. The most common causes of secondary amenorrhoea (or the absence of menses once they have commenced) are pregnancy and anorexia nervosa (see the discussion related to puberty later in the chapter); some diseases may cause the cessation of menstruation too, for example tumours of the hypothalamus or anterior pituitary, endocrine disturbances (hyperthyroidism or post-pill amenorrhoea).

Some women experience mood changes and unpleasant physical symptoms during the 10 days prior to the onset of menstruation. This has been given the name **premenstrual tension (PMT)** or, more commonly, the **premenstrual syndrome (PMS)**. The clinical features can include a varying and complex range of symptoms (Table 6.3.3).

**Table 6.3.3** Signs and symptoms of the premenstrual syndrome

Lower abdominal discomfort and distension
Nausea, giddiness or vertigo
Breast discomfort
General 'bloated' feeling
Weight gain of up to 3 kg
Frequency of micturition
Cystitis and urethritis
Change of bowel habit; food cravings
Increase in acne
Swelling of ankle and hands
Darkening of the skin under the eyes or red eyes
Headache, chest pain, joint and muscle pains
Increased emotional lability, especially increased irritability, depression, fatigue, loss of concentration
Decreased libido

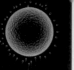

In the past it was thought that there was a considerable emotional component to premenstrual syndrome but now it is generally accepted that there is a physiological basis, although the exact nature of this is unknown. The definition of premenstrual syndrome is the presence of any symptoms or complaints that appear regularly just before or during early menstruation but are absent at other times of the cycle. Premenstrual syndrome has a complex aetiology and is likely to be the result of some form of endocrine disturbance. The precise cause (or causes) remains elusive: studies have shown that there is no simple relationship with blood levels of hormones such as progesterone, oestrogen, follicle stimulating hormone, luteinizing hormone or prolactin.

Whatever the physiological basis for premenstrual syndrome, it is undoubtedly the cause of much suffering in women and it has been estimated that several million working days are lost each year in the United Kingdom because of it. There are other problems beside absenteeism: it has also been associated with increased accidents and decreased ability to concentrate. Exam performance during this period can be impaired and a handicap of as much as 5% has been found. There is an increased admission rate to psychiatric hospitals during this period and suicide rates in women of reproductive age are seven times higher in the second half of the menstrual cycle than in the first. In the premenstrual and menstrual phases, the incidence of all types of crime committed by women increases. The United Kingdom and France have recognized the significance of premenstrual syndrome to such an extent that, in some criminal trials allowance has been made for the fact that the women were premenstrual.

The other common problem is **dysmenorrhoea**, or painful menstruation. Some pain at the time of menstruation is almost universal but a few women have severe and disabling pain. About 45% of menstruating women report moderate or severe dysmenorrhoea. The pain is lower abdominal, either suprapubic or lateralized. Dysmenorrhoea is described as being cramp-like or as a dull ache. It is most severe on the first day of bleeding and in some young women may be associated with faintness, nausea and vomiting. The incidence decreases with age and after childbearing. Sufferers can be reassured that dysmenorrhoea is usually experienced only in cycles in which ovulation occurs, although the reason for this remains obscure.

Dysmenorrhoea is classified in two categories. Primary dysmenorrhoea refers to painful menstrual cramps occurring in the absence of a pelvic abnormality, whereas secondary dysmenorrhoea is associated with pelvic pathology, such as endometriosis or pelvic inflammatory disease. There are differences in the presentation of primary and secondary dysmenorrhoea and so taking a careful menstrual history is important to help distinguish between them.

The origin of the pain is almost certainly within the uterus, but again the exact mechanism is unknown. The type of pain may be ischaemic, due to uncoordinated uterine contractions caused by hypersensitivity of nerve endings within the uterus. It is thought likely that the release of prostaglandins from the disintegrating endometrium may play a major part in the causation of dysmenorrhoea. Non-steroidal anti-inflammatory drugs such as aspirin, or ibuprofen, inhibit prostaglandin synthesis and are therefore effective in reducing pain.

Vasopressin (antidiuretic hormone) and leukotrienes have also been implicated in the aetiology of dysmenorrhoea. Leukotrienes increase smooth muscle activity and increased levels have been found in the endometrium of dysmenorrhoeic women compared to pain-free women. Antidiuretic hormone stimulates myometrial activity and increased levels have again been found in women who are dysmenorrhoeic.

## Other changes associated with the ovarian and menstrual cycles

Changes occur in other regions of the reproductive system, also under the influence of the ovarian hormones. During the follicular phase the epithelium of the uterine tubes proliferates and during the luteal phase the secretory cells become more active, presumably to supply nutrients for the ovum as it moves to the uterus. There are changes in the motility of the muscular elements of the uterine tubes and uterus: tubal movements and myometrial contractions predominate under oestrogenic influence, whilst progesterone decreases the motility. Again it has been suggested that prostaglandins may be involved in tubal contractility and ovum transport.

Cyclical changes are seen in the composition of the mucus secreted by the cervix (the cervix itself does not exhibit marked cyclical activity). As a result of the oestrogen secretion at the time of ovulation, the water and electrolyte content of the mucus increases. This thinner mucus, produced around the time of ovulation, is thought to allow easier penetration of the cervix by spermatozoa. During the luteal phase, under the influence of progesterone, the volume of mucus decreases and it becomes thicker.

These changes in the cervical mucus form the basis of some tests to ascertain whether ovulation has

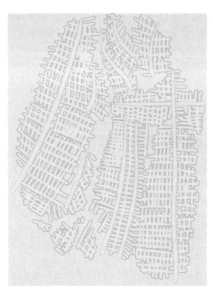

**Figure 6.3.24** 'Ferning' pattern of cervical mucus at the time of ovulation

occurred, and also its timing. If a cervical smear of mucus is taken around the time of ovulation, allowed to dry on a glass slide and examined under a microscope, a characteristic pattern of crystallization occurs, known as ferning or a fern-leaf pattern **(Fig. 6.3.24)**. This is indicative of well-oestrogenized cervical mucus. This phenomenon disappears after ovulation due to the effects of progesterone and it is absent during pregnancy. Also at the time of ovulation, the mucus develops the property of 'spinnbarkheit', which means that it can be drawn out into long threads. Monitoring the stretchiness of vaginal mucus is used by some women as a natural method of family planning.

There are marked changes in the squamous epithelial cells of the vagina during the menstrual cycle. Under oestrogenic stimulation, there is an increased tendency to cornification (an increase in 'horny' tissue) of the cells, which decreases under the influence of progesterone. This change may increase the vagina's resistance to trauma.

The breasts may increase in size and tenderness in the premenstrual week, due to oedema and hyperaemia (increased blood flow) in the intralobular connective tissue. There is often an increase in skin pigmentation premenstrually, especially around the eyes but also in the areola of the nipple. These changes may be due to an increase in the level of melanocyte-stimulating hormone from the anterior pituitary, and are similar to those seen in pregnancy, but less marked.

## The integration of the hormonal systems: the hypothalamic–pituitary–ovarian axis

Several components of the hormonal systems involved in female reproductive physiology have been discussed in isolation but it is crucial to understand the integration and interrelationships of these systems. Gonadotrophins (follicle stimulating hormone and luteinizing hormone) from the anterior pituitary induce both ovulation and the secretion of the ovarian hormones, and these in turn have widespread effects on the body. But how are all these events coordinated?

The hypothalamus is the vital integrating centre. The release of gonadotrophins follicle stimulating hormone and luteinizing hormone from the pituitary is controlled by a releasing hormone produced in the median eminence of the hypothalamus. There appears to be only one hormone produced and this one hormone stimulates the release of both follicle stimulating hormone and luteinizing hormone at the same time. Hence it is given the name gonadotrophin releasing hormone (GnRH) or sometimes luteinizing hormone releasing hormone (LH-RH).

**The release of gonadotrophin releasing hormone from the hypothalamus causes the release of follicle stimulating hormone and luteinizing hormone from the anterior pituitary, which in turn causes development of the ovarian follicles, release of an ovum, maintenance of the corpus luteum and, as a result, the secretion of oestrogens, progesterone and inhibin.** The regulation and integration of this system are complicated, involving fine balances between the levels of gonadotrophins and ovarian hormones, and incorporating both negative and positive feedback pathways and influences from other parts of the brain. Other locally acting hormones, cytokines and growth factors are also involved. One important sensor in the system is the part of the hypothalamus that is sensitive to circulating levels of oestrogens. It is logical for oestrogen to be the important factor, as oestrogen levels give a direct indication of the stage of follicular development and are also responsible for producing most of the preparatory changes necessary to ensure fertilization.

When there are low levels of circulating oestrogens, during and following menstruation, a negative feedback system operates, i.e. the hypothalamus detects the low oestrogen levels and release of gonadotrophin releasing hormone is increased. This in turn increases secretion of follicle stimulating hormone, which stimulates follicular development (in the presence of basal levels of luteinizing hormone). Several follicles begin to develop during each cycle under the influence of follicle stimulating hormone and they all contribute initially to the increasing oestrogen levels. The higher level of oestrogen is then detected by the hypothalamus and levels of follicle stimulating hormone are subsequently reduced; only the most mature follicle will be able to complete its development without the follicle stimulating hormone stimulus, the other follicles degenerate

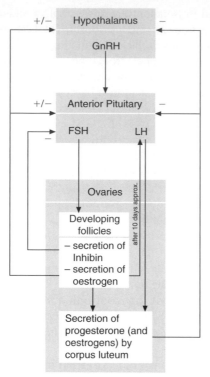

**Figure 6.3.25** Possible pathways controlling the release of female reproductive hormones. FSH, follicle stimulating hormone; GnRH, gonadotrophin releasing hormone; LH, luteinizing hormone

(**Fig. 6.3.25**). Follicle stimulating hormone levels also decline due to the negative feedback effects of inhibin.

Oestrogen probably affects both the anterior pituitary and the hypothalamus, although the latter is thought to be the main site of action. There may also be a short feedback loop, with levels of luteinizing hormone and follicle stimulating hormone directly influencing release of gonadotrophin releasing hormone.

However, a simple negative feedback loop is not an adequate explanation. The luteinizing hormone surge that produces ovulation (**see Fig. 6.3.21**) is due to a positive feedback mechanism, that is, *high* oestrogen levels, acting on the hypothalamus and anterior pituitary, produce the surge in luteinizing hormone secretion (the second surge of follicle stimulating hormone is presumably a result of the surge in releasing hormone and is of secondary importance to the luteinizing hormone surge). The precise mechanisms for this paradoxical negative/positive feedback system require confirmation by further research. The proposed mechanism stated here is no doubt a gross simplification of the complex monitoring system involved. Coad & Dunstall (2001) give a more detailed analysis of the hormonal control mechanisms.

External stimuli are also known to affect the occurrence and timing of ovulation and menstruation. Ovulation is commonly delayed in females subject to

mild stress, for example when taking examinations, and it may cease altogether under conditions of severe stress, for example some women in prisoner-of-war camps have been found to cease to menstruate. Synchronization of menstrual cycles is also sometimes seen (see p. 747).

### CLINICAL APPLICATIONS

Even though our knowledge of the control mechanisms in the human reproductive system is far from complete, the use of fertility drugs involves the hypothalamic–pituitary–ovarian axis. Gonadotrophins are sometimes administered directly, with good results, in the treatment of infertility and gonadotrophin releasing hormone is also used. The intended result is that, with raised levels of gonadotrophins, ovulation will occur. In fact, often multiple ovulation, or **superovulation** as it is sometimes called, occurs. This may result in multiple pregnancies.

Some cases of anovulation have been associated with high prolactin levels. Bromocriptine, a dopamine antagonist, has been found to inhibit the release of excessive prolactin from the anterior pituitary and to correct anovulatory cycles (this mechanism is also implicated in the lactational postpartum amenorrhoea).

The female reproductive system is thus governed by very complex control systems, the main points of which can be summarized as follows (**Fig. 6.3.26**).

1.  Falling oestrogen and progesterone levels initiate menstruation and also relieve the inhibition on follicle stimulating hormone secretion; thus follicle stimulating hormone levels rise and follicles begin to develop.
2.  As the follicles mature, increasing levels of oestrogen are secreted which in turn inhibits the secretion of follicle stimulating hormone (the negative feedback in operation); inhibin also suppresses follicle stimulating hormone secretion. Oestrogen also prepares the uterus and the rest of the body for ovulation.
3.  As a result of optimum follicular maturation, oestrogen levels rise high enough at midcycle to stimulate the release of sufficient luteinizing hormone to result in ovulation. This forms the positive feedback mechanism of oestrogen on the hypothalamus/anterior pituitary.
4.  A corpus luteum forms spontaneously from the collapsed follicle after ovulation and secretes progesterone and oestrogen, which maintain the suppression of the gonadotrophins and prepare the body for possible pregnancy.

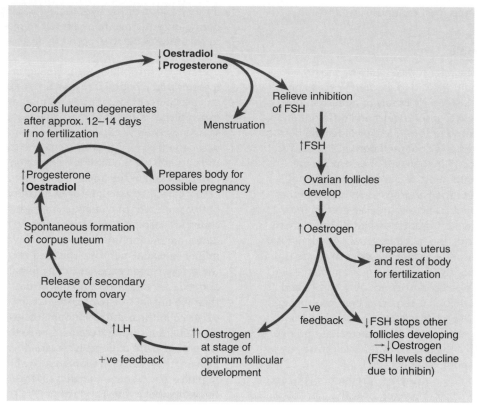

**Figure 6.3.26**    Summary of the events occurring in the female reproductive system

5. In the absence of fertilization and the implantation of the embryo, the corpus luteum degenerates and the levels of ovarian hormones fall, inducing endometrial breakdown.

6. The cycle is repeated.

## DEVELOPMENTAL ISSUES

### PUBERTY

The ovaries and testes are not active during childhood; the reproductive system becomes functional only during adolescence. Adolescence covers the time from the end of childhood to the beginning of adulthood and is a period of maturation, development and growth. Puberty occurs during the adolescent phase and is the point at which the reproductive organs become physically mature and capable of reproduction. During the later stages of childhood there is normally a slow increase in the secretion rates of oestrogens and androgens but the levels are not sufficient to promote the development of secondary sexual characteristics. At the start of puberty in both sexes the hypothalamus begins to release gonadotrophin releasing hormone, which in turn causes the release of follicle stimulating hormone and luteinizing hormones and these hormones stimulate the gonads to secrete their hormones (oestrogens and androgens).

The sequence of body changes during adolescence usually occurs in a definite pattern and is discussed separately for males and females.

### In the male

In the male, the testes increase rapidly in size and spermatogenesis commences. The Leydig cells secrete more androgens and the accessory organs of reproduction (e.g. penis and prostate gland) begin to grow. The higher androgen levels are responsible for the development of secondary sexual characteristics (e.g. hair grows on the face, trunk, axillae and pubic region); the larynx enlarges and, as a consequence, the voice 'breaks' or deepens; considerable muscle development starts and the male experiences occasional ejaculations. In boys, some growth of the testes takes place between 6 and 10 years of age but marked changes start to occur at a mean age of approximately 11½ years (in the United Kingdom and the United States), followed a year later by penile growth. During puberty there is a general growth spurt, with a peak at about 14 years. The onset of pubertal changes and the rate of progress vary from one individual to another and puberty is insidious in nature; indeed, hair

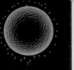

growth on the chest continues into the mid-twenties.

### In the female

In the female, breast development and growth of sexual hair occur first, the former commonly beginning just after 11 years of age. As in the male, there is a growth spurt and differentiation of the skeleton to form the typical female pelvis, and fatty tissue is deposited both in the breasts and buttocks. Higher levels of oestrogen are responsible for most of the female's pubertal changes but raised androgen levels lead to the growth of pubic and axillary hair even in the female. The most dramatic event during puberty is the **menarche**, the first menstrual period, but it is only one event in a complex series of changes that occur at puberty. The mean age of menarche in most developed countries lies between 12 and 13 years, although it can occur between the ages of 9 and 17 years. In Western Europe and the United States the age of menarche has declined steadily since the middle of the last century by as much as 4 months per decade.

Ovulation is normally an infrequent occurrence during the first 2 or 3 years after the menarche. Menstruation itself may be irregular during adolescence and intervals of 4–6 months between periods are not uncommon, especially during the first five cycles or so.

However, some mature gametes are produced from the time of puberty onwards; simultaneously, there are changes in the levels of reproductive hormones secreted by the gonads. The actual onset of puberty, in both sexes, is thought to be due to a significant fall in the sensitivity of the hypothalamus to the sex hormones. In the prepuberty period, *small* amounts of the sex hormones of adrenal origin are sufficient to suppress the activity of those parts of the central nervous system responsible for the synthesis and/or release of gonadotrophin releasing hormone. However, at puberty there is a decreased sensitivity to the negative feedback effect of the sex hormones in some hypothalamic neural 'centres'; thus the pituitary gonadotrophin levels increase, leading to an increase in the secretion of the gonadal sex hormones. Changes in pituitary sensitivity to gonadotrophin releasing hormone and adrenal androgens may also be involved.

After puberty, male and female gonadotrophin secretion differs: the sexually mature female exhibits marked fluctuations in an approximately monthly cycle **(see Fig. 6.3.21)**, whereas in the sexually mature male there is a relatively constant overall mean level of gonadotrophins. This difference is governed by the sexual differentiation of the hypothalamus, established during intrauterine life as a result of male and female fetuses being exposed to different hormones.

Other factors influence the timing of puberty. It seems that a critical body weight (or possibly a critical percentage of body fat or energy expenditure) is essential for sexual maturation. This 'body weight' concept may account for the decline in the mean age of menarche seen over the past 100 years, which is now flattening out. This reduction in the age at which menarche occurs coincides with improved nutrition and better standards of hygiene in developed countries, leading to improved growth and development and this, in turn, could well influence sexual maturity. This idea also explains the amenorrhoea experienced by females with anorexia nervosa, who stop menstruating once their weight falls below a critical point, about 42–47 kg in the United Kingdom. Menstruation recommences during treatment once the 'critical weight' of these patients is regained. This cannot explain, however, how women near starvation in famine areas manage to maintain their high fecundity (birth rates).

A relationship between the pineal gland and puberty has been speculated for many years. The **pineal gland** (a small reddish-grey structure on the dorsal surface of the midbrain) produces melatonin and serotonin. However, normal pubertal development does not appear to be linked to melatonin profiles, although there is some evidence that delayed puberty, precocious puberty and hypothalamic amenorrhoea may have altered melatonin profiles. The knowledge concerning puberty is extensive but far from complete, and the relationships between the hypothalamus and other regions, such as the pineal gland, are largely unexplained. Something holds the reproductive system in check during childhood and precisely what causes its activation is not yet known.

### The menopause

The menopause is a single event occurring during the **climacteric**, a period which extends for some years either side of the menopause. The menopause is the permanent cessation of menstruation resulting from loss of ovarian activity, but the term 'menopause' is frequently used to embrace both the last menses and the changes that occur around the same time. The length of this transition is usually about 4 years but is shorter in smokers than non-smokers. Twelve months of amenorrhoea are needed before fertility can safely be assumed to have ceased.

The human is probably the only animal which has a significant period of life beyond the cessation of reproductive ability. In the majority of women, the menopause occurs between the ages of 45 and 55 years (the median age being 51 years in the United Kingdom) but it can occur anywhere between 39 and 59 years (Royal College of Nursing, 2003). Pregnancy resulting in a spontaneous abortion has been reliably reported as late as the age of 56 years, and assisted reproductive technologies can lead to pregnancies in older women.

During the climacteric, ovulation ceases and there is a deficiency of oestrogen and progesterone. The hypothalamus and anterior pituitary respond to this deficiency by increasing secretions of gonadotrophin releasing hormone, and follicle stimulating hormone and luteinizing hormone, respectively. This increased output of gonadotrophins, which can reach ten times the level in a normal menstruating woman, remains raised for some 20 years or so until senescence occurs. The menopausal symptoms are caused by the deficiency of ovarian hormones and the increase in follicle stimulating hormone and luteinizing hormone. For reasons not yet understood, the ovary becomes resistant to stimuli from the pituitary gland and oestrogen levels fall. In its efforts to stimulate the ovary to work, increased levels of human menopausal gonadotrophin (hMG) are produced by the pituitary gland. Follicle stimulating hormone and human menopausal gonadotrophin are very similar. Every day during the menopausal transition, the levels of follicle stimulating hormone and luteinizing hormone fluctuate markedly from pre- to postmenopausal values. The decline in oestrogen is normally gradual, although it is rapid where a premenopausal woman has her ovaries removed surgically. Oestrogen is still produced after the menopause, not in the ovaries but in glands such as the adrenal gland and also in adipose tissue.

The years preceding the menopause show increasing irregularity of menstruation and the incidence of ovulatory cycles decreases. The usual pattern of events is a decrease in the frequency of menstruation, the amount of blood lost, or both. It is *not* normal for a woman to experience an increased loss or irregularity resulting in more frequent menstruation. It is also usual to regard episodes of bleeding occurring more than 1 year after the menopause as abnormal. Women who present with either of these two sets of symptoms need careful investigation, as there is an increased incidence of genital cancer in women with postmenopausal bleeding.

The effects of oestrogen deficiency can be considered in three categories – immediate effects, medium-term and longer-term effects (Royal College of Nursing, 2003).

**Immediate effects** include vasomotor symptoms including hot flushes, night sweats, palpitations and headaches. Vasomotor symptoms are at their worst in the 2 or 3 years before periods stop, but may continue for years afterwards. Psychological problems and emotional instability are common, including loss of confidence, depressed mood, irritability, forgetfulness, difficulty in concentrating and panic attacks (Royal College of Nursing, 2003). The precise aetiology for these changes is unknown but may be associated with changes in hypothalamic neurotransmitters, most probably due to an increase in the noradrenaline (norepinephrine) : dopamine ratio, which has an effect on thermoregulation thus resulting in the hot flush. Endogenous opioids might also be involved.

**Medium-term effects** of oestrogen deficiency. The low oestrogen levels are responsible for the atrophy of the breasts, labia, uterus and vaginal epithelium that occurs. Atrophy of the vaginal epithelium results in dryness and there is an increase in vaginal pH (it becomes less acidic), which together render the vagina more susceptible to infection, particularly *Candida* (vaginal thrush). Other commonly associated symptoms are pruritus (itching), dyspareunia (painful or difficult coitus) and the urinary problems (such as frequency, urgency and dysuria).

There is also generalized connective tissue atrophy. The skin may become thinner, causing wrinkles; there is thinning of the distribution of hair too, both on the head and in the pubic region. Other symptoms of connective tissue atrophy are brittle nails, muscular aches, and bone and joint pain. The changes in connective tissue can also lead to vaginal prolapse and this in term can be one factor in the development of stress incontinence.

**Longer-term effects:** over a longer period, the fall in oestrogen levels causes thinning of the bones, making them more fragile, and so after the menopause there is an increase in the incidence of **osteoporosis** (and so of fractures) in women. It is important to remember that oestrogen is only one of the factors involved in determining whether a woman develops osteoporosis: a low body mass index, smoking and an inherited tendency to osteoporosis are also significant influencing factors.

Falling oestrogen levels also change lipid metabolism, and the protective influence of oestrogens against ischaemic heart disease is removed. This is because oestrogens can lower total cholesterol and low-density lipoprotein (LDL) levels and raise high-density lipoprotein (HDL) levels. The high-density lipoproteins, which are protective against heart disease (anti-atherogenic), are reduced and the low-density lipoproteins, which are atherogenic, predominate. Other factors, such as diet and smoking, also influence the risk of heart disease. Non-specific symptoms including fatigue, insomnia, depression and headaches are common. These may have a hormonal basis but the menopause can take place at a time of significant psychological and sociological changes for some women. For example, perceptions of loss of sexual attractiveness, redundancy in a mothering role and increasing dependence of elderly parents undermine some women's well-being. Cultural differences are also apparent.

Many women have menopausal symptoms that they can tolerate, perhaps with advice and education; other (lucky!) women will have no symptoms but others will have such severe symptoms that treatment is necessary. General health advice for women at the time of the menopause is the same as for other stages of life, but with more emphasis on factors such as stopping smoking, having a healthy, balanced diet with 700 mg recommended calcium intake, and regular exercise, especially weight-bearing exercises.

## CLINICAL APPLICATIONS

In some instances, **hormone replacement therapy (HRT)** is prescribed for a woman during or after the menopause. It is debatable whether this should be used to maintain 'youthfulness' but it is certainly justified for the relief of distressing symptoms caused by falling oestrogen levels or for prophylaxis against the long-term effects of oestrogen withdrawal. Hormone replacement therapy usually comprises two hormones – oestrogen and progestogen or synthetic hormones. Women who have had a hysterectomy will probably use oestrogen on its own, whereas women with an intact uterus use a combination of the two: this is to prevent endometrial hyperplasia that could occur with oestrogen-only therapy.

Much research has been done and much is underway looking at the benefits and risks of hormone replacement therapy. However, the long-term effects of hormone replacement therapy are still being fully evaluated and studies are giving contradictory findings. Hormone replacement therapy does provide relief of vasomotor symptoms, and has a definite positive

effect in preventing osteoporosis. There is a known risk of developing endometrial cancer with oestrogen-only therapy and an increased risk of breast cancer with prolonged use (Bush et al., 2001). There is conflicting evidence surrounding the use of hormone replacement therapy and the incidence of breast cancer and also its effects on the cardiovascular system. The whole area of hormone replacement therapy and heart disease is currently under review. If the major menopausal problems are vaginal, application of a topical oestrogen cream is often helpful.

Some women are advised to undergo a **hysterectomy** (removal of the uterus) at some stage for problems such as fibroids or uterine prolapse. Premenopausal women who undergo a hysterectomy do not experience an 'artifical' menopause straightaway because their ovaries are not normally removed. However, if it is necessary to remove the ovaries at the same time (**oophorectomy**) the woman will experience an artificial menopause within days of the operation.

After a simple hysterectomy, pregnancy is impossible and monthly menstruation will stop but there should be no other significant changes. The uterus itself does not produce any sex hormones, therefore a woman's femininity or enjoyment of sex should not be altered. In most instances, the vagina is not made smaller by the operation and so normal intercourse is possible. Advice as to the resumption of sexual intercourse should be given postoperatively: it is advisable to wait 4–6 weeks before having gentle intercourse, particularly if there are internal sutures. Similarly, energetic sports should not be recommended until the same time. Intercourse may be uncomfortable at first and use of a lubricant such as KY Jelly or 'Senselle' may be helpful. The vagina may temporarily 'shrink' in size but intercourse will actually help the tissues to stretch and become supple again.

If the patient has had a hysterectomy for carcinoma of the uterus, some of the vagina may have been removed. However, intercourse will stretch the vagina again, although in this case it is advisable to wait longer (possibly 3 months) before resuming sexual activities. Radiotherapy to the genital region will probably decrease the lubricant properties and decrease the possible expansion and lengthening capacity of the vagina, but coitus is still usually feasible.

Patients should be encouraged to voice their anxieties at all stages of treatment. Practical points to help the patient include the giving of accurate and detailed information; seeing and talking with both partners together and providing privacy for them to talk to each other.

There is no equivalent climacteric in males to that occurring in females – males retain their fertility for a longer period and there are well-authenticated cases of men in their eighties becoming fathers. Male hormonal output shows a gradual decline between the ages of 20 and 70 years, although they continue to produce fertile sperm well past 70 years. The age at which an individual male loses his sexual drive has come to be called, quite wrongly, the male menopause. Loss of sexual drive, in either sex, can result from many causes and may occur at any age.

## The physiology of sexual intercourse

The male and female gametes are brought together by the act of sexual intercourse (**coitus**). A brief description of the events of coitus will now be given.

## The male

The normal state of the penis is flaccid but, under conditions of sexual excitement, it becomes erect. **Erection** is purely a vascular phenomenon: during sexual excitement, the arterioles in the erectile tissue of the penis (corpus spongiosum and corpora cavernosa, **see Fig. 6.3.5**) dilate and become engorged with blood. As the erectile bodies are surrounded by a strong fibrous coat, the penis becomes rigid, elongated and increases in girth. As the erectile tissue expands, the veins emptying the corpora are compressed and thus the outflow of blood is minimal. The process occurs rapidly, in 5–10 seconds. Erection is controlled primarily by a spinal reflex but other neurotransmitters are also involved in mediating the erectile response.

The erection reflex (**Fig. 6.3.27**) can start from direct stimulation of the genitals – the glans penis or the skin around the genitals. There are highly sensitive mechanoreceptors located in the tip of the penis. The afferent synapse in the lower spinal cord and the efferent flow, via the nervi erigentes, produce relaxation of the arterioles in the penis. The smooth muscle response in the blood vessels is mediated by a number of neurotransmitters, including nitric oxide. The higher brain centres, via descending pathways, can have profound facilitative or inhibitory effects. Thoughts, visual cues or emotions can cause erection in the complete absence of any mechanical stimulation.

The parasympathetic nerves simultaneously stimulate the urethral glands to secrete a mucoid-like material, which aids lubrication. Erection allows entry of the penis into the female vagina, and the angle the erect penis makes with the male's trunk closely follows the angle of the vagina in the female's pelvis.

After intromission (the insertion of the erect penis into the vagina), **ejaculation of semen** into the female vagina may occur. This is again basically a spinal reflex and the afferent pathway is the same as for erection. When the level of stimulation reaches a critical peak, a patterned automatic sequence of efferent discharge is elicited to the smooth muscle of the genital ducts and to the skeletal muscle at the base of the penis. The exact nature of the nervous pathways involved is complex but includes sympathetic stimulation to the ducts, via L1 and L2 nerve roots. The first stage is known as emission, and the genital ducts and accessory glands empty their contents into the posterior urethra. During the second stage, ejaculation proper, the semen is expelled from the penis, by a series of rapid muscle contractions, into the female genital tract.

During ejaculation, the sphincter at the base of the bladder is closed, therefore no spermatozoa can enter the bladder nor can urine be voided. This again is under the control of the sympathetic nervous system.

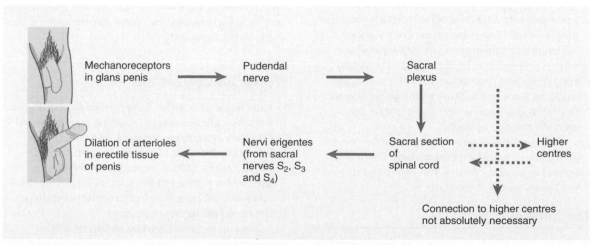

**Figure 6.3.27**   The nervous pathways (simplified) involved in the erection reflex

A feeling of intense pleasure arises with ejaculation and the event is referred to as an **orgasm**. There is simultaneously a noticeable skeletal muscle contraction throughout the body, which is rapidly followed by muscular and psychological relaxation. After ejaculation there is a **latent period** during which time a second erection is not possible. The latent period varies from individual to individual but can range from a few minutes to several hours in 'normal' men. Loss of erection occurs due to vasoconstriction of the arterioles in the penis, hence venous compression is reduced.

## CLINICAL APPLICATIONS

Any interference with the spinal reflexes may result in **impotence** or other sexual dysfunction (although libido is unaffected). For example, ejaculation is usually not possible after a bilateral lumbar sympathectomy below L2. Erection may not be possible after an abdominoperineal resection due to damage to the nervi erigentes. Administration of drugs that inhibit the release of noradrenaline (norepinephrine) from postganglionic sympathetic nerve endings, e.g. methyldopa and reserpine, can lead to ejaculatory failure, although erection and sensation would be normal.

Much erectile dysfunction is due to vascular disease (Crouch, 2003b): the blood vessels in the penis are affected by the same disease processes (e.g. atherosclerosis) as elsewhere in the body and so inevitably affects their function. Some hypertensive individuals report few problems in sexual performance whilst undiagnosed, and thus untreated, but once hypotensive therapy has been initiated, the incidence of impotence and erection failure increases considerably due to the nature of the drugs prescribed. Diabetic patients also suffer from problems with impotence, although the cause is probably a result of metabolic, neuropathological and vascular disturbance. Some patients who have spinal cord injuries have problems too. The prescription drug Viagra (sildenafil) has been found to be very useful in treating many cases of impotence; it works by enhancing and prolonging the effects of nitric oxide on the erectile tissue of the penis. Vacuum devices and intracorporeal injections to aid erection are also available.

Information and counselling for patients with all types of disability are important. There are several organizations that can help patients (see the Useful websites section).

## The female

In the female, sexual excitement is characterized by erection of the clitoris and labia minora, both of which are largely composed of erectile tissue. The tip of the clitoris that is visible externally connects to an internal pyramid-shaped mass of erectile tissue. The neural control of erection is the same as for the male. The breasts may enlarge during sexual excitement and the nipples become erect. As the sexual tension increases, there may be a flushing of the skin, which begins on the chest and spreads upwards over the breasts, neck and up to the face.

The female provides most of the lubrication for coitus by the transudation of fluid through the vaginal walls. The exact source of the mucus is unclear as there are no glands in the vagina. Additional secretions may come from the glands in the vulva and from the Bartholin's glands.

The movement of the penis in and out of the vagina causes pleasure in both the male and female. The female may experience a climax (or orgasm) similar to that of the male. Stimulation of the clitoris may heighten the state of excitement and contributes to the orgasm of the female. The female is potentially capable of several orgasms within a short period of time, unlike the male. During coitus and orgasm the uterus may contract rhythmically and this may serve to aspirate the semen into the uterine lumen. Females do not always experience orgasm and it is not necessary for successful fertilization; for example, orgasm does not occur in artificial insemination. Orgasm may, however, contribute to fertilization in some cases of subfertility where uterine aspirations hasten the movement of spermatozoa towards the ovum.

## Cardiovascular and respiratory changes during coitus

During orgasm in both the male and female there is a marked increase in the heart rate, blood pressure and respiratory rate. The respiratory rate may rise to 40 respirations/minute, the heart rate to between 100 and 170 beats/minute and the systolic blood pressure may be increased by 30–80 mmHg and the diastolic by 20–40 mmHg.

## CLINICAL APPLICATIONS

Individuals who suffer from cardiovascular disease are often anxious about resuming normal sexual activities after, for example, a myocardial infarction, because of the extra strain it might cause. Crouch (2003b) reports that the energy used in sex with a regular partner is roughly the same as walking a mile in 15 minutes and then climbing two flights of stairs.

Thus, in individuals who can tolerate light exercise, sexual activities are perfectly feasible. In a few patients, the effort tolerance is more limited and may be exceeded during sexual intercourse, and coital or postcoital angina or arrhythmias may be precipitated, but this does not rule out coitus, as glyceryl trinitrate or some similar drug could be taken beforehand. There may be a greater demand on the cardiovascular system, i.e. showing increased signs of physiological stress, if intercourse is being performed with a new partner.

Both the patient and his or her partner should be given advice on discharge from hospital, whether or not they verbally express anxieties.

## SEXUAL HEALTH

Sexual health is an important part of general health of individuals. Sexual activity carries with it the risk of infection from a number of microorganisms, including bacterial (e.g. *Chlamydia*, *Gonorrhoea*), viral (genital herpes and warts) and fungal infections. Sexually transmitted infections (STIs) are transferred from individual to individual by sexual intercourse. The consequences of infections can range from short-term inconvenience to serious permanent problems (such as pelvic inflammatory disease, infertility) up to life-threatening (e.g. HIV and AIDS). The incidence of sexually transmitted infections has been increasing in recent years.

## Conception

The egg is released from the ovary at the second metaphase stage of meiosis and it enters the uterine tube still surrounded by follicular cells. If **fertilization** occurs, it does so in the ampulla of the uterine tube.

Normally, the spermatozoa reach the oocyte by traversing the lumen of the uterus and moving along the uterine tubes. Estimates vary, but spermatozoa on their own can probably move only a few millimetres per hour, by propelled movement of their tails. The fact that after coitus spermatozoa can reach the ampulla of the uterine tube within 30 minutes or so implies that their movement is assisted. As already discussed, coitus provides the initial impetus to spermatozoa in their journey. After coitus, the primary transport mechanism is contraction of the musculature in the uterus and uterine tubes. Prostaglandins present in the semen may cause the smooth muscle to contract. The wastage rate of spermatozoa is huge: of the several hundred million spermatozoa deposited in the vagina, only a few thousand actually reach the uterine tubes. Fructose present in the semen provides an important energy source for the spermatozoa.

As the spermatozoa are transported to the site of fertilization, they undergo their final maturation, which enables them to pass through the follicular cells and zona pellucida and penetrate the oocyte. The maturation processes are known as **capacitation** and the **acrosome reaction**. These processes involve changes in the acrosome and the release of hyaluronidase and other proteolytic enzymes, which assist the passage of the spermatozoa through the layers of cells around the oocyte. It has been postulated that a high density of spermatozoa is required to produce sufficient hyaluronidase to remove most of the follicular cells. However, only one spermatozoon is able to enter one egg. The entry of additional spermatozoa is blocked in some way.

The time available for fertilization of the oocyte in the female is approximately 24 hours after ovulation, after which time the egg begins to degenerate. Spermatozoa maintain their fertilizing ability for up to 48 hours (some suggest even as long as 72 hours) inside the female genital tract, so there is only a limited period when fertilization is possible at all.

The penetration of the oocyte by the head of the spermatozoon is followed by completion of the second meiotic division of the ovum and the formation of the second polar body. The nuclei of the spermatozoon and ovum, containing the maternal and paternal haploid sets of chromosomes, come together on the mitotic spindle (**Fig. 6.3.28**). Fertilization is completed with the restoration of the diploid complement of chromosomes.

The role of the uterine or Fallopian tubes is much more than that of a simple muscular tube – they play an important part not only in ensuring fertilization occurs, but also in the first few days after fertilization. For example, appropriate muscular contraction and ciliary movement are necessary and there needs to be the correct volume and concentration of fluid in the tubes; this fluid probably has some nutritional role and may also convey biochemical signals, which condition subsequent events such as capacitation and cleavage in the gametes. It is thought that tubal activities are probably controlled by the ovary.

The fertilized ovum, usually referred to as the **embryo** (or **zygote**), continues a series of mitotic divisions as it passes along the uterine tube, although it does not increase in size. A round mass of cells is formed, still surrounded by the zona pellucida, known as a **morula** (Fig. 6.3.29). A central cavity develops in the morula so that a fluid-filled cyst is formed called the **blastocyst**. The cells of the blastocyst become arranged into an outer layer, the **trophoblast**, and an inner cell mass bulging into the central fluid-filled cavity.

Normally, only one oocyte is released during each cycle. Sometimes, however, two or more oocytes are released almost simultaneously. When this is the case, and two oocytes are fertilized, non-identical

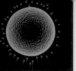

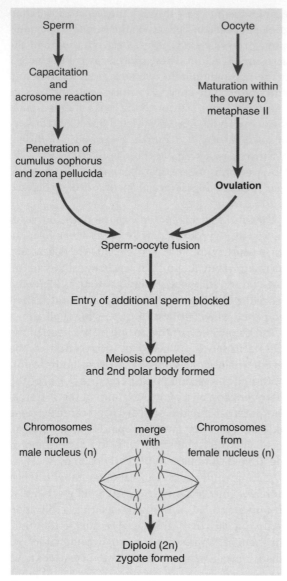

**Figure 6.3.28** Events in the female reproductive tract leading up to fertilization

(dizygotic) twins will develop. Identical (monozygotic) twins result when a single fertilized ovum, at a very early stage of development, becomes completely divided into two independently growing cell masses.

The developing zygote normally reaches the uterus approximately 3–5 days after fertilization, at the morula stage, and lies free within the lumen of the uterus for a short time. Chemical substances are capable of passing from the embryo to the mother and vice versa when the embryo is free living in the uterus, that is, before attachment or implantation.

By the sixth or seventh day after fertilization, the process of **implantation**, or embedding, into the oestrogen and progesterone primed endometrium occurs. The trophoblast lies next to the uterine epithelium and the two layers of cells become intimately associated as the cell boundaries between the

trophoblast and uterine epithelial cells disappear. This probably occurs as a result of cellular phagocytosis by the trophoblast. The cells of the trophoblast actively invade the endometrium, which responds by undergoing a hypertrophic reaction which converts the endometrium into the **decidua**. The trophoblast plays an active part in the nutrition of the inner cell mass from which the embryo and associated structures, such as the amnion, develop. The blastocyst becomes completely embedded in the decidua.

## CLINICAL APPLICATIONS

Occasionally, the embryo becomes implanted in the uterine tube and this is known as an **ectopic pregnancy**. It is not known why ectopic pregnancies occur but the incidence is increasing and it is a potentially life-threatening condition if the pregnancy is not terminated quickly. Ectopic pregnancies are significantly more common among women who have undergone treatment for infertility.

The **placenta** is derived from maternal (decidual) and embryonic (trophoblastic) components **(Fig. 6.3.30)**. After embedding, the trophoblast proliferates and divides into two layers, an inner one where the cell structure persists, called the **cytotrophoblast**, and an outer one where the cell boundaries largely break down, called the **syncytiotrophoblast**. In the embedding process endometrial capillaries are broken down and so maternal blood oozes around the trophoblast. Initial nutrition of the embryo is provided from the cell debris produced by the trophoblastic phagocytosis, with the placenta and fetal circulation taking over this role after a few weeks. During the first month of life, the embryo develops a comprehensive blood supply, including arteries and veins in the umbilical cord that connects the embryo and mother. Five weeks after implantation this system has become well established; the fetal heart has begun to pump blood and the entire mechanism for nutrition of the fetus is functional. Nutrients move from the maternal blood, across the placental membranes into the fetal blood; waste products move in the opposite direction. Oxygen and carbon dioxide move by simple passive diffusion whereas other substances are carried mainly by active transport mechanisms in the placental membranes. It is now recognized that conditions or experiences in the uterus not only restrict the normal growth of the fetus, but also probably 'programme' the baby to develop chronic diseases in later life (fetal programming). If a pregnant woman is stressed or malnourished, the fetus's development may be upset, increasing the chances of diabetes, heart disease and

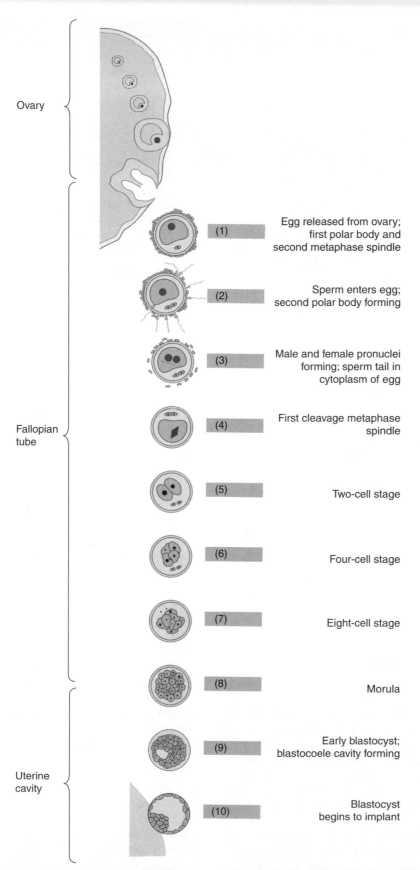

Ovary

Fallopian tube

Uterine cavity

(1) Egg released from ovary; first polar body and second metaphase spindle

(2) Sperm enters egg; second polar body forming

(3) Male and female pronuclei forming; sperm tail in cytoplasm of egg

(4) First cleavage metaphase spindle

(5) Two-cell stage

(6) Four-cell stage

(7) Eight-cell stage

(8) Morula

(9) Early blastocyst; blastocoele cavity forming

(10) Blastocyst begins to implant

**Figure 6.3.29** Diagrammatic representation of follicular growth, ovulation, fertilization and preimplantation

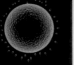

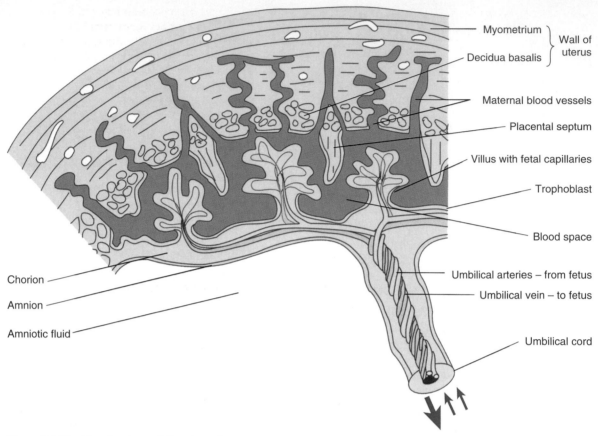

**Figure 6.3.30**    The structure of the placenta

high blood pressure when the offspring reaches middle age (Schmidt, 1999).

The fetus remains connected to the mother via the umbilical cord for the whole period of **gestation**. The average duration of pregnancy is 266 days (38 weeks) from conception and 280 days (40 weeks) from the date of the last menstrual period in a woman with a 26–32-day cycle.

### CLINICAL APPLICATIONS

Some drugs taken by the mother can reach the fetus via the placenta; thalidomide is an example of a drug transmitted to the embryo with disastrous effects, as affected children were born with grossly deformed or absent limbs. Physiologically, some chemicals may cause in the fetus exactly what they would do in the mother, for instance narcotics not only induce sleep in the mother but also make the fetus sleepy. Nicotine and lead can cross the placenta too; the former has been associated with 'small-for-dates' babies and a reduction in placental size. Montgomery & Ekbom (2002) suggest that in utero exposure to the effects of smoking results in life-long metabolic dysregulation, possibly due to fetal

malnutrition or toxicity: smoking during pregnancy should always be strongly discouraged. Even salicylates, taken as aspirin, may cause neonatal bleeding at term, alter the prothrombin time of the fetus and delay mechanisms of haemostasis. Pregnant women should be warned against taking drugs unless prescribed by the doctor, and this information should be included in the health education given to women during pregnancy. Large quantities of alcohol, especially binge drinking, should be avoided. Certain live viruses can also cross the placenta, for example the rubella virus (German measles). There is no direct mixing of the fetal and maternal blood during pregnancy; thus it is feasible for a Rhesus-negative mother to carry to term a Rhesus-positive fetus.

The fetus floats in a completely fluid-filled cavity. Specimens of this amniotic fluid can be removed during the second trimester by a technique called **amniocentesis**, which is usually carried out around the 15th week of pregnancy. This process can be used to diagnose certain congenital defects, for example Down syndrome and neural tube defects, as the fluid contains some fetal cells and fetal products, for example α-fetoproteins. The sex of the fetus can be determined from chromosomal examination. As the fetal cells have to be cultured, the complete results from amniocentesis are often not available for 3 or 4 weeks. There is a miscarriage risk of between 0.5 and 2% with amniocentesis, so the procedure should not be undertaken lightly. A method for first trimester prenatal diagnosis is available involving chorionic villus sampling (CVS) – the chorion is part of the embryonic sac (see Fig. 6.3.30). Chorionic villus sampling can be performed between 8 and 11 weeks of pregnancy, using either the transcervical or trans-abdominal route, and would allow a much earlier termination of pregnancy if necessary. However, the miscarriage rate with chorionic villus sampling is approximately twice that of amniocentesis. Non-invasive methods of fetal diagnosis, such as nuchal translucency by ultrasound scans, and blood tests, do not carry the same risks. Nuchal scans detect the presence of excess fluid which tends to collect behind the neck of a fetus partly because of its tendency to lie on its back; this accumulation of fluid can indicate possible problems, such as in Down syndrome and cardiac abnormalities.

A detailed description of embryological changes in pregnancy can be found in any textbook of human embryology (see Suggestions for further reading). The maintenance of pregnancy and changes in the mother are under hormonal influences and these will be considered shortly, but first there will be a brief discussion of methods of preventing conception, that is contraception, and methods that assist conception for couples with infertility problems.

## CLINICAL APPLICATIONS

### CONTRACEPTION

Conception refers to both the fertilization of the oocyte by a spermatozoon and the successful implantation (nidation) of the embryo into the endometrium. Thus contraceptive methods aim to prevent fertilization and/or implantation from occurring. Some contraceptives work by preventing fertilization, that is, preventing the male and female gametes uniting. Examples of these include simple mechanical barriers, e.g. the cap, sheath and spermicides, that interfere with spermatozoa viability. Sterilization by vasectomy and cutting of the uterine tubes are further examples. Intrauterine devices (IUDs), i.e. small plastic and copper devices, or small T-shaped plastic devices, also known as the coil, act by slowing ovum transport along the uterine tubes and also by preventing implantation of the embryo into the endometrium if fertilization

occurrs. The exact mechanism by which intrauterine devices act is not certain, but it is known that foreign bodies within the uterus will prevent implantation. The endometrium of women with intrauterine devices has been found to contain more leucocytes, which could be responsible for preventing the development of the blastocyst.

The combined oral contraceptive pill acts by a combination of both previously described methods. The various types of pill contain oestrogen and progestogen (a synthetic progesterone). Tablets are usually taken for 21 days, with a break of 7 days during which time there is a withdrawal bleed, i.e. simply due to the withdrawal of the hormonal support (some varieties of pill are taken for 28 days). The raised levels of these hormones disrupt the normal hypothalamus–pituitary–ovarian axis and its feedback system, with the consequence that no ovulation occurs. Higher levels of oestrogen and progestogen have other effects on the woman too: the cervical mucus remains viscid due to the progestogen, and penetration of it by the spermatozoa is difficult; the endometrium is altered and is not in a state capable of accepting any embryo, and the tubal transport mechanism is altered, interfering with the transport of the oocyte from the ovary to the uterus. These combined effects account for the almost complete effectiveness of combined oral contraceptives (providing that they are taken as prescribed). Thus, if ovulation were to take place, pregnancy would be unlikely to occur because conditions in the reproductive tract are unfavourable for spermatozoa and ovum transport and also for implantation. The pill thus seems to be an ideal contraceptive, but it does have some serious side-effects, for example in some individuals there is an increased risk of thromboembolus formation. Some high-risk factors have been identified and these include increasing age, obesity and cigarette smoking in the pill user.

Other steroid contraceptives can be prescribed, such as the progestogen-only pill. This is not as effective as the combined pill because ovulation still occurs in many cycles and it is essential that the pill is taken very regularly. It acts primarily by inducing unfavourable conditions for fertilization and implantation. There are also phased pills, where each phase contains a different proportion of an oestrogen and progestogen. The aim is to provide a hormonal balance that more closely resembles the fluctuations of a normal menstrual cycle.

Slow-release depot injections of progestogen can also be used. An intramuscular injection of the drug, e.g. Depo-Provera, can be given to a woman, giving her protection from pregnancy for

2–3 months while the hormones are released. Contraceptive implants that are placed under the skin and release progestogen over a number of years are available but tend to have a more restricted use. Under some circumstances, it is possible to take special doses of hormones (either progestogen only or a combined oestrogen–progestogen) as a postcoital or emergency contraceptive, within 72 hours of unprotected intercourse. The exact mode of action of the postcoital 'pill' is not fully understood but it has an effect between fertilization and implantation. Insertion of a copper-containing intrauterine device up to 5 days after intercourse can also be effective as emergency contraception, by interfering with implantation of the fertilized ovum.

Some couples rely on natural family planning methods, which rely on careful observation of the changes in the women throughout the menstrual cycle. Recording body temperature on waking is one such method as the body temperature rises slightly (by approximately 0.2°C) after ovulation. Some women also monitor the changes in cervical mucus (see earlier).

## ASSISTED REPRODUCTION

Infertility affects one in six couples in the United Kingdom (although many of these couples will conceive naturally within 2 years). There are many potential causes for infertility or failure to conceive and the problem can originate from either the male or female. Male infertility is the primary reason for failure to conceive in approximately 25% of childless couples. Pelvic inflammatory disease, endometriosis and polycystic ovary syndrome result in reduced fertility but the cause of many couple's infertility often remains unexplained. Some of the causes of infertility are now amenable to intervention either by treatment of the problem itself or by bypassing the problem with the use of assisted reproductive technology.

Damaged or blocked uterine tubes, possibly as a result of salpingitis (inflammation of the uterine tubes), is an important cause of infertility. Surgery to improve blocked or damaged tubes is sometimes possible. In November 1977, Patrick Steptoe, an obstetrician, and Robert Edwards, a physiologist, made history with the first successful human **in vitro fertilization** (IVF) (i.e. in artificial conditions). An oocyte that had undergone its initial maturation in vivo (i.e. within the ovary) was removed by laparoscopy, fertilized in vitro and the resultant embryo was transferred back to the uterus of the mother. Thus the mother's blocked uterine tubes were

bypassed. In July 1978, a perfectly healthy female infant weighing 2.7 kg was born. With in vitro fertilization, following a period of hormone stimulation, a number of eggs are collected from the woman and mixed with the man's sperm. Fertilization occurs in the culture dish. Up to three (this number is under review) of the resultant embryos can be transferred into the uterus. In vitro fertilization can be used with donated eggs, sperm or embryos. Since the first successful human in vitro fertilization, techniques have improved and around 6000 in vitro fertilization babies a year are born in the United Kingdom; however only 20–25% of women become pregnant after in vitro fertilization, with the success rate dropping dramatically after the age of 35.

In vitro fertilization with embryo transfer (ET) is one form of assisted conception but others are also available. Other processes include ovulation induction with hormone therapy and artificial insemination, when sperm (either from the woman's partner or a donor) are placed directly into the cervix. Gamete intrafallopian transfer (GIFT) is a form of therapy for infertile women with at least one anatomically and functionally intact Fallopian tube. The main theoretical advantage of this method lies in the assumption that fertilization of the oocyte and early development takes place as in spontaneous human conception in the ampullary–isthmus junction of the Fallopian tube, overcoming any defects in tubal transport. As its name suggests, gamete intrafallopian transfer involves transfer of preovulatory oocytes and washed sperm into the Fallopian tube. This process ensures that microscopically normal oocytes and motile sperm reach the normal site of fertilization, and placement into the Fallopian tube increases the chance of implantation.

The main treatment for couples affected by severe male factor infertility is intracytoplasmic sperm injection (ICSI). This involves fertilization by injection of a single sperm directly into an oocyte using micromanipulation techniques.

Some people have sperm and ova taken and then frozen for medical reasons, for example if the person needs chemotherapy for cancer, or if there is a family history of early menopause or endometriosis. In this way some viable gametes remain for use at a later stage. Embryos can also be frozen. If a couple fail to achieve a pregnancy with their own ova or sperm, donated sperm or ova can be used. Developments in this field are carefully controlled in the United Kingdom by the Human Fertilisation and Embryology Authority (HFEA). The success rates of these techniques varies with the regime adopted and the centre performing the treatment. The Human

Fertilisation and Embryology Authority gives details of these (see Useful websites).

Beside the financial cost of these treatments there are also great emotional and physical demands on the couple as well as the potential problems of coping with failure. Patients undergoing investigations and treatment for infertility are in particular need of sensitive interventions and support from those caring for them professionally.

## Hormone changes during pregnancy

The hormone changes during pregnancy are many and complex, and much remains to be learned about them. Progesterone and oestrogen are essential for the initiation and continuance of pregnancy. Fertilization results in the persistence of the corpus luteum, which continues to develop and increases its secretion of these hormones. Progesterone maintains the endometrium in its 'progestational' state essential for pregnancy, and is necessary to depress the contractile activity of the uterus, thus allowing the blastocyst to implant and preventing its expulsion. Oestrogens are necessary for uterine growth, which involves both general protein synthesis and the production of specific enzymes necessary for muscular contraction and energy mechanisms – these are important during parturition.

The non-pregnant corpus luteum is maintained by the gonadotrophin luteinizing hormone from the anterior pituitary. However, luteinizing hormone levels fall 12–14 days after ovulation. The corpus luteum is maintained in a pregnant woman by a hormone called **human chorionic gonadotrophin (hCG)**, produced by the trophoblast of the developing blastocyst. Human chorionic gonadotrophin is a glycoprotein very similar in structure to luteinizing hormone and is found only in the presence of a trophoblast. It can be detected in maternal blood and urine about 10 days after ovulation, i.e. 5 days before the next menstrual period would have occurred. Thus the blastocyst must begin to produce human chorionic gonadotrophin very soon after fertilization and before implantation is complete. Human chorionic gonadotrophin maintains the secretion of progesterone and oestrogen from the corpus luteum in early pregnancy. This is an amazing process, as all humans owe their lives to the fact that when they were little larger than a pin's head, they were capable of producing and sending a biological signal so potent that it was able to influence the mother's physiology to stop the menstrual cycle.

Secretion of human chorionic gonadotrophin reaches a peak 8–9 weeks after the last menstrual period and then the level drops dramatically to a lower one that is maintained until the end of pregnancy (**Fig. 6.3.31**). Thus the function of the corpus luteum also begins to decline after 8 weeks of pregnancy. Oophorectomy (excision of an ovary) before the sixth week leads to abortion, but after that time has no effect on pregnancy.

### CLINICAL APPLICATIONS

The presence of human chorionic gonadotrophin in the maternal urine forms the basis of the immunological **pregnancy test**. This will give a reliable positive result approximately 28 days after conception but human chorionic gonadotrophin can be detected as early as 14 days after conception with some tests. Recent development of a radioimmunoassay technique to detect the presence of a subunit of human chorionic gonadotrophin in maternal serum now allows diagnosis of pregnancy even before the first missed menstrual period.

In humans, the placenta takes over steroid production from the corpus luteum by the twelfth week of pregnancy. Oestrogen, particularly oestriol, and progesterone are synthesized in the placenta from precursors originating mainly from the fetal adrenal glands and liver and from the maternal adrenal glands. It is likely that the placental hormones are synthesized and released by the syncytiotrophoblast, the outer layer of the trophoblast. The interdependence of fetal and placental tissues for the production of oestrogen in particular has given rise to the concept of the **fetoplacental unit**, the term implying that both are necessary and neither can function in isolation.

Progesterone and oestrogen levels rise throughout pregnancy until just prior to delivery and these elevated levels inhibit the release of follicle stimulating hormone and luteinizing hormone. Another hormone produced by the fetoplacental unit is **human placental lactogen (hPL)**, also known as human chorionic somatomammotrophin (hCS). Levels of human placental lactogen rise steadily throughout pregnancy, with the curve flattening off towards term (**see Fig. 6.3.31**). Human placental lactogen is structurally very similar to growth hormone. The effect of this in terms of its effect on glucose metabolism and its antagonistic effect on insulin is discussed later (see Physiological effects associated with pregnancy). Human placental lactogen is also involved in the proliferation of alveoli in the breast tissue in preparation for lactation.

The role of the placenta in producing other hormones is uncertain; it has been proposed that relaxin, renin and possibly a substance similar to

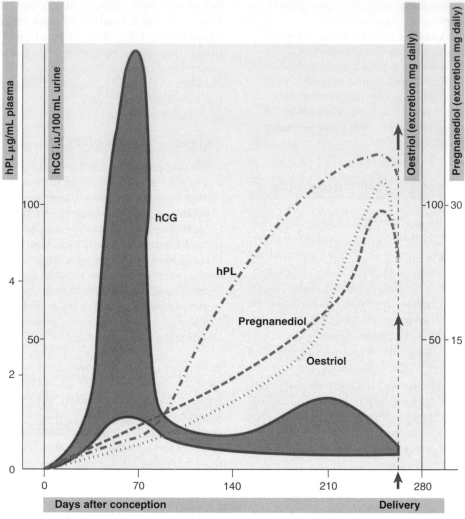

**Figure 6.3.31** Changes in hormone levels during pregnancy. hCG, human chorionic gonadotrophin; hPL, human placental lactogen

thyroid-stimulating hormone are also produced by the placenta. **Relaxin** has also been isolated from the corpora lutea; it is now thought that it may be synthesized in the ovaries and simply stored in the placenta. Relaxin has been shown to be similar in structure to insulin and so is likely to have growth controlling effects similar to insulin. As knowledge of relaxin has advanced, its role has been upgraded. Relaxin is thought to cause the softening of the elastic ligaments of the symphysis pubis and pelvic joints so that the fetal head can descend through the bony arch at delivery without damage. Relaxin also exercises restraint on myometrial contractility, is a potent stimulator of uterine growth and possibly fetal growth too and finally may play a role in the onset of labour. Relaxin has also been found to have a positive effect on sperm motility. So relaxin is a good example of a hormone that has many functions.

Maternal oxytocin levels rise throughout pregnancy. **Oxytocin**, secreted from the posterior pituitary gland, stimulates the contraction of the smooth muscle of the pregnant uterus and lactating mammary glands, but this effect is held in check by the high levels of progesterone that inhibit uterine motility. Only at parturition is oxytocin left unopposed to act on the smooth muscle of the uterus.

Many other physiological changes occur in the mother during pregnancy. A few of these changes are given below.

## Physiological changes in pregnancy

Pregnancy is very well described as 'a normal, if altered state of health'. For example, it is normal for the fetal blood pH in labour to be at levels of 7.25–7.35, i.e. significantly below that compatible with healthy adult life. The healthy fetus is thus well prepared for the rigors of labour.

Significant changes associated with pregnancy affect different body systems to a varying degree. The important aim is to understand what is normal for pregnancy, rather than viewing such changes as pathological. At the same time, pathological changes can develop associated with pregnancy. These include conditions such as pre-eclampsia, which are outside the scope of this book. Such conditions, while they can be very mild, warranting only greater vigilance, can also be life threatening.

## Cardiovascular and haematological systems

Pregnancy is associated with significant changes in haemodynamics and cardiac function that specifically meets the haemodynamic demand of the (separate) fetoplacental circulation. Circulating blood volume increases by 40–60%, and up to 100% in multiple pregnancies. This increase occurs gradually up to just over 20 weeks of gestation.

Higher levels of circulating oestrogens, progesterone and some prostaglandins effectively reduce systemic vascular resistance, thus blood pressure remains largely stable, although it is normal to find a slight lowering of the pressures in early pregnancy and a slight, steady rise in the third trimester. The increase in cardiac output of approximately 30% actually part-precedes the increase in blood volume. Both components of cardiac output, i.e. heart rate and stroke volume, increase although the heart rate increase is dominant towards term. In late pregnancy, uterine enlargement restricts diaphragm movement, increases intra-abdominal pressure and alters the position of the heart. This is of no consequence in healthy women but may severely compromise women with pre-existing severe cardiac disease. Many heart anomalies and conditions are successfully managed with surgery early in life and may place relatively little haemodynamics strain. However all such women require preconception counselling and direct management by the cardiologist and obstetrician during their pregnancy.

In late pregnancy the cardiac output is heavily dependent on the woman's position, and it is important to avoid supine hypotension. This occurs when the gravid uterus compresses the inferior vena cava. For this reason, heavily pregnant women should never be placed in this position unless a wedge is placed under their lower right back/hip to tilt the uterus to the left.

Increased plasma volume accounts for 75% of the total blood volume increase. Although red blood cells also increase by 18% there remains a haemodilution (reduced haematocrit) that has previously been viewed wrongly as an 'anaemia' rather than a normal physiological lowering of the red blood cell percentage. Advice on foods containing iron, folic acid and vitamin C is appropriate, with iron supplementation reserved only for women with haemoglobin

levels below 10.5 g/dL. Oversupplementation with iron in the past resulted in some women having abnormally high haemoglobin levels in pregnancy, which were associated with poorer fetal outcome. This is assumed to have been due to the greater viscosity of maternal blood resulting in poorer perfusion of the placental site.

Haemodilution also accounts for the lower body oedema seen in the majority of healthy pregnant women, particularly in the summer and later in the day. It occurs as a result of reduced colloid osmotic pressure and is not pathological. The heavy uterus may also contribute to poor venous return. While it is true that oedema may be associated with pre-eclampsia, greatest vigilance is required in terms of monitoring rises in blood pressure and identifying proteinuria.

Changes in haemostasis in pregnancy result in a hypercoagulable state. Both the balanced fibrin forming and fibrinolytic systems are associated with multiple and interrelated changes, but the net result is the clotting time is reduced, i.e. the blood clots more quickly. This begins in early pregnancy. Deep vein thromboses and pulmonary emboli are thus an increased risk in pregnancy. At the same time, this physiological adaptation serves to protect women to some extent in respect of the normal blood loss associated with childbirth (approximately 300 mL) or in the event of haemorrhage.

Among the white blood cells, neutrophils in particular increase. However, a woman's response to infection varies more in relation to the type of pathogen encountered and no overall conclusions as to her susceptibility to infection can be drawn. The greatest impact may occur at different times in pregnancy, e.g. Rubella in early pregnancy and varicella (chicken pox) at term. There are also significant altered effects depending on whether the infection is primary or secondary. To avoid unnecessary risk of infection early in pregnancy, women need specific advice on diet and management of pets and animals.

## Gastrointestinal system and the liver

There are marked changes in this system from early in pregnancy. Appetite change and cravings occasionally occur. The nausea and occasional vomiting that is slightly more common on waking appears to be associated with the presence of human chorionic gonadotrophin. These rather normal distressing symptoms appear largely hormonally induced. Should vomiting become uncontrolled, hyperemesis gravidarum may develop. In this condition woman's fluid and electrolyte balance is lost and the condition is potentially life threatening.

Hormonal changes also account of many of the other associated discomforts. Oestrogen is largely

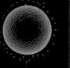

responsible for gingivitis, in which increased vascularization of gum tissue leads to increased risk of trauma. The increase in progesterone levels account for many of the other associated problems in the gut. Poor oesophageal sphincter tone and widening of the hiatus of the stomach may result in reflux of gastric acid and heartburn. Where hiatus hernia pre-exists there is potential risk of oesophageal rupture. Decreased intestinal tone facilitates an enhanced absorption of nutrients but is also associated with constipation. Advice with regard to adequate dietary fibre intake, especially fruit and vegetables, and fluids and exercise is important.

Liver function is also altered in pregnancy affecting bile production (slightly increased risk of gallstone formation) and changes in enzyme levels. This makes evaluation of liver enzyme function and liver-derived clotting factors potentially difficult because of the change in norms and the reduced reliability of some function tests. Pathological conditions associated with pregnancy in which diagnosis may be difficult include cholestiasis, HELLP syndrome (**h**ypertension, **e**levated **l**iver enzymes and **l**ow **p**latelets), preeclampsia, acute fatty liver and DIC (**d**isseminated **i**ntravascular **c**oagulation).

## Metabolism

Normal thyroid function is necessary for the normal pubertal developments and fertility to occur. The basal metabolic rate in pregnancy increases by 20–25% but most of this is associated with the increased work required, and the changes mimic hyperthyroidism. Only in Graves' disease is there a significant risk of affecting the fetus through growth retardation or pre-term labour. In pregnancy, human chorionic gonadotrophin and oestrogen increase production of thyroxine binding globulin (TBG) by the liver. This in turn influences complex alterations in thyroxine ($T_3$ and $T_4$) levels that increase the difficulty of diagnosis of any thyroid pathology in childbearing. Suboptimal thyroid function can be associated with hyperemesis gravidarum (mentioned earlier) and, as the return to prepregnant function takes some weeks postpartum, is also associated with some cases of postnatal depression.

Carbohydrate, protein and lipid metabolism in the pregnant woman and her fetus are essentially linked. They are focused on fetal growth and the provision of energy stores for extrauterine life and meeting the needs of pregnancy and the demands of labour. The placenta itself is a complex organ involved in hormone production, metabolism and transport. It therefore has precursor and energy demands of its own. In terms of transport, the usual active and passive transport mechanisms into and out of cells apply.

It therefore acts as a selective 'sieve' between mother and fetus, with (in general) smaller molecules such as some drugs, viruses and immunoglobulins passing through, whereas larger ones such as insulin do not.

In pregnancy, human placental lactogen, oestrogen and progesterone secretion alter maternal glucose utilization and insulin action. The mother's need for insulin nearly triples by the third trimester. This increase is partly due to the insulin resistance that develops in maternal cells. Where a woman is unable to meet this insulin demand her blood glucose rises and reversible gestational diabetes occurs. Women with insulin-dependent diabetes mellitus have gradually increasing insulin requirements. Women in these groups need the combined care of a diabetologist and a specialist midwife/nurse, together with an obstetrician. There are potentially significant implications for the fetus and preconceptual care for diabetic women is essential.

As with the liver function and haematological laboratory tests, the glucose tolerance test results lack reliability in pregnancy and need interpretation. It is therefore essential that when pregnant women are being investigated for any condition and tests are requested, information specifying gestation and any additional clinical features are given on the request form. This will enable appropriate clinical judgements to be made.

## Renal system

The increased circulating blood volume results in a 40–50% higher glomerular filtration rate. In turn this means that the rapid flow of primary urine does not allow full reabsorption of some substances, such as certain drugs. The result is that relevant drug dosages often need to be increased (appropriate for pregnancy), e.g. epilepsy medication. Similarly, glucose reabsorption in the proximal convoluted tubule is reduced. This may result in glycosuria. Blood glucose estimations are therefore required should glycosuria be identified.

In pregnancy, the kidneys enlarge through hypertrophy to meet the additional demands. Women with one kidney normally have no problems with the demands of pregnancy, but women with pre-existing disease require guidance from a nephrologist.

Progesterone dilates the renal pelvises, lengthening and dilating and reducing the tonicity of the ureters. Stasis is compounded in late pregnancy by pressure compression between the gravid uterus and the pelvis. Urinary tract infection risks are therefore much higher in pregnancy. Frequency of micturition is common in early pregnancy due to the growing uterus within the pelvis, and in late pregnancy as the presenting part descends into the pelvis. Urinalysis therefore requires observations for cloudiness and offensiveness, and dipstick assessment of leucocytes.

## The integumentary system

**Chloasma**, tanned areas of pigmentation of the face may be seen with oral contraceptive use but more commonly in pregnancy. In pregnancy, a linea negra forms as a darkened line between the umbilicus and the symphysis pubis and the areola around the nipples similarly darkens. Striae gravidarum (stretch marks) may appear on the abdomen. These are linear tears in the collagen in opposition to the tension lines. Their wrinkly purple hue ultimately fades, leaving small white streaks. The 'stretching of collagen fibres' explanation has been discounted but the precise roles of relaxin and increased oestrogen and corticosteroid levels, together with a possibly inherited tendency, have yet to be determined.

For a more detailed discussion of the physiological changes the reader is referred to Blackburn & Loper (2002) and Coad & Dunstall (2001).

In addition to the physiological changes discussed above, it should be remembered that pregnancy is a highly emotional time, too: there are psychological changes and wide mood swings that probably have, at least in part, a hormonal causation. Antepartum depression is frequently seen, as well as postnatal depression. Lack of social support and relationship difficulties may exacerbate the situation. Pre-existing mental health problems must be taken into account and a multiprofessional approach adopted.

## Parturition (childbirth) (Fig. 6.3.32)

The length of gestation is variable; the mean length is 40 weeks but there is considerable individual variability and a range of 250–285 days after presumed ovulation gives a broader spread of normal gestation. A term pregnancy is defined as one lasting between 37–42 weeks.

## Preparation for labour

Throughout pregnancy, the placenta produces increasingly high levels of progesterone. This results in the development of the thickened myometrial layer through the hypertrophy and hyperplasia of myometrial muscle cells. At the same time, progesterone

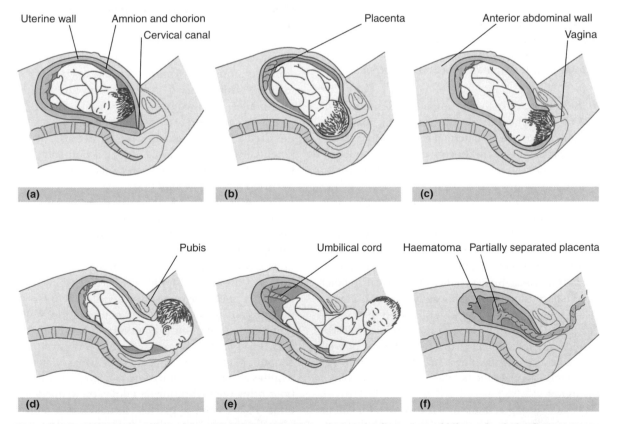

**Figure 6.3.32** The birth process. (a) and (b) The cervix dilates during the first stage of labour. (c–e) The fetus passes through the cervix and vagina during the second stage of labour. During the third stage of labour the uterus contracts and the placenta folds upon itself and detaches from the uterine wall. Bleeding from the large blood vessels forms a haematoma

causes the myometrium to be unresponsive to nervous stimuli, and this maintains the uterus in a quiescent state, despite the stimulus of oxytocin. However, increasingly during the third trimester it is normal for occasional, irregular painless contractions (known as Braxton Hicks contractions) to occur.

### CLINICAL APPLICATIONS

Unlike in other mammals, human oestrogen levels rise continually to term. Oestrogen is essential in the formation of gap junctions between the myometrial fibres that are required for coordinated uterine contractions in labour. They also stimulate the production of prostaglandins, the local hormones that stimulate powerful contractions in labour. Interestingly, these oestrogens are made from fetal rather than maternal precursors and the effect of a particular fetal congenital abnormality on the initiation of labour illustrates this. A fetus with anencephaly (absence of the cerebrum and overlying skull bones) produces less oestrogen from its adrenal gland and liver as a direct result of lack of hypothalamic and pituitary stimulation. This results in the delayed onset in labour. Such cases are rarely seen today because many women choose a termination of pregnancy because the condition is incompatible with life. Preconception care in terms of taking folic acid is aimed at reducing the risk of this and other neural tube defects, such as spina bifida and hydrocephaly.

As the fetus matures there is an increased secretion of various substances from the fetus (e.g. oxytocin, antidiuretic hormone, epidermal growth factor, platelet activating factor and advenocorticotrophic hormone). These factors secreted by the fetus are indicators of fetal maturity and it is thought that these, together with maternal stimuli, work synergistically, triggering the onset of labour.

In the normal fetus, the adrenal glands produce cortisol during the third trimester. The effects of this over such a long period is that the human fetus has, in relative terms, a much higher chance of survival than other mammals when born significantly preterm. This is therefore the basis for the administration of dexamethazone to pregnant women in preterm labour. These steroid injections enhance the development of fetal organs, particularly the lungs, and their production of surfactant. This gives the neonate an enhanced chance of survival.

Physiological preparation of the woman for labour also occurs through the presence of relaxin that softens the symphysis pubis and pelvic ligaments thereby enlarging the pelvis.

## The onset of labour

### Contractions

There is no one, precise trigger for the onset of labour. The fetal oestrogen levels (mentioned above) are perhaps the most significant. In addition, there is an increase in prostaglandin synthesis, particularly by the amniotic membranes. However, there appears to be more than one activating mechanism for this, and it has been the subject of considerable research. Other factors such as the stretching of the uterus by its contents sound plausible when multiple pregnancies have an increased chance of preterm labour. However, many twin pregnancies go to term with both babies weighing more than 3500 g, so this is not a significant factor.

An artificial way of ripening the cervix and/or inducing labour is the administration of prostaglandin $E_2$ in the form of pessary or gel into the posterior fornix of the vagina. Sexual intercourse with the deposition of prostaglandin-rich semen may similarly stimulate the cervix, but usually only when the woman is at term. Sexual intercourse during pregnancy is not contraindicated. The exceptions to this advice apply in the early weeks of pregnancy only in women who have suffered two or more miscarriages. Later in pregnancy abstinence may be appropriate when the woman has given birth significantly preterm previously.

The second method of inducing or accelerating labour is the administration of an intravenous infusion containing the synthetic form of oxytocin, syntocinon. This is used only after rupture of the membranes. Both require specific monitoring of the woman's condition and particularly the effects on the uterus by the midwife. This is because of the potential risk of hypertonic uterine action and deleterious effects on the fetal heart patterns as a result of restricted placental blood flow.

The onset of the uterine contractions may not signal the onset of labour immediately. It is very common for women to have several hours of irregular contractions with breaks in-between. These contractions help 'ripen' the cervix, making it softer and thinner, usually without any actual dilatation. Labour is said to have begun when the uterine contractions are associated with dilatation of the cervix. Whereas descent of the presenting part (normally the fetal head) can be assessed most effectively by abdominal palpation, assessment of actual dilatation requires a vaginal examination. However, all contractions bring the presenting part down on to the pelvic floor. This creates a positive feedback mechanism whereby the pressure stimulates *greater* production of oxytocin by the posterior pituitary. Use of a positive feedback mechanism is unusual in the human

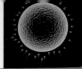

body where nearly all metabolic regulation normally occurs through negative feedback mechanisms.

The effect of increasing oxytocin levels is to increase the length, strength and frequency of the uterine contractions, from lasting approximately 20 seconds and occurring every 15–20 minutes, to lasting 1–1.5 minutes and occurring every 1–2 minutes close to birth. The cervix that has 'ripened' during the days preceding labour, or in labour, becomes dilated up to the maximum of about 10 cm. The cervix itself becomes 'taken-up' and contributes to the relatively thin lower segment of the uterus.

## The 'show'

An additional prerequisite for labour to commence is the coming away of the 'show'. Within the cervical canal, this mucoid plug provided protection against ascending infection in pregnancy. It comes away as the cervix ripens, and particularly as it dilates. The show is stained with fresh blood and may happen either prior to or at any time during labour. Occasionally, a show is not seen, having been passed in the toilet unnoticed.

## The rupture of the membranes

The fetus lies within the fluid-filled amniotic sac that is made up of the two membranes, the amnion and the chorion. Amniotic fluid is produced by the amnion and later in pregnancy by the fetal kidneys and lungs. Circulation and renewal occurs in part through swallowing by the fetus. The volume increases up to approximately 800 mL at 36 weeks gestation, declining a little towards term. This clear fluid, 98% water and solutes, gives space for fetal growth and development, and provides protection from trauma and ascending infection. Adequate amniotic fluid volume in pregnancy is essential for fetal lung development. The membranes may rupture spontaneously, either prior to labour or at any time during labour. The amount of liquor seen may vary from a small and persistent trickle to a considerable gush.

---

### CLINICAL APPLICATIONS

#### PLACE OF BIRTH

Having discussed the triggers for labour and how onset can be determined in the biological context, it is important to view labour and childbirth as acutely and inextricably involving the woman's emotional and social well-being. Among mammals it is widely known that many delay the onset of labour until the environment is conducive. This probably accounts for the cessation of contractions that occurs so frequently in women arriving at maternity units in early labour! It also provides the basis for the preference by some women for a home birth. Most importantly, women should be supported to give birth where they choose, whether it is in an obstetric unit, a birth centre or at home. At the same time it is essential that risk factors are identified promptly and women are referred for obstetric care as appropriate.

---

Labour is described as having three stages:

- **First stage of labour**: this begins with the onset of regular uterine contractions *and* the dilatation of the cervix. It ends when the cervix is fully dilated, 10 cm. It lasts very varying lengths of time but approximately 15 hours for a woman having her first baby (a primigravida).
- **The second stage of labour**: this follows the first stage and comes to an end with the birth of the baby. It takes approximately 1–2 hours. The woman generally has a spontaneous and increasing urge to bear down with the contractions as the fetal head becomes visible at the vulva.
- **The third stage of labour**: this begins following the birth. It involves the delivery of the placenta and membranes *and* the control of bleeding, which does not normally exceed 300 mL. It represents the time of greatest risk for the woman. Delivery of the placenta and membranes can occur spontaneously, taking anything from 5 minutes to an hour; the woman expels them by her own efforts. This requires 'physiological management' by the midwife. The myometrial fibres contract, acting as 'living ligatures' and sealing off the maternal blood flow that had been approximately 500 mL/min in blood vessels to the placenta. The non-elastic placenta is then sheared off the uterine wall and a retroplacental clot forms, further aiding separation.

This process can be hastened by 'active management' in which an oxytocic drug and ergometrine together are administered intramuscularly. The former contracts the uterus within 2–3 minutes, whereas the latter provides sustained contraction for 2–4 hours. This management significantly reduces the risk of postpartum haemorrhage. However, the ergometrine component is a potent vasoconstrictor and associated with a high incidence of nausea, vomiting and raised blood pressure, and some low-risk women choose not to have the drugs. The placenta and membranes are checked for completeness following the birth because any products of conception remaining in the uterus may reduce its ability to contract, resulting in haemorrhage and possible infection.

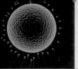

In the 6–8 weeks following birth, known as the **puerperium**, the mother's body returns to its non-pregnant state. The uterus and vagina both revert to their normal sizes about 6 weeks after childbirth. If the mother is not breastfeeding the baby, menstruation will recommence between 6 weeks and 6 months after the birth; a woman who is breastfeeding will have a delayed onset of menstruation, although she can become pregnant before the first normal period is observed.

## The breasts and lactation

The paired mammary glands (breasts) are specialized skin derivations that produce milk during the lactation period following childbirth. They exist in the male too, but only in the rudimentary state. The female breasts have a composite structure in which a radiating compound alveolar gland is embedded in a mound of fat and connective tissue in the pectoral region. The nipple of each gland is surrounded by an area of pigmented skin, known as the **areola**, which changes from pink to brown during the first pregnancy and remains so thereafter.

Each breast consists of between 15 and 25 independent glandular units called breast lobes. The lobes are arranged radially at different depths around the nipple. A single large duct, the **lactiferous duct**, drains each lobe via a separate opening on the surface of the nipple. Just before each duct opens onto the surface, it forms a dilation called the **lactiferous sinus (Fig. 6.3.33)**. Each breast lobe is divided into a variable number of lobules; the lobules consist of a system of alveolar ducts from which large numbers of secretory alveoli develop during pregnancy.

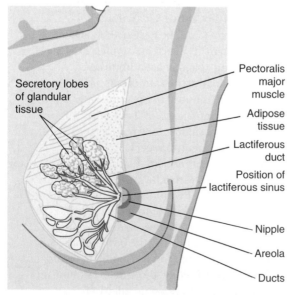

Secretory lobes of glandular tissue

Pectoralis major muscle

Adipose tissue

Lactiferous duct

Position of lactiferous sinus

Nipple

Areola

Ducts

**Figure 6.3.33** The mature female breast

The rudimentary breast in the female enlarges under hormonal influences during puberty and undergoes slight cyclical changes throughout the menstrual cycle.

The true transformation from an inactive to an active gland occurs during pregnancy and the breasts become fully functional only at parturition. Many hormones are involved in the transformation; oestrogen, in the presence of adrenal steroids and growth hormone, stimulates the development of the duct system, and progesterone stimulates growth of the secretory alveoli. Insulin, thyroid hormones, human placental lactogen and prolactin from the anterior pituitary are also required for complete development.

The breasts enlarge from the fifth week of pregnancy onwards. They receive an increased blood flow, the nipples increase in size, the areolae extend and become darker, and small cutaneous glands – the glands of Montgomery – which open onto the areola, become more prominent and appear as small tubercles. In the last 3 months of pregnancy, growth of the breasts slows down and **colostrum**, a fluid precursor of milk, is secreted. Colostrum is also secreted in the immediate postpartum days until replaced by milk. Colostrum is deep yellow in colour and rich in protein and salts, with less lactose than milk; it also carries some immunoglobulins (antibodies).

**Prolactin** exerts a major influence on the initiation and maintenance of lactation. During pregnancy, the level of prolactin begins to rise after about the eighth week and continues to rise until delivery. The release of prolactin is due partly to the inhibition of prolactin inhibitory factor from the hypothalamus; it may also be due to the stimulation of some, as yet unknown, hypothalamic releasing factor. If suckling does not follow parturition, prolactin levels fall to prepregnancy values within a few weeks. Prolactin primarily stimulates milk production in the alveoli. The milk produced consists of water, lactose, fat, protein (casein and lactalbumin) and electrolytes (sodium, potassium, calcium, chloride and hydrogen carbonate ions). A number of hormones with general metabolic effects, for instance insulin and corticosteroids, also influence lactation. Human milk contains considerably less protein, fewer salts and more carbohydrate than cow's milk.

Milk does not flow out of the nipple unless suckling takes place. The tactile stimulation of the nipple sets up a neuroendocrine reflex releasing oxytocin; this in turn stimulates the contraction of the myoepithelial cells surrounding the alveoli and the smooth muscle of the ductile system. Milk is forced into the main ducts of the breast, which ultimately connect to the nipple, and the milk is ejected. This is sometimes known as the 'let-down' reflex. Suckling also stimulates prolactin release, thus neuroendocrine reflexes are responsible for the secretion of both oxytocin and prolactin. Secretion and expulsion of milk from lactating breasts occur simultaneously. Breastfeeding can cause uterine contractions to occur at the same time, due to the effect of oxytocin on the uterine musculature. This helps to involute (reduce the size of) the uterus after the pregnancy.

If suckling does not occur, milk production diminishes. Oestrogen given in large doses postpartum effectively blocks lactation, indicating that oestrogen itself may act directly on mammary tissue. At the end of the lactation period the breasts return to their resting condition as quiescent glands.

Prolactin levels are higher at night, and higher with frequent feeding. This physiological understanding underpins the recommendations for establishing breastfeeding. On-demand breastfeeding, including feeding at night, is very important in the establishment of lactation. Attention to positioning detail to enable the baby to latch on at the breast is essential. Such detail is outside the scope of this text.

If a baby is poorly, in the special or intensive care unit and unable to feed, a breastfeeding mother needs to express her breasts six times in 24 hours to stimulate lactation and provide the breast milk. This will optimize nutrition for her baby, who is already at increased risk. Currently, the World Health Organization recommends exclusive breastfeeding for 6 months after birth, unless contraindicated.

The high prolactin level that occurs as a result of exclusive breastfeeding is associated with the likelihood of lactational amenorrhoea, but it is not a reliable form of contraception! However, in less developed countries it appears to be responsible for greater birth spacing, thereby indirectly reducing maternal mortality and morbidity.

High blood levels of prolactin are closely associated with both lactational and some pathological forms of amenorrhoea, although the exact linking mechanism is uncertain. There are adequate levels of luteinizing hormone and follicle stimulating hormone in the pituitary during lactation, but oestrogen fails to induce a positive feedback release of luteinizing hormone and the hypothalamic–pituitary axis appears to be more sensitive to the negative feedback effects of oestrogen.

## Benign breast disease

Benign breast disease is very common, with up to 30% of women requiring treatment for a benign condition at some time in their lives (Harmer, 2001). Some problems result from abnormalities of development, to inflammations and infections. These include mastalgia (breast pain), fibroadenomas and cysts and are often hormone dependent. Breast cancer is also on the increase in the United Kingdom, with one in nine women now developing breast cancer at some time in their life. The reasons for this high incidence are not fully understood (see Chapter 6.4).

## Conclusion

This chapter has introduced the reader to some key concepts in the field of reproduction and sexual health. After this discussion of reproductive physiology, the reader may now appreciate that there are many aspects of the subject that remain to be more fully researched and explained. However, progress in understanding all aspects of reproductive physiology is certainly leading to more effective treatment and care on an individual basis. With the relevant knowledge and attitudes, nurses and midwives are in a position to foster a positive culture of sexual health information amongst their clients (Fitzpatrick, 2002).

## Clinical review

In addition to the Learning Outcomes at the beginning of this chapter, the reader should be able to:

- Relate any altered physiology to the treatment of common health problems, particularly in the fields of obstetrics, gynaecology, urogenital medicine and surgery, family planning, well-women and infertility clinics

- Base the planning, delivery and evaluation of nursing care in the above fields on sound physiological principles

- Give patients adequate and comprehensible explanations of normal and abnormal conditions

- Compare and contrast gamete production in males and females

- Explain the relationship between the hypothalamic, pituitary and ovarian hormones. Describe the function of each hormone

- Describe the 'normal' menstrual cycle. Explain pre-menstrual syndrome and dysmenorrhoea

- Explain the terms **'conception'**, **'contraception'**, **'hormone replacement therapy'** and **'in vitro fertilization'**

- Discuss the biological differences between the sexes and the possible aetiology of these differences

- Describe and explain the changes that occur in the reproductive system (and associated structures) across the life span in a female from 10 to 70 years, paying particular emphasis to the implications these changes have for nurses working with either adolescents **or** women approaching the menopause **or** healthcare for elderly people

- Discuss what biological/physiological information would be relevant to promoting 'reproductive system health' in either women **or** men

## Review questions

1 Which chromosome is unique to the male?
2 What are the gonads?
3 Why do the testes descend out of the abdomen during development?
4 Where is the site of spermatogenesis?
5 Why might the acrosome contain digestive enzymes?
6 Why is semen slightly alkaline?
7 What effect does testosterone have on its target cells?
8 There is an essential difference between spermatogenesis and oogenesis. What is it?
9 What determines the survival of the corpus luteum?
10 What are the stages of the menstrual cycle?
11 Where are the cyclical changes in female reproductive hormones controlled?
12 How does gonadotrophic hormone secretion differ in males and females after puberty?
13 Where does fertilization take place?
14 What does fertilization achieve?
15 When does implantation take place?
16 What function does oxytocin fulfil?

## Suggestions for further reading

Blackburn, S.T. & Loper, D.L. (2002) *Maternal, Fetal and Neonatal Physiology: A Clinical Perspective*, 2nd edn. Philadelphia: W.B. Saunders.
*A large and comprehensive textbook for specialty and advanced practitioners – very detailed coverage of material (good to borrow from a library!).*

Brinsden, P.R. (ed) (1999) *A Textbook of In Vitro Fertilisation and Assisted Reproduction.* London: Parthenon Publishers.
*Good detailed coverage of this rapidly developing field of care*

Burnet, K. (2001) *Holistic Breast Care.* Philadelphia: W.B. Saunders.
*This book provides a wealth of information for any woman who wishes to know more about her breasts and for health professionals caring for breast problems, especially breast cancer.*

Coad, J. & Dunstall, M. (2001) *Anatomy and Physiology for Midwives.* Edinburgh: Mosby.
*An excellent, readable, but very thorough and detailed textbook covering all relevant biological science topics in the*

areas relating to reproduction, including immunology, genetics, pregnancy, neonates. Good value for money!

Johnson, M. & Everitt, B. (2000) *Essential Reproduction*, 5th edn. Oxford: Blackwell Scientific.
*A comprehensive research-based overview of reproductive physiology.*

Larsen, W.J. (2001) *Human Embryology*, 3rd edn. Edinburgh: Churchill Livingstone.
*This book addresses the relationship between basic science and embryology as well as clinical disorders arising out of embryological problems. Readable and large clear diagrams.*

Moore, K.L. & Persaud, T.V.N. (1998) *The Developing Human*, 6th edn. Philadelphia: W.B. Saunders.
*Clinically orientated embryology, a detailed but very readable book. Good colour diagrams and useful case studies are included.*

Sinclair, D. (1991) *Human Growth after Birth*, 5th edn. Oxford: Oxford University Press.
*A classic book covering all aspects of growth and development in an integrated way.*

## Useful websites/addresses

www.breastcancercare.org.uk
*National organization offering information and advice to those affected by breast cancer.*

www.hfea.gov.uk
*Human Fertilisation and Embryology Authority: statutory body that regulates fertility treatments.*

www.fpa.org.uk
*Information on family planning – formerly the Family Planning Association.*

The Impotence Association: www.impotence.org.uk

Prostate cancer charity: www.prostate-cancer.org.uk

The Prostate Help Associaton: www.bph.org.uk

The Association to Aid the Sexual and Personal Relationships of People with a Disability (formerly SPOD): www.spod-uk.org
*On-line resource explaining issues of personal and sexual relationships of people with a disability.*

## References

Adams, L.A. & Steiner, R.A. (1988) Puberty. In: Clarke, J.R. (ed) *Oxford Review of Reproduction Biology*, Vol. 10. Oxford: Oxford University Press.

Amias, A.G. (1975) Sexual life after gynaecological operations I and II. *British Medical Journal*, **2**; 608–609, 680–681.

Barlow, D., Egan, D. & Ross, F. (1990) In: Matson, P. & Lieberman, B. (eds) *The Outcome of IVF Pregnancy in Clinical IVF Forum*. Manchester: Manchester University Press.

Blackburn, S.T. & Loper, D.L. (2002) *Maternal, Fetal and Neonatal Physiology: A Clinical Perspective*, 2nd edn. Philadelphia: W.B. Saunders.

Bush, T.L., Whiteman, M. & Flaws, J.A. (2001) Hormone replacement therapy and breast cancer – a qualitative review. *Obstetrics and Gynaecology*, **98**; 498–508.

Coad, J. & Dunstall, M. (2001) *Anatomy and Physiology for Midwives*. Edinburgh: Mosby.

Crouch, D. (2003a) Does screening save lives? *Nursing Times*, **99**(19); 22–25.

Crouch, D. (2003b) Building hope, breaking taboos. *Nursing Times*, **99**(16); 38–39.

Fitzpatrick, J. (2002) Bringing it out into the open – sexual health. *Nursing Times*, **98**(31); 16.

Harmer, V. (2001) Benign breast disease. *Nursing Times*, **97**(47); 32–33.

Lewey, J. (2002) Prostate cancer update. *Nursing Times*, **98**(28); 56–57.

Montgomery, S. & Ekbom, A. (2002) Smoking during pregnancy and diabetes mellitus in a British longitudinal birth cohort. *British Medical Journal*, **324**(7328); 26–27.

Royal College of Nursing (2003) *Health and The Menopause*. RCN Guidelines for Nursing, Midwifery and Health Visitors. London: RCN.

Schmidt, K. (1999) Programmed at birth. *New Scientist*, **17 July**; 26–31.

Whiteford, A. & Wordley, J. (2003) Raising awareness and detection of testicular cancer in young men. *Nursing Times*, **99**(1); 34–36.

Wilcox, A.J. et al. (2000) The timing of the fertile window in the menstrual cycle: day specific estimates from a prospective study. *British Medical Journal*, **321**(7271); 1259–1262.

Wilson, E.W. & Rennie, P.I.C. (1976) *The Menstrual Cycle*. London: Lloyd-Luke.

Willard, H.F. (2003) Genome biology: Tales of Y chromosome. *Nature*, **423**; 810–813.

# Genetics

*Christine Patch   Heather Skirton*

## LEARNING OBJECTIVES

After studying this chapter the reader should be able to:

- Explain the mechanisms involved in inheritance
- Describe characteristics of different patterns of inheritance
- Discuss how mutations might occur and their consequences

- Explain the genetic basis of some common diseases
- Describe the stages of meiosis and the formation of gametes
- Explain the differences between genetic screening and genetic counselling

## INTRODUCTION

Genetics is a relatively new field of specialist health care. **Clinical genetic** services were first established in the United Kingdom and the United States about 60 years ago, when services for families were limited. Since the advent of recombinant **DNA** technology, options for families affected by rare genetic conditions have vastly expanded. Although understanding of genetics in the past has focused on disease or variation from the 'norm', advances in genetic science have also led to a greater understanding of the mechanisms that are involved in the maintenance of health, growth and development. Increasingly, genetics is relevant to the diagnosis and management of many common diseases and all healthcare professionals require a basic knowledge of genetic principles. The language and concepts used in genetics may be unfamiliar to the reader and a glossary of important terms is provided at the end of the chapter. These terms are in bold in the text the first time they are introduced.

The structure and function of every cell in the human body is controlled by the genetic material, most of which is located within the cell nucleus. At present, the number of human **genes** is believed to be approximately 30 000. The genes in the nucleus are arranged along **chromosomes**. There are a small number of additional genes located in the mitochondria of the cell, these and other nuclear genes organize mitochondrial activity (see Chapter 1.3).

In a normal human cell, there are 46 chromosomes, comprising 22 pairs of **autosomes** and two sex chromosomes. The autosomes are common to both males and females. The male has an X and a Y chromosome and the female has two X chromosomes. **Figure 6.4.1** shows the chromosome complement of a male. The determination of the child's sex is described in Chapter 6.3.

Each chromosome is formed by a length of DNA, with genes arranged along the chromosome in a specific sequence. For each pair of chromosomes, an individual will have inherited one from his or her mother and one from his or her father. This means that half of the genetic material is inherited from each parent. In addition, during **meiosis** (the cell division that forms the gametes, i.e. eggs and sperm) there is a further rearrangement of genetic material within each pair of chromosomes. The process by which this happens is discussed further on p. 789. This ensures that, apart from identical twins, every individual human has a unique combination of genes and genetic variation that they inherit from their parents.

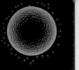

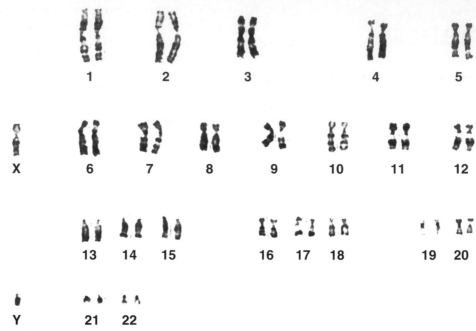

**Figure 6.4.1** The chromosome complement of a normal human male (46,XY) (courtesy of the Paediatric Research Unit, Guy's Hospital Medical School, London)

## The structure of DNA

The double helical structure of DNA was first described by Watson and Crick in 1953. Chemical bases called cytosine (C), thymine (T), adenine (A) and guanine (G) are arranged in strands in a definite sequence along each chromosome. Each triplet of bases provides the code for one amino acid. Specific sequences of bases also signal the beginning or end of a gene in the DNA molecule. Within the gene, there are **introns** (that function as non-coding sequences) and **exons** (that function as coding sequences).

The DNA is arranged along chromosomes within the cell nucleus. For the genetic code to be translated into protein products, the coding sequences of the DNA are transcribed into messenger RNA, which passes out of the nucleus and provides the template for amino acid formation in the cytoplasm (the process of protein synthesis is described in greater detail in Chapter 1.3 and it is recommended that the reader refer to this chapter before continuing).

Individuals inherit their DNA from their parents and the unit of DNA that codes for a specific protein product is normally referred to as a **gene**. The inheritance and development of specific characteristics may be controlled by a single gene or by many different genes; this will be discussed further in the following section.

## Single genes

Patterns of inheritance had been inferred from examining family trees or **pedigrees** long before developments

in molecular genetics made it possible to examine DNA, genes and **mutations** (alterations in DNA sequences) directly. These patterns had been predicted by Gregor Mendel in his experiments with pea plants two hundred years ago. This was many years before the current understanding of genetics and the sequencing of the human genome; these patterns are consequently described as **Mendelian**. Over 10 000 Mendelian conditions or characteristics are known and are catalogued in the Online Mendelian Inheritance in Man (OMIM, 2002) internet database.

Mendelian inheritance patterns are observed when the presence or absence of a characteristic is dependent on the actual DNA code at a specific position on the DNA sequence (known as a **locus**). At a specific position on the DNA sequence (locus) the sequence of bases may exist in a number of forms called **alleles**. These alleles comprise the genotype. Although people often refer to 'the gene for a condition', it is important to understand that in reality the **phenotype** (the characteristic that is actually manifested, for example blue eyes or brown eyes, extra fingers or blood groups) that is evident in the individual may be the result of several different events. For example, the characteristic may occur as a result of one type of mutation in one gene, the absence of a specific genetic sequence or a combination of genetic sequences, alterations and environmental changes. Particular genetic conditions will not be discussed in detail in this chapter but examples will be included. For sources of further information, see the Suggestions for further reading.

# Dominant and recessive inheritance

Mendel demonstrated that if a characteristic was dependent on what he called a single unit of heredity (and what are now termed genes) then these characteristics could be inherited in a dominant or recessive manner. Most of the analysis of patterns of inheritance focuses on disease or obvious variation from the norm, such as extra fingers and toes, sickle-cell anaemia, muscular dystrophy. This is because these are the situations that have come to medical attention and are the most obvious when looking at family trees. These disorders are caused by alterations or mutations in single genes, which disrupt the 'normal' function of the gene. In general, the disorders that follow classical patterns of inheritance tend to be rare, although the principles of single-gene inheritance apply to any characteristic that is under the control of a single gene and principles of the inheritance of genes are important to understand.

As is discussed later in this chapter, many characteristics of humans are not under the control of single genes but are the end result of multiple genetic and environmental factors. For example, type 2 diabetes is known to have an inherited component. However, it is not caused by a single gene and modifiable environmental factors such as diet or exercise may be more relevant when considering public health initiatives to reduce the disease burden. Hereditary haemochromatosis is a condition of progressive iron overload, which can lead to end-organ damage. The major genetic risk factor has been identified, however, even in siblings with the same genotype, one may develop the disease and another may not. Some of the other factors are known: alcohol consumption, gender, previous history of blood loss, but there are still undetermined genetic and environmental factors that influence the risk of actually developing the disease (Imperatore et al., 2003). It is crucial for the practitioner to understand that any phenotype or disease is the end result of a complex pathway involving an interaction between genetic and environmental factors.

As chromosomes exist in pairs (apart from the X and Y chromosomes), DNA sequences also exist in pairs. The sequence at any specific locus may be identical (**homozygous**) or different (**heterozygous**). A characteristic that can be seen within a family tree is dominant if it is present in the heterozygous state and recessive if it is present only in the homozygous state. In simple terms, in a dominant condition, only one copy of the gene is necessary for the condition to be manifest; in a recessive condition, two copies of the gene are necessary. In humans, most of the conditions that are referred to as dominant (from the pattern seen in families) are heterozygous. This is because

homozygotes for the particular gene may have a much more severe condition that is incompatible with life. For example, achondroplasia (short-limbed dwarfism) is caused by a single dominant gene mutation. If two affected people have children, there is the possibility that the fetus will inherit two copies of the mutated gene, and be homozygous. This results in a severe skeletal dysplasia, with the baby having extremely deformed bones, which means that it will not normally survive. However, in a condition such as Huntington's disease, homozygote individuals appear to be no different to heterozygotes. This is sometimes known as true dominance. As males have only one X chromosome and females have two, and since most genes on the X-chromosome are not carried on the Y chromosome, males are hemizygous (they only have one copy of each locus instead of two) for most loci on the X chromosome.

## Mendelian patterns of inheritance

There are five basic Mendelian inheritance patterns. **Figure 6.4.2** shows the symbols that are commonly used for drawing a family tree and the characteristics of each pattern are outlined below. Patterns of inheritance observed in the family structure refer to observable characteristics or diseases that are assumed to be caused by single genes. In medical genetics, the term 'affected' is used to describe an individual who has signs and symptoms of the condition. A **carrier** is an individual who has no signs and symptoms, but has one mutated copy of the relevant gene.

### Characteristics of inheritance patterns

#### Autosomal dominant (Fig. 6.4.3)
- One copy of the genetic mutation is sufficient to cause the condition.
- Either sex may be affected.
- The characteristic may be transmitted by a parent of either sex.
- An affected person has a 50%, or a 1 in 2, chance of passing the condition to each of his or her offspring.
- Unless the condition is caused by a new mutation, an affected child will have an affected parent.

#### Autosomal recessive (Fig. 6.4.4)
- Two copies of the genetic mutation are required to cause the condition.
- Either sex may be affected.
- Affected children are normally born to unaffected parents.
- Each parent of an affected child will have one copy of the mutated gene and one normal copy, and will therefore be asymptomatic **carriers**.

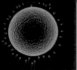

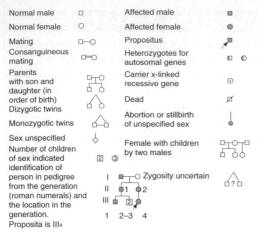

**Figure 6.4.2** Symbols used in pedigree charts (adapted from Mueller, R.F. & Young, I.D. (2001) *See* reference list

- If a couple are both carriers, they have a 25%, or 1 in 4, chance of having an affected child in each pregnancy.
- An affected person will have an affected child only if his or her partner is a carrier of the same recessive mutation.

## X-linked recessive (Fig. 6.4.5)

- The genetic mutation is within a gene on the X chromosome.
- Affects mainly males (occasionally females will be affected, see section later).
- The mother of an affected male will usually be an asymptomatic carrier (show no or minimal signs of the condition) but may have affected male relatives.
- No male to male transmission is seen on the family tree.
- All the daughters of affected males will be carriers.
- All sons of an affected male will be unaffected.

## X-linked dominant (Fig. 6.4.6)

- The genetic mutation is on the X chromosome.
- Females are more mildly affected than males.
- Most X-linked dominant conditions are lethal in males, so in family trees there is an excess of females.
- Any child of an affected female will have a 50%, or 1 in 2, chance of inheriting the genetic mutation.

## Y linked inheritance

- The genetic mutation is on the Y chromosome.
- Only males are affected.
- All sons of affected males will also be affected.

**Table 6.4.1** gives examples of conditions following specific Mendelian inheritance patterns.

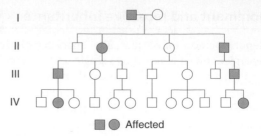

**Figure 6.4.3** Pedigree pattern of an autosomal dominant trait (adapted from Mueller, R.F. & Young, I.D. (2001) *See* reference list

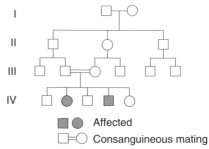

**Figure 6.4.4** Pedigree pattern of an autosomal recessive trait (adapted from Mueller, R.F. & Young, I.D. (2001) *See* reference list

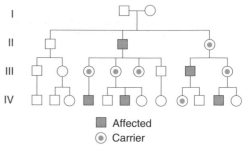

**Figure 6.4.5** Pedigree pattern of an X-linked recessive trait in which affected males reproduce (adapted from Mueller, R.F. & Young, I.D. (2001) *See* reference list

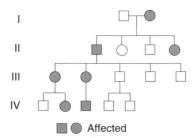

**Figure 6.4.6** Pedigree pattern of an X-linked dominant trait (adapted from Mueller, R.F. & Young, I.D. (2001) *See* reference list

## CLINICAL APPLICATIONS

### TAKING A FAMILY HISTORY

Despite the number of genetic tests that are now possible, the single most important tool and test in clinical genetics is the family history. Taking an

| **Table 6.4.1** | Conditions following specific Mendelian inheritance patterns | | |
|---|---|---|---|
| **Autosomal dominant** | **Autosomal recessive** | **X-linked recessive** | **X-linked dominant** |
| Huntington's disease | Cystic fibrosis | Duchenne muscular dystrophy | X-linked ichthyosis |
| Adult polycystic kidney disease | Phenylketonuria | Fragile X syndrome | Golz syndrome |
| Christmas disease | Thalassaemia | G6PD | |
| Achondroplasia | Recessive albinism | X-linked ocular albinism | |
| Dominant polydactyly | Sickle-cell disease | Haemophilia | |

accurate family history gives the genetic counsellor a wealth of information about the likelihood of a genetic condition in the family, the probable inheritance pattern and recurrence risks for family members. The ability to take a family history should be an essential skill for most health professionals but it is important to remember the ethical aspects of taking the family tree and recording details of the family. Some of the information may be highly confidential and should not be shared with other family members unless consent is expressly given. A common set of symbols are used to denote the family tree **(see Fig. 6.4.2)**.

The family tree is normally built up by first asking the patient about his or her immediate family, children, siblings and parents. It is sometimes necessary to phrase questions so that people who have died are still included. For example, how many brothers and sisters did you have? Did your mother have any more babies? Pregnancy losses may be important but not revealed unless specifically asked about. For example, did you lose any babies? The exact information recorded and how far the family tree is extended will vary but a minimum is probably three generations, with information recorded on serious illnesses, causes and ages of death and pregnancy losses. Further information on how to take a family tree can be found in Skirton & Patch (2002).

## Complications to single gene inheritance patterns

Classical Mendelian genetics explains patterns of inheritance of disorders caused by single genes. In reality, assessing the recurrence risk in a family may not be quite so simple. This section outlines some of the complications to these patterns of inheritance.

It is important to understand the section on **expression** and **penetrance**, and to be aware that:

- not all genes are in the nucleus (mitochondrial inheritance)
- in some conditions, a disease may be manifested in a more severe form as it is passed on (anticipation)
- it may make a difference if a gene is inherited from the mother or the father (imprinting).

Further details of mitochondrial inheritance, anticipation and imprinting are included for the interested reader.

### Expression and penetrance

The definition of **penetrance** of a genetic condition is the probability that an individual who has the mutation will develop the condition. The term **expression** relates to how the condition manifests in different individuals from one family who have inherited the same mutation. Non-penetrance and variable expression are particular features of autosomal dominant conditions.

In practice, it is not uncommon to see the following pedigree in a family who have a dominant condition **(Fig. 6.4.7)** the condition appears to have 'skipped a generation'. Individual 3.2 (June), despite having an affected parent and children, does not appear to have the condition herself. In conditions such as Huntington's disease (HD), the disorder does not normally present until later in life. If the family tree is taken before the disorder has had time to develop, then it is possible that she has not yet developed the condition but will do so in time. This is called age-related penetrance. In Huntington's disease it is considered that the penetrance is 100% if the person with the gene lives long enough. However, in other

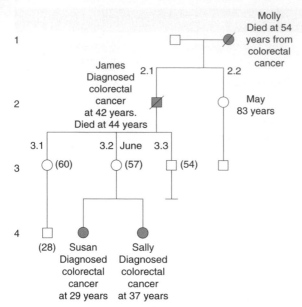

**Figure 6.4.7** Dominant pedigree with apparent non-penetrance in one generation

conditions, such as dominantly inherited breast and ovarian cancer, the age-related penetrance is less than 100% and depends on other genetic and environmental factors.

If age-related penetrance does not explain the apparent 'skipping of the generations' in this family, an alternative explanation might be variable expression of the gene mutation. This is where the phenotype that is observed can be very different in different individuals. For example, in neurofibromatosis type 1 (an autosomal dominant condition) some individuals have flat, light-brown patches on their skin (café au lait patches), freckles in their armpits (axillary freckling) and a few small skin lumps (neurofibromas) and may never have come to medical attention. Others may present at birth with disfiguring growths (plexiform neuromas), which are difficult to remove surgically and may cause considerable permanent damage.

## Mitochondrial inheritance

Mendelian patterns of inheritance relate to alterations in the DNA that forms the chromosomes in the nucleus of the cell. Mutations in the mitochondrial genome are also an important cause of human disease. Cells contain many mitochondria, each with their own self replicating DNA. The two unusual features about the pattern of inheritance that is associated with mitochondrial mutations are

- the disease is inherited through the maternal line only (matrilineal) and
- there is considerable variability in how the disease is manifested.

Inheritance is matrilineal because only the ovum contributes mitochondria to the developing embryo (the zygote). It is assumed that, apart from very rare situations, sperm do not contribute mitochondria because the mitochondria in the sperm are carried in the tail, which does not penetrate the ovum at fertilization. Therefore, a mitochondrial condition can affect both sexes but will only be inherited from an affected mother. The variability of the condition is partly because the DNA sequence in each individual mitochondrion within a cell may not be identical. In some mitochondrial diseases, all the mitochondrial genomes may be identical and may all carry the causative mutation (i.e. homoplasmy). In other cases there may be a mixed population of normal and mutant genomes (i.e. heteroplasmy). Mitochondrial heteroplasmy can be transmitted from mother to child but there can be considerable variation in the proportion of mutant and normal mitochondrial genomes. For example, a woman may have a child who presents with a severe encephalopathy and dies. The child is subsequently found to have a mitochondrial mutation in a muscle biopsy and in blood. When the mother is tested, she is shown to have no mutation in her blood but a muscle biopsy does demonstrate the mutation at a low level. However, for future pregnancies, all that can be said is that the child will inherit the mutation; the level of mutation cannot be determined.

## Anticipation

Another type of variable expression is anticipation. This is where a genetic condition appears to be more severe in successive generations. This had previously been thought to be due to variable expression, as discussed above and in the following situation. A family may come to medical attention when a child presents with severe problems but then a careful examination of the parents shows that one of them has very mild signs of the condition. This is called **ascertainment bias** and it was thought that the observation that genetic conditions may become more severe as they are passed on was explained by chance. However, it is now known that some diseases are caused by a particular type of mutation that can become more severe as it is passed down the family. The normal version of the gene that causes Huntington's disease has a section of DNA that consists of a number of repeated elements. These repeats are composed of three bases, CAG, and each CAG sequence is called a **triplet**. The usual number of these triplets in the gene is variable but, as long as the number does not exceed a certain limit, the gene works normally. However, if the number of repeats increases above a certain number, the protein the gene produces is altered and the result is a mutation in the gene which causes Huntington's disease. This causative mutation is called an expansion. Juvenile Huntington's disease (where the age of onset is in childhood rather than adulthood) is caused when this expansion becomes very large. Interestingly, this increase tends to occur only when the gene is inherited from the father.

## Parental origin effects – imprinting

In juvenile Huntington's disease, the parental origin effect is explained by the mutation behaving differently depending on whether it is maternally or paternally transmitted, i.e. whether it is inherited from the mother or the father. Parental origin effects are also observed in other conditions. Imprinting is a poorly understood mechanism by which portions of the genome are activated only if they are inherited from a parent of one particular sex. For example, there are families with autosomal dominant glomus tumours (a particular type of non-malignant growth of vascular origin) where the gene is only expressed if it is inherited from the father. If it is inherited by a male from his mother he will not express the condition, but his children will have a 50% chance of inheriting the gene and expressing the condition. If his daughters inherit the gene, they will express the condition but their children will not. As well as single genes being subject to imprinting, whole regions of chromosomes may be subject to the same effect. For example, Prader–Willi syndrome (a syndrome of excessive appetite, learning difficulties and short stature) is caused by a lack of a specific region of the paternally inherited copy of chromosome 15. One of the mechanisms that cause Prader–Willi is an imprinting mutation that 'switches off' the region, resulting in failure of expression of critical genes. Cloning embryos means that the 'normal' processes of imprinting do not occur. This is thought to explain the high embryo and fetal loss rate in cloned embryos.

## Pseudodominant inheritance

If a recessive gene is very common in a population, it is possible by chance for an affected person to have children with an individual who carries the recessive gene and have affected children. The condition in the family might then appear dominant. This can also happen in communities where many people are related and consanguineous marriages are common. If a couple have a common ancestor, then the chance that both partners have inherited the same gene mutation is greater than if they were unrelated. For example, first cousins have a common grandparent and will therefore share approximately 25% of their genes. If there is multiple **consanguinity** in the family, the number of people affected by a recessive genetic condition will increase, making interpretation of the pattern of inheritance more difficult (see Fig. 6.4.8).

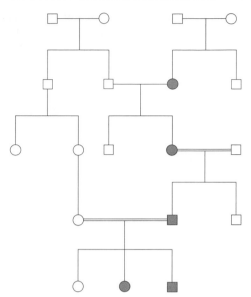

**Figure 6.4.8** Pseudodominant inheritance in a family with multiple consanguinity

## New mutations

Many causes of genetic disease are new mutations presenting with no family history of the condition. If a genetic disease is serious enough to prevent reproduction, then the gene mutation can only remain within a population if new mutations occur. This can cause difficulties in predicting recurrence risks when a family present with a child with severe abnormalities with no family history and normal chromosomes. The mode of inheritance may be autosomal recessive, autosomal dominant with a new mutation, X-linked recessive (if male) or non-genetic. There are some genetic conditions where it is well recognized that new mutations occur, for example it is common for the parents of a child born with achondroplasia to be of normal height. Mutations are random events and, although it is theoretically possible for a disease causing genetic mutation to revert to the normal DNA sequence, the chances are so remote that it would be considered to be impossible.

## Mosaicism

Mutations can occur in a single cell at any time after fertilization; such an alteration is called a **somatic** mutation. A somatic mutation affects only a proportion of the cells in the body. Mosaicism occurs when an individual has two (or more) genetically different cell lines. This can apply to chromosomes or single gene mutations. Mosaicism may cause problems in specific circumstances:

- The mutation causes abnormal growth and proliferation of cells, triggering malignancy (see section on Familial cancer, p. 795).

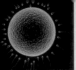

- The mutation happens early enough in embryonic development to affect a substantial proportion of the cells. The individual will then have clinical manifestations of the disease.
- The mutation affects a number of the cells that will produce the eggs or sperm. This may explain why two children with a new dominantly inherited condition might be born to parents who do not have the condition. This is occasionally seen clinically. For example, a grandmother was shown not to have a mutation in the Duchenne muscular dystrophy gene on a blood sample; however both her daughters were carriers of a mutation. This indicated that there was a mutation in a proportion of the egg-producing cells in her ovary.

## Non-Mendelian inheritance

Mendelian inheritance is based on an underlying assumption that a condition is either present or absent (e.g. an individual has brown eyes or blue eyes, or has cystic fibrosis or does not have cystic fibrosis). In reality, many human characteristics cannot be described in this way because they are continuous or quantitative (e.g. height, IQ, body size) and inheritance of this type of characteristic would be non-Mendelian. An observable phenotype is rarely the consequence of the action of one DNA variant but is the consequence of a pathway that may include many genes, proteins and other environmental mediators. For example, a person's final height will be determined by the combination of genes inherited from his or her parents; growth and development in fetal life; and nutrition, health, growth and development during childhood.

Common birth defects such as neural tube defects, cleft lip and palate and congenital heart disease rarely follow Mendelian patterns of inheritance, but clearly genetic factors are involved because there are more frequent recurrences within families than would be expected due to chance. Non-Mendelian characteristics may depend on interactions between many genetic loci (they are said to be controlled by many genes, i.e. are **polygenic**) together with smaller or larger environmental components and these are referred to as **multifactorial** conditions. The concept of a threshold effect is used to explain the presence or absence of a characteristic such as cleft lip and palate. The formation of a normal lip and palate is the end result of a complex developmental pathway. If enough genetic and environmental factors are present then the pathway can be disrupted and clefting occurs. In one case, the factors may be more genetic than environmental, in another, environmental influences may predominate. However, if enough of these small individual effects accumulate a threshold is reached where the developmental pathway is disrupted.

In genetic counselling for multifactorial conditions the risk that is given is not based on the theoretical risk derived from Mendelian theory but on empirical risks, which are derived from large observational surveys. Recent developments in genetics, computing and bioinformatics are making it possible to do large-enough studies to elucidate associations between genetic variation and complex human phenotypes. These tools are being applied in large-scale epidemiological studies to dissect-out the genetic component of complex human diseases such as cancer, diabetes and coronary heart disease. Many studies have been done in high-risk families or selected groups and have identified genetic variants that contribute to these diseases. These studies have had the advantage that they focus on one phenotype, for example asthma, and look for areas of genetic variation that people with asthma share in common. Once an area is identified the search for candidate genes can begin. This approach has been successful in identifying the major disease genes responsible for classic genetic diseases such as Huntington's disease, cystic fibrosis and dominantly inherited breast cancer.

As a result of these sorts of techniques, genetic factors have been implicated in many different conditions – such as cancer, diabetes, asthma and Alzheimer's disease – and in our susceptibility to infectious diseases. However, identifying the genetic contribution to these conditions is complicated by the number of different factors involved both genetic and environmental, by the small effect of each individual factor, by the differing contribution each factor makes to the end result of disease and because of the multiple possible interactions that may exist between factors. It is recognized that large population-based studies are needed to try to tease out all these things. In the United Kingdom, the research councils, charities and government propose setting up a large DNA database and linking it to medical records to facilitate such studies; this has been the subject of much discussion. A similar database has also been established in Iceland and has been the subject of some controversy. At the current time, the scientific advances from these sort of endeavours has yet to be translated into treatment or prevention strategies that improve health.

## Numerical calculations of risk

One of the commonly asked questions in clinical genetic practice is 'What are the chances of this happening again or what are the chances of this happening to me?' If a condition follows a Mendelian inheritance pattern then determining the risk from the family tree (the *a priori* risk) is straightforward, as shown in **Fig. 6.4.9**.

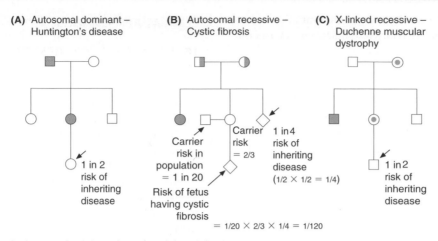

**(A)** Autosomal dominant – Huntington's disease

**(B)** Autosomal recessive – Cystic fibrosis

**(C)** X-linked recessive – Duchenne muscular dystrophy

1 in 2 risk of inheriting disease

Carrier risk in population = 1 in 20

Risk of fetus having cystic fibrosis

Carrier risk = 2/3

1 in 4 risk of inheriting disease (1/2 × 1/2 = 1/4)

= 1/20 × 2/3 × 1/4 = 1/120

1 in 2 risk of inheriting disease

**Figure 6.4.9** Calculation of risk based on Mendelian inheritance patterns

In practice, this risk can be modified by combining risk from the family tree with other information using simple statistical techniques. Before it became possible to test directly for many genes, clinical genetic practice frequently involved these mathematically derived assessments of risk. These techniques are now used more rarely, but are still occasionally necessary when direct mutation testing is not possible.

## Mutations

Every time a cell divides, the DNA sequence has to be copied. The DNA is therefore undergoing a constant process of replication and synthesis and there is always the possibility of error in this process. Although there are robust mechanisms for repairing DNA, some of these mistakes or alterations may persist and be passed on to future generations, i.e. be inherited. The difference between mutations and genetic variation is becoming less clear as more is discovered about genetics. A distinction that is sometimes made is that mutations are inheritable variations that occur in less than 1% of the population, whereas normal variations, or **polymorphisms**, are variants occurring in more than 1% of the population that can also be passed on. Alterations in DNA sequences occur in both coding and non-coding portions of the DNA. Mutations in coding portions of DNA can be neutral (i.e. have no overall effect on the sequence of the gene product or organism), beneficial, detrimental (resulting in disease) or lethal.

Disease-causing mutations usually affect the protein sequence produced by the gene and can be categorized in the following ways:

### Single **base-pair** substitutions or point mutations

As each protein may be coded for by several different combinations of base pairs (i.e. the code is redundant), single base-pair substitutions may change the triplet code but produce the same amino acid. For example, leucine may be encoded by CUC or CUA. A change in the last base from C to A would therefore be neutral. As discussed previously, the code for each amino acid in the protein string is composed of three base pairs called a **codon**. A substitution may change the codon to a stop codon, which would stop translation and lead to the production of the protein being terminated prematurely. This is commonly called a **nonsense mutation** and would have a significant effect on the final protein structure.

A **missense mutation** occurs when the substitution and subsequent altered codon specifies a different amino acid. So it can be seen that whereas some substitutions will have little effect on the final protein structure, others will have major effects.

### Insertions and deletions

Insertion or deletion of one or more bases may also cause mutant phenotypes. The effect of insertions or deletions depends on whether the number of bases involved is a multiple of three or not. As each amino acid is coded by a multiple of three bases, the way in which the DNA is read remains constant, although there may be one missing or one extra amino acid. The way this is normally referred to is that the reading frame of the DNA sequence remains constant and the mutation is said to be 'in frame'. The exact phenotypic effects of these in frame mutations will depend on the effect of the mutation on the structure of the encoded protein, i.e. whether the alteration seriously disrupts the final protein.

If the numbers of bases inserted or deleted are not multiples of three then the reading frame is disrupted and the sequence of amino acids downstream from the mutation will be read differently. These frameshift mutations usually have a serious effect on the eventual protein. **Figure 6.4.10** shows some examples of the consequences of insertions and deletions of bases on the protein code.

## Gross mutations

When large sections of DNA are altered, the mutation normally disrupts the amino acid sequence. Deletions are a loss of a portion of DNA that may be part of the gene or the entire gene sequence. There may be sequences of DNA inserted either from another region of the genome or as duplications. A novel mutation responsible for a number of human diseases such as Huntington's disease and fragile X syndrome is an expansion of triplet repeats (Fu et al., 1991). As mentioned previously, some parts of the DNA sequence consist of a series of repeats of bases. If the normal number of repeats is increased or expanded this mutation can cause disease (**Fig. 6.4.11**).

Disease-causing mutations are not inevitably in the coding portion of a gene. A mutation may affect the part of the sequence that starts RNA transcription and protein translation (the promoter region), causing failure of transcription. A gene is composed of exons (the coding portion of the gene) and introns (the non-coding portion of the gene). The RNA transcript undergoes processing to remove these unwanted segments (RNA splicing). If a mutation alters a splice site, the RNA product will be disrupted affecting the final protein structure.

| | |
|---|---|
| CUU AUG CAG GGA CGG | *original code* |
| CUU AUG GGA CGG | *in frame deletion* |
| CUU AUG CAG **AAA** GGA CGG | *in frame insertion* |
| CUU   UGC AGG GAC GG | *frameshift deletion* |
| CUU AU**U** GCA GGG ACG G | *frameshift insertion* |

**Figure 6.4.10**   Examples of the consequences of insertions and deletions of bases on the protein code

### CLINICAL APPLICATIONS

#### TISSUES FOR CLINICAL GENETIC ANALYSIS

As DNA is present in all cells with a nucleus, many types of tissue can be used for genetic analysis. In prenatal diagnostic testing, a sample of the chorionic villi can be taken at about 10 weeks of pregnancy and analysed. This is the preferred source of material for prenatal diagnosis, rather than cells from the amniotic fluid (amniocytes). Amniocentesis is usually not performed until about 16 weeks of gestation and the yield of DNA for analysis is much lower than that obtained from chrorionic villus sampling. It is also possible to perform analysis of genes at a very early stage of development before the cells implant. This is known as preimplantation genetic diagnosis and involves taking one cell from a blastocyst created using in vitro fertilization technology and analysing it for a specific genetic mutation. This technique is used by couples who are at risk of a recurrence of a genetic disease and who wish to implant only healthy embryos, thus avoiding the recurrence of a known problem.

Blood from adults, children and occasionally fetuses is the most common source of material for genetic analysis and DNA is easily extracted from white blood cells. Non-invasive sources of cells for DNA extraction are the buccal cells from the inside of the cheek, collected either through saliva samples or through buccal scrapings. These samples can be collected by the patient and posted to a laboratory and may be a source of DNA for large population surveys.

Structural abnormalities of the chromosomes are commonly found in tumour tissue or in the bone marrow of patients with leukaemia. These abnormalities have arisen in the tumour cells or are somatic (rather than being part of the person's genetic make-up) and are in fact part of the disease process. Much progress has been made in classifying these abnormalities and using the information to make treatment decisions and monitor disease progression or remission.

#### DNA analysis

Molecular genetic laboratories use a variety of techniques to detect mutations or to track genes

| | |
|---|---|
| AGC **CAG CAG CAG CAG** AAA CTG | *Normal sequence* |
| AGC **CAG CAG CAG CAG CAG CAG CAG** AAA CTG | *Expanded triplet repeat* |

**Figure 6.4.11**   Example of a gross mutation from an increase in the normal number of triplet repeats

through families. The basis of much genetic testing currently in clinical genetics is the **polymerase chain reaction (PCR)**. Using this technique, specific DNA sequences can be copied many times to yield large quantities of the particular portion of DNA corresponding to genes or fragments of genes. These can then be analysed or manipulated. The exact method of analysis used will depend on the characteristics of the DNA sequence of interest and the type of potential mutations. Polymerase chain reaction has also been important in the development of forensic DNA analysis. It has allowed the amplification of small amounts of DNA to provide a unique DNA 'fingerprint', which can be used as evidence. Once sufficient quantities of target DNA have been generated, it can be used for clinical analysis or research.

Techniques used to identify specific known gene mutations depend on the nature of the mutation. Analysis of specific mutations often utilizes DNA probes that match the mutation and stick to it (hybridize). DNA probes are single-stranded specific DNA sequences; they are radioactively or fluorescently labelled. If a probe is specific for a mutation then it will show a signal if the mutation is present and will not show a signal if it is absent. Probes may be designed to detect either normal or mutated sequences [for further details see Skirton & Patch (2002) and Strachan & Read (1999)].

## Factors affecting gene frequencies

Population geneticists estimate the frequency of specific genes or genetic variation within populations using mathematical means. Although details are beyond the scope of this chapter, it is important for health professionals to understand some of the reasons why genes vary within populations. This is needed to assess carrier status and new mutation rates for single gene disease. It also explains why gene frequencies vary between populations and is helpful to understand when trying to appraise the evidence from scientific research that claims to have identified an association between a genetic factor and a disease.

The relationship between gene frequencies in a population and genotype frequencies is described by the Hardy–Weinberg distribution:

$$p^2 + 2pq + q^2 = 1$$

where p is the frequency of the normal allele and q is the frequency of the mutated allele of a particular gene. The assumption underpinning this distribution is that populations are stable and the genes are independent. It can be used to calculate population carrier frequencies based on the observed number of cases. Thus, if q is a mutated recessive gene then the frequency of carriers of the recessive gene is 2 pq. In reality, because the population sample is so large, the frequency of the normal allele (p) is regarded as 1. Therefore, for practical purposes the carrier rate in the population (frequency of heterozygotes) is 2 q. The frequency of homozygotes (number of affected people) in a population is usually known, and this figure can be used to calculate carrier frequency.

Medically important Mendelian diseases are normally serious and would affect the ability to reproduce. However, as the diseases can be observed in a population, the maintenance of these disease genes within the population has to be explained. Natural selection would tend to remove harmful genes because they would affect the ability to have children. The gene would therefore not be passed on and would become extinct from the gene pool (the gene pool being all the genes within a population). The rate at which a genetic mutation disappears is balanced by the new mutation rate, therefore, for a disease to remain in the population there must be some mechanism by which this happens. This mechanism may be:

- a high new mutation rate, as happens in Duchenne muscular dystrophy
- onset of symptoms after reproductive age, as in Huntington's disease
- maintenance of a premutation stage in the population (fragile X syndrome)
- heterozygote advantage, which occurs in some recessive conditions, e.g. in sickle-cell disease.

Sickle-cell disease is a recessive disorder common in populations from equatorial Africa. The carrier frequency is greater than 1 in 10 (i.e. more than 1 in 10 people carry the recessive gene for sickle cell). The reason that this frequency remains so high is because carriers of the mutation (the recessive gene) have a selective advantage and are more resistant to malaria and therefore more likely to have children and pass the gene on. There will always be many more carriers than affected people and the gene therefore becomes common in the population.

New mutation rates for specific conditions can be derived using the Hardy–Weinberg distribution but give a surprisingly high new mutation rate for some autosomal recessive conditions when there is evidence that they are in fact very rare events. However, if carriers of the condition possess some kind of advantage that means they are more likely to reproduce, a particular allele will remain common within the population in the heterozygous state, as in sickle-cell disease.

Natural selection explains why some alleles become more common in a population. Other explanations are that some alleles become common simply by chance. Alternatively, if the population originates from a small number of individuals and there is little mixture with other populations then the genotypes of those individuals will be overrepresented, a so-called **founder effect**. This is the situation for Tay–Sachs disease, a devastating neurodegenerative recessive disorder of children that occurs predominantly in the Ashkenazi Jewish population. This population arose from a small original population that tended to marry within the culture. By chance, one (or more) of the founders of the original population carried the gene for Tay–Sachs disease, and it therefore became common.

## Genetic influences on common diseases

The sequence of DNA in any species is called the genome and the variability of the human genome has been used to map and describe most of the major Mendelian disease-causing genes. Interest is now focusing on looking for associations between patterns of genetic markers and more common diseases. This is a far more complex task than looking for single-gene disease association as many of these diseases will depend on complex gene–gene and gene–environment interactions.

The media is constantly reporting that the 'gene' for some particular condition has been discovered, but care must be taken in interpreting these results. What has been discovered very often is an association between particular genotypes and the disease. These genotypes may simply be markers of the disease and may have no functional significance: often more research is necessary before causation can be established. For example, there have been many reports relating to a 'gene' for schizophrenia. What has in fact been discovered is that individuals with schizophrenia have DNA sequences at particular loci in common, and each study tends to report a different association. At the time of publication of this chapter, a gene that codes for a protein that has biological importance in most cases of schizophrenia has not yet been discovered. The reader may recollect that there was a debate about a 'gene' for homosexuality being discovered. Again, this was a report of an association study. In addition, there are many possibilities for error in these types of studies, including misclassification of genotypes, errors in the biochemical techniques and errors in study design. It is likely, however, that such studies will yield important results that extend the understanding of the genetic mechanisms underpinning health and disease. Collaboration between geneticists, genetic epidemiologists, classical epidemiologists, statisticians, computing scientists, protein scientists, public health experts and others are necessary to maximize the benefits and minimize the harm of these scientific endeavours.

## CLINICAL APPLICATIONS

### GENETIC TESTING AND GENETIC SCREENING

There is a clear distinction between genetic testing and genetic screening. On the one hand, genetic testing refers to the situation where there is a known genetic risk and a test can be used to demonstrate the presence or absence of a disease-causing gene. Usually this is a direct mutation test, but it may be an investigation that reveals the phenotype, e.g. a renal ultrasound to check for cysts in an individual who is at 50% risk of inheriting autosomal dominant polycystic kidney disease. Particular protocols have been developed when testing for adult onset diseases such as Huntington's disease (International Huntington's Disease Association, 2002). A test for the Huntington's gene mutation will demonstrate its presence or absence. It is a predictive test because the presence of the Huntington's disease gene predicts that the person will develop Huntington's disease if they live long enough. However, the test cannot determine when the disease will start and does not lead to any therapeutic possibilities, as there are none available at present. People who have these sorts of predictive tests are aware of their risk and should be fully informed as to the nature, implications and outcomes of the tests.

Genetic screening, on the other hand, is a public health initiative. Individuals from a population (who are not aware they are at risk) are offered a test that will identify those who are at risk. Further diagnostic tests are necessary to clarify the extent of the risk. Genetic screening has received particular attention because it is claimed that genetic information has different implications to other medical information, in that it has implications for extended family members who might not have sought the information, it raises particular concerns about insurance issues and confidentiality, and it is concerned with prediction of disease rather than diagnosis. To date, genetic screening programmes have either been neonatal (e.g. phenylketonuria) or antenatal (e.g. maternal serum screening to detect pregnancies at risk of Down syndrome).

### REPRODUCTIVE OPTIONS FOR COUPLES AT RISK OF HAVING A CHILD WITH A GENETIC CONDITION

Couples who have an increased risk of having a child with a genetic disease will sometimes be referred to the clinical genetic team for discussion of their risks and options. If they wish to try to have a child, a number of options may be available to them:

- Natural conception with no intervention and accepting the risk of having a child with the disorder.

- Natural conception and prenatal diagnosis, therefore becoming pregnant naturally but opting to have the baby tested in utero. The offer of a test does not presuppose that an affected pregnancy would be terminated; some individuals choose to continue with a pregnancy knowing the child had the condition, although many do take the difficult decision to have a termination. To pursue this option there must be a test available to identify the gene or chromosome abnormality in an affected child.
- Conception using donor sperm or ovum: this may be relevant in recessive conditions, when the use of ovum or sperm from a non-carrier of either sex would avoid the risk of the condition, or in a dominant or X-linked condition when the gamete from the parent who carries the gene mutation is replaced by ova or sperm from a donor.
- Preimplantation genetic diagnosis: reproductive medicine technology (such as in vitro fertilization) is used to produce a number of fertilized ova. At the eight-cell stage, one cell is removed from the blastocyst for genetic testing. Only blastocysts that are not affected by the condition are re-introduced into the uterus. This technique is available in a limited number of conditions.
- Adoption: couples who do not wish to undertake these techniques could consider adopting a child as an alternative way of creating a family.

In each case, the choice will depend on the couples' beliefs and values, the extent to which they feel the condition is burdensome, along with the availability of the technology. The techniques and the decision-making process are discussed in depth in other texts (Abramsky & Chapple, 2003; Skirton & Patch, 2002).

## The chromosomes

The previous discussions have related to changes in the genes themselves. It is now appropriate to consider the changes that can affect chromosomes. As mentioned at the beginning of this chapter, the DNA in the nucleus of the cell is organized into 46 chromosomes: 22 autosomal pairs and a pair of sex chromosomes. Some of the problems that develop with chromosomes occur during cell division and gamete formation, and so it is relevant to consider these at this point. The process of cell division that occurs during growth and development is **mitosis**; during mitosis the chromosomes are replicated, and each daughter cell has 46 chromosomes (mitosis is described in Chapter 1.3). The cell division that forms the gametes (germ cells)

is called **meiosis**, and is discussed below. Meiotic cell division is unique to reproductive cells and gamete production. Meiosis does, however, have some features in common with mitosis. Meiosis begins in immature reproductive cells and involves two successive nuclear divisions, unlike mitosis, which involves one nuclear division. The end result is four haploid daughter cells, each containing 23 chromosomes, i.e. one of each of the 23 pairs.

## Meiosis and the formation of gametes

Like mitosis, meiosis is divided into stages. However, as the prophase stage in the first division is considerably longer than that in mitosis, this stage is further subdivided into recognizable phases.

Before meiosis begins, the chromatin material in the nucleus doubles in quantity (again like mitosis). Chromosomes are not clearly visible between cell divisions (**Fig. 6.4.12i**).

### Prophase I

In the **leptotene** phase of prophase I, the chromosomes are in the form of very fine single threads, hence the derivation of the name of this phase, meaning 'slender ribbon'. The chromosomes become clearly visible (**Fig. 6.4.12ii**).

In **zygotene**, the homologous, or paired, chromosomes (one from each parent) come together. This is called synapsis or pairing. An **homologous pair** is also known as a bivalent (**Fig. 6.4.12iii**).

In **pachytene**, the two chromosomes become coiled around each other and also become shorter and thicken (pachytene means 'thick ribbon') (**Fig. 6.4.12iv**).

In **diplotene**, the two chromosomes in each pair begin to part. With microscopes it is possible to see that each chromosome has itself divided into two daughter chromatids and so each unit now has four units, that is, it is quadrivalent. The separation of the homologous pairs is incomplete: some of the chromatids remain attached at one or more points along their length. These 'crossing-overs', or chiasmata (singular, chiasma), allow exchange of chromatin between chromatids (**Fig. 6.4.12v**). This is an important stage because it is one of the mechanisms by which genetic variation between parents and offspring is produced (**recombination**). The resultant chromatid is not identical to either of the two parent chromosomes but a mixture of the two. This is described more fully later in this section. It is during this stage that the female gametes go into a prolonged resting phase (see Chapter 6.3).

In **diakinesis**, the two bivalents continue to contract and move away from each other. The nucleolus also disappears at this point.

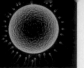

## Metaphase I

The nuclear membranes break down and the spindle apparatus, composed of contractile protein, appears. The bivalents arrange themselves on the spindle so that the centromeres of the two homologous chromosomes lie on either side of the equator of the spindle (**Fig. 6.4.12vi**). This arrangement is important because it ensures that each daughter cell receives only one of the chromosome pair (in contrast to the arrangement of the chromosomes during mitosis where each chromosome lies independently on the equator of the spindle).

## Anaphase I

The chromosomes move to opposite poles of the spindle but the centromeres do not divide as they do during mitosis. The remaining chiasmata slip apart and free the homologous chromosomes from each other (**Fig. 6.4.12vii**). Thus, at each pole there are 23 chromosomes, that is, half the total complement of 46 chromosomes. The total complement (46) is referred to as the **diploid** (2n) number of chromosomes.

## Telophase I

The nuclear membrane forms around the **haploid** (n) set of chromosomes at each pole (**Fig. 6.4.12viii**). At this stage there are two daughter cells, each containing 23 chromosomes.

There is then a short interphase period during which no DNA synthesis occurs.

**The second meiotic division** (starting with prophase II) closely resembles mitotic division because the units involved are chromosomes, not bivalents, and the centromere takes up a position on the equatorial plate at metaphase II. It differs from mitosis in that only half the normal number of chromosomes are present. During anaphase II, the centromeres divide and the daughter chromatids go to opposite poles. During telophase II the nuclear membranes reform.

Thus, at the end of meiosis, four haploid nuclei have been produced, each containing 23 individual chromosomes (22 autosomes and one sex chromosome), from the original diploid (23 pairs) parent nucleus. One of the most important aspects of meiosis is the halving of the chromosome number: each gamete must contain the haploid number of chromosomes so that when the male and female gametes fuse the resulting zygote will have the full complement of 46 chromosomes – the same number as each parent.

In the first stage of meiosis (**Fig. 6.4.12v**), the two copies of each autosome link at cross-over points known as chiasmata and there is an exchange of genetic material between the two, resulting in two completely different chromosomes. This is described as **recombination** and is illustrated in **Fig. 6.4.13**. The sex chromosomes do also pair up. In males the X and the Y chromosomes pair at specific small regions called pseudoautosomal regions where the DNA sequences are homologous.

The separation of the two copies of each chromatid into the daughter cells is termed **disjunction**. However, if disjunction does not occur cleanly, cells may be

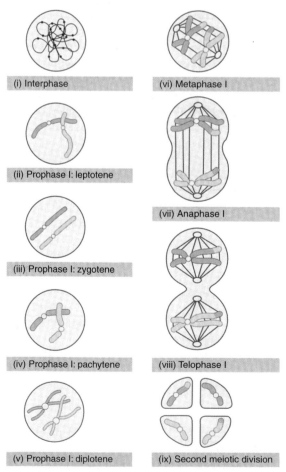

(i) Interphase

(ii) Prophase I: leptotene

(iii) Prophase I: zygotene

(iv) Prophase I: pachytene

(v) Prophase I: diplotene

(vi) Metaphase I

(vii) Anaphase I

(viii) Telophase I

(ix) Second meiotic division

**Figure 6.4.12**  The stages of meiosis. For explanation, see text; only one chromosome pair is shown for clarity

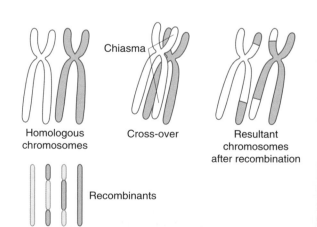

Homologous chromosomes

Chiasma

Cross-over

Resultant chromosomes after recombination

Recombinants

**Figure 6.4.13**  Recombination during meiosis

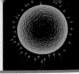

formed with an abnormal number of chromosomes. This is termed non-disjunction. **Non-disjunction** can also occur during the first stage of meiosis when the paired chromosomes fail to separate.

Most ova or spermatazoa that form with an unbalanced amount of chromosomal material will not successfully fertilize, but if fertilization does occur the embryo will not form normally. Frequently, the pregnancy will spontaneously abort but in some cases the abnormalities caused by the imbalance are not necessarily life threatening and the fetus will be viable. Non-disjunction is the most common cause of **trisomy** 21 (Down syndrome) and sex chromosome aneuploidies such as 47,XXY (Klinefelter syndrome) and 45,X (Turner syndrome).

## Chromosome nomenclature

An accepted international nomenclature is used to express the chromosome number and structure in a cell. Chromosomes have been allocated a number according to length, the largest chromosome being given the number 1. The total number of chromosomes in the cell is stated first, followed by the number and type of sex chromosomes. If there is an abnormality of the chromosome structure, this is signified after the sex chromosomes are listed. Hence, the normal male and female arrangements are written as 46,XY and 46,XX respectively. The chromosome arrangement usually associated with Down syndrome is written as 47,XX, +21 (for a female) or 47,XY, +21 (for a male).

The short arm of the chromosome is termed p (for petit) and the long arm q.

## Chromosome rearrangements

Rearrangements of chromosomes may occur during cell division in either a balanced or an unbalanced form. If the position of a chromosome or part of a chromosome is altered but there is no overall change in the amount of genetic material, there are unlikely to be any health implications for the carrier. However, if chromosomal imbalance occurs, the affected person is likely to have a range of physical and learning problems. Even a small section of a chromosome will contain many genes and therefore, if there are chromosome changes, multiple body systems are likely to be affected.

## Specific chromosomal rearrangements

### Balanced **reciprocal translocation**

When sections of two different chromosomes break and parts of each chromosome change positions, this is known as a **translocation**. In a balanced translocation the usual location of a part of at least two chromosomes may simply be altered, with no loss of genetic material. If the breakpoint of the translocation occurs through a gene there may be health implications, but this is not usually the case and the carrier may be unaware of the rearrangement. However, when the translocation carrier creates gametes, an unbalanced amount of chromosomal material may be passed to the embryo in the ovum or sperm **(Fig. 6.4.14)**.

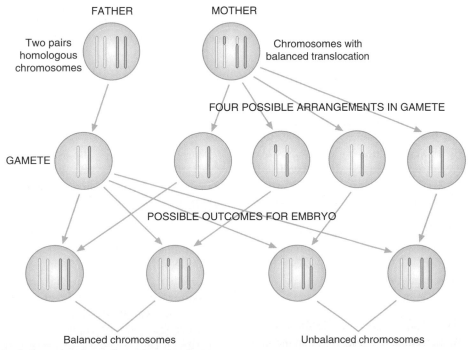

**Figure 6.4.14**   Balanced reciprocal translocation in one parent

An embryo with an unbalanced translocation will usually not survive and spontaneous abortion is common in these circumstances. If the fetus is viable, the resulting child will usually have serious physical and mental problems.

For example, a mother has a balanced translocation of the short arm of chromosome 5 and the short arm of X chromosome. This is written 46,XX t(5:X) (p15.3:p11.3). The fetus inherits the normal X chromosome and the translocated chromosome 5. Part of the short arm of chromosome 5 is deleted. The consequence of these changes is that the child has the condition cri du chat syndrome.

## Balanced Robertsonian translocation

Some chromosomes have no unique genetic material beyond the centromere (on the p arm); these are called **acrocentric chromosomes**. Two acrocentric chromosomes can join at their centromeres, forming one larger chromosome with effectively two long (q) arms. This type of translocation is called Robertsonian, and the **karyotype** of a person with a balanced Robertsonian translocation will be reported as having one less chromosome than usual, even though the individual has the necessary amount of genetic material to develop normally. The embryo of a person who carries a balanced Robertsonian translocation is at increased risk of inheriting an abnormal amount of genetic material. For example, if a parent has a balanced Robertsonian translocation of chromosomes 14 and 21, the embryo could inherit that parent's normal copy of chromosome 14 and the Robertsonian chromosome, with a copy of chromosome 21 and an additional copy of 14. This is illustrated in **Figs 6.4.15** and **6.4.16**.

## Deletion

When the chromosomes are copied during meiosis, it is possible for a portion of the chromosome to be deleted, resulting in the loss of genes. The deletion may not be visible by microscopy and specific techniques may be used in the laboratory to detect a small deletion known as a microdeletion. Conditions caused by a microdeletion are velocardiofacial syndrome (chromosome 22 q), Williams syndrome (chromosome 7 q) and Prader–Willi syndrome (chromosome 15 q). In all these conditions, the person may have learning difficulties as well as physical structural abnormalities. For example, a person who has a microdeletion of chromosome 22 q may have learning difficulties, a congenital heart defect, high arched palate and immune deficiency.

## Inversion

Inversion occurs when a part of a chromosome is reversed within the same chromosome, changing the order of the genetic material. An inversion that occurs

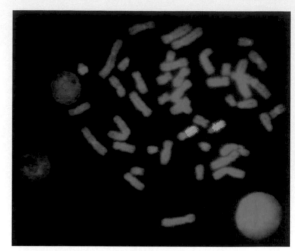

**Figure 6.4.15**   Karyotype of a child with Downs syndrome caused by a 14, 21 Robertsonian translocation (arrowed) (adapted from Mueller, R.F. & Young, I.D. (2001) *See* reference list

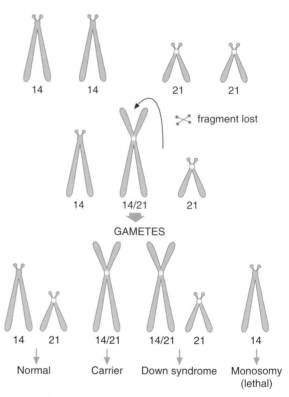

**Figure 6.4.16**   Translocation mechanism in Down syndrome (adapted from Mueller, R.F. & Young, I.D. (2001) *See* reference list

exclusively on one side of the centromere, within the p or q arm of that chromosome, is termed a **paracentric inversion (Fig. 6.4.17b)**. If it involves the centromere, the term pericentric inversion is used (**Fig. 6.4.17a**).

If there is no loss or duplication of chromosomal material, the person who has an inversion will probably be unaware of it. However, the presence of an inversion

## Pericentric inversions

**(a)**

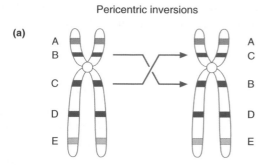

## Paracentric inversion

**(b)**

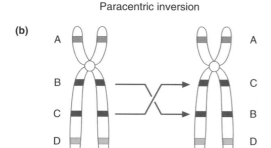

**Figure 6.4.17** (a) Diagrammatic representation of a pericentric inversion. (b) Diagrammatic representation of a paracentric inversion (adapted from Mueller, R.F. & Young, I.D. (2001) *See* reference list) (courtesy of J. Delhanty, Galton Laboratory, London)

in a parent will usually increase the risk of an unbalanced chromosome structure in his or her offspring.

## Chromosome analysis

The description of the chromosome structure of an individual is termed the **karyotype**. To study the human chromosome structure, a sample of cells is required. Although cells from any area of the body could be used, in practice karyotyping is usually done on samples of blood, skin or the chorionic villi of the placenta (for fetal testing) (the method of obtaining cells from the chorionic villi is described in Chapter 6.3).

Leucocytes (from blood) or fibroblasts (from skin) are grown in a culture medium. When mitosis is at the stage of metaphase, the process is 'frozen' by adding a chemical such as colchicine and the cells are viewed under the microscope. The cells are stained and the characteristic staining pattern of each chromosome aids the cytogeneticist in differentiating between chromosomes of similar length. A trained cytogeneticist is able to distinguish a normal chromosome pattern from the abnormal.

In the case of a microdeletion, the abnormality may be too small to be seen through the microscope. Techniques such as **fluorescent in situ hybridization** (**FISH**) may then be used to examine the chromosome structure. Before the test is done, the suspected area of

the microdeletion must be identified. The patient is examined carefully by an appropriate medical specialist (such as a geneticist or paediatrician). The pattern of physical features in the affected person will suggest the possible diagnosis. The microdeletion area associated with that diagnosis is identified. A radioactive probe is attached to a portion of DNA that matches the DNA sequence in the area of the suspected microdeletion. If the probe attaches to a chromosome, the fluorescent marker will be seen on that chromosome. However, if part of the chromosome is deleted, the marker will not attach and a microdeletion is diagnosed.

It is important to note that this type of diagnostic test cannot be done without use of advanced clinical skills of a medical specialist in the field to indicate the potential site of the microdeletion. For example, a child of 3 years is referred to the genetic clinic. She has delayed speech development and a cardiac defect. Her mother feels she has reached her developmental milestones at a much later age than her older brother. The girl has a facial appearance consistent with a microdeletion of chromosome 22 q. A blood sample is taken from the child, with the mother's consent, and the laboratory identifies a 22 q microdeletion.

## X-inactivation and methylation

In males and females, the dosage (amount) of genes is the same except for the genes carried on the sex chromosomes. Some genes are common to both the X and Y chromosomes but the majority of genes on the X chromosome do not occur elsewhere. In effect, females have twice the dosage of genes on the X chromosome when compared to males (see Chapter 6.3). To counteract this effect, a process known as X-inactivation occurs early in embryonic life. In each cell in the female embryo, one of the two X chromosomes is 'switched off', leaving only one active X in each cell. The initiation of X-inactivation is controlled by the *XIST* gene on the X chromosome, but other genes are known to affect the function of *XIST*. The X-inactivation should occur randomly, with 50% of each of the maternally and paternally derived X chromosomes inactivated throughout the body. The inactivation of the X chromosome is achieved by methylation, a chemical process whereby methyl groups are added to the DNA molecule at the site to be inactivated.

### Skewed X-inactivation

If a female is a carrier of an X-linked condition (described on p. 780), such as haemophilia or Duchenne muscular dystrophy, the X chromosome with the normal copy of the gene may be preferentially activated in the majority of cells, leading to a skewing of the X-inactivation pattern. Females who 'carry' an X-linked condition have one normal X chromosome and one X chromosome with a mutation on the relevant gene. Potential carriers may ask for tests to determine whether they could pass the gene mutation to their children. The phenomenon of skewed X-inactivation is sometimes used as a test for carrier status when other tests are inconclusive. In a woman who suspects she may be a carrier of an X-linked condition, a skewed pattern will increase the probability that she is a carrier. For example, a woman whose brother died of Duchenne muscular dystrophy may request a carrier test. If samples are not available from her sibling or parents, studying her X-inactivation pattern may provide some information about her status. If she has a skewed inactivation pattern, she is more likely to be a carrier of the condition and her children more likely to inherit it.

## Dysmorphology

An alteration in the normal chromosomal pattern, or even a change in a single gene, may alter the genetic code influencing a number of the body organs or systems. This may result in a child having unusual physical characteristics, termed **dysmorphic features**. Many normally functioning individuals have at least one dysmorphic feature, but where the features fit a recognized pattern that has been previously documented in other individuals, the child is said to have a dysmorphic syndrome.

The most common dysmorphic syndrome seen in live born children is Down syndrome. Ninety-five per cent of all cases of Down syndrome are caused by nondisjunction. In this case, the two chromosomes (bivalents) of pair 21 do not part during meiosis. Thus, if this 'imperfect' gamete is fertilized, the zygote will have three chromosome 21s and a total complement of 47 chromosomes. This example is known as **trisomy** 21. The incidence of Down syndrome is approximately 1 in 600 live births but the occurrence varies with the age of the mother: it occurs in mothers of 25 years of age once in every 2000 births but the risk rises 40-fold for mothers aged 45 years. The maternal age factor is thought to be associated with the increased length of time that a oocyte remains dormant in prophase I (an oocyte remains dormant from before birth until just prior to ovulation). In oocytes, that are dormant for 30–40 years, there is a greater risk of exposure to events that may bring about nondisjunction, e.g. radiation, toxins, viruses.

An individual with Down syndrome will usually have all or some of the following features:

- short stature
- upslanting palpebral (eyelid) fissures
- webbed neck
- small, broad hands and feet
- brachycephaly (broad short head)
- congenital heart defect
- hypotonia (lack of muscle tone)
- learning difficulties.

Other trisomies are also seen, for example trisomy 13 (Patau's syndrome) and trisomy 18 (Edwards' syndrome). However, there are thousands of dysmorphic syndromes and a genetic cause should generally be suspected only if a baby is born with a number of different unusual features.

## Cancer genetics

The number of families referred to a genetic service because of concern about a family history of cancer has increased dramatically over the past decade. As it is relatively common in the general population, it is discussed here as a model for managing aspects of care such as genetic testing and presymptomatic screening for other common conditions in the future.

Cancer is a term that is used to refer to literally hundreds of different conditions in which uncontrolled cell division (or mitosis) occurs, where that process results in malignant cell growth. In one sense, all malignancies have a genetic basis, as genes control the replication, differentiation and programmed death (apoptosis) of cells. Malignancy occurs when the normal balance of cell growth and differentiation is altered. However, in most cases the disruption to the process of cell replication, differentiation and apoptosis is a sporadic occurrence due to an accumulation of somatic gene mutations (a gene mutation that occurs accidentally in a particular cell in a tissue or organ; a germline mutation is present in all cells from conception).

In a small proportion of families, some individuals inherit a predisposition to develop cancer. Except in exceedingly rare cases, this is not a general predisposition to cancer but an increased tendency to develop cancer in specific organs. Familial predisposition to cancer is due to the inheritance of a mutation in a specific gene.

### Two-hit theory

There are several theories concerning the onset of cancerous changes in a tissue. One strong theory proposes that development of cancer is a result of mutations in both copies of a particular gene and is called the two-hit theory (Knudson, 1971). This theory was first applied to cancer genetics in 1971, when it became clear that retinoblastoma (a rare cancer affecting the eye) was caused by separate mutations in both copies of the same gene, known as the Rb gene. In some children, the mutations occur sporadically (randomly) but others inherit one mutated gene and a sporadic change in the other copy triggers the formation of the retinoblastoma. A proportion of children who inherit a mutation from a parent develop tumours in both eyes due to their highly increased susceptibility. **Figure 6.4.18** shows the two-hit theory.

The two-hit theory helps to explain the earlier onset of cancer in individuals who inherit a mutation. During the lifetime of any individual, two somatic mutations may occur in a cell line (all the daughter cells produced from a particular parent cell but not in the gametes), increasing the likelihood of cancer in that area of the body. However, if an individual inherits a gene mutation in a tumour suppressor gene or an oncogene (see below), then all cells in the body will have a fault in one copy of the gene. It then only requires a somatic mutation to occur in the other copy of the gene in a single cell for normal gene function to be inhibited.

### CLINICAL APPLICATIONS

If a child is diagnosed with retinoblastoma, the parents and other children in the family are investigated for any sign of retinoblastoma, since they will be at increased risk. The affected child is monitored throughout life because there is a risk of a second retinoblastoma occurring and siblings of an affected child continue to be screened regularly until adulthood.

The more common familial cancer syndromes are caused by alterations in several groups of genes.

## Oncogenes

**Oncogenes** are created when genes that normally initiate and control new cell growth (proto-oncogenes)

are permanently switched on. In the normal state, the gene will activate proteins that trigger cell growth intermittently, whenever new cells are required. However, a mutation in the proto-oncogene produces an 'oncogene', which continuously triggers new cell growth. One product of such a gene is the ras protein, which exists in normal cells and relays signals by acting as a switch. In response to the presence of a trigger that indicates a need for new cell growth (such as a change in hormone level), the ras protein is produced. However, when there is a mutation in the *ras* gene, ras protein may be continually produced, even in the absence of the trigger. These types of genetic mutation are called gain-of-function mutations.

Oncogenes can be created by exposure of the cell to drugs, chemicals or radiation, or the gene mutation may be inherited. Cancer is not usually due to a single mutation in one oncogene, it may be the result of a number of different mutations in a number of genes.

### The Philadelphia chromosome

One example illustrating an oncogene is the Philadelphia chromosome. When the chromosomes of patients who have chronic myeloid leukaemia are examined, a small chromosome – the Philadelphia chromosome – is almost inevitably detected. This abnormal chromosome is formed when the long arms of two chromosomes, 9 and 22, break off and the two tips of the chromosomes exchange places. This is a form of reciprocal translocation. A fusion gene is formed in the Ph chromosome (the translocated chromosome 9) and an abnormal protein is produced that is thought to have a role in the development of leukaemia (Rowley, 1996).

### *Tumour suppressor genes*

When tissue damage or loss occurs due to trauma or natural cell death, rapid cell replication is triggered by genes that control mitosis. After the requisite number

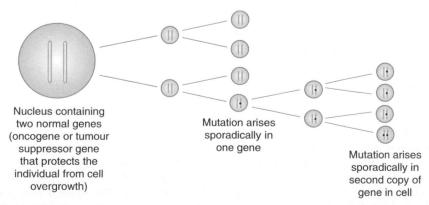

**Figure 6.4.18** The two-hit theory

Nucleus containing two normal genes (oncogene or tumour suppressor gene that protects the individual from cell overgrowth)

Mutation arises sporadically in one gene

Mutation arises sporadically in second copy of gene in cell

of cells have been produced, the process of cell growth is normally inhibited by genes that are known as tumour suppressor genes (TSG). Generally, only one intact tumour suppressor gene is required to ensure normal function, however, if both copies are faulty, cell replication will continue without the normal control (or 'brake'), and the growth of additional cells will result in formation of a tumour. This is termed a loss-of-function mutation.

## Mismatch repair genes

Mismatch repair genes can be thought of as caretaker genes that maintain the integrity of the genome. During mitosis, the full complement of DNA is copied into each new daughter cell. Both strands of DNA forming the double helical structure of the molecule are required to 'match', so that the gene structure of one strand mirrors the sequence of the opposite strand. If disruption occurs when the process of replication takes place, the genes designed to repair any mismatch come into play, and adjust the sequence to ensure the match is correct. When there are faults in both copies of a mismatch repair (MMR) gene, this adjustment does not occur and the genetic code for cell growth in those particular cells may be altered, enabling excessive growth to occur.

## Cancer-predisposing syndromes

Some cancer predisposing syndromes have a recognizable phenotype. In this category are the single-gene disorders known to almost inevitably cause cancer in the affected individual. These are usually rare syndromes such as ataxia telangectasia (which causes chromosome breakage) or Li Fraumeni syndrome (caused by a fault in a tumour suppressor gene called p53), where a genetic alteration may cause disruption to cell growth in any area of the body and multiple episodes of malignancy are inevitable. In this group there are also conditions caused by dominant gene mutations that allow rapid cell division, where the risk of cancer is almost 100% unless preventative treatment is undertaken. One of these conditions is familial adenomatous polyposis (FAP), in which hundreds of polyps develop in the colon. The polyps have a strong tendency to become malignant and treatment is by removal of polyps and eventual removal of the colon.

Some common forms of cancer may involve an inherited factor. Cancers of the breast and colon are common in the general population and only about 5% of cancers of these organs will be due to an inherited predisposition. In this small percentage of families, some individuals inherit an autosomal dominant gene mutation, but this mutation alone does not cause cancer. Other (as yet unidentified) events, either genetic or environmental, are required for cancer to develop. The genes BRCA1 and BRCA2 (mutations that contribute to breast or ovarian cancer) are in this category, as are the MLH2 and MSH2 genes that increase the risk of hereditary non-polyposis colon cancer.

In many families that are referred to the genetic service, the family history of cancer will be strong, with a number of relatives affected. However, a slightly increased susceptibility to cancer is shown in individuals who have one first-degree relative with either breast or colorectal cancer. In these families, a clear inheritance pattern cannot be demonstrated but empirical data indicate that there must be some increased genetic risk, perhaps because of the individual inheriting a certain gene or combination of genes that interact with environmental factors.

The assessment of an individual's cancer risk is based on his or her family tree. The history is carefully taken and the cases of cancer in the family are examined according to the following criteria:

1. **Location of the malignancy:** if the tumours have occurred in the same organ, or in organs that are known to be affected by the same gene mutation (e.g. breast and ovarian cancer), this increases the suspicion that there is an inherited cancer syndrome in the family.
2. **Evidence of inheritance from one generation of the family to the next:** when three or more generations of a family are affected by related cancers, this markedly increases the chance of an inherited predisposition to cancer.
3. **Age of diagnoses:** cancer is a common condition in the elderly but where individuals have been diagnosed with cancer at a younger age than would be expected (e.g. breast cancer diagnosed before 40 years of age) this may be evidence that the person was born with a gene mutation that contributed to the formation of cancer.

Unusual occurrences, such as a male in the family having breast cancer or a woman having primary tumours in both breasts, increases the chance of an inherited gene mutation in the family.

### CLINICAL APPLICATIONS

#### ROLE OF THE GENETIC NURSE OR COUNSELLOR IN CANCER GENETIC COUNSELING

When a client is concerned about a family history of cancer, the genetic nurse or counsellor can play a key role in explaining the risks and options but may also be able to support the family during periods of adjustment and decision-making. In practical terms, the counsellor will:

1. Take an accurate family history, noting the types of disease and age of diagnosis in each case.
2. Confirm each diagnosis, if possible, using medical records or death certificates. Informed consent is required from affected relatives before their medical history can be confirmed.
3. Make a genetic risk assessment for the client.
4. Make recommendations for cancer screening if indicated.

Further explanation of the role of genetic services can be found later in the chapter. Additional cancer screening will usually be advised only if the client's risk of developing cancer is significantly higher than the general population risk, if there is a reliable screening method and if the screening method is not associated with significant morbidity or mortality.

In the case of colorectal cancer, screening by regular colonoscopy may be indicated if the lifetime risk of colorectal cancer for the client is assessed as greater than a risk of 1 in 10 (Vasen et al., 1991). There is a risk associated with colonoscopy, an invasive test, but it is highly reliable as a method of detecting tumours. For women at increased risk of breast cancer, mammography may be advised. This test is not as reliable in premenopausal women as it is for women after the menopause, so mammography is not an ideal screening method. Magnetic resonance imaging (MRI) and ultrasound scanning are being investigated as possible alternatives. Although there is evidence that population breast cancer screening for postmenopausal woman is effective in reducing cancer morbidity and mortality, the evidence for screening those at higher than population risk is still awaited.

## Testing for gene mutations in familial cancer

At the present time, genetic testing for familial cancers is not always possible within a family. Before a test can be offered to an individual who is unaffected, the gene mutation must be identified in an affected person. As numbers of genes are known to be implicated in both breast and colorectal cancer, a number of genes may have to be investigated. In addition to this factor, the mutation in the gene may be individual to a certain family, so finding the pathogenic sequence in the gene may not be possible. When a gene mutation is found in an affected family member, presymptomatic testing can be offered to relatives who are at risk. This will confirm the need for screening in those who carry the mutation, while at the same time

removing the need for screening from those who have not inherited the gene mutation. Some of those who choose to be tested may opt for prophylactic surgery (such as prophylactic oopherectomy or mastectomy), to reduce the risk of developing cancer if they are found to be gene-mutation-positive. In practical terms, it may take several years to identify a gene mutation in a family member. Once a mutation is identified, the testing of further members usually takes several months. It is vital that supportive counselling is offered prior to presymptomatic testing, to ensure the client understands the implications of such a test and is psychologically prepared for the result.

## Gene testing for an affected individual

In any family consultation where genetic testing is discussed, the needs of the affected family member should be considered. Although the affected person has had a diagnosis of cancer, the confirmation that he or she does have a gene mutation, and therefore an increased genetic predisposition to cancer, may be an additional burden. This will be especially so if it brings a realization that they will be prone to further episodes of cancer. The affected family member may also feel guilt at having possibly passed on a gene mutation, thus increasing risks to his or her offspring. Informed consent for testing is essential. Thorough explanations are needed to ensure that difficult concepts are understood. The results should be conveyed in person and additional counselling support offered if a mutation is found.

---

### CLINICAL APPLICATIONS

#### FAMILY HISTORY OF BREAST AND/OR OVARIAN CANCER – REFERRAL GUIDELINES

Because many women will be concerned about a family history of breast and/or ovarian cancer, guidelines have been produced to assist primary care practitioners in assessing the need for a genetics referral (Eccles et al., 2000). These may alter as research evidence on genetic predisposition to breast/ovarian cancer accumulates and the websites of reputable organizations (such as Cancer UK) can provide reliable, updated information.

A woman should be referred for a genetic risk assessment if she has a family history of any of the following:

- three close relatives from the same side of the family diagnosed with breast cancer at any age
- two close relatives from the same side of the family with an average age of diagnosis of breast cancer under 60 years

- a mother or sister diagnosed with breast cancer at less than 40 years of age
- a father or brother with breast cancer diagnosed under 60 years
- one close relative with bilateral breast cancer, with the first cancer diagnosed under the age of 50 years.

## Current and future developments in genetics

Much of the promise of genetics in terms of treatment or therapy is as yet unrealized. For most genetic disease or congenital abnormality the treatment is conventional, such as surgery for repairing cleft lip and palate, replacement therapies, such as factor VIII in haemophilia, and drug and lifestyle modification, as in familial hyperlipidaemia. In reality, most healthcare workers will be applying principles that they already are familiar with to the treatment and management of genetic disease. Many of these interventions will not cure the disease but will ameliorate symptoms and improve quality of life.

## Pharmacogenomics

The term **pharmacogenomics** refers to a new area of development in the production of drug therapies, related to the genetic basis of disease and the genetic make-up of the individual. Discoveries about the underlying genetic basis of some diseases are enabling drugs to be developed that are based upon the effect of the gene, rather than in response to the clinical manifestations of the condition. Using this approach, a drug may correct the altered protein product of the mutated gene, or counteract the gene effect upon the cell at the protein level. Research is currently being undertaken to develop such drugs for use in conditions such as Huntington's disease, where glutamine clumps invade the nucleus of the cell, causing premature cell death.

Understanding the genetic basis of a condition may also indicate the correct therapy for each individual, for example identifying those clients who have a type of diabetes caused by a particular gene mutation that does not respond to insulin therapy. Another aspect of pharmacogenomics relates to the effective usage of particular drugs. It is known that individuals respond to certain therapies in different ways, according to polymorphic variations in different relevant genes that affect metabolism of drugs. If the genetic variant in the individual is identified through a genetic test, the drug therapy for that person can be tailored to his or her own needs, thus reducing the need to identify the correct drug and

dosage by trial and error. This also has the potential for reducing the incidence of side-effects and complications, as it may be possible to identify individuals who are at risk of a reaction to a specific drug and avoid administering it.

## Gene therapy

Gene therapy refers to any procedure that is intended to modify or treat disease by genetically modifying the cells of the patient. A distinction is made between therapy affecting the general body tissues (somatic gene therapy) and that affecting the ovary or sperm (germ cell therapy). Modifying genetic material in the ova or sperm is considered unacceptable and is not sanctioned since this would have effects on future, as yet unborn, individuals.

Genes may be introduced into cells to:

- produce a protein that patients cannot produce themselves, which is the situation in many inherited diseases (such as cystic fibrosis transmembrane receptor)
- kill diseased cells directly by producing a toxin (this is one approach to gene therapy for cancer)
- activate the body's own defence systems (such as the immune system)
- inhibit the expression of genes associated with a particular disease restoring normal function (such as the excess glutamine in the cells in Huntington's disease).

Genes can be inserted directly into the cells of patients (e.g. via a nebulizer into the lungs of a patient with cystic fibrosis) or cells (e.g. bone marrow) can be taken and modified in the laboratory and transplanted into the patient. The promise of gene therapy has not yet been realized either in the treatment of inherited disorders or in the development of novel therapeutics. However, trials are being conducted particularly in cancer and advances are being made.

## The Human Genome Project

In the 1980s, researchers began using techniques from molecular biology to map genes that cause disease. This led to enthusiasm from some scientists for the proposal to determine the DNA sequence of the entire human genome (i.e. all the genetic material) and the human genome project was inaugurated in 1990. At that time the technology was not available for the large-scale sequencing of DNA that was required. Initial energy focused on creating genetic and physical maps to provide a scaffold for the sequencing initiative. From the outset, the sequencing project was an international initiative and, in addition, 3–5% of the budget was set aside to look at the ethical, legal and social implications of the project. The original plan was to complete the sequence in the year 2005. However, developments in sequencing technology, bioinformatics and computing meant that a draft sequence was published in June 2000 (Collins & McKusick, 2001). The Human Genome Project agreed from the beginning that all map and sequence data should remain in the public domain and this was an undoubted factor in the rapid progress of the project. The working draft was published simultaneously by the publicly funded international sequencing consortium and a private-sector company (Lander et al., 2001; Venter et al., 2001).

This published sequence is purely a working draft and it is necessary to complete the sequence by filling the gaps and resolving ambiguities: it is also only the first step. Further work is needed to:

- characterize human variation and its relationship with disease
- determine the function of genes and the functional consequences of variation
- develop the bioinformatic and computational tools to examine complex relationships and associations
- develop new sciences of functional genomics and proteomics (proteins are the functional units of the genotype phenotype pathway). Gene expression patterns are the first step in the pathway to protein expression but there is not always a direct relationship. Proteomics is concerned with protein expression in different tissues, determination of protein structure, modification of protein structure after translation, protein–protein and protein–drug interactions.

The human genome project has been described as 'the end of the beginning'. The next phase is to develop an understanding of the major pathways involved in homeostasis of the human organism and how those pathways are maintained or disrupted in health and disease.

## Clinical genetic services

Clinical genetic services were first established for families in the United Kingdom and in North America in the late 1940s. Services now exist throughout most areas of Europe, Australasia and Asia. Genetic services are commonly provided by a professional team that includes medically qualified doctors and genetic nurses or counsellors. The clinical services must of necessity work in close contact with laboratory scientists who provide the facility for genetic testing.

The definition of genetic counselling published by the American Society of Human Genetics (1975) emphasizes that genetic counselling is a process of communication that addresses the problems and challenges that accompany the risk of a genetic condition in the family. Although specialist genetic services primarily serve families who are at high risk of genetic conditions, genetics is increasingly becoming an integral part of many other specialties and the way in which services are delivered will therefore have an impact in a wider context in future. This is especially true in the field of cancer services. The number of referrals for individuals who are concerned about an increased risk of cancer (due to family history) has risen sharply over the last 5 years and is expected to increase still further.

A family may benefit from contact with the genetics service:

- If a genetic condition is known or suspected in a family. These may include the more common genetic diseases such as Huntington's disease, cystic fibrosis, muscular dystrophy, fragile X or Marfan syndrome, or may be one of the extremely rare conditions.
- After the birth of a baby who has health problems caused by a genetic condition.
- After recurrent miscarriage, stillbirth, or death of a baby, particularly if the baby was found to have physical problems.
- When a child within the family has learning difficulties, particularly if the child also has other health problems or unusual physical features.
- When individuals are concerned about a strong family history of cancer.

The aims of genetic counselling are to help the individual or family:

- understand the information about the genetic condition
- appreciate the inheritance pattern and risk of recurrence
- understand the options available
- make decisions appropriate to their personal and family situation
- make the best possible adjustment to the disorder or risk.

Genetic counselling may change the client's quality of life, either positively or negatively. For a positive change to occur, a good relationship between client and genetic counsellor is necessary. Providing factual information is an integral part of genetic counselling but the counsellor should also enable the client to place the information into the context of their family, and integrate their own ideas and experience of the condition with the scientific information.

## What occurs when a family is referred?

In many genetic teams, the first contact with the client will be made by a genetic nurse or counsellor. A full family history is taken. As explained earlier, the family tree is the most important tool in making a genetic risk assessment. Medical history may need confirmation and the consent of relatives is needed before their records can be accessed by genetics staff. In many cases, a diagnostic opinion is required from the medical staff; this will usually necessitate a hospital clinic appointment.

Genetic testing may be requested but in the majority of cases the genetic consultation pivots on a clinical opinion and in-depth discussion with families. As genetic conditions often affect multiple family members and may remain an issue for a client's life time, long-term contact with families is an integral part of the service.

Genetic nurses or counsellors require training and education in both genetics and counselling, and are professionally prepared to offer families reliable information and psychosocial support. However, although there is a distinction between genetic counsellors, who work primarily with families at high genetic risk, and other health professionals who may need a basic knowledge of genetics to practise in their own settings, genetics is no longer a specialty that exists in isolation (Skirton & Patch, 2000). It is a subject that will eventually provide insight into virtually all aspects of human health and disease. There is therefore a need for all nurses, midwives and health visitors to attain genetic literacy, that is, to understand and be able to explain genetic concepts to be able to offer competent care to patients and their families in all healthcare settings.

---

### Clinical review

In addition to the Learning Objectives at the beginning of this chapter, the reader should be able to:

- Describe the differences between autosomal and sex-linked inheritance, phenotype and genotype, and dominant and recessive characteristics
- Understand the key issues involved in taking a family history
- Discuss the role of genetics in cancer
- Consider the advantages and disadvantages of gene testing
- Discuss possible advances in gene therapies

---

### Review questions

1. What is a gene?
2. What is a chromosome?
3. What is an allele?
4. What is meant by Mendelian inheritance?
5. Describe the features of autosomal recessive inheritance.
6. Draw the symbols used when compiling family pedigrees.
7. Draw a family tree demonstrating X-linked inheritance.
8. List the stages of meiosis.
9. Give two examples of types of mutations.
10. What is the human genome project?

# Glossary of terms

**Allele/alleles:** a copy of the gene at a particular locus. One allele is inherited from each parent.

**Autosomal dominant inheritance pattern:** the inheritance pattern whereby one copy of a gene is mutated, this is sufficient to cause the disease to be manifest.

**Autosomal recessive inheritance pattern:** the inheritance pattern whereby both copies of the gene are mutated and the person develops the condition because they have no normal copy. Carriers of recessive conditions are usually unaffected.

**Autosomes:** the chromosomes that are present in equal numbers in both male and female of the species (in humans, the chromosomes 1 to 22).

**Base pair:** a pair of nucleotides positioned opposite each other on the two strands of the DNA double helix. Adenine always pairs with thymine, and guanine with cytosine.

**Carrier:** a person who is generally not affected with the condition but carries one faulty copy of a gene. Generally relates to heterozygotes in recessive or X-linked conditions.

**Chromosome:** the physical structures into which the DNA is packaged within the nucleus of cells. The usual number of chromosomes in humans is 46.

**Clinical genetics:** the branch of the health service that is chiefly involved in diagnosis of genetic conditions and genetic counselling for families.

**Codon:** a triplet in the messenger RNA that provides the code for one amino acid.

**Consanguinity:** the biological relationship between two individuals who have a common ancestor.

**Diploid:** having two copies of each autosome.

**DNA:** deoxyribonucleic acid. The biochemical substance that forms the genome. It carries in coded form the information that directs the growth, development and function of physical and biochemical systems. It is usually present within the cell as two strands with a double helix conformation.

**Dysmorphic features:** physical features that are outside of the variability of the normal population. They may occur because of a change in the genetic code providing instructions for those features.

**Exon:** a sequence of DNA that contributes to the protein product of a gene (see also *intron*).

**Expression:** the way in which the gene mutation manifests within an individual.

**FISH (fluorescent in situ hybridization):** a technique that uses both cytogenetics and molecular biology to identify subtle changes in chromosome structure.

**Gene:** the fundamental physical and functional unit of heredity consisting of a sequence of DNA.

**Haploid:** having one copy of each autosome.

**Heterozygous:** having two different alleles at a genetic locus, usually one normal and one faulty copy of a gene (see also *homozygous*).

**Homologous pair:** two copies of the same chromosome.

**Homozygous:** having two identical alleles at a genetic locus. In Mendelian diseases these may be copies of a gene that are either both normal or both faulty.

**Intron:** a sequence of DNA that does not contribute to the code for protein product, as the genetic sequence within introns is omitted when the mRNA is made.

**Karyotype:** a description of the chromosome structure of an individual (assessed during metaphase), including the number of chromosomes and any variation from the normal pattern.

**Locus:** the position of a gene, a genetic marker or a DNA marker on a chromosome.

**Meiosis:** the production of gametes (haploid cells).

**Mendelian disorder or Mendelian condition:** a genetic disorder caused by a single gene fault, following a dominant, recessive or X-linked pattern of inheritance.

**Mitosis:** the production of somatic diploid cells.

**Multifactorial:** a condition is said to be multifactorial if both genetic and environmental influences are thought to be causative.

**Mutation:** a gene sequence variation that is found in less than 1% of the population. The mutation may cause a change in the protein product of the gene, and therefore cause health problems for the person concerned.

**Non-disjunction:** failure of the two copies of chromosomes to separate effectively into the two daughter cells.

**(polymerase chain reaction) PCR:** a laboratory method of manufacturing many copies of a sequence of DNA.

**Pedigree:** family tree.

**Penetrance:** the extent to which specific gene mutations are manifested within an individual.

**Phenotype:** the observable characteristic, e.g. brown eyes, blood group, height.

**Polygenic:** relating to a number of different genes, e.g. a disorder is polygenic if it could be caused by a combination of mutations in several different genes.

**Polymorphism:** normal variation in sequence of DNA in a gene, differs from *mutation* in that it is usually found in more than 1% of the population.

**Reciprocal translocation:** exchange of chromosomal material between at least two chromosomes.

**Recombination:** the creation, during meiosis, of a new chromosome or sequence of DNA that is a unique combination of the parent's maternal and paternal DNA.

**Somatic:** relating to cells other than the germ line.

**Trisomy:** having three copies of a particular chromosome.

**X-linked inheritance pattern:** a pattern of inheritance whereby the mutated gene is on the X chromosome, of which males have one copy and females have two.

## Suggestions for further reading

Gardner, A., Howell, R. T. & Davies, T. (2000) *Human Genetics*. London: Arnold.
*An excellent text on the scientific aspects of genetics and the way they are applied in the laboratory when testing patients. Very suitable for nurses.*

Harper, P.S. (1998) *Practical Genetic Counselling*, 5th edn. Oxford: Butterworth-Heinemann.
*A comprehensive text with short references to a huge number of genetic conditions. Good reference for any ward or primary care centre.*

Mueller, R.F. & Young, I.D. (2001) *Emery's Elements of Medical Genetics*, 11th edn. Edinburgh: Churchill Livingstone.

*A comprehensive, detailed but understandable text covering all aspects of medical genetics.*

Skirton, H. & Patch, C. (2002) *Genetics for Healthcare Professionals – A Lifestage Approach*. Oxford: BIOS.
*Written specifically for nurses and midwives. Explains the clinical applications of genetics in straightforward language and uses clinical cases to illustrate application of genetics in the health service.*

Strachan, T. & Read, A. P. (1999) *Human Molecular Genetics*, 2nd edn. Oxford: BIOS.
*Very advanced textbook on scientific aspects of molecular genetics.*

## Useful websites

Cancer and genetics: www.cancergenetics.org/
genetics.htm
*General information on cancer.*

Family Cancer and Genetic Testing: www.
familycancer.org/FamilyCancer/index_gene.stm
*Information, links and support groups for breast and
ovarian cancer.*

Hereditary colon cancer: www.mdacc.tmc.edu/~hcc/

Hereditary Nonpolyposis Colon Cancer (HNPCC):
www.penrosecancercenter.org/info-hnpcc.htm

National Institute of Health: www.nih.gov/
*General information on a huge variety of conditions.*

Cystic Fibrosis Foundation: www.cff.org/

National Association for Down Syndrome (NADS):
www.nads.org/
*Counselling and support service for parents of children with
Down syndrome.*

National Down Syndrome Society web site:
www.ndss.org/
*A comprehensive, on-line information source about Down
syndrome.*

Huntington's Disease Association site: www.hda.org.uk/

## References

Abramsky, L. & Chapple, J. (2003) *Prenatal Diagnosis:
The Human Side,* 2nd edn. Cheltenham, UK: Nelson
Thornes.

American Society of Human Genetics (Ad hoc
Committee on Genetic Counselling) (1975)
Genetic counselling. *American Journal of Human
Genetics,* **27**; 240–242.

Collins, F.S. & McKusick, V.A. (2001) Implications of
the Human Genome Project for medical science.
*Journal of the American Medical Association,* **285**(5);
540–544.

Eccles, D.M., Evans, D.G.R. & Mackay, J. (2002)
Guidelines for a genetic risk based approach
to advising women with a family history
of breast cancer. *Journal of Medical Genetics,* **37**;
203–209.

Fu, Y.H., Kuhl, D.P., Pizzuti, A. et al. (1991) *Variation of
the CGG repeat at the fragile X site results in genetic
instability: Resolution of the Sherman paradox.* Cell,
**67**(6); 1047–1058.

Imperatore, G., Pinsky, L.E., Motulsky, A. et al. (2003)
Hereditary hemochromatosis: Perspectives of public
health, medical genetics and primary care. *Genetics
and Medicine,* **5**(1); 1–8.

International Huntington's Disease Association
(2002) *Guidelines for the molecular genetic
predictive test in HD.* Online. Available:
www.huntington-assoc.com/guidel.htm

Knudson, A. (1971) *Proceedings of the National Academy
of Science. USA,* **68**; 820–823.

Lander, E.S., Linton, L.M., Birren, B. et al. (2001)
Initial sequencing and analysis of the human
genome. *Nature,* **409**(6822); 860–921.

Mueller, R.F. & Young, I.D. (2001) *Emery's Elements of
Medical Genetics,* 11th Edn. Edinburgh: Churchill
Livingstone.

Online Mendelian Inheritance in Man (2002)
National Centre for Biotechnology Information.
Online. Available: www3.ncbi.nlm.nih.gov/Omim/

Rowley, J. (1996) Leukaemias, lymphomas, and other
related disorders. In: Rimcin, D., Connor, M. &
Pyeritz, R.E. (eds) *Emery and Rimoin's Principles and
Practice of Medical Genetics.* New York: Churchill
Livingstone.

Skirton, H. & Patch, C. (2000) The new
genetics – what's it got to do with me? *Nursing
Standard,* **14**(19); 42–46.

Skirton, H. & Patch, C. (2002) *Genetics for healthcare
professionals – a lifestage approach.* Oxford: BIOS.

Strachan, T. & Read, A.P. (1999) *Human Molecular
Genetics,* 2nd edn. Oxford: BIOS.

Vasen, H.F.A., Mecklin, J.P., Meera Khan, P. &
Lynch, H.T. (1991) Hereditary non-polyposis
colorectal cancer. *Lancet,* **338**; 877.

Venter, J.C., Adams, M.D., Myers, E.W. et al. (2001) The
sequence of the human genome. *Science,* **291**(5507);
1304–1351.

Watson, J.D. & Crick, F.H. (1953) Molecular structure
of nucleic acids: A structure for deoxyribonucleic
acid. *Nature,* **4356**; 737–738.

# Index

Pancreatitis 341
Pancuronium 201, 279
Papanicolaou (Pap) test *see* Cervical
smears
Papillae, tongue 175, *175*, 471, *471*
Papillary muscles 390
Papilloedema 151, 161
Paracasein 482
Paracentesis, ascites 530
Paracetamol 659
  osteoarthritis 326
  overdose 534
Paracrine control 209
Paraesthesia 236
Paraesthesiae 350
Paralysis agitans *see* Parkinson's disease
Paralytic ileus 506
Paramesonephric ducts 727, *727*
Paraphimosis 729
Paraplegia 147
Parasympathetic nervous system (PNS)
  74, 183, *187*, 187–8
  blood vessel 428
  cholinergic receptors 190
  cranial nerves 188
  development 189
  drugs affecting 201–2
  erection control 757
  functions **184**, 195–6
  ganglionic synapses 188
  gastrointestinal tract 476
  heart rate 414–15, 449, *450*
  kidney 599
  micturition 623
  sacral outflow 188
Parasympathetic tone 193–4
Parathormone *see* Parathyroid hormone
Parathyroid glands **212**, 235
  overactivity 235
Parathyroid hormone **212**, 235–6, 237,
  302
  action 235
  calcium/phosphate homeostasis 302
  excess 304
  growth **66**
  half life 235
  secretion regulation 235
  synthesis 235
Paraventricular nucleus 129
Paravertebral ganglia 184, 185, *187*
Paracentric inversion 792, *793*
Parenchyma 6
Parietal cells *479*, 481
Parietal lobe 108
Parietal lobe lesions 113
Parietal lobe tumours **84**
Parietal pleura 549
Parkinson's disease 118–19
  clinical features 118–19
  nursing management 119
Paronychia 647
Parotid glands 472
Paroxysmal nocturnal dyspnoea
  418–19
Partial seizure
  complex 127
  simple 127
Partial thickness burns 654
Parturition *769*, 769–72
  stress incontinence 625
  *see also* Labour
Pascal 20, 420
Pascal's principle 420
Passive external rewarming **663**

Passive immunization 703
Passive transport 495, 606–7
  nephron reabsorption 608–9
Patau syndrome (trisomy 13) 794
Patent ductus arteriosus (PDA) 390
Pathogens, access to body 668–70
Patient-controlled analgesia (PCA) 144
Pavementing 675
Peak expiratory flow rate (PEFR) 562,
  563
Peak flow 546
Pedicels 596
Pedicle, of cone 155
Pedigree *see* Family tree
PEG tube **649**
Pelvic cavity 13, *16*
Pelvic inflammatory disease 750
Penetrance 781
Penile urethra 729
Penis 729, *730*
Pentagastrin 480, 482, 483
Pentoses 35, *36*
Pepsin 41, 482
Pepsinogen 482
Peptic ulcers 188, 246, 261
Peptide bond 40, *42*, **46**
Peptide hormones 213
Peptides 40–1
Percentile charts 62, *63*
Percutaneous transluminal coronary
  angioplasty (PTCA) 399
Perfusion 542
Pericardial cavity 13, 389
Pericardial fluid 389
Pericardial friction rub 389
Pericardial tamponade 399
Pericarditis 389
Pericardium 389
Periderm 645
Perilacunar bone 296
Perilymph 165
Perimetry 161–2
Perimysium 272
Perineurium 77
Periosteal arteries 297
Periosteum 296
Perioxisomes 54
Peripheral arterial disease 433
Peripheral neuropathy 85
Peripheral resistance 421
Peripheral temperature 655
  measurement 667
Peripheral vascular disease 256
Peristalsis
  colonic 504, 507
  gastric 480, 484
  innervation 478
  oesophagus *477*, 477–8
  ureters 622
Peritoneal cavity 13
Peritoneal dialysis **649**
Peritoneum 13, 486, *488*
  pain 511
Peritonitis 511
Periurethral/transurethral injection
  therapy 626
Pernicious anaemia 352, 470, 511
Persantin 361
Peyer's patches 486, 693
PH 33–4
  bile 491, 519
  blood 34, 587
  cerebrospinal fluid 102
  colonic 505

definition 33
gastric 487
scale **33**, 34
semen 737
Si units 19
skin secretions 668
urine **601**
vagina 741
Phaeochromocytoma 200, 244
Phagocytes **669**, 671–2, 687
  respiratory tract 547
Phagocytosis 52, 355, *356*, 671
Phagolysosome 671
Phagosome 671
Phantom limb pain 142
  sympathectomy 198
Pharmacogenomics 798
Pharmacokinetics, hypothermia **665**
Pharyngeal tonsil 544
Pharyngotympanic tube *163*, 164
Pharynx 473, *474*
Phenelzine 201
Phenergan 356
Phenindione 368
Phenotype 778
Phenoxybenzamine 200
Phenylalanine 40, *41*
Phenylbutazone 360
Phenylketonuria 60
Phenylthiourea 175
Phenytoin 85, 288, 535
Pheromones 747
  apocrine secretions 643
Philadelphia chromosome 795
Phosphataemia 608
Phosphate
  blood concentration 234, 302–3
  fluid compartment composition 8, *9*
  metabolism control 234–8
  nephron reabsorption 608
  role 235
Phosphate ester bonds **46**
Phosphatidylcholine 39, 525–6
Phosphodiesterase inhibitors 368
Phospholipids 39
  bile 525–6
  cell surface membrane 51
  structure *40*
Phosphorus 26, **26**, **27**
Phosphorylase 37
Photopic vision 157
Phototherapy, physiological jaundice
  523
Phrenic nerve 543, 578
Physiological jaundice 523
Physiotherapy
  airway secretion removal 548
  joint disorders 328
  muscle disorders 289
Physostigmine 202, 288
Phytate 506
Pia mater 102
Picogram **17**, 346
Piles 509
Pilocarpine 201
Piloerection 656
Piloerector muscles 195
Pineal body 111–12
Pineal glands 754
Pink puffers 573, 585
Pinnae 163
Pinocytosis 52
Pirenzepine 482
Pitch 166